**Local Anesthesia in Dentistry**

# Local Anesthesia in Dentistry

## A Locoregional Approach

**Jesús Calatayud, MD, PhD, DMD**
*Associate Professor (retired)
Pediatric Dentistry
School of Dentistry
Universidad Complutense. Madrid (Spain)*

**Mana Saraghi, DMD, DADBA**
*President, American Dental Board of Anesthesiology
Director, Dental Anesthesiology Residency Program, Jacobi Medical Center
Assistant Professor of Dentistry, Albert Einstein College of Medicine
Bronx, New York (United States)*

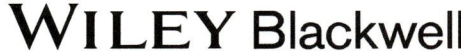

This edition first published 2024
© 2024 John Wiley & Sons Ltd

All rights reserved. No part of this publication may be reproduced, stored in a retrieval system, or transmitted, in any form or by any means, electronic, mechanical, photocopying, recording or otherwise, except as permitted by law. Advice on how to obtain permission to reuse material from this title is available at http://www.wiley.com/go/permissions.

The right of Jesús Calatayud and Mana Saraghi to be identified as the authors of the editorial material in this work has been asserted in accordance with law.

*Registered Offices*
John Wiley & Sons, Inc., 111 River Street, Hoboken, NJ 07030, USA
John Wiley & Sons Ltd, The Atrium, Southern Gate, Chichester, West Sussex, PO19 8SQ, UK

For details of our global editorial offices, customer services, and more information about Wiley products visit us at www.wiley.com.

Wiley also publishes its books in a variety of electronic formats and by print-on-demand. Some content that appears in standard print versions of this book may not be available in other formats.

Trademarks: Wiley and the Wiley logo are trademarks or registered trademarks of John Wiley & Sons, Inc. and/or its affiliates in the United States and other countries and may not be used without written permission. All other trademarks are the property of their respective owners. John Wiley & Sons, Inc. is not associated with any product or vendor mentioned in this book.

*Limit of Liability/Disclaimer of Warranty*
The contents of this work are intended to further general scientific research, understanding, and discussion only and are not intended and should not be relied upon as recommending or promoting scientific method, diagnosis, or treatment by physicians for any particular patient. In view of ongoing research, equipment modifications, changes in governmental regulations, and the constant flow of information relating to the use of medicines, equipment, and devices, the reader is urged to review and evaluate the information provided in the package insert or instructions for each medicine, equipment, or device for, among other things, any changes in the instructions or indication of usage and for added warnings and precautions. While the publisher and authors have used their best efforts in preparing this work, they make no representations or warranties with respect to the accuracy or completeness of the contents of this work and specifically disclaim all warranties, including without limitation any implied warranties of merchantability or fitness for a particular purpose. No warranty may be created or extended by sales representatives, written sales materials or promotional statements for this work. The fact that an organization, website, or product is referred to in this work as a citation and/or potential source of further information does not mean that the publisher and authors endorse the information or services the organization, website, or product may provide or recommendations it may make. This work is sold with the understanding that the publisher is not engaged in rendering professional services. The advice and strategies contained herein may not be suitable for your situation. You should consult with a specialist where appropriate. Further, readers should be aware that websites listed in this work may have changed or disappeared between when this work was written and when it is read. Neither the publisher nor authors shall be liable for any loss of profit or any other commercial damages, including but not limited to special, incidental, consequential, or other damages.

*Library of Congress Cataloging-in-Publication Data*

Names: Calatayud, Jesús, author. | Saraghi, Mana, author.
Title: Local anesthesia in dentistry: a locoregional approach / Jesús Calatayud, Mana Saraghi.
Description: Hoboken, NJ: Wiley-Blackwell, 2023. | Includes bibliographical references and index.
Identifiers: LCCN 2023007820 (print) | LCCN 2023007821 (ebook) | ISBN 9781394180158 (cloth) | ISBN 9781394180165 (adobe pdf) | ISBN 9781394180172 (epub)
Subjects: MESH: Anesthesia, Dental-methods | Anesthesia, Local-methods | Anesthesia, Dental-adverse effects | Anesthesia, Local-adverse effects | Anesthetics, Local
Classification: LCC RK510 (print) | LCC RK510 (ebook) | NLM WO 460 | DDC 617.9/676–dc23/eng/20230420
LC record available at https://lccn.loc.gov/2023007820
LC ebook record available at https://lccn.loc.gov/2023007821

Cover Design: Wiley
Cover Image: © Christine von Diepenbroek/Getty Images

Set in 9.5/12.5pt STIXTwoText by Straive, Pondicherry, India
Printed and bound by CPI Group (UK) Ltd, Croydon, CR0 4YY
C9781394180158_120124

# Contents

**Preface** *xxiii*
**About the Companion Website** *xxv*

1 **History of Local Anesthesia in Dentistry** *1*
   The Coca Leaf *1*
   Cocaine *2*
   The Development of the Syringe *3*
   The Dangers of Cocaine *4*
   Adrenaline and the Vasoconstrictive Effect *4*
   Novocaine or Procaine *5*
   The Development of Local Anesthesia in Dentistry *5*
      Local Anesthetics *5*
      Vasoconstrictors *6*
      Instruments *7*
      Anesthetic Techniques *7*
      Twenty-First Century Developments *8*
      Frequency of Use of Local Anesthesia in Dentistry *9*
   References *9*

**Applied Anatomy** *15*

2 **Applied Anatomy I: Maxillary Arch** *17*
   Introduction *17*
      The Trigeminal Nerve *17*
      Trigeminal Ganglion *17*
      Trigeminal Nerve: Functions *17*
   Maxillary Nerve ($V_2$) *17*
      Overview of Collateral Branches *18*
         Intracranial Zone *18*
         Pterygopalatine Fossa Zone *18*
         Infraorbital Zone *19*
      Palatine Nerves *19*
         Greater Palatine Nerve *20*
         Nasopalatine Nerve *20*
      Superior Alveolar Nerves *22*
         Posterior Superior Alveolar Nerve (PSAN) *22*
         Middle Superior Alveolar Nerve (MSAN) *22*
         Anterior Superior Alveolar Nerve (ASAN) *23*
      Superior Dental Plexus *23*
   Other Structures of Interest *24*

         Greater Palatine Canal and Foramen  24
            Greater Palatine Canal  24
            Greater Palatine Foramen  24
         Nasopalatine Canal and Foramen  24
            Nasopalatine Canal  24
            Nasopalatine Foramen  24
         Cortical Bone Thickness  25
         Pterygoid Venous Plexus  25
         Infraorbital Foramen  25
         Pterygopalatine Fossa  26
            Margins  26
            Content  27
      Glossary  27
      References  28

3  **Applied Anatomy II: Mandibular Arch**  31
      Mandibular Nerve ($V_3$)  31
         Overview  31
         Buccal Nerve  31
            Course  32
            Innervation  32
         Auriculotemporal Nerve  33
            Course  33
            Innervation  33
         Lingual Nerve  33
            Course  33
            Innervation  34
            Remarks  34
         Inferior Alveolar Nerve  34
            Course  34
            Innervation  35
            Remarks  35
         Mylohyoid Nerve  36
            Course  36
            Innervation  36
      Body of the Mandible  36
         Cortical Bone Thickness  36
         Retromolar Zone (Trigone and Fossa)  37
            Retromolar Trigone  37
            Retromolar Fossa  37
         Mandibular Canal  37
         Mental Foramen  38
      Ramus of the Mandible  39
         Divergent Angle  39
         Ramus Width  39
         Lingula  39
         Mandibular Foramen  39
         Sulcus colli  40
         Coronoid Notch  41
         Accessory Foramina  41
      Pterygomandibular Space  41
         Anatomic Boundaries of the Pterygomandibular Space  42
         Open/Closed Mouth and Pterygomandibular Space  44

    Contents of the Pterygomandibular Space   44
        Sphenomandibular Ligament   44
    Positive Aspirations and Hematomas   45
Glossary   46
References   46

## 4  The Peripheral Nerve and Local Anesthesia   50

Peripheral Nerve Microanatomy   50
  Neurons   50
  Sensory Neurons   50
  Axons   50
  Membranes   51
  Nerve Fibers and Myelin   51
    Myelinated Fibers   51
    Unmyelinated Fibers   52
    Nerve Fiber Classification   52
  Peripheral Nerve Structure   52
Basic Membrane Proteins   54
  Sodium–Potassium Pump   54
  Sodium Channels   54
  Potassium Channels   55
Peripheral Nerve Neurophysiology   56
  Fundamentals   56
  Membrane Potentials: Membrane at Rest (Polarized)   56
  Action Potentials: Excited Membrane   56
    Phase 1: Depolarization   57
    Phase 2: Repolarization   57
    Phase 3: Hyperpolarization   57
  Propagation of the Action Potential   58
Mechanisms of Local Anesthesia   58
  Mechanism   58
  Differential Nerve Block   58
  Tonic and Phase Block   59
  Critical Length   59
  Transient Receptor Potential Channel   60
Nerve Block Kinetics   60
  Induction Stage   60
  Recovery Stage   60
  Re-Injection   61
  Tachyphylaxis   61
  Resistance to Local Anesthetics   61
References   62

## Pharmacology   65

## 5  Local Anesthetics   67

Chemical Structure   67
Physical-chemical Characteristics of Local Anesthetics   67
  Dissociation Constant or pKa   68
  Partition Coefficient or Lipid Solubility   69
  Protein Binding   70
  Vasodilation   70

Assessment of Anesthesia and the Anesthetic Parameter  70
   Assessment of Local Anesthesia in Dentistry  70
   Anesthetic Parameter  72
Anesthetic Concentration  72
   Concentration and Volume  72
   Concentration and Safety  73
   Concentration and Anesthetic Potency  73
   Concentration and Tissue Irritation  73
Maximum Doses  74
Maximum Doses for Children  75
Pregnancy and Lactation  76
   Pregnancy  76
   Lactation  77
Mixing Local Anesthetics  77
Isomers  78
References  79

# 6 Vasoconstrictors  85

Introduction  85
   Advantages  85
   Disadvantages  85
   Dilutions and Concentrations  87
Catecholamines  87
   Isomers and Catecholamines  88
   Adrenergic Receptors  88
   Systemic Effects  90
     Heart  90
     Circulatory System  91
     Respiratory Tract  91
     Endocrine System and Metabolism  91
     Uterus  91
   Vasoconstrictive Effect  91
   Catecholamine Metabolism  92
   Epinephrine  92
   Norepinephrine  93
   Levonordefrin  94
Phentolamine (OraVerse®)  95
   OraVerse®  96
   Advantages and Indications  96
   Technique and Dose  96
   Clinical Efficacy  97
   Tolerance, Toxicity, and Adverse Side Effects  97
Felypressin (Octapressin®)  98
   Cardiovascular Effects  98
   Vasoconstrictive Effect  99
   Adverse Effects  100
   Contraindications  100
   Advantages and Disadvantages  100
   Maximum Doses  100
Combinations of Vasoconstrictors  101
References  101

**7 Injectable Anesthetic Solutions Used in Dentistry** *107*

Solution Composition *107*
  Local Anesthetic *107*
  Vasoconstrictor *107*
  Antioxidants (Sulfites) *107*
  Preservatives (Methylparaben) *108*
  pH Adjustment *108*
  Other Compounds *109*
Procaine (Novocaine) *109*
  Metabolism *109*
  Procaine with Epinephrine *109*
  Remarks *109*
Lidocaine (Lignocaine) *109*
  Metabolism *111*
  Remarks *111*
  Indications *111*
    Standard 2% Lidocaine: L-100 with 1:100 000 (10 μg/ml) Epinephrine or L-80 with 1:80 000 (12.5 μg/ml) Epinephrine *111*
    L-50, 2% Lidocaine with 1:50 000 (20 μg/ml) Epinephrine *113*
Articaine *113*
  Metabolism *115*
  Remarks *115*
    Maximum Dose and Toxicity *115*
    Anesthetic Potency *115*
    Anesthetic Effect *116*
  Indications *116*
    A-100, 4% Articaine with 1:100 000 (10 μg/ml) Epinephrine *116*
    A-200, 4% Articaine with 1:200 000 (5 μg/ml) Epinephrine *117*
Mepivacaine *117*
  Metabolism *117*
  Remarks *119*
    Maximum Doses *119*
    Mepivacaine Solutions *119*
  Indications *119*
Prilocaine (Propitocaine) *120*
  Metabolism *120*
  Remarks *120*
    Toxicity and Safety *120*
    Clinical Efficacy *122*
    Prilocaine Solutions *122*
  Indications and Contraindications *122*
    Indications *122*
    Contraindications *123*
Bupivacaine *123*
  Metabolism *123*
  Remarks *123*
  Indications and Contraindications *125*
    Indications *126*
    Contraindications *126*
References *126*

**Contraindications** 133

**8 Contraindications for Local Anesthetic Techniques in Dentistry** 135
   Lack of Cooperation from the Patient  135
      Predisposing Factors  135
      Evaluation of Risk  136
      Approach to Behavioral Problems  136
   ASA IV Physical Status  137
      ASA I Patients  137
      ASA II Patients  137
      ASA III Patients  138
      ASA IV Patients  139
      ASA V Patients  140
   Clotting Abnormalities  140
      High-risk Anesthetic Techniques  140
      Systemic Causes of the Risk of Hemorrhage  140
         Antiplatelet Agents  140
         Oral Vitamin K Antagonists: Anticoagulants  141
         Direct Oral Anticoagulants  141
         Low Platelet Counts  142
         Hemophilia  142
      Alternatives and Recommendations  142
   Other Contraindications  142
      Injection Site Infection  142
      Impossible Physical Access  143
   Summary  143
   References  143

**9 Contraindications for Local Anesthetics** 148
   Relevant Contraindications  148
      Allergy to Local Anesthetics  148
      Long-acting Anesthetics  148
      Prilocaine, Benzocaine, and Methemoglobinemia  148
      Cholinesterase Deficiency and Esther Anesthetics  149
      Myasthenia Gravis and Esters  149
   Minor Contraindications  149
      Procaine and Sulfonamides  149
      Lidocaine and Cimetidine  150
      Lidocaine and Propranolol  150
      Lidocaine and Succinylcholine  150
      Bupivacaine and Cardiotoxicity  150
      Amide Anesthetics and Malignant Hyperthermia  151
   References  151

**10 Contraindications for Vasoconstrictors** 155
   Absolute Contraindications  155
      Uncontrolled Insulin-dependent Diabetes Mellitus  155
      Intolerance to Sulfites  156
      Asthma Controlled with Corticosteroids  156
      Pheochromocytoma-induced Arterial Hypertension  156
      Recent Consumption of Cocaine  157
      Patients with Cardiovascular Diseases Who Take Amphetamines and Psychostimulants  157

Allergy to Vasoconstrictors  *157*
Relative Contraindications  *158*
    Nonselective Beta-blockers  *158*
    COMT Inhibitor-type Antiparkinson Drugs  *160*
    ASA III Patients with Cardiovascular Conditions  *160*
    Digitalis Glycosides (Digoxin)  *160*
    Amphetamines and Psychostimulants  *161*
    Tricyclic Antidepressants  *161*
    Interactions Involving Drugs that are No Longer in Use  *162*
        Older Antihypertensive Agents (Anti-adrenergic Drugs)  *162*
        General Anesthesia (Halothane and Thiopental)  *162*
Contraindications of Little Relevance  *163*
    Uncontrolled Hyperthyroidism  *163*
    Phenothiazines and Antipsychotic Drugs  *163*
    Vasoconstrictors and Osteoradionecrosis  *164*
Contraindications of Felypressin  *164*
References  *165*

## Instruments and Topical Anesthesia  171

## 11 Instrument Set and Equipment  173
Needles  *173*
    Parts of a Needle  *173*
        Anterior Part  *173*
        Middle Part  *174*
        Posterior Part  *174*
        Protective Sheath  *175*
    Lengths and Gauges  *175*
    Needles: Critical Aspects  *175*
        Aspiration and Gauge  *176*
        Pain and Gauge  *176*
        Deflection of the Needle and Gauge  *176*
        Lesions Caused by a Barbed Needle  *177*
        Breakage of Needles  *177*
    Criteria for the Selection of Needles  *177*
Cartridges  *177*
    Parts of a Cartridge  *178*
        Anterior Part or Needle Adapter  *178*
        Neck  *178*
        Cylindrical Body  *178*
        Posterior Part  *179*
        Other Elements  *179*
    Storage of Cartridges  *179*
        Norms for All Cartridges  *179*
        Norms for Cartridges Containing Catecholamines  *179*
    Problems Affecting Cartridges  *180*
    Degradation of Drugs in the Cartridge  *180*
        Local Anesthesia  *181*
        Sympathomimetic Vasoconstrictors (Epinephrine)  *181*
        Sulfites  *181*
Syringes  *181*

Parts of a Cartridge-type Syringe  *181*
   Anterior Part or Needle Adapter  *181*
   Syringe Barrel or Body of the Syringe  *182*
   Posterior Part (Back)  *182*
   Piston  *182*
Using the Syringe  *182*
   Set-up  *182*
   Dismantling  *182*
   Cleaning and Sterilization  *183*
Self-aspirating Syringes  *183*
   Characteristics  *183*
   Mechanism of Action  *184*
   Advantages and Disadvantages  *184*
Variants of Cartridge-type Syringes  *184*
   Plastic Syringes  *184*
   Uniject-type Syringes  *184*
   Disposable Antineedle Stick Syringes  *184*
   Power-operated Syringes  *185*
   Other Injection Devices  *185*
Additional Instruments  *185*
   Complementary Devices  *185*
   Alkalinization System (pH Onset System®)  *186*
     Advantages  *186*
     Mechanism of Action  *186*
     Cartridges for the Device  *187*
     Mixing Pen  *187*
     Mixing  *188*
     pH  *188*
   Vibrating Devices  *188*
     Gate Control Theory  *189*
     VibraJect  *189*
     DentalVibe  *189*
   Cartridge Heaters  *190*
References  *190*

## 12 Topical Anesthesia  *195*

Factors Affecting Topical Anesthesia with Local Anesthetics  *195*
   Local Anesthetic  *195*
   Application Time  *195*
   Method of Application  *195*
   Amount Administered  *196*
   Types of Pain  *196*
   Area of the Mouth  *197*
Effect of Topical Anesthesia  *197*
Topical Anesthetics in Dentistry  *197*
   Benzocaine  *197*
     Maximum Dose  *197*
     Advantages and Disadvantages  *197*
     Specific Adverse Effects  *198*
   Lidocaine  *199*
     Maximum Dose  *199*
     Advantages and Disadvantages  *199*

        Specific Adverse Effects  *199*
      Lidocaine Adhesive Patches (DentiPatch®)  *199*
        Maximum Dose  *199*
        Advantages and Disadvantages  *199*
        Specific Adverse Effects  *200*
      EMLA Cream  *200*
        Advantages of the Structure and Composition of EMLA  *200*
        Maximum Dose  *200*
        Advantages and Disadvantages  *200*
        Specific Adverse Effects  *201*
      Tetracaine (Amethocaine)  *201*
        Maximum Dose  *201*
        Advantages and Disadvantages  *201*
        Specific Adverse Effects  *201*
      Cocaine  *203*
        Maximum Dose  *203*
        Advantages and Disadvantages  *203*
        Specific Adverse Effects  *203*
        Formulations for Use in Dentistry  *203*
      Topical Anesthetic Compounds  *203*
        Composition  *203*
        Advantages and Application  *205*
        Adverse Effects  *205*
        Clinical Efficacy  *205*
      Other Experimental Formulations  *205*
    Topical Cooling  *206*
      Cold Aerosols  *206*
      Refrigerants  *207*
      Topical Ice  *207*
    Indications for Topical Anesthetic  *208*
      For Symptomatic Relief of Pain  *209*
        Pain Resulting from Tooth Decay  *209*
        Painful Ulcers and Lesions on the Mucosa  *209*
      Indication as Anesthetic  *209*
        Minor Surgical Interventions  *209*
        Clinical Procedures  *209*
        Management of the Gag Reflex  *209*
    Periodontal Oraqix® Gel  *209*
      Oraqix System (Needle-free Anesthesia)  *210*
        Method of Application  *210*
        Efficacy  *211*
        Specific Adverse Effects  *211*
    References  *211*


## Local Anesthetic Techniques in Dentistry  217

### 13 Basic Injection Technique  *219*
    Comment on Retraction  *219*
    Phases of the Injection  *219*
      Initial Preparation  *219*
      Preparation Phase  *220*

Application of Topical Anesthetic  *222*
  Method of Application  *222*
  Observations on Aerosols  *223*
Transfer of the Syringe  *223*
Insertion of the Needle  *225*
Aspiration  *226*
  False Positives and Negatives  *226*
  How to Interpret a Positive Aspiration  *227*
  Aspiration Technique  *227*
  Remarks  *228*
Injection  *228*
Final Phase  *229*
Evaluation of Anesthesia  *230*
Post-treatment Phase  *231*
Causes of Pain During the Injection  *232*
  Factors That Cause Pain  *232*
  Factors That Play a Role in Pain  *232*
  Unimportant Causes (Myths)  *233*
Terminology  *234*
Appendix  *235*
References  *235*

## 14 Maxillary Anesthesia I: Pulpal Anesthesia  *241*

Introduction  *241*
  Maxilla  *241*
  Maxillary Nerve ($V_2$)  *241*
  Buccal Anesthesia of the Upper Molars  *241*
Buccal Infiltration  *242*
  Zones Anesthetized  *242*
  Technique  *242*
  Efficacy of this Technique  *245*
  Complications Specific to this Technique  *245*
  Factors That Lead to Success  *245*
  Modified Cotton Roll Approach  *245*
Infraorbital Nerve Block  *245*
  Uses  *246*
  Zones Anesthetized  *246*
  Intraoral Technique  *246*
  Extraoral Technique  *248*
  Efficacy of this Technique  *249*
  Complications Specific to this Technique  *249*
  Remarks  *250*
Posterior Superior Alveolar Nerve Block  *251*
  Zones Anesthetized  *251*
  Technique  *251*
  Efficacy of this Technique  *252*
  Complications Specific to this Technique  *253*
  Modified Adatia Technique  *253*
High Tuberosity Approach  *253*
  Uses  *253*
  Zone Anesthetized  *254*
  Technique  *254*

Efficacy of this Technique  *256*
Complications Specific to this Technique  *256*
Remarks  *256*
Transpalatal Technique  *256*
Uses  *257*
Zone Anesthetized  *257*
Technique  *257*
Efficacy of this Technique  *260*
Complications Specific to This Technique  *261*
Factors That Lead to Success  *263*
Final Remarks  *263*
References  *263*

## 15 Maxillary Anesthesia II: Complementary Anesthesia of the Palate  *267*
Introduction  *267*
The Nasopalatine Nerve Innervates Less than Previously Thought  *267*
The Potency of the Anesthetic is not Important  *267*
Anesthesia of the Palate Without Complementary Palatal Anesthesia  *267*
Indications  *268*
Methods for Reducing Pain in Palatal Techniques  *269*
Topical Anesthesia  *269*
Pressure Techniques  *270*
Topical Cooling  *270*
Periodontal Ligament Technique  *270*
Minimal Intervention Technique  *271*
Nasopalatine Nerve Block  *271*
Anesthetized Area  *271*
Technique  *271*
Specific Complications of This Technique  *273*
Intranasal Variant  *274*
Technique  *274*
Greater Palatine Nerve Block  *274*
Area Anesthetized  *274*
Technique  *275*
Specific Complications of This Technique  *276*
Partial Variant of the Palate  *276*
Transpapillary Technique in Children  *276*
Technique  *277*
References  *278*

## 16 Mandibular Anesthesia I: Pulpal Anesthesia  *281*
Mandibular Block: General Remarks  *281*
Zone Anesthetized  *282*
Factors to Consider for the Mandibular Block  *282*
Efficacy is Correlated to the Location of Tooth in the Mandible  *282*
High Failure Rate  *283*
Unreliability of Lower Lip Anesthesia  *283*
Sequential Nature  *283*
The Longer the Time, the More Intense the Anesthesia  *283*
Minor Effect of the Type of Anesthetic  *283*
Impact of the Volume Injected  *284*
Minor Effect of the Specific Mandibular Block Technique  *284*

  Bilateral Mandibular Blocks *284*
  Long, Caliber 25G Needles *284*
  Slow Injection *285*
 Mandibular Block: Conventional or Direct Technique *285*
  Distribution of the Anesthetic Solution *285*
  Zone Anesthetized *286*
  Technique *286*
  Efficacy of this Technique *291*
  Complications Specific to this Technique *291*
 Mandibular Block: Gow-Gates Technique *292*
  Mechanism *292*
  Advantages, Disadvantages, and Non-advantages *294*
   Advantages *294*
   Disadvantages *294*
   Non-advantages *295*
  Zone Anesthetized *296*
  Technique *296*
  Efficacy of this Technique *299*
  Complications Specific to this Technique *299*
  Remark on the Gow-Gates Technique *300*
 Mandibular Block: Laguardia–Akinosi Technique *300*
  Advantages and Disadvantages *300*
  Use *301*
  Distribution of the Anesthetic Solution *301*
  Zone Anesthetized *301*
  Technique *301*
  Efficacy of this Technique *303*
  Complications Specific to this Technique *303*
 Double Infiltration in Anterior Teeth *304*
  Keys to Success *304*
  Zone Anesthetized *304*
  Technique *304*
  Efficacy of this Technique *306*
  Complications Specific to this Technique *306*
 References *307*

## 17 Mandibular Anesthesia II: Complementary Anesthesia *312*
 Introduction *312*
 Indications *312*
 Lingual Nerve Block *312*
  Anesthetized Area *312*
  Technique *312*
  Complications of this Technique *314*
  Partial Variant as Complementary Anesthesia *314*
 Buccal Nerve Block *314*
  Anesthetized Area *315*
  Technique *315*
  Specific Complications of this Technique *316*
 References *316*

## 18 Supplementary Techniques in Cases of Failure *318*
 Introduction *318*
 Intrapulpal Anesthesia *318*

Traditional Technique  *318*
    Keys to a Successful Approach  *318*
        Intrapulpal Technique  *319*
    Topical Anesthetic Technique  *319*
        Technique  *319*
Periodontal Ligament Technique (PDL)  *320*
    Indications and Contraindications  *320*
        Indications  *320*
        Contraindications  *320*
    Diffusion of the Solution  *320*
    Factors that Determine Efficacy  *321*
        Major Factors  *321*
        Minor Factors  *321*
    Instrument Set  *322*
        Syringes  *322*
        Needles  *324*
        Cartridges  *324*
    Anesthetized Area  *324*
    Technique  *324*
    Efficacy of This Technique  *326*
    Specific Complications of the Technique  *326*
        Complications Due to Performance of the Technique  *326*
        Periodontal Abnormalities  *326*
        Pulpal Abnormalities  *327*
        Cardiovascular Abnormalities  *328*
Intraseptal Technique  *328*
    Factors Underlying a Successful Technique  *328*
    Contraindications  *328*
    Anesthetized Area  *328*
    Technique  *328*
    Specific Complications of the Technique  *329*
Intraosseous Technique  *329*
    Indications, Contraindications, and Disadvantages  *330*
    Instrument Set  *330*
        Stabident®  *330*
        X-Tip®  *331*
    Anesthetic Solutions  *331*
    Anesthetized Area  *331*
    Intraosseous Technique  *332*
    Efficacy  *336*
    Specific Complications  *336*
        Complications Due to Mechanical Aspects  *336*
        Postoperative Complications  *337*
        Pulpal Abnormalities  *338*
Final Remarks  *338*
References  *339*

## 19 Failure of Dental Local Anesthesia  *344*

Frequency  *344*
Consequences of Failure  *344*
Failures: General Causes  *345*
    Highly Anxious Patients  *345*
    Patients with Drug Addiction and Alcoholism  *346*

Teeth Affected by Irreversible Acute Pulpitis  *346*
      Reasons for Failure of Anesthesia in Acute Pulpitis  *346*
      Approach  *347*
   Resistance to Local Anesthetics  *348*
   Other Causes of Failure  *348*
  Specific Failures After Maxillary Infiltration  *348*
   Causes of Maxillary Failure  *348*
   Approach  *349*
  Specific Failures After Mandibular Block  *349*
   Reasons for Failure After Mandibular Block  *349*
      Failure Owing to Inappropriate Technique  *349*
      Failure for Anatomical Reasons  *349*
      Failure Arising from Accessory Innervation  *350*
   Approach  *354*
  References  *354*

# 20 Alternatives to Conventional Techniques  *360*
  Jet Injection  *360*
   Distribution of the Solution  *360*
   Indications  *361*
   Disadvantages  *361*
   Advantages  *361*
   Equipment  *361*
      Syrijet®  *361*
      Injex®  *362*
   Technique  *362*
   Complications of this Technique  *363*
  Electronic Anesthesia: Electronic Dental Anesthesia  *364*
   Mechanism of Action  *364*
   Indications  *364*
   Disadvantages  *366*
   Advantages  *366*
   Contraindications  *366*
   Equipment  *367*
   Technique  *367*
   Complications of this Technique  *368*
  Computer-Controlled Injection Systems (The Wand®)  *368*
   Description of the Device  *369*
      Central Processing Unit  *369*
      Foot Control  *370*
      Handpiece  *370*
      Needles  *370*
      Set-up  *370*
      Advantages and Disadvantages  *371*
   P-AMSA  *371*
      Anesthetized Area  *371*
      Technique  *371*
      Efficacy of the P-AMSA Technique  *373*
      Specific Complications of this Technique  *373*
      Advantages of the P-AMSA Technique  *373*
   P-ASA  *373*
      Anesthetized Area  *373*

Technique  *374*
  Efficacy of P-ASA  *375*
  Specific Complications with this Technique  *375*
  Advantages of P-ASA  *375*
 The Wand and Conventional Techniques  *375*
  Periodontal Ligament Technique  *375*
  Mandibular Block  *376*
Other Computer-controlled Injection Systems  *376*
 Comfort Control Syringe from Midwest  *376*
 Quicksleeper  *377*
  Equipment  *377*
  Anesthetized Area  *377*
  Transcortical Technique  *377*
  Efficacy of QuickSleeper  *378*
  Disadvantages  *379*
Intranasal Maxillary Local Anesthesia (Kovanaze®)  *379*
 Composition of the Solution  *379*
 Zone Anesthetized  *379*
 Indications and Contraindications  *379*
  Indications  *379*
  Contraindications  *380*
 Equipment  *380*
  Preparation  *380*
 Technique  *380*
 Efficacy of the Technique  *381*
 Complications Specific to this Technique  *381*
 Advantages and Disadvantages  *383*
  Advantages  *383*
  Disadvantages  *384*
 References  *384*

## 21 Local Anesthesia in Children  *389*
The Problem with Children and Adolescents  *389*
Local Anesthetic Solutions  *389*
Anesthetic Technique in Children  *390*
Anesthesia of the Primary Mandibular Molars  *391*
 Needles and Mandibular Block  *392*
 Remarks on Buccal Infiltration  *392*
References  *392*

## Complications  395

## 22 Local Complications of Dental Local Anesthesia  *397*
Persistent Post-injection Pain  *397*
Self-inflicted Injury  *397*
Facial Blanching  *398*
 Anesthetic Techniques Involved  *399*
 Clinical Manifestations  *399*
 Causes and Pathophysiology  *399*
  Proposed Causes  *399*
  Pathophysiology  *400*

- Localized Late-onset Skin Lesion  *400*
  - Clinical Manifestations  *400*
  - Causes and Pathophysiology  *400*
    - Ischemic Necrosis Due to Vasospasm  *400*
    - Type III Allergic Reaction  *401*
- Facial Hematomas  *401*
  - Technical Factors Contributing to Hematomas  *401*
  - Clinical Manifestations  *401*
  - Management by the Dentist  *402*
- Nerve Lesions  *402*
  - Anatomical Lesions  *402*
  - General Causes  *402*
  - Immediate Electric Shock Sensation  *403*
    - Electric Shock Sensation After the Transpalatal Approach  *403*
  - Long-Term Paresthesia  *404*
    - Causes of Long-term Lesions  *404*
    - Clinical Manifestations  *404*
    - Management by the Dentist  *406*
  - Alterations of the Sense of Taste  *407*
  - Hoarseness  *407*
- Trismus  *407*
  - Local Anesthetic Techniques Implicated in the Development of Trismus  *407*
  - Causes of Trismus  *408*
  - Clinical Types of Trismus  *408*
    - Acute Early-onset Trismus  *408*
    - Chronic Late-onset Trismus Due to Fibrous Band Formation  *408*
    - Chronic Late-onset Trismus Due to Infection  *408*
  - Treatment of Trismus  *408*
    - Conservative Treatment (Mechanical Therapy)  *408*
    - Forced Opening Under General Anesthesia  *409*
    - Surgical Drainage  *409*
- Facial Palsy  *409*
  - Clinical Manifestations  *410*
  - Facial Palsy Associated with Mandibular Block  *410*
    - Immediate Onset and Short Duration  *410*
    - Late Onset and Long Duration  *411*
  - Facial Palsy Associated with Maxillary Infiltration  *412*
- Ocular Complications  *412*
  - Anesthetic Techniques Involved  *412*
  - Clinical Manifestations  *412*
  - Other Clinical Aspects of Interest  *413*
  - Onset and Duration  *413*
  - Predictors of Sequelae  *414*
  - Management by the Dentist  *414*
  - Pathophysiology of Complications  *414*
    - Retrograde Arterial Flow  *414*
    - Retrograde Venous Flow  *414*
    - Passive Diffusion to the Orbit  *417*
    - Irritation of the Sympathetic System  *417*
    - Sympathetic System Block (Horner-like Syndrome)  *418*
    - Other Proposed Causes  *418*
- Needle-induced Infection  *418*

Clinical Manifestations  *418*
    Management by the Dentist  *419*
  Post-injection Mucosal Ulceration  *419*
    Clinical Manifestations  *419*
    Proposed Causes  *419*
    Management by the Dentist  *419*
  Breakage of the Needle  *419*
    Anesthetic Techniques Involved  *420*
    Causes of Needle Breakage  *420*
    Associated Factors of Interest  *420*
    Clinical Manifestations  *421*
    Decision to Retrieve (or Not)  *421*
    Management by the Dentist  *421*
    Preventive Measures  *422*
  Breakage of the Cartridge in the Mouth  *423*
  Aural Complications  *423*
    Techniques Responsible  *423*
    Clinical Manifestations  *423*
    Management by the Dentist  *424*
  References  *424*

## 23 General Complications of Dental Local Anesthesia  *433*

  Preventive Measures  *435*
  Basic Management of Complications  *435*
    Initial Measures  *435*
    Unconscious Patient  *436*
      P: Posture  *436*
      A: Airway  *436*
      B: Breathing  *437*
      C: Circulation  *438*
    Routes of Administration of Drugs  *438*
    Calling the Emergency Services  *439*
  Psychogenic Reactions  *439*
    General Causes  *439*
    Vasovagal Syncope  *439*
      Pathophysiology  *439*
      Predisposing Factors  *440*
      Clinical Manifestations  *440*
      Management by the Dentist  *441*
      Prevention  *442*
    Hyperventilation Syndrome  *442*
      Pathophysiology  *442*
      Clinical Manifestations  *443*
      Differential Diagnosis  *443*
      Management by the Dentist  *443*
    Allergic-like Reactions  *444*
  Toxicity Induced by Sympathomimetic Vasoconstrictors  *444*
    Pathophysiology  *444*
    Symptoms of Reaction to Epinephrine  *444*
    Symptoms of Reaction to Norepinephrine  *445*
    Management by the Dentist  *445*
  Systemic Toxicity Induced by Local Anesthetics  *445*

Pathophysiology  *445*
  Causes of Local Anesthetic-induced Toxicity  *446*
    Inadvertent Intravascular Injection  *446*
    Overdose  *447*
    Rapid Absorption  *447*
  Clinical Manifestations  *447*
    First Phase: Initial  *447*
    Second Phase: Advanced  *448*
    Third Phase: Convulsions  *448*
    Fourth Phase: Final  *448*
  Clinical Variations  *449*
  Management by the Dentist  *449*
  Recovery and Discharge  *450*
  Prevention  *450*
Toxic Methemoglobinemia  *450*
  Local Anesthetics Involved  *451*
    Benzocaine  *451*
    Prilocaine  *451*
    Other Anesthetics  *451*
  Aggravating Factors  *452*
  Clinical Manifestations  *452*
  Management by the Dentist  *453*
Allergy  *453*
  Allergy to the Components of Local Anesthetic Solution  *455*
    Local Anesthetic  *455*
    Esters  *455*
    Amides  *455*
    Vasoconstrictor  *456*
    Antioxidants (Sulfites)  *456*
    Preservative (Methylparaben)  *457*
  Confusion with Other Reactions  *457*
  Clinical Manifestations  *458*
    Minor Manifestations  *458*
    Major Manifestations  *458*
  Diagnosis  *459*
  Management by the Dentist  *459*
    Treatment of Minor Manifestations  *459*
    Treatment of Major Manifestations  *459*
    Support Measures for Major Manifestations  *460*
    Recovery and Discharge  *460*
  Prevention  *460*
References  *461*

**Index**  *469*
**For Annexes: Refer Online**

# Preface

Dental local anesthesia is the principal means at our disposal for controlling the pain caused by our treatments and procedures. The importance of dental local anesthesia is so profound that it is impossible to imagine carrying out our work without it. This approach has considerable advantages and an excellent safety profile over other techniques for managing pain in our day-to-day activity as compared to sedation and general anesthesia. Furthermore, administration of local anesthesia is one of the most common procedures in clinical practice and is generally the first treatment administered. If its effect is inadequate, our work is complicated enormously.

Correct application of local anesthesia is very important in adults, since many patients may refuse to undergo dental treatment owing to their fear of needles and injections. Paradoxically, the method we use to control pain causes most anxiety for patients. Correct application is even more important in children, since traumatic experiences in childhood can be carried forward to adulthood: poor control of dental pain in children is one of the main factors underlying the development of anxiety over dental treatment at older ages.

We highlight a series of peculiar aspects in this book. Almost all of the techniques discussed are intraoral, and while extraoral techniques that cross the skin are used occasionally – mainly in hospitals – they have a negligible role in modern dentistry. In addition, many chapters and sections provide simple and practical quantitative data (percentages, means, ranges, etc.). This information has been obtained from many sources and studies with the aim of guiding dentists in the situations that arise in daily practice. The annexes found at the end of the book provide abundant information based on specific and practical data. They are presented separately so as not to interrupt the flow and reduce the effectiveness of this textbook.

The images and illustrations aim to explain concepts as clearly as possible. Consequently, most drawings are more schematic than strictly topographic, much in the same style as that of the famous illustrator Frank H. Netter, who expressed the idea perfectly: "Clarification of a subject is the aim and goal of illustration. No matter how beautifully painted, how delicately and subtly rendered a subject may be, it is of little value as a medical illustration if it does not serve to make clear some medical point." Of course, we do not aim to surpass the artistic quality of Dr. Netter, although we do hope to follow his approach. We have endeavored to provide clear criteria and practice guidelines. While these may occasionally be debatable, we believe that one criterion is better than none. In any case, every effort has been made to present practical and actionable information.

We would like to express our gratitude to Hilding Björn, lecturer at the Universities of Malmo and Lund, for providing us with studies on dental local anesthesia. We are also grateful to his son, Lars Olof Björn, for providing us with information on his father. We thank Professors Rafael Rioboo and Antonio Bascones of Universidad Complutense for their inspiration and example over so many years. We appreciate the help provided by all of the libraries involved in the search for documentation, namely, the Kungliga Biblioteket in Stockholm, the Library of the Academy of Sciences in Saint Petersburg, the British Library, the Centro de Información y Documentación Científica (Spain), and, in particular, the Library of the School of Dentistry of Universidad Complutese and its directors Rosa Mª Rodríguez Durántez and Marian de la Casa, as well as all their staff. Special mention must be made of all those students from the School of Dentistry, Universidad Complutense de Madrid who, over the years, provided information, documents, and studies on dental local anesthesia

Finally, we would like to stress that the information we provide is the fruit of enormous efforts made by many. Therefore, we wish to thank all those great professionals who have played a key role in the history of dentistry, as well as the thousands of specialists (chemists, physicians, and dentists) who, while not part of this history, made essential contributions to the development of techniques that provide relief for millions of people every day throughout the world. We thank them all.

*Jesús Calatayud*
Associate Professor, School of Dentistry
Universidad Complutense, Madrid, Spain

*Mana Saraghi*
Director, Dental Anesthesiology Residency Program,
Jacobi Medical Center
Assistant Professor of Dentistry,
Albert Einstein College of Medicine
Bronx, New York

## About the Companion Website

This book is accompanied by a companion website:

www.wiley.com/go/Calatayud/local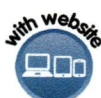

The website includes:

- The Annexes 1 to 42

# 1

# History of Local Anesthesia in Dentistry

The development of anesthesia in general and local anesthetics in particular required a cultural change. The concept of pain (especially obstetrical pain) was linked to the concept of original sin, and the ability to endure pain was regarded as a sign of character and, in men, was even associated with virility (Greene 1971).

The changes taking place in Western Europe between 1750 and 1850, with the enlightenment, industrialization, progressive democratization, and humanization of society, created an atmosphere favorable to the discovery of anesthetics. Nothing comparable occurred in Asia, Russia, or the Islamic countries, where feudalism persisted in a variety of forms. This general process altered the cultural, political, and religious climate, affecting a significant number of individuals (Greene 1971).

Dentists, not medical doctors, were responsible for the discovery of anesthesia, given their close day-to-day contact with pain and hence their motivation to seek the means to alleviate it (Greene 1971). Doctors focused more on infections than on pain, for people were dying of pneumonia, diphtheria, gangrene, tuberculosis, tetanus, puerperal fever, and appendicitis (Greene 1971; Vandam 1973). Two dentists were the first to introduce anesthesia: Horace Wells (1815–1848), with nitrous oxide in 1844 (Wells 1847; Menczer and Jacobsohn 1992; Jacobsohn 1994), and William Thomas Green Morton (1819–1868), with ether in 1846 (Greene 1979).

Local anesthesia, the basis of modern local anesthetics for dentistry, developed later. This chapter reviews the discovery and evolution of local anesthesia from the Spanish discovery of the coca leaf in America to recently established forms of local anesthesia in dentistry.

## The Coca Leaf

Coca leaves are taken from a shrub of the genus *Erythroxylum*, a member of the Erythroxylaceae family, so named by Patricio Browne because of the reddish hue of the wood of the main species (Loza-Balsa 1992). Of the various species in this genus, *Erythroxylum coca* contains the highest concentration of the alkaloid known as cocaine in its leaves, up to 0.7–1.8% by weight (Caldwell and Sever 1974; Van Dyke and Byck 1982). Many species of this genus have been grown in Nicaragua, Venezuela, Bolivia, and Peru since pre-Columbian times (Loza-Balsa 1992).

The earliest cultivation and use of the coca leaf in the Bolivian and Andean region date back to 700 BCE (Loza-Balsa 1992), although recent discoveries in Ecuador indicate human usage more than 5000 years ago (Van Dyke and Byck 1982). Alfred Bühler premised that the Arhuaco, a tribe from the Negro River region, were the first to discover the properties of the drug and spread this knowledge to neighboring peoples (Bülher 1944a,b).

Sixteenth century Spanish chroniclers associated the appearance of coca with Francisco Pizarro's (1475–1541) conquest of the Inca or Tahuantinsuyo empire in 1532. The earliest chroniclers made no mention of the plant. The reason for the belated mention of the coca leaf and its consumption may lie, as the sixteenth century Spanish chroniclers aver, in the fact that its use was restricted to the ruling class of the Inca Empire and to certain religious rites, but did not extend to the population as a whole (Calatayud and González 2003). Modern authors have verified those assumptions; noting that after the fall of the empire in 1532 coca consumption became popular among the population at large (Gutierrez-Noriega and Zapata 1947; Loza-Balsa 1992) as the entire social system underwent drastic change, particularly after 1540 (Loza-Balsa 1992).

The first reliable account of coca leaf consumption is a manuscript letter from the Bishop of Cuzco, Friar Vicente de Valverde (15..–1542), to Emperor Charles V in 1539 (*Carta* 1864). His letter is important because Valverde accompanied Francisco Pizarro throughout the conquest of Peru and was present at all the significant events. The second reliable reference is another manuscript, also a letter, from the President of the Peruvian Assembly, member

*Local Anesthesia in Dentistry: A Locoregional Approach*, First Edition. Jesús Calatayud and Mana Saraghi.
© 2024 John Wiley & Sons Ltd. Published 2024 by John Wiley & Sons Ltd.
Companion website: www.wiley.com/go/Calatayud/local

of the clergy and man of letters Pedro de la Gasca (1485–1567), to the Council of the Indies in 1549, in which he described the measures taken by Francisco Pizarro to distribute coca (Carta 1954). The third reference, and the first to be published in print, is attributed to traveler Pedro Cieza de León (1520–1554) whose chronicle of Peru, published in Seville in 1553, refers to the chewing of coca leaves with a chalk-like powder to assuage hunger, and increase strength and stamina (Cieza de Leon 1553). Pedro Cieza traveled through America between 1530 and 1550, and lived in Peru from 1548 to 1550 (Cieza de Leon 1984). All these chroniclers observed that coca consumption was widespread throughout the population (Table 1.1).

The first reference to the anesthetic effects of coca is attributed to Spanish Jesuit Bernabé Cobo (1582–1657) (Torres 1943), who, in his 1653 manuscript work on the new world, mentioned that toothaches could be alleviated by chewing coca leaves (Cobo 1890).

In subsequent centuries, most writers tended to be apologists, stressing the stimulant effects of coca but paying little or no heed to its dangers. Physicians such as Peruvian José Hipólito Unanúe (1755–1833) (Vicuña-Mackenna 1914) recommended the use of coca leaves in 1794 (Unanúe 1914) while Austrian physician Sigmund Freud (1856–1939) recommended cocaine itself in 1884. Scholar Francisco Falcon draw attention to the dangers of coca for the first time, in 1582, on the grounds of the mortality it produced among the aboriginal peoples (although this was mainly due to disease acquired during its cultivation) and the difficulty of ridding oneself of the "custom" of using it. The choice of that word in sixteenth century usage is indicative of certain characteristics of addiction. Falcon also recommended measures to restrict its consumption (*Representación* 1946), but it was not until the nineteenth century that the voice of alarm was sounded about the negative effects of coca abuse. German doctor Eduard Friedrich Pöppig (1798–1868), who drew a detailed picture of coca leaf addiction after a voyage to the Amazon in 1827–1832, stressed the digestive changes, migraine, weakness, weight loss, and alterations of personality it induced and the low public opinion of coca consumption and its consumers, who were more poorly regarded than alcoholics in Europe, and unable to give up their habit (Poeppig 1836). The most important landmarks in connection with the coca leaf are outlined in Table 1.1.

## Cocaine

The active principle of the coca leaf was first isolated in 1860 at Friedrich's laboratory in Göttingen by German chemist Albert Niemann (1834–1861) (Niemann 1860; Bühler 1944b), who called it "cocaine." Although Niemann unfortunately died the following year, his work was carried on by his disciple Wilhelm Lossen (1838–1906) (Bühler 1944b), who determined the correct molecular formula, $C_{17}H_{21}NO_4$, in 1865 (Lossen 1865). The structural formula of the new alkaloid was far from obvious and in fact was not fully known until chemist Richard Willstätter (1872–1942) analyzed it successfully in 1898 (Figure 1.1). He and his colleagues in Munich, and the Merck Laboratory in Darmstadt, synthesized artificial cocaine in 1923 (Willstätter 1898; Willstätter et al. 1923).

From the time cocaine was isolated, steps were taken to apply it as the first local anesthetic. Nothing had changed since the early reference to the anesthetic effect of the coca leaf by Jesuit Bernabé Cobo in 1653 (Cobo 1890). In 1860, Niemann reported and clearly demonstrated numbness of the tongue caused by the new alkaloid, an observation corroborated by Lossen in his 1865 paper (Lossen 1865). The first experimental study on cocaine, however, was conducted by Peruvian Thomas Moreno y Maïz, ex-naval surgeon, as part of his doctoral thesis published in Paris in 1868. While observing that injecting a cocaine solution in animals induced insensitivity to pain, he made no mention of its use in surgery (Moréno y Maïz 1868). In 1880, Russian aristocrat and physician Vassily von Anrep of the University of Würzburg published a paper on his experiments on animals, animal tissues and organs, and, especially, himself and recommended the use of cocaine as a surgical anesthetic (Anrep 1880).

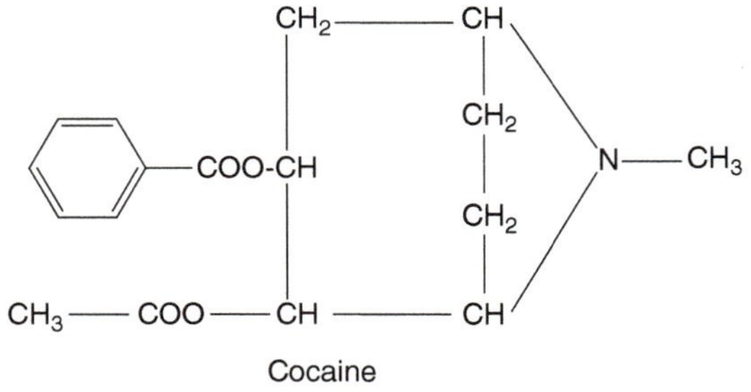

**Table 1.1** Earliest descriptions of the coca leaf, its anesthetic effect, and harmful side effects.

| |
|---|
| Earliest writings on the coca leaf |
| • 1539 Friar Vicente de Valverde. Manuscript letter |
| • 1549 Pedro de la Gasca. Manuscript letter |
| • 1553 Pedro Cieza de León. First book in print |
| First description of the anesthetic effect |
| • 1653 Bernabé Cobo. Manuscript |
| First references to harmful effects |
| • 1582 Francisco Falcon |
| • 1836 Eduard Friedrich Pöppig |

**Figure 1.1** Structural formula for cocaine.

The ground was laid but the final step had yet to be taken when Viennese ophthalmologist Carl Koller (1857–1944) rose to the challenge (Liljestrand 1967). Koller was working in the Wiener Allgemeines Krankenhaus (Viennese General Hospital) where he got to know and become friends with Sigmund Freud. Freud, interested in the stimulant effects of cocaine to overcome morphine addiction, encouraged Koller to participate in a series of experiments with cocaine during the spring and summer of 1884 (Buess 1944; Liljestrand 1967). Koller noted the numbing effect on his tongue when he swallowed the cocaine (Koller 1928). In July 1884, Freud published a review on cocaine and his experiments, again noting but without lending any particular attention to the alkaloid's anesthetic effect on mucous membranes (Freud 1884). It was Koller who grasped its importance, experimenting with animal corneas (Leonard 1998) as well as on himself and on patients (Koller 1884a). On 11 September 1884, he performed the first operation using local anesthetic on a patient suffering from glaucoma (Fink 1985). The German Ophthalmologyt Society Congress met in Heidelberg on 15–16 September 1884, but Koller was unable to attend. However, he asked Dr. Josef Brettauer, an ophthalmologist from Trieste passing through Vienna on his way to Heidelberg, to read his paper at the Congress (Fink 1985). The impact was instantaneous. Koller himself read his paper on 17 October in the Wiener Medizinische Gesellschaft (Vienna's medical society) (Koller 1884a, 1928; Liljestrand 1967) and it was published on 25 October (Leonard 1998). Dr. Henry D. Noyes of New York, who attended the Heidelberg Congress, sent a summary highlighting Koller's work to the *New York Medical Record*, who published it on 11 October (Noyes 1884). Dr. Bloom translated Koller's article into English and had it published in *The Lancet* on 6 December (Koller 1884b). The news of Koller's findings appeared in other publications of the time and sparked the development of regional and local anesthesia. Between September 1884 and late 1885, 60 publications concerning local anesthesia using cocaine appeared in the United States and Canada (Matas 1934a).

Vassily von Anrep (1852–1927) published the first report of a truncal block in an intercostal nerve on 15 November (Yentis and Vlassakov 1999) and Dr. William Stewart Halsted (1852–1922) and his co-worker Richard John Hall (1856–1897) read Noyes's report and immediately became interested in local anesthesia (Olch and William 1975). On 6 December 1884, Hall published a report on the first mandibular block. Dr. Nash of New York was able to block the infraorbital plexus with 8 minims (about 0.5 ml) of 4% cocaine hydrochloride to obturate an upper incisor, while Dr. Halsted performed a mandibular block of the inferior alveolar nerve in a medical student using 9 minims of the same solution (Hall 1884). In 1892, François Franck coined the term "block" to describe this type of local anesthesia (Matas 1934b). The most significant milestones in the discovery of local anesthesia based on cocaine in late 1884 are listed in Table 1.2.

**Table 1.2** Stages in the discovery of the local anesthetic effect of cocaine in late 1884.

| Month and day in 1884 | Landmark |
|---|---|
| July | • Sigmund Freud publishes his paper on cocaine (Freud 1884) |
| 11 September | • First operation using cocaine as a local anesthetic, performed by Carl Koller on a glaucoma patient (Fink 1985) |
| 15–16 September | • German Ophthalmological Society congress at Heidelberg (Liljestrand 1967) |
| 11 October | • Henry D. Noyes publishes a summary of the Heidelberg proceedings in the *New York Medical Record* (Noyes 1884) |
| 17 October | • Carl Koller reads his paper at the Vienna Medical Society (Koller 1928; Liljestrand 1967) |
| 25 October | • Carl Koller publishes his paper in the *Wiener Medizinische Wochenschrift* (Koller 1884a) |
| 15 November | • von Anrep reports implementing the first intercostal block (Yentis and Vlassakov 1999) |
| 6 December | • J.N. Bloom translates Koller's paper and publishes it in *The Lancet* (Koller 1884b) |
| | • Richard John Hall describes the first application of local anesthesia in dentistry and the first mandibular block, effected by William Stewart Halsted (Hall 1884) |

## The Development of the Syringe

The development of local anesthesia was contingent on the invention of the hypodermic syringe for subcutaneous injections. Subcutaneous administration of medication had already begun by way of incisions in the skin. Von Neuner developed an early syringe in 1827 to introduce fluids into animals (McAuley 1966), and in 1841 the American firm Zophar Jayne, working out of Illinois, began to market its syringe, but to be used it required a prior incision in the skin (McAuley 1966). According to Charles Pfender's studies of the origin of hypodermic medication (Pfender 1911) the first to use injection by syringe was Irish surgeon Francis

Rynd (1801–1861) of Meath Hospital. In 1845, he reported two cases of morphine acetate injection (Rynd. 1845). One of the cases was an injection in the vicinity of the supraorbital nerve to treat neuralgia. Rynd failed to publish the design of his syringe until 1861 (Rynd 1861). In 1853, veterinary surgeon Charles Gabriel Pravaz (1791–1855) of Lyon developed a syringe to inject iron perchloride into animals to treat aneurysm (Pravaz 1853). At almost at the same time, in 1855, the Scottish physician Alexander Wood (1817–1884) (Pfender 1911) published a report of nine cases treated with muriate of morphia, which he had injected via a syringe (Wood 1855). From then on, the hypodermic syringe was readily available to the medical community. Wood was instrumental in the extension of its use, although it was Charles Hunter who first used the term "hypodermic" to refer to these subcutaneous methods of injection in 1859 (Pfender 1911; Matas 1934a).

## The Dangers of Cocaine

After Koller's discovery of its local anesthetic powers, the use of cocaine spread rapidly, but since it was administered in high concentrations, on the order of 10–30% (Pernice 1890; Mayer 1924; McAuley 1966), practitioners soon began to report its alarming side-effects. Between 1884 and 1891, 200 cases of systemic intoxication and 13 deaths attributable to the drug were recorded (Anonymus 1979), quenching enthusiasm for it and prompting physicians to turn to gases such as nitrous oxide and ether, particularly for minor surgical procedures, including dentistry (Sauvez 1905). Around this time, the dependence liability of cocaine also began to emerge as several early users, Freud and Halsted among them, fell victims to it (Liljestrand 1967; Olch and William 1975).

The credit for making the infiltration of cocaine safer is shared by a number of researchers. In Germany, Maximilian Oberst of Halle (1849–1925) (Buess 1944) applied low concentrations of cocaine to the fingers, compressing them for slower release of the drug into the bloodstream, a technique that proved to be effective, as reported on 3 April 1890 by another scientist from Halle, Ludwig Pernice, who had worked with Oberst (Pernice 1890). On 11 June 1892, Carl Ludwig Schleich (1859–1922), a surgeon from Berlin, published the results of a study using a solution of 0.1–0.2% cocaine hydrochloride, infiltrating it under several layers of skin and chilling the area with an ether aerosol (to fix the drug and enhance its effects) (Schleich 1892). Parisian surgeon Paul Reclus (1847–1914), in turn, published a paper in 1895 in which he described the use of low concentrations of cocaine (from 2% to 0.5%) to achieve a good local anesthetic which, though slower in taking hold, caused no side effects (Reclus 1895). The operations described in Reclus's work included dental extractions and pulpotomies.

Today we know that around the same time Halsted was working with solutions containing low cocaine concentrations, to be applied by compression, but he unfortunately became addicted to cocaine and morphine, and was unable to publish his results (Matas 1934b; Olch and William 1975; Fink 1985). The maximum cocaine dosage for infiltration was eventually established at 50 mg (Fischer 1912; Bieter 1936).

## Adrenaline and the Vasoconstrictive Effect

From the outset, as discussed above, the development of local anesthesia went hand in hand with studies to improve its effectiveness and safety. The clinical experiments reported by Leonard Corning on 19 September 1885 are a case in point. Corning showed that using compression and a tourniquet on the limbs prevented cocaine from diffusing from the injection site, thereby increasing and deepening its anesthetic effect, in turn making it possible to reduce the dose administered (Corning 1885).

Toward the end of the nineteenth century, the Polish researcher Napoleon Cybulski (1854–1919) (Grybowski and Pietrzak 2013) unsuccessfully attempted to isolate the active principle of the suprarenal medulla, which increased arterial pressure (Cybulski 1895). A similar attempt was made by Dr. John Jacob Abel (1857–1938), a researcher from the Johns Hopkins hospital, who while coming very close, always isolated contaminated forms (Abel and Crawford 1897; Abel 1898, 1899). Abel named his substance "epinephrine" (from the Greek *epi* and *nephros* "on top of the kidneys") (Abel 1899). In that same time frame, Austrian physician Otto Ritter von Fürth (1867–1938) also unsuccessfully attempted to isolate the substance, which he called "suprarenin" (von Fürth 1900). In 1901 two researchers, Jokichi Takamine (1854–1922) (Takamine 1901a,b) and Thomas Bell Aldrich (1861–1939) (Aldrich 1901), did isolate the compound, which Takamine called "adrenalin" (from the Latin *ad* and *renal* "near the kidney") and for which Aldrich determined the correct molecular formula, namely $C_9H_{13}NO_3$. In 1904, German Friedrich Stolz (1860–1936) synthesized adrenaline or epinephrine in its two isomeric forms levo (L) and dextro (D) (Stolz 1904). At present, only the more powerful levo form is used.

The clinical application of adrenaline as a local anesthetic is attributed to Leipzig surgeon Heinrich Braun (1862–1934) (Braun 1903a). Braun obtained epinephrine from the London Parke Davies laboratories and added it to a cocaine solution in 1903, achieving a deeper and longer-lasting anesthetic effect, which he called a chemical tourniquet (Braun 1903a,b). Braun subsequently conducted a series of experiments with animals and patients to evaluate different cocaine and epinephrine concentrations (Braun 1903b).

Today, for reasons traceable to its history, this vasoconstrictor is known as epinephrine in the United States and adrenaline in Europe and the rest of the world. Takamine patented the technique and marketed the product with Parke Davis as "adrenalin" (without the final "e") (Navarro 2003). Inasmuch as Adrenalin was a registered trade name in the United States, the American Medical Association's Council on Pharmacy and Chemistry chose epinephrine as the generic name for the active principle (Smith 1920). Chemists and physicians in the rest of the world, however, not subject to such pharmaceutical company interests, chose the name "adrenaline" (with the final "e"), which is now the term used by the European Pharmacopoeia, the World Health Organization (WHO) and the International Union of Pure Applied Chemistry (IUPAC) (Navarro 2003).

## Novocaine or Procaine

As soon as the undesirable effects of cocaine began to appear (such as cardiovascular toxicity and dependence liability), attempts were made to find new drugs with anesthetic properties to replace it. However, none of these attempts were very successful until 27 November 1904, when German chemist Alfred Einhorn (1856–1917) (Link 1959) patented 18 derivatives of para-aminobenzoic acid, developed in the Meister Lucius und Brüning factories at Höchst. Composition number two was to bring radical change (Farbwerke vorm 1904).

Professor Heinrich Braun published the first paper on what he called novocaine (Figure 1.2) in 1905, comparing it to other promising local anesthetics such as stovaine and alypin (Braun 1905). Braun compared different concentrations of novocaine with adrenaline and obtained excellent results (Braun 1905). In 1909, Einhorn and his disciple Emil Uhlfelder published a paper outlining the properties and chemical characteristics of novocaine (Einhorn and Uhlfelder 1909).

Novocaine was introduced in North America by W.S. Schley in 1907 and more specifically into dentistry by Hermann Prinz in 1910 (Rahart 1972). In 1910, German dentist Guido Fischer (1877–1959) published the first book on local anesthesia in dentistry, in which he described the novocaine-based local anesthetic techniques already in use in dentistry as opposed to the anesthetic gases applied until then (Fischer 1910). The book was enormously successful, with a second edition translated into English by Richard Riethmüller in 1912 (Fischer 1912) and the fifth edition translated into Spanish in 1924 (Fischer 1924). A number of editions of Fischer's work were published in the early twentieth century and translated into various languages. The second major text to appear on local anesthesia in dentistry, authored by Kurt Hermann Thoma of Harvard in 1914, was likewise based on novocaine (Thoma 1914). Novocaine replaced cocaine, ushering in the modern era of local anesthesia and allowing for the development of new, more effective, and safer techniques (Matas 1934b).

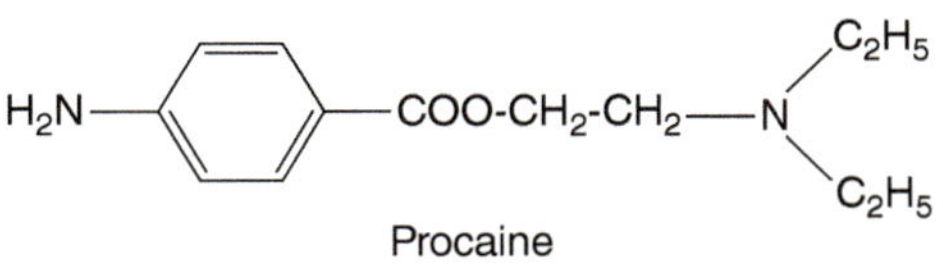

As the patent for novocaine was German, during the First World War the United States Government provided its chemical industry with the formula to manufacture the drug without having to depend on the German license and, in an attempt to protect their product, changed the name to procaine. When the war ended, Germany lost the patent (Smith 1920; Benedict et al. 1932; Nevin and Puterbaugh 1949; Link and Alfred Einhorn 1959). Today novocaine is more commonly known as procaine (Figure 1.2).

## The Development of Local Anesthesia in Dentistry

Much progress has been made since local anesthesia first came into general use. The following discussion, not intended to be exhaustive, highlights the major twentieth and twenty-first century developments in anesthesia, vasoconstriction, instruments, and techniques used in dentistry.

### Local Anesthetics

As discussed above, the first local anesthetic was cocaine, but the risks it entailed soon prompted the pursuit of other drugs. In 1890 Eduard Ritsert (1859–1946) developed benzocaine, sold under the trade name "Anësthesin." As it is scantly water-soluble however, it was used as a topical anesthetic (Nueve Arneimittel 1902). Novocaine, as noted earlier, was synthesized in 1904. It was safe, but since its effects were weak, it called for the addition of large quantities of adrenaline, especially for infiltration. To overcome the problem, in 1919 Alfred Kneucker of Vienna began to use 4% instead of 2% novocaine (Kneucker 1919). These concentrations were marketed in the United States beginning

$H_2N-\langle\rangle-COO-CH_2-CH_2-N\langle\begin{array}{c}C_2H_5\\C_2H_5\end{array}$

Procaine

**Figure 1.2** Structural formula for novocaine, labeled procaine.

in 1941 (Dobbs 1965). In 1944, however, the American Dental Association's Council on Dental Therapeutics disallowed them (Council on Dental Therapeutics 1944) on the grounds that toxicity increased geometrically with linear increases in concentration. In other words, 1 ml of 2% novocaine is four times as toxic as 1 ml of a 1% solution (Waters 1933). Their decision was also influenced, no doubt, by the reminiscence of the tragic consequences in the late nineteenth century of high concentrations (10–30%) of cocaine and the safety afforded by diluted doses (Pernice 1890; Schleich 1892; Reclus 1895). In 1949, Frank Everett not only showed that 4% novocaine solutions were indeed more effective than 2% solutions (both mixed with epinephrine) but that the 50% lethal dose (LD50), administered intravenously in rabbits and subcutaneously in rats, varied very little with concentration and, in fact, only depended on the total dose administered (Everett 1949). The Council on Dental Therapeutics has accepted the use of 4% novocaine ever since (Dobbs 1965).

In 1928, Otto Eisleb (1887–1948) synthesized a new local anesthetic, tetracaine, distributed under the trade name Pantocaine (Eisleb 1934). Tetracaine is very powerful but unfortunately also very toxic and its effects are delayed. The 2% novocaine and 0.15% tetracaine solution introduced by Cook-Waite in 1940 was intended to prolong and intensify the effects of the anesthetic (Dobbs 1965).

Novocaine, however, posed new problems, in the form of allergic reactions in patients and dentists (Guptill 1920; Klauder 1922). Since cartridge syringes were not in use at the time and dentists did not use gloves, the skin on their fingers was frequently in contact with the anesthetic. In 1920, Arthur Guptill reported the first case of allergic dermatitis in one such professional (Guptill 1920).

These developments led to a search for an alternative to novocaine, but of the many developed in the first half of the twentieth century, none proved to be clearly better. In 1943, Swedish chemists Nils Isak Löfgren (1913–1967) and Bengt Lundqvist (1922–1953) synthesized a xylidine derivative called lidocaine, chemically very different from novocaine, but safe, more powerful, and virtually allergy-free (Löfgren and Lundqvist 1946; Gordh et al. 2010). On the grounds of the studies conducted by Hilding Björn (1907–1995) and Sven Huldt, it came to be considered the standard local anesthetic and remains the standard to this day (Björn and Huldt 1947). Around that time Björn authored another breakthrough, a method to assess the efficacy of local anesthetic solutions in dental practice by electrically stimulating teeth with a pulp tester, which delivers objective data on pulpal anesthesia and its duration, overcoming the bias inherent in earlier, more subjective methods (Björn 1946, 1947). In 1948, Astra Pharmaceutical Products Inc. introduced lidocaine in the United States and Sweden (Gordh et al. 2010). New amide-type anesthetics began to make their appearance soon after. In 1957, for instance, mepivacaine and bupivacaine were developed by Bo af Ekenstam et al. (1957) and the former was marketed in the United States by Cook-Waite in 1960 (Dobbs 1965). Nils Löfgren and Cläes Tegner synthesized prilocaine in 1960 (Löfgren and Tegner 1960) and in 1972 Adams et al. developed etidocaine (Adams et al. 1972). Articaine was synthesized in 1969 (Frenkel 1989; Rahn and Ball 2001; Malamed 2004) by Roman Muschaweck (Rahn and Ball 2001; Vogel 2007) at Hoechst AG, Frankfurt, and Winther and Nathalang (1972) published the first paper on the substance in 1972.

One characteristic development in the history of local anesthetics is the steady downward trend in the recommended doses used in dentistry. Thus, for instance, the maximum dose of novocaine recommended by Fischer in 1910 was 500 mg (Fischer 1910), whereas today it is 400 mg (American Dental Association 1984). The 1000 mg maximum dose of lidocaine initially recommended (Lozier 1949; Gordh et al. 2010) has now been lowered to 300 mg (American Dental Association 1984). With mepivacaine the original recommendation for 7.9 mg/kg was later reduced to 6.6 mg/kg (Zinman 1976) and today stands at 4.3 mg/kg (American Dental Association 1984).

## Vasoconstrictors

The first and to date the best vasoconstrictor, epinephrine, continues to be widely used, although maximum concentrations and doses have changed. In 1910, Fisher recommended maximum doses of 312 μg (Fischer 1912) and Mayer no more than 1000 μg (Mayer 1924). The concentrations used in those days were on the order of from 1:20 000 (50 μg/ml) to 1:40 000 (25 μg/ml) (Fischer 1912; Thoma 1914; Hein 1917; Smith 1920; Steadman 1923). The aim of these high concentrations was to strengthen the weak effects of novocaine.

In 1938, Tainter showed that 2% novocaine solutions together with 1:25 000 (40 μg/ml) epinephrine caused nervous reactions such as shaking and sweating in 42% of patients and dizziness in 9%, due to high concentrations of epinephrine. Reducing the concentration to 1:50 000 (20 μg/ml) led to a significant decline in such reactions (Tainter et al. 1938). In 1953, the Council of the New York Institute of Clinical Oral Pathology sought an official report from the New York Heart Association (NYHA) on the administration of epinephrine to cardiovascular patients. In October 1954, the NYHA recommended a maximum concentration of 1:50 000 (20 μg/ml) and an absolute maximum dose of 200 μg (Report of the Special Committee of the New York Heart Association 1955). In 1964, the

American Dental Association, in conjunction with the American Heart Association, confirmed the NYHA recommendations for the maximum epinephrine concentration and dose (ADA-AHA 1964).

Until 1931, epinephrine was the only vasoconstrictor allowed by the Council on Dental Therapeutics (1931), although nordefrin hydrochloride (cobefrin, corbadrine, or corbasil) was introduced in 1933 at concentrations of 1:10000 (100 μg/ml) by Cook-Waite laboratories (Dobbs 1965). In 1940, Mizzy Laboratories Inc. introduced phenylephrine (neosynephrine) at concentrations of 1:2500 (400 μg/ml) (Dobbs 1965). Levonordefrin, the levo isomer of nordefrin, was proven to be more powerful than the dextro form in 1957 (Moose 1959). In 1946, Swedish researcher Ulf Svante von Euler (1905–1983) (Gordh et al. 2010) was the first to isolate norepinephrine (Von Euler 1946a, 1946b), the more potent levo form of which was introduced in the 1950s (Dobbs and de Vier 1950; Epstein et al. 1951; Berling and Björn 1951). In the end, however, of all the sympathomimetic vasoconstrictors developed, the original, epinephrine, has proved to be the safest and most powerful. Noradrenaline is not only less effective in anesthetizing pulp with different local anesthetics (Berling and Björn 1951; Brown 1968), but more dangerous insofar as it may provoke blood pressure spiking (Boakes et al. 1972; Okada et al. 1989).

Felypressin (octapressin), a vasopressin (a hormone produced by the posterior lobe of the pituitary gland) derivative synthesized by Vigneaud et al. in 1953, constitutes a wholly different approach to vasoconstrictors (Du Vigneaud et al. 1953). As a polypeptide unrelated to sympathetic-mimetic substances governed by an entirely different mechanism, it can be used where the latter are contraindicated. Felypressin is used at concentrations of 0.03 International Units, i.e. a concentration of 1:1850000 (0.54 μg/ml), with 3% prilocaine. It was studied in 1966 by Cläes Berling with satisfactory results, although not as good as 2% lidocaine with 1:80000 (12.5 μg/ml) epinephrine (Berling 1966). Felypressin is presently marketed in a number of European countries, but not in the United States.

## Instruments

Early in the use of local anesthesia, and especially in the first few decades of the twentieth century, needles were re-usable, thick (Fischer 1912; Smith 1920), and made of platinum, steel, or a platinum–iridium alloy (Fischer 1912; Thoma 1914; Tompkins 1921). They broke easily (Blum 1919; Tompkins 1921) and the steel models corroded with use (Fischer 1912; Thoma 1914; Tompkins 1921). Needles made of new stainless-steel alloys were introduced in the 1940s and were not only stronger but finer in caliber, down to 25-gauge (25G) (Harrison 1948; Bump and Roche 1973). In 1959, the Cook-Waite and Roehr laboratories introduced disposable, sterilized needles to prevent viral hepatitis (Dobbs 1965). Modern disposable needles with new alloys are highly resistant to breakage and come in even finer calibers, 27G or 30G, although they tend to bend rather easily (Robison et al. 1984).

Becton and Dickinson glass syringes appeared in 1897 and glass ampoules of novocaine and epinephrine solution were introduced in 1914 (Dobbs 1965). Prior to their appearance, dentists had to mix the solution themselves by dissolving anesthetic tablets in distilled water with salts (Fischer 1912). Around 1920, military surgeon and World War I veteran Harvey S. Cook devised the cartridge system (a cartridge containing the anesthetic attached to a syringe) which, much like a rifle cartridge, could be loaded and injected into a single patient (Dobbs 1965), enhancing safety, sterilization, and speed (Nevin and Puterbaugh 1949). Later, Cook-Waite introduced a cartridge he called a "carpule," a name that became so popular that even today cartridges are known as carpules in many dental clinics (Nevin and Puterbaugh 1949). In 1935, the Novocol Chemical Company brought out vacuum-packed cartridges, extending the shelf life of solutions, and in 1947 the same company introduced a kind of screw at the upper end of the syringe plunger and a thumb ring for aspiration (Nevin and Puterbaugh 1949; Dobbs 1965).

The first papers on aspiration prior to injection appeared at the end of the 1950s (Harris 1957; Seldin 1958) and in 1957 the Council on Dental Therapeutics recommended routine aspiration before any injection (Council on Dental Therapeutics 1957). Self-aspirating, cartridge-type syringes appeared in the early 1970s (Evers 1971; Cowan 1972; Corkery and Barret 1973), although the first self-aspirating cartridge, attributed to Niels Bjorn Jorgensen (1894–1974), was designed in the early 1960s (Monheim 1965).

## Anesthetic Techniques

US surgeon William Stewart Halsted (1852–1922) was the first to block the mandibular nerve in 1884 (Hall 1884), although he left no record of whether the technique used was intra- or an extra-oral. In his 1910 book, German dentist Guido Fischer (1877–1959) (Groß 2018) described and popularized the indirect mandibular nerve block, otherwise known as the 1-2-3 technique (Fischer 1912) attributed to Braun in 1904 (Lindsay 1929). In 1924, Boris Levitt of New York developed the direct technique (Levitt 1924), also known as the conventional technique because it is the one most commonly used even today. In 1940, Laguardia of Montevideo developed a closed-mouth mandibular block technique (Laguardia 1940), which was rediscovered by

Akinosi of Lagos in 1977 (Akinosi 1977). In 1973, a new mandibular block technique was described by Australian dentist George Albert Edward Gow-Gates (1910–2001), which he had been perfecting since 1947 but which had not been published earlier (Gow-Gates 1973; Gow-Gates and Watson 1989).

Intraligamentary injection, one of the oldest techniques known, was first described by Emilie Sauvez of Paris in 1905 (Sauvez 1905), but as he did not lay claim to it as an original technique, it may have been in use prior to that date, perhaps in 1904 by Guido Fischer. Although Cassamani of Paris wrote his doctor's thesis on this technique in 1924 (Cassamani 1924), it was not included in the scientific literature until the 1970s, when it was described by Robert Lafargue (1973) and Chenaux et al. (1976). In 1981, a paper by Richard Walton et al. retrieved the method for the English-speaking world (Walton and Abbott 1981). According to Mendel Nevin and Pliny Guy Puterbaugh, the intra-pulp technique was first used in 1895 (Nevin and Puterbaugh 1949).

The foremost technique for blocking the upper maxillary nerve behind the tuberosity (high tuberosity approach) was developed after 1913 by Arthur Ervin Smith and described in 1920 (Smith 1920). The greater palatine foramen technique was first described by Juan Ubaldo Carrea (1883–1956) of Buenos Aires in 1921 (Carrea 1921).

Another technique for administering anesthetic solutions is high-pressure jet injection, based on high-pressure injection of a flow of very fine droplets which penetrate the skin and mucus and get into the tissues. It was used on human beings for the first time in 1947 by Frank Figge et al. (Figge and Scherer 1947). That same year, another paper describing a device called hypospray (Hingson and Hughes 1947) was published, but this device was not used in dentistry until Margetis et al. implemented it in 1958 (Margetis et al. 1958). The dermojet, an instrument specifically designed for dentistry, was developed in 1960 (Roberts and Sowray 1987). New and improved devices continued to be developed, the most prominent of which is the syrijet introduced in 1971 (Bennett and Monheim 1971; Epstein 1971).

Power-operated injection systems constitute another group of techniques for administering anesthetics. The history of the use of electricity has been revised (Kane and Taub 1975; Malamed and Joseph 1987), with the consensus being that the first reference was authored by Scribonius Largus, a Roman physician during the period of Tiberius and Claudius (first century) (Chinchilla 1841). In his treatise *de Compositionibus Medicamentorum* (Scribonii 1529) Largus described the use of an electric fish [the marbled electric ray (*Torpedo marmorata*): Kane and Taub 1975] to alleviate pain. Centuries later, in Wesley 1760, Methodism founder John Wesley (1703–1791) published *The Desideratum*, in which he addressed the application of electrodes to relieve pain. The first reference in the application of electrodes to alleviate tooth-related pain was penned by another British scientist, James Ferguson, in 1770 (Ferguson 1770). In 1858, Jerome B. Francis reported 164 cases of electricity-mediated painless tooth extractions after the application of electrodes to the teeth in an article published in *The Dental Reporter* (Francis 1858). The impact of Francis's paper in the United States and Europe was enormous in the years thereafter, but its influence declined due to the poor results obtained in the late nineteenth and early twentieth centuries. As early as 1858, the London College of Dentists advised against its use because electricity was found to have no anesthetic effects and heighten pain and the few favorable results were attributable to "distraction" (Kane and Taub 1975). With the description of gate control theory (Melzack and Wall 1965) in 1965 and the mechanisms of pain modulation, truly operative systems have begun to be developed. In medicine, a technique known as TENS (transcutaneous electrical nerve stimulation) is used, whose equivalent in dentistry is called EDA (electronic dental anesthesia) (Malamed et al. 1989). The first practical system to be marketed for use in dentistry was Ultracalm in 1989 (Silverstone 1989) and more recently in 1994, 3M brought out a smaller and more accessible piece of equipment specifically applicable to dentistry, which goes by the name of Dental Electronic Anesthesia System, 8670 3M Dental (Croll and Simonsen 1994).

Power-driven injection systems are yet another technique for administering anesthetic solutions. Spring-driven or gas-actuated syringes introduced in the 1970s were designed to inject solutions while maintaining a constant pressure and hence a more uniform injection flow (Roberts and Sowray 1987). In 1997 a new, even more sophisticated apparatus called "the Wand" appeared, a computerized injection system developed by Dr. Mark Hochman of New York that automatically adapts the pressure to ensure a slow and constant flow at all times (Friedman and Hochman 1997) and separating injection rate from pressure. All these systems have built-in aspiration.

## Twenty-First Century Developments

*Oraqix® gel* was introduced to the market in 2005. As a derivative of eutectic mixture of local anesthetic (EMLA) cream it contains 5% topical anesthetic in a 1:1 eutectic blend of 2.5% lidocaine and 2.5% prilocaine, but designed for use in the oral cavity. It is a noninjectable, thermoreversible anesthetic gel characterized by low viscosity at ambient temperature. When introduced into the periodontal pockets, however, the body temperature converts it into an elastic gel that remains at the application site, which it anesthetizes with low risk of dissemination to other areas of the mouth (Friskopp and Huledal 2001; Friskopp et al. 2001; Herdevall et al. 2003; Magnusson et al. 2003) (see Chapter 12).

In 2008 the US Food and Drug Administration (FDA) authorized the inclusion of phentolamine mesylate in dentistry cartridges under the trade name *OraVerse*® for administration in standard syringes to reduce the duration of anesthesia in soft tissue (Tavares et al. 2008; Malamed 2008).

As a nonselective α-adrenergic antagonist, phentolamine neutralizes the vasoconstrictive effect of epinephrine and the other vasoconstrictive sympathomimetics (norepinephrine and levonordefrin). It was synthesized in 1950 at the CIBA laboratory in Basel, Switzerland, by Urech et al. (1950) and marketed in the United States in 1952 (Hersh et al. 2008) under the trade name Regitine® (Weaver 2008).

Phentolamine is injected into the same site as the vasoconstrictive sympathomimetic-bearing local anesthetic to block the effect on the α-adrenoreceptors. The outcome is vasodilation that increases the local blood flow, carrying the local anesthetic from the oral submucosa into the bloodstream to restore normal sensation in the oral and perioral tissues much more quickly, reducing the duration of soft tissue anesthesia by half (Hersh et al. 2008; Tavares et al. 2008) (see Chapter 6).

The *pH Onset System* developed by Dr. Mic Falker (Malamed and Falkel 2013), appeared in the United States in 2010, although much earlier papers on the method can be found in the literature (Davies 2003). Automated, speedy, and sterile, this device is highly practical for alkalinizing local dental anesthetic cartridges bearing sympathomimetic vasoconstrictors such as epinephrine, which usually have a pH of around 4 (Annex 14). The device raises the pH to a value very close to the physiological 7.4, reducing the burning, stinging, or pain attendant on the initial insertion of these solutions. It also aims to reduce anesthetic latency (Malamed et al. 2013) (see Chapter 11).

*Intranasal maxillary local anesthesia Kovanaze*™ (intranasal 3% tetracaine and 0.05% oxymetazoline spray) is a needle-free means of achieving dental local anesthesia and was approved by the US FDA in June 2016 for anesthesia of the anterior teeth and maxillary premolars (Saraghi and Hersh 2017). Kovanaze® is a formulation of two well-known medications: local anesthetic (tetracaine) and vasoconstrictor (oxymetazoline) for intranasal administration were combined based on the fact that these medications have been used for many years to provide local anesthesia for surgical and diagnostic procedures in the nasal cavity (Hersh et al. 2017) (see Chapter 20).

### Frequency of Use of Local Anesthesia in Dentistry

In the United States the number of cartridges/injections per year grew from 30 million in 1950 to 300 million in 2010, while worldwide the number rose from 730 million in 1980 to 1 billion in 2000. Around 30% can be estimated to consist of mandibular blocks (Annex 1).

According to these data, local anesthesia is the most prominent tool at dentists' disposal to control the pain induced by their treatments. The anesthetics involved are widely used by dentists the world over and in their absence, practice of the profession is simply unthinkable.

## References

Abel, J.J. (1898). Further observations on the chemical nature of the active principle of the suprarenal capsule. *Johns Hopkins Hosp. Bull.* 9 (90–91): 215–218.

Abel, J.J. (1899). Ueber den blutdruckerregenden Bestandteil der Nebenniere, das Epinephrin. *Hoppe-Seyler's Z. Physiol. Chem.* 28: 318–362.

Abel, J.J. and Crawford, A.C. (1897). On the blood-pressure-raising constituent of the suprarenal capsule. *Johns Hopkins Hosp. Bull.* 8 (76): 151–156.

ADA-AHA (American Dental Association and American Heart Association (1964). Management of dental problems in patients with cardiovascular diseases. *J. Am. Dent. Assoc.* 68 (3): 333–342.

Adams, H.J., Kronberg, G.H., and Takman, B.H. (1972). Local anesthetic activity and acute toxicity of (±)-2-(N-ethylpropylamino)-2′,6′-butyroxylidide, a new long-acting agent. *J. Pharm. Sci.* 61 (11): 1829–1831.

Akinosi, J.O. (1977). A new approach to the mandibular nerve block. *Br. J. Oral Surg.* 15 (1): 83–87.

Aldrich, T.B. (1901). A preliminary report on the active principle of the suprarenal gland. *Am. J. Phys.* 5: 457–461.

American Dental Association (1984). *Accepted Dental Therapeutics*, 40e. Chicago: Council on Dental Therapeutics. Chicago: American Dental Association. 185.

Annex 1. Frequency of use of local anesthesia in dentistry.

Annex 14. Injectable anesthetic solutions pH.

Anonymus (1979). Cocaine. *Br. Med. J.* 1 (6169): 971–972.

Anrep, B.v. (1880). Ueber die physiologische Wirkung des Cocaïn. *Pflügers Arch. Ges. Physiol.* 21 (1): 38–77.

Benedict, H.C., Clark, S.W., and Freeman, C.W. (1932). Studies in local anesthesia. *J. Am. Dent. Assoc.* 19 (12): 2087–2105.

Bennett, C.R. and Monheim, L.M. (1971). Production of local anesthesia by jet injection. A clinical study. *Oral Surg. Oral Med. Oral Pathol.* 32 (4): 526–530.

Berling, C. (1966). Octapressin(R) as a vasoconstrictor in dental plexus anesthesia. *Odontol. Revy* 17 (4): 369–385.

Berling, C. and Björn, H. (1951). Noradrenalin (Norexadrin) som vasokonstringens vid xylocainanästesi i tandläkarpraxis. En experimetell och klinisk undersökning, omfattande 677 dentala anästesier. *Odontol. Revy* 2: 153–164.

Bieter, R.N. (1936). Applied pharmacology of local anesthetics. *Am. J. Surg.* 34: 500–510.

Björn, H. (1946). Electrical excitation of teeth and its application to dentistry. *Sven. Tandläk.-Tidskr.* 39 (Suppl): 7–101.

Björn, H.I. (1947). The determination of the efficiency of dental local anesthetics. *Sven. Tandläk.-Tidskr.* 40 (6): 771–796.

Björn, H. and Huldt, S. (1947). IV The efficiency of xylocaine as a dental terminal anesthetic compared to that of procaine. *Sven. Tandläk.-Tidskr.* 40 (6): 831–851.

Blum, T. (1919). Failures and accidents with mandibular injections. *Dent. Cosmos* 61 (4): 275–292.

Boakes, A.J., Laurence, D.R., Lovel, K.W. et al. (1972). Adverse reactions to local anaesthetic/vasoconstrictor preparations. A study of the cardiovascular responses to xylestesin and hostacain-with-noradrenaline. *Br. Dent. J.* 133 (4): 137–140.

Braun, H. (1903a). Zur Anwendung der Adrenalins bei anästhesierenden Gewebsinjektionen. *Zentralbl. Chir.* 38: 1025–1028.

Braun, H. (1903b). Ueber den Einfluss der Vitalität der gewebe auf die örtlichen und allgemeinen Giftwirkungen Localanästhesirender mittel und über die Bedeutung des Adrenalins für die Localanästhesie. *Arch. Klin. Chir.* 69 (29): 541–591.

Braun, H. (1905). Ueber einige neue örtliche anaesthetica (Stovain, Alypin, Novocain). *Dtsch. Med. Wochenschr.* 31 (42): 1667–1671.

Brown, G. (1968). The influence of adrenaline, noradrenaline vasoconstrictors on the efficiency of lidocaine. *J. Oral Ther. Pharmacol.* 4 (5): 398–405.

Buess, H. (1944). Über die Anwendung der Koka und des Kokains in der Medizin. *Ciba Z* 8 (94): 3362–3365.

Bühler, A. (1944b). Zur erforschung des Kokagenusses. *Ciba Z* 8 (94): 3353–3359.

Bülher, A. (1944a). Die Koka bei den Indianern südamerikas. *Ciba Z* 8 (94): 3338–3351.

Bump, R.L. and Roche, W.C. (1973). A broken needle in the pterygomandibular space. Report of a case. *Oral Surg. Oral Med. Oral Pathol.* 36 (5): 750–752.

Calatayud, J. and González, A. (2003). History of the development and evolution al local anesthesia since the cocoa leaf. *Anestehsiology* 98 (6): 1503–1508.

Caldwell, J. and Sever, P.S. (1974). The biochemical pharmacology of abused drugs I. Anfetamines, cocaine, and LSD. *Clin. Pharm. Ther.* 16 (4): 625–638.

Carrea, J.U. (1921). Anestesia troncular del nerviomaxilar superior por el conductopalatino posterior. *La Odontología (Madrid)* 30 (6): 266–271. (Note: the author's name was misspelled in the original paper, as "Carrba").

Carta del licenciado Gasca al Consejo de Indias avisando las disposiciones que se habían adoptado respecto al repartimiento de la coca que tuvo Francisco Pizarro. Lima (Perú). 16 de septiembre de 1549. Publicada por: María del Carmen Pescador del Hoyo. Documentos de Indias. Siglos XV–XIX. Catálogo de la serie existente en la sección diversos. Madrid: Dirección General de Archivos y Bibliotecas. Servicio de Publicaciones. 1954: 40 (microfilm n° 97).

Carta del Obispo del Cuzco al Emperador sobre asuntos de su iglesia y otros de la gobernación general de aquel pais. Cuzco (Perú), 20 de marzo de 1539. Publicada en: Colección de documentos inéditos relativos al descubrimiento, conquista y colonización de las posesiones españolas de América y Oceanía, sacados en su mayor parte del Real Archivo de Indias. Bajo la dirección de Joaquín F. Pacheco, Francisco de Cardenas y Luis Torres de Mendoza. Madrid: Imprenta de Manuel B. de Quiros. 1864; Vol III: 92–137.

Cassamani, C. (1924). Une nouvelle technique d'anesthesia intraligamentaire. Doctoral thesis, Paris.

Chenaux, G., Castagnola, L., and Colombo, A. (1976). L'anesthesie intraligamentaire avec la jeringue "Peripress". *Scheweiz. Monatsschr. Zahnheilkd.* 86 (11): 1165–1173.

Chinchilla, A. (1841). *Anales históricos de la medicina en general y biográfico-bibliográficos de la española en particular*. Valencia: Imprenta de López y Compañía: 180.

Cieza de Leon, P. (1553; Capítulo XCVI). *Parte primera de la crónica del Perú. Que trata de la demarcacion de sus provincias: La descripcion de ellas. Las fundaciones de las nuevas ciudades. Los ritos y costumbres de los indios. Y otras cosas extrañas dignas de ser sabidas*. Sevilla: Impresa en casa de Martin de Montesdoca: 111–112.

Cieza de Leon, P. (1984). *La crónica del Perú*, 10. Madrid: Edición de Manuel Ballesteros. Crónicas de América 4. Edita Historia 16: 10, 17, 19, 21, 346–347.

Cobo, B. (1890). *Historia del Nuevo Mundo. Manuscrito en Lima (Perú). 1653*; libro 5, capítulo XXIX. Bernabe Cobo. Historia del Nuevo Mundo. Sociedad de Bibliófilos Andaluces. Con notas de Marcos Jiménez de la Espada. Sevilla: Impreso por E. Rasco. Tomo I, Libro 5, Capítulo XXIX: 473–477.

Corkery, P.F. and Barret, B.E. (1973). Aspiration using local anaesthetic cartridges with an elastic recoil diaphragm. *J. Dent.* 2 (2): 72–74.

Corning, J.L. (1885). On the prolongation of the anaesthetic effects of the hydrochlorate of cocaine when subcutaneously injected. An experimental study. *N.Y. Med. J.* 42: 317–319.

Council on Dental Therapeutics (1931). Epinephrin. *J. Am. Dent. Assoc.* 18 (4): 744–745.

Council on Dental Therapeutics (1944). Four per cent procaine solutions – not acceptable for ADR. *J. Am. Dent. Assoc.* 31 (3): 278–279.

Council on Dental Therapeutics (1957). Chicago: American Dental Association. 109.

Cowan, A. (1972). A new aspirating syringe. *Br. Dent. J.* 133 (12): 547–548.

Croll, T.P. and Simonsen, R.J. (1994). Dental electronic anesthesia for children: technique and report of 45 cases. *J. Dent. Child* 61 (2): 97–104.

Cybulski, N. (1895). Ueber die function der Nebenniere. *Cetralblatt für Physiologie* 9 (4): 172–176.

Davies, R.J. (2003). Buffering the pain of local anaesthetics: a systematic review. *Emerg. Med. (Fremantle)* 15 (1): 81–88.

Dobbs, E.C. (1965). A chronological history of local anesthesia in dentistry. *J. Oral Ther. Pharmacol.* 1 (5): 546–549.

Dobbs, E.C. and de Vier, C. (1950). L-arterenol as a vasoconstrictor in local anesthesia. *J. Am. Dent. Assoc.* 40 (4): 433–436.

Du Vigneaud, V., Ressler, C., Swan, J.M. et al. (1953). The synthesis of an octapeptide amide with the hormonal activity of oxitocin. *J. Am. Chem. Soc.* 75 (19): 4879–4880.

Einhorn, A. and Uhlfelder, E. (1909). Ueber den p-Aminobenzoësäurediäthylamino- und -piperidoäthylester. *Justus Liebig's Ann. Chem.* 371 (2): 131–142.

Eisleb, O. (1934). Vom cocain zum pantocain. Der Werdegang der örtlichen Betäubung. *Med. Chem. (Leverkusen)* 2: 364–376.

Ekenstam, B., Egner, B., and Pettersson, G. (1957). Local anaesthetics I. N-alkyl pyrrolidine and N-alkyl piperidine carboxylic acid amides. *Acta Chem. Scand.* 11 (11): 1183–1190.

Epstein, S. (1971). Pressure injection of local anesthetics. Clinical evaluation of an instrument. *J. Am. Dent. Assoc.* 82 (2): 374–377.

Epstein, S., Throndson, A.H., and Schmitz, J.L. (1951). Levo-arterenol (levophed) as a vasoconstrictor in local anesthetic solutions. *J. Dent. Res.* 30 (6): 870–873.

Everett, F.G. (1949). A comparison of depth of anesthesia and toxicity of two and four per cent procaine hydrochloride solution. *J. Dent. Res.* 28 (3): 204–218.

Evers, H. (1971). Ett nytt injektionssystem. *Tandlaek. Tidn.* 63 (22): 834–837.

Farbwerke vorm (1904). Meister Lucius und Brüning in Höchst a. M. Verfahren zur Darstellung von p-aminobenzoësäurealkaminestern. Kaiserliches Patentamt. Patentschrift nr 179 627. Klasse 12q. Gruppe 6.

Ferguson, J. (1770). An introduction to electricity. In: *Six Sections*. London: printed for W. Straham and T. Cadell: 73.

Figge, F.H.J. and Scherer, R.P. (1947). Anatomical studies on jet penetration of human skin for subcutaneous medication without the use of needles. *Anat. Rec.* 97 (3): 335. (Abstract nº 17).

Fink, B.R. (1985). Leaves and needles: the introduction of surgical local anesthesia. *Anesthesiology* 63 (1): 77–83.

Fischer, G. (1910). *Di lokale Anästhesie in der Zahanheilkunde, mit spezieller Berücksichtingung der Schleimhaut und Leitungsanästhesie. Kurz gefaßtes lehrbuch für zahnärte, Ärzte und Studierende*. Berlin: Hermann Meusser.

Fischer, G. (1912). *Local Anesthesia in Dentistry. With Special Reference to the Mucous and Conductive Methods. A Concise Guide for Dentists, Surgeons and Students*. Philadelphia: Lea and Febiger: 37, 42–6, 64–5, 176–87.

Fischer, G. (1924). *Anestesia local en odontología para odontólogos, médicos y estudiantes*. Madrid: Edita sucesores de Rivadeneyra SA.

Francis, J.B. (1858). Extracting teeth by galvanism. *Dent. Rep.* 1: 65–69.

Frenkel, G. (1989). Opening of the symposium (Foreword). In: *Local anesthesia in dentistry today. Two decades of articaine*. Symposium 1–2 November 1989. Bad Nauheim (Germany): Meducation Up-Date Hoechst, 5–6.

Freud, S. (1884). Ueber coca. *Centralbl. Gesamte Ther.* 2: 289–314.

Friedman, M.J. and Hochman, M.N. (1997). A 21st century computerized injection system for local pain control. *Compend. Cont. Educ. Dent.* 18 (10): 995–1003.

Friskopp, J. and Huledal, G. (2001). Plasma level of lidocaine and prilocaine after application of Oraqix®, a new intrapocket anesthetic, in patients with advanced periodontitis. *J. Clin. Periodontol.* 28 (5): 425–429.

Friskopp, J., Nilsson, M., and Isacsson, G. (2001). The anesthetic onset and duration of a new lidocaine/prilocaine gel intra-pocket anesthetic (Oraqix®) for periodontal scaling/root planing. *J. Clin. Periodontol.* 28 (5): 453–458.

Gordh, T., Gordh, T.E., and Lindqvist, K. (2010). Lidocaine: the origin of a modern local anesthetic. *Anesthesiology* 113 (6): 1433–1437.

Gow-Gates, G.A.E. (1973). Mandibular conduction anesthesia: a new technique using extraoral landmarks. *Oral Surg. Oral Med. Oral Pathol.* 36 (3): 321–328.

Gow-Gates, G. and Watson, J.E. (1989). Gow-Gates mandibular block – applied anatomy and histology. *Anesth. Prog.* 36 (4–5): 193–195.

Greene, N.M. (1971). A consideration of factors in the discovery of anesthesia and their effects on its development. *Anesthesiology* 35 (5): 515–522.

Greene, N.M. (1979). Anesthesia and the development of surgery (1846–1896). *Anesth. Analg.* 58 (1): 5–12.

Groß, D. (2018). Guido Fischer – Pionier der Lokalanästhesie. *Zahnärztliche Mitteilungen* 108 (6): 100–101.

Grybowski, A. and Pietrzak, K. (2013). Napoleon Cybulski (1854–1919). *J. Neurol.* 260 (11): 2942–2943.

Guptill, A.E. (1920). Novocain as a skin irritant. *Dent. Cosmos* 62 (12): 1460–1461.

Gutierrez-Noriega, C. and Zapata, V. (1947). *Estudios sobre la coca y la cocaína en el Perú*. Lima (Perú): Ediciones de la Dirección de Educación Artística y Extensión Cultural del Ministerio de Educación Pública: 21.

Hall, R.J. (1884). Hydrochlorate of cocaine. *N.Y. Med. J.* 40: 643–644.

Harris, S.C. (1957). Aspiration before injection of dental local anesthetics. *J. Oral Surg.* 15 (4): 299–303.

Harrison, S.M. (1948). Regional anaesthesia for children. *Dent. Rec.* 68: 146–155.

Hein, G.N. (1917). Local anesthesia, infiltration, conductive and intraosseus methods. *Dent. Items Interest* 39 (11): 852–853.

Herdevall, B.-M., Klinge, B., Persson, L. et al. (2003). Plasma levels of lidocaine, o-toluidine, and prilocaine after application of 8.5 g Oraqix® in patients with generalized periodontitis: effect on blood methemoglobin and tolerability. *Acta Odontol. Scand.* 61 (4): 230–234.

Hersh, E.V., Moore, P.A., Papas, A.S. et al. (2008). Reversal of soft-tissue local anesthesia with phentolamine mesylate in adolescents and adults. *J. Am. Dent. Assoc.* 139 (8): 1080–1093.

Hersh, E.V., Saraghi, M., and Moore, P.A. (2017). Two recent advances in local anesthesia: intranasal tetracaine/oxymetazoline and liposomal bupivacaine. *Curr. Oral Health Rep.* 4: 189–196.

Hingson, R.A. and Hughes, J.G. (1947). Clinical studies with jet injection. A new method of drug administration. *Anesth. Analg.* 26 (6): 221–230.

Jacobsohn, P.H. (1994). Dentistry's answer to "the humiliating spectacle" Dr. Wells and his discovery. *J. Am. Dent. Assoc.* 125 (12): 1576–1581.

Kane, K. and Taub, A. (1975). A history of local electrical analgesia. *Pain* 1 (2): 125–138.

Klauder, J.V. (1922). Novocain dermatitis. *Dent. Cosmos* 64 (3): 305–309.

Kneucker, A. (1919). Weitere Bemerkungen zur Verwendung der 4Prozentigen Novokain-suprarreninlösung in der Zahnchirurgie. *Osterr. Z. Stomatol.* 17: 107–113.

Koller, K. (1884a). Ueber die Verwendung des Cocaïn zur Aanästhesirung am Auge. *Wien. Med. Wochenschr.* 34, (43): 1276–1278 and 1884 (44): 1309–1311.

Koller, C. (1884b). On the use of cocaine for producing anaesthesia on the eye. *Lancet* 2: 990–992.

Koller, C. (1928). Historical notes on the beginning of local anesthesia. *J. Am. Med. Assoc.* 90 (21): 1742–1743.

Lafargue, R. (1973). Anesthésie intraligamentaire possibilities d'une nouvelle technique. *Actual Odontoestomatol. (Paris)* 27 (103): 551–573.

Laguardia, H.J. (1940). Ueber die Leitungsanaesthesie und eine neue Methode der Mandibularanaesthesie. *Korrespondezblatt. Zahnärzte (Berlin)* 64 (9): 283–291.

Leonard, M. (1998). Carl Koller: mankind's greatest benefactor? The story of local anesthesia. *J. Dent. Res.* 77 (4): 535–538.

Levitt, B. (1924). A few departures from the standard technique in conduction anesthesia. *Dent. Cosmos* 66 (11): 1168–1176.

Liljestrand, G. (1967). Carl Koller and the development of local anesthesia. *Acta Physiol. Scand. Suppl.* 299: 3–30.

Lindsay, A.W. (1929). The direct approach technic in mandibular block anesthesia. *J. Am. Dent. Assoc.* 16: 2284–2286.

Link, W.J. (1959). Alfred Einhorn, Sc. D. Inventor of novocaine. *Dent. Radiog. Photog.* 32: 1–20.

Löfgren, N. and Lundqvist, B. (1946). Studies on local anaesthetics II. *Svenks. Kem. Tidskr.* 58 (8): 206–217.

Löfgren, N. and Tegner, C. (1960). Studies on local anaesthetics XX. Synthesis of some α-monoalkylamino-2-methylpropionanilides. A new useful local anaesthetic. *Acta Chem. Scand.* 14 (2): 486–490.

Lossen, W. (1865). Ueber das Cocain. *Justus Liebig's Ann. Chem. Pharm.* 133 (3): 351–371.

Loza-Balsa, G. (1992). *Monografia sobre la coca*, ix. La Paz (Bolivia): Edita Sociedad Geográfica de la Paz, x, xiv, xv and 3.

Lozier, M. (1949). The evaluation of xylocaine as a new local anesthetic. *Oral Surg. Oral Med. Oral Pathol.* 2 (11): 1460–1468.

Magnusson, I., Geurs, N.C., Harris, P.A. et al. (2003). Intrapocket anesthesia for scaling and root planing in pain-sensitive patients. *J. Periodontol.* 74 (5): 597–602.

Malamed, S.F. (2004). *Handbook of Local Anesthesia*, 5e. St. Louis (Missouri): Elsevier-Mosby. 71.

Malamed, S.F. (2008). Reversing local anesthesia. *Inside. Dentistry* (July/August): 2–3.

Malamed, S.F. and Falkel, M. (2013). Buffered local anaesthetics: the importance of pH and $CO_2$. *SAAD Dig.* 29 (January): 9–17.

Malamed, S.F. and Joseph, C. (1987). Electricity in dentistry. The shocking concept of using electricity had its begining in socratic times. *J. Can. Dent. Assoc.* 15 (6): 12–14.

Malamed, S.F., Quinn, C.L., Torgersen, R.T., and Thompson, W. (1989). Electronic dental anesthesia for restorative dentistry. *Anesth. Prog.* 36 (4–5): 195–198.

Malamed, S.F., Tavana, S., and Falkel, M. (2013). Faster onset and more comfortable injection with alkalinized 2% lidocaine with epinephrine 1:100,000. *Compend. Contin. Educ. Dent* 34 (Special 1): 10–20.

Margetis, P.M., Quarantillo, E.P., and Lindberg, R.B. (1958). Jet injection local anesthesia in dentistry: a report of 66 cases. *U.S. Armed Forces Med. J.* 9: 625–634.

Matas, R. (1934a). Local and regional anesthesia: a retrospect and prospect. Part I. *Am. J. Surg.* 25: 189–196.

Matas, R. (1934b). Local and regional anesthesia: a retrospect and prospect. Part II. *Am. J. Surg.* 25: 362–379.

Mayer, E. (1924). The toxic effects following the use of local anesthetics. *JAMA* 82 (11): 876–885.

McAuley, J.E. (1966). The early development of local anaesthesia. *Br. Dent. J.* 121 (3): 139–142.

Melzack, R. and Wall, P.D. (1965). Pain mechanisms: a new theory. *Science* 150 (3699): 971–979.

Menczer, L.F. and Jacobsohn, P.H. (1992). Dr Horace Wells: the discoverer of general anesthesia. *J. Oral Maxillofac. Surg.* 50 (5): 506–509.

Monheim, L.M. (1965). *Local Anesthesia and Pain Control in Dental Practice*, 3e. St. Louis: The CV Mosby Co. 261.

Moose, S. (1959). Clinical evaluation of levo-nordefrin in local anesthetics. *Oral Surg. Oral Med. Oral Pathol.* 12 (7): 838–845.

Moréno y Maïz, T. (1868). *Recherches chimiques et physiologiques sur l'erythroxylum coca du Perou et la cocaïne*. Paris: Louis Leclerc Libraire-Editeur. 76–79.

Navarro, F.A. (2003). ¿Quién lo usó por vez primera? Adrenalina. *Panacea (revista de medicina, lenguaje y traducción)* 4 (12): 142. (Open Access).

Nevin, M. and Puterbaugh, P.G. (1949). *Conduction, Infiltration and General Anesthesia in Dentistry*, 5e. New York: Dental Items of Interest Publishing Co Inc., 254–255, 272–273, 296–297.

Niemann, A. (1860). Ueber eine neue organische Base in den Cocablättern. *Arch. Pharm.* 153 (129–155): 291–308.

Noyes, H.D. (1884). The ophthalmological congress in Heidelberg. *Med. Rec.* 26: 417–418.

Nueve Arzneimittel und pharmaceutische Spezialitäten (1902). *Dr. Ritsert''s Anästhesin. Pharm. Ztg.* 47: 356.

Okada, Y., Suzuki, H., and Ishiyama, I. (1989). Fatal subarachnoid haemorrhage associated with dental local anaesthesia. *Aust. Dent. J.* 34 (4): 323–325.

Olch, P.D. and William, S. (1975). Halsted and local anesthesia: contributions and complications. *Anesthesiology* 42 (4): 479–486.

Pernice, L. (1890). Ueber Cocainanästhesie. *Dtsch. Med. Wochenschr.* 16 (14): 287–289.

Pfender, C.A. (1911). Historical synopsis of the development of hypodermic medication. *Washington Med. Ann.* 10: 346–359.

Poeppig, E. (1836). *Reise in Chile, Peru und auf dem Amazonenstrome während der Jahre 1827–1832*, vol. II. Leipzig: Friedrich Fleischer, JC Hinrichssche Buchhandlung. 209–217.

Pravaz, C.G. (1853). Sur un nouveau moyend'opérer la coagulation du sang dans les artères, applicable à la guérison des anéurismes. *Comp. Rend. Acad. Sci. (Paris)* 36: 88–91. (Note: first and middle initial not cited in the paper; name, Charles Gabriel).

Rahart, J.P. (1972). A short history of local anesthesia. *Bull. Hist. Dent.* 20 (1): 27–31.

Rahn, R. and Ball, B. (2001). Articaine and epinephrine for dental anesthesia. In: *Local anesthesia in dentistry*. Seefeld (Germany): 3M ESPE AG. 6.

Reclus, P. (1895). *La cocaine en chirurgie*, 69–91. Paris: G Masson Editeurs et Gauthier-Villars et Fils Imprimeurs-Editeurs, 172–175.

Report of the Special Committee of the New York Heart Association (1955). On the use of epinephrine in connection with procaine in dental procedures. *J. Am. Dent. Assoc.* 50 (1): 108.

Representación hecha por el licenciado Falcón en concilio provincial sobre los daños y molestias que se hacen a los indios. Lima (Perú). 1582. Arreglos, introducción, notas y comentarios de Francisco A. Loayza. Lima (Peru): Publicado en los pequeños grandes libros de la historia Americana. 1946; Serie I, Vol X: 123–164.

Roberts, D.H. and Sowray, J.H. (1987). *Local Analgesia in Dentistry*, 3e. Bristol: Wright. 37–52.

Robison, S.F., Mayhew, R.B., Cowan, R.D., and Hawley, R.J. (1984). Comparative study of deflection characteristics and fragility of 25-, 27-, and 30-gauge short dental needles. *J. Am. Dent. Assoc.* 109 (6): 920–924.

Rynd (1845). Neuralgia – introduction of fluid to the nerve. *Dublin Med. Press* 13 (March 12): 167–168.

Rynd, F. (1861). Description of an instrument for the subcutaneous introduction of fluids in affections of the nerves. *Dublin Q. J. Med. Sci.* 32: 13. (and plate III).

Saraghi, M. and Hersh, E.V. (2017). Intranasal tetracaine and oxymetazoline spray for maxillary local anesthesia without injections. *Gen. Dent.* 65 (2): 16–19.

Sauvez, E. (1905). *L'anesthésie locale pour l'extraction des dents*. Paris: Vigot Fréres Editeurs, 1–34, 178. (Note: first initial missing from paper; name is Emil).

Schleich, C.L. (1892). Infiltrationsanästhesie (locale anästhesie) und ihr Verhältniss zur allgemeinen Narcose (inhalationsanästhesie). *Verh. Dtsch. Ges. Chir.* 21: 121–127.

Scribonii Largii de compositionibus medicamentorum liber unus (1529). Chapter XI and CLXII. Aurelii Cornelii Celsi de re medica libri octo, inter latinos eius professionis autores facile principis: ad ueterum et recentiu exemplarium fidem, necnon doctorum hominum indicium, summa diligentia excusi. Apud Christianum Vuechel, sub scuto Basilerensi. Paris.

Seldin, H.M. (1958). Survey of anesthetic fatalities in oral surgery and a review of the etiological factors in anesthetic deaths. *J. Am. Dent. Soc. Anesth.* 5 (2): 5–12.

Silverstone, L.M. (1989). Electronic dental anaesthesia. *Dent. Pract.* 27 (11): 1–2.

Smith, A.E. (1920). *Block Anesthesia and Allied Subjects. With Special Chapters on the Maxillary Sinus, the Tonsils, and Neuralgias of the Nervous Trigeminus for Oral Surgeons, Dentists, Laryngologists, Rhinologists, Otologists, and Students.* St. Louis, MO: CV Mosby Co., 234, 264, 270–271, 286–327, 380–386.

Steadman, F.S.J. (1923). *Local Anesthesia in Dental Surgery.* Philadelphia: Blakiston's Son and Co. 84–85.

Stolz, F. (1904). (n° 647) Ueber Adrenalin und Alkylaminoacetobrenzcatechin. *Ber. Dtsch. Chem. Ges.* 37 (15): 4149–4154.

Tainter, M.L., Throndson, A.H., and Moose, S.M. (1938). Vasoconstrictors on the clinical effectiveness and toxicity of procaine anesthetic solutions. *J. Am. Dent. Assoc. Dent. Cosmos* 25 (8): 1321–1334.

Takamine, J. (1901a). Adrenalin the active principle of the suprarenal glands and its mode of preparation. *Am. J. Pharm.* 73: 523–531.

Takamine, J. (1901b). The blood-pressure-raising principle of the suprarenal glands – a preliminary report. *Ther. Gaz.* 25 (4): 221–224.

Tavares, M., Goodson, J.M., Student-Pavlovich, D. et al. (2008). The soft tissue anesthesia recovery group. Reversal of soft-tissue local anesthesia with phentolamine mesylate in pediatric patients. *J. Am. Dent. Assoc.* 139 (8): 1095–1104.

Thoma, K.H. (1914). *Oral Anaesthesia. Local Anaesthesia in the Oral Cavity. Technique and Practical Application in the Different Branches of Dentistry.* Boston: Ritter and Flebbe. 54, 58–59.

Tompkins, H.E. (1921). How to avoid breaking of needles in local anesthesia (letter). *Dent. Cosmos* 63 (11): 1148–1149.

Torres, E. (1943). Prólogo. In: *Historia del Nuevo Mundo. Colección Cisneros* (ed. P.B. Cobo). Madrid: Editorial Atlas. 5–6.

Unanúe, J.H. (1914). *Disertación sobre el cultivo, comercio y las virtudes de la famosa planta del Perú nombrada "coca". Al Excelenetisimo Señor Don Luis Fermín Carbajal y Vargas, Conde de la Unión. Lima (Perú), 1794. En: Obras científicas y literarias del Doctor J. Hipólito Unanúe*, Tomo II. Barcelona: Tipografía la Academia de Serra Hermanos y Russell. 90–125.

Urech, E., Marxer, A., and Miescher, K. (1950). 182. 2-Aminoalkyl-imidazoline. *Helv. Chim. Acta* 33 (5): 1386–1407.

Van Dyke, C. and Byck, R. (1982). Cocaine. *Sci. Am.* 246 (3): 128–141.

Vandam, L.D. (1973). Early American anesthetists. The origins of professionalism in anesthesia. *Anesthesiology* 38 (3): 264–274.

Vicuña-Mackenna, B. (1914). Hipólito Unanúe. In: *Obras científicas y literarias del Doctor J. Hipólito Unanúe.* Barcelona: Tipografía la Academia de Serra Hermanos y Russell. Tomo I: ix–xxiv.

Vogel, H.G. (2007). Nachruf für Dr. med. Roman Muschaweck. *BIOspektrum* 13 (5): 547. http://www.biospektrum.de/blatt/d_bs_pdf&_id=932179.

Von Euler, U.S. (1946a). A substance with sympathin E properties: spleen extracts. *Nature* 157 (3986): 369.

Von Euler, U.S. (1946b). A sympathomimetic ergone in adrenergic nerve fibers (sympathin) and its relations to adrenaline and noradrenaline. *Acta Physiol. Scand.* 12 (1): 73–97.

Von Fürth, O. (1900). Zur Kenntniss der brenzcatechinähulichen Substanz der Nebennieren. III. Mittheilung. *Hoppe-Seyler's Z. Physiol. Chem.* 29 (2): 105–123.

Walton, R.E. and Abbott, B.J. (1981). Periodontal ligament injection: a clinical evaluation. *J. Am. Dent. Assoc.* 103 (4): 571–575.

Waters, R.M. (1933). Procaine toxicity: its prophylaxis and treatment. *J. Am. Dent. Assoc.* 20 (12): 2211–2215.

Weaver, J.M. (2008). New drugs on the horizon may improve the quality safety of anesthetic (editorial). *Anesth. Prog.* 55 (2): 27–28.

Wells, H. (1847). *A History of the Discovery of the Application of Nitrous Oxide Gas, Ether and Other Vapors to Surgical Operations.* Hartford: J Gaylord Wells.

Wesley, J. (1760). *The Desideratum: Or Electricity Made Plain Useful. By Lover of Mankind and of Common Sense.* London: W. Flexney.

Willstätter, R. (1898). (n° 254) Ueber die constitution der Spaltungsproducte von Atropin und Cocaïn. *Ber. Dtsch. Chem. Ges.* 31 (10): 1534–1553.

Willstätter, R., Wolfes, D., and Mäder, H. (1923). Synthese des natürlichen Cocaïns. *Justus Liebig's Ann. Chem.* 434 (2): 111–139.

Winther, J.E. and Nathalang, B. (1972). Effectivity of a new local analgesic Hoe 40 045. *Scand. J. Dent. Res.* 80 (4): 272–278.

Wood, A. (1855). New method of treating neuralgia by the direct application of opiates to the painful points. *Edinburg Med. Surg. J.* 82 (203): 265–281.

Yentis, S.M. and Vlassakov, K.V. (1999). Vassily von Anrep, forgotten pioneer of regional anesthesia. *Anesthesiology* 90 (3): 890–895.

Zinman, E.J. (1976). Toxicity and mepivacaine (letter). *J. Am. Dent. Assoc.* 92 (5): 858.

**Applied Anatomy**

# 2

# Applied Anatomy I: Maxillary Arch

## Introduction

This chapter aims not to review the anatomy of the orofacial region, for which there are excellent books and atlases (DuBrul 1988; Olson 1996; Brand and Isselhard 2003; Norton 2011; Schünke et al. 2012), but to address the aspects most pertinent to local anesthesia in dentistry. A number of sensory nerves are lodged in the region (Sanz et al. 1995):

- The glossopharyngeal nerve (cranial nerve IX) innervates the tongue behind the uvula and the tonsillar fossa.
- The cervical plexus innervates the skin at the angle of the mandible, as well as the ear and its canal.
- The vagus nerve (cranial nerve X) also innervates the ear and its canal.

The major nerve in the mouth and face, however, and the one of greatest interest in dentistry, is the trigeminal nerve (cranial nerve V), addressed in this chapter along with the respective osseous and adjacent structures.

Federative Committee on Anatomical Terminology (FCAT 1998) anatomic terminology is used throughout, although occasional reference is made to certain classical names (listed in the glossary) to help the reader recognize anatomic structures discussed in older texts or articles.

## The Trigeminal Nerve

The trigeminal is the fifth of the 12 pairs of cranial nerves (CN V). It arises by from two roots, a larger sensory root and a smaller motor root, on the ventral side of the pons. From there it courses anterolaterally and inferiorly to the trigeminal ganglion (Figure 2.1).

## Trigeminal Ganglion

Traditionally known as the semilunar or Gasserian ganglion, the trigeminal ganglion is kidney- or crescent-shaped, i.e. anterolaterally convex. The posterior concave part receives both the larger sensory root with its 170000 fibers and the motor root with its 7700 (Pennisi et al. 1991). Three divisions proceed from the anterior convex border (Figure 2.2):

- $V_1$ or first division, the exclusively sensory ophthalmic nerve.
- $V_2$ or second division, the exclusively sensory maxillary nerve.
- $V_3$ or third division, the sensory and motor mandibular nerve, the largest of the three.

The intracranial trigeminal ganglion is lodged near the apex of the petrous part of the temporal bone in the middle cranial fossa (Figure 2.3).

### Trigeminal Nerve: Functions

At least five functions are attributed to the trigeminal nerve (cranial nerve V) (Jastak et al. 1995):

- Sensory: touch, pressure, heat/cold, and pain.
- Proprioceptive: position and movement of the masticatory apparatus.
- Motor: innervation of masticatory and similar facial muscles.
- Neurovegetative: vasomotor or secretory action or visual accommodation due to the presence in its channels of branches of cranial nerves VII and IX carrying sympathetic and parasympathetic system fibers.
- Gustatory: sense of taste via connections with cranial nerve VII (facial nerve).

## Maxillary Nerve ($V_2$)

The medial branch of the trigeminal nerve (cranial nerve V) is exclusively sensory. It travels forward, outward, and downward from the skull to the pterygopalatine fossa through the foramen rotundum in the greater wing of the sphenoid bone. From that fossa it enters the orbit through the inferior orbital

*Local Anesthesia in Dentistry: A Locoregional Approach*, First Edition. Jesús Calatayud and Mana Saraghi.
© 2024 John Wiley & Sons Ltd. Published 2024 by John Wiley & Sons Ltd.
Companion website: www.wiley.com/go/Calatayud/local

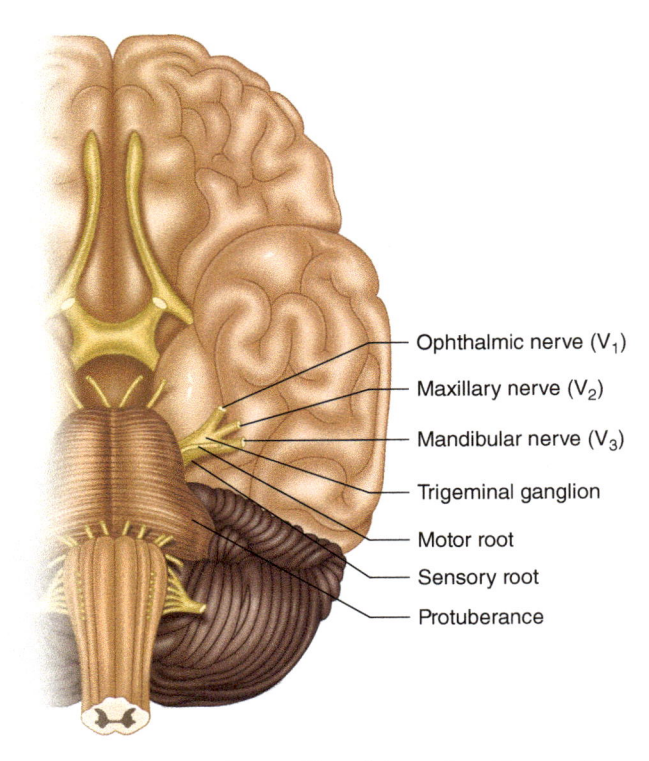

**Figure 2.1** Trigeminal nerve (V cranial nerve) and its ganglion arising from the pons (view from base of brain).

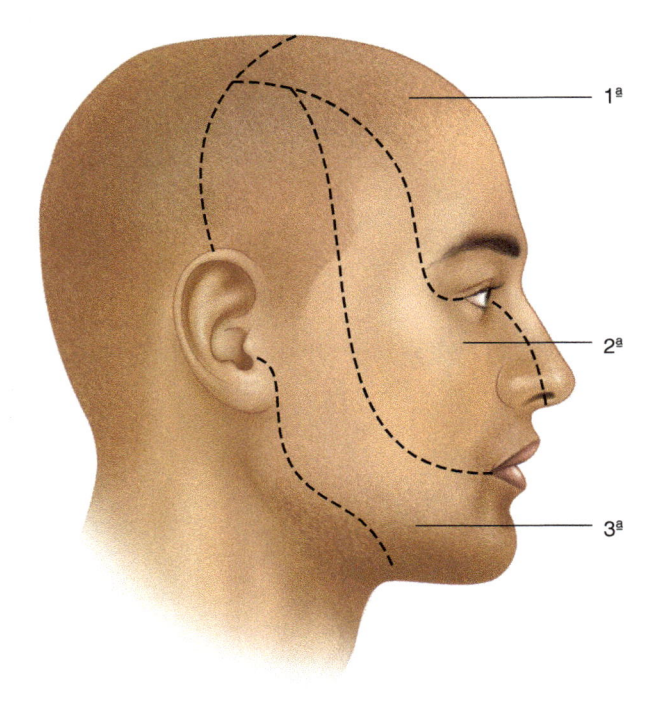

**Figure 2.2** Areas of the face innervated by each of the three branches of the trigeminal nerve: (1) ophthalmic nerve ($V_1$); (2) maxillary nerve ($V_2$); (3) mandibular nerve ($V_3$).

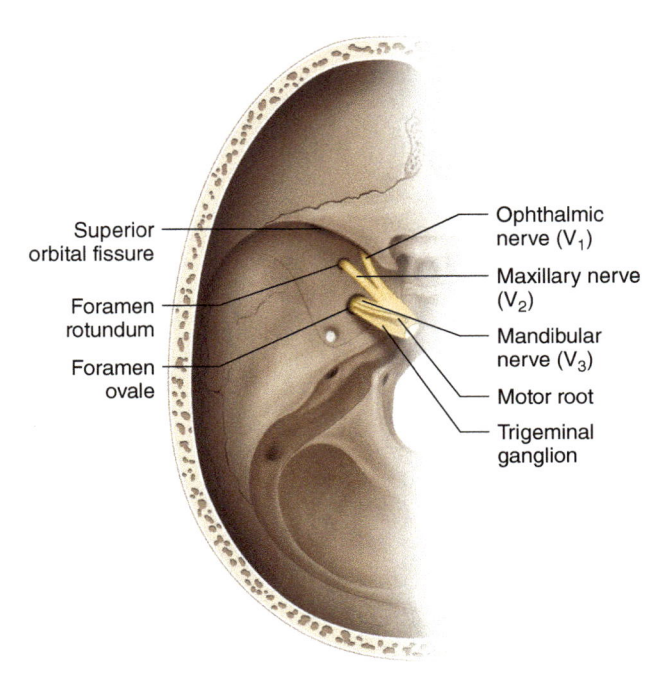

**Figure 2.3** Trigeminal ganglion, lodged intracranially in the middle cranial fossa in the petrous part of the temporal bone, and branches.

fissure and courses along the roofless infraorbital groove on the floor of the orbit. It subsequently traverses the roofed infraorbital canal (continuous with the groove), changing its name from maxillary ($V_2$) to infraorbital nerve, to the infraorbital foramen where it distributes its terminal branches.

## Overview of Collateral Branches

The maxillary nerve ($V_2$) distributes collateral branches in four areas along its course (Figure 2.4).

### Intracranial Zone
As it exits the ganglion, the maxillary nerve gives off the meningeal branch that innervates areas of the dura mater.

### Pterygopalatine Fossa Zone
Located within the infratemporal fossa (formerly the zygomatic fossa), the pterygopalatine fossa is an inverted pyramid. It is bound posteriorly by the pterygoid apophysis in the sphenoid bone and anteriorly by the maxillary tuberosity. The anterior–posterior distance at the base (upper side) is 12–15 mm (Cook 1950a; Canter et al. 1964; von Arx et al. 2020). The following branches proceed from this fossa:

1) The zygomatic nerve, which penetrates the orbit through the inferior orbital fissure, branching into:
    - The zygomaticotemporal nerve, which innervates the skin on the forehead and eyelid.

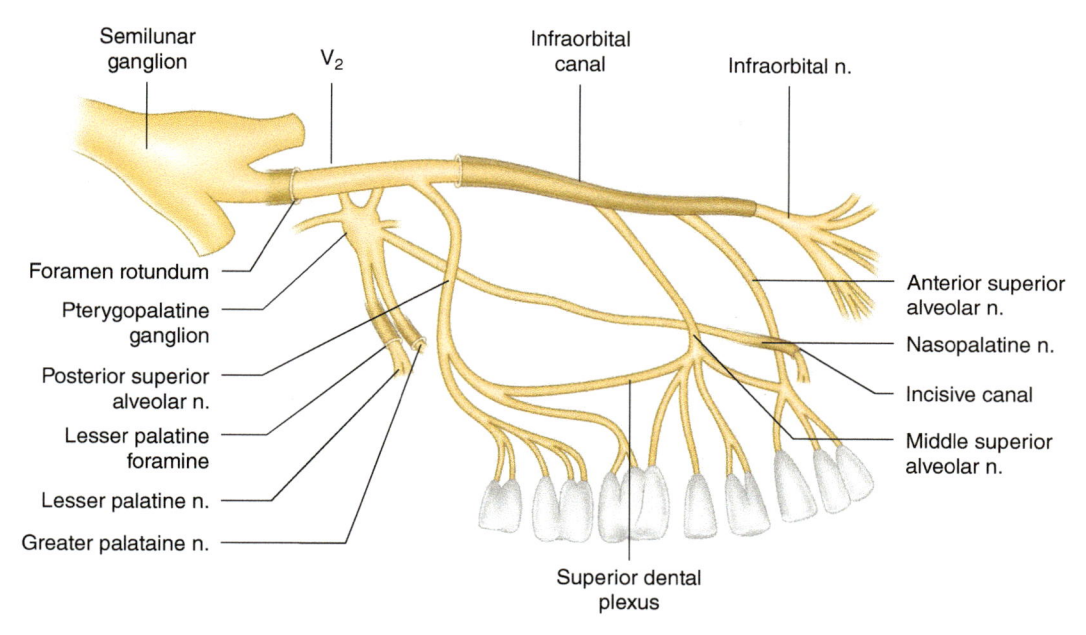

**Figure 2.4** Schematic representation of maxillary nerve (V₂), origin and distribution of branches. Semilunar ganglion is trigeminal ganglion. *Source:* Redrawn with modifications from Allen (1979).

- The zygomaticofacial nerve, which innervates the skin in the malar and temporal zones.
2) The pterygopalatine nerves, generally two trunks that fuse at the pterygopalatine ganglion (former Meckel's sphenopalatine ganglion), which they merely traverse with no synapse. Six branches proceed from this ganglion:
    - The orbital branches, which enter the orbit through the inferior orbital fissure, innervating the orbital bone and sphenoidal sinus.
    - The middle and lateral nasal branches, which innervate the nasal mucosa and posterior ethmoidal air cells.
    - The *nasopalatine nerve*, discussed in detail in a later section.
    - The *greater palatine nerve*, discussed in detail in a later section.
    - The lesser palatine nerves, which proceed through the lesser palatine foramen, innervating the soft palate mucosa, uvula, and (partially) the superior part of the tonsils.
    - The pharyngeal nerve, which proceeds from the posterior part of pterygopalatine ganglion that innervates the posterior nasal mucosa, roof of the pharynx, and auditory tube.
3) The *posterior superior alveolar nerve* (PSAN), discussed in detail in a later section.

### Infraorbital Zone

When the maxillary nerve (V₂) penetrates the orbit via the inferior orbital fissure its name changes to the infraorbital nerve, which travels across the infraorbital groove and the infraorbital canal at the base of the orbit, which also roofs the maxillary sinus. It gives off two branches:

1) The *middle superior alveolar nerve* (MSAN), discussed in detail in a later section.
2) The *anterior superior alveolar nerve*, discussed in detail in a later section.

In the elderly, when the infraorbital nerve courses through the infraorbital groove and canal it often runs above the maxillary sinus because the osseous base disappears with the bone, leaving the nerve in superficial contact with the maxillary sinus.

*Terminal zone and facial branches.* The infraorbital nerve, transmitted to the face by the infraorbital foramen under the inferior margin of the orbit, branches into the:

1) Branches for the lower eyelid.
2) External nasal branches for the outer skin of the nose and internal branches for the nostril mucosa.
3) Superior labial branches, for the skin and mucosa on the upper lip, traveling as far as the gingival-labial sulcus.

### Palatine Nerves

These two pairs of nerves (two on the right and two on the left), which are particularly pertinent to local-regional anesthesia in dentistry, arise from the pterygopalatine ganglion in the pterygopalatine fossa.

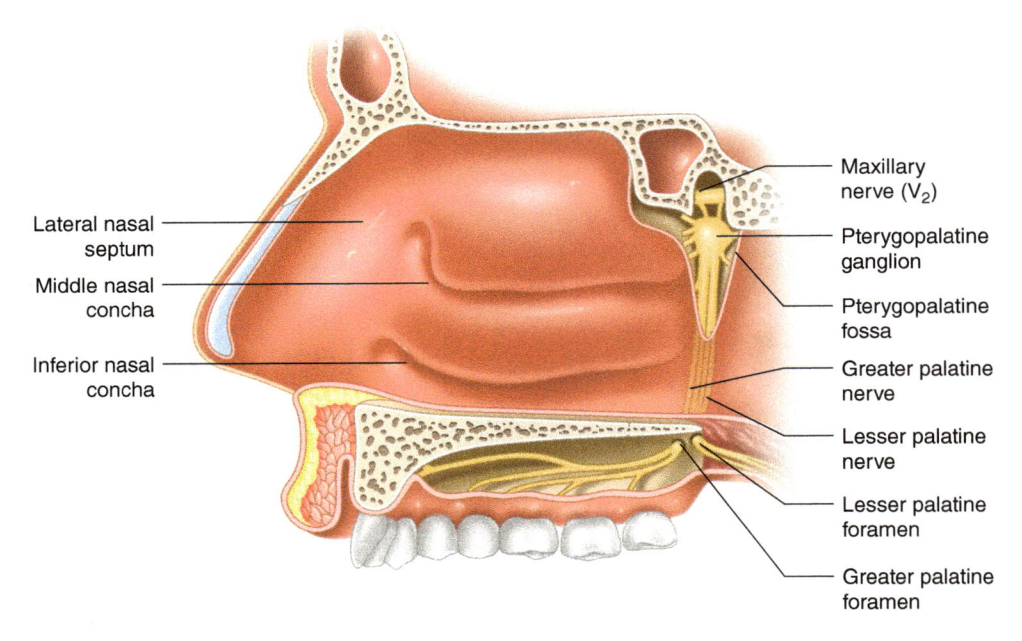

**Figure 2.5** Course of greater palatine nerve from pterygopalatine fossa, across pterygopalatine ganglion to palate.

### Greater Palatine Nerve

After traversing the pterygopalatine ganglion without exchanging fibers, the greater palatine nerve enters the pterygopalatine fossa, descending along the greater palatine canal (Figure 2.5), which opens into the pterygopalatine fossa vertex (Cook 1950b; von Arx et al. 2020). Initially formed as a vertical groove on the maxillary surface of the palatine, it is converted into a canal by articulation with the maxillary tuberosity and pterygoid process of the sphenoid. Here the nerve distributes a branch to innervate the inferior nasal concha. The canal also transmits the descending palatine artery (branch of the maxillary).

The greater palatine nerve arises in the hard palate after crossing the greater palatine foramen (Figure 2.6), accompanied by its artery, here named the greater palatine artery. It passes forward in the hard palate between the periosteum and the fibromucosa to the canine and lateral incisor zone, where it runs across the nasopalatine nerve. It innervates:

- The anterior-most part of the soft palate fibromucosa.
- The fibromucosa, periosteum, and hard palate from the molars up to the second premolar (100%), as far forward as the midline of the palate and the first premolar (95%), canine (75%), or lateral incisor (50%) (Langford 1989; Calatayud 2001) (Figure 2.7).
- Rarely, the pulp of the upper molars at the palate root (Ulusoy and Alacam 2014).

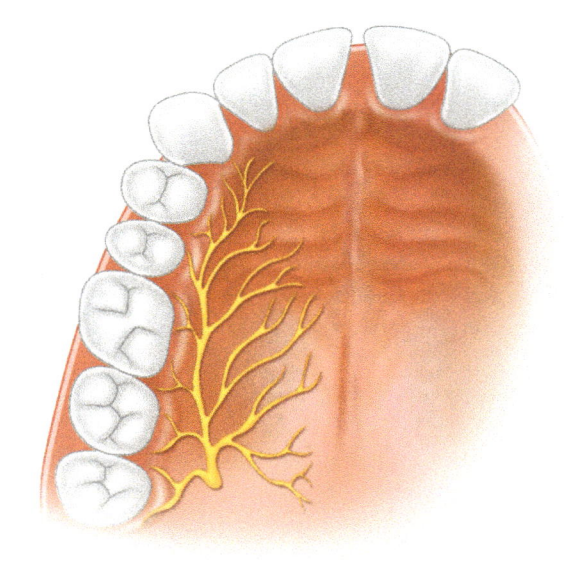

**Figure 2.6** Origin of greater palatine nerve and distribution in hard palate. *Source:* Redrawn from Roberts and Sowray (1987).

### Nasopalatine Nerve

Also known as Scarpa's nerve, or nervus incisivus, the nasopalatine nerve, after traversing the pterygopalatine ganglion where no fibers are exchanged, travels through the sphenopalatine foramen (space between the palatine bone, orbital apophysis, and sphenoidal process of the palatine bone) to the posterior part of the nasal cavity

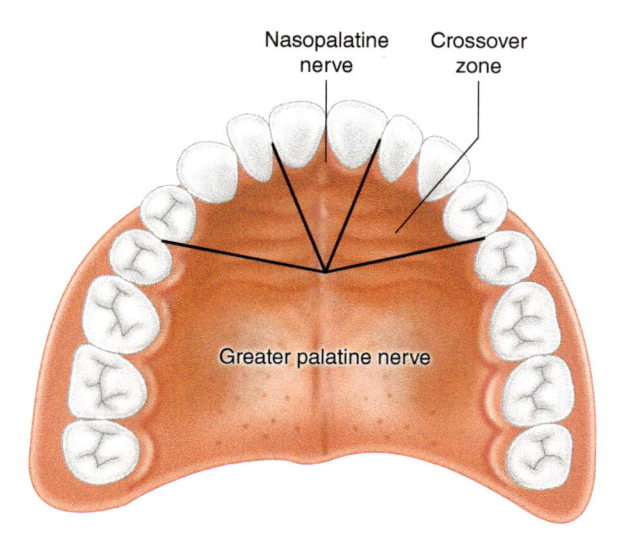

**Figure 2.7** Areas of palate innervated by nasopalatine and greater palatine nerves, and crossover zone.

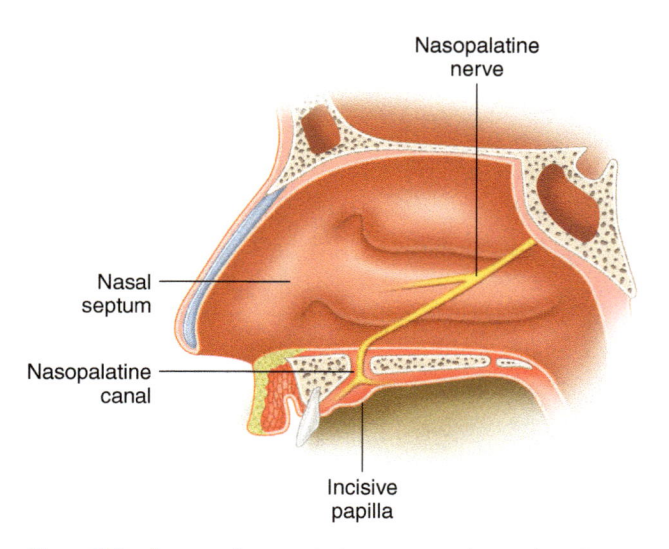

**Figure 2.8** Course of nasopalatine nerve and entry in palate across maxillary incisive canal.

(Cook 1949). It then passes forward and downward (Figure 2.8) between the mucosa and periosteum of the nasal septum (formed by the inferior side of the sphenoid, the vomer, and the nasal wall), distributing two branches:

- The external branches that innervate the nasal mucosa.
- The *internal branch*, known as the nasopalatine nerve, which reaches the floor of the nasal fossa and enters the nasopalatine canal (or maxillary incisive canal) via the foramina of Stensen before emerging in the oral cavity via the nasopalatine (or incisive) foramen (located at the midline of the palate, about 3 mm behind the central incisors) immediately below the incisive or interincisive papilla (Figure 2.9) (Annex 41). This branch innervates:

  - The fibromucosa, periosteum, and bone around the incisive papilla, the central incisors (100%), the lateral incisors (nearly 50%), and canines (25%) (Table 2.1 and Figure 2.7).
  - In some individuals it gives off a branch that contributes to incisor pulp innervation (Hofer 1922; Phillips and Maxmen 1941; Phillips 1943; Cook 1949, 1950b), although that assertion has been challenged by other authors (Olsen et al. 1955; FitzGerald and Scott 1958; Westwater 1960).
  - It may often fuse with the anterior superior alveolar nerve plexus (Roda and Blanton 1994).

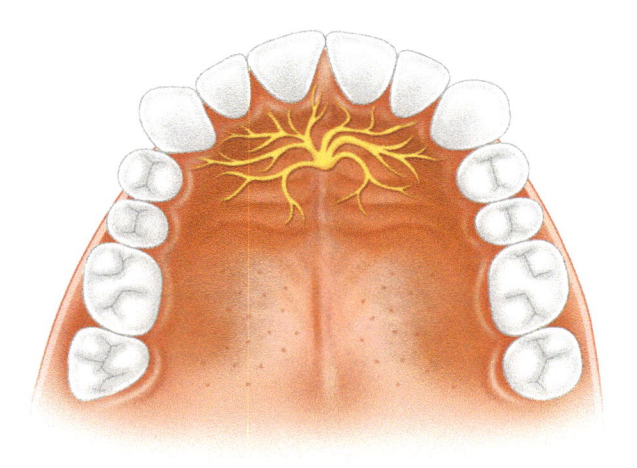

**Figure 2.9** Course of nasopalatine nerve through maxillary incisive canal and distribution in palate. *Source:* Redrawn from Roberts and Sowray (1987).

**Table 2.1** Nasopalatine nerve innervation of the palatal marginal gingiva (%).

| Tooth | Langford 1989 ($n = 20$) | Calatayud 2001 ($n = 24$) | Rounded mean |
|---|---|---|---|
| CI | 100 | 96 | 100% |
| LI | 50 | 38 | 50% |
| C | 25 | 28 | 25% |
| First PM | 5 | 4 | 5% |
| Second PM | 0 | 0 | 0% |

CI, central incisor; LI, lateral incisor; C, canine; First PM, first premolar; Second PM, second premolar.

## Superior Alveolar Nerves

These three nerve pairs are particularly pertinent to local-regional anesthesia in dentistry. They innervate:

- Teeth, pulp, and periodontal ligament.
- Interdental papillae, including fibromucosa, bone, and periosteum.
- Buccal, fibromucosa (alveolar mucosa, attached gingiva, and interdental papillae), bone, and periosteum.

### Posterior Superior Alveolar Nerve (PSAN)

This nerve is present in 100% of maxillary dissections (Heasman 1984; Loestscher and Walton 1988). It arises from the main trunk of the maxillary nerve ($V_2$) at the pterygopalatine fossa immediately before entering the infraorbital groove (Jones 1939; McDaniel 1956; Heasman 1984). It consists of one to four branches (two to three branches in 95%) that descend and traverse the posterior wall of the maxilla (maxillary tuberosity) across foramina located, in 90% of individuals, at a height of 10–40 mm over the posterior maxillary alveolar bone (Heasman 1984). At that level they pass through the posterior external wall of the maxillary sinus to fuse with the superior alveolar nerve plexus (Figure 2.10), innervating:

- The posterior wall of the maxillary sinus.
- The third, second, and first molars except the mesiobuccal root (Jones 1939) where the MSAN is present.
- The second and first premolars in the absence of the MSAN (Sicher 1950; Cook 1950a; FitzGerald and Scott 1958; Hayden 1965; Loestcher and Walton 1988).
- The canine, on occasion (Cook 1950a).
- In children, the first and second primary molars, which coexist with the MSAN (FitzGerald 1960; Roberts and Jorgensen 1961).

### Middle Superior Alveolar Nerve (MSAN)

Present in a little over 50% of dissections (Table 2.2), the MSAN arises from a long stretch of the infraorbital nerve that may extend from the posterior-most preorbital zone to the middle third of its course (FitzGerald and Scott 1958; Heasman 1984; Hindy and Raouf 1993). Depending on whether its origin is more posterior or more medial, the

**Table 2.2** Dissections where the middle superior alveolar nerve was present.

| Reference | Size | Percentage |
| --- | --- | --- |
| Szabó (1948) | 14 | 25 |
| Cook (1950a) | 10 | 70 |
| Olsen et al. (1955) | 26 | 47 |
| FitzGerald (1956) | 100 | 82 |
| McDaniel (1956) | 50 | 30 |
| Gaballah et al. (1973) | 28 | 89 |
| Heasman (1984) | 19 | 37 |
| Loestscher and Walton (1988) | 29 | 72 |
| Hindy and Raouf (1993) | 15 | 47 |
| | Mean | **55%** |

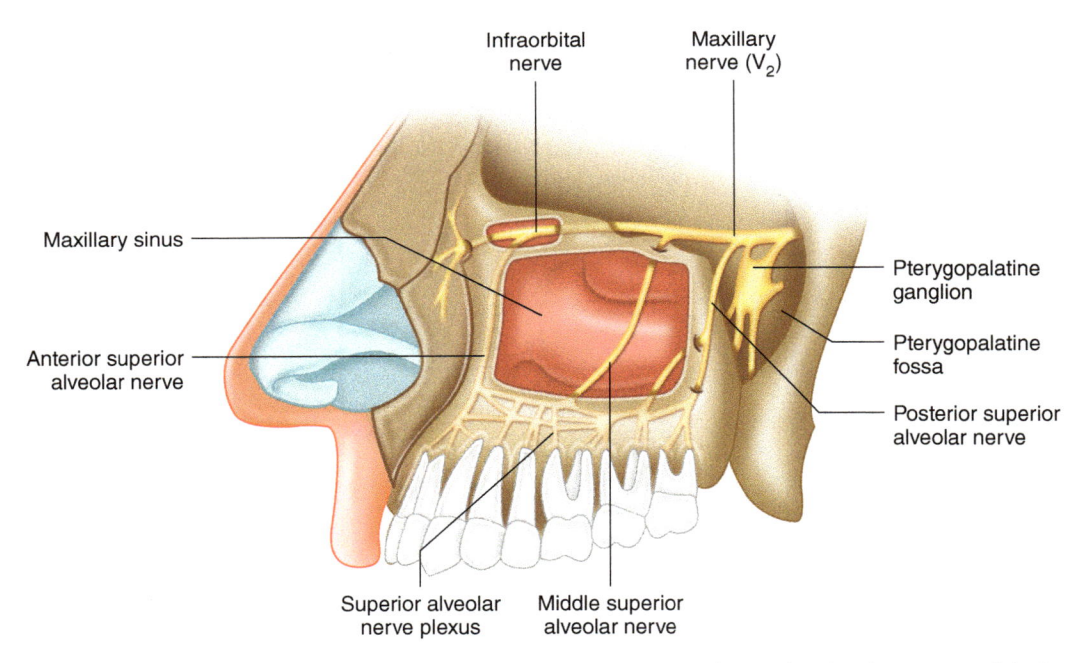

**Figure 2.10** Schematic representation of anterior superior, middle, and posterior alveolar nerves, origin from maxillary nerve ($V_2$), course, and fusion in superior alveolar nerve plexus or superior dental plexus and innervation of maxillary teeth.

MSAN descends along the posterior or anterior external wall of the maxillary sinus to fuse with the superior alveolar nerve plexus (Figure 2.10). It innervates:

- The lateral wall near the posterior and the maxillary sinus near the anterior part.
- The first and second premolars and the mesiobuccal root of the first molar (Jones 1939; Szabó 1948).
- In children, the first and second primary molars, which may coexist with the PSAN (FitzGerald 1960; Roberts and Jorgensen 1961).

**Anterior Superior Alveolar Nerve (ASAN)**

This nerve is present in 100% of maxillary anatomical dissections (McDaniel 1956; Heasman 1984; Loetscher and Walton 1988; von Arx and Lozanoff 2015). It arises from the infraorbital nerve at a mean of 10–15 mm from the infraorbital foramen (Table 2.3), although in 20% of individuals it may originate at more than 20 mm from the foramen (FitzGerald and Scott 1958; Heasman 1984). It consists of one to four branches (Jones 1939; Olsen et al. 1955) that descend along the anterior wall of the maxillary sinus, bordering the nasal fossa to the floor of the sinus and fusing there with the superior alveolar nerve plexus (Figure 2.10). This nerve, accompanied by its vessels, is the largest of the superior alveolar nerves, since the whole curse is some 55 mm in length (Jones 1939) in its bony canal, the *canalis sinuosus* (because it exhibits a tortuous course) (FitzGerald and Scott 1958; von Arx et al. 2013; Ferlin et al. 2019; Rusu et al. 2019); this canal has a small diameter <1 mm (von Arx et al. 2013; Ferlin et al. 2019) (Figure 2.11). It innervates:

- The anterior wall of the maxillary sinus.
- The incisors and the maxillary canine.

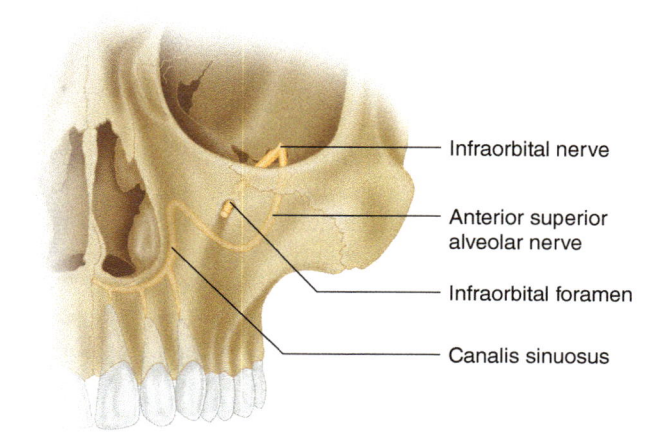

**Figure 2.11** Anterior superior alveolar nerve and *canalis sinuosus*.

- The premolars, particularly the first in the absence of the MSAN (Szabó 1948; Sicher 1950; FitzGerald and Scott 1958).

**Superior Dental Plexus**

The superior dental plexus or superior alveolar nerve plexus lies on the maxilla at or above the teeth apices in over 80% of individuals (Table 2.4). As a result, it is often impossible to determine which of the superior alveolar nerves (posterior, middle, or anterior) actually innervates a given tooth, for the three converge at and fuse in this plexus (Cook 1950a; FitzGerald and Scott 1958; Heasman 1984; von Arx and Lozanoff 2015) (Figure 2.10), even when the nasopalatine nerve is anteriorly located (Roda and Blanton 1994).

Some authors have reported nerve and branch fusions like tiny sensory ganglia in 6% of dissections of this plexus, denominated Valentin's ganglion when in the posterior part and Bochdalek's ganglion when in the anterior part, near the canine (McDaniel 1956).

**Table 2.3** Distance from the anterior superior alveolar nerve to the infraorbitral foramen when it arises from the infraorbital nerve.

| Reference | Size | Population | Distance to infraorbital foramen |
|---|---|---|---|
| Jones (1939) | — | UK | 15 |
| Heasman (1984) | 19 | UK | 11 (<5 to >20)[a] |
| Von Arx and | 5 | United States | 12.2 ± 5.8 (3–19) |
| | | Mean | 12.7 |
| | | Rounded mean | **10–15 mm** |

Studies in cadavers and length in millimeters (mm).
[a] Mean estimated from class interval.

**Table 2.4** Dissections where the superior alveolar nerve plexus was present.

| Reference | Size | Percentage |
|---|---|---|
| Olsen et al. (1955) | 26 | 100 |
| McDaniel (1956) | 50 | 48 |
| Heasman (1984) | 19 | 100 |
| Mean | | **83%** |

## Other Structures of Interest

### Greater Palatine Canal and Foramen

**Greater Palatine Canal**

The greater palatine canal starts at the lower vertex of the pterygopalatine fossa. It runs between the maxilla and the vertical lamina of the palatine bone, where the vascularnervous package (greater palatine nerve and artery accompanied by the descending palatine vein) descends until it enters the hard palate across the greater palatine foramen. The canal is angled at 50–60° relative to the occlusal plane of the upper molars (Table 14.7, Chapter 14) and the mean diameter is 2–3 mm (Rapado-González et al. 2015).

The mean length between the greater palatine foramen in the palate and the roof of the pterygopalatine fossa is around 35 mm, ranging from 20 to 45 mm (Annex 42). At the age of 10 the mean length is around 30 mm, rising by only 2–3 mm up to the age of 18 (Slavkin et al. 1966).

The characteristics of the greater palatine canal are pertinent to transpalatal maxillary nerve ($V_2$) block, also known as the greater palatine canal technique.

**Greater Palatine Foramen**

The greater palatine foramen is found at the junction of the horizontal hard palate with the vertical alveolar process (Westmoreland and Blanton 1982; Malamed and Trieger 1983). It is 3–4 mm in diameter, with an oval shape in 75% of cases and round in 15% of cases. It opens anterolaterally in the posterior part of the palate in 45% of cases and anteriorly in 25% of cases (Annex 42). Its location varies in adults with permanent teeth or children with temporary teeth: in approximately 85% of adults, it is found around the third molar (by "around," we understand the space between the second and third molars, the third molar itself, and the space that is behind the third molar) (Annex 42) (Figure 2.6). In children with temporary teeth, the foramen opens behind the last molar, irrespective of whether it is permanent or temporary (Slavkin et al. 1966) (Table 2.5).

In edentulous patients, it is important to know the position of the greater palatine foramen with respect to the posterior limit of the hard palate, which is approximately 4 mm, and the distance that separates it from the midline of the palate, which is approximately 15 mm (Annex 42).

The position of the greater palatine foramen is important not only for transpalatal maxillary nerve ($V_2$) block, as noted, but also to block the greater palatine nerve in the palate.

### Nasopalatine Canal and Foramen

**Nasopalatine Canal**

The nasopalatine canal, which is also known as the maxillary incisive canal, connects the floor of the nasal cavity with the roof of the oral cavity.

The canal arises on the floor of the nasal cavity at each side of the septum approximately 20 mm inside each nostril (Lake et al. 2018) from the foramina of Stensen, which are bilateral and symmetrical (Jacobs et al. 2007; Song et al. 2009). It finishes in the anterior part of the hard palate in the nasopalatine foramen, or maxillary incisive foramen, which is situated some 3 mm behind the maxillary central incisors (Chatriyanuyoke et al. 2012).

*Note*: Please consult Bahsi et al. (2017) and www.whonamedit.com, which provide information on doubts surrounding the spelling of the name Stensen or Stenson.

The nasopalatine canal is around 3 mm in diameter and 10–15 mm in length (Annex 41). It is formed by one (55% of cases) up to four channels that are completely or partially separated (Song et al. 2009; Al-Amery et al. 2015). *This canal is almost parallel to the axis of the maxillary central incisors* (Liang et al. 2009; Jornet et al. 2015; Matsumura et al. 2017), with an angle of ~70° between the axis of the canal and the floor of the nasal fossa (Annex 41).

The canal contains the neurovascular bundle, with the nasopalatine nerve or maxillary incisive nerve (Fitzpatrick and Downs et al. 2019), which is a myelinated nerve (Liang et al. 2009) formed by at least two bundles found in the central area and are surrounded by vessels (Song et al. 2009). The artery is relatively large and is surrounded by small veins (Liang et al. 2009). It also contains seromucous glands (Liang et al. 2009) and some fat (Fitzpatrick and Downs 2019).

Curiously, the nasopalatine nerve is found not only in the canal or channels, but also at the level of the median intermaxillary suture (Song et al. 2009).

**Nasopalatine Foramen**

The nasopalatine foramen, which is also known as the maxillary incisive foramen, arises in the medial area of the anterior hard palate (Jacobs et al. 2007) about 3 mm behind the maxillary central incisors (Chatriyanuyoke et al. 2012)

Table 2.5 Distance behind molars of greater palatine foramen by age (Slavkin et al. 1966).

| Age (years) | Behind | Distance (mm) |
| --- | --- | --- |
| 3–6 | Primary second molar | 8–12 |
| 7–10 | Permanent first molar | 4–6 |
| 11–14 | Permanent second molar | 2–5 |

Table 2.6  Mean (mm) thickness of cortical and medullary bone (Medulla.) over buccal and palatine sides of maxillary tooth apices.

| Tooth | Buccal | | | | Palatine | | | |
|---|---|---|---|---|---|---|---|---|
| | Cortical | Medullary | C+M[a] | Max. | Cortical | Medullary | C+M | Max. |
| Incisiors | <1 | 0 | 1 | — | 2 | 3–5 | 4–6 | — |
| Canine | <1 | 0 | 1 | — | 2 | 3–5 | 4–6 | — |
| Premolars | <1 | 1 | 2 | 11 | 2 | 4 | 6 | 10 |
| Molars | 1–2 | 2 | 3–4 | 11 | 2 | 1–2 | 3–4 | 9 |

A column with maximum value (Max.). Values rounded to the nearest unit.
[a] C + M = cortical plus medullary.
*Source:* Data from Arens et al. (1984) and Jang et al. (2017).

and below the incisive papilla. This foramen is 4–5 mm in diameter and round or oval in 80% of cases (Annex 41).

In 15–30% of cases, we can find small accessory foramina measuring 1–2 mm in diameter close to the location of the foramen in the palate. In more than 50% of cases, these foramina enter into contact with the *canalis sinuosus*, along which the anterior superior alveolar nerve courses (de Oliveira-Santos et al. 2013; Von Arx et al. 2013).

## Cortical Bone Thickness

As Table 2.6 shows, the cortical bone over the dental apex is thinner on the buccal than on the palatine side and is generally scant in the former, favoring buccal infiltration techniques. In addition, the maxilla is more porous in this area, where it features many foramina, further enhancing diffusion of the anesthetic solution (DuBrul 1988). Nonetheless, buccal may be greater than palatine cortical thickness in the molar zone, possibly prompting buccal infiltration failure.

The incisor apex may lie below the floor of the nasal fossae and the premolar and molar underneath the floor of the maxillary sinus; the alveolar nerves course along its anterior, external, and posterior walls. The canine, with its socket behind the canine eminence (DuBrul 1988), is the boundary between them.

## Pterygoid Venous Plexus

The pterygoid venous plexus is a network of up to 15 or more intertwined veins of some size (Murphy and Grundy 1969) forming anastomoses located in the infratemporal (formerly zygomatic) fossa in the posterior part of the maxilla (around the tuberosity) between the lateral pterygoid and temporal muscles (Archer and Zubrow 1954; Murphy and Grundy 1969; Shaw and Fierst 1988). At times the former muscle may be traversed by vessels (Murphy and Grundy 1969).

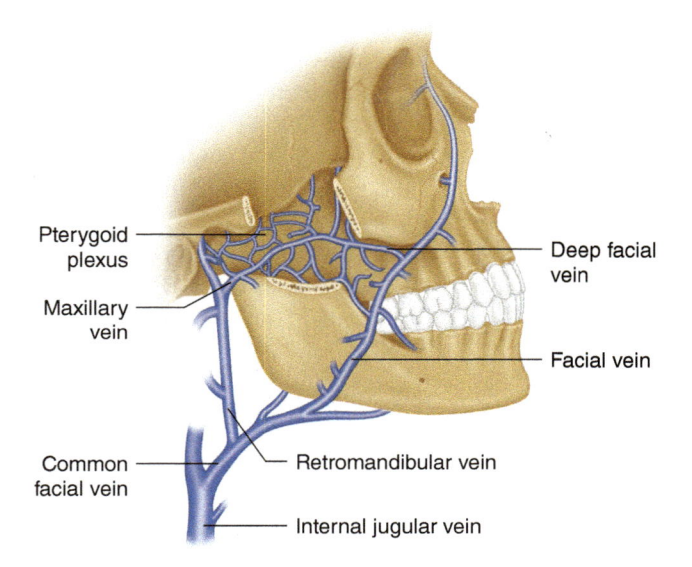

Figure 2.12  Pterygoid venous plexus and drainage system.
*Source:* Redrawn with modifications from Brand and Isselhard (2003).

This posterior part of the complex drains blood into the maxillary vein and the anterior part into the facial vein across a number of branches, with the deep facial vein generally collecting the greatest share. The maxillary vein, in turn, drains into the retromandibular vein and the latter into the common facial vein (Figure 2.12), which also collects blood from the facial vein and drains into the internal jugular vein (Brand and Isselhard 2003).

An understanding of the pterygoid plexus is important as bleeding may occur during local anesthesia in this area.

## Infraorbital Foramen

The infraorbital foramen is ovoid in around half of individuals, although it may be crescent-shaped or rounded with a diameter on the order of 3–4 mm. It is located about

5–10 mm underneath the infraorbital margin (Annex 2), normally at the depression in the margin resulting from the zygomaticomaxillary suture that lies at about two-fifths of the width from the inside edge (Figure 14.8, Chapter 14).

This foramen opens downwardly and medially (toward the nose) in nearly 60% of individuals and downwardly only in 20% (Annex 2), forming a 20–30° vertical angle with the occlusal plane (Agthong et al. 2005; Lopes et al. 2009; Karkut et al. 2010). It is covered by a layer about 7 mm thick consisting of soft tissue, subcutaneous tissue, and skin (Kleier et al. 1983).

Horizontally it lies above the *second premolar zone in 85% of individuals* (Figure 2.13). By second premolar zone is meant the area ranging from a point slightly forward of the second premolar (between it and the first premolar) to a point slightly posterior to the second premolar (between it and the first molar) and including the second premolar zone (Annex 2). Vertically it is positioned around 30–35 mm above the amelocemental junction of the second premolar (Feige 1978; Annex 2).

Fifteen percent of individuals have been shown to have accessory foramina, bilateral in 20% of those and multiple (up to three or four foramina) in 15% (Annex 2) (Riesenfeld 1956; Kadanoff et al. 1970). These accessory foramina may be located at a considerable distance from the main infraorbital foramen (Kadanoff et al. 1970; Leo et al. 1995) in up to 40% of individuals in some series (Kadanoff et al. 1970). These important findings may explain why, when such structures lie outside the range of the anesthetic, infraorbital foramen block may fail (Leo et al. 1995; Canan et al. 1999).

## Pterygopalatine Fossa

The pterygopalatine fossa (formerly pterygomaxillary fossa) (Figure 2.10), which lies within the infratemporal fossa (formerly zygomatic fossa), is a quadrangular, inverted pyramid, which, in panoramic X-rays, typically looks like an upside-down droplet (Erdogan 2003; Roberti 2007; von Arx et al. 2020). It is 17–24 mm high (Douglas and Wormald 2006; Gibelli et al. 2019; Vuksanovic-Bozaric et al. 2019; von Arx et al. 2020), with an anteroposterior distance of 12–15 mm on the upper part (base) (Cook 1950a; Canter et al. 1964; von Arx et al. 2020) and a volume 0.7–1.2 ml (Gibelli et al. 2019; von Arx et al. 2020).

### Margins

- The base lies in the superior zone. Formed from the pterygomaxillary face of the greater wing of the sphenoid bone, it lodges on its outer/lateral-most side the inferior orbital fissure that connects to the orbit.
- The vertex lies in the inferior zone. Formed by the sphenoidal process, the pyramidal apophysis of the maxilla and the maxillary tuberosity, it lodges the beginning of the greater palatine canal and the lesser canals that open onto the palatal vault.
- The anterior wall is formed by the maxillary tuberosity, with foramina that transmit the branches of the PSAN.
- The posterior wall, formed by the anterior side of the pterygoid process of the sphenoid, lodges three superior foramina:
  - The greater foramen rotundum for the maxillary nerve ($V_2$) and its venous plexus.
  - The pterygoid (formerly Vidian) canal for the nerve of the pterygoid canal (formerly Vidian nerve) and its artery and vein.
  - The pterygopalatine foramen for the pterygopalatine (Bock's) nerve and pterygopalatine artery.
- The internal wall forms from the vertical lamina of the palatine bone that separates it from the nasal fossae. Superiorly it lodges the sphenopalatine foramen, formed by the body of the sphenoid, and the orbital and sphenoidal processes of the palatine bone. This foramen transmits the nasopalatine nerve and its vessels to the nasal cavity.
- The external wall is a large opening or cleft that connects with the infratemporal fossa.

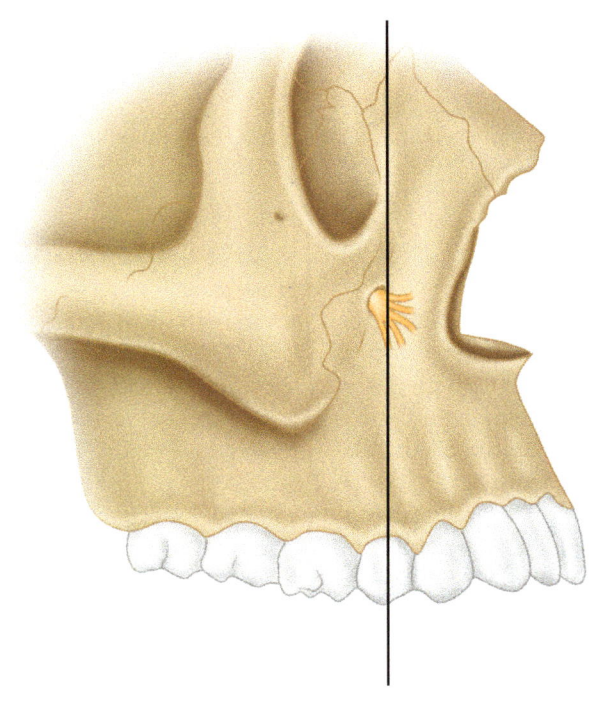

**Figure 2.13** Site of infraorbital foramen relative to maxillary second premolar axis.

### Content

- The maxillary nerve ($V_2$), after crossing the foramen rotundum, traverses the pterygopalatine fossa obliquely from back to front and inside out, then enters the orbit through the inferior orbital fissure, distributing in its course the branches described under the heading "Pterygopalatine fossa zone."
- The pterygopalatine (Meckel's) ganglion lies in the pterygopalatine fossa.
- The maxillary artery gives off the following branches at its terminus:
  - The infraorbital artery, which enters the orbit through the inferior orbital fissure and passes along the infraorbital groove, accompanied by the infraorbital nerve.
  - The descending palatine artery, which runs downward through the greater palatine canal with the greater palatine nerve.
  - The artery of the pterygoid canal (formerly Vidian artery), which feeds the pterygoid canal and accompanies the pterygoid canal nerve.
  - The sphenopalatine artery, which traverses the sphenopalatine foramen and enters the nasal fossae with the nasopalatine nerve.
- The middle and lower parts of the pterygoid venous plexus also lie in the fossa.

## Glossary

*Note*: The terms in bold are those which are popular in the profession and therefore often used instead of the formal terms.

| Anatomic terminology[a,b] | Other terminology used |
|---|---|
| Trigeminal ganglion | Semilunar/Gasserian ganglion |
| Pterygopalatine ganglion | Sphenopalatine/Meckel's ganglion |
| Greater palatine nerve | Anterior palatine nerve |
| Infraorbital nerve | Suborbital nerve |
| Lesser palatine nerves | Middle and posterior palatine nerves |
| Nasopalatine nerve | Nasopalatine nerve of Scarpa |
| | Incisive nerve |
| | Internal sphenopalatine nerve of Hirschfeld |
| | Long sphenopalatine nerve[c] |
| Nerve of the pterygoid canal | Vidian nerve |
| Pharyngeal nerve | Bock's nerve/pharyngeal nerve of Bock |
| Pterygopalatine nerves | Sphenopalatine nerves |
| Superior alveolar nerves | Superior dental nerves |
| Temporal zygomatic nerve | Palpebral lacrimal nerve |
| Zygomatic nerve | Orbital nerve |
| Zygomatic facial nerve | Temporomalar nerve |
| Greater palatine foramen | Posterior palatine foramen |
| Greater palatine canal | Pterygopalatine canal |
| | Posterior palatine canal |
| | Pterygomaxillary canal |
| Incisive canal (maxilla) | **Nasopalatine canal** |
| | Anterior palatine canal |
| Incisive foramen (maxilla) | Sphenopalatine foramen |
| | **Nasopalatine foramen** |
| | Anterior palatine foramen |
| | Scarpa's foramen[d] |
| | Retroincisive foramen |
| Incisive papilla | Interincisive papilla |
| | Anterior palatine papilla |
| | Retroincisive papilla |
| Inferior orbital fissure | Sphenomaxillary fissure |
| Infraorbital foramen | Suborbital foramen |
| Infraorbital groove | Infraorbital canal |
| Infratemporal fossa | Zygomatic fossa |
| Pterygoid canal | Vidian canal |
| Pterygopalatine fossa | Pterygomaxillary fossa |
| | Sphenomaxillary fossa |
| Auditory tube | Eustachian tube |
| Maxillary artery | Internal maxillary artery |

[a] FCAT (Federative Committee on Anatomical Terminology). Terminologia Anatomica. International Anatomical Terminology. Stuttgart. George Thieme Verlag. 1998.
[b] FCAT (Comité Federal sobre Terminología Anatómica). Terminología anatómica. Terminología anatómica internacional. Madrid. Editorial Panamericana SA. 2001.
[c] FitzGerald MJT, Scott JH. Observations on the anatomy of the superior dental nerves. Br Dent J 1958; 104 (6): 205–208.
[d] Phillips WH. Anatomic considerations in local anesthesia. J Oral Surg (Chicago) 1943; 1: 112–121.

## References

Agthong, S., Huanmanop, T., and Chentanez, V. (2005). Anatomical variations of the supraorbital, infraorbital, and mental foramina relation to gender and side. *J. Oral Maxillofac. Surg.* 63 (6): 800–804.

Al-Amery, S., Nambiar, P., Jamaludin, M. et al. (2015). Cone beam computed tomography assessment of maxillary incisive canal and foramen: considerations of anatomical variations when placing immediate implants. *PloS One* 10(2): e0117251.

Allen, G.D. (1979). *Dental Anesthesia and Analgesia (Local and General)*, 2e. Baltimore: Williams and Wilkins. 79.

Annex 2. Infraorbital foramen.

Annex 41. Nasopalatine canal and foramen.

Annex 42. Greater palatine canal and foramen.

Archer, W.H. and Zubrow, H.J. (1954). Fatal hemorrhage following regional anesthesia for operative dentistry in a hemophiliac. *Oral Surg. Oral Med. Oral Pathol.* 7 (5): 464–470.

Arens, D.E., Adams, W.R., and de Castro, R.A. (1984). *Endodontic Surgery*. New York: Harper and Row. 30–38.

Bahsi, I., Orhan, M., and Kervancioglu, P. (2017). A sample of morphological eponym confusion: foramina of Stenson/Stensen. *Surg. Radiol. Anat.* 39 (8): 935–936.

Brand, R.W. and Isselhard, D.E. (2003). *Anatomy of Orofacial Structures*, 7e. St. Louis: Mosby-Elsevier. 203.

Calatayud, J. (2001). *Información no publicada*. Madrid: Universidad Complutense.

Canan, S., Asim, O.M., Okan, B. et al. (1999). Anatomic variations of the infraorbital foramen. *Ann. Plast. Surg.* 43 (6): 613–617.

Canter, S.R., Slavkin, H.C., and Canter, M.R. (1964). Anatomical study of pterygopalatine fossa and canal: considerations applicable to the anesthetization of the second division of the fifth cranial nerve. *J. Oral Surg. Anesth. Hosp. Dent. Serv.* 22 (4): 318–323.

Chatriyanuyoke, P., Lu, C.-I., Suzuki, Y. et al. (2012). Nasopalatine canal position relative to the maxillary central incisors: a cone beam computed tomography assessment. *J. Oral Implantol.* 38 (6): 713–717.

Cook, W.A. (1949). The nerve supply to the maxillary incisors. *J. Oral Surg. (Chicago)* 7 (2): 149–154.

Cook, W.A. (1950a). The nerve supply to the maxillary bicuspid teeth. *Dent. Items Interest*.

Cook, W.A. (1950b). The anterior superior alveolar nerve and its control with local anesthetics. *Dent. Items Interest* 72 (10): 1021–1028.

Douglas, R. and Wormald, P.J. (2006). Pterygopalatine fossa infiltration through the greater palatine foramen: where to bend the needle. *Laryngoscope* 116 (7): 1255–1257.

DuBrul, E.L. (1988). *Sicher and Dubrul's Oral Anatomy*, 8e. St. Louis: Ishiyaku EuroAmerica Inc. 257, 260.

Erdogan, N., Unur, E., and Baykara, M. (2003). CT anatomy of pterygopalatine fossa and its communications: a pictorical review. *Comput. Med. Imaging Graph.* 27 (6): 481–487.

FCAT (Comité Federal sobre Terminología Anatómica). Terminología anatómica (2001). *Terminología anatómica internacional*. Madrid: Editorial Panamericana SA.

FCAT (Federative Committee on Anatomical Terminology) (1998). *Terminologia Anatomica. International Anatomical Terminology*. Stuttgart: George Thieme Verlag.

Feige, V.I. (1978). Technik un Erfolgesbewertung der Infraorbitalanästhesie be idem Zugangsweg eutlang der Achse des 2. Prämolaren. *Stomatol. DDR* 28 (9): 649–653.

Ferlin, R., Pagin, B.S.C., and Yaedú, R.Y.F. (2019). Canalis sinuosus: a systematic review of the literature. *Oral Surg. Oral Med. Oral Pathol.* 127 (6): 545–551.

FitzGerald, M.J.T. (1956). The occurrence of middle superior alveolar nerve in man. *J. Anat. (Lond.)* 90 (4): 520–522.

FitzGerald, M.J.T. (1960). The pattern of superior dental nerves in relation the growth changes in the upper jaw. *Br. Dent. J.* 108 (7): 265–269.

FitzGerald, M.J.T. and Scott, J.H. (1958). Observations on the anatomy of the superior dental nerves. *Br. Dent. J.* 104 (6): 205–208.

Fitzpatrick, T.H. and Downs, B.W. (2019). *Anatomy, Head and Neck, Nasopalatine Nerve. StatPearls [Internet]*. Treasure Island (FL): StatPearls Publishing.

Gaballah, M.F., Rakhawy, M.T., and Badawy, Z.H. (1973). On the course of the posterior and the middle superior alveolar canals. *Acta Anat. (Basel)* 86 (1): 151–156.

Gibelli, D., Cellina, M., Gibelli, S. et al. (2019). Anatomy of the pterygopalatine fossa: an innovative metrical assessment based on 3D segmentation on head CT-scan. *Surg. Radiol. Anat.* 41 (5): 523–528.

Hayden, J. Jr. (1965). The innervation of the maxillary first permanent and primary molars a determinate by the deposition of local anesthetic solutions. A preliminary report. *Acta Odontol. Scand.* 23 (2): 147–162.

Heasman, P.A. (1984). Clinical anatomy of the superior alveolar nerves. *Br. J. Oral Maxillofac. Surg.* 22 (6): 439–447.

Hindy, A.M. and Raouf, F.A. (1993). A study of infraorbital foramen, canal and nerve in adult Egyptians. *Egypt. Dent. J.* 39 (4): 573–580.

Hofer, O. (1922). Die Leitungsästhesie des Nervus nasopalinus Scarpae bei stomatologischen Eingriffen. *Z. Stomatol.* 20: 411–416.

Jacobs, R., Lambrichts, I., Liang, X. et al. (2007). Neurovascularization of the anterior jaw bones revisited using high-resolution magnetic resonance imaging. *Oral Surg. Oral Med. Oral Pathol.* 103 (5): 683–693.

Jang, J.K., Kwak, S.W., Ha, J.H., and Kim, H.C. (2017). Anatomical relationship of maxillary posterior teeth with the sinus floor and buccal cortex. *J. Oral Rehabil.* 22 (8): 617–625.

Jastak, J.T., Yagiela, J.A., and Donaldson, D. (1995). *Local Anesthesia of the Oral Cavity*. Philadelphia: WB Saunders Company. 169.

Jones, F.W. (1939). The anterior superior alveolar nerve and vessels. *J. Anat. (Lond.)* 73 (Pt 4): 583–591.

Jornet, P.L., Boix, P., Perez, A.S., and Boracchia, A. (2015). Morphological characterization of the anterior palatine region using cone beam computed tomography. *Clin. Implant Dent. Relat. Res.* 17 (Suppl 2): e459–e464.

Kadanoff, D., Mutafov, S.T., and Jordanov, J. (1970). Über die Hauptöffunngen resp. Incisurae des Gesichtsschädels (Incisurae frontalis seu Foramen frontale, Foramen supraorbitale seu Incisurae supraorbitalis, Foramen infraorbitale, foramen mentale). *Gegenbaurs Morphol. Jahrb.* 115 (1): 102–118.

Karkut, B., Teader, A., Drum, M. et al. (2010). A comparison of the local anesthetic efficacy of the extraoral versus the intraoral infraorbital nerve block. *J. Am. Dent. Assoc.* 141 (2): 185–192.

Kleier, D.J., Deeg, D.K., and Auerbach, R.E. (1983). The extraoral approach to the infraorbital nerve block. *J. Am. Dent. Assoc.* 107 (5): 758–760.

Lake, S., Iwanaga, J., Kikuta, S. et al. (2018). The incisive canal: a comprehensive review. *Cureus* 10 (7): e3069.

Langford, R.J. (1989). The contribution of the nasopalatine nerve to sensation of the hard palate. *Br. J. Oral Maxillofac. Surg.* 27 (5): 379–386.

Leo, J.T., Cassell, M.D., and Bergman, R.A. (1995). Variation in human infraorbital nerve, canal and foramen. *Ann. Anat.* 177 (1): 93–95.

Liang, X., Jacobs, R., Martens, W. et al. (2009). Macro- and micro-anatomical, histological and computed tomography scan characterization of the nasopalatine canal. *J. Clin. Periodontol.* 36 (7): 598–603.

Loestscher, C.A. and Walton, R.E. (1988). Patterns of inervation of the maxillary first molar: a dissection study. *Oral Surg. Oral Med. Oral Pathol.* 65 (1): 86–90.

Lopes, P.T.C., Pereira, G.A.M., Santos, A.M.P.V. et al. (2009). Morphometric analysis of the infraorbital foramen related to gender and laterality in dry skulls of adult individuals in southern Brazil. *Braz. J. Morphol. Sci.* 26 (1): 19–22.

Malamed, S.F. and Trieger, N. (1983). Intraoral maxillary nerve block: an anatomical and clinical study. *Anesth. Prog.* 30 (2): 44–48.

Matsumura, T., Ishida, Y., Kawabe, A., and Ono, T. (2017). Quantitative analysis of the relationship between maxillary incisors and the incisive canal by cone beam computed tomography in an adult Japanese population. *Prog. Orthod.* 18: 24.

McDaniel, V.M.L. (1956). Variations in nerve distributions of the maxillary teeth. *J. Dent. Res.* 35 (6): 916–921.

Murphy, T.R. and Grundy, E.M. (1969). The inferior alveolar neurovascular bundle at the mandibular foramen. *Dent. Pract. Dent. Rec.* 20 (2): 41–48.

Norton, N.S. (2011). *Netter's Head and Neck Anatomy for Dentistry (Netter Basic Science)*, 2e. St. Louis: Elsevier Health Science Division.

de Oliveira-Santos, C., Rubira-Bullen, I.R.F., Monteiro, S.A.C. et al. (2013). Neurovascular anatomical variations in the anterior palate observed on CBCT images. *Clin. Oral Implant. Res.* 24 (9): 1044–1048.

Olsen, N.H., Tenscher, G.W., and Vehe, K.L. (1955). A study of the nerve supply to the upper anterior teeth. *J. Dent. Res.* 34 (4): 413–420.

Olson, T.R. (1996). *ADAM Student Atlas of Anatomy*. Baltimore: Williams and Wilkins, 386, 432, 446.

Pennisi, E., Gruccu, G., Manfredi, M., and Palladini, G. (1991). Histometric study of myelinated fibers in the human trigeminal nerve. *J. Neurol. Sci.* 105 (1): 22–28.

Phillips, W.H. (1943). Anatomical considerations in local anesthesia. *Anesth. Analg.* 22 (1): 5–14.

Phillips, W.H. and Maxmen, H.A. (1941). The nasopalatine block injection as an aid in operative procedures for maxillary incisors. *Am. J. Orthod. Oral Surg.* 27 (8): 426–434.

Rapado-González, O., Suárez-Quintanilla, J.A., Otero-Cepeda, X.L. et al. (2015). Morphometric study of the greater palatine canal: cone-beam computed tomography. *Surg. Radiol. Anat.* 37 (10): 1217–1224.

Riesenfeld, A. (1956). Multiple infraorbital, ethmoidal and mental foramina in the races of man. *Am. J. Phys. Anthropol.* 14 (1): 85–100.

Roberti, F., Boari, N., Mortini, P., and Caputy, A.J. (2007). The pterygopalatine fossa: an anatomic report. *J. Craniofac. Surg.* 18 (3): 586–590.

Roberts, W.H. and Jorgensen, N.B. (1961). A note on the distribution of the superior alveolar nerves in relation to the primary teeth. *Anat. Rec.* 141 (2): 81–84.

Roberts, D.H. and Sowray, J.H. (1987). *Local Analgesia in Dentistry*, 3e. Bristol (UK): Wright. 98–101.

Roda, R.S. and Blanton, P.L. (1994). The anatomy of the local anesthesia. *Quintessence Int.* 25 (1): 27–38.

Rusu, M.C., Iacov-Craitoiu, M.-M., Sandulescu, M. et al. (2019). Constant features of the adult maxillary bone in the site of the premaxillary suture: the *sutura notha*, Macalister's foramina, Parinaud's canal, and the second angle of the *canalis sinuosus* of Wood Jones. *Roman. J. Morphol. Embryol.* 60 (4): 1097–1103.

Sanz, J.V., Esporrin, J., Marco, J. et al. (1995). Vías del dolor desde la región orofacial. *Av. Odontoestomatol. (Madrid)* 11 (Suppl A): 13–18.

Schünke, M., Schulte, E., and Schumacher, U. (2012). *Prometheus. LernAtlas der Anatomie. Kopf, Hals und neuroanatomie*, 3e. Stuttgart: Georg Thieme Verlag KG.

Shaw, M.D. and Fierst, P. (1988). Clinical prosection for dental gross anatomy: a medial approach to the pterygomandibular space. *Anat. Rec.* 222 (3): 305–308.

Sicher, H. (1950). Aspects in the applied anatomy of local anesthesia. *Int. Dent. J.* 1 (1): 70–82.

Slavkin, H.C., Canter, M.R., and Canter, S.R. (1966). An anatomic study of the pterygomaxillary region in the craniums of infants and children. *Oral Surg. Oral Med. Oral Pathol.* 21 (2): 225–235.

Song, W.-C., Jo, D.-I., Lee, J.-Y. et al. (2009). Microanatomy of the incisive canal using three-dimensional reconstruction of microCT images: an ex vivo study. *Oral Surg. Oral Med. Oral Pathol.* 109 (4): 583–590.

Szabó, E. (1948). Variationen der Nervi alveolares superiors. *Schweiz. Monatsschr. Zahnheil.* 58 (9): 819–829.

Ulusoy, Ö.I.A. and Alacam, T. (2014). Efficacy of single buccal infiltrations for maxillary first molars in patients with irreversible pulpitis: a randomized controlled trial. *Int. Endod. J.* 47 (3): 222–227.

Von Arx, T. and Lozanoff, S. (2015). Anterior superior alveolar nerve (ASAN). A morphometric-anatomical analysis. *Swiss Dent. J.* 125 (11): 1202–1209.

Von Arx, T., Lozanoff, S., Sendi, P., and Bornstein, M.M. (2013). Assessment of bone channels other than the nasopalatine canal in the anterior maxilla using limited cone beam computed tomography. *Surg. Radiol. Anat.* 35 (9): 783–790.

Von Arx, T., Lozanoff, S., and Bornstein, M.M. (2020). Extraoral anatomy in CBCT – a literature review. *Swiss Dent. J.* 130 (3): 216–228.

Vuksanovic-Bozaric, A., Vukcevic, B., Abramovic, M. et al. (2019). The pterygopalatine fossa: morphometric CT study with clinical implications. *Surg. Radiol. Anat.* 41 (2): 161–168.

Westmoreland, E.E. and Blanton, P.L. (1982). An analysis of the variations in position of the greater foramen in the adult human skull. *Anat. Rec.* 204 (4): 383–388.

Westwater, L.A. (1960). The innervation of the pulps of the teeth. *Br. Dent. J.* 109 (10): 407–410.

# 3

## Applied Anatomy II: Mandibular Arch

This anatomical review of the mandibular arch addresses the anatomic areas of interest for local anesthesia in dentistry, divided into three subchapters: the mandibular nerve ($V_3$), the mandible, and the pterygomandibular space.

A glossary of presently accepted terms (FCAT 1998) is listed at the end of the chapter with equivalent terminology (current and past) to enable the reader to recognize the anatomical structures referenced in other texts and older scientific articles.

The names of three anatomical structures that are not widely utilize in the current vernacular are used here as they are highly practical to explain lower arch anesthetic techniques, i.e. the mandibular incisive nerve, the *sulcus colli* (groove of the mandibular neck), and the coronoid notch.

## Mandibular Nerve ($V_3$)

This is the third and largest branch of the trigeminal nerve. It arises from the middle fossa of the skull, traveling forward, outward, and downward across the *foramen ovale* with the middle meningeal artery and associated veins toward the lower surface of the infratemporal fossa that borders the pterygomandibular space. The small motor root of this nerve passes beneath the trigeminal ganglion (semilunar ganglion or Gasserian ganglion) and joins the large sensory root just outside the skull (Figures 2.1 and 2.3, Chapter 2).

### Overview

Three branches can be distinguished in the mandibular nerve ($V_3$) after it exits the skull.

*Pre-division.* After crossing the *foramen ovale* it distributes:

- Branches to the otic and peripheral parasympathetic ganglia, the latter, just beyond the *foramen ovale*, traveling with branches of the glossopharyngeal nerve (CN IX).
- The meningeal (recurrent) branch or *nervus spinosus*, a sensory nerve that re-enters the skull through the *foramen spinosum* with the middle meningeal artery to innervate the *dura mater*.
- A motor nerve to the medial (internal) pterygoid muscle
- A motor nerve to the *tensor veli palatini*.

*Anterior division.* The following emerge from this primarily motor division:

- *Buccal nerve*, a sensory nerve particularly relevant in anesthesia.
- Masseteric nerve, which innervates the masseter muscle.
- Deep temporal nerves, which innervate the temporal muscle.
- Nerve to the lateral (external) pterygoid muscle.

*Posterior division.* This primarily sensory division, which is larger than the anterior division or trunk, gives off:

- The *auriculotemporal nerve*.
- A nerve to supply the temporomandibular joint (TMJ).
- A nerve from the common motor trunk that innervates the medial (internal) pterygoid, *levator veli palatini*, and *malleus* (tensor tympani) muscles.
- The *lingual nerve*.
- The *inferior alveolar nerve* and its branches:
  - *Mylohyoid nerve*.
  - *Branch to the third molar*.
  - *Mental nerve*.
  - *Mandibular incisive nerve*.

As the targets of local anesthesia in dentistry, the sensory nerves are the ones most relevant to this discussion (Figure 3.1).

### Buccal Nerve

Although this sensory nerve is usually regarded as a branch of the anterior division of the mandibular nerve (third branch of the trigeminal nerve), variations have been reported.

*Local Anesthesia in Dentistry: A Locoregional Approach*, First Edition. Jesús Calatayud and Mana Saraghi.
© 2024 John Wiley & Sons Ltd. Published 2024 by John Wiley & Sons Ltd.
Companion website: www.wiley.com/go/Calatayud/local

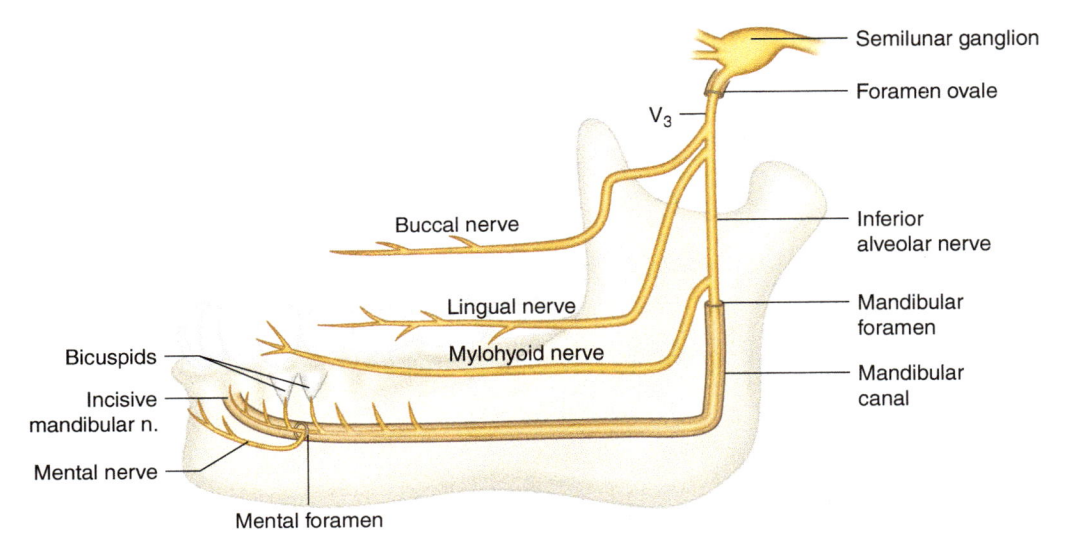

**Figure 3.1** Schematic representation of emergence and distribution of the branches of the mandibular nerve (V₃). *Source:* Redrawn from Allen (1979), with changes.

## Course

From the upper pterygomandibular space (lower infratemporal fossa) the buccal nerve passes downward between the two bellies/fascicles/heads of the lateral (external) pterygoid muscle (Figure 3.13) toward the external surface of the muscle. From there it may subsequently course downward with the deep tendon of the temporal muscle or its fascia (Barker and Davies 1972) and along the outer surface of the temporal crest (Sicher 1950).

In an open mouth, at the height of the lower molar occlusal plane the buccal nerve crosses outward beyond the anterior border of the ramus of the mandible and the temporal muscle (Phillips 1943) (Figures 3.2 and 3.14). It may also course at a higher level, however, defined by the upper molar occlusal plane (Roda and Blanton 1994). Significantly, the nerve is very close to the surface here, at only about 2 mm beneath the mucosa (Phillips 1943).

The buccal nerve subsequently enters but does not innervate the buccinator muscle of the cheek (which is innervated by the facial nerve, CN VII), distributing sensory fibers to the retromolar zone, the buccal mucosa, and the mucosa on the buccal side of the lower molars.

The buccal nerve may, albeit rarely, start at a very low position inside the mandibular canal, entering the buccinator muscle through a foramen in the retromolar fossa (Turner 1864; Singh 1981; Jablonski et al. 1985).

## Innervation

- The buccal nerve innervates the fibromucosa (alveolar mucosa and gum), bone, and periosteum of the buccal side of the lower molars, although that may vary. In 10% of cases it innervates only the vestibule of the retromolar trigone (Hendy and Robinson 1994), whereas in under 1% it may reach as far forward as the buccal side of the lower canines (Stewart and Wilson 1928; Stewart 1932; Sicher 1950; Singh 1981) (Figure 3.3).
- The buccal nerve supplies the buccal mucosa in the posterior, as well in many cases as the upper, mouth.
- In 80–90% of cases, this primarily sensory nerve carries motor innervation to the lateral (external) pterygoid muscle (Kim et al. 2003).
- It may occasionally give off branches that supply the pulp of the mandibular molars (Schejtman et al. 1967; Sutton 1974; Ossenberg 1986).

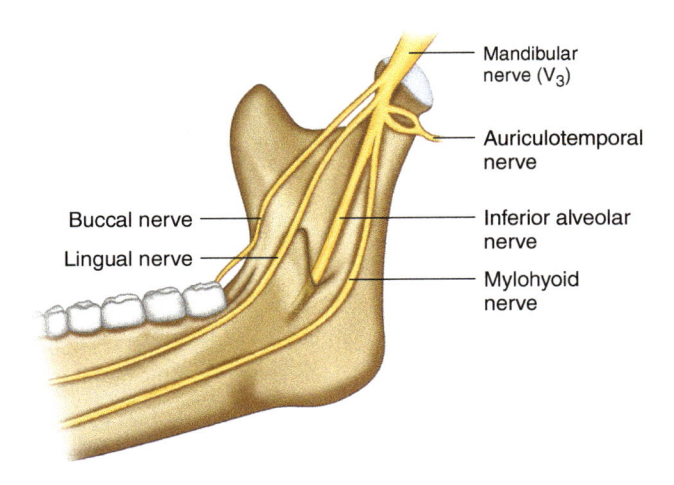

**Figure 3.2** Position in the mandible of the main sensory nerves in the lower arch that are anesthetized.

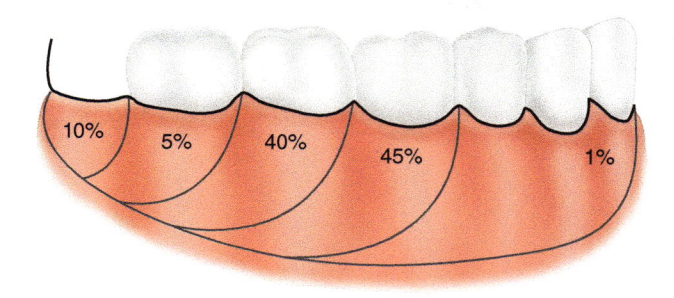

**Figure 3.3** Vestibular areas provided sensation by the buccal nerve. *Source:* Data rounded from Stewart (1932), Sicher (1950), Singh (1981), and Hendy and Robinson (1994).

## Auriculotemporal Nerve

### Course

This nerve is given off from the posterior division of the mandibular nerve ($V_3$) in the interpterygoid region. It normally has a superior and an inferior root, which run backward, enveloping the middle meningeal artery (branch of the maxillary artery) and uniting shortly thereafter to form a V-shaped interval (Figure 3.2). This description matches 30–50% of cases, whereas in the rest there may be one to four roots that surround the middle meningeal artery medially and laterally in every possible combination (Baumel et al. 1971; Gülekon et al. 2005). The inferior root may also branch off from the upper end of the inferior alveolar nerve (Baumel et al. 1971) (Table 3.1), where it receives postganglionic fibers from the otic ganglion (peripheral parasympathetic ganglion connected to the glossopharyngeal nerve, CN IX).

After uniting, the auriculotemporal nerve passes backward, outward, and downward, brushing against the condylar neck, continuing behind the capsule of the TMJ, distributing two branches toward the facial nerve (CN VII) and perforating the parotid fascia to enter the upper part of the parotid gland. Variations on this standard scheme include the distribution of one to three branches toward the facial nerve, even after the auriculotemporal nerve enters the parotid gland (Namking et al. 1994).

**Table 3.1** Number of roots forming the auriculotemporal nerve.

| No. of roots | Baumel et al. (1971) n = 85 (%) | Gülekon et al. (2005) n = 32 (%) |
| --- | --- | --- |
| 1 | 12 | 50 |
| 2 | 73 | 37 |
| 3 | 14 | 10 |
| 4 | 2 | 3 |

Ultimately the nerve crosses the zygomatic arch posteriorly and turns upward at a right angle, passing between the tragus and the auditory meatus, and terminating in the temporal region.

### Innervation

The auriculotemporal nerve supplies:

- The *auricula*, tragus and to a lesser extent the helix.
- The *skin in the temporal region*, in some cases reaching as far as the border of the parietal, masseteric, frontal, and supraorbital regions.
- The external auditory meatus.
- The posterior part of the articular capsule of the TMJ.

The auriculotemporal nerve carries otic ganglion secretory and vascular fibers to the parotid gland.

On occasion branches of the auriculotemporal nerve supply the pulp of the mandibular molars, entering the mandible through the foramina near the condylar neck and the retromolar zone (Carter and Keen 1971; Sutton 1974).

## Lingual Nerve

### Course

The lingual nerve passes through two zones, the pterygomandibular space and the floor of the mouth.

*Pterygomandibular space.* The lingual nerve originates in from the upper pterygomandibular space, branching off the posterior division of the mandibular nerve ($V_3$). It runs between the medial (internal) side of the lateral (external) pterygoid muscle and the interpterygoid aponeurosis. There, posteriorly, it receives the *chorda tympani* nerve (a branch of facial nerve – CN VII – that carries parasympathetic nerve fibers for submandibular gland secretion and also sensory fibers for taste for the anterior two-thirds of the tongue). It then passes downward along the anterior pterygomandibular space parallel to but in a more anterior and medial (interior) course than the inferior alveolar nerve (Shaw and Fierst 1988). It reaches the lower pterygomandibular space between the exterior (lateral) surface of the medial (internal) pterygoid muscle and the internal surface of the ramus of the mandible (Sicher 1946) (Figure 3.14).

*Floor of the mouth and submandibular zone.* The lingual nerve enters the floor of the mouth underneath the lower border of the superior pharyngeal constrictor muscle and the pterygomandibular raphe or ligament, coursing adjacent to the (osseous) lingual alveolar crest in the retro- and third molar zones (Annex 3). There it is usually round or oval, although in 20% of cases it may be flat and ribbon-like (Kiesselbach and Chamberlain 1984) with a diameter of 2–3 mm (Annex 3). In >30% of cases it may touch the

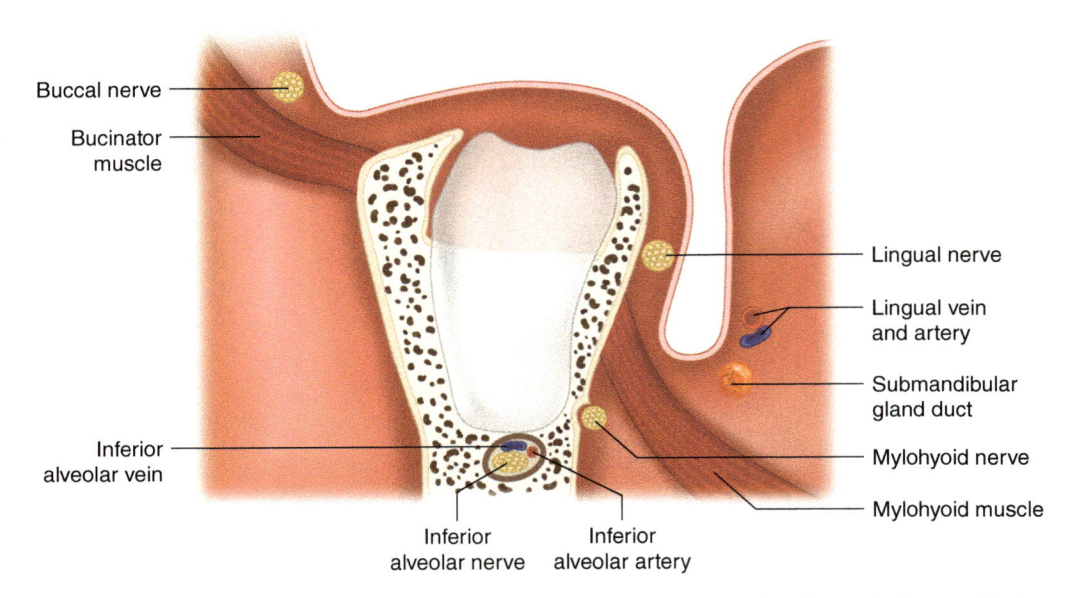

**Figure 3.4** Sagittal section of the floor of the mouth through the third molar. *Source:* Redrawn with changes from Andreasen et al. (1997).

alveolar process (Figure 3.4), in 10% it may lie over the lingual alveolar crest at the third molar and in one in 300 cases it may run above the soft retromolar tissue (Annex 3).

The lingual nerve passes very near the surface here, underneath the mucosa of the floor of the mouth and over the mylohyoid muscle (Figure 3.4), separating off the bone toward the medial zone and running deeper as it progresses forward (Annex 3). This is a good area to block the lingual nerve.

Here it distributes branches to the submandibular ganglion, a peripheral parasympathetic ganglion that receives fibers from the *chorda tympani*. Its course subsequently deepens, crossing medially beneath the submandibular or Wharton's duct. It then rises medially (internally), entering the tongue where its branches communicate with the hypoglossal nerve (CN XII). It terminates at the sublingual gland, where it gives off its terminal branches.

### Innervation

The lingual nerve supplies:

- The fibromucosa (alveolar mucosa and gums), bone, and periosteum of the lingual zone of the lower arch on the same side to the midline.
- The fibromucosa of the floor of the mouth on the same side to the midline.
- The anterior two-thirds of the tongue to the midline.

The lingual nerve supplies some proprioception to the muscles of the tongue (Barker and Davies 1972) and some gustatory perception to the anterior tongue (Malamed 2004; Jastak et al. 1995).

### Remarks

At the lingula, the lingual nerve is multifascicular, with one to eight (mean = three) fascicles, although in 30% of cases it has only one, making it vulnerable to irreversible damage in the event of trauma caused by needle impact during the mandibular block procedure (Pogrel et al. 2003). Moreover, in the retromolar and third molar zones it may adopt a ribbon-like shape with a diameter of 0.5 mm in less than 10% of cases according to some authors (Kiesselbach and Chamberlain 1984). Since, as noted, it courses adjacent to the lingual alveolar process (Annex 3), it is vulnerable there also (given that the diameter of a 25G needle is 0.5 mm).

### Inferior Alveolar Nerve

#### Course

The inferior alveolar nerve, the largest of the three branches of the posterior division of the mandibular nerve, arises around 4–5 mm under the *foramen ovale*, descends along the pterygomandibular space between the internal surface of the lateral (external) pterygoid muscle and the interpterygoid aponeurosis, and courses obliquely (posteriorly-anteriorly, interiorly-exteriorly) from there parallel to but following a more posterior and external course than the lingual nerve. In this downward length it gives off the *mylohyoid nerve* (Figure 3.2).

In its descent it converges with the internal surface of the ramus of the mandible as far as the mandibular foramen (Sicher 1946; Barker and Davies 1972), through which it passes with the inferior alveolar artery (branch of the maxillary artery) and associated veins (tributaries of the pterygoid plexus; Archer and Zubrow 1954; Khoury et al. 2010), which are usually located behind the inferior alveolar nerve (Murphy and Grundy 1969; Roda and Blanton 1994). In this area, where its diameter is 2–3 mm (Annex 3), it gives an *accessory branch for the wisdom tooth* in 10–40% of cases just before or after entering the mandibular canal (Sicher 1946; Barker and Davies 1972).

The inferior alveolar nerve runs across the body of the mandible through the mandibular canal, usually under the mandibular molar apexes, close to the mental foramen (normally located near the second premolar apex) where, around half the time, it courses further, forming a 2–3 mm long *anterior loop* (Annex 4) that takes an abrupt posterior and vestibular turn, rising until it abuts with the mental foramen. At this point it distributes two branches (Figure 3.5).

1) The internal branch or *mandibular incisive nerve* proceeds in more 85% of cases from a forward-running, 10–15 mm long mandibular incisive canal, coursing adjacent to the buccal surface of the mandible (Annex 4) and through the trabecular or medullary bone under the apexes of the anterior teeth (Mardinger et al. 2000; Pires et al. 2012; Apostolakis and Brown 2013; Huang et al. 2013) to supply the mandibular first premolar, canine, and incisors on that side. In the few cases where there is no mandibular incisive canal, the mandibular incisive nerve forms a plexus in the trabecular or spongy bone to substitute for it, but in neither case does it cross the midline (Olivier 1927; Sicher 1946), site of the intermandibular cartilage in the embryo.

2) The external branch or *mental nerve* initially runs upward and backward after exiting the mental foramen to then turn forward and form the *labial plexus* in the soft tissue mucosa, which does cross the midline (Figure 19.9, Chapter 19). It subsequently anastomoses with fibers from the other side, passing in some cases through foramina of the body of the mandible and at times innervating the pulp of the contralateral incisors (Starkie and Stewart 1931; Rood 1977).

### Innervation

The inferior alveolar nerve supplies:

- The molar and premolar pulp and periodontal ligament, and via the mandibular incisive nerve, canines and incisors.
- Interdental papillae as well as molar and premolar (and via the mandibular incisive nerve, also canine and incisor) fibromucosa, bone, and periosteum.
- Buccal, via the mental nerve; fibromucosa (alveolar mucosa and attached gums), bone, and periosteum of the entire zone between the premolars and the lower central incisor, although this may vary depending on the area covered by the buccal nerve (Sutton 1974), with extremes ranging from the entire molar zone (10% of cases) to the canines and incisors only (1%) (Hendy and Robinson 1994).
- Tip of the chin and its skin, lower lip, likewise via the mental nerve.

### Remarks

When the mouth is closed the inferior alveolar nerve is folded and lies very medially (internally) in the pterygomandibular space, separated from the ramus of the mandible. When the mouth is wide open, the nerve stretches and is positioned posteriorly, coursing adjacent to the internal surface of the ramus (Sicher 1950) near the *sulcus colli* (Bremer 1952; Via 1953).

The inferior alveolar nerve comprises several fascicles whose composition tends to change along its course (Rood 1978a). Its myelinated fibers exhibit a node of Ranvier every 0.5–1.8 mm (Rood 1977, 1978b) and given that to anesthetize a nerve of these characteristics at least three such nodes must be blocked (Blair and Erlanger 1939), around 6 mm of the inferior alveolar nerve must be bathed in the anesthetic (Rood 1977, 1978b). The myelin sheaths around the axons of this nerve bear Schmidt–Lantermann clefts. These oblique inclusions communicate the axon with the exterior and afford the nerve greater elasticity when the mouth is wide open, facilitating application of the anesthetic through the clefts (Heasman and Beynon 1987).

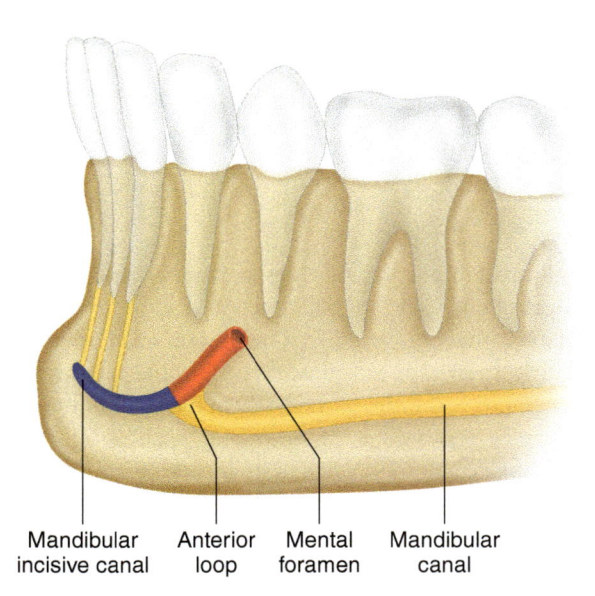

**Figure 3.5** Termination of the mandibular canal at the mandibular incisive canal, mental foramen, and anterior loop.

Since at the lingula the inferior alveolar nerve is multifascicular, with three to 14 fascicles (mean = 7), it is less likely to be injured by needle trauma during mandibular block as it is highly unlikely that all the fascicles would be injured (Pogrel et al. 2003).

### Mylohyoid Nerve

#### Course
Motor fibers predominate in this mixed nerve. The mylohyoid nerve branches from the inferior alveolar nerve around 15 mm (range 4–23 mm) before entering the mandibular foramen (Wilson et al. 1984; Bennett and Townsend 2001; Stein et al. 2007) (Figure 3.2). It runs against the ramus of the mandible in the mylohyoid groove, an osseous groove located beneath the mandibular foramen, crosses the sphenomandibular ligament and the medial (internal) pterygoid muscle insertion to then enter the floor of the mouth or submandibular region (Archer and Zubrow 1954; Roberts and Harris 1973; Madeira et al. 1978). It passes under the mylohyoid muscle (Figure 3.4), coursing along and adjacent to the internal surface of the body of the mandible, just below the mylohyoid line, which in 15% of cases may form a canal for the mylohyoid nerve as the ligaments and periosteum that cover it ossify (Arensburgh and Nathan 1979).

#### Innervation
- The motor part of the nerve supplies the mylohyoid muscle and the anterior belly of the digastric muscle.
- The sensory fibers innervate the skin at the tip of the chin (Roberts and Harris 1973) and the dental pulp of molars, premolars, canines, and incisors (Novitzky 1938; Sicher 1946; Carter and Keen 1971; Frommer et al. 1972; Madeira et al. 1978; Chapnick 1980; Bennett and Townsend 2001), as well as the contralateral incisors (Madeira et al. 1978).

*Note*: Exceptionally, the mylohyoid nerve may proceed from the inferior end of the lingual nerve (Jablonski et al. 1985).

## Body of the Mandible

The mandible is the largest, strongest, and lowest facial bone. It is horseshoe-shaped, with a horizontally curved body (body of the mandible) flanked posteriorly by two ascending branches (rami of the mandible). The body of the mandible, also known as the horizontal ramus of the mandible, features several characteristics of interest here (Figures 3.6 and 3.7).

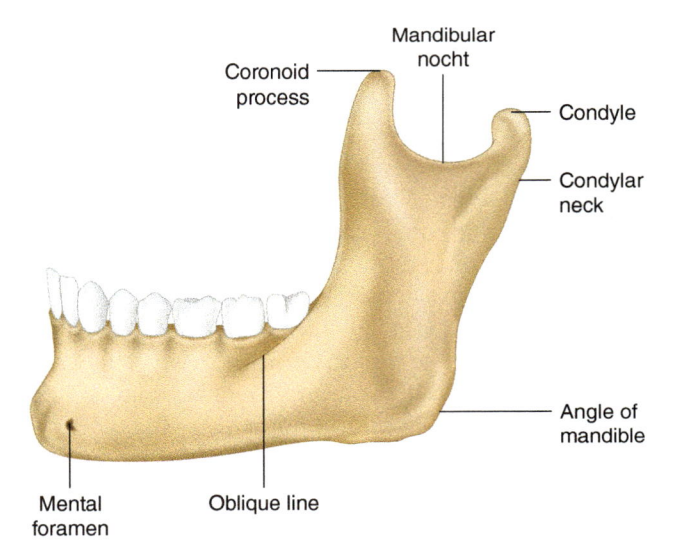

**Figure 3.6** Predominant anatomical features on the external surface of the mandible.

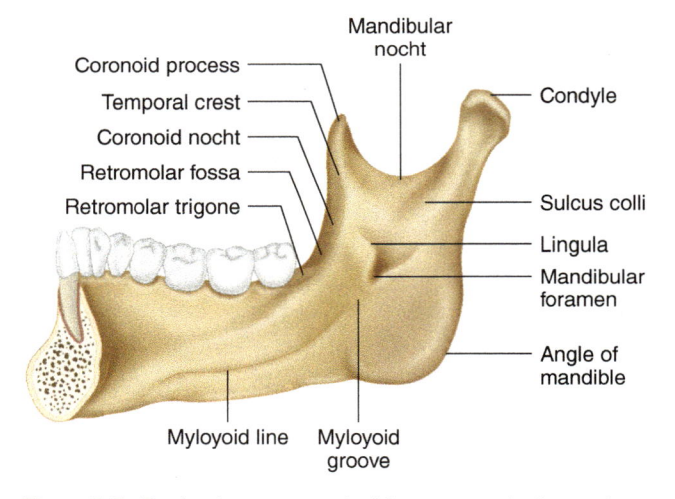

**Figure 3.7** Predominant anatomical features on the internal surface of the mandible.

### Cortical Bone Thickness

The teeth are housed in the alveolar part, on the upper border of the body of the mandible. The mandible or lower jaw is denser than the maxillary bone and, as shown in Table 3.2, at the apex the cortical, as well as the spongy or medullary bone, is thicker, particularly in the posterior vestibule, due in part to the more lingual position of the molars (Denio et al. 1992). For that reason, mandibular block is required in pulpal anesthesia of the molars.

Buccal infiltration techniques can be used in the anterior mandible, which is less dense than the posterior bone. In contrast, the cortical bone is even thicker in the lingual region.

Table 3.2 Mean vestibular and lingual height (mm) of cortical and medullary bone over apexes of mandibular teeth.

|  | Buccal | | Lingual | |
| --- | --- | --- | --- | --- |
| Tooth | Cortical | Medullary | Cortical | Medullary |
| Incisors | 1–2 | 2–3 | 3–4 | 2–3 |
| Canines | 1–2 | 3–5 | 2–3 | 4–5 |
| Premolars | 0–5 | 0.5–5 | 3.5 | 1–3 |
| Molars | 2–5 | 2–6 | 3–4 | 1–2 |

*Source*: From data published by Arens et al. (1984), Denio et al. (1992) and Gowgiel (1992).

## Retromolar Zone (Trigone and Fossa)

This zone has significant practical implications in light of the presence of accessory innervation, primarily in the dental pulp of the mandibular molars very likely due to: (i) the high frequency (45%, ranging from 12% to 92%) of mandibles with accessory foramina (Löfgren 1957; Carter and Keen 1971; Haveman and Tebo 1976), the largest diameter foramina in the mandible (Haveman and Tebo 1976), and the presence, confirmed by anatomic dissections and histological studies, of many nerve fibers (Schejtman et al. 1967; Sutton 1974; Singh 1981); and (ii) the existence of dual (bifid) mandibular canals, here denominated retromolar canals (Table 3.3), detected with modern cone beam computed tomographic techniques in 15% of cases. The retromolar zone consists in two structures, the retromolar trigone and fossa (Figure 3.8).

### Retromolar Trigone

The retromolar trigone is a triangular depression located behind the wisdom teeth. It has no muscular insertions (Sicher 1946) and is bounded laterally (externally) by the alveolar crest and medially (internally) by the temporal crest in the ramus of the mandible (Löfgren 1957). Its internal surface is the attachment of the pterygomandibular raphe or ligament, the reference point for direct or conventional mandibular block.

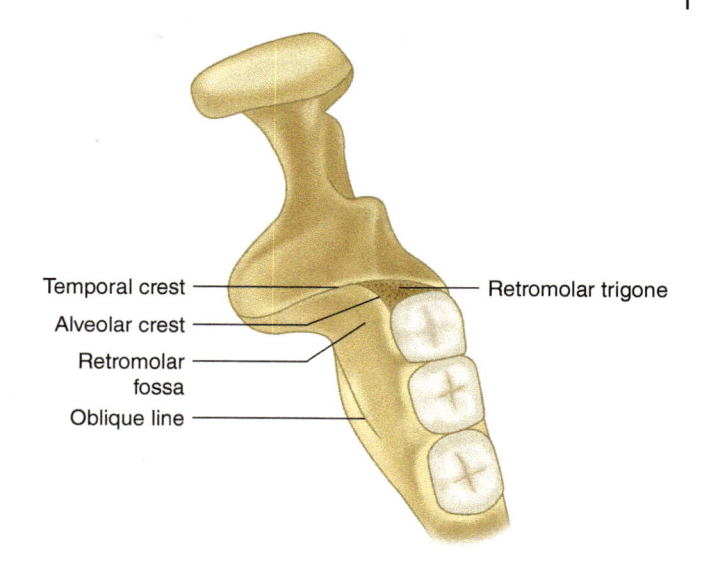

**Figure 3.8** Retromolar trigone and fossa.

### Retromolar Fossa

This depression, the insertion of the buccinator muscle, is lodged in the lateral (external)-most part of the retromolar trigone. It is bounded medially (internally) by the alveolar crest.

## Mandibular Canal

After entering the mandibular foramen the inferior alveolar vascular-nerve package passes through this canal, also formerly known as the inferior dental canal, across the entire body of the mandible to the mental foramen (Figure 3.9). The nerve lies in the center of the canal while the veins (Figure 3.4) normally run along its ceiling and the artery courses lingually to the nerve (Pogrel et al. 2009) or

Table 3.3 Percentage of retromolar (bifid) canals discovered with cone beam computerized tomography.

| Reference | No. of patients | No. of hemimandibles | No. of retromolar canals | Percentage (%) |
| --- | --- | --- | --- | --- |
| Naitoh et al. (2009) | 122 | 244 | 29 | 12.0 |
| Kuribayashi et al. (2010) | 252 | 301 | 5 | 1.7 |
| Naitoh et al. (2010) | 28 | 56 | 3 | 5.4 |
| Orhan et al. (2011) | 242 | 484 | 78 | 16.1 |
| Correr et al. (2013) | 75 | 150 | 80 | 53.3 |
| Kang et al. (2014) | 1933 | — | 104 | 5.4 |
|  |  |  | Rounded mean | **15%** |

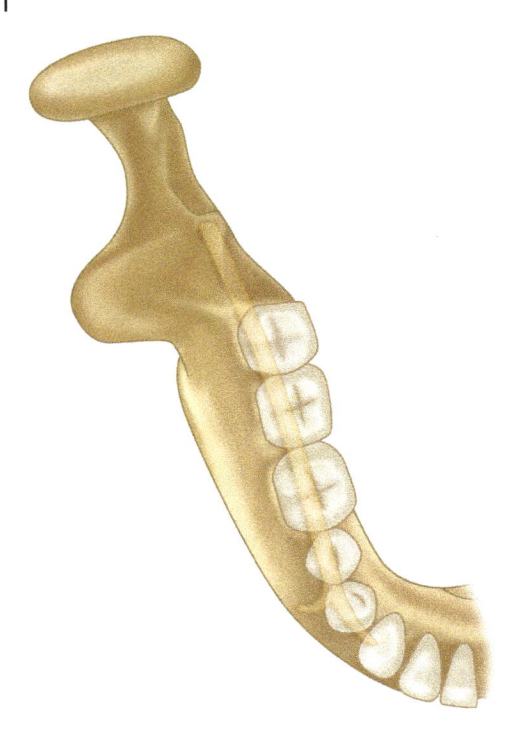

Figure 3.9 Position of mandibular canal relative to the posterior mandibular teeth.

Table 3.4 Diameter of mandibular canal.

| Reference | Diameter (mm) |
| --- | --- |
| DuBrul (1988) | 4 |
| Gowgiel (1992) | 3 |
| Ikeda et al. (1996) | 3.4 ± 0.5 |
| Kilic et al. (2010) | 2.5 ± 0.8 |
| Kuribayashi et al. (2010) | 3.3 (2–4.6) |
| Oliveira-Santos et al. (2012) | 2–4 |
| Kang et al. (2014) | 2.8 (1.5–4.3) |
| Yu et al. (2015) | 2.8 ± 0.5 (2.1–3.7) |
| Koivisto et al. (2016) | 3 |
| Mean | 3.1 |
| Rounded mean | 2–4 mm |

Table 3.5 Percentage of poorly defined mandibular canals.

| Reference | Number | Method | Percentage (%) |
| --- | --- | --- | --- |
| Olivier (1927) | 50 | Dissection | 40 |
| Carter and Keen (1971) | 92 | X-rays | 11 |
| Heasman (1988) | 80 | X-rays | 25 |
| Denio et al. (1992) | 22 | Dissection | 28 |
| | | Rounded mean | 25 |

superolingually (Lee et al. 2015). The canal is 2–4 mm in diameter (Table 3.4), around 60 mm long (Liu et al. 2009), and consists of a thin layer of condensed trabecular or spongy bone (Gowgiel 1992; Denio et al. 1992; Kilic et al. 2010). Nonetheless, in around 25% of cases, the mandibular canal is not clearly defined (Table 3.5).

The mandibular canal passes under the apexes of the posterior teeth 95% of the time and over them in less than 5%, coursing vestibularly in 60% of cases (Littner et al. 1986). It sometimes passes lingually to the first molars and exactly at the apex in less than 5% of cases (Littner et al. 1986; Denio et al. 1992).

The canal runs downward, gradually separating off the third, second, and first molar apexes. It turns slightly upward near the premolars (Littner et al. 1986; Denio et al. 1992), coursing adjacent to the lingual surface of the cortical bone and then shooting abruptly upward and toward the vestibule and often backward toward the mental foramen (Gowgiel 1992). Half of the time the backward bend forms the so-called (2–3 mm long) *anterior loop*, forward of the mental foramen (Annex 3) (Figure 3.5).

In the anterior area, forward of the anterior loop and the mental foramen, the mandibular canal disappears, forming in over 85% of cases a mandibular incisive canal around 2 mm in diameter and 10–15 mm long (Annex 4), which tends to course adjacent to the vestibular cortical bone (Starkie and Stewart 1931; Gowgiel 1992; Annex 4), favoring infiltration-mediated pulpal anesthesia in the incisor–canine area.

## Mental Foramen

The mandibular canal terminates at the mental foramen before becoming the mandibular incisive canal. The mental foramen is round or oval, normally with a diameter of 2–4 mm and in 70% of cases opening toward the rear (Annex 5).

In 95% of cases, its horizontal position relative to the mandibular teeth is above the *zone of the second premolar apex* (Figure 3.10). The zone of the second premolar apex is defined here to start slightly anterior to the second premolar, between the first and second premolar, and end slightly posterior to the second premolar, between the second premolar and the mesial root of the first molar. Vertically, it is positioned 10–15 mm above the lower ridge of the mandible (Annex 5).

In 5% of cases, the mental foramen has accessory foramina, 25% of which are multiple (Annex 5). These accessory foramina are smaller than the main foramen and there is usually only one, although cases of up to three or four have been reported (Martani and Stefanini 1964; Kadanoff

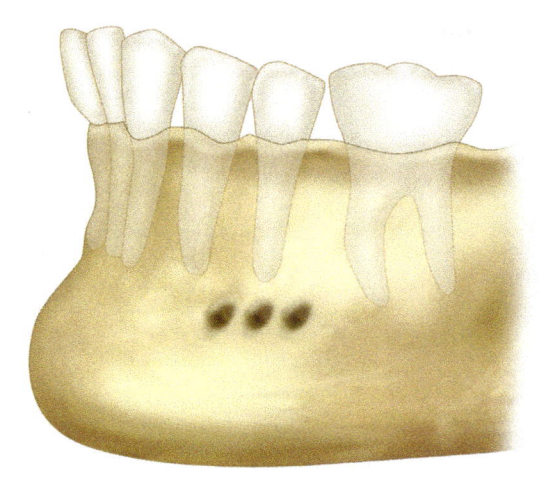

**Figure 3.10** The most likely (95%) positions of the mental foramen relative to the apex of the second mandibular premolar.

et al. 1970; Gershenson et al. 1986; Askar et al. 2018). Mandibles lacking the mental foramen have exceptionally been observed (Annex 5).

## Ramus of the Mandible

The ramus of the mandible was formerly also known as the ascending ramus of the mandible (Figures 3.6 and 3.7).

### Divergent Angle

The divergent angle of the ramus of the mandible is formed by the line defining its axis (the most prominent anterior and posterior points of its margins) and the median (or mid-sagittal) plane. It varies from 0° or nearly parallel to 27°, or very open (Simon and Kömives 1938) (Figure 3.11).

In around 90% of cases the angle ranges from 0° to 18°, providing access to the *sulcus colli* from the antagonist mandibular premolars in direct or conventional mandibular block. In the 10% of cases with a very open angle (18–27°), the syringe must rest on a very posterior area, around the contralateral mandibular molars, to reach the *sulcus colli* when performing a mandibular block (Simon and Kömives 1938).

### Ramus Width

The width helps determine the depth of the insertion of the needle to reach the *sulcus colli*, where the inferior alveolar nerve lies when the mouth is wide open for a direct mandibular block. This anterior-posterior *width ranges from 20 to 40 mm* (Table 3.6) with a *mean of around 30 mm*.

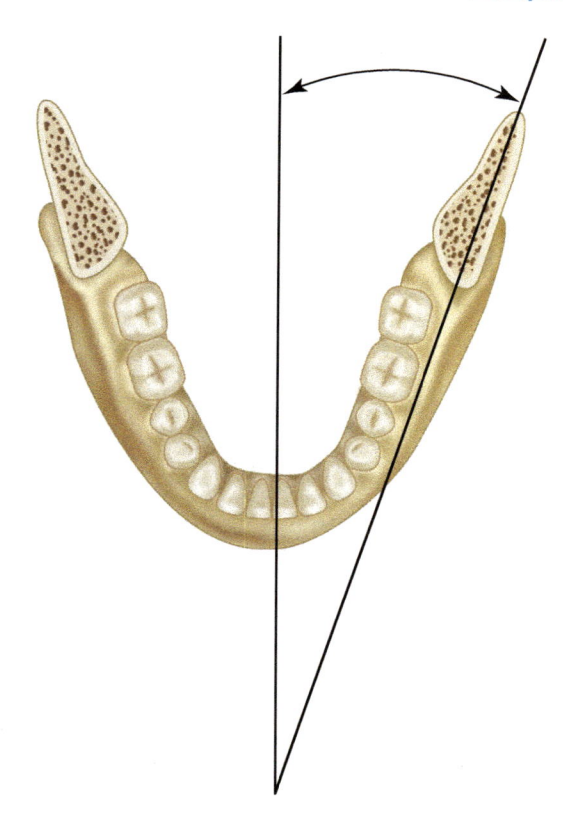

**Figure 3.11** Divergent angle of the ramus of the mandible. *Source:* Simon and Kömives (1938).

### Lingula

The lingula, formerly also known as the Spix spine, lies on the inner part of the ramus of the mandible forward of (Hayward et al. 1977) and 5–9 mm above (Bremer 1952; Harvey 1970) the mandibular foramen (Figure 3.12). The lingula gives attachment to the wide, thin sphenomandibular ligament that runs from the lingula upward and backward along the internal surface of the medial (internal) pterygoid muscle to the spine of the sphenoid (Angelman 1945).

The height of the lingula relative to the occlusal plane varies. In nearly 100% of adults it lies on average around 5 mm above the plane (Table 3.7) (Bremer 1952). The height varies with age in children and is usually below the plane in the youngest (Via 1953; Benham 1976). The factor that conditions the vertical position of the lingula is the eruption of the permanent teeth: as the permanent dentition erupts, the lingula will gradually move above the occlusal plane (Table 3.8).

### Mandibular Foramen

This is the foramen through which the inferior alveolar nerve and its vascular bundle enter the mandibular canal. It lies on the internal surface of the ramus of the mandible,

**Table 3.6** Anterior–posterior width of the ramus of the mandible.

| Reference | Value $\bar{x}$ | Range (mm) | Sample Number | Origin |
|---|---|---|---|---|
| Simon and Kömives (1938) | 30 | 20–44 | 750 | Multi-ethnic |
| Nevin and Putterbaugh (1949) | — | 18–44 | — | United States |
| Bremer (1952) | 33 | 24–43 | 100 | — |
| Harvey (1970) | 30 | 24–43 | 316 | UK |
|  | 31 | — | 332 | India |
|  | 34 | — | 46 | Multi-ethnic |
| Kay (1974) | 34 | 18–50 | 451 | — |
| Hayward et al. (1977) | 30 | — | 107 | Multi-ethnic |
| Menke and Gowgiel (1979) | 31 | 24–38 | 35 | Europe and Africa United States |
| Nicholson (1985) | 30 | 22–37 | 80 | India |
| Hetson et al. (1988) | 30 | 23–37 | 317 | — |
| Ashkenazi et al. (2011) | 30 | — | 21 | Israel (Bedouin) |
| Ashkenazi et al. (2011) | 32 | — | 38 | Israel (Bedouin) |
| Sittitavornwong et al. (2017) | 32 | 27–38 | 28 | United States |
|  | 31.3 | 21.3–41.8 | Mean |  |
|  | **30** | **20–40 mm** | Rounded means |  |

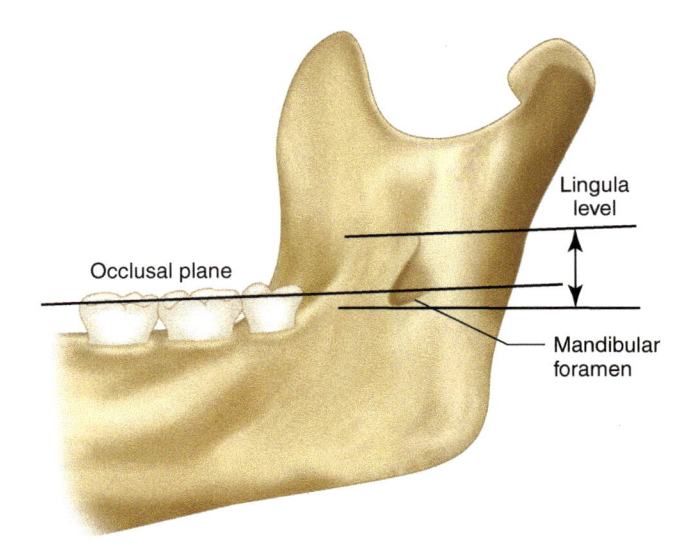

**Figure 3.12** Position of the lingula and mandibular foramen relative to the mandibular occlusal plane.

**Table 3.7** Height of lingula relative to occlusal plane in adults

| Height (mm) | Bremer (1952) n = 399 (%) | Kay (1974) n = 963 (%) |
|---|---|---|
| −3 | 0.25 | 2.5 |
| 1–5 | 63 | 91 |
| 6–10 | 31 | 6.5 |
| 11–20 | 5 | 0.1 |

**Table 3.8** Position of lingula over occlusal plane by age

| Age (years) | Number | Over occlusal plane (%) | Cause |
|---|---|---|---|
| 2.5–5 | 6 | 50 | Stabilization primary teeth |
| 5–9 | 11 | 80 | Eruption first permanent molar |
| 9–11 | 24 | 100 | Eruption first and second premolars |
| >12 | 13 | 100 | Eruption second permanent molar |

*Source:* From Benham (1976).

located anterior-posteriorly (from the oblique line to the posterior border) backward of mid-width (Via 1953; Benham 1976; Hayward et al. 1977; Menke and Gowgiel 1979; Hetson et al. 1988). In dry skulls it exhibits a wide, 8–10 mm (range 6–12 mm) diameter (Hayward et al. 1977), although dimensions of around only 5 mm appear on (admittedly deformed) panoramic X-rays (Liu et al. 2009).

As noted, the mandibular foramen lies backward of and under the lingula (Figure 3.12) and in around 75% of cases, and under the occlusal plane and above it in only 5% (Table 3.9).

## Sulcus colli

The *sulcus colli* or groove of the mandibular neck (Sicher 1946) is a depression located in the distal third of the internal surface of the ramus of the mandible (at times just barely visible) that descends obliquely forward toward the internal condylar neck to the mandibular foramen (Figure 3.7).

While not included in anatomical terminology (FCAT 1998), this anatomical structure is important for clinicians because in a wide open mouth the inferior alveolar nerve, which is targeted by the needle in direct or

Table 3.9 Position of mandibular foramen relative to occlusal plane.

| Reference | Number | Population | Below (%) | Flush (%) | Above (%) |
|---|---|---|---|---|---|
| Lotric (1956) | 200 | Yugoslavia | 82 | 13 | 5 |
| Harvey (1970) | 210 | India | 84 | 9 | 7 |
| Harvey (1970) | 158 | Britan | 70 | 24 | 6 |
| Nicholson (1985) | 80 | India | 75 | 23 | 2 |
| Mwaniki and Hassanali (1992) | 79 | Kenia | 65 | 31 | 5 |
| Palma et al. (2020) | 82 | Brazil | 84 | 1 | 15 |
| | | Means | 76.7 | 16.7 | 6.7 |
| | | Round means | 75 | 20 | 5 |

conventional mandibular block, stretches and tends to run inside this groove (Bremer 1952; Via 1953).

## Coronoid Notch

The coronoid notch is a depression where the mandible meets the anterior border of the ramus of the mandible located below the coronoid process and between the most anterior and lateral (external) parts of the ramus, a continuation of the oblique line, and the medial (internal)-most part of the temporal crest (Figure 3.7).

Although this structure is not found in the anatomical terminology (FCAT 1998) either, it has practical significance because in this depression clinicians rest their finger or mirror to guide the needle and stretch the mucosa to access the pterygotemporal depression, the site for needle penetration in a direct or conventional mandibular block.

## Accessory Foramina

The accessory foramina, 0.2–1.5 mm diameter holes on the surface of the mandible, provide passage to nutritional vessels and nerves (Shiller and Wiswell 1954; Carter and Keen 1971; Barker and Davies 1972; Sutton 1974; Haveman and Tebo 1976; Chapnick 1980). Eight to 36 foramina per mandible are located in both the ramus of the mandible and its body, predominantly (80–85% of cases) on the internal surface (Sutton 1974; Haveman and Tebo 1976), where the largest lie (Carter and Keen 1971; Haveman and Tebo 1976; Chapnick 1980) (Table 3.10). The practical significance of these foramina is that they may favor accessory innervation of the dental pulp.

The foramina on the external surface tend to cluster around incisors and canines (Sutton 1974). Their practical implications stem not only from their role in the passage of accessory innervation (Starkie and Stewart 1931; Sutton 1974), but also in favoring the diffusion of anesthetic solutions, rendering local buccal infiltration effective in that region.

## Pterygomandibular Space

The pterygomandibular space (formerly known as the pterygomaxillary space) is a narrow groove between the medial (internal) pterygoid muscle and the internal surface

Table 3.10 Percentage of dry mandibles with foramina on the internal surface.

| | | Ramus of mandible | | | Body of mandible | |
|---|---|---|---|---|---|---|
| Reference | Number | Condylar neck (%) | Mandibular foramen (%) | Retromolar fossa (%) | Mylohyoid line under premolar (%) | Genial spine (%) |
| Carter and Keen (1971) | 62 | 20 | Yes | 33 | — | — |
| Barker (1972) | 122 | 40 | Yes | — | — | — |
| Haveman and Tebo (1976) | 150 | 100 | 100 | 92 | — | — |
| Bilecenoglu and Tuncer (2006) | 80 | — | — | 25 | — | — |
| Shiller and Wiswell (1954) | 126 | — | — | — | 63 | 90 |
| Zivanovic (1970) | 335 | — | — | — | — | 100 |
| Sutton (1974) | 300 | — | — | — | 80 | 85 |
| Chapnick (1980) | 122 | — | — | — | 69 | — |

Yes, foramina present but % of mandibles bearing them not specified; —, no data.

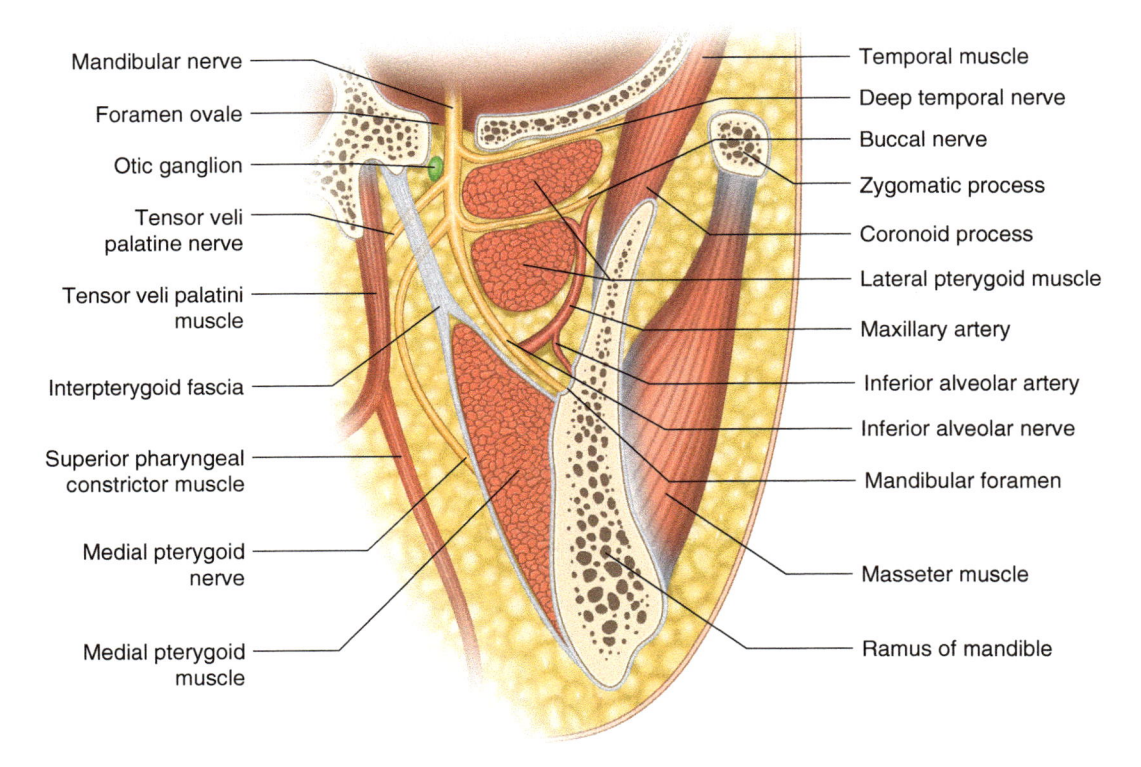

**Figure 3.13** Sagittal/frontal section of pterygomandibular space. *Source:* Redrawn with changes from Rouviere (1976).

of the ramus of the mandible. It lies in the lower infratemporal fossa (formerly the zygomatic fossa) (Galbreath and Eklund 1970) (Figures 3.13 and 3.14).

### Anatomic Boundaries of the Pterygomandibular Space

- *External/lateral*. This boundary, formed by the internal surface of the ramus of the mandible, features, from back to front, the *sulcus colli*, the mandibular foramen, and the lingula (forward of and above the mandibular foramen) (Sicher 1946; Barker and Davies 1972; Shaw and Fierst 1988).
- *Internal/medial*. In the medial to external direction this boundary consists of: the *tensor veli palatini*, the interpterygoid fascia or aponeurosis (a layer of fibrous tissue that prevents the diffusion of the anesthetic solution to the most medial/internal part of the pterygomandibular space) (Barker and Davies 1972; Watson 1973), and the medial (internal) pterygoid muscle under the interpterygoid fascia in the lower pterygomandibular space (Sicher 1946; Murphy and Grundy 1969; Shaw and Fierst 1988). The interpterygoid fascia is partially thickened, especially this part which is attached to the spine of the sphenoid, on the skull base and the lingual of the mandible; this segment is named the sphenomandibular ligament (Barker and Davies 1972; Lipski et al. 2013; Khoury et al. 2011).
- *Anterior/ventral* (Murphy and Grundy 1969; Galbreath and Eklund 1970).
  o The structures at the two ends of these boundaries are as follows (Figure 3.14).
    - In the lateral (external)-most region, the space is bounded by the *temporal crest* that gives attachment to the *deep tendon of the temporal muscle*.
    - The medial (internal)-most boundary is the *pterygomandibular raphe or ligament*, a fibrous band that joins the posterior and most aponeurotic part of the buccinator muscle to the anterior-most part of the superior pharyngeal constrictor muscle (buccino-pharyngeal aponeurosis) and lies forward of the medial (internal) pterygoid muscle. This ligament runs from the internal flange of the pterygoid process to the posterior-most part of the mylohyoid line.

    The *pterygotemporal depression*, elliptical and elongated in shape that is pierced by the needle and hence of critical significance in direct or conventional mandibular block, lies between these two extremes (Figure 16.7, Chapter 16).
  o From the external-most to the internal-most part of the pterygotemporal depression (Angelman 1945) lie the

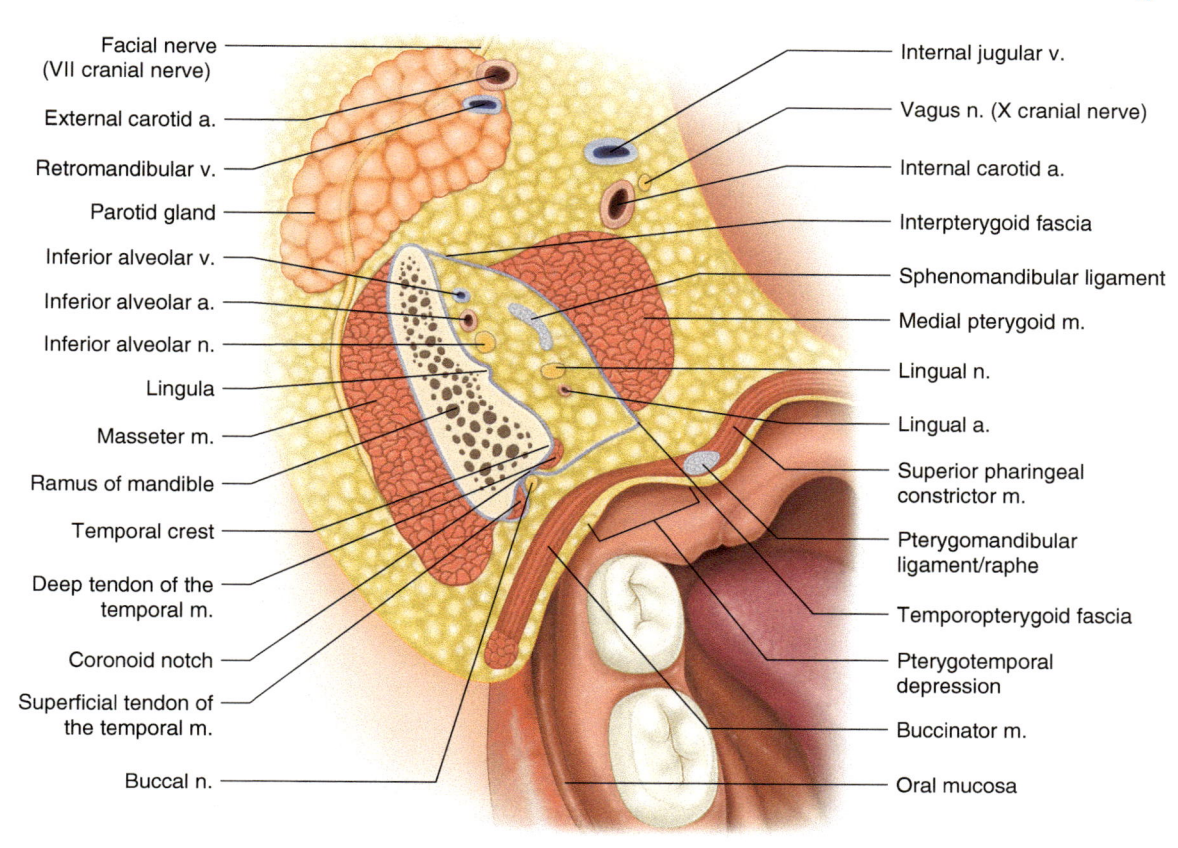

**Figure 3.14** Schematic representation in cross-section of the pterygomandibular space at a medium height. a., artery; m., muscle; n., nerve; v., vein. *Source:* Based on data from Sicher (1946), Murphy and Grundy (1969) and Barker and Davies (1972).

oral mucosa, the most aponeurotic part of the buccinator muscle, small adipose bodies, and the temporopterygoid fascia. That aponeurosis, like the interpterygoid aponeurosis or fascia of which it is a continuation, prevents the diffusion of the local anesthetic solution to the anterior and outer pterygomandibular space (Barker and Davies 1972; Watson 1973).

- *Posterior/dorsal* (Berns and Sadove 1962; Murphy and Grundy 1969; Galbreath and Eklund 1970; Petersen 1971; Shaw and Fierst 1988). Here the boundary is the posterior border of the ramus of the mandible and the distalmost part of the parotid gland with its capsule (Angelman 1945). The facial nerve (CN VII) (Petersen 1971) and the retromandibular vein (Murphy and Grundy 1969) lie in the parotid (Figure 3.14).

Behind and medially (internally) to the pterygomandibular space lies the parapharyngeal space, which houses the external and the (more posterior and medial) internal (common) carotid artery, the (more medial) jugular vein and the (more posterior) vagus nerve (CN X), and their fascia (Murphy and Grundy 1969; Petersen 1971). The internal carotid artery, internal jugular vein, and vagus nerve run inside the carotid sheath (Kafalias et al. 1987).

- *Superior/cranial* (Sicher 1946; Galbreath and Eklund 1970; Coleman and Smith 1982; Shaw and Fierst 1988). A frontal cross-section of the pterygomandibular space reveals its triangular shape, with the widest base at the top (Sicher 1946; Petersen 1971). It houses the condylar neck and the inferior surface of the lateral (external) pterygoid muscle, through whose bellies/fascicles/heads the buccal nerve runs (Figure 3.13), and the descending loop of the maxillary artery (internal maxillary artery), where present (Lacouture et al. 1983).
- *Inferior/caudal* (Sicher 1946; Bremer 1952; Galbreath and Eklund 1970). The vertex and narrowest part of the triangle mentioned in the preceding bullet point lie at the bottom, where the following are found: the medial (internal) pterygoid muscle at its insertion into the internal surface of the ramus of the mandible (Figure 3.13) and the lingual nerve exit to the floor of the mouth and submandibular (submaxillary) space (Via 1953).

## Open/Closed Mouth and Pterygomandibular Space

In a closed mouth the medial (internal) pterygoid and temporal muscles are relaxed and the pterygomandibular space is a very narrow groove. In a wide open mouth the coronoid process moves forward and downward, and the medial (internal) pterygoid and temporal muscles contract, elongating the pterygomandibular raphe or ligament. Under these circumstances the pterygomandibular space grows, adopting a triangular shape and filling up with areolar and adipose tissue transferred under pressure from the maxillary tuberosity and adjacent regions (Angelman 1945).

## Contents of the Pterygomandibular Space

This space, with a volume of around 2 ml with an open mouth (Murphy and Grundy 1969; Takeuchi 1993), is a groove about 3–4 mm wide in its anterior (entrance) side and around 30 mm long in the anterior–posterior direction (Murphy and Grundy 1969). It contains primarily lax, adipose connective tissue (Sicher 1946; Bremer 1952; Via 1953; Murphy and Grundy 1969) suspended from the planes of several fascias (Galbreath and Eklund 1970) (Figure 3.14). By region (high, medium, and low), its content is as follows.

- *High/cranial region.* Here, nearly in the infratemporal fossa (zygomatic fossa), the contents include the following (Berns and Sadove 1962; Galbreath and Eklund 1970; Shaw and Fierst 1988; Pretterklieber et al. 1991).
  - Arteries: They are robust in this region and are not in a restricted space but move very freely (Watson 1973; Coleman and Smith 1982). The arteries present include the maxillary artery (internal maxillary artery), a branch of the external carotid artery and its descending loop where present (Lacouture et al. 1983), the accessory meningeal artery, and behind it the middle meningeal artery.
  - The veins constitute the most inferior branches of the pterygoid venous plexus (Via 1953; Archer and Zubrow 1954).
  - The nerves present include the lingual nerve, attached to the *chorda tympani* (branch of the facial nerve, CN VII), the buccal nerve that passes between the two bellies/fascicles/heads of the lateral (external) pterygoid muscle (Figure 3.13), and the auriculotemporal nerve.
- *Central/middle region.* From front to back this region houses the following (Barker and Davies 1972) (Figure 3.14).
  - The lingual artery and vein, located in front on the lingual nerve (Harn and Durham 2003), separate from the alveolar artery and vein around 5–15 mm before entering the mandibular foramen (Archer and Zubrow 1954).
  - The lingual nerve lies around 7–10 mm from the entrance to the pterygomandibular space along the anterior (ventral) part of the pterygotemporal depression (Murphy and Grundy 1969; Barker and Davies 1972).
  - The inferior alveolar nerve also lies in this central region.
  - In 10% of cases the inferior alveolar artery may lie forward of the inferior alveolar nerve, but it is always much closer to the bone (Roda and Blanton 1994; Khoury et al. 2011).
  - The veins associated with the inferior alveolar nerve (one to four veins) are tributaries of the pterygoid venous plexus (Archer and Zubrow 1954; Khoury et al. 2010).
- *Lower region.* This region houses:
  - The inferior alveolar nerve before it enters the mandibular foramen.
  - The mylohyoid nerve after its separation from the inferior alveolar nerve around 15 mm before the latter enters the mandibular foramen (Wilson et al. 1984; Bennett and Townsend 2001).
  - The mylohyoid artery and vein, behind the mylohyoid nerve (Archer and Zubrow 1954).
  - The lingual artery and vein that separate from the associated veins around 5–15 mm before the inferior alveolar artery enters the mandibular foramen (Archer and Zubrow 1954).

## Sphenomandibular Ligament

The sphenomandibular ligament is located mainly in the central (middle) and lower region of the pterygomandibular space. It is a fibrous band that originates in the spine of the sphenoid bone and the petrotympanic fissure (upper attachment), and runs into the posterior border and medial aspect of the lingula of the mandible (lower attachment) (Barker and Davies 1972; Garg and Townsend 2001; Shiozaki et al. 2007; Khoury et al. 2011) (Figure 3.14). The shape, size, and nature of its attachments vary significantly from one person to another (Garg and Townsend 2001; Shiozaki et al. 2007; Khoury et al. 2010). The interpterygoid fascia covers the entire medial aspect of the mandibular ramus and sphenomandibular ligament (Garg and Townsend 2001). The ligament may even be considered a thickening of the interpterygoid fascia (Barker and Davies 1972; Khoury et al. 2011; Lipski et al. 2013).

It is interesting note that the mylohyoid nerve emerges from behind the postero-inferior mandibular attachment of the sphenomandibular ligament before inserting in the mylohyoid groove (Barker and Davies 1972; Garg and Townsend 2001).

Given its density and shape, the sphenomandibular ligament has the potential to impede diffusion of local anesthetic solution to the inferior alveolar nerve (Barker and Davies 1972; Garg and Townsend 2001; Shiozaki et al. 2007; Khoury et al. 2010, 2011), especially if the tip of the needle is placed too far medially or inferiorly with respect to the ligament (Khoury et al. 2010, 2011).

## Positive Aspirations and Hematomas

In the highly vascularized pterygomandibular space, the likelihood of piercing a vessel during the mandibular block procedure is high, inducing positive aspiration or hemorrhage (especially where an artery is involved) due to intravascular injection (Roda and Blanton 1994). The vessels that may be impacted, depending on where the needle is inserted, are as follows.

- Injection too high
  - The lowest branches of the pterygoid venous plexus may be pierced (Archer and Zubrow 1954; Roda and Blanton 1994).
  - The maxillary artery (internal maxillary artery) or its descending loop: in 60% of cases this artery runs very superficially and laterally relative to the lateral (external) pterygoid muscle (Pretterklieber et al. 1991) (Figure 3.13). Under these circumstances, in around 90% of cases (possibly equivalent to 50% of patients), a descending loop lies close to the mandibular foramen (Lacouture et al. 1983) (Figure 3.15) and may be pierced. Moreover, the diameter of the loop at this point varies substantially, from 2 to 6 mm (Biermann 1943).
  - The inferior alveolar artery and vein may be pierced where they course near the condyle (Archer and Zubrow 1954).
  - The intramuscular vessels of the lateral (external) pterygoid muscle are vulnerable.
- Even when the needle is introduced at a suitable height, it may pierce the artery and veins that accompany the inferior alveolar nerve. Given that these vessels normally lie closer to the bone than to the nerve and the artery is forward of the nerve in only 10% of cases, it is not readily pierced (Roda and Blanton 1994; Khoury et al. 2011). However, as the veins are located further back, they are more easily injected (Khoury et al. 2010). The same is true of the lingual artery, which lies in front of the lingual nerve and is therefore the first artery encountered as the needle enters the pterygomandibular space (Harn and Durham 2003).

(a)

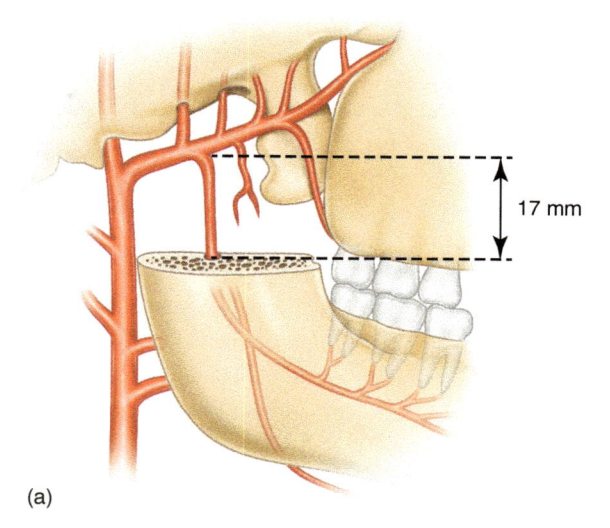

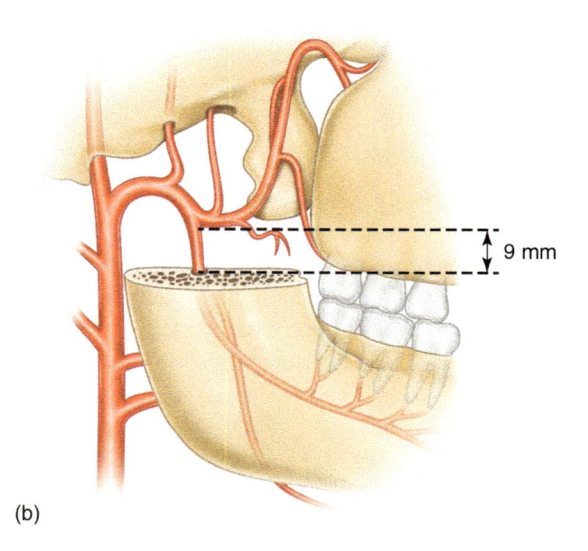

(b)

Figure 3.15 Maxillary artery and its descending loop, where present: (a) most frequent location of descending loop; (b) another configuration with descending loop.

- Injection too low
  - The mylohyoid artery and vein are vulnerable, although it would take a deep injection to pierce them (Archer and Zubrow 1954).
  - The lingual artery and vein are vulnerable.
  - The medial (internal) pterygoid muscle intramuscular vessels are vulnerable.
- An overly medial (internal) injection, even inside the pterygomandibular raphe or ligament, may pierce the intramuscular vessels of the medial (internal) pterygoid muscle.

## Glossary

| Anatomical terminology | Other terminology used |
|---|---|
| Otic ganglion | Arnold's ganglion |
| Submandibular node | Submaxillary ganglion/node |
| Auriculotemporal nerve | Superficial temporal nerve |
| Buccal nerve | Buccinator nerve |
|  | Long buccal nerve |
| Inferior alveolar nerve | Inferior dental nerve |
| Mandibular nerve | Inferior maxillary nerve |
| Meningeal branch or *nervus spinosus* | Recurrent meningeal nerve |
|  | Recurrent meningeal branch of spinal nerves |
| Angle of mandible | Gonial angle |
| Coronoid process | Coronoid apophysis |
| External acoustic meatus | Acoustic meatus |
| Infratemporal fossa | Zygomatic fossa |
| Lingula | Spix spine |

| Anatomical terminology | Other terminology used |
|---|---|
| Mandibular canal | Inferior dental canal |
| Mandibular notch | Sigmoid notch |
| Mylohyoid line | Internal oblique line |
|  | Mylohyoid crest |
| Oblique line | External oblique line |
| Pterygomandibular space | Pterygomaxillary space |
| Retromolar trigone | Retromolar triangle |
| Lateral pterygoid muscle | External pterygoid muscle |
| *Levator veli palatini* | Internal peristaphylin muscle |
| *Malleus* muscle | *Tensor tympani* muscle |
| Medial pterygoid muscle | Internal pterygoid muscle |
| *Tensor veli palatine* | External peristaphylin muscle |
| Maxillary artery | Internal maxillary artery |
| Buccal | Vestibule |
| Premolars | Bicuspids |

## References

Allen, G.D. (1979). *Dental Anesthesia and Analgesia (Local and General)*, 2e. Baltimore: Williams and Wilkins. 83.

Andreasen, J.O., Petersen, J.K., and Laskin, D.M. (1997). *Textbook and Color Atlas of Tooth Impactations. Diagnosis, Treatment and Prevention*. Copenhagen: Munksgaard. 266.

Annex 3. Lingual nerve and inferior alveolar nerve.

Annex 4. Mandibular incisive canal and anterior loop.

Annex 5. Mental foramen.

Angelman, J. (1945). The inferior dental injection. *Br. Dent. J.* 79 (2): 31–37.

Apostolakis, D. and Brown, J.E. (2013). The dimensions of the mandibular incisive canal and its spatial relationship to various anatomical landmarks of the mandible: a study cone beam computed tomography. *Int. J. Oral Maxillofac. Implants* 28 (1): 117–124.

Archer, W.H. and Zubrow, H.J. (1954). Fatal hemorrhage following regional anesthesia for operative dentistry in a hemophiliac. *Oral Surg. Oral Med. Oral Pathol.* 7 (5): 464–470.

Arens, D.E., Adams, W.R., and De Castro, R.A. (1984). *Cirugía en endodoncia*. Barcelona: Ed Doyma. 38–50.

Arensburgh, B. and Nathan, H. (1979). Anatomical observation on the mylohyoid groove, and the course of the mylohyoid nerve and vessels. *J. Oral Surg.* 37 (2): 93–96.

Ashkenazi, M., Taubman, L., and Gavish, A. (2011). Age-associated changes of the mandibular foramen position in anteroposterior dimension and the mandibular angle in dry human mandibles. *Anat. Rec.* 294 (8): 1319–1325.

Askar, H., Di Gianfilippo, R., Askar, G. et al. (2018). Morphometric analysis of the mental foramina, accessory mental foramina, and anterior loops. *Acta Sci. Dent. Sci.* 2 (1): 126–132.

Barker, B.C.W. (1972). Multiple canals in the rami of mandible. *Oral Surg. Oral Med. Oral Pathol.* 34 (3): 384–389.

Barker, B.C.W. and Davies, P.L. (1972). The applied anatomy of the pterygomandibular space. *Br. J. Oral Surg.* 10 (1): 43–55.

Baumel, J.J., Vanderheiden, J.P., and McElenney, J.E. (1971). The auricolotemporal nerve of man. *Am. J. Anat.* 130 (4): 431–440.

Benham, N.R. (1976). The cephalometric position of the mandibular foramen with age. *J. Dent. Child.* 43 (4): 233–237.

Bennett, S. and Townsend, G. (2001). Distribution of the mylohyoid nerve: anatomical variability and clinical implications. *Aust. Endod. J.* 27 (3): 109–111.

Berns, J.M. and Sadove, M.S. (1962). Mandibular block injection: a method of study using an injected radiopaque material. *J. Am. Dent. Assoc.* 65 (6): 735–745.

Biermann, H. (1943). Die chirurgische Bedentung der Lagevariationen der Arteria maxillaries. *Anat. Anz.* 94 (18–19): 289–309.

Bilecenoglu, B. and Tuncer, N. (2006). Clinical and anatomical study of the retromolar foramen and canal. *J. Oral Maxillofac. Surg.* 61 (10): 1493–1497.

Blair, E.A. and Erlanger, J. (1939). Propagation and extension of the excitatory effects on the nerve action potentials across nonresponding internodes. *Am. J. Physiol.* 126 (1): 97–108.

Bremer, G. (1952). Measurements of special significance in connection with anesthesia of the inferior alveolar nerve. *Oral Surg. Oral Med. Oral Pathol.* 5 (9): 966–988.

Carter, R.B. and Keen, E.N. (1971). The intramandibular course of the inferior alveolar nerve. *J. Anat.* 108 (3): 433–440.

Chapnick, L. (1980). A foramen on the lingual of the mandible. *J. Can. Dent. Assoc.* 46 (7): 444–445.

Coleman, R.D. and Smith, R.A. (1982). The anatomy of mandibular anesthesia: review and analysis. *Oral Surg. Oral Med. Oral Pathol.* 54 (2): 148–153.

Correr, G.M., Iwankod, D., Leonardi, D.P. et al. (2013). Classification of bifid mandibular canals using cone beam computed tomography. *Braz. Oral Res.* 27 (6): 510–516.

Denio, D., Torabinejad, M., and Bakland, L.K. (1992). Anatomical relationship of the mandibular canal to its surrounding structures in mature mandibles. *J. Endod.* 18 (4): 161–165.

DuBrul, E.L. (1988). *Sicher and Dubrul's Oral Anatomy*, 8e. St. Louis: Ishiyaku EuroAmerica Inc. 257–260.

FCAT (Federative Committee on Anatomical Terminology) (1998). *Terminologia Anatomica. International Anatomical Terminology*. Stuttgart: George Thieme Verlag.

Frommer, J., Mele, F.A., and Monroe, C.W. (1972). The possible role of the mylohioid nerve in mandibular posterior tooth sensation. *J. Am. Dent. Assoc.* 85 (1): 113–117.

Galbreath, J.C. and Eklund, M.K. (1970). Tracing the course of the mandibular block injection. *Oral Surg. Oral Med. Oral Pathol.* 30 (4): 571–582.

Garg, A. and Townsend, G. (2001). Anatomical variation of the sphenomandibular ligament. *Aust. Endod. J.* 27 (1): 22–24.

Gershenson, A., Nathan, H., and Luchang, K.E. (1986). Mental foramen and mental nerve: changes with age. *Acta Anat. (Basel)* 126 (1): 21–28.

Gowgiel, J.M. (1992). The position and course of the mandibular canal. *J. Oral Implamtol.* 18 (4): 383–385.

Gülekon, N., Anil, A., Poyraz, A. et al. (2005). Variations in the anatomy of the ariculotemporal nerve. *Clin. Anat.* 18 (1): 15–22.

Harn, S.D. and Durham, T.M. (2003). Anatomical variations and clinical implications of the artery to the lingual nerve. *Clin. Anat.* 16 (4): 294–299.

Harvey, W. (1970). The mandibular foramen and its position in relation to anaesthesia of the inferior alveolar nerve. *Glasgow Dent. J.* 1 (2): 22–27.

Haveman, C.W. and Tebo, H.G. (1976). Posterior accessory foramina of the human mandible. *J. Prosth. Dent.* 35 (4): 462–468.

Hayward, J., Richardson, E.R., and Malhotra, S.K. (1977). The mandibular foramen: its anteroposterior position. *Oral Surg. Oral Med. Oral Pathol.* 44 (6): 837–843.

Heasman, P.A. (1988). Variation in the position of the inferior dental canal and its significance to restorative dentistry. *J. Dent.* 16 (1): 36–39.

Heasman, P.A. and Beynon, A.D.G. (1987). Clinical considerations from axon–myelin relationship in human inferior alveolar nerve. *Int. J. Oral Maxillofac. Surg.* 16 (3): 346–351.

Hendy, C.W. and Robinson, P.P. (1994). The sensory distribution of the buccal nerve. *Br. J. Oral Maxillofac. Surg.* 32 (6): 384–386.

Hetson, G., Share, J., Frommer, J., and Kronman, J.H. (1988). Statistical evaluation of the position of the mandibular foramen. *Oral Surg. Oral Med. Oral Pathol.* 65 (1): 32–34.

Huang, H., Liu, P., Li, X. et al. (2013). Mandibular incisive canal by cone beam CT (English abstract). *Hua Xi Kon Quiang Yi Xue Za Zhi* 31 (5): 479–482.

Ikeda, K., Ho, K.-C., Nowicki, B.H., and Haughton, V.M. (1996). Multiplanar MR and anatomic study of the mandibular canal. *Am. J. Neuroradiol.* 17 (3): 579–584.

Jablonski, N.G., Cheng, C.M., and Cheung, H.M. (1985). Unusual origins of the buccal and mylohioid nerves. *Oral Surg. Oral Med. Oral Pathol.* 60 (5): 487–488.

Jastak, J.T., Yagiela, J.A., and Donaldson, D. (1995). *Local Anesthesia of the Oral Cavity*. Philadelphia: WB Saunders Company. 119.

Kadanoff, D., Mutafou, S.T., and Jordanov, J. (1970). Über die Hauptöffunungen resp. Incisure des Gesichtsschädels (Incisura frontalis sen Foramen frontale, Foramen supraorbitale sen Incisura supraorbitalis, Foramen infraorbitale, Foramen mentale). *Gegenbaurs Morphol. Jahrb.* 115 (1): 102–118.

Kafalias, M.C., Gow-Gates, G.A.E., and Saliba, G.J. (1987). The Gow–Gates technique for mandibular block anesthesia. A discussion and mathematical analysis. *Anesth. Prog.* 34 (4): 142–149.

Kang, J.-H., Lee, K.-S., Oh, M.-G. et al. (2014). The incidence and configuration of the bifid mandibular canal in Koreans by using cone beam computed tomography. *Imaging Sci. Dent.* 44 (1): 53–60.

Kay, L.W. (1974). Some anthropologic investigation of interest to oral surgeons. *Int. J. Oral Surg.* 3 (6): 363–379.

Khoury, J.N., Mihailidis, S., Ghabriel, M., and Townsed, G. (2010). Anatomical relationship within the human pterygomandibular space: relevance to local anesthesia. *Clin. Anat.* 23 (8): 936–944.

Khoury, J.N., Mihailidis, S., Ghabriel, M., and Townsed, G. (2011). Applied anatomy of the pterygomandibular space: improving the success of inferior alveolar nerve blocks. *Aust. Dent. J.* 56 (2): 112–121.

Kiesselbach, J.E. and Chamberlain, J.G. (1984). Clinical and anatomic observations on the relationship of the lingual nerve to the mandibular third molar region. *J. Oral Maxillofac. Surg.* 43 (9): 565–567.

Kilic, C., Kamburogluk, K., Ozen, T. et al. (2010). The position of the mandibular canal and histologic feature of the inferior alveolar nerve. *Clin. Anat.* 23 (1): 34–42.

Kim, H.J., Kwak, H.H., Hu, K.S. et al. (2003). Topographic anatomy of the mandibular nerve branches distributed on the two heads of the lateral pterygoid. *Int. J. Oral Maxillofac. Surg.* 32 (4): 408–413.

Koivisto, T., Chiona, D., Milroy, L.L. et al. (2016). Mandibular canal location: cone-beam computed tomography examination. *J. Endod.* 42 (7): 1018–1021.

Kuribayashi, A., Watanabe, H., Imaizumi, A. et al. (2010). Bifid mandibular canals: cone beam computed tomography. *Dentomaxillofac. Radiol.* 39 (4): 235–239.

Lacouture, C., Blanton, P.L., and Hairston, L.E. (1983). The anatomy of the maxillary artery in the infratemporal fossa in relationship to oral injections. *Anat. Rec.* 205 (3): 104A.

Lee, M.-H., Kim, H.-J., Kim, D.K., and Yu, S.-K. (2015). Histologic features and fascicular arrangement of the inferior alveolar nerve. *Arch. Oral Biol.* 60 (12): 1736–1741.

Lipski, M., Lipska, W., Motyl, S. et al. (2013). Anatomy of the pterygomandibular space – clinical implication and review. *Folia Med. Cracov.* 53 (1): 79–85.

Littner, M.M., Kaffe, I., Tamse, A., and Dicapua, P. (1986). Relationship between the apices of the lower molars and mandibular canal – a radiographic study. *Oral Surg. Oral Med. Oral Pathol.* 62 (5): 595–602.

Liu, T., Xia, B., and Gu, Z. (2009). Inferior alveolar canal course: a radiographic study. *Clin. Oral Implant. Res.* 20 (11): 1212–1218.

Löfgren, A.B. (1957). Foramina retromolaria mandibulae. A study on human skulls of nutrient foramina situated in the mandibular retromolar fossa. *Odontol. Tidskr.* 65: 552–573.

Lotric, N. (1956). Foramen mentale. Morphological and topographical investigations. *Excerpta Med. (Sect. 1)* 10 (6): 236. (abstract 1093).

Madeira, M.C., Percinoto, C., and Silva, M.C. (1978). Clinical significance of supplementary innervations of the lower incisor teeth: a dissection study of the mylohyoid nerve. *Oral Surg. Oral Med. Oral Pathol.* 46 (5): 608–614.

Malamed, S.F. (2004). *Handbook of Local Anesthesia*, 5e. St. Louis (MI): Elsevier-Mosby. 183.

Mardinger, O., Chaushu, G., Arensburg, B. et al. (2000). Anatomic and radiographic course of the mandibular incisive canal. *Surg. Radiol. Anat.* 22 (3–4): 157–161.

Martani, F. and Stefanini, F. (1964). Contributio statistico, morfologico e topográfico allo studio del foro mentoniero in mandibole umane non vitali. *Mondo Odontostomatol.* 6: 705–717.

Menke, R.A. and Gowgiel, J.M. (1979). Short-needle block anesthesia at the mandibular foramen. *J. Am. Dent. Assoc.* 99 (1): 27–30.

Murphy, T.R. and Grundy, E.M. (1969). The inferior alveolar neurovascular bundle at the mandibular foramen. *Dent. Pract. Dent. Rec.* 20 (2): 41–48.

Mwaniki, D.L. and Hassanali, J. (1992). The position of mandibular and mental foramina in Kenyan African mandibles. *East Afr. Med. J.* 69 (4): 210–213.

Naitoh, M., Hiraiwa, Y., Aimiya, H., and Ariji, E. (2009). Observation of bifid mandibular canal using cone-beam computed tomography. *Int. J. Oral Maxillofac. Implants* 24 (1): 155–159.

Naitoh, M., Nakahara, K., Snenaga, Y. et al. (2010). Comparison between cone-beam and multislice computed tomography depicting mandibular neurovascular canal structures. *Oral Surg. Oral Med. Oral Pathol.* 109 (1): e25–e31.

Namking, M., Boonruangsri, P., Woraputtaporn, W., and Güldner, F. (1994). Communication between the facial and auriculotemporal nerves. *J. Anat.* 185 (Pt 2): 421–426.

Nevin, M. and Putterbaugh, P.G. (1949). *Conduction, Infiltration and General Anesthesia in Dentistry*, 5e. New York: Dental Items of Interest Publishing Co. Inc. 179.

Nicholson, M.L. (1985). A study of the position of the mandibular foramen in the adult human mandible. *Anat. Rec.* 212 (1): 110–112.

Novitzky, J. (1938). Sensory nerves and anesthesia of the teeth and jaws. *Mod. Dent.* 5 (1): 5–10.

Oliveira-Santos, C., Souza, P.H.C., Berti-Couto, S.A. et al. (2012). Assessment of variations of the mandibular canal through cone beam computed tomography. *Clin. Oral Invest.* 16 (2): 387–393.

Olivier, E. (1927). Le canal dentaire inferiour et son nerf chez l'adulte. *Ann. Anat. Path. Anat. Norm. Med-Chir (Paris)* 4 (9): 975–987.

Orhan, K., Aksoy, S., Bilecenoglu, B. et al. (2011). Evaluation of bifid mandibular canals with cone-beam computed tomography in a Turkish adult population: a retrospective study. *Surg. Radiol. Anat.* 33 (6): 501–507.

Ossenberg, N.S. (1986). Temporal crest canal: case report and statistics on a rare mandibular variant. *Oral Surg. Oral Med. Oral Pathol.* 62 (1): 10–12.

Palma, L.F., Almeida, F.S.O., Lombardi, L.A. et al. (2020). Is inferior oclusal plane a reliable anatomic landmark for inferior alveolar nerve block? A study on dry mandibles of Brazilian adults. *Morphologie* 104 (344): 59–63.

Petersen, J.K. (1971). The mandibular foramen block. A radiographic study of the spread of the local analgesic solution. *Br. J. Oral Surg.* 9 (21): 126–138.

Phillips, W.H. (1943). Anatomic considerations in local anesthesia in dental surgery. *Anesth. Analg.* 22 (1): 5–14.

Pires, C.A., Bissada, N.F., Becker, J.J. et al. (2012). Mandibular incisive canal: cone beam computed tomography. *Clin. Implant Dent. Relat. Res.* 14 (1): 67–73.

Pogrel, M.A., Schmidt, B.L., Sambajon, V., and Jordan, R.C.K. (2003). Lingual nerve damage due to inferior alveolar nerve blocks. A possible explanation. *J. Am. Dent. Assoc.* 134 (2): 195–199.

Pogrel, M.A., Dorfman, D., and Fallah, H. (2009). The anatomic structure of the inferior alveolar neurovascular bundle in the third molar region. *J. Oral Maxillofac. Surg.* 67 (11): 2452–2454.

Pretterklieber, M.L., Skopakoff, C., and Mayr, R. (1991). The human maxillary artery reinvestigated: I. Topographical relations in the infratemporal fossa. *Acta Anat.* 142 (4): 281–287.

Roberts, G.D. and Harris, M. (1973). Neuropraxia of the mylohyoid nerve and submental analgesia. *Br. J. Oral Surg.* 11 (2): 110–113.

Roda, R.S. and Blanton, P.L. (1994). The anatomy of local anesthesia. *Quintessence Int.* 25 (1): 27–38.

Rood, J.P. (1977). Some anatomical and physiological causes of failure to achieve mandibular analgesia. *Br. J. Oral Surg.* 15 (1): 75–82.

Rood, J.P. (1978a). The organization of the inferior alveolar nerve and its relation to local anesthesia. *J. Dent.* 6 (4): 305–310.

Rood, J.P. (1978b). The diameters and intermodal lengths of the myelinated fibers in human inferior alveolar nerve. *J. Dent.* 6 (4): 311–315.

Rouviere, H. (1976). *Compendio de anatomía y disección. Ediciones Científico Técnicas.* Barcelona: Masson-Salvat (Reprint of the 3rd edition, 1959). 160.

Schejtman, R., Devoto, F.C.H., and Arias, N.H. (1967). The origin and distribution of the elements of the human mandibular retromolar canal. *Archs. Oral Biol.* 12 (11): 1261–1267.

Shaw, M.D. and Fierst, P. (1988). Clinical prosection for dental gross anatomy: a medial approach to the pterygomandibular space. *Anat. Rec.* 222 (3): 305–308.

Shiller, W.R. and Wiswell, O.B. (1954). Lingual foramina of the mandible. *Anat. Rec.* 119 (3): 387–390.

Shiozaki, H., Abe, S., Tsumori, N. et al. (2007). Macroscopic anatomy of the sphenomandibular ligament related to the inferior alveolar nerve block. *Cranio* 25 (3): 160–165.

Sicher, H. (1946). The anatomy of the mandibular anesthesia. *J. Am. Dent. Assoc.* 33 (23): 1541–1557.

Sicher, H. (1950). Aspects in the applied anatomy of local anesthesia. *Int. Dent. J.* 1 (1): 70–82.

Simon, B. and Kömives, O. (1938). Dimensional and positional variations of the ramus of the mandible. *J. Dent. Res.* 17 (2): 125–149.

Singh, S. (1981). Aberrant buccal nerve encountered at the third molar surgery. *Oral Surg. Oral Med. Oral Pathol.* 52 (2): 142.

Sittitavornwong, S., Babston, M., Denson, D. et al. (2017). Lingual nerve measurements in cadaveric dissections: clinical applications. *J. Oral Maxillofac. Surg.* 75 (6): 1104–1112.

Starkie, C. and Stewart, D. (1931). The intra-mandibular course of the inferior dental nerve. *J. Anat.* 65 (Pt 3): 319–323.

Stein, P., Brueckner, J., and Milliner, M. (2007). Sensory innervations of mandibular teeth by the mylohyoid nerve: implications in local anesthesia. *Clin. Anat.* 20 (6): 591–595.

Stewart, D. (1932). The innervations of the dental tissues and its importance in regional anaesthesia. *Br. Dent. J.* 53 (6): 277–284.

Stewart, D. and Wilson, S.L. (1928). Regional anaesthesia and innervations of the teeth. *Lancet* 212 (5486): 809–811.

Sutton, R.N. (1974). The practical significance of mandibular accessory foramina. *Aust. Dent. J.* 19 (3): 167–173.

Takeuchi, T. (1993). The study of volume and shape of pterygomandibular space by computed tomography. *J. Jpn. Dent. Soc. Anesthesiol.* 221: 293–310. (In Japanese).

Turner, M.B. (1864). LXXIII. On some variations in the arrangement of the nerves of the human body. *Nat. Hist. Rev.* 4: 612–617.

Via, W.F. (1953). The pterygomandibular space in relation to effective mandibular block anesthesia for children. *J. Dent. Child* 20: 105–110.

Watson, J.F. (1973). Appendix: some anatomic aspects of the Gow–Gates technique for mandibular anesthesia. *Oral Surg. Oral Med. Oral Pathol.* 36 (3): 328–330.

Wilson, S., Johns, P., and Fuller, P.M. (1984). The inferior alveolar and mylohioid nerves: an anatomical study and relationship to local anesthesia of the anterior mandibular teeth. *J. Am. Dent. Assoc.* 108 (3): 350–352.

Yu, S.-K., Kim, S., Kang, S.G. et al. (2015). Morphological assessment of the anterior loop of the mandibular canal in Koreans. *Anat. Cell Biol.* 48 (1): 75–80.

Zivanovic, S. (1970). Some morphological characters of the East African mandible. *Acta Anat.* 77 (1): 109–119.

# 4

# The Peripheral Nerve and Local Anesthesia

This chapter reviews the microanatomy of peripheral nerves, nerve cell membranes, neurophysiology, and the mechanism governing local anesthetic action.

## Peripheral Nerve Microanatomy

### Neurons

Nerve cells, called neurons, are the anatomic and functional units of the nervous system. While all human cells are characterized by a difference in potential (voltage) across their membranes, with a negatively charged interior and positively charged exterior near the surface, only muscle and nerve cells are excitable, meaning that they are able to alter that potential in response to a stimulus. Neurons, moreover, can convey electrical impulses along their membranes between the central nervous system (CNS) and the rest of the body, and *vice versa*. Neurons have three main constituents.

- The body, soma, neurocyton, or perikaryon (*peri* = around, *karyon* = nucleus), the bulbous part of the cell that contains the nucleus and subcellular organelles (endoplasmic reticulum [ER], Golgi apparatus, mitochondria, etc.), provides vital metabolic support for the entire neuron.
- The dendrites (*dendron* = tree branch) are thin cytoplasmic filaments projecting off the cell body. They receive electrochemical impulses that they propagate to the soma.
- The axon, a longer and thicker extension than the dendrites, carries electrochemical impulses from the soma to other organs and nerves.

Depending on function and morphology, neurons can be divided into three basic types: (i) motor or efferent (typically multipolar) neurons that conduct impulses from the Central Nervous System (CNS) to effectors (such as muscles); (ii) sensory or afferent (pseudo-unipolar or unipolar) neurons, discussed below; and (iii) association or interneurons.

### Sensory Neurons

These cells are also known as unipolar or pseudo-unipolar neurons because the single axon (trunk or extension) that projects off the body subsequently divides into two. One part courses to the periphery, ending in this case in the gums, teeth, or bones, where sensory receptors capture stimuli for propagation to the soma, while the other carries stimuli to other CNS neurons. Although anatomically the former would be a dendrite and the latter an axon, as functionally they act as a single long axon, thus that is the term used for both (Figure 4.1).

The body of these neurons lies not in the CNS but in the dorsal root ganglion (spinal cord), while the maxillofacial sensory nerves lie in the semilunar or trigeminal (Gasserian) ganglion.

### Axons

Axons are the trunks or axis cylinders that extend off the bodies of sensory nerves. They are sheathed by a series of cells known as Schwann cells. Although the functions of the latter are not fully understood, they are associated with the modulation of nervous conduction, the provision of direct metabolic support in the form of energy or protein synthesis, and the release of trophic factors to enhance axon function. Together the axon and its Schwann cells, called *nerve fibers*, constitute a functional element separated from the surrounding tissue by a basal lamina. Axons consist essentially of two parts.

- The axoplasm or neuron cytoplasm, like the cytoplasm in the soma, is a viscous liquid five times denser than water. It contains subcellular organelles such as

---

*Local Anesthesia in Dentistry: A Locoregional Approach*, First Edition. Jesús Calatayud and Mana Saraghi.
© 2024 John Wiley & Sons Ltd. Published 2024 by John Wiley & Sons Ltd.
Companion website: www.wiley.com/go/Calatayud/local

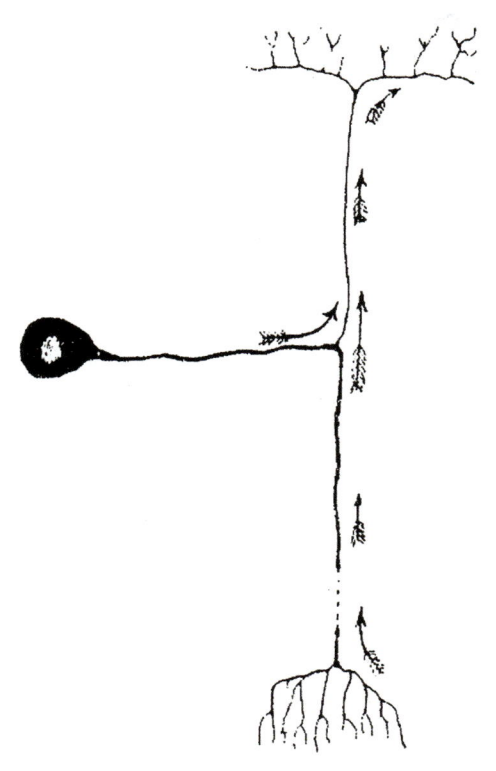

**Figure 4.1** Sensory or unipolar neuron. *Source:* Redrawn from Cajal (1899).

mitochondria or the ER and provides the cell membrane with metabolic support (Meymaris 1975).
- The nerve membrane or axolemma or neurilemma that separates the axoplasm from extracellular liquids is the element around which this discussion revolves as it is where nervous excitation and electrochemical conduction take place. It is discussed in detail below.

## Membranes

The cell membrane is a semipermeable structure just 7–10 nanometers (nm) thick that separates the axoplasm from extracellular fluids. Although the molecular organization of the membrane is not understood in full detail, a number of important features have been described (Singer and Nicolson 1972; Meymaris 1975; Wildsmith 1986; Guyton and Hall 2007).

1) It has a phospholipid bilayer (25%) in which each layer consists of (i) polar (hydrophilic) phosphate groups oriented toward the membrane surface, in other words, in the inner layer toward the axoplasm and in the outer toward the extracellular fluids, and (ii) apolar or nonpolar (hydrophobic) fatty acid groups in the center, oriented inward in both layers and attracted to one another. The hydrophobic part blocks the flow of water and hydrosoluble ions such as sodium ($Na^+$) and potassium ($K^+$) while allowing the flow of liposoluble compounds.
2) Cholesterol and neutral lipids (13%) dissolved in the phospholipid bilayer.
3) Proteins (55%) distributed along and across the membrane. There are two types: (i) integral or intrinsic proteins spanning the entire width of the membrane from the axoplasm to the extracellular fluids; (ii) peripheral or extrinsic proteins found only on either the inner or outer surface that do not penetrate the entire membrane. All these proteins have many functions, such as antigen or other markers, receptors (for hormones for instance), enzymatic control of reactions on the membrane surface or molecular transport across the membrane. The fourth is the type of protein of major interest here.
4) Small amounts (3%) of carbohydrates on the outer surface only, bound to lipids (glycolipids) or proteins (glycoproteins).

As the membrane is not solid its constituent phospholipids and proteins can move laterally. The proteins, which float in a "sea" of phospholipids, are not uniformly distributed (Figure 4.2) but change constantly in keeping with the so-called "fluid mosaic model of the plasma membrane" (Singer and Nicolson 1972). Some however, bound to the cytoskeletal proteins, help maintain the general shape of the cell.

## Nerve Fibers and Myelin

Schwann cells may surround the axon in one of two ways, either forming myelin or not.

### Myelinated Fibers

Myelinated fibers are enveloped in a layer of myelin, a substance comprising alternating concentric layers of lipids and proteins. These layers are actually the Schwann cell

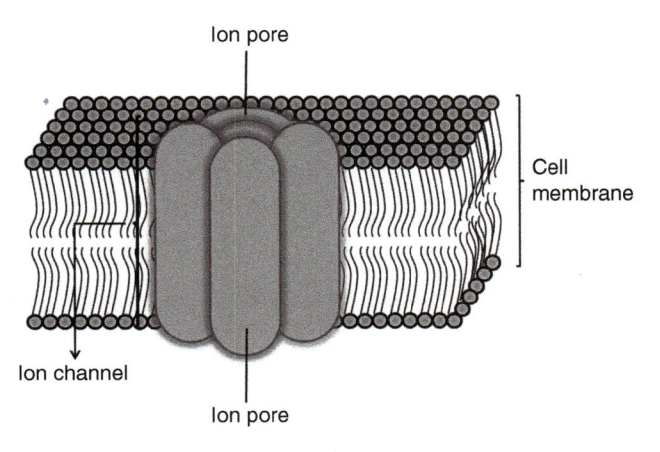

**Figure 4.2** Diagram of cell membrane.

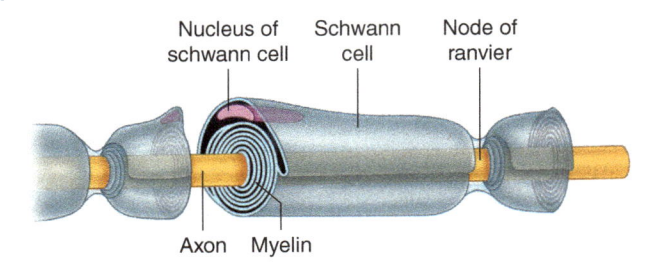

**Figure 4.3** Myelinated fiber, Schwann cell, and nodes of Ranvier. *Source:* Redrawn from De Jong (1977).

membrane that winds around the axon with scarcely any cytoplasm between layers (Figure 4.3).

The most peripheral layer of the myelin sheath, the Schwann cell cytoplasm where the nucleus is located, is called the neurilemma or neurolemma (Jastak et al. 1995). At regular 0.2–0.3-mm intervals in myelinated fibers, the neurilemmas of adjacent Schwann cells interconnect. As there is no myelin in this region the cover narrows, exposing the axon directly to extracellular fluids. Myelin affords powerful insulation that drastically reduces ion flow in the membrane by impeding contact between it and extracellular fluids because it leaves a tiny extracellular space, measuring barely 10–15 nm.

These gaps in the myelin layer, known as the *nodes of Ranvier* (Figure 4.3), while just 0.5–1.5 microns (μm) long, are extraordinarily important. It is here that ionic exchange takes place between the axoplasm close to the membrane and the extracellular fluids and where local anesthetics act.

The larger the diameter of the axon the thicker the myelin sheath and the greater the internodal distance (distance from one node of Ranvier to the next). Accordingly, the nodes of Ranvier are spaced at a fairly constant 100–200 times the axon diameter (Jastak et al. 1995). In myelinated fibers the nervous impulse jumps from node to node of Ranvier (Tasaki 1953) in "saltatory conduction", accelerating propagation speed and requiring less ion movement. This arrangement is more efficient than conduction in unmyelinated axons because it calls for less energy and less metabolic activity.

The myelin sheath itself is interrupted at intervals by oblique incisions, Schmidt–Lantermann clefts, that connect it to the exterior and enhance elasticity by stretching the nerve (Heasman and Beynon 1987).

### Unmyelinated Fibers

Unmyelinated fibers have an axon surrounded by the myelin-free part of Schwann cells. In these fibers the Schwann cell membrane and cytoplasm normally sheathe several axons (Wildsmith 1986). Nerve impulse conduction in smaller diameter unmyelinated fibers is continuous, slower, and more energy-intensive than in myelinated axons.

### Nerve Fiber Classification

Table 4.1 lists the three main categories, A, B, and C, of peripheral nerve fibers and their subdivisions. Axon diameter, location, and function are also given in the table, along with the presence or otherwise of myelination.

Nerve impulse conduction depends primarily on two factors (Jack 1975): diameter, the greater the speedier, and the presence of myelin, which enhances speed. Myelinated A fibers, which are the thickest, exhibit the highest conduction speed. Conversely, C fibers are the thinnest and slowest. A delta (Aδ) and B fibers are often nearly undistinguishable and can only be differentiated on the grounds of electrophysiological properties not shown in the table (Jastak et al. 1995). The following are the fibers of greatest interest here.

- Myelinated Aδ fibers conduct first (sharp, immediate, and localized) pain that disappears with the pain stimulus.
- Type IV sensorial unmyelinated polymodal C fibers transmit second (diffuse or scantly localized, dull) pain that persists beyond the duration of the stimulus.

The first mandibular premolar dental pulp has been shown to have around 300–500 Aδ fibers and 1500–1800 polymodal C fibers (Johnsen et al. 1983). While the electrical pulp tester stimulates the former, it barely affects the latter (Lin and Chandler 2008; Abd-Elmeguid and Yu 2009; Sampaio et al. 2012). Furthermore, polymodal C fibers seems more resistant to the effects to local anesthetics (Saha et al. 2016).

### Peripheral Nerve Structure

Peripheral nerve trunks comprise hundreds or thousands of myelinated and unmyelinated nerve fibers, supported and protected by surrounding connective tissue (Figure 4.4) consisting of the following structures starting from the innermost layer (closest to the nerve) to the outermost layer (Sunderland 1965; Wildsmith 1986):

- The *endoneurium*, the innermost sheath of connective tissue, runs parallel to, bathes, and separates the nerve fibers, and its capillaries provide nutrients for the tissues (Wildsmith 1986). These blood vessels form the intrinsic system, are mainly nutritive, and have minimal adrenergic receptors (Myers and Heckman 1989).
- The *perineurium* is connective tissue surrounding the endoneurium that runs concentrically, obliquely, and parallel to nerve fibers, bundling from 500 to 1000 axons known as a *fascicle*. The perineurium carries blood vessels (vasa nervorum) which, in the form of a terminal capillary and precapillary network, penetrate the

**Table 4.1** Classification of peripheral nerve fibers.

| Type of fiber | Myelin | Diameter (μm) | Speed (m/s) | Location | Function |
|---|---|---|---|---|---|
| Aα | +++ | | | | |
| Motor | | 12–20 | 65–120 | Muscle | Motor |
| Ia sensorial | | 13–22 | 70–130 | Muscle spindle | Proprioceptive |
| Ib sensorial | | 12–120 | 65–120 | Tendon | Proprioceptive |
| Aβ | ++ | | | | |
| Motor | | 7–14 | 40–80 | Muscle | Motor |
| II sensorial[a] | | 5–15 | 20–80 | Tendon | Proprioceptive |
| Aγ | ++ | | | | |
| Motor | | 2–10 | 10–50 | Muscle | Motor |
| II sensorial[a] | | 5–15 | 20–80 | Tendon | Proprioceptive |
| Aδ | + | | | | |
| III sensorial | | 1–7 | 5–40 | Various | **First pain** Temperature Pressure |
| B | + | | | | |
| Preganglionic autonomic (sympathetic) | | 1–5 | 4–25 | Heart Smooth muscle Gland | Motor Motor Secretion |
| C | – | | | | |
| Postganglionic autonomic (sympathetic) | | 0.2–2 | 0.2–2 | Heart Smooth muscle Gland | Motor Motor Secretion |
| IV sensorial | | 0.2–2 | 0.2–2 | Various | **Second pain** Temperature Pressure Visceral |

[a] Not distinguishable from one another.
Source: Data from Jastak et al. (1995).

endoneurium. These blood vessels form the extrinsic system and are under adrenergic control (Myers and Heckman 1989). The innermost layer of the perineurium consists of a sort of membrane with several layers of cells known as the *perilemma* or perineural epithelium *that hampers the diffusion of the anesthetic solution* into nerve fascicles (Sunderland 1965; Shanthaveerappa and Bourne 1966).

- The *epineurium*, lax connective tissue containing some fatty cells, surrounds fascicles and holds them together. Its blood vessels form a vascular network (an extrinsic system) that responds to adrenergic stimulation and anastomose with intrinsic vessels (Myers and Heckman 1989). Its dense, thick outermost layer, the external epineurium, does not interfere with local anesthetic diffusion. The epineurium accounts for 30–75% of the total cross-section of peripheral nerves (Sunderland 1965).

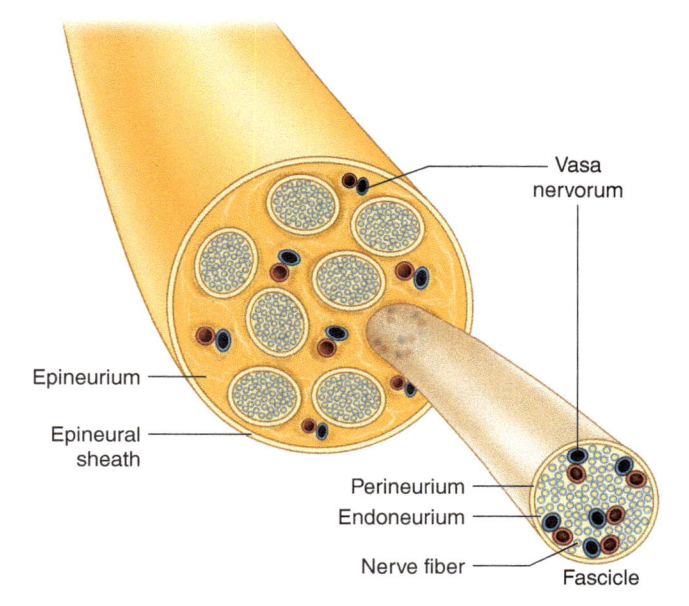

**Figure 4.4** Peripheral nerve structure.

All these vasa nervorum absorb local anesthetic molecules, removing them from the nerve trunk. Lymphatic vessels also participate in this process, albeit minimally (<1%) (Asher 1892; Schou 1961).

## Basic Membrane Proteins

Three membrane proteins are essential to conducting electrochemical impulses, the sodium–potassium pump, and the sodium and potassium channels. All three are integral membrane proteins (spanning the entire cell membrane) which, as their names infer, transport sodium ($Na^+$) and potassium ($K^+$) ions.

### Sodium–Potassium Pump

The sodium–potassium pump ($Na^+/K^+$ pump) was discovered in 1957 by Skou, although there were precedents. Initially called the sodium pump (Skou 1957), it is an enzyme (sodium–potassium ATPase, $Na^+/K^+$ ATPase) essential to all animal cell membranes (Scheiner-Bobis 2002). This bulbous integral protein transports $Na^+$ and $K^+$ ions and has three subunits (Scheiner-Bobis 2002):

- The alfa ($\alpha$) subunit, with a molecular mass of 100–113 kiloDaltons (kDa) and four isoforms ($\alpha_1$, $\alpha_2$, $\alpha_3$, and $\alpha_4$), is where adenosine triphosphate (ATP) bonds to the $Na^+$ and $K^+$ ions.
- The beta ($\beta$) subunit, with a molecular mass of 60 kDa and three isoforms ($\beta_1$, $\beta_2$, and $\beta_3$), apparently stabilizes $\alpha$.
- The gamma ($\gamma$) subunit, with a molecular mass of 7–11 kDa, is believed to modulate $Na^+/K^+$ pump activity, although its exact function is not known.

$Na^+/K^+$ ATPase pumps three $Na^+$ ions out and two $K^+$ ions into the cell per ATP molecule hydrolyzed (Guyton 1987; Butterworth and Strichartz 1990; Scheiner-Bobis 2002). As the enzyme pumps both ions against their respective electrochemical gradients, the process is active, i.e. it consumes energy. Interestingly, the $Na^+/K^+$ pump can increase its activity as circumstances require (Guyton and Hall 2007).

The function of the $Na^+/K^+$ pump is essential to the osmotic regulation of cell volume (Scheiner-Bobis 2002), for the cell contains sizeable quantities of negatively charged organic proteins and other molecules too large to flow out of the cell. They consequently attract positively charged ions such as $Na^+$, although as three $Na^+$ ions are pumped out per every two $K^+$ ions pumped in, inducing a net ionic loss, there is less water in the cell (Guyton and Hall 2007).

Another essential $Na^+/K^+$ pump function is its role in nerve impulse conduction, which is of particular interest in the present context, as discussed later.

### Sodium Channels

Sodium channels ($Na^+$ channels) are glycoproteins (Catterall 1984, 1988) with three subunits, $\alpha$, $\beta_1$, and $\beta_2$ (Table 4.2). Their glycosylated groups are located on the outer surface of the cell membrane (Butterworth and Strichartz 1990). The structure–function relationship is still poorly understood (Ulbricht 2005). As these proteins are 11.8 nm in diameter (Catterall 1984), they span and project beyond the cell membrane, which is just 7–10 nm thick (Catterall 1984; Butterworth and Strichartz 1990).

The $\alpha$ subunit has four domains (D1–D4) with six membrane-spanning helicoid $\alpha$ segments (S1–S6) (Ulbricht 2005). These segments are connected by intra- and extracellular loops (Catterall 2000; Ulbricht 2005) (Figure 4.5). The local anesthetic receptor is located in domain D4, segment 6, concurring with amino acids phenylalanine and tyrosine, the sites of which vary with sodium channel isoform or subtype. Segment S4 is positively charged and the pore lies between S5 and S6 (Ulbricht 2005). The $Na^+$ ions, with a 0.095-nm radius (Scheiner-Bobis 2002; Lockless et al. 2007), or 0.19 nm when hydrated (Lipscombe 2005), flow through the pore, which on the outer end has a diameter of 0.3–0.5 nm (Catterall 1984, 1988; Fozzard et al. 2005).

Subunits $\beta_1$ and $\beta_2$ are long, glycosylated extracellular domains with folds reminiscent of those in immunoglobulins or myelin (Catterall 2000; Ulbricht 2005), a single transmembrane segment, and a small intracellular domain (Catterall 2000).

To date nine $Na^+$ channel subtypes or isoforms have been identified, which differ in structure, expression pattern, biophysical properties, and location (Lai et al. 2004; Ulbricht 2005). Local anesthetics, which are scantly specific in this regard, block all nine (Lai et al. 2004; Fozzard et al. 2005). The subtypes of greatest relevance here are sited on the sensory neurons that propagate nociceptor (pain) signals, such as $Na_v$ 1.8, $Na_v$ 1.9 (Lai et al. 2004; Wells et al. 2007), and in the dental pulp, especially $Na_v$ 1.7 (Luo et al. 2008). Molecules may be developed in the future to

Table 4.2 Atomic mass and percentage of carbohydrates in sodium channel subunits.

| Subunit | Atomic mass (kDa) | Carbohydrates (%) |
|---|---|---|
| $\alpha$ | 260 | 15–30 |
| $\beta_1$ | 36 | 25 |
| $\beta_2$ | 33 | 25 |
| Reference | Catterall (2000) Lai et al. (2004) | Catterall (1988) |

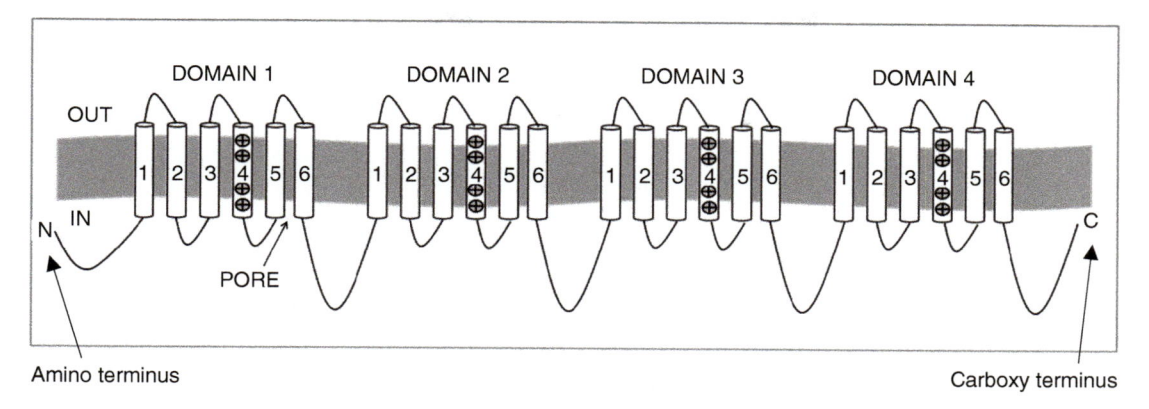

Figure 4.5 Structure of sodium channel alpha (α) protein. N is the amino terminus and C is the carboxy terminus.

act specifically on certain types of sodium channels, thereby reducing risks such as cardiotoxicity.

As inflammatory mediators such as prostaglandins sensitize sodium channels, inducing depolarization with less intense stimuli (hyperalgesia), local anesthetics block sodium channels less effectively under those circumstances (Lai et al. 2004).

Sodium channels play a pivotal role in nerve impulse formation and propagation. They are normally closed, but when stimulated they open (Figure 4.6) to allow the passive inward flow of extracellular $Na^+$ further to a concentration gradient, for $Na^+$ concentration is greater in extracellular (150 mEq/l) than intracellular (15 mEq/l) fluids (Elmslie 2001; Lipscombe 2005) (Figure 4.7).

## Potassium Channels

Potassium channels ($K^+$ channels), studied by the MacKinnon group, are protein structures with two functional subunits (Doyle et al. 1998; Lee et al. 2005).

1) The 1.2-nm long, 0.35-nm diameter pore (at its narrowest) (MacKinnon 2003) is the site of the selectivity filter that governs which $K^+$ ions flow out of the open channel (Lee et al. 2005). The filter is sited at a quarter of the length from the extracellular edge, opening on to the central cavity prior to the end of the pore. Upstream of the filter the cavity widens to 1 nm (MacKinnon 2003). The determining factor for ion selection would appear to be size (Lockless et al. 2007) and potassium, at 0.133 nm (Doyle et al. 1998; MacKinnon 2003; Lockless et al. 2007) and 0.266 nm when hydrated (Lipscombe 2005), is larger than the 0.095-nm $Na^+$.
2) The voltage sensor around the pore is a structure that when stimulated by alterations in membrane voltage opens the pore by changing the configuration of the top of the central cavity.

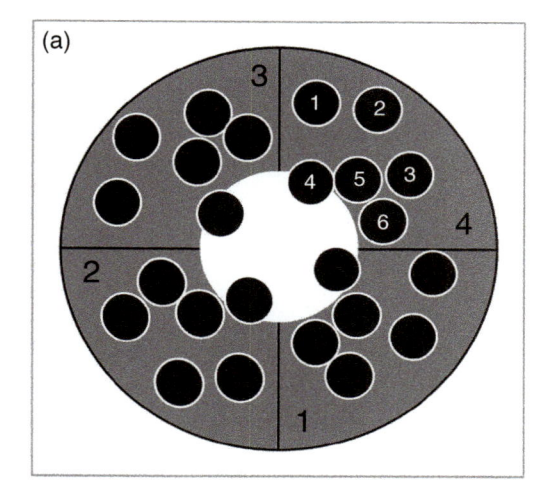

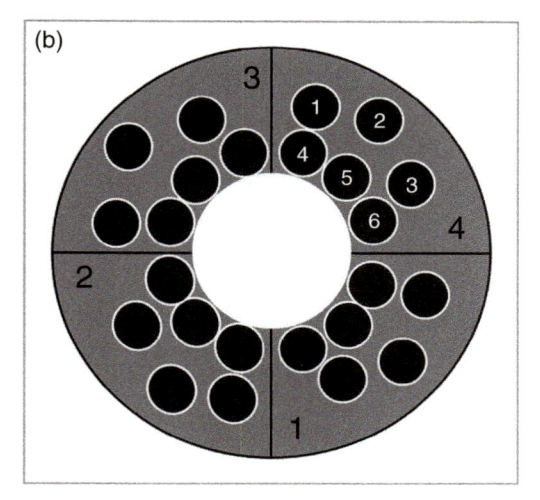

Figure 4.6 Sodium channel pore: (a) closed; (b) open.

The two subunits have different structures and properties and as they bond only loosely, they must be anchored in the membrane to perform their functions (Lee et al. 2005).

|  | Extracellular | Intracellular |
|---|---|---|
| Na⁺ | 150 mEq/l | 15 mEq/l |
| K⁺ | 5 mEq/l | 150 mEq/l |

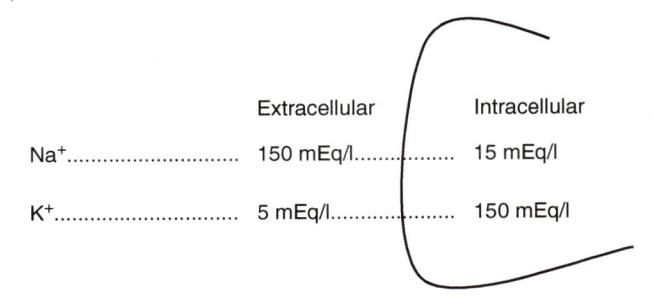

**Figure 4.7** Intra- and extracellular Na⁺ and K⁺ concentrations (rounded values).

Potassium channels play a secondary role in nerve impulse formation and propagation. They are normally closed and open later and longer than sodium channels to help recover the resting potential by allowing K⁺ ions to flow passively (without consuming energy) from the axoplasm, where they are highly concentrated (150 mEq/l), to the cell exterior, where concentration is lower (5 mEq/l) (Elmslie 2001; Lipscombe 2005) (Figure 4.7).

## Peripheral Nerve Neurophysiology

The basic texts on peripheral nerve neurophysiology were published in 1952 by Hodgkin and Huxley, who worked with giant (0.4–0.8 mm in diameter), unmyelinated Atlantic squid (*Loligo pealeii* and *Loligo forbesii*) axons. These were large enough for the thinnest (0.15 mm) and most precise electrodes available at the time to penetrate the axon through the membrane (Hodgkin and Huxley 1952a,b) and measure the action potential and intra- and extracellular ion exchange (Hodgkin and Huxley 1952b; Hodgkin et al. 1952c). In the following description of peripheral nerve physiology, some of the data initially reported by Hodgkin and Huxley (Hodgkin and Huxley 1952b) are adapted to results in mammals, and corrected and rounded.

### Fundamentals

A number of preliminaries are in order for a clearer understanding of the process described below.

- Intra- and extracellular fluids are electrolytic solutions carrying positively charged ions (cations) such as sodium (Na⁺), potassium (K⁺), or calcium (Ca⁺) or negatively charged (anions) such as organic phosphates, sulfates, or protein ions. Most anions are bound to molecules too large to exit the cell.
- To pump three Na⁺ ions out of and two K⁺ ions into the cell against the concentration gradient, the cell membrane's Na⁺/K⁺ATPase consumes energy.

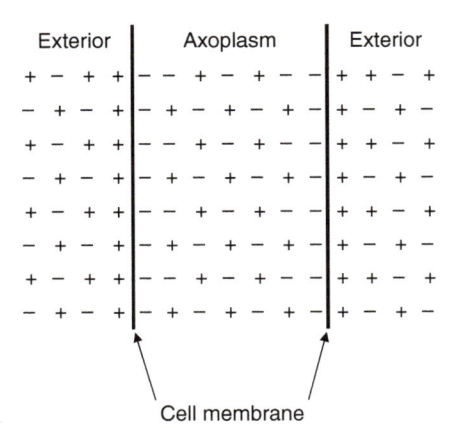

**Figure 4.8** Electrochemical imbalance adjacent to intercellular side of cell membrane.

- When at rest, the cell membrane Na⁺ channel is closed, but when stimulated it opens to allow the passive (without energy) inflow of extracellular Na⁺ in keeping with the concentration gradient.
- When at rest, the cell membrane K⁺ channel is closed, but when stimulated it opens to allow the passive (without energy) outflow of intracellular K⁺, likewise in keeping with the concentration gradient.
- Despite the presence of large numbers of positively or negatively charged ions along the membrane, imbalance is in fact minimal. Only a small proportion of axoplasmic ions (from 1 per 3 million to 1 per 100 million) (Guyton and Hall 2007) moves to create a negative potential of around −70 mV adjacent to the intracellular side of the membrane (Figure 4.8). As such electrochemical imbalance occurs only around the membrane, the potential of −70 mV is present there and absent in the rest of the axoplasm and extracellular fluids.

### Membrane Potentials: Membrane at Rest (Polarized)

The axon membrane exhibits a negative electrical imbalance of −70 mV along its entire surface due to the prevalence of negative charges, but only on *the inner side*. This interior/exterior charge differential is called the membrane potential or resting potential and the membrane is said to be polarized.

Such polarization is maintained by the Na⁺/K⁺ pump which, as noted, extrudes three Na⁺ ions for every two K⁺ ions imported into the axoplasm, creating a standing charge imbalance (Butterworth and Strichartz 1990; Scheiner-Bobis 2002).

### Action Potentials: Excited Membrane

The membrane is excited by electrical, chemical, mechanical (pressure, squeezing, etc.) or thermal (heat, cold) stimulants. By exciting the membrane these

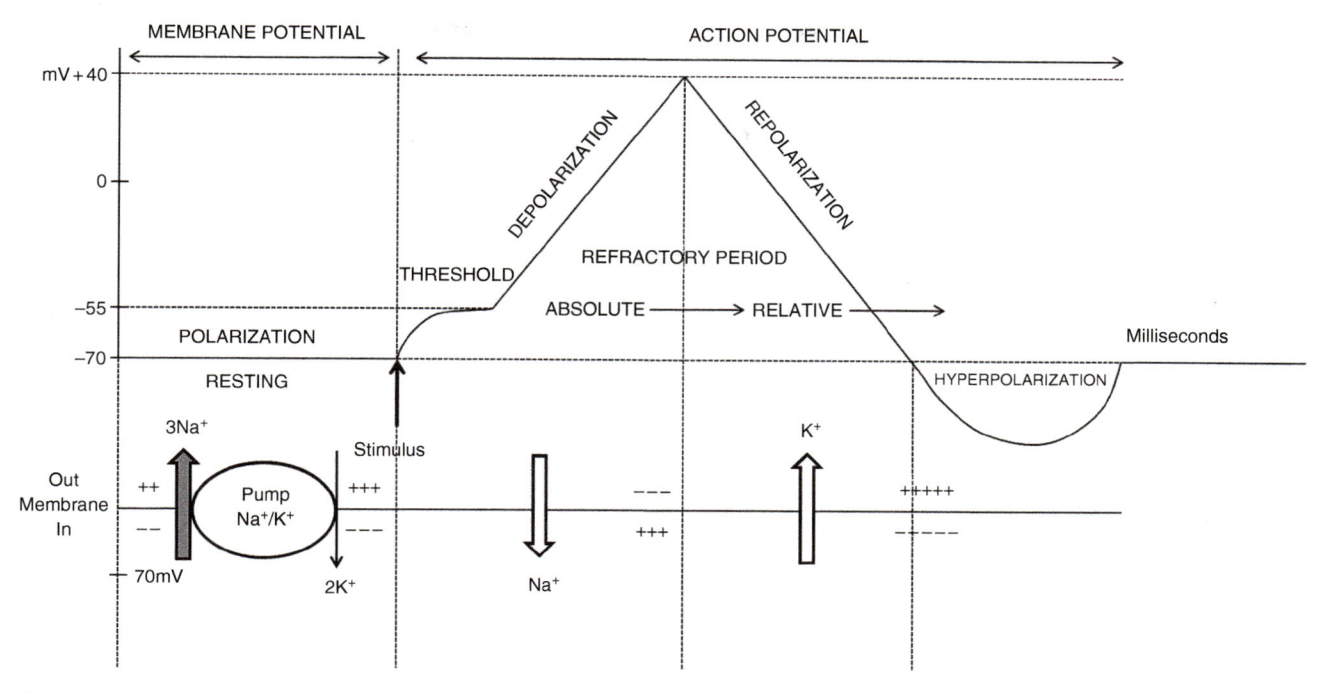

**Figure 4.9** Action potential showing the variations in mV and ion ($Na^+$ and $K^+$). Movements and changes in membrane charge with $Na^+/K^+$ pump operating and $Na^+$ and $K^+$ channels open. Schematic drawn.

stimulants disrupt the resting balance, changing the voltage from −70 to +40 mV adjacent to the inner surface of the membrane due to the predominance of positive ions, after which the resting status is restored. This process, known as the action potential, lasts for only a few, normally 2–4, milliseconds (ms), but may vary with circumstances and type of nerve fiber. Its three phases are described below (Figure 4.9).

### Phase 1: Depolarization

Any of the stimuli mentioned opens the sodium channels (closed in the resting position), with the passive inward flow of $Na^+$ ions induced by the electrochemical gradient (low concentration and prevalence of negative charges inside). The voltage inside the axon therefore starts to change to less negative values.

This process is initially fairly slow, but when the differential reaches around −15 mV (de Jong 1977; Malamed 2004; Guyton and Hall 2007), varying from −70 to −55 mV, *the excitation threshold is crossed*. Irrespective of the stimulus and its intensity, in keeping with the *all or nothing law*, full depolarization is triggered and the $Na^+$ channels are opened wide with a massive inward flow of $Na^+$ until the electric charge is neutralized (0 mV) or a maximum of +40 mV is reached alongside the inner surface of the membrane.

From the excitation threshold (−55 mV) to maximum depolarization (+40 mV), and even briefly during the repolarization phase, the voltage-gated sodium channel is inactivated. During this *absolute refractory period* the membrane fails to react to any further stimulus, no matter how intense.

### Phase 2: Repolarization

Two events taking place during repolarization govern the membrane recovery of its resting potential after maximum depolarization (+40 mV).

- The $Na^+$ channels close to stop the inward flow of $Na^+$. For a short time, these channels are inactive (not only closed) and cannot open.
- The $K^+$ channels open more slowly and for a longer time, allowing $K^+$ ions to flow from the axoplasm outward, where the $K^+$ concentration is lower, helping to offset and reduce depolarization.

$Na^+/K^+$ATPase pumps throughout, intensifying its activity (pumping $Na^+$ in and $K^+$ out) to restore the resting status (−70 mV) (Guyton and Hall 2007).

The *relative refractory period*, which appears during the repolarization period, lasts through hyperpolarization, and only very intense stimuli can re-trigger depolarization and re-open the closed $Na^+$ channels after inactivation.

### Phase 3: Hyperpolarization

This phase is known as hyperpolarization because after reaching its resting level (−70 mV), the membrane becomes slightly more negative for a few milliseconds (because the K$^+$ channels remain open longer than the Na$^+$ channels), after which the Na$^+$/K$^+$ pump restores resting status.

Curiously, hyperpolarization is also called "more positive after action potential" instead of the more logical "more negative after action potential". Tradition has maintained that apparent misnomer, which stems from the practice of the earliest researchers to measure voltage outside the cell (−70 mV is the inside value). Sodium channel inactivation during the refractory period ensures that nerve impulses can be propagated in one direction only (Wildsmith 1986).

### Propagation of the Action Potential

In the presence of an action potential the adjacent parts of the axon membrane are excited/stimulated and the electrochemical impulses spread swiftly along the nerve fiber in the form of a depolarization–repolarization–hyperpolarization wave.

Once initiated, the impulse travels constantly along the nerve fiber irrespective of the power or the nature of the stimulus that prompted it, for the propagation energy is released by the axon itself along its entire length. A very intense stimulus is expressed by a higher frequency of action potential and the enlistment of more axons to carry the impulse.

Action potentials are propagated differently in unmyelinated and myelinated nerve fibers.

- In the former the depolarization–repolarization–hyperpolarization wave (electrochemical impulse) travels continuously at a lower speed because more energy is needed to surmount the resistance encountered.
- In the latter the depolarization–repolarization–hyperpolarization wave (the action potential) jumps from one node of Ranvier to the next (saltatory conduction), where the axon membrane is in contact with extracellular fluids, establishing ion exchange. For that reason, many fewer net Na$^+$ and K$^+$ ions move along the myelinated than the unmyelinated fibers, raising the propagation speed and lowering the energy required. Nonetheless, ion activity and the number of Na$^+$ channels are much greater in the nodes of Ranvier than on the surface of unmyelinated nerves (110 Na$^+$ channels per µm$^2$ in unmyelinated fibers versus 2000–12 000 in nodes of Ranvier) (Catterall 1984).

## Mechanisms of Local Anesthesia

Widely accepted evidence now available shows that local anesthetics act by temporarily blocking Na$^+$ channels, inducing the membrane to remain at its resting potential. That prevents stimuli from triggering the action potential and consequently inhibits the propagation of the nerve impulse (Hille 1966; de Jong 1977; Strichartz 1981).

Although the K$^+$ channels are also blocked by local anesthetics, the effect is less intense, particularly as regards inhibition of nerve impulse conduction (Ritchie 1975).

### Mechanism

Local anesthetic action appears to be governed by the mechanism described below (Ritchie 1975; Strichartz 1981; Wildsmith 1986; Butterworth and Strichartz 1990). When the local anesthetic reaches the extracellular surface of the axon, its ionized (cationic, BH$^+$) and neutral base (salt, B) states are in equilibrium. Their respective proportions depend on the local anesthetic's pKa value.

The liposoluble neutral base (B) can penetrate the phospholipid bilayer in the axon membrane, particularly the apolar zone in the hydrophobic, liposoluble center (Ritchie 1975). With that inflow a new BH$^+$ − B equilibrium is reached. The local anesthetic receptor in the Na$^+$ channel to which the anesthetic bonds can be reached in one of two ways (Strichartz 1981; Wildsmith 1986; Butterworth and Strichartz 1990; Fozzard et al. 2005).

1) The quickest is via B, once in the cell membrane (hydrophobic or external path).
2) The most powerful way to block the Na$^+$ channel is from the axoplasm via BH$^+$, which flows into the open pore in the Na$^+$ channel (hydrophilic or internal path).

The local anesthetic penetrates the axon membrane differently depending on whether it is myelinated or unmyelinated.

- In unmyelinated fibers the local anesthetic bathes the entire surface of the nerve fiber along the axon, although its distribution is not wholly uniform (Franz and Perry 1974).
- In myelinated fibers the local anesthetic only penetrates and acts on the axon membrane at the nodes of Ranvier, where there is no myelin and the axon is in contact with extracellular fluids.

### Differential Nerve Block

Local anesthetics have been shown to anesthetize different nerve fibers with unequal efficacy. The factors conditioning efficacy are listed below:

1) The first is nerve fiber thickness. Logically, fibers with a smaller diameter are more readily anesthetized (Gasser and Erlanger 1929; Franz and Perry 1974) because the smaller the diameter, the fewer the Na$^+$ channels that need to be blocked (de Jong 1977).

2) The second is the presence or otherwise of myelin. Unmyelinated fibers are anesthetized more readily than myelinated fibers, particularly where the myelin layer is thick (Franz and Perry 1974).
3) The third is the frequency of the stimuli transmitted by the nerve fibers and therefore the type of stimulus. Fibers carrying stimuli such as pain have a high action potential frequency per second and consequently are anesthetized more easily (frequency- or use-dependent or phase block). Fibers carrying motor stimuli, with a lower action potential frequency, are less readily anesthetized (Franz and Perry 1974).

A review of the classification of nerve fibers in Table 4.1 shows the following (Wildsmith 1986):

- Smaller, unmyelinated or scantly myelinated fibers carrying high-frequency stimuli are readily anesthetized:
  - Small, free nerve endings usually carrying *pain*.
  - Polymodal C fibers carrying *second*, burning, diffuse, persistent *pain*.
  - Sympathetic postganglionic fibers of the autonomic nervous system, such as polymodal C fibers.
  - Sympathetic preganglionic fibers of the autonomic nervous system, such as B fibers.
- Anesthetization is also attained fairly readily in somewhat thicker, scantly myelinated fibers, including:
  - Polymodal C and Aδ fibers carrying temperature sensitivity (heat, cold).
  - Polymodal C and Aδ fibers carrying sensitivity to pressure.
  - Aδ fibers carrying *first*, sharp, fast, localized *pain*.
- The fibers most difficult to block, typically A alfa (Aα), A beta (Aβ), and A gamma (Aγ), are thick and heavily myelinated, with a longer internodal distance (between nodes of Ranvier) and carrying lower frequency (motor and proprioceptive) impulses.

Despite the morphological differences in polymodal C and Aδ fibers, local anesthetics can effectively anesthetize both (de Jong 1977).

### Tonic and Phase Block

Both the ionized and neutral forms of local anesthetics can produce "tonic" and "phase" block in $Na^+$ channels, although the characteristics differ (Strichartz 1981; Wildsmith 1986; Butterworth and Strichartz 1990; Fozzard et al. 2005).

- When the membrane is kept at resting potential with the $Na^+$ channels closed, local anesthetics are said to effect *tonic block*, primarily via the neutral base lodged within the membrane.
- When the membrane is excited, with action potentials present and the $Na^+$ channels open, the local anesthetic is said to induce *phase* (or *frequency-* or *use-dependent*) *block*. Such blocks, which are more powerful, are primarily produced by the ionized (cationic) form that bonds to the receptor at the inner side of the pore from the axoplasm (Fozzard et al. 2005).

### Critical Length

This section addresses the question of the length of nerve fiber that should be coated by local anesthetics to block nerve impulse conduction. It is pertinent because depolarization activates the membrane several millimeters beyond the initiation site (de Jong 1977). Experimental research has established that distance for myelinated and unmyelinated fibers, as follows:

- In unmyelinated fibers the local anesthetic should coat and block around 3–4 mm (de Jong 1977).
- In myelinated fibers at least three successive nodes of Ranvier should be blocked (Blair and Erlanger 1939; Tasaki 1953) (Figure 4.10).

One of the thickest nerve trunks requiring dental block is the myelinated inferior alveolar nerve, in which the nodes of Ranvier are spaced at 0.5–1.8 mm (Rood 1978a, 1978b). Blocking three nodes consequently calls for coating around 6 mm of nerve trunk with the anesthetic

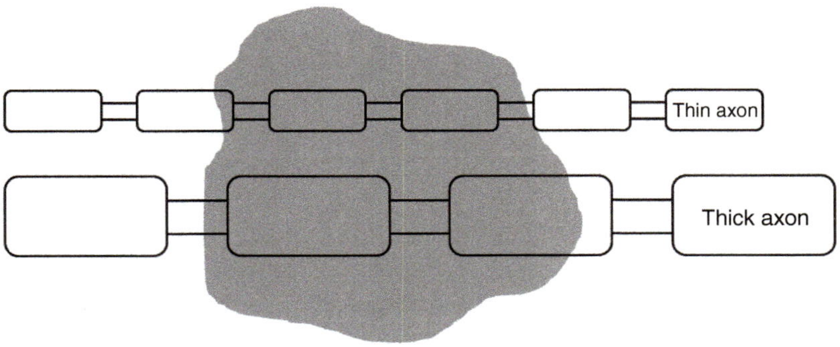

Figure 4.10 Comparison of anesthetic coverage of nodes of Ranvier in thin and thick axons.

(Rood 1978a, 1978b). In practice, however, since the anesthetic does not diffuse regularly, to guarantee a minimum block the distance to be coated should be somewhat longer than the experimental value (de Jong 1977).

## Transient Receptor Potential Channel

The function of TRPV1, the transient receptor potential cation channel, subfamily V, member 1, was discovered in the twenty-first century. The first breakthrough came with the identification of capsaicin receptors and their role in pain mechanisms (Caterina et al. 1997). Capsaicin is the active ingredient in hot peppers such as chili, cayenne, and wasabi. This family of receptors is presently referred to as vanilloid receptors (transient receptor potential vanilloide [TRPV]), six of which have been discovered. The first is the formerly labeled capsaicin receptor, now known as TRPV1.

Found on the membranes of pain neurons (nociceptors), TRPV1 is an integral protein similar to $K^+$ channels. This receptor is a nonselective cation channel, allowing the inflow of $Ca^{++}$, $Na^+$ and so on, although it is five to nine times more permeable to $Ca^{++}$ ions (Butterworth and Oxford 2009).

Recent research appears to show that when this channel is stimulated its filter opens, *allowing the inflow of the cationic form ($BH^+$) of local anesthetic molecules such as lidocaine*, which block the $Na^+$ channels from the axoplasm (Butterworth and Oxford 2009). As the selective filter in this channel is 0.6–1.0 nm and lidocaine molecules are estimated to measure $3 \times 0.68 \times 0.47$ nm (Glówka et al. 1996), the entry pore may expand dynamically to allow anesthetic inflow (Butterworth and Oxford 2009). The actual significance of this mechanism has yet to be determined.

## Nerve Block Kinetics

Local anesthetics differ from most drugs used in medicine in that they are deposited near the target structures. When a local anesthetic solution is injected periorally, the subcutaneous deposit diffuses from the injection site to the surrounding tissues. If, for instance, 1 ml of a 2% local anesthetic is injected, the space occupied is a sphere with a radius of 0.62 cm. As the solution diffuses concentrically (ideally), the anesthetic molecules spread and the sphere grows. The concomitant dilution lowers the initial concentration: when the radius of the sphere is 2.62 cm the volume is 76 ml and the concentration 0.026% (Schilli 1977) (Table 4.3).

As local anesthetic solutions diffuse along the least resistant pathways, they do not spread uniformly, as mentioned earlier, for the soft and hard tissues in the mouth constitute more or less compact barriers. They can be penetrated by the local anesthetic but at the expense of lowering its concentration even further. In addition, some of the molecules are captured non-nervous (such as adipose) tissues and others are absorbed and removed from the area by blood and (to a lesser extent) lymph vessels. Some of the anesthetic molecules nonetheless reach the nearby nerve trunks and nerve endings.

**Table 4.3** Sphere-like diffusion of 1 ml of 2% anesthetic.

| Sphere radius (cm) | Anesthetic (%) | Volume (ml) |
| --- | --- | --- |
| 0.62 | 2 | 1 |
| 1.12 | 0.34 | 6 |
| 2.62 | 0.062 | 76 |

*Source:* Data from Schilli (1977).

### Induction Stage

Once in the nerve trunk, the anesthetic molecules spread in two stages (de Jong 1977). They reach and hence anesthetize the fascicles nearest the surface of the nerve trunk first. Given the greater distance, wider diffusion and larger number of barriers to be permeated to reach the fascicles in the center of the nerve trunk, anesthetization there takes longer. As a result anesthesia is *somatotopic*, for the fascicles on the surface of the nerve trunk normally innervate the closest, and the fibers in the center the more distant tissues and organs. In inferior alveolar nerve block, for instance, the first lower molar is anesthetized before the mandibular incisors, which are located farther from the mandibular block site (Table 4.4).

Other factors impacting the time to onset or the time it takes to numb tissues include the *concentration of the anesthetic* (the higher the concentration, the earlier is onset) and *nerve trunk thickness* (the thinner, the earlier). The anesthetic concentration in- and outside the nerve trunk ultimately reaches equilibrium.

### Recovery Stage

Recovery from nerve trunk block follows the same pathway as the induction stage, but in reverse order. The extraneural store of local anesthetic continues to decline due to dispersion, capture by connective and adipose tissue, and vessel absorption, lowering the concentration to below the value inside the nerve trunk. The anesthetic seeps out of the fascicles nearest the outer surface of the nerve trunk first, inducing early recovery in these fibers. As the concentration of the anesthetic is higher in the central fascicles, anesthesia lasts longer in the more distant tissues.

*Recovery is slower* than induction, for once the anesthetic binds to the nerve fibers its release takes time. The pattern

Table 4.4 Mean onset (in minutes) of pulpal anesthesia after mandibular block with 2% lidocaine, 1:100 000 epinephrine.

| Tooth | Chaney et al. (1991) | Hinkley et al. (1991) | McLean et al. (1993) | Kanaa et al. (2006) | Goldberg et al. (2008) |
|---|---|---|---|---|---|
| First molar | 8.2 | 8.8 | 10.8 | 5.4 | 8.0 |
| First premolar | 10.2 | 10.6 | 11.8 | 8.9 | 7.0 |
| Lateral incisor | 13.0 | 14.3 | 17.2 | 13.3 | 12.0 |

See Table 16.2, Chapter 16.

involved is approximately exponential, with initial speedy recovery gradually slowing through the end of the process. Recovery time is impacted by a number of factors.

1) A higher anesthetic concentration entails longer duration.
2) The thinner the nerve trunk, the longer the duration of the effect.
3) Nerve function also affects duration, for anesthesia lasts longer in pain than in motor fibers. That effect is associated with the thinner diameter, lack of myelin and the type of block (phase or use-dependent) involved.

### Re-Injection

If more anesthesia is injected before the peripheral fascicles recover their resting potential, re-block is nearly immediate, with no somatotopic phasing between near and far tissues (de Jong 1977). Moreover, the effect is attained with smaller amounts of anesthetic than initially, since the fibers are already coated with anesthetic.

### Tachyphylaxis

Tachyphylaxis, in this context the loss of anesthetic efficacy in successive injections immediately after the anesthetic effect reverts, is a manner of tolerance (de Jong 1977; Choi et al. 1997; Vadhanan et al. 2015). Surprisingly, however, its presence cannot be proven in laboratory studies.

Tachyphylaxis (Greek: *tachys* = fast and *phylaxis* = protection) to local anesthetics has been known since the 1960s (Kongsgaard and Wemer 2016). However, in a systematic review in 2016 it was noted that the number of documented cases was very low and mainly in epidural, intrathecal anesthesia, or in regional blocks with continuous anesthesia, but there were no registered cases of regional blocks in dentistry (Kongsgaard and Wemer 2016).

Although not fully understood, the possible causes of this condition are as follows (Vadhanan et al. 2015):

1) The nerves may be altered by edema or microhemorrhaging due to the toxicity of local anesthetics (de Jong 1977; Vadhanan et al. 2015).
2) Successive injections may cause acidosis. Local anesthetic solutions with sympathomimetic vasoconstrictors, such as epinephrine, have an acidic pH. After injection this pH is neutralized by tissue fluids. Nonetheless, successive injections in the same site may saturate the buffer capacity of the fluids, in which case acidity persists. At acid pH the cationic form ($BH^+$) prevails over the neutral form (B) of the anesthetic, retarding and reducing penetration across cell membranes (Cohen et al. 1968; de Jong 1977; Vadhanan et al. 2015).
3) Successive injections may induce hypernatremia. Local anesthetic solutions contain sodium chloride (NaCl) to balance tissue osmolarity and prevent tissular irritation. Repeated injections in the same site may raise $Na^+$ concentration and lower the effect of the anesthetic on sodium channels (de Jong 1977; Vadhanan et al. 2015), although this has not been proven.
4) Pharmacokinetics may reduce the intranervous concentration of the local anesthetic significantly (Vadhanan et al. 2015), an effect observed in experiments with rats *in vivo* (Choi et al. 1997). The mechanism possibly involved is vasodilation as the initial anesthetic action recedes, hastening the removal of further doses of the solution.

Re-injection of the local anesthetic 15 minutes after the effect of the local anesthetic reverts should be avoided, for otherwise 25–35% more solution is required to attain the same efficacy (de Jong 1977).

### Resistance to Local Anesthetics

Some cases of resistance to the action of local anesthetics have been described in medical (Miller et al. 1981; Kavlock and Ting 2004) and dental (Beckett and Gilmour 1990) practice. The symptoms are short duration or insufficient effect attributable not to conventional causes of failure (Chapter 19) but to genetic alterations that induce structural variations in some sodium channel isoforms (Panigel and Cook 2011; Clendenen et al. 2016). Although the frequency of such anomalies is presently unknown, it is assumed to be low.

# References

Abd-Elmeguid, A. and Yu, D.C. (2009). Dental pulp neurophysiology: part 1. Clinical and diagnostic implications. *J. Can. Dent. Assoc.* 75 (1): 55–59.

Asher, L. (1892). Ein Beitrag zur Resorption durch die Blutgefässe. *Z. Biol.* 29: 247–255.

Beckett, H.A. and Gilmour, A.G. (1990). Resistance to local analgesia – report of a case treated using 5% lignocaine solution. *Br. Dent. J.* 169 (10): 327–328.

Blair, E.A. and Erlanger, J. (1939). Propagation, and extension of excitatory effects of the nerve action potential across nonresponding internodes. *Am. J. Physiol.* 126 (1): 97–108.

Butterworth, J. and Oxford, G.S. (2009). Local anesthetics. A new hydrophilic pathway for the drug-receptor reaction (editorial). *Anesthesiology* 111 (1): 12–14.

Butterworth, J.F. and Strichartz, G.R. (1990). Molecular mechanism of local anesthesia: a review. *Anesthesiology* 72 (4): 711–734.

Cajal, S.R. (1899). *Textura del sistema nervioso del hombre y de los vertebrados. Tomo I*. Madrid: Editorial Nicolás Moya. 94.

Caterina, M.J., Schumacher, M.A., Tominaga, M. et al. (1997). The capsaicin receptor: a heat-activated ion channel in the pain pathway. *Nature* 389 (6653): 816–824.

Catterall, W.A. (1984). The molecular basis of neuronal excitability. *Science* 223 (4637): 653–661.

Catterall, W.A. (1988). Structure and function of voltage-sensitive ion channels. *Science* 242 (4675): 50–61.

Catterall, W.A. (2000). From ionic currents to molecular mechanisms: structure and function of voltage-gated sodium channels. *Neuron* 26 (1): 13–25.

Chaney, M.A., Kerby, R., Reader, A. et al. (1991). An evaluation of lidocaine hydrocarbonate compared with lidocaine hydrochloride for inferior alveolar nerve block. *Anesth. Prog.* 38 (6): 212–216.

Choi, R.H., Birknes, J.K., Popitz-Bergez, A. et al. (1997). Pharmacokinetic nature of tachyphylaxis to lidocaine: peripheral nerve blocks and infiltration anesthesia in rats. *Life Sci.* 61 (12): PL 177–184.

Clendenen, N., Cannon, A.D., Porter, S. et al. (2016). Whole-exome sequencing of a family with local anesthetic resistance. *Minerva Anesthesiol.* 82 (10): 1089–1097.

Cohen, E.N., Levine, D.A., Colligs, J.E., and Gunther, R.E. (1968). The role of pH in the development of tachyphylaxis to local anesthetic agents. *Anesthesiology* 29 (5): 994–1001.

De Jong, R.H. (1977). *Local Anesthetics*, 2e. Springfield (IL): Charles C Thomas Publisher. 9, 18–20, 30, 57–60, 74–77.

Doyle, D.A., Cabral, J.M., Pfuetzner, R.A. et al. (1998). The structure of the potassium channel: molecular basis of $K^+$ conduction and selectivity. *Science* 280 (5360): 69–77.

Elmslie, K. (2001). *Membrane Potential. Encyclopedia of Life Sciences*. Wiley (Cell Biology → cell membranes) (www.els.net).

Fozzard, H.A., Lee, P.J., and Lipkind, G.M. (2005). Mechanism of local anesthetic drug action on voltage-gated sodium channels. *Curr. Pharm. Des.* 11 (21): 2671–2686.

Franz, D.N. and Perry, R.S. (1974). Mechanisms for differential block among single myelinated and nonmyelinated axons by procaine. *J. Physiol. (London)* 236 (1): 193–210.

Gasser, H.S. and Erlanger, J. (1929). The role of fiber size in the establishment of a nerve block by pressure or cocaine. *Am. J. Physiol.* 88 (4): 581–591.

Glówka, M.L., Olczak, A., Kwapiszewski, W., and Bialasiewicz, W. (1996). Geometry of lidocaine-like molecules. 1. Crystal structure of tocainide. *J. Chem. Crystallogr.* 26 (7): 515–518.

Goldberg, S., Reader, A., Drum, M. et al. (2008). Comparison of the anesthetic efficacy of the conventional inferior alveolar, Gow-gates, and Vazirani-Akinosi technique. *J. Endod.* 34 (11): 1306–1311.

Guyton, A.C. (1987). *Basic Neuroscience. Anatomy and Physiology*. Philadelphia: WB Saunders Co. 67, 68.

Guyton, A.C. and Hall, J.E. (2007). *Tratado de fisiología médica*, 11e. Madrid: Elsevier. 12, 54, 59, 65, 66.

Heasman, P.A. and Beynon, A.D.G. (1987). Clinical considerations from axon-myelin relationship in human inferior alveolar nerve. *Int. J. Oral Maxillofac. Surg.* 16 (3): 346–351.

Hille, B. (1966). Common mode of action of three agents that decrease the transient change in sodium permeability in nerves. *Nature* 210 (5042): 1220–1222.

Hinkley, J.A., Reader, A., Beck, M., and Meyers, W.J. (1991). An evaluation of 4% prilocaine with 1:200,000 epinephrine and 2% mepivacaine with 1:20,000 levonordefrin compared with 2% lidocaine with 1:100,000 epinephrine for inferior alveolar nerve block. *Anesth. Prog.* 38 (3): 84–89.

Hodgkin, A.L. and Huxley, A.F. (1952a). The dual effect of membrane potential on sodium conductance in the giant axon of Loligo. *J. Physiol. (London)* 116 (4): 497–506.

Hodgkin, A.L. and Huxley, A.F. (1952b). A quantitative description of membrane current and its application to conduction and excitation in nerve. *J. Physiol. (London)* 117 (4): 500–544.

Hodgkin, A.L., Huxley, A.F., and Katz, B. (1952c). Measurement of current-voltage relations in the membrane of the giant axon of Loligo. *J. Physiol. (London)* 116 (4): 424–448.

Jack, J.J.B. (1975). Physiology of peripheral nerves fibers in relation to their size. *Br. J. Anaesth.* 47 (Suppl): 173–182.

Jastak, J.T., Yagiela, J.A., and Donaldson, D. (1995). *Local Anesthesia of the Oral Cavity*. Philadelphia: WB Saunders Co., 3, 5, 6, 20.

Johnsen, D.C., Harshbarger, J., and Rymer, H.D. (1983). Quantitative assessment of neuronal development in human premolars. *Anat. Rec.* 205 (4): 421–429.

Kanaa, M.D., Meechan, J.G., Cobertt, I.P., and Whitworth, J.M. (2006). Speed injection influences efficacy of inferior alveolar nerve blocks: a double-blind ramdomized controlled trial in volunteers. *J. Endod.* 32 (10): 919–923.

Kavlock, R. and Ting, P.H. (2004). Local anesthetic in a pregnant patient with lumbosacral plexopathy. *BMC Anesthesiol.* 4: 1.

Kongsgaard, U.E. and Werner, M.U. (2016). Tachyphylaxis to local anaesthetics. What is the clinical evidence? A systematic review. *Acta Anaesthesiol. Scand.* 60 (1): 6–14.

Lai, J., Porreca, F., Hunter, J.C., and Gold, M.S. (2004). Voltage-gated sodium channels and hyperalgesia. *Annu. Rev. Pharmacol. Toxicol.* 44: 371–397.

Lee, S.-Y., Lee, A., Chen, J., and MacKinnon, R. (2005). Structure of the KvAP voltage-dependent$^+$ K$^+$ channel and its dependence of the lipid membrane. *PNAS* 102 (43): 15441–15446.

Lin, J. and Chandler, N.P. (2008). Electric pulp testing: a review. *Int. Endod. J.* 41 (5): 265–374.

Lipscombe, D. (2005). *Ion Channels. Encyclopedia of Life Sciences*. Wiley (Cell biology → cell membrane) (www.els.net).

Lockless, S.W., Zhou, M., and MacKinnon, R. (2007). Structural and thermodynamic properties of selective ion binding in a K$^+$ channel. *PLoS Biol.* 5 (5): e 121. 1079–1088.

Luo, S., Perry, G.M., Levinson, S.R., and Henry, M.A. (2008). Na$_v$ 1.7 expression is increased in painful human dental pulp. *Mol. Pain* 4: 16–29.

MacKinnon, R. (2003). Potassium channels. *FEBS Lett.* 555 (1): 62–65.

Malamed, S.F. (2004). *Handbook of Local Anesthesia*, 5e. St. Louis: Elsevier-Mosby. 8.

McLean, C., Reader, A., Beck, M., and Meyers, W.J. (1993). An evaluation of 4% prilocaine and 3% mepivacaine compared with 2% lidocaine (1:100,000 epinephrine) for inferior alveolar block. *J. Endod.* 19 (3): 146–150.

Meymaris, E. (1975). Chemistry and physiology of local anaesthesia. Chemical anatomy of the nerve membrane. *Br. J. Anaesth.* 47 (Suppl): 164–172.

Miller, G.L., Scurlock, J.E., Covino, B.G. et al. (1981). Letters to the editor. *Reg. Anesth.* 6 (3): 122–125.

Myers, R.R. and Heckman, H.M. (1989). Effects of local anesthesia on nerve blood flow: studies using lidocaine with and without epinephrine. *Anesthesiology* 71 (5): 757–762.

Panigel, J. and Cook, S.P. (2011). A point mutation at F1737 of the human Na$_v$ 1.7 sodium channel decreases inhibition by local anesthetics. *J. Neurogenet.* 25 (4): 134–139.

Ritchie, J.M. (1975). Mechanism of action of local anesthetics agents and biotoxins. *Br. J. Anaesth.* 47 (Suppl): 191–198.

Rood, J.P. (1978a). Some anatomical and physiological causes of failure to achieve mandibular analgesia. *Br. J. Oral Surg.* 15 (1): 75–82.

Rood, J.P. (1978b). The diameters on intermodal lengths of the myelinated fibers in human inferior alveolar nerve. *J. Dent.* 6 (4): 311–315.

Saha, S.G., Jain, S., Dubey, S. et al. (2016). Effect of oral premedication on the efficacy of inferior alveolar nerve block in patients with symptomatic irreversible pulpitis: a prospective, double-blind, randomized controlled trial. *J. Clin. Diagn. Res.* 10 (2): ZC25–ZC29.

Sampaio, R.M., Carvanal, T.G., Lanfredin, C.B. et al. (2012). Comparison of the anesthetic efficacy between bupivacaine and lidocaine in patients with irreversible pulpitis of mandibular molar. *J. Endod.* 38 (5): 594–597.

Scheiner-Bobis, G. (2002). The sodium pump. Its molecular properties and mechanism of ion transport. *Eur. J. Biochem.* 269 (10): 2424–2433.

Schilli, W. (1977). Vasoconstrictors in local anesthetics. *Quintessence Int.* 8 (12): 15–18.

Schou, J. (1961). Absorption of drugs from subcutaneous connective tissue. *Pharmacol. Rev.* 13 (3): 441–464.

Shanthaveerappa, T.R. and Bourne, G.H. (1966). Perineural epithelium: a new concept of its role in the peripheral nervous system. *Science* 154 (3755): 1464–1467.

Singer, S.J. and Nicolson, G.L. (1972). The fluid mosaic model of the structure of cell membranes. *Science* 175 (4023): 720–731.

Skou, J.C. (1957). The influence of some cations on adenosine-triphosphatase from peripheral nerves. *Biochim. Biophys. Acta* 23 (2): 394–401.

Strichartz, G.R. (1981). Current concepts of the mechanism of action of local anesthetics. *J. Dent. Res.* 60 (8): 1460–1467.

Sunderland, S. (1965). The connective tissues of peripheral nerves. *Brain* 88 (4): 841–854.

Tasaki, I. (1953). Saltatory transmission (chapter III). In: *Nervous Transmission* (ed. I. Tasaki). Springfield (IL): Charles C Thomas Publisher. 37–50.

Ulbricht, W. (2005). Sodium channel inactivation: molecular determinants and modulation. *Physiol. Rev.* 85 (4): 1271–1301.

Vadhanan, P., Tripaty, D.K., and Adinarayanan, S. (2015). Physiological and pharmacological aspects of peripheral nerve blocks. *J. Anesthesiol. Clin. Pharmacol.* 31 (3): 384–393.

Wells, J.E., Bingham, V., Rowland, K.C., and Hatton, J. (2007). Expression of Nav1.9 channels in human dental pulp and trigeminal ganglion. *J. Endod.* 33 (10): 1172–1176.

Wildsmith, J.A.W. (1986). Peripheral nerve and local anesthetic drugs. *Br. J. Anaesth.* 58 (7): 692–700.

# Pharmacology

# 5

# Local Anesthetics

Local anesthetics differ from most other drugs in that they are applied very close to the site where they are intended to act. Consequently, they travel across very short distances and their effects are felt in a matter of minutes. Their action consists of reversibly blocking the transmission of peripheral nerve impulses, an essential feature in local anesthesia.

Local anesthetics are weak bases in the form of oily liquids or low melting point solids. They are scantly water soluble and highly soluble in lipids and organic solvents. They are very unstable, readily decomposing when exposed to heat, light, or oxidation. When anesthetics are combined with strong acids such as hydrochloric acid, they form hydrochloride salts: white, crystalline, water-soluble powders that are very stable and compatible with epinephrine (Bonica 1959). The local anesthetics most commonly used in dentistry are listed in Table 5.1, together with the molecular weights of their bases and salts.

## Chemical Structure

The chemical structure of the local anesthetics presently used in dentistry, which is always basically the same, consists of the following three components (Löfgren and Lundquist 1946; Löfgren 1948; de Jong 1977) (Figure 5.1):

1) *Aromatic ring.* This is the lipid-soluble portion of the molecule that governs local anesthetic penetration into cell membranes. It may also help block nerve impulse transmission (Ritchie and Ritchie 1968). While the ring is normally a benzene, it may also be a thiophene, as in articaine.
2) *Intermediate aliphatic chain.* This is what determines the type of biotransformation and metabolic breakdown of the anesthetic. There are two types (Figure 5.2):
   - Ester or amino-ester chains are rapidly broken down via plasma cholinesterase (also known as plasma pseudocholinesterase, plasma esterase, or butyrylcholinesterase)-mediated hydrolysis.
   - Amide or amino-amide bonds are broken down more slowly in the liver, first via N-dealkylation of their tertiary amino terminus and subsequently by other mechanisms.
3) *Amino terminus.* This is the hydrophilic component and active principle in anesthetics. It exists in two forms (Figure 5.1):
   - The cationic, ionized (positive electric charge: $BH^+$), quaternary amine (the amino terminus has four bonds) or acid form is water-soluble and binds to the transmembrane protein receptor. It blocks the sodium channels and subsequently prevents depolarization of the neuron and the eventual transmission of the nerve impulse (Ritchie et al. 1965a, b; Wildsmith 1986; Butterworth and Strichartz 1990), intensifying the effect of the aromatic ring (Ritchie and Ritchie 1968).
   - The free, nonionized or uncharged and consequently electrically neutral (free neutral base: B) or tertiary amine (the amino terminus has three bonds) is lipid soluble and drives diffusion of the local anesthesia across the cell membranes and even to the protein receptor (Ritchie et al. 1965a, b). This form also blocks the transmission of nerve impulses, although less effectively than the cationic form (Ritchie and Ritchie 1968; Wildsmith 1986; Butterworth and Strichartz 1990).

## Physical-chemical Characteristics of Local Anesthetics

As local anesthetics act on a transmembrane receptor located in the sodium channel within the cell membrane, their effectiveness depends on the four main physical-chemical properties that govern their anesthetic activity.

---

*Local Anesthesia in Dentistry: A Locoregional Approach*, First Edition. Jesús Calatayud and Mana Saraghi.
© 2024 John Wiley & Sons Ltd. Published 2024 by John Wiley & Sons Ltd.
Companion website: www.wiley.com/go/Calatayud/local

**Table 5.1** Molecular weight (in International Units) of local anesthetics: bases and salts (hydrochlorides).

| | Local anesthetic | Base | Salt |
|---|---|---|---|
| Esters | Benzocaine | 165.2 | — |
| | Procaine | 236.3 | 272.8 |
| | Tetracaine | 264.4 | 300.8 |
| | Cocaine | 303.4 | 339.8 |
| Amides | Prilocaine | 220.3 | 256.8 |
| | Lidocaine | 234.3 | 270.8 |
| | Mepivacaine | 246.2 | 282.8 |
| | Ropivacaine | 274.4 | 310.8 |
| | Etidocaine | 276.0 | 312.9 |
| | Articaine | 284.4 | 320.9 |
| | Bupivacaine | 288.0 | 324.9 |

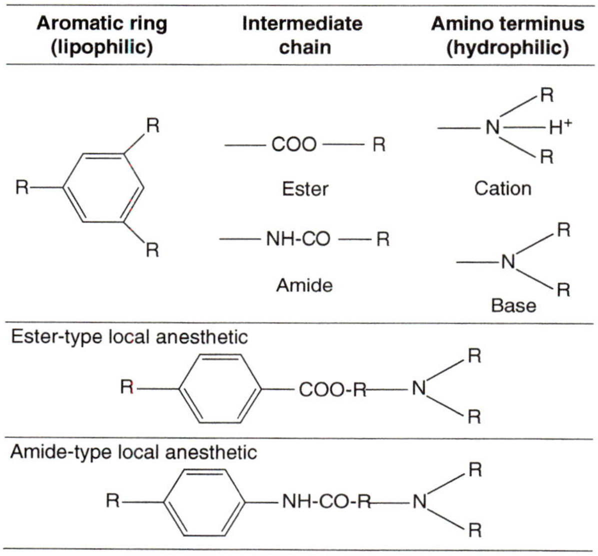

**Figure 5.1** Three components of the chemical structure of local anesthetics and basic or cationic amino terminus.

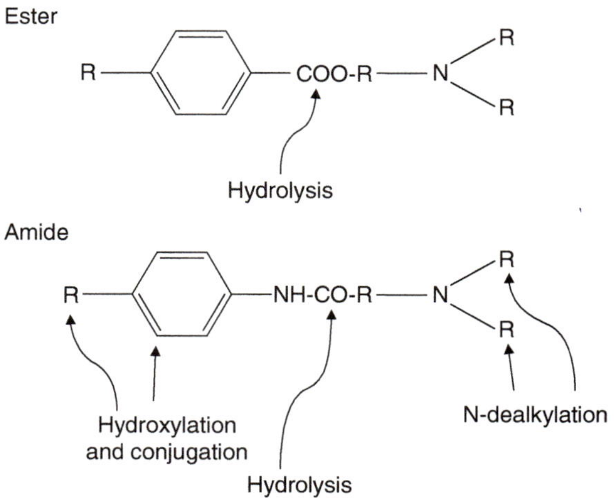

**Figure 5.2** Standard metabolism of ester- and amide-type local anesthetics, catabolic action. *Source:* Redrawn from Jastak et al. (1995).

**Table 5.2** pKa, proportions of cationic (BH$^+$), and free base (B) forms at physiological pH (7.4) and 25 °C, and relative onset for 10 local anesthetics.

| pKa | BH$^+$/B ratio | %BH$^+$ | %B | Anesthetic | Onset |
|---|---|---|---|---|---|
| 7.6 | 1.6/1 | 61 | 39 | — | Early |
| 7.7 | 2/1 | 65 | 35 | Mepivacaine Etidocaine | |
| 7.8 | 2.5/1 | 71 | 29 | Articaine | |
| 7.9 | 3.2/1 | 76 | 24 | Lidocaine Prilocaine | |
| 8.0 | 4/1 | 80 | 20 | — | Intermediate |
| 8.1 | 4.8/1 | 83 | 17 | Bupivacaine Ropivacaine | |
| 8.5 | 6.3/1 | 92 | 8 | Tetracaine | Late |
| 8.8 | 25/1 | 96 | 4 | Cocaine | |
| 9.0 | 40/1 | 97 | 3 | Procaine | |

pKa values as in Annex 6.

## Dissociation Constant or pKa

The dissociation constant or pKa, also known as the ionization constant, is related to the amino terminus. As noted above the N-terminus has two forms, cationic (BH$^+$) and free base (B), that are in equilibrium, although the proportion of one and the other depends on the following two factors (Covino 1972).

1) The dissociation constant or pKa specific to each anesthetic is defined as the pH at which 50% of the molecules in the local anesthetic adopt the BH$^+$ form and the other 50% the B form (Table 5.2).

2) The pH of the tissues because this modifies the proportion of the dissociated forms in keeping with the Henderson–Hasselbalch equation (Henderson 1908; Hasselbalch 1917):

$$pKa - pH\,tissues = \log\frac{BH^+}{B}$$

whereby

$$pH\,tissues = \log\frac{BH^+}{B} + pKa$$

Although the physiological pH is 7.4, the pH in tissues may drop to 6 or lower in the presence of inflammation or pus (Schade et al. 1921; De Jong and Cullen 1963). The proportion of the B form, which diffuses across cell membranes, consequently declines, rendering the anesthetic less effective since a smaller amount reaches the axon interior.

The pKa value effects two properties of local anesthetics: the onset of action and anesthetic potency.

1) *Onset of local anesthetic action.* The lower the pKa, the greater the proportion of free base (B) in the anesthetic in tissues at physiological pH (7.4) and the speedier its diffusion inside the axon after crossing the cell membrane. In the axon interior (axoplasm) it reaches a new B $\leftrightarrow$ BH$^+$ equilibrium, enabling the cationic form (BH$^+$) to act on the protein receptor (Ritchie et al. 1965a, b), blocking the sodium channels and with them the nerve impulse. This is the property that pKa affects most significantly.

2) *Anesthetic potency.* The lower the pKa, the higher the potency of the local anesthetic, as more anesthetic penetrates the membrane more quickly, leaving less outside to be captured by the bloodstream (Courtney 1980; Wildsmith et al. 1987). The effect of pKa is minor here, acting merely as a coadjutant. As discussed below, other factors such as lipid solubility have a heavier impact on the potency of local anesthetics.

## Partition Coefficient or Lipid Solubility

The partition coefficient or lipid solubility, also known as the diffusion coefficient, a measure of the relative penetration of drugs in biological membranes, is closely related to drug–cell membrane component binding. While the partition coefficient is actually a measure of lipid solubility, in practice the two terms are used indistinctly (Tucker et al. 1970). The two best-known methods for determining lipid solubility yield very different values, although as the data in Table 5.3 shows, they exhibit a consistent pattern.

Lipid solubility affects a number of properties of local anesthetics, as discussed below.

1) *Relative anesthetic potency.* The higher the lipid solubility, the higher the anesthetic potency. Although it is the single most important factor in anesthetic potency (Courtney 1980; Wildsmith et al. 1987), others act as coadjutants: (i) as noted earlier, pKa impacts potency, which is greater at lower pKa values; (ii) binding to blood plasma proteins also plays a role, for the more strongly the anesthetic binds, the higher is it potency (Truant and Takman 1959; Tucker et al. 1970); and (iii) the larger the size of the drug molecule, the higher the potency (Courtney 1980; Butterworth and Strichartz 1990). The reference for anesthetic potency, procaine, is assigned a value of 1 and all other anesthetics are measured against that standard.

2) *Relative toxicity.* Lipid solubility is closely related to toxicity (Covino 1987; Garfield and Grugino 1987), such that the higher the former the higher the latter (Covino 1972; Gangorosa 1981). Procaine, which is also the reference for toxicity, is assigned a value of 1 and all other anesthetics are measured against that standard.

3) *Topical anesthetic effectiveness* (Gangorosa 1981). Although topical anesthesia depends on both the lipid solubility and anesthetic concentration, a certain level

Table 5.3 Relationship between lipid solubility (calculated with two methods) and properties of local anesthetics.

| | Lipid solubility | | Anesthetic property | | |
|---|---|---|---|---|---|
| Anesthetic | N-heptane | N-octanol | Topical anesthesia | Relative potency | Relative toxicity |
| Procaine | 0.02 | 2 | No | 1 | 1 |
| Articaine | 0.7 | 15 | No | 2 | 2 |
| Mepivacaine | 0.8 | 20 | No | 2 | 2 |
| Prilocaine | 0.9 | 25 | No | 1.5 | 1.5 |
| Lidocaine | 2.9 | 45 | Yes | 2 | 2 |
| Benzocaine | 3.1 | 80 | Yes | — | — |
| Ropivacaine | 3.4 | 115 | Yes | — | — |
| Tetracaine | 4.1 | 220 | Yes | 8 | 8 |
| Bupivacaine | 27.5 | 350 | Yes | 8 | 8 |
| Etidocaine | 141.0 | 800 | Yes | 6 | 6 |

Lipid solubility as in Annex 7; relative toxicity as in Annex 8.

of lipid solubility can be defined that ensures good topical anesthetic action with no need to increase the concentration to intolerably high proportions (Table 5.3).

### Protein Binding

The ability of local anesthetics to bind to plasma proteins has been studied primarily for $\alpha_1$-acid glycoprotein (Routledge et al. 1980; Meunier et al. 2001) and to a lesser extent, albumin (Mather et al. 1971; Meunier et al. 2001). An equilibrium between the fraction of anesthetic bound to proteins and the free portion is reached in a matter of microseconds (Widman 1975), the latter being the pharmacologically active fraction (Tucker et al. 1970; Tucker and Mather 1975).

Anesthetic binding to proteins *conditions the duration of their effect*: the more strongly they bind, the longer the duration (Covino 1981; Milam and Giovannitti Jr. 1984). That is because the transmembrane receptors for local anesthetics are also proteins (Covino 1981). These considerations are summarized in Table 5.4.

### Vasodilation

Nearly all local anesthetics generate vasodilation in two ways: (i) they cause the smooth muscle cells lining the vessels to relax (Aps and Reynolds 1976; Covino and Giddon 1981) and (ii) they block sympathetic type B nerve fibers that control vasoconstriction. However, exceptions exist.

- Cocaine has an indirect vasoconstrictive effect because it blocks mono-amine-oxidase (MAO), an enzyme, preventing the recapture of nerve ending norepinephrine, which is a vasoconstrictor (Muscholl 1961; Covino and Giddon 1981).

Table 5.4 Percentage of local anesthetics bound to proteins and duration of anesthetic effect.

| Anesthetic | Binding to proteins (%) | Duration of anesthetic |
|---|---|---|
| Procaine | 5 | Short |
| Prilocaine | 55 | Medium |
| Articaine | 60 | |
| Lidocaine | 65 | |
| Mepivacaine | 75 | |
| Tetracaine | 85 | Long |
| Ropivacaine | 95 | |
| Etidocaine | 95 | |
| Bupivacaine | 95 | |

Data on protein bonds as in Annex 9.

- Mepivacaine is slightly vasoconstrictive (Du Mesnil de Rochemont and Hensel 1960; Lindorf et al. 1974; Lindorf 1979; Vongsavan et al. 2000), as is ropivacaine (Iida et al. 2001; Timponi et al. 2006), although the effect is less widely acknowledged in the latter (De Oliveira et al. 2014).

Vasodilation increases blood flow and with it, anesthetic transport, which in turn lowers anesthetic potency and duration (Widman 1975; Aps and Reynolds 1976). One curious effect is that the higher the concentration of the drug, the greater is its vasodilatory effect, partially offsetting the increase in potency afforded by higher concentrations (Aps and Reynolds 1976; Reynolds et al. 1976). The clinical conclusion is that the greater the vasodilatory effect of an anesthetic, the greater the benefit to be administered with a vasoconstrictor, which enhances anesthetic potency and duration, hindering vascular absorption of the local anesthetic and thereby lowering the risk of systemic toxicity. Further to the data listed in Table 5.5, in amide-type anesthetics, the vasodilatory effect rises with anesthetic potency (Covino and Giddon 1981).

## Assessment of Anesthesia and the Anesthetic Parameter

A number of methods have been deployed to assess the efficacy of local anesthetic solutions. The earliest involved *in vitro* trials with the sciatic nerves from frogs (Truant and Takman 1959; Bianchi and Strobel 1968) or the pneumogastric nerves from rabbits (Wildsmith et al. 1987). In humans, efficacy has been assessed via needle prick after dermal infiltration or (more sophisticated) ulnar nerve infiltration (Löfström 1975), in addition to evaluation using the various local anesthetic techniques.

### Assessment of Local Anesthesia in Dentistry

Such methods are insufficient in dentistry, as the dental pulp is an organ not present in any other part of the body and which is very difficult to anesthetize. Unlike readily anesthetized soft tissues where the effect is long-lasting, the duration of pulpal anesthesia is much shorter (Björn 1946; Björn and Huldt 1947) (Figure 5.3).

An effective assessment method was developed in 1946 by Hilding Björn (1907–1995), who used an electric pulp tester (EPT) to study the efficacy of anesthetic solutions. The device may be applied repeatedly to assess the duration of pulpal anesthesia, the criteria for which is if the tooth fails to respond to the maximum stimulus of the EPT. The reasoning behind this is that if the patient feels discomfort at less than the maximum stimulus, then there is a risk that

Table 5.5 Vasodilatory effect of local anesthetics.

| Anesthetic | Type | Vasodilatory effect | Intensity of effect | Reference |
|---|---|---|---|---|
| Procaine | Ester | +++ | Very high | Du Mesnil de Rochemont and Hensel (1960), Lindorf et al. (1974), Lindorf (1979) |
| Tetracaine | Ester | ++ | High | Martindale (1982) |
| Bupivacaine | Amide | ++ | | Aps and Reynolds (1976), Reynolds et al. (1976) |
| Etidocaine | Amide | ++ | | Eicholizer and Feldman (1976) |
| Lidocaine | Amide | + | Moderate | Du Mesnil de Rochemont and Hensel (1960), Lindorf et al. (1974), Lindorf (1979), Muschaweck and Rippel (1974), Aps and Reynolds (1976), Reynolds et al. (1976) |
| Articaine | Amide | + | | Muschaweck and Rippel (1974) |
| Prilocaine | Amide | ± | Dilation, weak | Aström and Persson (1961), Akerman et al. (1966), Lindorf et al. (1974), Lindorf (1979), Reynolds et al. (1976), Chng et al. (1996) |
| Mepivacaine | Amide | − | Weak | Du Mesnil de Rochemont and Hensel (1960), Lindorf et al. (1974), Lindorf (1979), Vongsavan et al. (2000) |
| Ropivacaine | Amide | − | | Iida et al. (2001), Timponi et al. (2006) |
| Cocaine | Ester | − | High | Muscholl (1961) |

+ vasodilation; − vasoconstriction.

Figure 5.3 Concentration required to anesthetize soft tissue and pulp, showing much lower concentration and much longer duration in soft tissue. *Source:* Redrawn from Haglund and Evers (1985).

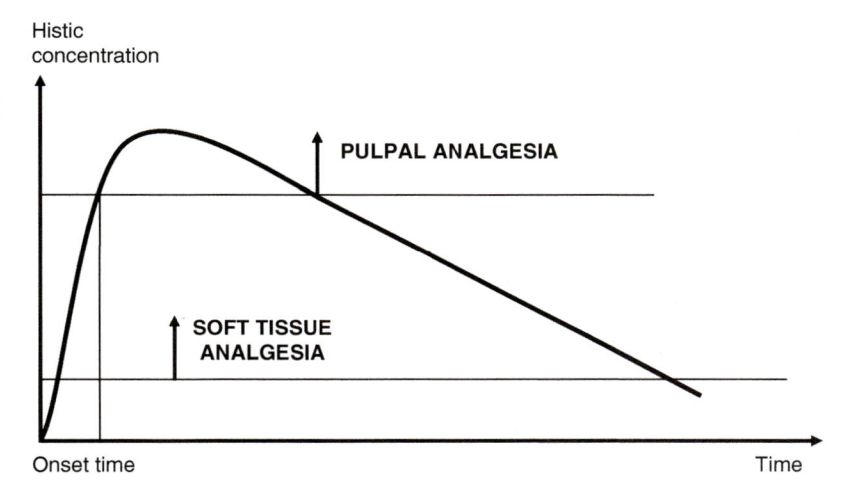

the patient may respond to stimuli during the dental procedure (Björn 1946; Björn and Huldt 1947; Certosimo and Archer 1996). Moreover, successive electrical testing over a given time has been shown to induce no harm in the dental pulp (McDaniel et al. 1973). Recent research has found that the myelinated Aδ fibers in the pulp are stimulated by the EPT, whereas the unmyelinated polymodal C fibers are not (Lin and Chandler 2008; Sampaio et al. 2012).

Björn standardized the procedure by selecting the maxillary lateral incisor (LI) as the target, as this tooth exhibits scant anatomical variations and can be anesthetized with buccal infiltration, a simple technique which also limits individual variation. By injecting 1 ml of solution, Björn ensured that the experimental conditions were standardized and reproducible in all the series studied (Björn 1947; Björn and Huldt 1947). Such standardization is lacking in other methods (i.e. restorations, scaling, root canals, extractions) and uniform pain stimulus is difficult to attain and assess, and such methods furnish no information on the anesthetic effect in the pulp.

Mandibular block studies are useful for obtaining clinical information on that anesthetic technique and its limitations, but are of scant utility in assessing the effectiveness of local anesthetic solutions for a number of reasons.

1) Technique sensitivity: As the technique is more difficult, failures due to technical errors are common. High interindividual variability, in turn, renders it more difficult to standardize.
2) Accessory innervations: Despite a successful block indicated by an anesthetized lower lip, the patient may still

have sensation in the pulp due to the high frequency of accessory innervation in the lower arch such as the buccal nerve and mylohyoid nerve (see Chapter 19).
3) Anatomic variation: Anatomic variation in the mandible such as double mandibular foramen, accessory canals, high lingula, and variable gonial angle may result in anesthetic failure despite the use of correctly implemented standardized techniques to fail (see Chapter 19).

All the above-mentioned variables are difficult to control and standardize, and thus reduce the utility of using mandibular block injections to assess local anesthetic solution efficacy.

### Anesthetic Parameter

Certain variables, listed below, may be used as surrogate indicators of the clinical efficacy of anesthetic solutions, and these indicators may vary depending on the specific local anesthetic and vasoconstrictor, and their respective concentrations.

- Of the four variables selected here (Annexes 21 and 27), three are related to buccal infiltration of the maxillary lateral incisor (LI) with 1 ml of the local anesthetic solution (Annex 21):
  1) The percentage of LI pulpal anesthesia, i.e. the % of times the tooth is successfully anesthetized: 95%, for example.
  2) The mean duration in minutes of pulpal anesthesia in the LI: 45 minutes (written as 45′), for example.
  3) The mean duration in minutes of soft tissue anesthesia (upper lip anesthesia): 190 minutes (190′), for example.
- The fourth is related to mandibular block with 1.8 ml (equivalent to one cartridge) of the solution using the direct or conventional technique (Annex 27):
  4) The mean duration in minutes of lower lip anesthesia (soft tissue anesthesia): 200 minutes (200′), for example.

These four variables were used to build the anesthetic parameter, as follows: *95%-45′/190′-200′*. This is the parameter for the standard solution, 2% lidocaine with 1:100 000 epinephrine (10 µg/ml) (L-100) or 1:80 000 epinephrine (12.5 µg/ml) (L-80). It means that injection of 1 ml of this solution in the maxillary lateral incisor ensures pulpal anesthesia in 95% of individuals that lasts on average for 45 minutes. In addition, soft tissue anesthesia lasts 190 minutes in the upper lip and 200 minutes in the lower, in the latter case after mandibular block with 1.8 ml of anesthetic solution. The first two values (% of anesthesia and duration in minutes of pulpal anesthesia) assess the potency and efficacy of the local anesthetic solution and the other two (duration of upper and lower lip anesthesia) provide information that can be conveyed to patients about the approximate post-procedure duration of the perceivable effects (Figure 5.3).

The main advantage to this approach is that different solutions can be compared in a standard format, helping to choose the anesthetic solution best suited to the circumstances and to predict the expected results.

## Anesthetic Concentration

Concentration is a factor particularly relevant to the efficacy and toxicity of local anesthetics, which are typically available in a number of dilutions.

### Concentration and Volume

Medical practice often calls for anesthetizing large areas of (readily anesthetized) soft tissue, which in turn requires large volumes of anesthetic solution (20–30 ml for caudal or epidural block and up to 60 ml for intercostal or brachial plexus block). More diluted solutions are used under such conditions, with a lower concentration of anesthetic (Moore et al. 1972, 1977) and a standard epinephrine concentration of 1:200 000 (5 µg/ml) (Bonica 1959; Moore et al. 1972).

In dentistry, by contrast, the area involved is small and the target tissue is the dental pulp, which is very difficult to anesthetize. As a result, small volumes of more highly concentrated anesthetic solutions and vasoconstrictors are used (note: doses of over 5–7 ml per session, equivalent to three to four 1.8 ml cartridges, are rare) (Table 5.6). In dentistry, the standard epinephrine concentration is 1:100 000 (10 µg/ml), double the standard value applied in other areas of medical practice.

Table 5.6 Most commonly used concentrations of local anesthetics and epinephrine in medical and dental practice.

| Drug | Medicine | Dentistry |
| --- | --- | --- |
| Lidocaine | 1–2% | 2% |
| Mepivacaine | 1–2% | 2–3% |
| Prilocaine | 2% | 3–4% |
| Epinephrine Standard concentration | 1:200 000 (5 µg/ml) | 1:100 000 (10 µg/ml) |

## Concentration and Safety

In the early twentieth century the systemic toxicity of anesthetics was believed to rise exponentially with linear increases in their concentration, so that 1 ml of 2% procaine was deemed to be four times more toxic than 1 ml of a 1% solution (Waters 1933). That notion was accepted by the Council on Dental Therapeutics, which prohibited the use of 4% procaine (Council on Dental Therapeutics 1944).

Everett was the first to prove that in laboratory animals the median lethal dose, $LD_{50}$, barely varied with concentration, but depended critically on the total dose administered (Everett 1949) (Table 5.7). Those findings were confirmed by clinical studies: the blood levels of local anesthetics are directly related to the amount administered and not to the concentration at which they are administered (Campbell and Adriani 1958; Braid and Scott 1965; Jebson 1971; Rood and Cannell 1978).

## Concentration and Anesthetic Potency

Anesthetic potency has long been known to rise with concentration in animals (Gasser and Erlanger 1929; Campbell and Adriani 1958). In clinical dental studies 5% lidocaine was observed to yield better results than the 2% solution (Eldridge and Rood 1977; Rood and Sowray 1980; Lambrianidis et al. 1980). Clinical trials using the Björn EPT also proved that more highly concentrated solutions anesthetized dental pulp more effectively (Table 5.8).

The reason is that a more highly concentrated local anesthetic tends to maintain a higher concentration is some of the injected local anesthetic may diffuse away from the initial injection site. Starting off with a more concentrated local anesthetic will result in more of the local anesthetic reaching the nerve fibers, thus translating into greater efficacy (Tainter et al. 1953; Schilli 1977).

## Concentration and Tissue Irritation

At higher concentrations of local anesthetics, the post-injection damage to subcutaneous tissue is more likely to rise. For reasons of tissue toxicity, bupivacaine cannot be administered at concentrations of over 1%, for instance, and is consequently used at 0.25–0.75% (Ekblom and Widman 1966; Henn and Brattsand 1966). Similarly, an increase in concentration can be correlated with an increased risk of tissue irritation for other local ansesthetics (Bennett et al. 1971).

Animal experiments have shown that the neurotoxicity of anesthetic solutions rises with concentration (Lundy et al. 1933; Tui et al. 1944; Skou 1954; Fink and Kish 1976; Kalichman et al. 1993).

These results are also confirmed in clinical studies. In medical practice, spinal anesthesia with 5% lidocaine or 1% tetracaine solutions (high concentrations) increases the risk of producing cauda equina syndrome because of its neurotoxic effect (Ringler et al. 1991).

Long-term paresthesia after mandibular block with high concentrations of local anesthesia is a risk in dentistry.

Table 5.7 Lethal dose ($LD_{50}$, mg/kg) of local anesthetics in animals.

| Anesthetic | Ad. | Animal | Concentration (%) | $LD_{50}$ (mg/kg) | Reference |
|---|---|---|---|---|---|
| Procaine | SC | Mouse | 2 | 900 | Everett (1949) |
| | | | 4 | ±890 | |
| | IV | Rabbit | 2 | 50 | |
| | | | 4 | ±49 | |
| Mepivacaine | IV | Mouse | 2 | 31 | Luduena et al. (1960) |
| | | | 3 | 32 | |
| | IV | Rabbit | 2 | 21 | |
| | | | 3 | 22 | |
| | IV | Guinea pig | 2 | 24.5 | |
| | | | 3 | 20.0 | |
| | SC | Guinea pig | 2 | 93 | |
| | | | 3 | 94 | |
| Articaine | IV | Rabbit | 3 | 20.6 | Baeder et al. (1974) |
| | | | 4 | 19.6 | |

Ad, administered; SC, subcutaneous; IV intravenous.

Table 5.8 Percentage of pulpal anesthesia and duration in minutes after buccal infiltration of 1 ml of anesthetic (without vasoconstrictor) in maxillary lateral incisor.

| Anesthetic | Concentration (%) | Pulpal anesthesia (%) | Duration pulpal anesthesia (min) | Reference |
| --- | --- | --- | --- | --- |
| Lidocaine | 1 | 60 | <1 | Feldman and Nordenram (1959) |
| | 3 | 95 | 3 | Feldman and Nordenram (1959) |
| Mepivacaine | 1 | 85 | 2 | Feldman and Nordenram (1959) |
| | 3 | 91 | 15 | Annex 21 |
| Articaine | 2 | 63 | 7 | Winther and Nathalang (1972) |
| | 4 | 76 | 11 | Winther and Nathalang (1972) |
| Prilocaine | 2 | 74 | 9 | Berling and Björn (1960) |
| | 4 | 87 | 12 | Annex 21 |

With 4% articaine and 4% prilocaine (Haas and Lennon 1995; Pogrel and Thambys 2000) the risk is 22–35 times greater than with standard 2% lidocaine (Table 22.8, Chapter 22). Fortunately, however, such complications are very rare (see Chapter 22).

One may conclude that a more highly concentrated local anesthetic will deliver better clinical results for the comfort of the dental patient. An important caveat is that smaller volumes of solution must be administered to avoid exceeding the maximum recommended dose, and preventing systemic toxicity or local neurotoxicity. In short, a balance must be consistently pursued between maximum efficacy and minimum risk.

## Maximum Doses

A standard maximum dose cannot be determined because conditions vary widely between individuals and even in one and the same person under different circumstances. Nonetheless, maximum doses based on animal experiments and clinical experience afford very useful guidelines for preventing toxicity in dental procedures (Campbell and Adriani 1958; Adriani and Zepernick 1966).

The absolute maximum doses for adults weighing 70 kg or over differ in dental and medical practice. In the early 1980s, the American Dental Association's Council on Dental Therapeutics recommended lower maximum doses for dental applications of lidocaine, mepivacaine, and prilocaine than established by the United States Food and Drug Administration (US FDA) and the pharmaceutical industry for applications in other types of medical practice (Table 5.9) (American Dental Association 1984). At around the same time, the FDA authorized 1.8-ml cartridges of bupivacaine for dental use, likewise a lower maximum dose than used in medicine (Dean 1983; ADA Guide 2003). This criterion was justified by the greater frequency of local anesthetic administration in dentistry, most of which are performed in the office setting, making the recognition and management of adverse reactions less predictable (Moore 1984). This lower dose criterion has always been regarded as one of the factors contributing to the extreme safety of dental anesthesia (Seldin 1958). Such prudence in using lower maximum doses than established for medical practice is recommended here as well as by other authors (Jeske and Blanton 2002).

*Articaine*, a local anesthetic, was approved by the FDA in 2000 for dental use at a concentration of 4%, double the concentration approved for 2% lidocaine (Weaber 1999; Malamed et al. 2001). Articaine and lidocaine have similar characteristics. *In vitro* studies have shown articaine to be slightly more effective (Den Hertog 1974; Borchard and Drouin 1980; Potocnik et al. 2006) and in clinical trials to yield similar or slightly better results with or without epinephrine at a given concentration (Winther and Nathalang 1972; Winther and Patirupanusara 1974). Performance was also better in animal experiments studying acute toxicity (Annex 8).

Further to the Council on Dental Therapeutics' prudent criterion, the absolute maximum dose of articaine in dentistry would be 300 mg (4.3 mg/kg) (Table 5.9). However, the pharmacokinetic properties of articaine differ from those of lidocaine and mepivacaine. At 4.17 l/min, its clearance level is much higher than the 0.83 l/min for lidocaine and 0.74 l/ml mepivacaine. Articaine's half-life is much shorter: 25 minutes compared to 110 minutes for lidocaine and 120 minutes for mepivacaine (Annex 11). The reason for the above behavior is that 85–95% of the ester side chain on the thiophene ring in articaine is rapidly hydrolyzed by plasma cholinesterases (Figure 5.4). The result is the rapid

Table 5.9 Absolute maximum doses in milligrams (mg/kg in parentheses) recommended by different sources for medical and dental practice for adults weighing 70 kg or over.

| Anesthetic | Medical practice | | | Dental practice | |
|---|---|---|---|---|---|
| | Without vasoconstrictor | With vasoconstrictor | Reference | With and without vasoconstrictor | Reference |
| Lidocaine | 300 (4.3) | 500 (7.1) | a,b,c | 300 (4.3) | d |
| Articaine | 300 (4.3) | 500 (7.1) | b | 500 (7) | c,e,f |
| | — | 500 (7.1) | c | | |
| Mepivacaine | 400 (5.7) | 400 (5.7) | a,c | 300 (4.3) | d |
| | 300 (4.3) | 500 (7.1) | b | | |
| Prilocaine | 600 (8.5) | 600 (8.5) | a,c | 400 (5.7) | d |
| | 400 (5.7) | 600 (8.5) | b | | |
| Bupivacaine | 175 (2.5) | 225 (3.2) | a,d | 90 (1.3) | c,e |
| | — | 225 (3.2) | c | | |
| | 150 (2.1) | 150 (2.1) | b | | |

[a] AMA Drug Evaluation (1983).
[b] Die Arzneimittelkommission (1985).
[c] ADA Guide (2003).
[d] American Dental Association (1984).
[e] AAPD (2020).
[f] Council on Clinical Affairs (2015).

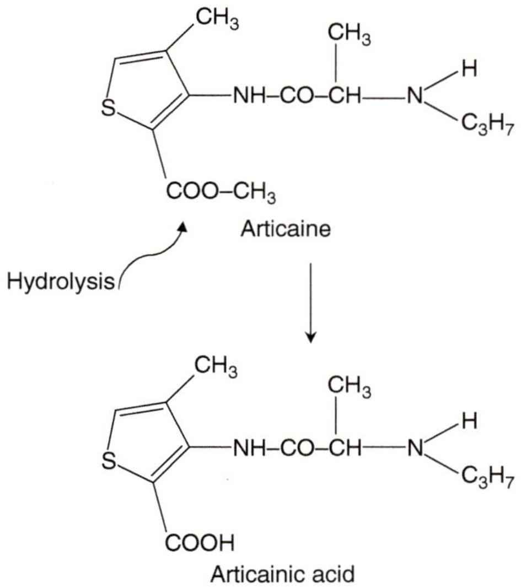

Figure 5.4 Hydrolysis of the ester side chain on the thiophene ring in articaine and its conversion to articainic acid.

inactivation of articaine and conversion to articainic acid, which lacks anesthetic or CNS effects. Moreover, as in lidocaine, only 5–15% of the drug is broken down in the liver (Isen 2000; Rahn and Ball 2001). Consequently, clinical trials have shown articaine doses of 7 mg/kg to be well tolerated in both adults (Hersh et al. 2006) and children (Dudkiewiez et al. 1987; Malamed et al. 2000).

In spite of articaine's rapid metabolic inactivation and safety profile, the provider must be cognizant of the potential for this metabolism to be affected in individuals with a hereditary defect in plasma cholinesterase, either quantitatively or qualitatively. One in every 3000 individuals is known to have a hereditary deficit of or alteration in plasma cholinesterase (Kalow and Gunn 1959). In those cases, like lidocaine, the metabolism of articaine would rely on the liver. The maximum dose of articaine in dentistry is deemed here to be higher than 300 mg (4.3 mg/kg), and as signs of toxicity may appear at 500–800 mg (Rahn and Ball 2001), the absolute maximum dose proposed is 500 mg (7 mg/kg), which at 4% is equivalent to seven 1.8-ml or seven and a half 1.7-ml cartridges (Council on Clinical Affairs 2015; AAPD 2020) (Table 5.9).

## Maximum Doses for Children

The maximum doses for adults must be corrected for children for several reasons:

1) Children have less body mass and hence a lower capacity to metabolize drugs.
2) Children's organ systems are immature and in children under 3 years enzymatic capacity is relatively lower.
3) The distribution of total body water differs between children and adults. Children around 7 years old have

(proportionately) 5% more body water than adults and medication is distributed primary in the extracellular space.
4) Many drugs tend to be stored in adipose tissue, of which children have approximately 10% less than adults.

Ritschel (1992) reviewed 24 methods for calculating pediatric doses, examining a total of 52 equations as well as adjustment tables on body surface area, age, and weight in an attempt to draw some relationship between body mass and maturity. The three methods used in dentistry are:

1) Body surface area, such as the Butler–Ritchie (Butler and Ritchie 1960) method, which specifies the highest dose for each pediatric age group (Calatayud et al. 1996).
2) Age, such as the Bastedo (1918) or Young (Ritschel 1992) methods, which specify the lowest doses for each pediatric age group (Calatayud et al. 1996). That approach is in line with growth trends over the last 100 years, according to which children are now taller and heavier (Tanner 1966) due to improved nutrition, medical progress (fewer infections thanks interventions such as to antibiotics and vaccinations), and higher standards of living (housing, clothing, etc.). Many authors consequently prefer weight-based over age-based methods (Goodson and Moore 1983).
3) Weight, such as the Clark weight method (American Dental Association 1984; Ritschel 1992; Anderson et al. 1994). This method, the one most commonly applied, consists of dividing the absolute maximum dose by 70 (weight in kilograms of a standard adult) and multiplying the quotient by the child's weight in kilograms. The resulting dose is an intermediate value for each pediatric age group specified in the two preceding methods. Weight, moreover, has proven to be the factor with the greatest effect on oxygen consumption, biochemical activity, physiological activity, and the size and activity of the body's organs and viscera (Adolph 1949).

*Annex 10 is based on weight* (Council on Clinical Affairs 2015; AAPD 2020), although adapted to the number of cartridges. It includes a very useful table for determining the number of (1.8-ml) cartridges of a given local anesthetic solution that can be administered to a child or small adult depending on their weight.

## Pregnancy and Lactation

Pregnant and breastfeeding women require special consideration because some drugs may have an adverse effect on the fetus or breastfed infant.

### Pregnancy

Most drugs cross the placental barrier during pregnancy and can consequently affect the fetus. The first quarter (15th–90th day of gestation), characterized by organogenesis, is regarded as the period when the fetus is most vulnerable to possible drug-induced congenital alterations (Ouanounou and Haas 2016).

In 2014 the FDA published its new "pregnancy and lactation labeling rule" (PLLR) (also know as the "final rule"), which entered into force on June 30, 2015. The timelines for implementing the final rule are variable. Prescription drugs submitted for FDA approval after June 30, 2015 will use the new format, while drugs approved prior to June 30, 2001 will be phased in gradually (Department of Health and Human Services, Food and Drug Administration 2014). Local dental anesthetics and vasoconstrictors are consequently still subject to the 1979 FDA "pregnancy risk classification" rule with five categories: A, B, C, D, and X (Department of Health, Education, and Welfare, Food and Drug Administration 1979; FDA 1979; Millstein 1980) (Table 5.10). The 0.7% of medications are classified in category A and the 19% in B are deemed safe (Haas et al. 2000). Two-thirds (66%, Haas et al. 2000) are classified in category C, further divided into two subcategories: (i) those that have proven to induce fetal alternations in animals and (ii) those for which no data is in place for animals or humans, a finding difficult to interpret. Moreover, the alterations in animals vary widely, from clearly teratogenic (birth defects) to merely toxic (Hubbard 1997). Even when listed under category C, however, the local anesthetics and vasoconstrictors used in dentistry can be regarded as safe (Haas et al. 2000; Donaldson and Goodchild 2012; Ouanounou and Haas 2016) (Table 5.11). A trial study with 351 women at 13–21 weeks' gestation (Michalowicz et al. 2008), and a cohort study with over 1000 pregnant women (Hagai et al. 2015) showed that *neither dental local anesthesia nor dental treatment during pregnancy raise the newborn malformation rate (teratogenic risk) or serious adverse events* (spontaneous abortions).

Epinephrine can alter the blood flow to the uterus, although at the doses used in dentistry the effect is negligible (Stepke et al. 1994; Haas et al. 2000). Felypressin however, as a derivative of vasopressin and oxytocin, not only reduces the blood flow to the uterus as a result of vasoconstriction, but also increases contraction in the organ, which may raise the risk of premature delivery or miscarriage (Oliver 1974; Stepke et al. 1994). It is consequently contraindicated during pregnancy, as is norepinephrine, which has effects on the uterus not generated by epinephrine (Stepke et al. 1994).

Lastly, a reminder: the fetal–maternal equilibrium is only affected by the free form of drugs circulating in the

Table 5.10 US FDA pregnancy risk classification.

| Risk category | Definition | Clinical guidelines, dentistry |
|---|---|---|
| A | The results of controlled studies in women fail to demonstrate a risk to the fetus in the first trimester (and there is no evidence of risk in later trimesters), and the possibility of fetal harm appears remote | Very safe |
| B | Either the results of animal reproduction studies have not demonstrated a fetal risk but there are no controlled studies in pregnant women<br>Or<br>The results of animal reproduction studies have shown an adverse effect (other than a decrease in fertility) that was not confirmed in controlled studies in women in the first trimester and there is no evidence of risk in later trimesters | Safe |
| C | Either the results of studies in animal have reveled adverse effects (teratogenic, embryocidal, or other) on the fetus and there are no controlled studies in women<br>Or<br>Results of studies in women and animals are not available; drug should be given only if the potential benefit justifies the potential risk to the fetus | Uncertain |
| D | There is positive evidence of human fetal risk, but the benefits of use in pregnant women may be acceptable despite the risk (e.g., if the drug is needed in a life-threatening situation or for a serious disease for which safer drugs cannot be used or are ineffective) | Contraindicated |
| X | Results of studies in animals or humans have demonstrated fetal abnormalities or evidence of fetal risk based on human experience, or both, and the risk of the use of the drug in pregnancy women clearly outweighs any possible benefit; use of the drug is contraindicated in women who are or may become pregnant | Contraindicated |

*Source*: Department of Health, Education, and Welfare, Food and Drug Administration (1979), FDA (1979), Millstein (1980), Donaldson and Goodchild (2012), Ouanounou and Haas (2016).

bloodstream unbound to plasma proteins and therefore able to cross the placenta (Poppers 1975).

## Lactation

For most drugs, the infant is exposed to a much higher concentration during pregnancy than during lactation. Therefore, if a drug is considered acceptable for use during pregnancy, it usually is reasonable to continue its use during breast-feeding (Donaldson and Goodchild 2012). As a general rule, the infant ingests approximately 1% of the maternal dose, although that percentage may vary depending on blood flow in the mammary gland, blood, or milk pH, drug molecular weight, lipid solubility, etc. (Haas et al. 2000).

Clinical studies (Lebedevs et al. 1993; Ortega et al. 1999; Giuliani et al. 2001) have shown that local anesthetics can be administered to nursing mothers because at the doses normally applied in dentistry they are safe for the baby (Haas et al. 2000; Donaldson and Goodchild 2012) (Table 5.11).

## Mixing Local Anesthetics

Local anesthetics may be mixed to combine a long duration, late onset solution (tetracaine, bupivacaine) with an anesthetic with a medium or short duration and rapid onset time (procaine, lidocaine, mepivacaine, prilocaine). Theoretically, the result is a quick-acting, long-lasting anesthetic solution, usable subject only to possible rises in toxicity.

Clinical studies have delivered uneven findings. Some authors have observed advantages (Moore et al. 1972; Cunningham and Kaplan 1974) while others the contrary: Oka et al. (1997) found a bupivacaine-lidocaine mix to be long-lasting but with a delayed onset. Animal experiments involving a mix of bupivacaine and chloroprocaine showed early onset but a short duration (Galindo and Witcher 1979). In such cases mixes afford no advantage: the effects would appear to depend on only one of the anesthetics. The explanation suggested is that the use of two local anesthetics at the same site might induce competition for the transmembrane receptor, with one of the two effects prevailing to the detriment of the other (Grima et al. 1985; Oka et al. 1997).

Toxicity experiments in animals also yield contradictory results. According to some studies toxicity is merely the sum of the effects of the solutions involved (Munson et al. 1977), whereas others report a higher value (Daos et al. 1962; Akamatsu and Siebold 1967).

In light of that data and in the absence of further information, mixing local anesthetics at the same injection site is not recommended here. The following alternatives are suggested.

Table 5.11 FDA pregnancy risk category and possible use of dentistry anesthetics and vasoconstrictors during pregnancy and lactation.

| Drug | FDA category | Can be used in pregnancy | Can be used in lactation |
|---|---|---|---|
| **Injectable local anesthetic** | | | |
| Lidocaine | B[a-f] | Yes[a,c-f] | Yes[a,c-e,g] |
| Articaine | C[b,d-f] | Yes[f] <br> With caution[d,e] | Yes[a] <br> With caution[d,e] |
| Mepivacaine | C[a,f] | Yes[a,f] <br> With caution[c-e] | Yes[a,c-e] |
| Prilocaine | B[a-f] | Yes[a,c-f] | Yes[a,c-e] |
| Bupivacaine | C[a-f] | Yes[a,f] <br> With caution[c-e] | Yes[a,c-e] |
| **Vasoconstrictor** | | | |
| Epinephrine 1:100 000 1:200 000 | C[a,e] | Yes[a] <br> With caution[e] | Yes[a,e] |
| Levonordefrin 1:20 000 | Unclassified | Yes[a] | Yes[a] |
| Felypressin 0.03 UI/ml | Unclassified | No[h,i] | ? |
| Norepinephrine 1:30 000 1:50 000 | Unclassified | No[i] | ? |
| **Topical local anesthetic** | | | |
| Benzocaine | C[a,b,f] | Yes[a] <br> With caution[e,f] | Yes[a] <br> With caution[e] |
| Lidocaine | B[a,b,e,f] | Yes[a,e,f] | Yes[a,e] |
| Tetracaine | C[a,b,e,f] | Yes[a] <br> With caution[e,f] | Yes[a] <br> With caution[e] |
| Cocaine | C[b] | ? | ? |

[a] Haas et al. (2000).
[b] ADA Guide (2003).
[c] Suresh and Radfar (2004).
[d] Fayans et al. (2010).
[e] Donaldson and Goodchild (2012).
[f] Ouanounou and Haas (2016).
[g] American Academy of Pediatrics (2001).
[h] Oliver (1974).
[i] Stepke et al. (1994).

1) If periapical infiltration with 2% lidocaine and 1:100 000 epinephrine (10 μg/ml) fails in a maxillary tooth, it can be reinforced with a second injection of 2% lidocaine and 1:50 000 epinephrine (20 μg/ml). Note that the reinforcement consists of injecting a larger volume of the same local anesthetic while enhancing its potency by administering a higher concentration of the vasoconstrictor (epinephrine).
2) Mandibular block with 2% lidocaine and 1:100 000 epinephrine can be used to anesthetize mandibular molars, reinforced with periapical infiltration on the buccal side of these teeth with 4% articaine and 1:100 000 epinephrine. Note that although different anesthetics are used, they are not mixed, but administered at different sites.

By way of summary, as the data available are inconclusive, until further research findings are forthcoming, *mixing local anesthetics at the same site is not recommended here.*

## Isomers

The chemical structure of most local anesthetics is characterized by isomers or enantiomers, i.e. compounds with the same chemical structure but a different configuration, in which atoms or groups of atoms occupy different spatial positions. Because such substances rotate polarized light in opposite directions, they are also called optical isomers (Calvey 1995).

Table 5.12 Local anesthetics and optical isomers.

| Achiral[a] (non-isomers) | Racemic[a] (isomers) | Levoisomers[a] |
|---|---|---|
| Lidocaine[a,b] | Procaine | Levobupivacaine |
| Tetracaine | Articaína[c,d] | Ropivacaine |
| | Mepivacaine | |
| | Prilocaine | |
| | Bupivacaine | |
| | Etidocaine | |
| | Cocaine[e,f] | |

[a] Calvey (1995).
[b] Tucker (1986).
[c] Van Oss et al. (1989).
[d] Vree et al. (1988).
[e] Mather and Chang (2001).
[f] de Jong (1977).

There are two optical isomers (Cahn et al. 1956; Calvey 1995). Dextro (d) or (+) or R, from the Latin *rectus*, isomers rotate plane-polarized light clockwise or to the right, while the levo (l) or (−) or S, from the Latin *sinister*, counterparts rotate it to the left or counter-clockwise. Most local anesthetics adopt a *racemic form*, which means that 50% of their molecules are dextro and the other 50% levo. However, a few are achiral or not optically active because their chemical structure can only exist in one configuration, with no isomers (Table 5.12). Both lidocaine and tetracaine are achiral.

In some cases, one isomeric form may behave like an independent chemical structure, featuring higher activity or lower toxicity than the other isomer or the racemic mix. In such cases the more active isomer is dubbed the "eutomer" and the less active the "distomer" (Calvey 1995). Some long-lasting local anesthetics have been developed with the levo isomer only because it is more active, less toxic (Luduena 1969; Luduena et al. 1972; Aberg 1972; Foster and Markham 2000), or (especially) less cardiotoxic (Mather and Chang 2001). These include:

1) Levobupivacaine or S-bupivacaine is the pure levo isomer of bupivacaine. Its clinical use was introduced in 1999 and while its efficacy is similar to that of bupivacaine, it appears to be less cardiotoxic (Bardsley et al. 1998; Branco et al. 2006).
2) Ropivacaine is the pure levoisomer of propivacaine, a long-lasting local anesthetic very similar to bupivacaine. It differs in that instead of a four-carbon atom terminus (butyl, hence bupivacaine) in the piperdine ring, it has a three-C terminus (propyl, hence propivacaine). This shorter chain lowers its potency (Aberg et al. 1977) but also its toxicity for the nervous system and the heart (Akerman et al. 1988; Scott et al. 1989; Knudsen et al. 1997; Simpson et al. 2005). This anesthetic was first used in clinical practice in 1997 (Malamed 2004).

Although neither of these medications is presently marketed in cartridge form for use in dentistry, they may be a substitute for bupivacaine in the future.

# References

AAPD (American Academy of Pediatric Dentistry) (2020). *Use of Local Anesthesia for Pediatric Dental Patients. The Reference Manual of Pediatric Dentistry*. Chicago IL: American Academy of Pediatric Dentistry. 318–323.

Aberg, G. (1972). Toxicological and local anaesthetic effects of optically active isomers of two local anesthetic compounds. *Acta Pharmacol. Toxicol.* 31 (4): 273–286.

Aberg, G., Dhuner, K.-G., and Sydnes, G. (1977). Studies on the duration of local anesthesia: structure/activity relationships in a series of homologous local anesthetics. *Acta Pharmacol. Toxicol.* 41 (5): 432–443.

ADA Guide (2003). *ADA Guide to Dental Therapeutics*, 3e. Chicago: American Dental Association. 1–16 and 611.

Adolph, E.F. (1949). Quantitative relations in the physiological constitutions of mammals. *Science* 109 (2841): 579–585.

Adriani, J. and Zepernick, R. (1966). Influence of the status of the patient on systemic effects of local anesthetic agents. *Anesth. Analg.* 45 (1): 87–92.

Akamatsu, T.J. and Siebold, K.H. (1967). The synergist toxicity of local anesthetics. *Anesthesiology* 28 (1): 238.

Akerman, B., Aström, A., Ross, S., and Telc, A. (1966). Studies on the absorption, distribution and metabolism of labeled prilocaine and lidocaine in some animal species. *Acta Pharmacol. Toxicol.* 24 (4): 389–403.

Akerman, B., Hellberg, I.B., and Trossvik, C. (1988). Primary evaluation of the local anesthetic properties of the amino amide agent ropivacaine (LEA 103). *Acta Anaesth. Scand.* 32 (7): 517–518.

AMA Drug Evaluation (1983). *American Medical Association*, 5e. Philadelphia: WB Saunders Co. 373–394.

American Academy of Pediatrics Committee on Drugs (2001). The transfer of drugs and other chemicals into human milk. *Pediatrics* 108 (3): 776–789.

American Dental Association (1984). *Accepted Dental Therapeutics*, 40e. Chicago: Council on Dental Therapeutics, American Dental Association. 124–133, 185, 193.

Anderson, J.A., Dilley, D.C., and Vann, W.F. Jr. (1994). Pain and anxiety control (part I: pain perception control). In: *Pediatric Dentistry. Infancy Through Adolescence*, 2e (ed. J.R. Pinkham). Philadelphia: WB Saunders Co. 98–105.

Annex 6. Dissociation constant or pKa.

Annex 7. Partition coefficient or lipid solubility.

Annex 8. Acute experimental toxicity of local anesthetics.

Annex 9. Local anesthetic bonding to plasmatic proteins.

Annex 10. Maximum doses of dental local anesthetics solutions.

Annex 11. Pharmacokinetics of local anesthetics and vasoconstrictors.

Annex 21. Maxillary pulpal anesthesia. Buccal infiltration.

Annex 24. Mandibular block I. Efficay of standard solution L-100 or L-80.

Annex 27. Mandibular block IV. Anesthesia of the lower lip and time to first pain.

Aps, C. and Reynolds, F. (1976). The effect of concentration on vasoactivity of bupivacaine and lignocaine. *Br. J. Anaesth.* 48 (12): 1171–1174.

Aström, A. and Persson, N.H. (1961). Some pharmacological properties of o-methyl-α-propylaminopropionanilide, a new local anesthetic. *Br. J. Pharmacol.* 16 (1): 32–44.

Baeder, C., Bähr, H., Benoit, W. et al. (1974). Untersuchungen zur Verträglichkeit von Carticaine, einem neuen Lokalanästhetikum. *Prakt. Anästh.* 9 (3): 147–152.

Bardsley, H., Gristwood, R., Baker, H. et al. (1998). A comparison of the cardiovascular effects of levobupivacaine and rac-bupivacaine following intravenous administration to healthy volunteers. *Br. J. Clin. Pharmacol.* 46 (3): 245–249.

Bastedo, W.A. (1918). *Materia Medica. Pharmacology: Therapeutics Prescription Writing for Students and Practitioners*, 2e. Philadelphia: WB Saunders Co.

Bennett, C.R., Mundell, R.D., and Monheim, C.D. (1971). Studies on tissue penetration characteristics produced by jet injection. *J. Am. Dent. Assoc.* 83 (3): 625–629.

Berling, C. and Björn, C. (1960). L-67-ettnytt lokalbedövningsmedel av anilidtyp. Experimetell bes tämning av effektiviteten vid plexusa nestesi pa homo. *Sven. Tandläk-Forb. Tidn.* 52 (19): 511–522.

Bianchi, C.P. and Strobel, G.E. (1968). Modes of action of local anesthetics in nerve and muscle in relation to their uptake and distribution. *Trans. N.Y. Acad. Sci.* 30 (8): 1082–1092.

Björn, H. (1946). Electrical excitation of teeth and its application to dentistry. *Sven. Tandläk.-Tidskr.* 39 (Suppl): 7–101.

Björn, H.I. (1947). The determination of the efficiency of dental local anesthetics. *Sven. Tandläk.-Tidskr.* 40 (6): 771–796.

Björn, H. and Huldt, S. (1947). IV. The efficiency of xylocaine as a dental terminal anesthesia compared to the procaine. *Sven. Tandläk.-Tidskr.* 40 (6): 831–851.

Bonica, J.J. (1959). *Tratamiento del dolor con estudio especial del empleo del bloqueo analgésico en el diagnóstico, pronóstico y terapeútica*. Barcelona: Salvat Editores SA. 160. (Original title: The management of pain. Philadelphia: Lea and Febiger. 1953).

Borchard, U. and Drouin, H. (1980). Carticaine: action of the local anesthetic on myelinated nerve fibers. *Eur. J. Pharmacol.* 62 (1): 73–79.

Braid, D.P. and Scott, D.B. (1965). The systemic absorption of local analgesic drugs. *Br. J. Anaesth.* 37 (6): 394–404.

Branco, F.P., Ranaldi, J., Ambrosano, G.M.B., and Volpato, M.C. (2006). A double-blind comparison of 0.5% bupivacaine with 1:200,000 epinephrine and 0.5% levobupivacaine with 1:200,000 epinephrine for the inferior alveolar nerve block. *Oral Surg. Oral Med. Oral Pathol.* 101 (4): 442–447.

Butler, A.M. and Ritchie, R.H. (1960). Simplification and improvement in estimating drug dosage and fluid dietary allowances for patients of varying sizes. *N. Engl. J. Med.* 262 (18): 903–908.

Butterworth, J.F. and Strichartz, G.R. (1990). Molecular mechanism of local anesthetic: a review. *Anesthesiology* 72 (4): 711–734.

Cahn, R.S., Ingold, C.K., and Prelog, V. (1956). The specification of asymmetric configuration in organic chemistry. *Experientia (Basel)* 12 (3): 81–94.

Calatayud, J., Ceron, J., and Cacho, A. (1996). Cálculo de las dosis farmacológicas en odontopediatría. Los anestésicos locales. *Prof. Dent. (Madrid)* 10: 20–23.

Calvey, T.N. (1995). Isomerism and anesthetic drugs. *Acta Anaesthesiol. Scand.* 39 (Suppl. 106): 83–90.

Campbell, D. and Adriani, J. (1958). Absorption of local anesthetics. *J. Am. Med. Assoc.* 168 (7): 873–877.

Certosimo, A.J. and Archer, R.D. (1996). A clinical evaluation of the electric pulp tester as an indicator of local anesthesia. *Oper. Dent.* 21 (1): 25–30.

Chng, H.S., Pitt Ford, T.R., and McDonald, T. (1996). Effects of prilocaine local anaesthetic solutions on pulpal blood flow in maxillary canines. *Endod. Dent. Traumatol.* 12 (2): 89–95.

Council on Clinical Affairs (2015). Guideline on use of local anesthesia for pediatric dental patients. *Pediatr. Dent.* 37 (Special issue): 199–205.

Council on Dental Therapeutics (1944). Four per cent procaine solutions – not acceptable for ADR. *J. Am. Dent. Assoc.* 31 (3): 278–279.

Courtney, K.R. (1980). Structure–activity relations for frecuency-dependent sodium channel block in nerve by local anesthetics. *J. Pharmacol. Exp. Ther.* 213 (1): 114–119.

Covino, B.G. (1972). Local anesthesia (first part). *N. Engl. J. Med.* 286 (18): 975–983.

Covino, B.G. (1981). Physiology and pharmacology of local anesthetic agents. *Anesth. Prog.* 28 (4): 98–104.

Covino, B.G. (1987). Toxicity and systemic effects of local anesthetic agents (Chapter 6). In: *Local Anesthetics*, Handbook of Experimental Pharmacology (ed. G.R. Strichartz). Berlin: Springer-Verlag. Vol. 81: 187–212.

Covino, B.G. and Giddon, D.B. (1981). Pharmacology of local anesthetic agents. *J. Dent. Res.* 60 (8): 1454–1459.

Cunningham, N.L. and Kaplan, J.A. (1974). A rapid-onset long-acting regional anesthesia technique. *Anesthesiology* 41 (5): 509–511.

Daos, F.G., Lopez, L., and Virtue, R.W. (1962). Local anesthetic toxicity modified by oxygen and combination of agents. *Anesthesiology* 23 (6): 755–761.

De Jong, R.H. (1977). *Local Anesthetics*, 2e. Springfield (Illinois): Charles C Thomas Publisher, 39–43 and 223.

De Jong, R.H. and Cullen, S.C. (1963). Buffer-demand and pH of local anesthetic solutions containing epinephrine. *Anesthesiology* 24 (6): 801–807.

De Oliveira, A.C.A., Britto, A.C.S., Souza, L.M.A. et al. (2014). Avaliacao dos efeitos da ropivacaína sobre a reatividade vascular em arteria mesentérica de rato. *Rev. Odontol. UNESP* 43 (4): 258–264.

Dean, M. and Cook-Waite Laboratories Inc. Communication to: Moore PA, Dunsky JL (1983). Bupivacaine anesthetic – a clinical trial for endodontic therapy. *Oral Surg. Oral Med. Oral Pathol.* 55 (2): 176–179.

Den Hertog, A. (1974). The effect of carticain on mammalian non-myelinated nerve fibers. *Eur. J. Pharmacol.* 26 (2): 175–178.

Department of Health and Human Services, Food and Drug Administration (2014). Content and format of labeling for human prescription drug and biological products: requerirments for pregnancy and lactation labeling. *Fed. Register* 79 (233): 72064–72103.

Department of Health, Education, and Welfare, Food and Drug Administration (1979). Labeling and prescription drug advertising; content and format for labeling for human prescription drugs. *Fed. Register* 44 (124): 37434–37467.

Die Arzneimittelkommission der Deutschen Ärzteschaft Informiert (1985). Lokalanästhetika: Bei Anwendung in der Praxis beachten. *Dtsch. Arztebl.* 82 (3): 100–101.

Donaldson, M. and Goodchild, J.H. (2012). Pregnancy, breast-feeding and drugs used in dentistry. *J. Am. Dent. Assoc.* 143 (8): 858–871.

Dudkiewiez, A., Schwartz, S., and Laliberte, R. (1987). Effectiveness of mandibular infiltration in children using the local anesthetic Ultracain®. *J. Can. Dent. Assoc.* 53 (1): 29–31.

Du Mesnil de Rochemont, W., and Hensel, H. (1960). Messung der hautdurchblutung am menschen bei Einwirkung verscheidener lokalanasthetica. *Naunyn-Schmiedeberg Arch. Exp. Path. Pharmakol.* 239 (5): 464–474.

Eicholizer, A.W. and Feldman, H.S. (1976). Acute toxicity of etidocaine following various routes of administration in the dog. *Toxicol. Appl. Pharmacol.* 37 (1): 13–21.

Ekblom, L. and Widman, B. (1966). LAC-43 and tetracaine in spinal anaesthesia. A controlled clinical study. *Acta Anaesthesiol. Scand. (Suppl.)* 23: 419–425.

Eldridge, D.J. and Rood, J.P. (1977). A double-blind trial of 5 per cent lignocaine solution. *Br. Dent. J.* 142 (4): 129–130.

Everett, F.G. (1949). A comparison of depth of anesthesia and toxicity of two and four per cent procaine hydrochloride solution. *J. Dent. Res.* 28 (3): 204–218.

Fayans, E.P., Stuart, H.R., Carsten, D. et al. (2010). Local anesthetic use in pregnant and postpartum patient. *Dent. Clin. N. Am.* 54 (4): 697–713.

FDA (1979). Pregnancy labeling. *FDA Drug Bull.* 9 (4): 23–24.

Feldman, G. and Nordenram, A. (1959). Carbocainets och lidocainets anästetiskc effect. En jämforande experimentell undersökning. *Sven. Tandläk.-Tidskr.* 52 (11): 531–545.

Fink, B.R. and Kish, S.J. (1976). Reversible inhibition of rapid axonal transport in vivo by lidocaine hydrochloride. *Anesthesiology* 44 (2): 139–146.

Foster, R.H. and Markham, A. (2000). Levobupivacaine. A review of its pharmacology use as a local anesthetic. *Drugs* 59 (3): 551–579.

Galindo, A. and Witcher, T. (1979). Mixtures of local anesthetics: bupivacaine – chloroprocaine. *Anesthesilogy* 51 (3): S213.

Gangorosa, L.P. (1981). Newer local anesthetics and techniques for administration. *J. Dent. Res.* 60 (8): 1471–1480.

Garfield, J.M. and Grugino, L. (1987). Central effects of local anesthetic agents (Chapter 8). In: *Local Anesthetics. Handbook of Experimental Pharmacology* (ed. G.R. Strichartz). Berlin: Springer-Verlag. Vol. 81: 253–284.

Gasser, H.S. and Erlanger, J. (1929). The role of fiber size in the establishment of a nerve block by pressure or cocaine. *Am. J. Phys* 88: 581–591.

Giuliani, M., Grossi, G.B., Pileri, M. et al. (2001). Could local anesthesia while breast-feeding be harmful to infants? *J. Pediatr. Gastroenterol. Nutr.* 32 (2): 142–144.

Goodson, J.M. and Moore, P.A. (1983). Life-threatening reactions after pedodontic sedation: an assessment of narcotic, local anesthetic, and antiemetic drug interaction. *J. Am. Dent. Assoc.* 107 (2): 239–245.

Grima, M., Schwartz, J., Spach, M.-O., and Velly, J. (1985). [$^3$H]-tetracaine binding on rat synaptosomes and sodium channels. *Br. J. Pharmcol.* 86 (1): 125–129.

Haas, D.A. and Lennon, D. (1995). A 21 years retrospective study of reports of paresthesia following local anesthetic administration. *J. Can. Dent. Assoc.* 61 (4): 319–330.

Haas, D.A., Rynn, B.R., and Sands, T.D. (2000). Drug use for the pregnant or lactating patient. *Gen. Dent.* 48 (1): 54–60.

Hagai, A., Diav-Citrin, O., Shechtman, S., and Ornoy, A. (2015). Pregnancy outcome after in utero exposure to local anesthetics as part of dental treatment. *J. Am. Dent. Assoc.* 146 (8): 572–580.

Haglund, J. and Evers, H. (1985). *Local Anaesthesia in Dentistry*, 6e. Södertälje (Sweden): Astra Läkemedel AB. 14.

Hasselbalch, K.A. (1917). Die Berechnung der Wasserstoffzahl des Blutes aus der freien und gebundenen kohlensäure desselben, und die Sauerstoffbindung des Blutes als Funktion der Wasserstoffzahl. *Biochem. Z.* 78: 112–144.

Henderson, L.J. (1908). Concerning the relationship between the strength of acids and their capacity to preserve neutrality. *Am. J. Phys* 21 (2): 173–179.

Henn, F. and Brattsand, R. (1966). Some pharmacological and toxicological properties of a new long-acting long analgesic, LAC-43 (Marcaine®), in comparison with mepivacaine and tetracaine. *Acta Anaesthesiol. Scand.* 21 (suppl): 9–30.

Hersh, E.V., Ginnakopoulos, H., Levin, L.M. et al. (2006). The pharamacokinetics and cardiovascular effects of high-dose articaine with 1:100,000 and 1:200,000 epinephrine. *J. Am. Dent. Assoc.* 137 (11): 1562–1571.

Hubbard, W.K. (1997). Content and format of labeling for human prescription drugs; pregnancy labeling; public hearing. *Fed. Regist.* 62 (147): 41061–41063.

Iida, H., Ohta, H., Iida, M. et al. (2001). The differential effects of steroisomers of ropivacaine on cerebral pial arterioles in dogs. *Anesth. Analg.* 93 (6): 1552–1556.

Isen, D.A. (2000). Articaine: pharmacology and clinical use of a recently approved local anesthetic. *Dent. Today* 19 (11): 72–77.

Jastak, J.T., Yagiela, J.A., and Donaldson, D. (1995). *Local Anesthesia of the Oral Cavity*. Philadelphia: WB Saunders Co. 53.

Jebson, P. (1971). Intramuscular lignocaine 2% and 10%. *Br. Med. J.* 3 (5774): 566–567.

Jeske, A.H. and Blanton, P.L. (2002). Misconceptions involving dental local anesthesia. Part 2: Pharmacology. *Tex. Dent. J.* 119 (4): 310–314.

Kalichman, M.W., Moorehouse, D.F., Powell, H.C., and Myers, R.R. (1993). Relative neural toxicity of local anesthetics. *J. Neurophatol. Exp. Neurol.* 52 (3): 234–240.

Kalow, W. and Gunn, D.R. (1959). Some statistical data on atypical cholinesterase of human serum. *Ann. Hum. Genet.* 23 (3): 239–250.

Knudsen, K., SuurKüla, M.B., Blomberg, S. et al. (1997). Central nervous and cardiovascular effects of i.v. infusion of ropivacaine, bupivacaine and placebo in volunteers. *Br. J. Anaesth.* 78 (5): 507–514.

Lambrianidis, T., Rood, J.P., and Sowray, J.H. (1980). Dental analgesia by jet injection. *Br. J. Oral Surg.* 17: 227–231.

Lebedevs, T.H., Wojnar-Horton, R.E., Yapp, P. et al. (1993). Excretion of lignocaine and its metabolite monoethylglycinexylidide in breast milk following its use in dental procedure. A case report. *J. Clin. Periodontol.* 20 (8): 606–608.

Lin, J. and Chandler, N.P. (2008). Electric pulp testing: a review. *Int. Endod. J.* 41 (5): 265–374.

Lindorf, H.H. (1979). Investigation of the vascular effect of newer local anesthetics and vasoconstrictors. *Oral Surg. Oral Med. Oral Pathol.* 48 (4): 292–297.

Lindorf, H.H., Ganssen, A., and Mayer, P. (1974). Thermographic representation of vascular effects of local anaesthetics. *Electromedica* 42 (4): 106–110.

Löfgren, N. (1948). *Studies on Local Anesthetics: Xylocaine, a New Synthetic Drug*. Stockholm: Ivar Hoeggerströms. 13–16.

Löfgren, N. and Lundquist, B. (1946). Studies on local anaesthetics II. *Svenks Kem. Tidskr.* 58 (8): 206–217.

Löfström, J.B. (1975). Ulnar nerve blockade for the evaluation of local anesthetic agents. *Br. J. Anaesth.* 47 (suppl): 297–300.

Luduena, F.P. (1969). Duration of local anesthesia. *Ann. Rev. Pharmacol.* 9: 503–520.

Luduena, F.P., Hope, J.O., Coulston, F., and Drobeck, H.P. (1960). The pharmacology and toxicology of mepivacaine, a new local anesthetic. *Toxicol. Appl. Pharmacol.* 2 (3): 295–315.

Luduena, F.P., Bogado, E.F., and Tullar, B.F. (1972). Optical isomers of mepivacaine and bupivacaine. *Arch. Int. Pharamacodyn. Ther.* 200 (2): 359–369.

Lundy, J.S., Essex, H.E., and Kernohan, J.W. (1933). Experiments with anesthetics. IV. Lesions produced in the spinal cord of dogs by a dose of procaine hydrochloride sufficient to cause permanent and fatal paralysis. *J. Am. Med. Assoc.* 101 (20): 1546–1550.

Malamed, S.F. (2004). *Handbook of Local Anesthesia*, 5e. St. Louis (Missouri): Elsevier Mosby. 31, 62–73 and 146–147.

Malamed, S.F., Gagnon, S., and Leblanc, D. (2000). A comparison between articaine HCl and lidocaine HCl in pediatric dental patients. *Pediatr. Dent.* 22 (4): 307–311.

Malamed, S.F., Gagnon, S., and Leblanc, D. (2001). Articaine hydrochloride: a study of the safety of a new amide local anesthetic. *J. Am. Dent. Assoc.* 132 (2): 177–185.

Martindale (1982). *The Extrapharmacopeia*, 28e (ed. R. JEF). London: The Pharmaceutical Press. 899–923.

Mather, L.E. and Chang, D.H.-T. (2001). Cardiotoxicity with modern local anesthetics. Is there a safer choice? *Drugs* 61 (3): 333–342.

Mather, L.E., Long, G.J., and Thomas, J. (1971). The binding of bupivacaine to maternal and foetal plasma proteins. *J. Pharm. Pharmacol.* 23 (5): 359–365.

McDaniel, K.F., Rowe, N.H., and Charbenau, G.T. (1973). Tissue response to an electric pulp test. *J. Prosthet. Dent.* 29 (1): 84–87.

Meunier, J.-F., Goujard, E., Dubousset, A.-M. et al. (2001). Pharmacokinetics of bupivacaine after continuous epidural infusion in infants with and without biliary atresia. *Anesthesiology* 95 (1): 87–95.

Michalowicz, B.S., DiAngelis, A.J., Novak, J. et al. (2008). Examining the safety of dental treatment in pregnant woman. *J. Am. Dent. Assoc.* 139 (6): 685–695.

Milam, S.B. and Giovannitti, J.A. Jr. (1984). Local anesthetics in dental practice. *Dent. Clin. N. Am.* 28 (3): 493–508.

Miller, P.A. and Haas, D.A. (2000). Incidence of local anesthetic-induced neuropathies in Ontario from 1994–1998. *J. Dent. Res.* 79: (IADR abstracts): 627 (abstract no. 3869).

Millstein, L.G. (1980). FDA's pregnancy categories. *N. Engl. J. Med.* 303 (12): 706.

Moore, P.A. (1984). Bupivacaine: a long-lasting local anesthetic for dentistry. *Oral Surg. Oral Med. Oral Pathol.* 58 (4): 369–374.

Moore, D.C., Bridenbaugh, L.D., Bridenbaugh, P.O. et al. (1972). Doses compounding of local anesthetic agents increase their toxicity in humans? *Anesth. Analg.* 51 (4): 579–585.

Moore, D.C., Mather, L.E., Bridenbaugh, L.D. et al. (1977). Bupivacaine (Marcaine®) an evaluation of its tissue and systematic toxicity in humans. *Acta Anaesth. Scand.* 21 (2): 109–121.

Munson, E.S., Paul, W.L., and Embro, W.J. (1977). Central-nervous-system toxicity of local anesthetic mixtures in monkeys. *Anesthesiology* 46 (3): 179–183.

Muschaweck, R. and Rippel, R. (1974). Ein neues lokalanästhetikum (Carticain) aus der Thiophenreihe. *Prakt. Anästh.* 9 (3): 135–146.

Muscholl, E. (1961). Effect of cocaine and related drugs on the uptake of noradrenalina by heart and spleen. *Br. J. Pharmacol.* 16 (3): 352–359.

Oka, S., Shimamoto, C., Kyoda, N., and Misaki, T. (1997). Comparison of lidocaine with and without bupivacaine for local dental anesthesia. *Anesth. Prog.* 44 (3): 83–86.

Oliver, L.P. (1974). Local anaesthesia – a review of practice. *Aust. Dent. J.* 19 (5): 313–319.

Ortega, D., Viviand, X., Lorec, A.M. et al. (1999). Excretion of lidocaine and bupivacaine in breast milk following epidural anesthesia for cesarean delivery. *Acta Anaesthesiol. Scand.* 43 (4): 394–397.

Ouanounou, A. and Haas, D.A. (2016). Drug therapy during pregnancy: implications for dental practice. *Br. Dent. J.* 220 (8): 413–417.

Pogrel, M.A. and Thambys, S. (2000). Permanent nerve involvement resulting from inferior alveolar nerve blocks. *J. Am. Dent. Assoc.* 131 (7): 901–907.

Poppers, P.J. (1975). Evaluation of local anesthetic agents for regional anaesthesia in obstetrics. *Br. J. Anaesth.* 47 (Suppl): 322–327.

Potocnik, I., Tomsic, M., Sketelj, J., and Bajrovic, F.F. (2006). Articaine is more effective than lidocaine or mepivacaine in rat sensory nerve conduction block in vitro. *J. Dent. Res.* 85 (2): 162–166.

Rahn, R. and Ball, B. (2001). Local anesthesia in dentistry. Articaine and epinephrine for dental anesthesia. In: *3M ESPE AG*. Seefeld (Germany). 13–18.

Reynolds, F., Bryson, T.H.L., and Nicholas, A.D.G. (1976). Intradermal study of a new local anaesthetic agent: aptocaine. *Br. J. Anaesth.* 48 (4): 347–354.

Ringler, M.L., Drasner, K., Krejcie, T.C. et al. (1991). Cauda equina syndrome after continuous spinal anesthesia. *Anesth. Analg.* 72 (3): 275–281.

Ritchie, J.M. and Ritchie, B. (1968). Local anesthetics: effect of pH on activity. *Science* 162 (3869): 1394–1395.

Ritchie, J.M., Ritchie, B., and Greengard, P. (1965a). The active structure of local anesthetics. *J. Pharmacol. Exp. Ther.* 150 (1): 152–159.

Ritchie, J.M., Ritchie, B., and Greengard, P. (1965b). The effect of the nerve sheath on the action of local anesthetics. *J. Pharmacol. Exp. Ther.* 150 (1): 160–164.

Ritschel, W.A. (1992). *Handbook of Basic Pharmacokinetics, Including Clinical Applications*. Hamilton (IL): Drug Intelligence Publications Inc. 365–380.

Rood, J.P. and Cannell, H. (1978). Plasma levels of lignocaine after perioral injections of two different concentrations. *Pharmacol. Ther. Dent.* 3 (1): 45–47.

Rood, J.P. and Sowray, J.H. (1980). Clinical experience with 5 per cent lignocaine solution. *J. Dent.* 8 (2): 128–131.

Routledge, P.A., Barchowsky, A., Bjornsson, T.D. et al. (1980). Lidocaine plasma protein binding. *Clin. Pharmacol. Ther.* 27 (3): 347–351.

Sampaio, R.M., Carvanal, T.G., Lanfredin, C.B. et al. (2012). Comparison of the anesthetic efficacy between bupivacaine and lidocaine in patients with irreversible pulpitis of mandibular molar. *J. Endod.* 38 (5): 594–597.

Schade, H., Neukrich, P., and Halpert, A. (1921). Ueber lokale Acidose des Gewebes und die Methodik ihner intravitalen Messung, zugleich ein Beitrag zur Lehre der Entzündung. *Z. Gesamte Exp. Med. (Berlin)* 24 (1–4): 11–56.

Schilli, W. (1977). Vasoconstrictors in local anesthetics. *Quintessece Int.* 8 (12): 15–18.

Scott, D.B., Lee, A., Fagan, D. et al. (1989). Acute toxicity of ropivacaine compared with that of bupivacaine. *Anesth. Analg.* 69 (5): 563–569.

Seldin, H.M. (1958). Survey of anesthetic fatalities in oral surgery and review of the etiological factors in anesthetic deaths. *J. Am. Dent. Soc. Anesth.* 5 (2): 5–12.

Simpson, D., Curran, M.P., Oldfield, V., and Keating, G.M. (2005). Ropivacaine. A review of its use in regional anaesthesia and acute pain management. *Drugs* 65 (18): 2675–2717.

Skou, J.C. (1954). Local anesthetics. II. The toxic potencies of some local anesthetics and of butyl alcohol, determined on peripheral nerves. *Acta Pharmacol. Toxicol.* 10 (3): 292–296.

Stepke, M.T., Schwenzer, N., and Eichhorn, W. (1994). Vasoconstrictors during pregnancy – in vitro trial on pregnant and non pregnant mouse uterus. *Int. J. Oral Maxillofac. Surg.* 23 (6 Pt 2): 440–442.

Suresh, L. and Radfar, L. (2004). Pregnancy and lactation. *Oral Surg. Oral Med. Oral Pathol.* 97 (6): 672–682.

Tainter, M.L., Luduena, F.P., and Hoppe, J.O. (1953). The trend to more potent local anesthetic solutions in dentistry. *Oral Surg. Oral Med. Oral Pathol.* 6 (5): 645–661.

Tanner, J.M. (1966). Galtonian eugenics and the study of growth: the relation of body size, intelligence test score and social circumstances in children and adults. *Eugen Rev.* 58 (3): 122–135.

Timponi, C.F., Oliveira, N.E., Arruda, R.M.P. et al. (2006). Effects of the local anaesthetic ropivacaine on vascular reactivity in the mouse perfused mesenteric arteries. *Basic Clin. Pharmacol. Toxicol.* 98 (5): 518–520.

Truant, A.P. and Takman, B. (1959). Differential physical–chemical and neuropharmacologic properties of local anesthetic agents. *Anesth. Analg.* 38 (6): 478–484.

Tucker, G.T. (1986). Pharmacokinetics of local anesthetics. *Br. J. Anaesth.* 58 (7): 717–731.

Tucker, G.T. and Mather, L.E. (1975). Pharmacology of local anesthetic agents. Pharmacokinetics of local anaesthetic agents. *Br. J. Anaesth.* 47 (suppl): 213–224.

Tucker, G.T., Boyes, R.N., Bridenbaugh, P.O., and Moore, D.C. (1970). Binding of anilide-type local anesthetics in human plasma I. Relationships between binding, physicochemical properties, and anesthetic activity. *Anesthesiology* 33 (3): 287–303.

Tui, C., Press, A.L., Barcham, I., and Nevin, M.I. (1944). Local nervous tissue changes following spinal anesthesia in experimental animals. *Pharmacol. Exp. Ther.* 81 (3): 209–217.

Van Oss, G.E.C.J.M., Vree, T.B., Baars, A.M. et al. (1989). Pharmacokinetics, metabolism, and renal excretion of articaine and its metabolite articainic acid in patients after epidural administration. *Eur. J. Anaesthesiol.* 6 (1): 49–56.

Vongsavan, N., Soo-Ampon, S., Mathews, R.W., and Mathews, B. (2000). Effects of some local anaesthetic solutions on blood flow. *J. Dent. Res.* 79. (IADR abstracts): 491 (abstract no. 2778).

Vree, T.B., Baars, A.M., Van Oss, G.E.C.J.M., and Booij, L.H.D. (1988). High-performance liquid chromatography and preliminary pharmacokinetic of articaine and its 2-carboxy metabolite in human serum and urine. *J. Chromatogr.* 424 (2): 440–444.

Waters, R.M. (1933). Procaine toxicity: its prophylaxis and treatment. *J. Am. Dent. Assoc.* 20 (12): 2211–2215.

Weaber, J.M. (1999). Articaine, a new local anesthetic for American dentists: will it superade lidocaine? (Editorial). *Aneth. Prog.* 49 (4): 111–112.

Widman, B. (1975). Plasma concentration of local anaesthetic agents in regard to absorption, distribution and elimination, with special reference to bupivacaine. *Br. J. Anaesth.* 47 (suppl): 231–236.

Wildsmith, J.A.W. (1986). Peripheral nerve and local anaesthetic drugs. *Br. J. Anaesth.* 58 (7): 692–700.

Wildsmith, J.A.W., Gissen, A.J., Takman, B., and Covino, B. (1987). Differential nerve blockade: esters v. amides and the influence of pKa. *Br. J. Anaesth.* 59 (3): 379–384.

Winther, J.E. and Nathalang, B. (1972). Effectivity of a new local analgesic Hoe 10 045. *Scand. J. Dent. Res.* 80 (4): 272–279.

Winther, J.E. and Patirupanusara, B. (1974). Evaluation of carticaine—a new local analgesic. *Int. J. Oral Surg.* 3 (6): 422–427.

# 6

# Vasoconstrictors

## Introduction

Blood vessel constrictors, the second most important drugs in local anesthesia, enhance the efficacy and safety of the primary drug, the local anesthetic itself.

Two families of blood vessel constrictors or vasoconstrictors are presently used in dentistry:

1) Sympathomimetics or catecholamines, so-called because they share a catechol core, including the natural hormones and neurotransmitters epinephrine and norepinephrine, and the synthetic drug levonordefrin.
2) Felypressin, a polypeptide derived from the posterior pituitary hormone vasopressin.

The most effective and by far most commonly used vasoconstrictor is epinephrine, oddly enough the first vasoconstrictor ever to be used.

## Advantages

As noted, vasoconstrictors heighten local anesthetic effects and safety.

1) In dentistry that enhanced efficacy and potency translate into a higher percentage of successful anesthetization of dental pulp, the most difficult tissue to numb (Table 6.1). The mass-volume-time effect attributable to the vasoconstrictor's ability to hold the local anesthetic in place raises the potency of lower doses (1–2% for action comparable to 6–7%).
2) Vasoconstrictors lengthen anesthesia duration in both pulp and soft tissues (Table 6.1), likewise as a result of the mass-volume-time effect.
3) Both epinephrine (Curtis et al. 1966; Meyer and Allen 1968; Hecht and App 1974; Sveen 1979; Buckley et al. 1984; Moore et al. 2007) and felypressin (Shanks 1963; Light et al. 1965; Fisher et al. 1965) reduce hemorrhaging in surgeries by constricting blood vessels. An additional advantage is that they shorten the duration of oral surgeries by affording the surgeon a wider field of view (Hecht and App 1974; Buckley et al. 1984; Moore et al. 2007).
4) Vasoconstrictors reduce the toxicity of local anesthetics.
   - Experimental studies in animals have shown that the subcutaneous injection of a local anesthetic in conjunction with a vasoconstrictor such as epinephrine (Campbell and Adriani 1958; Henn 1960; Henn and Brattsand 1966) or felypressin (Akerman 1969) lowers the toxicity of the former (Table 6.2). The subcutaneous injection of 2% lidocaine in rats has been shown to disappear in 2 hours, whereas if administered with epinephrine it lasts more than 4 hours (Sung and Truant 1954).
   - Clinical studies have found that adding a vasoconstrictor lowers the anesthetic peak (Bromage and Robson 1961; Braid and Scott 1965; Lund and Cwik 1965; Cannell and Beckett 1975a; Perovic et al. 1980) (Table 6.3) and delays its appearance in plasma (Bromage and Robson 1961; Braid and Scott 1965; Lund and Cwik 1965) (Figure 6.1). This is because the slower absorption of the anesthetic (Campbell and Adriani 1958; Lund and Cwik 1965; Cannell and Beckett 1975a) reduces its capacity to reach toxic levels in the blood by giving the body more time to break the drug down.
   - The greater potency afforded local anesthetics by vasoconstrictors (see (1) above) also enhances safety indirectly because it enables clinicians to inject smaller quantities to achieve the same effect.

## Disadvantages

Vasoconstrictors are characterized by two major drawbacks.

1) They heighten the toxicity of intravascularly injected local anesthetics (hence the importance of aspirating

*Local Anesthesia in Dentistry: A Locoregional Approach*, First Edition. Jesús Calatayud and Mana Saraghi.
© 2024 John Wiley & Sons Ltd. Published 2024 by John Wiley & Sons Ltd.
Companion website: www.wiley.com/go/Calatayud/local

Table 6.1 Anesthetic efficacy of upper lip and maxillary lateral incisor pulp (measured with electric pulpometer), with and without vasoconstrictors.

| Variable | 2% lidocaine | 3% prilocaine | 2% mepivacaine |
|---|---|---|---|
| **No vasoconstrictor** | | | |
| Pulpal anesthesia | 58% | 85% | 83% |
| Duration pulpal anesthesia | 6 min | 11 min | 13 min |
| Duration lip anesthesia | 67 min | 86 min | 82 min |
| Reference | Annex 21 | Berling and Björn (1960) Berling (1966) | Berling (1958) |
| **Epinephrine 1:100 000** | | | |
| Pulpal anesthesia | 95% | 100% | 93% |
| Duration pulpal anesthesia | 45 min | 26 min | 35 min |
| Duration lip anesthesia | 190 min | 135 min | 160 min |
| Reference | Annex 21 | Berling and Björn (1960) | Annex 21 |
| **Felypressin** | 0.01 IU/ml | 0.03 IU/ml | |
| Pulpal anesthesia | 82% | 88% | — |
| Duration pulpal anesthesia | 15 min | 25 min | — |
| Duration lip anesthesia | 141 min | 180 min | — |
| Reference | Berling (1966) | Annex 21 | |

IU/ml, international units per milliliter.

Table 6.2 Lethal doses (LD$_{50}$, mg/kg) after subcutaneous or intravenous injection of anesthetic with or without epinephrine.

| Anesthetic | Animal | Subcutaneous injection | | Intravenous injection | | Reference |
|---|---|---|---|---|---|---|
| | | No epinephrine | With epinephrine | No epinephrine | With epinephrine | |
| Procaine | Mouse | — | — | 56 | 22 | Keil and Vieten (1952) |
| | Mouse | 620 | 670 | 59 | 17 | Henn (1960) |
| Lidocaine | Mouse | — | — | 30 | 14 | Keil and Vieten (1952) |
| | Mouse | 314 | 317 | 30 | 9 | Henn (1960) |
| | Rat | — | — | 28 | 16 | Hardin et al. (1981) |
| | Rat | — | — | 28 | 18 | Yagiela (1985) |
| Mepivacaine | Mouse | 285 | 320 | 40 | 20 | Henn (1960) |
| | Mouse | — | — | 40 | 23 | Henn and Brattsand (1966) |
| Tetracaine | Mouse | — | — | 9.5 | 4.2 | Keil and Vieten (1952) |
| | Mouse | 62 | 101 | 8 | 2.4 | Henn and Brattsand (1966) |
| Conclusion | | Higher toxicity with NO epinephrine, subcutaneous administration | | Higher toxicity WITH epinephrine, intravenous administration | | |

Using felypressin as the vasoconstrictor delivers very similar results (Akerman 1969).

after every injection). Experimental studies with animals show that if administered intravenously, anesthetic solutions are more toxic if they bear vasoconstrictors than if they do not (Table 6.2), i.e. exactly the opposite behavior as observed in subcutaneous injections.

2) Counterindications and interactions are discussed in Chapter 10.

**Table 6.3** Peak blood level of local anesthetic (ng/ml) and time to appearance (minutes) after perioral injection of 1.8-ml cartridge solutions of anesthetic with and without epinephrine and levonordefrin.

| Anesthetic[a] | Quantity | | No vasoconstrictor | | With vasoconstrictor[a] | | Reference |
|---|---|---|---|---|---|---|---|
| | mg | Number of cartridges | ng/ml | Minutes | ng/ml | Minutes | |
| Lidocaine | 36 | 1 | 310 | 15 | 220 | 30 | Goebel et al. (1979, 1980a,b) |
| Mepivacaine | 36 | 1 | 400 | 10 | 370 | 30 | Goebel et al. (1979, 1980a,b) |
| Lidocaine | 80 | 2.2 | 1000 | 10 | 800 | 30 | Cannell and Beckett (1975a) |
| Lidocaine | 160 | 4.5 | 1450 | 10 | 1150 | 60 | Cannell and Beckett (1975b) |

[a] 2% lidocaine with 1:80 000 (12.5 μg/ml) epinephrine; 2% mepivacaine with 1:20 000 (50 μg/ml) levonordefrin.

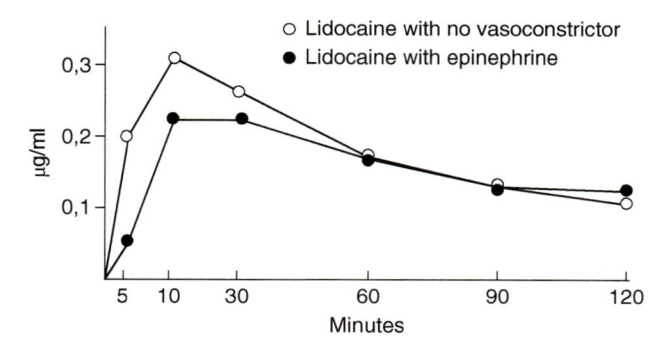

**Figure 6.1** Lidocaine vein blood levels with no vasoconstrictor and with epinephrine. *Source:* Data from Goebel et al. (1980b).

## Dilutions and Concentrations

Vasoconstrictor dilutions are measured as a ratio of parts per thousand, written as, for instance, 1:1000. Doses may also be expressed in milligrams (mg) or micrograms (μg). Concentrations are expressed in milligrams or micrograms per milliliter (mg/ml, μg/ml) or percentage (%). Some examples are listed below.

- A 1:1000 dilution is 1 g (1000 mg) of drug in 1000 ml of solution. Hence:
  1:1000 = 1 mg/ml = 1000 μg/ml = 0.1%
  One liter (1000 ml) contains 1000 mg (1 g) of drug
- A 1:100 000 dilution is 0.01 g (10 mg) of drug in 1000 ml of solution, whereby:
  1:100 000 = 0.01 mg/ml = 10 μg/ml = 0.001%
  One liter (1000 ml) contains 10 mg (0.01 g) of drug
- A 1:200 000 dilution is 0.005 g (5 mg) of drug in 1000 ml of solution, whereby:
  1:200 000 = 0.005 mg/ml = 5 μg/ml = 0.000 5%
  One liter (1000 ml) contains 5 mg (0.005 g) of drug

Table 6.4 lists examples of the vasoconstrictor concentrations most commonly used in dentistry, along with the maximum doses allowed.

## Catecholamines

These vasoconstrictors derive their name from the fact that they consist of a catechol group (a benzene ring with two adjacent hydroxy groups) and an amine side chain (Figure 6.2). They are also known as *sympathomimetic vasoconstrictors* because they act on the autonomic sympathetic nervous system or *adrenergic amines* because some of them (epinephrine and norepinephrine) are released by the adrenal medulla or are artificial derivatives of such substances (levonordefrin).

Vasoconstrictor sympathomimetics administered in dentistry anesthetic solutions are characterized by three properties.

1) In their basic form catecholamines are not water soluble. As hydrochloric salts they, like local anesthetics, dissolve in water, but are unfortunately not stable in that medium. They are consequently used as bitartrates, i.e. the *bitartrate salts* such as epinephrine bitartrate resulting from the reaction with two molecules of tartaric acid, which are both stable and water soluble (Smith 1920; Bonica 1959).
2) They are combined with *sulfites*, the antioxidizing action of which lengthens catecholamine life because these vasoconstrictors are highly vulnerable to oxidation (Milano et al. 1982; Klein 1983).
3) Vasoconstrictor solutions must have a *low pH of 2.7–5.5* (USP 38 2015) because otherwise they are oxidized and degraded (Fyhr and Brodin 1987): at a pH >6 epinephrine breaks down in a matter of hours (De Jong and Cullen 1963).

**Table 6.4** Maximum doses established for vasoconstrictors and routine concentrations and dilutions.

| | Vasoconstrictor | Maximum dose μg (mg) | Parts per thousand[a] | Percentage (%) | μg/ml | mg/ml | μg per 1.8-ml cartridge |
|---|---|---|---|---|---|---|---|
| Sympathomimetic | Levonordefrin | 1000 (1)[1]<br>500 (0.5)[7] | 1:20 000[1] | 0.005% | 50 | 0.05 | 90 |
| | Norepinephrine | 330 (0.33)[1] | 1:30 000[2] | 0.00333% | 33 | 0.033 | 59.4 |
| | Epinephrine | 200 (0.2)[3] | 1:50 000[2,3] | 0.002% | 20 | 0.02 | 36 |
| | | | 1:80 000 | 0.00125% | 12.5 | 0.0125 | 22.5 |
| | | | 1:100 000 | 0.001% | 10 | 0.01 | 18 |
| | | | 1:200 000 | 0.0005% | 5 | 0.005 | 9 |
| | Felypressin | 7.02 (0.00702)[4]<br>(0.39 IU)* | 1:185 0000[6] | 0.00000054% | 0.54[5]<br>(0.03 IU) | 0.00054 | 0.972<br>(0.054 IU) |

*IU, international units.
[a] References: 1, Jastak and Yagiela (1983); 2, ADA-AHA (1964); 3, Report of the Special Committee of the New York Heart Association (1955); 4, Dunlop Committee (Oliver 1974; Roberts and Sowray 1987); 5, Berling (1966), Goldman and Evers (1969); 6, Barnard et al. (1987); 7, Bennett (1984).

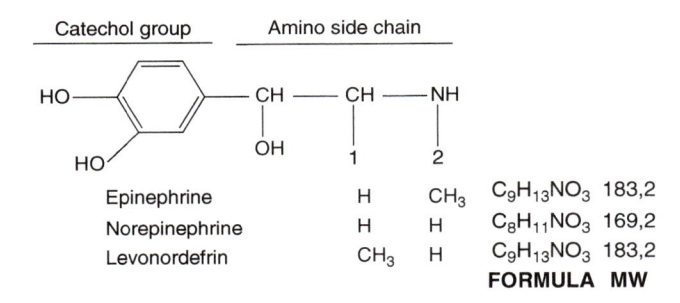

| | | | Formula | MW |
|---|---|---|---|---|
| | 1 | 2 | | |
| Epinephrine | H | $CH_3$ | $C_9H_{13}NO_3$ | 183.2 |
| Norepinephrine | H | H | $C_8H_{11}NO_3$ | 169.2 |
| Levonordefrin | $CH_3$ | H | $C_9H_{13}NO_3$ | 183.2 |

**Figure 6.2** Chemical structure common to all catecholamines, showing catechol group and amino side chain: vasoconstrictor drugs differ in side-chain terminations. *Source:* American Dental Association (1984).

## Isomers and Catecholamines

The three vasoconstrictive sympathomimetic amines used with local anesthetics in dentistry are isomeric or enantiomeric, i.e. they may present as either of two molecular configurations that differ in the positions of their atoms or atomic groups. As a result, a plane of polarized light can rotate in one of two opposite directions, hence the name optical isomers.

Unlike local anesthetics, most of which adopt racemic forms (DL or ± or RS), i.e. 50% of their molecules are dextrorotated (D or + or R, rectus) and 50% levorotated (L or − or S, sinister), *only levorotated catecholamines are used as vasoconstrictors*, resulting in a more potent effect (as well as higher toxicity). Levo epinephrine is 15–20 times more potent and more toxic than the dextro form (Table 6.5), while racemic forms are half as potent and toxic.

Hereafter, all references to epinephrine and norepinephrine are understood to be to L-epinephrine and L-norepinephrine, while nordefrin is referred to throughout as levonordefrin.

## Adrenergic Receptors

Dale (1906) was the first researcher to realize that epinephrine action is mediated by two receptors, although it was Raymond Ahlquist who actually typified the two types of adrenoreceptors: alpha (α) or stimulant and beta (β) or inhibitory receptors (Alquist 1948).

Each type was later subdivided, β receptors into $β_1$ receptors, located primarily in the heart as well as in adipose tissue and the intestine, and the more widely distributed $β_2$ receptors. Their purpose is to relax the smooth muscle in blood vessels and bronchi (Lands et al. 1967).

The α receptors were found to consist, firstly, of post-synaptic $α_1$ receptors located in the *tunica media* (edge of the *tunica adventitia*). Their vasoconstrictive action is triggered by the exogenous catecholamines carried in the bloodstream and the norepinephrine released by nerve endings. The pre-synaptic $α_2$ receptors in the sympathetic nerve endings block the release of norepinephrine on activation. When located in the *tunica intima* of vessels they constrict the blood vessels on activation, similar to the response to exogenous catecholamines carried in the bloodstream (Langer 1974; Langer and Hicks 1984).

Today, information deriving from the isolation of the pure proteins comprising adrenoreceptors and functional pharmacological studies suggests the existence of subtypes

Table 6.5 Potency and toxicity of levo over dextro isomers of epinephrine, norepinephrine, and levonordefrin.

| Catecholamine | Δ potency levo > dextro | Reference | Δ toxicity levo > dextro[a] | Reference |
|---|---|---|---|---|
| Epinephrine | 15–20 | Cushny (1909) | 15–20 | Launoy and Menguy (1920) |
|  |  | Welsh (1955) |  | Launoy and Menguy (1922) |
|  |  | Hondrum et al. (1993) |  | Hondrum et al. (1993) |
|  | 20 | Tye et al. (1967) |  |  |
| Norepinephrine | 25–33 | Tainter et al. (1949) | 10–15 | Hoppe et al. (1949) |
|  | 27 | Luduena et al. (1949) |  |  |
|  | 12–18 | Luduena et al. (1949) |  |  |
|  | 10–15 | Welsh (1955) |  |  |
|  | 40 | Tye et al. (1967) |  |  |
| Nordefrin | 100–200 | Luduena et al. (1958) | 10 | Hoppe and Seppelin (1953) |
|  | 35 | Tye et al. (1967) |  | Luduena et al. (1958) |

[a] Toxicity can be verified in Annex 18.

of $\alpha_1$ ($\alpha_{1a}$, $\alpha_{1b}$, $\alpha_{1c}$, $\alpha_{1d}$) and $\alpha_2$ ($\alpha_{2a}$, $\alpha_{2b}$, $\alpha_{2c}$) (Ruffolo Jr et al. 1991; Bylund et al. 1994; Hieble 2000; Goldstein 2001), as well as further β receptors, such as $\beta_3$ (Goldstein 2001; Bylund et al. 1994; Coman et al. 2009) and $\beta_4$ (Hieble 2000). The identification of adrenoreceptor subtypes and the characterization of their functions may clear the way for the design of future drugs with an optimal pharmacological spectrum (Bylund et al. 1994; Hieble 2000).

Adrenoreceptors are transmembrane receptors with an alpha-helix structure that span the cell membrane seven times. They are G protein-coupled receptors, i.e. they activate the G proteins, intracellular "switches" that help regulate cell function (Ostrowski et al. 1992). The various parts of this helix structure are depicted schematically in Figure 6.3 (Wolfe and Molinoff 1988; Ruffolo Jr et al. 1991; Ostrowski et al. 1992; Coman et al. 2009).

- The transmembrane segments or domains are the seven "pieces" that span the cell membrane. They are shown as tubes because each one is two to four amino acids thick and labeled with indoarabic numerals (Figure 6.3).
- Six hydrophilic connecting loops connect the seven transmembrane domains, three of which are extracellular (E) and the other three intracellular or cytoplasmic (C). They are shown as lines because each chain is just one amino acid thick.
- The COOH terminal is intracellular and the $NH_2$ terminal is extracellular.
- The extracellular segment has two glycosilation zones (Y).

Each adrenoreceptor, with around 400–560 amino acids, has a molecular weight of 45–70 kDa (Ruffolo Jr et al. 1991; Ostrowski et al. 1992; Coman et al. 2009). Adrenoreceptors

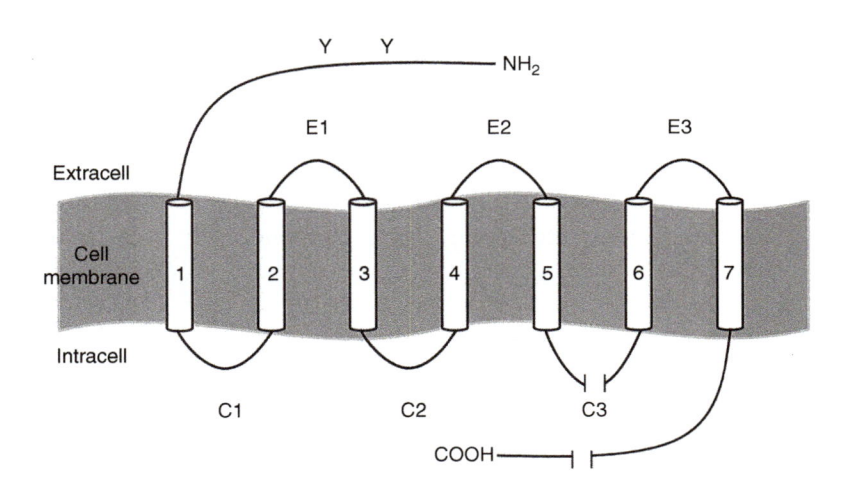

Figure 6.3 Basic structural model common to adrenoreceptors.

Table 6.6 Vasoconstrictor affinity for adrenoreceptors and relative potency (values for levo isomers).

| Vasoconstrictor | Adrenoreceptor | | | | Relative potency (%) |
|---|---|---|---|---|---|
| | $\alpha_1$ | $\alpha_2$ | $\beta_1$ | $\beta_2$ | |
| Epinephrine | + | + | + | + | 100 |
| Norepinephrine | + | + | + | − | 25 |
| Levonordefrin | − | + | + | − | 15 |

+, stimulates receptor;
− does not stimulate receptor.

differ primarily in the composition of their C3 and cytoplasmic terminal zones (Ruffolo Jr et al. 1991).

Today catecholamines are believed to bind to the extracellular portion of the receptors between transmembrane domains 3 and 4 (Ostrowski et al. 1992). The lipid solubility coefficient is consequently unimportant in vasoconstrictor sympathomimetics because contact is made on the surface of the membrane and not, as in local anesthetics, inside the sodium channel.

Not all receptors are stimulated by vasoconstrictive sympathomimetics, nor do all these vasoconstrictors exhibit the same potency. Table 6.6 summarizes their properties: as epinephrine is the most potent catecholamine and stimulates all four main receptors ($\alpha_1$, $\alpha_2$, $\beta_1$, and $\beta_2$), it is assigned an activity of 100%. It is fourfold more potent than norepinephrine (Furchgott 1972) and six to seven times more potent than levonordefrin (Robertson et al. 1984). Adrenoreceptor distribution and the major effects of their stimulation are given in Table 6.7 (Keiser 2001; Goldstein 2001). As these receptors tend to seek equilibrium (receptor dynamics), when large quantities of catecholamines are present in the blood for lengthy periods of time they adapt by becoming less sensitive to stimulation. In contrast, when the receptors are not exposed to catecholamines they tend to be overstimulated by adrenergic amines (Brown and Rhodus 2005).

## Systemic Effects

Of the many effects induced on the body by vasoconstrictive sympathomimetics (Keiser 2001; Goldstein 2001), the ones of greatest interest to dental clinicians are discussed below.

### Heart

The heart bears adrenoreceptors $\alpha_1$, $\alpha_2$, $\beta_1$, and $\beta_2$. Receptors $\alpha_1$ and $\alpha_2$ constrict the coronary vessels while receptor $\beta_2$ induces vasodilation. Receptors $\beta_1$ and $\beta_2$ raise heart frequency and strength.

Table 6.7 Adrenoreceptors: distribution and key responses.

| Receptor | Location | Response |
|---|---|---|
| $\alpha_1$ | Heart | ↑ Contraction strength |
| | Vessels, smooth muscle | Contraction |
| | Liver | Glycogenolysis, neoglucogenesis |
| | Genitourinary smooth muscle | Contraction |
| | Uterus | Pregnancy → contraction |
| | Sudoriparous glands | ↑ Perspiration |
| $\alpha_2$ | Vessels, smooth muscle | Contraction |
| | Pancreas (β cells) | ↓ Insulin secretion |
| | Platelets | Platelet aggregation |
| | Nerve endings | ↑ Norepinephrine release |
| $\beta_1$ | Heart | ↑ Contraction strength and frequency |
| | Juxtaglomerular cells | ↑ Renin secretion |
| $\beta_2$ | Heart | ↑ Contraction strength and frequency |
| | Vessels, smooth muscle | Relaxation |
| | Liver | Glycogenolysis, neoglucogenesis |
| | Pancreas | ↑ Insulin secretion |
| | Bronchi, smooth muscle | Relaxation |
| | Skeletal muscle | Glycogenolysis and $K^+$ capture |
| | Genitourinary smooth muscle | Relaxation |
| | Uterus | Pregnant or otherwise → relaxation |
| $\beta_3$ | Adipose tissue | Lipolysis |

*Source:* Data from Goldstein (2001) and Keiser (2001).

As epinephrine stimulates the four types of receptors it raises cardiac frequency or heart rate (tachycardia) and contraction strength ($\beta_1$ and $\beta_2$), and generates an oxygen deficit because the effect of $\beta_2$-induced vasodilation is offset by $\alpha_1$ and $\alpha_2$ vasoconstriction.

Norepinephrine, and to a lesser extent levonordefrin, induce coronary vessel vasoconstriction by stimulating $\alpha_1$ and $\alpha_2$, and although they stimulate $\beta_1$, as they do not bind to receptor $\beta_2$ the vasodilation effect is minor. The concomitant rise in blood pressure triggers the baroreflex, a feedback mechanism involving the baroreceptors located in the carotid sinus and aortic arch that ultimately reduces heart rate (bradycardia) (Annex 15).

### Circulatory System

The arteries and veins of organs, muscles, viscera (lungs, kidneys, genitourinary tract, etc.) have $\alpha_1$, $\alpha_2$, and $\beta_2$ receptors. As $\alpha_1$ and $\alpha_2$ receptors prevail in most of these vessels, they are constricted by sympathomimetic amines, raising (primarily systolic) blood pressure and peripheral resistance. Skeletal muscle and some abdominal viscera vessels bear readily stimulated vasodilating $\beta_2$ receptors that tend to lower (primarily diastolic) blood pressure.

Epinephrine stimulates $\alpha_1$ and $\alpha_2$ receptors, inducing vasoconstriction and raising (primarily systolic) blood pressure. It also stimulates vasodilating $\beta_2$ receptors in skeletal muscle, which tends to lower (primarily diastolic) blood pressure; by balancing systolic and diastolic, *it tends to stabilize blood pressure* (Annex 15). Systolic and diastolic blood pressure rise simultaneously only when large quantities of epinephrine are injected, stimulating skeletal muscle α receptors (Campbell 1977).

By stimulating only the α receptors, norepinephrine, and less intensely levonordefrin, induce a general rise in both systolic and diastolic blood pressure, given the absence or weakness of the compensatory vasodilating effect induced by $\beta_2$ (Annex 15).

### Respiratory Tract

Here the prevalent effect is receptor $\beta_2$ stimulation, with relaxation of the bronchial muscles and increased air ingress in the lungs attendant on bronchodilation. That effect is induced by epinephrine almost exclusively because it is the sole catecholamine that stimulates these receptors effectively (Himms-Hagen 1972).

### Endocrine System and Metabolism

Catecholamines stimulate bodily metabolism by raising the number of nutrients to the heart and skeletal muscle, increasing oxygen consumption by 15–30% via the β receptors to prepare the body for the fight-or-flight response.

Catecholamines activate glycogenolysis in the skeletal muscles ($\beta_2$) and glycogenolysis and neoglucogenesis in the liver ($\alpha_1$, $\beta_2$), releasing glucose into the blood and raising blood glucose levels, a condition that may be highly detrimental to uncontrolled diabetics. By stimulating the $\beta_2$ receptors in the pancreas, catecholamines intensify insulin release and subsequent glucose entry into the cells, although high levels of epinephrine activate the $\alpha_2$ receptors, notably reducing insulin release (Table 6.7) (Annex 16).

In adipose tissue, via $\alpha_2$, $\beta_1$, and especially $\beta_3$ receptors, sympathomimetics induce lipolysis, with the release of glycerol, free fatty acids, and even ketone bodies.

Another effect of stimulating $\beta_2$ receptors stimulation is hypokalemia, a reduction in plasma potassium levels. While under normal circumstances these actions are of no consequence, in patients taking digoxin (a cardiac stimulant) they may favor heart arrhythmias (Meechan and Rawlins 1988; Meechan et al. 1991).

### Uterus

This organ has $\alpha_1$ receptors that stimulate contraction and $\beta_2$ receptors that favor relaxation, although it is highly impacted by the menstrual cycle and pregnancy.

By acting on both types of receptors (contraction-simulating $\alpha_1$ and relaxation-stimulating $\beta_2$), epinephrine has a neutral effect on the uterus, inhibiting contraction during pregnancy.

As norepinephrine acts primarily on $\alpha_1$ contraction-stimulating receptors, it intensifies uterus contraction during pregnancy and with it the risk of premature labor or miscarriage (Stepke et al. 1994). As levonordefrin acts on neither receptor, it barely affects the uterus.

### Vasoconstrictive Effect

Like the vessels in the skin and mucosa, those in oral tissue (gums, alveolar mucosa, submucosa, periodontium, etc.) have $\alpha_1$ and $\alpha_2$ receptors (Goldstein 2001; Keiser 2001). That, together with the paucity of β receptors, explains why the vasoconstrictive effect of sympathomimetic amines prevails in these areas. These pharmaceuticals induce vasoconstriction defined by a series of special characteristics.

1) They act on the *entire microcirculatory system*, contracting arterioles, meta-arterioles, precapillary sphincters, and venules (Berde and Cerletti 1964; Altura et al. 1965; Burcher et al. 1977; Olgart and Gazelius 1977).
2) They penetrate tissues, in particular the *vasa nervorum* of nerve trunks, very effectively due to their low molecular weight (Burcher et al. 1977; Olgart and Gazelius 1977).
3) The *vasoconstrictive effect is immediate* (Burcher et al. 1977; Lindorf 1979), with the effect of epinephrine peaking in 3 minutes and lasting around 60 minutes (Lindorf 1979).
4) Hypoxia occurs in infiltrated tissue usually due to the rise in local oxygen consumption and decline in oxygen supply due to intense vasoconstriction (Klingenström and Westermar 1964). That in turn induces *rebound vasodilation*, mediated primarily by epinephrine and norepinephrine (Klingenström and Westermar 1964), which induces a response in 2–3 hours (Lindorf 1979).

Epinephrine has a vasoconstrictive effect four times more potent than that of norepinephrine (Furchgott 1972) and six to seven times more potent than that of levonordefrin (Robertson et al. 1984) (Table 6.6).

### Catecholamine Metabolism

Neural sympathomimetic amines (epinephrine and norepinephrine) are released into the circulatory system in two ways.

1) Norepinephrine originates primarily in sympathetic nerve endings, with only small amounts released by the adrenal medulla (Landsberg and Young 1980; Goldstein 2001).
2) Epinephrine is supplied almost exclusively by the adrenal medulla (Kopin 1989; Goldstein 2001). Of the catecholamines released by the medulla, around 80–85% are epinephrine and the rest norepinephrine.

In the circulatory system 50–60% of these amines bind to plasmatic proteins, primarily albumin (Landsberg and Young 1980), and have a very short (1 minute) mean half-life in the plasma (Lund 1951; Whitby et al. 1961). They are inactivated in two ways (Landsberg and Young 1980; Trendelenburg 1988; Goldstein 2001):

1) Uptake 1. After the post-synaptic release of norepinephrine, the noradrenergic nerve endings recapture over two-thirds of the neurotransmitter (Kopin 1989; Eisenhofer et al. 2004), storing it in cytoplasmic vesicles for reuse or metabolizing it by monoamino-oxidase (MAO)-mediated deamination in the ribosome membrane. Small amounts of exogenous epinephrine and norepinephrine administered with local anesthetics are also metabolized along this pathway.
2) Uptake 2. Non-nervous cells originating primarily in the liver, but also in the kidneys, lungs, intestines, and other organs, capture circulating catecholamines, which they metabolize by a number of pathways.
   - As noted, deamination is mediated by ribosomal MAO, converting catecholamines into aldehydes.
   - O-methylation is catalyzed by the cytoplasmic enzyme catechol-O-methyltransferase (COMT). COMT acts directly on the catecholamines or their MAO-deaminated metabolites by methylizing one of the catechol-OH groups to produce new methoxy derivatives. This is the predominant catabolic pathway for exogenous catecholamines (Eisenhofer et al. 2004).
   - Conjugation takes place primarily in the gastrointestinal tract and other mesenteric organs (Landsberg 1976; Eisenhofer et al. 2004).

Interestingly, levonordefrin, due to its methyl group in position 1 (Figure 6.1), is protected from MAO and can therefore only be inactivated by COMT (Jastak et al. 1995). There are two pathways for eliminating catecholamines and their metabolites.

1) Liver gall is the minority pathway (Landsberg and Young 1980).
2) Urine via the kidneys is the prevalent pathway and, as shown in Annex 12, only around 5% of epinephrine and norepinephrine are eliminated unchanged.

Annex 12 describes the metabolic pathways for epinephrine degradation and the formation of its metabolites, along with the enzymes involved, while Annex 11 lists the major pharmacokinetic variables.

### Epinephrine

Epinephrine was first isolated in 1901 by Jokichi Takamine and Thomas Aldrich (Takamine 1901; Aldrich 1901) and began to be used as a vasoconstrictor in local anesthetics in 1903 by Heinrich Braun (Braun 1903). Epinephrine is a natural hormone and neurotransmitter found in the brain (Mefford et al. 1978) and produced and released into the blood by the adrenal medulla (Kopin 1989; Goldstein 2001). Initially denominated epinephrine by John Jacob Abel (Abel 1899), it was renamed suprarenin by Austrian chemist Otto von Fürth (von Fürth 1900) and adrenalin by Takamine (Takamine 1901). Today it is known in US pharmacology (USP 38) as epinephrine, further to an American Medical Association Council on Pharmacy and Chemistry decision (Smith 1920), while in European pharmacology, the World Health Organization, and the International Union of Pure Applied Chemistry (IUPAC), it goes by the term adrenaline (Navarro 2003).

The levo isomer (levo-epinephrine = L-epinephrine) is used in clinical settings, as for all other catecholamines, because it has been observed to be 15–20 times more potent than the dextro form (Cushny 1909; Welsh 1955; Hondrum et al. 1993). Epinephrine stimulates $\alpha_1$, $\alpha_2$, $\beta_1$, and $\beta_2$ receptors (Table 6.8) intensely and in human beings it has been shown to induce metabolic and hemodynamic effects 10-fold more potent than norepinephrine (Clutter et al. 1980). Its vasoconstrictive effect in humans is around four times more potent than exhibited by norepinephrine. For that reason epinephrine is taken as the model and assigned a vasoconstrictive potency value of 100%, to which norepinephrine is normalized to 25% (Table 6.6).

The rise in epinephrine in the blood during dentistry treatments is associated not with stress or pain, but rather essentially with the amount contained in local anesthetic injections (Annex 16). A close relationship can be observed between the number of cartridges injected and the levels of epinephrine in the blood because, like the natural events that raise epinephrine levels, exogenous epinephrine is associated with metabolic and hemodynamic responses (Annex 16).

Table 6.8 Epinephrine: prominent pharmacological and clinical factors.

| Pharmacological factor | Reference |
|---|---|
| • Name and synonym: epinephrine, adrenaline, suprarenin | |
| • First isolated by Takamine in 1901 and Aldrich in 1901 | Takamine (1901)<br>Aldrich (1901) |
| • Chemical name 1,1-(3,4-dihydroxyphenyl)-2-methylaminoethanol | American Dental Association (1984) |
| • Formula: $C_9H_{13}NO_3$ | Aldrich (1901)<br>USP 38 |
| • Molecular weight: Baseline: 183.2<br>  As bitartrate: 333.3 | USP 38 |
| • pKa value or dissociation constant: 8.6 | Annex 6 |
| • Adrenoreceptors stimulated: $\alpha_1$, $\alpha_2$, $\beta_1$ and $\beta_2$ | Goldstein (2001) |
| • Vasoconstrictor potency: 100% | Furchgott (1972) |
| • Clearance (l/min): 6.8 | Annex 11 |
| • Volume of distribution (l): 86.5 | Annex 11 |
| • Elimination half-life (min): <1 | Annex 11 |
| **Clinical factor** | |
| • Usable during pregnancy: Yes (FDA category = C) | Haas et al. (2000)<br>Donaldson and Goodchild (2012) |
| • Usable during lactation: Yes | Haas et al. (2000)<br>Donaldson and Goodchild (2012) |
| • Absolute maximum dose in dentistry.<br>0.2 mg = 200 μg = 2.85 μg/kg | Report (1955) |
| • Maximum concentration in dentistry:<br>1:50 000 = 20 μg/ml = 0.002% | Report (1955) |
| • Other concentrations used in dentistry:<br>1:80 000 = 12.5 μg/ml = 0.00125%<br>1:100 000 = 10 μg/ml = 0.001%<br>1:200 000 = 5 μg/ml = 0.0005% | |

Table 6.8 lists the most salient pharmacological and clinical factors. The safety of administering local anesthesia containing epinephrine during pregnancy and lactation (Haas et al. 2000) and the establishment of the absolute maximum dose at 200 μg (2.85 μg/kg) for adults weighing 70 kg or over (Report of the Special Committee of the New York Heart Association 1955) are among the most prominent of the clinical indications. The maximum concentration authorized for dentistry is 1:50 000 (20 μg/ml), while in general concentrations of 1:100 000 (10 μg/ml) (10 μg/ml) and in some European countries as well as in India and Japan of 1:80 000 (12.5 μg/ml) are regarded as standard. A concentration of 1:200 000 (5 μg/ml) is regarded as low in clinical dentistry.

The world over, epinephrine continues to be the most commonly used vasoconstrictor by far in local anesthesia today because it is more effective and safer than other sympathomimetic amines.

### Norepinephrine

Chemically speaking, the difference between norepinephrine and epinephrine is the lack of a methyl group on the side chain nitrogen in the former (Figure 6.2). The prefix "nor" is taken from the German initials for "Nitrogenum ohne Radikal" (nitrogen without the radical). It was first isolated in 1946 in Sweden by Ulf Svante von Euler and named noradrenalin or arterenol (von Euler 1946a, 1946b). Today US pharmacology (USP 38) calls it norepinephrine while in Europe it is known as noradrenaline.

Norepinephrine is a natural hormone and neurotransmitter. It is released in all noradrenergic sympathetic nerve endings, with around 30% reaching the circulatory system (Kopin 1989; Eisenhofer et al. 2004). Norepinephrine is also released by the adrenal medulla, where it accounts for only 15–20% of the total released, while epinephrine accounts for the remaining 80–85% (Kopin 1989; Goldstein 2001). The levo isomer (levo-norepinephrine = L-norepinephrine = Levophed[1]) is used in clinical settings because, as for other catecholamines, it is much (10–40 times) more potent than the dextro form (Table 6.5).

In the earliest experimental studies with animals norepinephrine was observed to induce a vasoconstrictive effect less potent than but similar to that of epinephrine. Its softer effect on the heart, lower toxicity, and lack of the vasodilating effects compared with epinephrine (Luduena et al. 1949; Berling and Björn 1951; Tye et al. 1967) encouraged its use in local dental anesthetics. After promising results at concentrations of 1:30 000 (33 μg/ml) in early clinical trials (Dobbs and de Vier 1950; Epstein et al. 1951; Ekmanner and Persson 1951), it began to be preferred over epinephrine. Subsequent research and clinical practice revealed a number of discouraging findings, however.

---

[1] Levophed is the trade name for L-norepinephrine, which was brought to market in 1951 (Epstein 1951).

- Norepinephrine proved to be less effective than epinephrine in clinical experience (Persson 1969; Boakes et al. 1972) and clinical trials conducted to a more rigorous methodology. In 2% lidocaine with 1:50 000 (20 μg/ml) norepinephrine, pulp was found to be poorly anesthetized, with results comparable to those with 2% lidocaine and 1:200 000 (5 μg/ml) epinephrine (Annex 21).
- Toxicity was observed to be higher than in epinephrine. Clinical studies detected higher hypertension with norepinephrine (Annex 15), as well as substantial cerebral vasoconstriction rarely present with epinephrine (Hirota et al. 1992). Frequent adverse and at time severe reactions were observed, with hypertension crises leading to headaches (cephaleas) (Boakes et al. 1972; New Zealand 1974; Barnard et al. 1987). Extreme cases of death due to cerebral hemorrhaging (subarachnoid hemorrhage), arrhythmias, and heart failure were also reported (Boakes et al. 1972; Tomlin 1974; Cawson et al. 1983; Barnard et al. 1987; Okada et al. 1989).

Table 6.9 lists the main pharmacological and clinical properties of norepinephrine; note that its vasoconstrictive effect in humans is 25% of the epinephrine value and it is *contraindicated during pregnancy*, although during lactation we have no information. The contraindication during pregnancy is due to its stimulation of $\alpha_1$ receptors and hence uterus contraction, raising the risk of miscarriage or premature labor (Stepke et al. 1994). As noted earlier, norepinephrine has little impact on $\beta_2$ receptors, which relax the uterus.

Table 6.9 also shows that the maximum absolute dose of norepinephrine is 330 μg (4.7 μg/kg) for adults weighing 70 kg or more (Jastak and Yagiela 1983). The maximum concentration is 1:30 000 (33 μg/ml) (ADA-AHA 1964), while the standard concentration for local anesthesia in dentistry is 1:50 000 (20 μg/ml).

There are currently no commercially available local anesthetic formulations with norepinephrine in the United States, although it is available in a few European countries. Most authors presently advise against the use of norepinephrine as a vasoconstrictor because it is less effective and carries higher risk and more complications than epinephrine (Haglund and Evers 1985; Van der Bijl and Victor 1992; Jage 1993; Malamed 2004; Brown and Rhodus 2005).

## Levonordefrin

Nordefrin was introduced as a vasoconstrictor in dentistry in 1933 at a concentration of 1:10 000 (100 μg/ml) (Dobbs 1965). At the time it also went by the trade names of corbasil, cobefrin, corbadrine, and lirotil. In 1958 the levo isomer (levonordefrin) was found to be 100–200 times more active than the dextro form (Luduena et al. 1958) and began to be used instead of racemic nordefrin, at concentrations of 1:20 000 (50 μg/ml), half the dose of the latter, in the belief that the levo isomer generated the entire vasoconstrictive effect (Moose 1959).

Levonordefrin, a derivative of norepinephrine, is the primary alternative to epinephrine as a vasoconstrictor in the United States and Canada. This drug is not used in Europe. Moreover, unlike epinephrine and norepinephrine, which are natural hormones and neurotransmitters,

Table 6.9 Norepinephrine: prominent pharmacological and clinical factors.

| Pharmacological factor | Reference |
|---|---|
| - Name and synonym: noradrenaline, norepinephrine, levartrenol, levophed | |
| - First isolated by Euler in 1946 | Von Euler (1946a, b) |
| - Chemical name: 1,1-(3,4-dihydroxyphenyl)-2-aminoethanol | American Dental Association (1984) |
| - Formula: $C_8H_{11}NO_3$ | |
| - Molecular weight: Baseline 169.2 As bitartrate: 337.3 | American Dental Association (1984) |
| - pKa value or dissociation constant: 8.6 | Annex 6 |
| - Adrenoreceptors stimulated: $\alpha_1$, $\alpha_2$ and $\beta_1$ | Goldstein (2001) Langer and Hicks (1984) |
| - Vasoconstrictive potency: 25% | Furchgott (1972) |
| - Clearance (l/min): 5.6 | Annex 11 |
| - Elimination half-life (min): <1 | Annex 11 |
| **Clinical factor** | |
| - Usable during pregnancy: No (not classified by the FDA) | Stepke et al. (1994) |
| - Usable during lactation: ? | (Table 5.11) |
| - Absolute maximum dose in dentistry: 0.33 mg = 330 μg = 4.7 μg/kg | Jastak and Yagiela (1983) |
| - Maximum concentration in dentistry: 1:30 000 = 33 μg/ml = 0.0033% | ADA-AHA (1964) |
| - Other concentrations used in dentistry: 1:50 000 (20 μg/ml) = 0.002% 1:80 000 = 12.5 μg/ml = 0.00125% | |

levonordefrin is an artificial catecholamine designed to constrict blood vessels.

The earliest animal experiments appeared to suggest that the vasoconstrictive effect of levonordefrin was approximately half the value observed for epinephrine (Luduena et al. 1958; Tye et al. 1967) and the first clinical studies proved to be promising (Dobbs and de Vier 1950; Epstein et al. 1951; Moose 1959). As the vasoconstrictive effect was later found to be around 20% of the L-epinephrine value, a 1:20000 (50 μg/ml) concentration was used, as the theoretical equivalent of 1:100000 (10 μg/ml) of L-epinephrine (Robertson et al. 1984). Subsequent clinical experience and clinical research (Annex 21) has nonetheless shown that levonordefrin is approximately 15% as potent as L-epinephrine (Robertson et al. 1984).

The major pharmacological and clinical properties of levonordefrin are summarized in Table 6.10. It can be safely used during pregnancy and lactation (Haas et al. 2000) because it acts only weakly on the $\alpha_1$ receptors in the uterus (Langer and Hicks 1984). The absolute maximum dose for an adult weighing 70 kg or over is 1000 μg (14.3 μg/kg) (Jastak and Yagiela 1983). Levonordefrin is used in the United States and Canada with 2% mepivacaine at a fixed concentration of 1:20000 (50 μg/ml). It is less effective and more toxic than epinephrine, although not as toxic as norepinephrine (Barnard et al. 1987).

## Phentolamine (OraVerse®)

As a nonselective α-adrenergic antagonist, phentolamine neutralizes the vasoconstrictive effect of epinephrine and the other vasoconstrictive sympathomimetics (norepinephrine and levonordefrin). Phentolamine was synthesized in 1950 at the CIBA laboratory in Basel, Switzerland, by Urech et al. (1950) and marketed in the United States in 1952 (Hersh et al. 2008; Rutherford et al. 2009) under the trade name Regitine® (Weaver 2008). In medicine it is used to treat hypertension caused by pheochromocytoma, a rare chromaffin tissue tumor in the adrenal medulla that produces excess epinephrine and norepinephrine, or to extravasate injectable catecholamines administered intravenously to prevent them from inducing dermic necrosis (Hersh et al. 2008; Laviola et al. 2008; Saunders et al. 2011; Elmore et al. 2013).

In early dentistry phentolamine was used under a different formulation, phentolamine mesylate, experimentally known as NV-101 (Weaver 2008; Laviola et al. 2008). In 2008 the US Food and Drug Administration (FDA) authorized the inclusion of this drug in dentistry cartridges under the trade name OraVerse® (OraVerse 2015) for administration in standard syringes to *reduce the duration of anesthesia in soft tissue* (Tavares et al. 2008; Malamed 2008; Hersh et al. 2017).

**Table 6.10** Levonordefrin: prominent pharmacological and clinical factors.

| Pharmacological factor | Reference |
|---|---|
| • Name and synonym: levonordefrin, α-methylnorepinephrine (α-Me-Ne), α-methylnorepinephrine, neocobephrine, Corbadrine | |
| • First synthesized: ? | |
| • Chemical name: 1,1-(3,4-dihydroxyphenyl)-2-aminopropanol | American Dental Association (1984) |
| • Formula: $C_9H_{13}NO_3$ | USP38 |
| Levonordefrin structure | |
| • Molecular weight: Baseline 183.2 | USP 38 |
| • pKa value or dissociation constant: 8.6 | Annex 6 |
| • Adrenoreceptors stimulated: $\alpha_2$ and $\beta_1$ | Robertson et al. (1984) Langer and Hicks (1984) |
| • Vasoconstrictive potency: 15% | Robertson et al. (1984) |
| **Clinical factor** | |
| • Usable during pregnancy: Yes (not classified by the FDA) | Haas et al. (2000) |
| • Usable during lactation: Yes | Haas et al. (2000) |
| • Absolute maximum dose in dentistry: 1 mg = 1000 μg = 14.3 μg/kg 0.5 mg = 500 μg = 7.15 μg/kg | Jastak and Yagiela (1983) Bennett (1984) |
| • Sole concentration used in dentistry: 1:20 000 = 50 μg/ml = 0.005% | Jastak and Yagiela (1983) |

Phentolamine is injected into the same site as the vasoconstrictive sympathomimetic-bearing local anesthetic to block the effect on the α adrenoreceptors. The outcome is vasodilation that raises the local blood flow, carrying the local anesthetic from the oral submucosa into the bloodstream to restore normal sensation in the oral and perioral tissues much more quickly (Malamed 2008; Hersh et al. 2008; Tavares et al. 2008). Research has shown that after injecting phentolamine the level of the local anesthetic in the blood rises, an indication of speedier elimination from the injection site (Moore et al. 2008). The pharmacological and clinical characteristics are given in Table 6.11.

Table 6.11 Phentolamine: prominent pharmacological and clinical factors.

| Pharmacological factor | References |
|---|---|
| • Name and synonym: phentolamine | |
| • First synthesized by Urech et al. in 1950 | Urech et al. (1950) |
| • Chemical name: 3-[[(4,5-dihydro-1H-imidazol-2-yl)-methyl](4-methylphenyl)-amino]-phenol | |
| • Formula: $C_{17}H_{19}N_3O$ | |
| Phentolamine structure | |
| • Molecular weight: Baseline: 281.35  Mesylate: 377.46 | |
| • Clearance (l/min): 2.88 | Moore et al. (2008) |
| • Volume of distribution (l/min): 407 | Moore et al. (2008) |
| • Elimination half-life (min): 155 | Moore et al. (2008) |
| **Clinical factor** | |
| • Usable during pregnancy: ? (FDA category = C) | Malamed (2008) |
| • Usable during lactation: ? | |
| • Absolute maximum dose in dentistry: ? but 0.8 mg accepted, equivalent to two 1.7-ml cartridges containing 0.0235% = 0.4 mg per cartridge = 0.235 mg/ml | Tavares et al. (2008) Hersh et al. (2008) Fowler et al. (2011) |
| • Usable with children: Yes (but not authorized by the FDA in children under 3) | Hersh et al. (2019) |

## OraVerse®

This product comes in 1.7-ml cartridges with 0.4 mg (400 μg) of phentolamine mesylate, equivalent to a concentration of 0.235 mg (235 μg) per milliliter or 0.0235%. The glass cylinder cartridges bear a transparent green label and a blue aluminum ring at the mouth to ensure they are not mistaken for cartridges containing the local anesthetic.

This drug is made by two laboratories, Novolar Pharmaceuticals Inc. at San Diego, California and Septodont at Lancaster, Pennsylvania and New Castle, Delaware. The ingredients are (Moore et al. 2008):

- sterile water
- ethylene diamino tetraacetic acid (EDTA)
- D-manitol
- sodium acetate
- acetic acid
- sodium hydroxide to adjust the pH.

## Advantages and Indications

While most routine dental procedures take less than an hour, soft tissue (primarily lips and tongue) anesthesia may last for 3–4 hours (Annexes 21 and 27), hampering eating, drinking, speaking, and smiling and favoring self-inflicted injury as a result of biting lips, tongue, or cheeks, particularly in children. Moreover, as most procedures generate minimal post-operation pain, there is no advantage to prolonging the effect of anesthesia in the soft tissue (Malamed 2008; Hersh et al. 2008). In light of the foregoing, the indications for this drug are as follows:

1) Routine dentistry procedures such as obturation, scaling, root planning, etc.
2) Root canals in asymptomatic teeth (Fowler et al. 2011), which are not usually characterized by a painful prognosis (Mattscheck et al. 2001).
3) After installing implants in the posterior jaw for the early detection of lesions in the inferior alveolar nerve and, in the event, withdrawal of the implant as soon as possible to limit the lesion (Froum et al. 2010).
4) *In children to reduce the post-procedure duration* of the anesthesia in soft tissue and with it possible self-inflicted injury due to biting lips, tongue, or cheeks (Tavares et al. 2008; Zurfluh et al. 2015; Hersh et al. 2017, 2019).

## Technique and Dose

After completing the dental procedure, phentolamine is injected into the same site as the anesthetic solution containing the sympathomimetic vasoconstrictor (buccal infiltration, mandibular blockage, etc.) *at a proportion of 1:1* (1 ml of anesthetic per 1 ml of phentolamine) to block the vasoconstrictor effect (Tavares et al. 2008; Hersh et al. 2008; Fowler et al. 2011; Saunders et al. 2011). Phentolamine injection causes no pain because the soft tissues are still anesthetized (Malamed 2008; Fowler et al. 2011).

No maximum dose is presently in place for dental use, although there are recommended ceilings (Tavares et al. 2008; Hersh et al. 2008, 2019; Fowler et al. 2011; Saunders et al. 2011):

○ Children 3–6 years old (15–30 kg): half a cartridge
○ Children 6–12 years old (25–40 kg): one cartridge
○ Children over 12 and adults: two cartridges

The ratio of the amount to be injected is, as noted earlier, 1:1, although if a patient receives two cartridges of anesthesia for mandibular blockage and a third for buccal infiltration, just two cartridges of phentolamine would be injected, one in the mandibular blockage site and the other in the buccal infiltration site (Fowler et al. 2011).

## Clinical Efficacy

A number of clinical trials have shown that the duration of the anesthesia in soft tissue *is shortened by approximately 50%* (around 55% in the upper lip and 45% in the lower) to about 80 minutes after phentolamine injection (Table 6.12).

The duration depends on individual variations as well as on the time of the dental procedure. The shorter the procedure, the longer the post-procedure duration of the anesthetic in the soft tissue and therefore the more effective phentolamine is in reducing that time (Fowler et al. 2011).

According to an in-practice assessment, around 80% of patients are satisfied with phentolamine and about 50% of dentists contemplate using it in their treatments (Saunders et al. 2011).

## Tolerance, Toxicity, and Adverse Side Effects

In medical practice, phentolamine is administered intramuscularly or intravenously at doses of 1 mg in children and up to 15 mg in adults (Saunders et al. 2011; Hersh et al. 2019). In dentistry, the dose is half to two cartridges or 0.2–0.8 mg, i.e. about five to 19 times less, and this dose is not administered intravenously or systemically but rather is injected submucosally in the same site as the original infiltration or block injection. Therefore, the dental dose and method of administration result in hemodynamic stability, mitigating a potential decrease in blood pressure (in response to general vasodilation) as well as any potential reflexive increase in heart rate (Hersh et al. 2008; Tavares et al. 2008; Laviola et al. 2008; Fowler et al. 2011). Experiments in animals have shown phentolamine to have low local and systemic toxicity under the conditions used in dentistry (Rutherford et al. 2009).

Adverse side effects are infrequent and short-lived (a few hours or days) and barely differ from the discomfort reported by a placebo group (Tavares et al. 2008; Laviola et al. 2008; Fowler et al. 2011). They include the following.

Table 6.12 Clinical efficacy of phentolamine: clinical trials studying duration of anesthesia in soft tissues and percentage reduction after phentolamine injection.

| Location | Reference | Number | Treatment duration | Time (min) Control group | Phentolamine group | Reduction |
|---|---|---|---|---|---|---|
| Upper lip | Hersh et al. (2008) | 120 | 20–60[a] | 133 | 50 | 65% |
|  | Tavares et al. (2008) | 77 | 20–60[a] | — | — | 47% |
|  | Laviola et al. (2008) | 61 | 20–70 | 155 | 50 | 68% |
|  | Fowler et al. (2011)[b] | 85 | 67–71 | 224 | 136 | 38% |
|  |  |  |  |  | 79 | **54%** |
| Lower lip | Hersh et al. (2008) | 122 | 20–60 | 155 | 70 | 55% |
|  | Tavares et al. (2008) | 75 | 20–60 | — | — | 67% |
|  | Laviola et al. (2008) | 61 | 20–70 | 150 | 101 | 33% |
|  | Fowler et al. (2011) | 85 | 85 | 217 | 170 | 22% |
|  |  |  |  |  | 114 | **44%** |
| Global | Hersh et al. (2008) | 240 | 20–60 | 140 | 60 | 57% |
|  | Tavares et al. (2008) | 152 | 20–60 | 135 | 60 | 56% |
|  | Laviola et al. (2008) | 122 | 20–70 | 155 | 70 | 55% |
|  | Fowler et al. (2011) | 85 | 67–85 | 220 | 153 | 30% |
|  | Saunders et al. (2011) | — | — | — | 60 | — |
|  |  |  |  |  | 80 | **50%** |

[a] The time in minutes is the median except in the Fowler et al. (2011) paper, where it is the mean.
[b] Time estimated by Fowler et al. (2011).

1) Sensitivity may linger in the injection zone, with slight swelling and discomfort (Hersh et al. 2008; Laviola et al. 2008) in 4–6% of cases.
2) Some 2–4% of patients complain of headaches (cephalea) (Hersh et al. 2008; Elmore et al. 2013).
3) Around 3% of mandibular blockage patients report soreness on opening their mouths (Elmore et al. 2013).

## Felypressin (Octapressin®)

Felypressin (Octapressin or Octopressin®) was synthesized by Du Vigneaud et al. in 1953 (Du Vigneaud et al. 1953) as a derivative of the posterior pituitary hormones (oxytocin and vasopressin, the latter is also known as antidiuretic hormone or ADH) and more exactly as a derivative of vasopressin, replacing two amino acids: tyrosine with phenylamine in position 2 and arginine with lysine in position 8. The chemical name is consequently 2-phenylamine-8-lysine-vasopressin (PLV-2) (Berde and Cerletti 1964; Altura et al. 1965; Anonymous 1965) (Figure 6.4). This new compound is a vasoconstrictor, and the antidiuretic or oxytocin-like effects are not seen as it is injected in the oral mucosa (Berde and Cerletti 1964). The major pharmacological and clinical properties of felypressin are summarized in Table 6.13.

This vasoconstrictor is not marketed in the United States, although it is sold in several European Union countries under the trade name Octapressin, synthesized by Sandoz at Basel, Switzerland. Felypressin is measured in international units (IU) and used in dentistry at a fixed concentration of 0.03 IU/ml (0.54 µg/ml) in solution with 3% prilocaine.

### Cardiovascular Effects

Experimental studies in animals (Cecanho et al. 2006), children (Meechan et al. 2001), healthy adults (Aelling et al. 1970; Meechan and Rawlins 1988), hypertensive patients (Sunada et al. 1996), and patients with arrhythmias and coronary insufficiency (Caceres et al. 2008) show that felypressin induces very mild cardiovascular side effects, raising mean blood pressure very slightly and lowering heart rate barely perceptibly. These slight effects are observed when over three and a half cartridges of anesthesia are administered with the standard 0.03 IU/ml concentration of felypressin (Sunada et al. 1996).

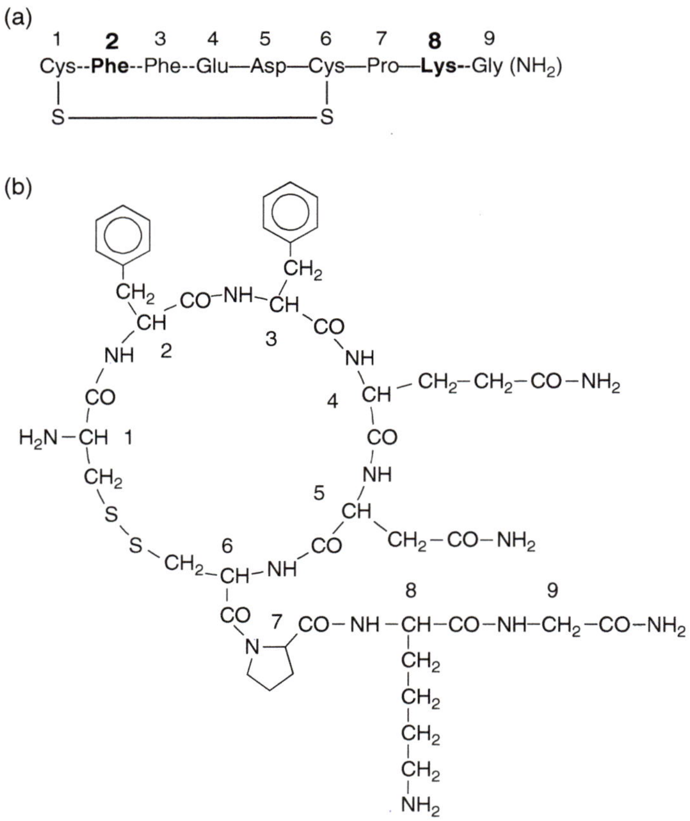

**Figure 6.4** Felypressin formula: (a) abbreviated formula; (b) full formula. *Source:* Modified from Berde and Cerletti (1964) and Anonymous (1965).

Table 6.13 Felypressin: prominent pharmacological and clinical factors.

| Pharmacological factor | Reference |
|---|---|
| • Name and synonym: felypressin, octapressin, PLV-2 <br> • First synthesized by Du Vigneaud et al. in 1952 <br> • Chemical name: 2-phenylalanine-8-lysine-vasopressin <br><br> • Formula: $C_{42}H_{65}N_{13}O_{11}S_2$ | Du Vigneaud et al. (1953) <br> Berde and Cerletti (1964) <br> Altura et al. (1965) <br> Anonymous (1965) |
| • Molecular weight: 1040.2 <br> • Receptors stimulated: $v_1$ <br> • Vasoconstrictive potency: less than in catecholamines | Cecanho et al. (2006) |
| **Clinical factor** | |
| • Usable during pregnancy: No (not classified by the FDA) <br><br> • Usable during lactation: ? <br> • Absolute maximum dose in dentistry: 7.02 μg = 0.39 IU[a] <br> 0.1 μg/kg = 0.0056 IU/kg <br> • Sole concentration used in dentistry: <br> 1:1 850 000 = 0.54 μg/ml (0.03 IU/ml) = 0.000 000 54% | Oliver (1974) <br> Stepke et al. (1994) <br> (Table 5.11) <br> Dunlop Committee[a] <br><br> Berling (1966) <br> Barnard et al. (1987) |

[a] See Tables 6.4 and 6.14. IU, international units.

As the side effects are much less intense in felypressin than in epinephrine (Aelling et al. 1970; Meechan et al. 2001; Cecanho et al. 2006), it is generally regarded as safe for patients with cardiovascular disease.

## Vasoconstrictive Effect

Felypressin induces vasoconstriction by binding to vasopressive and oxytocic $v_1$ receptors (Cecanho et al. 2006), while barely impacting antidiuretic $v_2$ receptors. Its vasopressive properties differ from those of catecholamines in a number of ways.

1) It acts essentially on the microcirculation venules, rarely affecting arterioles, metarterioles, or precapillary sphincters (Cerletti et al. 1963; Altura et al. 1965; Burcher et al. 1977).
2) It spreads to the tissues and penetrates the nerve trunk *vasa nervorum* less readily than epinephrine

due to its higher molecular weight (1040.2 vs. 183.2) (Burcher et al. 1977; Olgart and Gazelius 1977; Chng et al. 1996).
3) The vasoconstrictive effect is consequently slow, taking several minutes as opposed to the immediate action observed in epinephrine (Burcher et al. 1977; Lindorf 1979).
4) Hypoxia does not occur in the infiltrated tissue (Klingenström and Westermar 1964), making it less of an irritant for tissue than catecholamines, thereby eluding late-stage rebound vasodilation.

As a result of the above, felypressin is a less potent vasoconstrictor than catecholamines, epinephrine in particular (Fisher et al. 1965; Altura et al. 1965; Burcher et al. 1977). As the use of high felypressin concentrations does not deliver good results, concentrations of only 0.05–0.03 IU/ml are recommended (Berling 1966; Akerman 1969).

### Adverse Effects

Two adverse effects have been detected in connection with the use of felypressin in dentistry and medicine:

1) Pale skin on the face, neck, and arms due to cutaneous vasoconstriction (Shanks 1963; Light et al. 1965; Katz and Katz 1966; Berling 1966; Anonymous 1970).
2) Abdominal discomfort due to intestinal contraction and the sudden need to defecate (Light et al. 1965; Akerman 1969).

Adverse reactions are fewer, less frequent, and much less severe in felypressin than in the catecholamines, particularly norepinephrine and levonordefrin (Barnard et al. 1987).

### Contraindications

The two major contraindications for the use of felypressin in dentistry are discussed below.

1) It is *contraindicated in patients who have had a heart attack* (angina or myocardial infarction) *but only relatively so*, given that it is administered at very low doses.
    o Felypressin-induced vasoconstriction of the coronary vessels reduces the blood flow and the supply of oxygen to the heart (Light et al. 1965; Miyachi et al. 2003). Interestingly, however, doses equivalent to 14 cartridges of 0.03 IU/ml barely affect ischemia in hypertensive patients (Sunada et al. 1996).
    o The United Kingdom's Dunlop Committee on Safety of Drugs recommends a maximum dose of five 1.8-ml cartridges of 0.03 IU/ml felypressin for such patients (Oliver 1974; Roberts and Sowray 1987), while experimental data with dogs suggests similar values (Miyachi et al. 2003).
2) *It is absolutely contraindicated in pregnancy* (Anonymous 1970; Oliver 1974) because the residual oxytocic effect of felypressin resulting from stimulation of $v_1$ receptors may cause the pregnant uterus to contract, reducing the blood flow to the placenta and raising the risk of contraction, premature labor or miscarriage (Anonymous 1970; Oliver 1974; Stepke et al. 1994). Moreover, felypressin is used with prilocaine, a local anesthetic that can induce fetal methemoglobinemia, which would worsen the situation (Anonymous 1970; Oliver 1974).

### Advantages and Disadvantages

- Felypressin has three advantages over epinephrine.
    1) Its small cardiovascular effects make if safe for such patients, except those who have had a heart attack (as mentioned earlier), although even in such cases it can be used in small doses.
    2) It does not interact with:
        o tricyclic antidepressants (Goldman 1971; Persson and Siwers 1971; Boakes et al. 1973), eliminating the risk of prompting hypertension or arrhythmias
        o halothane (general anesthetic) (Shanks 1963; Light et al. 1965; Katz 1965; Katz and Katz 1966), eliminating the risk of arrhythmias
        o sodium thiopental, an ultra-speedy barbiturate used in general anesthesia induction (Light et al. 1965), eliminating the risk of arrhythmias.
    3) It is less irritating than epinephrine because it does not induce tissue hypotoxia (Klingenström and Westermar 1964).
- The disadvantages relative to epinephrine include the following.
    1) As its vasoconstrictive effect is less potent, it delivers poorer results:
        o lower percentage of pulpal anesthesia (Table 6.1)
        o shorter duration of pulpal anesthesia (Table 6.1)
        o less effective hemostasis (Fisher et al. 1965).
    2) It is wholly contraindicated during pregnancy, as noted above.

### Maximum Doses

Experimental studies on acute toxicity in animals have shown that felypressin is much safer than epinephrine and the tolerance levels are much higher (Annex 18). The absolute maximum doses cited in the literature vary across a wide spectrum (Table 6.14), a discrepancy possibly

Table 6.14 Maximum recommended doses for felypressin.

| | | | 0.03 IU/ml | | | |
| --- | --- | --- | --- | --- | --- | --- |
| | IU | μg | ml | 1.8-ml cartridges | Type of patient | Reference |
| Author | | | | | | |
| | 0.27 | 4.86 | 9.0 | 5 | Healthy | Jastak and Yagiela (1983) |
| | 16.70 | 300 | 555 | 308 | Healthy | Jage (1993) |
| Dunlop Committee | | | | | | |
| | 0.262 | 4.75 | 8.8 | 5 | **Ischemia** | Oliver (1974) |
| | | | | | | Roberts and Sowray (1987) |
| | 0.39 | 7.02 | 13.0 | **7.2** | **Healthy** | Oliver (1974) |
| | | | | | | Roberts and Sowray (1982) |

spawned by a fear of coronary vasoconstriction. The recommendations for healthy patients and those with ischemia (angina and myocardium infarction) cited here are taken from the United Kingdom's Dunlop Committee (full name: the Committee on Safety of Drugs).[2]

Further to the Committee's findings, the maximum recommended dose of 3% prilocaine with 0.03 IU/ml (0.54 μg/ml) is five 1.8-ml cartridges in patients with ischemia and 7.2 cartridges in healthy patients (Oliver 1974; Roberts and Sowray 1987).

## Combinations of Vasoconstrictors

The few papers published on the combination of two vasoconstrictors in the same anesthetic solution can be divided into two groups.

- The combination 1:100 000 (10 μg/ml) epinephrine and 1:100 000 (10 μg/ml) norepinephrine was introduced in Germany in the 1950s to reduce the palpitations (tachycardia) induced by epinephrine and the cephalea prompted by norepinephrine, initially with promising results (Holler 1954; Adler and Kelentey 1965). Today, however, most authors concur that these combinations of vasoconstrictors are contraindicated, in as much as they may have exactly the opposite effect: norepinephrine may cause rises in blood pressure (and concomitant cephalea) and epinephrine tachycardia (Reynolds 1972; Evers and Haegerstam 1981; Jage 1993; Malamed 2004).
- Epinephrine and felypressin combinations also fail to lower anesthetic solution toxicity as initially believed and are consequently not recommended either (Volpato et al. 1999).

In conclusion, based on the small amount of data available, combinations of vasoconstrictors not only afford no advantages but may have adverse effects and are therefore *not recommended at this time*.

## References

Abel, J.J. (1899). Ueber den blutdruckenrregeden Bestandtheil der Nebenniere, das Epinephrin. *Hoppe-Seyler's Z Physiol. Chem.* 28: 318–362.

ADA-AHA (American Dental Association and American Heart Association) (1964). Management of dental problems in patients with cardiovascular disease. *J. Am. Dent. Assoc.* 68 (3): 333–342.

Adler, P. and Kelentey, B. (1965). Über die Testung neuer lokalanästhetica. *Dtsch. Zahnartzl. Z.* 20 (2): 144–152.

Aelling, W.H., Laurence, D.R., O'Neill, R., and Verril, P.J. (1970). Cardiac effects of adrenaline and felypressin as vasoconstrictor in local anaesthesia for oral surgery under diazepam sedation. *Br. J. Anaesth.* 40 (2): 174–176.

Akerman, B. (1969). Effects of Felypressin (Octopressin®) on the acute toxicity of local anesthetics. *Acta Pharmacol. Toxicol.* 27 (5): 318–330.

Aldrich, T.B. (1901). A preliminary report on the active principle of the suprarenal gland. *Am. J. Phys.* 5: 457–461.

---

2 The Dunlop Committee was founded in 1964 under the chairmanship of Sir Derrick Dunlop (1902–1980). Its real name was the Committee on Safety of Drugs, but it was popularly identified with the name of its chairman. In 1970 the name was changed to Committee on Safety of Medicines and in 2005 to the Commission on Human Medicines.

Alquist, R.P. (1948). A study of the adrenotropic receptors. *Am. J. Phys.* 153 (3): 586–600.

Altura, B.M., Hershey, S.G., and Zweifach, B.W. (1965). Effects of a synthetic analogue of vasopressin on vascular smooth muscle (30152). *Proc. Soc. Exp. Biol. Med.* 119: 258–261.

American Dental Association (1984). *Accepted Dental Therapeutics*, 40e, 203–209. Chicago (IL): Council on Dental Therapeutics, American Dental Association.

Annex 6. Dissociation constant or pKa.

Annex 11. Pharmcokinetics of local anesthetics and vasoconstrictors.

Annex 12. Biotransformation of local anesthetics and vasoconstrictors.

Annex 15. Epinephrine I. Epinephrine and norepinephrine. Hemodynamic alterations in healthy dental patients.

Annex 16. Epinephrine II. Dose administered and plasma levels.

Annex 18. Acute experimental toxicity of vasoconstrictors.

Annex 21. Maxillary pulpal anesthesia. Buccal infiltration.

Annex 27. Mandibular blockage IV. Anesthesia of the lower lip and time to first pain.

Anonymous (1965). Über den Angriffspunkt vasokonstriktorischer Wirkstoffe im Gefäßgebiet der Mikrozirkulation. *Triangle (Sandoz, Basel)* 7 (2): 77–82.

Anonymous (1970). Felypressin – a new vasoconstrictor with prilocaine. *Drug Ther. Bull.* 8 (10): 38–40.

Barnard, D.P., Joubert, P.H., and Venter, C.P. (1987). Noradrenaline and local anesthesia: a review of the literature and clinical evaluation. *J. Dent. Assoc. S. Afr.* 42 (4): 185–191.

Bennett, C.R. (1984). *Monheim's Local Anesthesia and Pain Control in Dental Practice*, 7e. St Louis (MI): The CV Mosby Company. 178.

Berde, B. and Cerletti, A. (1964). Medizinische und biologische Aspeckte von pharmakologischen Arbeiten mit synthetischen Peptiden von neurohypophysärem Typus. *Klin. Wochenschr.* 42 (23): 1159–1165.

Berling, C. (1958). Carbocain in local anaesthesia in the oral cavity. *Odontol. Revy* 9: 254–267.

Berling, C. (1966). Octapressin® as a vasoconstrictor in dental plexus anesthesia. *Odontol. Revy* 17 (4): 369–185.

Berling, C. and Björn, H. (1951). Noradrenalin (norexadrin). En översikt. *Odontol. Revy* 2 (3): 147–152.

Berling, C. and Björn, H. (1960). L67-ett nytt lokalbedövningsmedel av anilidtyp. Experimentell bestämnig av effektiveten vid plexusanestesin pa homo. *Sven. Tandläk-Forb. Tidn.* 52 (19): 511–522.

Boakes, A.J., Laurence, D.R., Lovel, K.W. et al. (1972). Adverse reactions to local anaesthetic/vasoconstrictors preparations. A study of the cardiovascular response to xilestin and hostacain-with-noradrenaline. *Br. Dent. J.* 133 (4): 137–140.

Boakes, A.J., Laurence, D.R., Teoh, P.C. et al. (1973). Interactions between sympathomimetic amines and antidepressant agents in man. *Br. Med. J.* 1 (5849): 311–315.

Bonica, J.J. (1959). *Tratamiento del dolor, con estudio especial del empleo del bloqueo analgésico en el diagnóstico, pronóstico y terapéutica*. Barcelona (España): Salvat Editores SA. 159.

Braid, D.P. and Scott, D.B. (1965). The systemic absorption of local analgesic drugs. *Br. J. Anaesth.* 37 (6): 394–404.

Braun, H. (1903). Ueber den Einfluss der Vitalität der Gewebe auf die örtlichen und allgemeinen Giftwirkungen localanästhesirender mittel und über die Bedeutung des Adrenalins für die Localanästhesie. *Arch. Klin. Chir.* 69 (29): 541–591.

Bromage, P.R. and Robson, J.G. (1961). Concentrations of lignocaine in the blood after intravenous, intramuscular, epidural and endotracheal administration. *Anaesthesia* 16 (4): 461–478.

Brown, R.S. and Rhodus, N.L. (2005). Epinephrine and local anesthesia revisited. *Oral Surg. Oral Med. Oral Pathol.* 100 (4): 401–408.

Buckley, J.A., Ciancio, S.G., and McMullen, J.A. (1984). Efficacy of epinephrine concentration in local anesthesia during perioral surgery. *J. Periodontol.* 55 (11): 653–657.

Burcher, E., Olgart, L., and Gazelius, B. (1977). Comparative effects of adrenaline and felypressin (octapressin) on consecutive sections of the vascular bed in canine adipose tissue. *Acta Physiol. Scand.* 100 (2): 215–220.

Bylund, D.B., Eikenberg, D.C., Hieble, J.P. et al. (1994). IV. International Union of Pharmacology nomenclature of adrenoceptors. *Pharmacol. Rev.* 46 (2): 121–136.

Caceres, M.T.F., Ludovice, A.C.P.P., de Brito, F.S. et al. (2008). Effect of local anesthetics with and without vasoconstrictor agent in patients with ventricular arrhythmias. *Arq. Bras. Cardiol.* 91 (3): 128–133.

Campbell, R.L. (1977). Cardiovascular effects of epinephrine overdose. Case report. *Anesth. Prog.* 24 (6): 190–193.

Campbell, D. and Adriani, J. (1958). Absorption of local anesthetics. *J. Am. Med. Assoc.* 168 (7): 873–877.

Cannell, H. and Beckett, A.H. (1975a). Peri-oral injections of local anesthetic intro defined sites. *Br. Dent. J.* 139 (6): 242–244.

Cannell, H. and Beckett, A.H. (1975b). Circulating levels of lignocaine after peri-oral injections. *Br. Dent. J.* 138 (3): 87–93.

Cawson, R.A., Curson, I., and Whittington, D.R. (1983). The hazards of dental anesthetics. *Br. Dent. J.* 154 (8): 253–258.

Cecanho, R., de Luca, L.A., and Ranali, J. Jr. (2006). Cardiovascular effects of felypressin. *Anesth. Prog.* 53 (4): 119–125.

Cerletti, A., Weber, H., and Weidmann, H. (1963). Zur Wirkung von Phenylalanine 2-Lysin-Vasopressin (octapressin) auf den arteriellen und venösen Anteil eines peripheren Gefäßgebietes. *Helv. Physiol. Pharmacol. Acta* 21 (4): 394–401.

Chng, H.S., Pitt Ford, T.R., and McDonald, F. (1996). Effects of prilocaine local anaesthetic solutions on pulpal blood flow in maxillary canines. *Endod. Dent. Traumatol.* 12 (2): 89–95.

Clutter, W.E., Bier, D.M., Shah, S.D., and Cryer, P.E. (1980). Epinephrine plasma metabolic clearance rates and physiologic thresholds for metabolic and hemodynamic actions in man. *J. Clin. Invest.* 66 (1): 94–101.

Coman, O.A., Paunescu, H., Ghita, I. et al. (2009). Beta 3 adrenergic receptors: molecular, histological, functional and pharmacological approachs. *Rom. J. Morphol. Embryol.* 50 (2): 169–179.

Curtis, M.B., Gores, R.J., and Owen, C.A. Jr. (1966). The effect of certain hemostatic agents and the local use of diluted epinephrine on bleeding during oral surgical procedures. *Oral Surg. Oral Med. Oral Pathol.* 21 (2): 143–147.

Cushny, A.R. (1909). Further note on adrenalin isomers. *J. Physiol. (London)* 38 (4): 259–262.

Dale, H.H. (1906). One some physiological actions of ergot. *J. Physiol. (London)* 34 (3): 163–206.

De Jong, R.H. and Cullen, S.C. (1963). Buffer-demand and pH of local anesthetics solutions containing epinephrine. *Anesthesiology* 24 (6): 801–807.

Dobbs, E.C. (1965). A chronological history of local anesthesia in dentistry. *J. Oral Ther. Pharmacol.* 1 (5): 546–549.

Dobbs, E.C. and de Vier, C. (1950). L-arterenol as a vasoconstrictor in local anesthesia. *J. Am. Dent. Assoc.* 40 (4): 433–436.

Donaldson, M. and Goodchild, J.H. (2012). Pregnancy, breast-feeding and drugs used in dentistry. *J. Am. Dent. Assoc.* 143 (8): 858–871.

Du Vigneaud, V., Ressler, C., Swan, J.M. et al. (1953). The synthesis of an octapeptide amide with the hormonal activity of oxitocin. *J. Am. Chem. Soc.* 75 (19): 4879–4880.

Eisenhofer, G., Kopin, I.J., and Goldstein, D.S. (2004). Catecholamine metabolism: a contemporary view with implications for physiology and medicine. *Pharmacol. Rev.* 56 (3): 331–349.

Ekmanner, S. and Persson, H. (1951). Noradrenalin son vasokonstriktor i xylocain. En klinisk prövning i odontologisk praxis. *Sven. Tandlak. Tidskr.* 44 (6): 451–458.

Elmore, S., Nusstein, J., Drum, M. et al. (2013). Reversal of pulpal and soft tissue anesthesia by using phentolamine: a prospective, randomized, single-blind study. *J. Endod.* 39 (4): 429–434.

Epstein, S., Thromdson, A.H., and Schmitz, J.L. (1951). Levo-arterenol (levophed) as a vasoconstrictor in local anesthetic solutions. *J. Dent. Res.* 30 (6): 870–873.

Evers, H. and Haegerstam, G. (1981). *Handbook of Dental Local Anesthesia*. Copenhagen: Schultz Medical Information. 58.

Fisher, S.J., Gehrig, H., and Green, H. (1965). Non-catechol amine vasopressor (PLV-2) for use as adjunct to local anesthesia. *J. Am. Dent. Assoc.* 70 (5): 1189–1193.

Fowler, S., Nusstein, J., Drum, M. et al. (2011). Reversal of soft-tissue anesthesia in asymptomatic endodontic patients: a preliminary, prospective, randomized, single-blind study. *J. Endod.* 37 (10): 1353–1358.

Froum, S.J., Froum, S.H., and Malamed, S.F. (2010). The use of phentolamine mesylate to evaluate mandibular nerve damage following implant placement. *Compend. Contin. Educ. Dent* 31 (7): 520–528.

Furchgott, R.F. (1972). The classification of adrenoceptors (adrenergic receptors). An evaluation from the standpoint of receptor theory (Chapter 9). In: *Catecholamines. Handbook of Experimental Pharmacology (New Series)*, vol. 33 (ed. H. Blaschko and E. Muscholl). Berlin: Springer-Verlag. 283–335.

Fyhr, P. and Brodin, A. (1987). The effect of anaerobic conditions on epinephrine stability. *Acta Pharm. Suec.* 24 (3): 89–96.

Goebel, W.M., Allen, G., and Randall, F. (1979). Comparative circulating serum levels of mepivacaine with levo-nordefrin and lidocaine with epinephrine. *Anesth. Prog.* 26 (4): 93–97.

Goebel, W.M., Allen, G., and Randall, F. (1980a). Comparative circulating serum levels of 2 percent mepivacaine and 2 percent lignocaine. *Br. Dent. J.* 148 (11–12): 261–264.

Goebel, W.M., Allen, G., and Randall, F. (1980b). The effect of commercial vasoconstrictor preparations on the circulating venous serum level of mepivacaine and lidocaine. *J. Oral Med.* 35 (4): 91–96.

Goldman, V. (1971). Local anesthetics containing vasoconstrictors (letter). *Br. Med. J.* 1 (5741): 175.

Goldman, V. and Evers, H. (1969). Prilocaine-felypressin: a new combination for dental analgesia. *Dent. Prac. Dent. Rec.* 19 (7): 225–231.

Goldstein, D.J. (2001). Physiology of the adrenal medulla and the sympathetic nervous system (Chapter 85). In: *Principles and Practice of Endocrinology and Metabolism*, 3e (ed. K.L. Becker). Philadelphia: Lippincott Williams and Wilkins. 817–826.

Haas, D.A., Pynn, B.R., and Sands, T.D. (2000). Drugs use for the pregnant or lactating patient. *Gen. Dent.* 48 (1): 54–60.

Haglund, J. and Evers, H. (1985). *Local anaesthesia in dentistry*, 6e. Södertäle (Sweden): Astra Läkemedel AB. 59–60.

Hardin, R.L., Yagiela, J.A., Bilger, D.A.L., and Hunt, L.M. (1981). Influence of epinephrine on intravascular lidocaine toxicity. *J. Dent. Res.* 60 (Special issue): 463. (abstract n° 615).

Hecht, A. and App, G.R. (1974). Blood volume lost during gingivectomy using two different anesthetic techniques. *J. Periodontol.* 45 (1): 9–12.

Henn, F. (1960). Determination of the toxicological and pharmacological properties of carbocaine, lidocaine and procaine by means of simultaneous experiments. *Acta Anaesthesiol. Scand.* 4: 125–154.

Henn, F. and Brattsand, R. (1966). Some pharmacological and toxicological properties of a new long-acting local analgesic, LAC-43 (Marcaine®), in comparison with mepivacaine and tetracaine. *Acta Anesthesiol. Scand. Suppl.* 21: 9–30.

Hersh, E.V., Moore, P.A., Papas, A.S. et al. (2008). The Soft Tissue Anesthesia Recovery Group. Reversal of soft-tissue local anesthesia with phentolamine mesylate in adolescents and adults. *J. Am. Dent. Assoc.* 139 (8): 1080–1093.

Hersh, E.V., Lindemeyer, R., Berg, J.H. et al. (2017). Pediatric Soft Tissue Anesthesia Recovery Group. Phase four, randomized, double-blinded, controlled trial of phentolamine mesylate in two- to five-year-old patients. *Pediatr. Dent.* 39 (1): 39–45.

Hersh, E.V., Moore, P.A., and Saraghi, M. (2019). Phentolamine mesylate: pharmacology, efficacy, and safety. *Gen. Dent.* 67 (3): 12–17.

Hieble, J.P. (2000). Adrenoceptor subclassification: an approach to improved cardiovascular therapeutics. *Pharm. Acta Helv.* 74 (2–3): 163–171.

Himms-Hagen, J. (1972). Effects of catecholamines on metabolism (Chapter 11). In: *Catecholamines. Handbook of Experimental Pharmacology (New Series)*, vol. 33 (ed. H. Blaschko and E. Muscholl). Berlin: Springer-Verlag. 363–462.

Hirota, Y., Hori, T., Kai, K., and Matsuura, H. (1992). Effects of epinephrine and norepinephrine contained in 2% lidocaine on hemodynamica of the carotid and cerebral circulation in older and younger adults. *Anesth. Pain Control Dent.* 1 (3): 143–151.

Holler, W.V. (1954). Vergleichende Untersuchungen einiger Vasokonstringentien. *Dtsch. Zahnartzl. Z.* 9 (9): 505–511.

Hondrum, S.O., Seng, G.F., and Robert, N.W. (1993). Stability of local anesthetics in dental cartridge. *Anesth. Pain Control Dent.* 2 (4): 198–202.

Hoppe, J.O. and Seppelin, D.K. Unpublished data cited by: Tainter ML, Luduena FP, Hoppe JO.(1953). The trend to more potent local anesthetic solutions in dentistry. *Oral Surg. Oral Med. Oral Pathol.* 6 (5): 645–661.

Hoppe, J.O., Seppelin, D.K., and Lands, A.M. (1949). An investigation of the acute toxicity of the optical isomers of arterenol and epinephrine. *J. Pharmacol. Exp. Ther.* 95 (4): 502–505.

Jage, J. (1993). Circulatory effects of vasoconstrictors combined with local anesthetics. *Anesth. Pain Control Dent.* 2 (2): 81–86.

Jastak, J.T. and Yagiela, J.A. (1983). Vasoconstrictors and local anesthesia: a review and rationale for use. *J. Am. Dent. Assoc.* 107 (4): 623–630.

Jastak, J.T., Yagiela, J.A., and Donaldson, D. (1995). *Local Anesthesia of the Oral Cavity*. Philadelphia: WB Saunders Co. 81.

Katz, R.L. (1965). Epinephrine and PLV-2: cardiac rhythm and local vasoconstrictor effects. *Anesthesiology* 26 (5): 619–623.

Katz, R.L. and Katz, G.J. (1966). Surgical infiltration of pressor drugs and their interaction with volatile anesthetics. *Br. J. Anaesth.* 38 (9): 712–718.

Keil, W. and Vieten, H. (1952). Neue Geischtspunkte für die Anästhesie des tracheobronchialsystems, erisbesondere zur bronchographie. *Fortschr. Geb. Rontgenstr.* 77 (4): 409–425.

Keiser, H.R. (2001). Pheochromocytoma and related tumors (Chapter 135). In: *Endocrinology*, 4e (ed. L.J. DeGroot and J.L. Jameson). Philadelphia: WB Saunders Co. 1862–1883.

Klein, R.M. (1983). Components of local anesthetic solutions. *Gen. Dent.* 31 (6): 460–465.

Klingenström, P. and Westermar, K.L. (1964). Local tissue-oxygen tension after adrenaline, noradrenaline and Octapressin® in local anaesthesia. *Acta Anaesth. Scand.* 8: 261–266.

Kopin, I.J. (1989). Plasma levels of catecholamines and dopamine – β-hydroxilase (Chapter 15). In: *Catecholamines II. Handbook of Experimental Pharmacology*, vol. 90/II (ed. U. Trendelenburg and N. Weiner). Berlin: Springer-Verlag. 211–275.

Lands, A.M., Arnold, A., McAuliff, J.P. et al. (1967). Differentiation of receptor systems active by sympathomimetic amines. *Nature (London)* 214 (5088): 597–598.

Landsberg, L. (1976). Extraneuronal uptake and metabolism of [$^3$H] L-noerepinephrine by the rat duodenal mucosa. *Biochem. Pharmacol.* 25 (6): 729–731.

Landsberg, L. and Young, J.B. (1980). Catecholamines and the adrenal medulla (Chapter 24). In: *Metabolic Control and Disease*, 8e (ed. P.K. Bondy and L.E. Rosenberg). Philadelphia: WB Saunders Co. 1621–1693.

Langer, S.Z. (1974). Presynaptic regulation of catecholamine release. *Biochem. Pharmacol.* 23 (13): 1793–1800.

Langer, S.Z. and Hicks, P.E. (1984). Alpha-adrenoreceptor subtypes in blood vessels: physiology and pharmacology. *J. Cardiovasc. Pharmacol.* 6 (Suppl 4): S547–S558.

Launoy, L. and Menguy, B. (1920). Sur la sensibilité de l'essai physiologique de l'adrenaline: constantes d'action. *C. R. Seances Soc. Biol. (Paris)* 83: 1510–1511.

Launoy, L. and Menguy, B. (1922). Documents numeriques sur les adrenalines, droite, gauche et sur l'adrenaline. *C. R. Seances Soc. Biol. Fil. (Paris)* 87: 1066–1068.

Laviola, M., McGavin, S.K., Freer, G.A. et al. (2008). Randomized study of phentolamine mesylate for reversal of local anesthesia. *J. Dent. Res.* 87 (7): 635–639.

Light, G.A., Rattenborg, C., and Holaday, D.A. (1965). A new vasoconstrictor: preliminary studies of phelypressin. *Anesth. Analg.* 44 (3): 280–287.

Lindorf, H.H. (1979). Investigation of the vascular effect of newer local anesthetics and vasoconstrictors. *Oral Surg. Oral Med. Oral Pathol.* 48 (4): 292–297.

Luduena, F.P., Ananenko, E., Siegmund, O.H., and Miller, L.C. (1949). Comparative pharmacology of optical isomers of arterenol. *J. Pharmacol. Exp. Ther.* 95 (2): 155–170.

Luduena, F.P., Hoppe, J.O., Oyen, I.H., and Wessinger, G.D. (1958). Some pharmacologic properties of levo- and dextro-nordefrin. *J. Dent. Res.* 37 (2): 206–213.

Lund, A. (1951). Elimination of adrenaline and noradrenaline from the organism. *Acta Pharmacol. Toxicol.* 7 (4): 297–308.

Lund, P.C. and Cwik, J.C. (1965). Citanest®. . .a clinical and laboratory study. Part 1. *Anesth. Analg. Curr. Res.* 44 (5): 623–631.

Malamed, S.F. (2004). *Handbook of Local Anesthesia*, 5e. St. Louis (Mi): Elsevier-Mosby. 44, 48–49.

Malamed, S.F. (2008). Reversing local anesthesia. *Inside Dentist.* (july/august) 2–3.

Mattscheck, D.J., Law, A.J., and Noblett, W.C. (2001). Retratament versus initial root canal treatment: factor affecting posttreatment pain. *Oral Surg. Oral Med. Oral Pathol.* 92 (3): 321–324.

Meechan, J.G. and Rawlins, M.D. (1988). The effects of two different dental local anesthetic solutions on plasma potassium levels during third molar surgery. *Oral Surg. Oral Med. Oral Pathol.* 66 (6): 650–653.

Meechan, J.G., Thomson, C.W., Blair, G.S., and Rawlins, M.D. (1991). The biochemical and haemodynamic effects of adrenalin in lignocaine local anaesthetic solutions in patients having third molar surgery under general anaesthesia. *Br. J. Oral Maxillofac. Surg.* 29 (4): 263–268.

Meechan, J.G., Cole, B., and Welbury, R.R. (2001). The influence of two different dental local anaesthetic solutions on the haemodynamic responses of children undergoing restorative dentistry: a randomized, single-blind, split-mouth study. *Br. Dent. J.* 190 (9): 502–504.

Mefford, I., Oke, A., Keller, R. et al. (1978). Epinephrine distribution in human brain. *Neuro Sci. Lett.* 9 (23): 227–231.

Meyer, R. and Allen, G.D. (1968). Blood volume studies in oral surgery: I. Operative and postoperative blood losses in relation to vasoconstrictors. *J. Oral Surg.* 26 (11): 721–726.

Milano, E.A., Waraszkiewicz, S.M., and Dirubio, R. (1982). Aluminium catalysis of epinephrine degradation in lidocaine hydrochloride with epinephrine solutions. *J. Parenter. Sci. Technol.* 36 (6): 232–236.

Miyachi, K., Ichinohe, T., and Kaneko, Y. (2003). Effects of local injection of prilocaine-felypressin on the myocardial oxygen balance in dogs. *Eur. J. Oral Sci.* 111 (4): 339–345.

Moore, P.A., Doll, B., Delie, R.A. et al. (2007). Hemostatic and anesthetic efficacy of 4% articaine HCL with 1:200,000 epinephrine and 4% articaine HCL with 1:100,000 epinephrine when administered intraorally for periodontal surgery. *J. Periodontol.* 78 (2): 247–253.

Moore, P.A., Hersh, E.V., Papas, A.S. et al. (2008). Pharmacokinetics of lidocaine with epinephrine following local anesthesia reversal with phentolamine mesylate. *Anesth. Prog.* 55 (2): 40–48.

Moose, S. (1959). Clinical evaluation of levo-nordefrin in local anesthetics. *Oral Surg. Oral Med. Oral Pathol.* 12 (7): 838–845.

Navarro, F.A. (2003). ¿Quién lo usó por vez primera? Adrenalina. *Panacea (revista de medina, lenguaje y traducción)* 4 (12): 142. (Open Access).

New Zealand Committee (1974). New Zealand Committee on Adverse Drug Reactions: Eight annual report. *N. Z. Dent. J.* 70: 50–56.

Okada, Y., Suzuki, H., and Ishiyama, I. (1989). Fatal subaracnoid haemorrhage associated with dental local anaesthesia. *Aust. Dent. J.* 34 (4): 323–325.

Olgart, L. and Gazelius, B. (1977). Effect of adrenaline and felypressin (Octapressin) on blood flow and sensory nerve activity in the tooth. *Acta Odontol. Scand.* 35 (2): 69–75.

Oliver, L.P. (1974). Local anesthesia—a review of practice. *Aust. Dent. J.* 19 (5): 313–319.

OraVerse Prospecto: información para el usuario. Septodont. 2015.

Ostrowski, J., Kjelsberg, M.A., Caron, M.G., and Lefkowitz, R.J. (1992). Mutagenesis of the $\beta_2$-adrenergic receptor: how structure elucidates function. *Annu. Rev. Pharmacol. Toxicol.* 32: 167–183.

Perovic, J., Perovic, V., Obradovic, O., and Todorovic, L.J. (1980). The influence of vasoconstrictors in local anaesthetic solutions and injection sites on blood levels of lidocaine after intraoral application. *Bull Group Int. Rech. Sci. Stomatol. Odontol.* 23 (2): 113–117.

Persson, G. (1969). General side effects of local dental anesthesia: with special reference to catecholamines as vasoconstrictors and to the effects of some premedications. *Acta Odontol. Scand.* 27 (Suppl 53): 1–141.

Persson, G. and Siwers, B. (1971). The risk of potentiating effect of local anaesthesia with adrenalin in patients treated with trycyclic antidepressants. *Swed. Dent. J.* 68 (1): 9–18.

Report of the Special Committee of the New York Heart Association (1955). The use of epinephrine in connection with procaine in dental procedures. *J. Am. Dent. Assoc.* 50 (1): 108.

Reynolds, F. (1972). Vasoconstrictors in local anesthetic preparations (letter). *Lancet* 2 (7780): 764–765.

Roberts, D.H. and Sowray, J.H. (1987). *Local analgesia in dentistry*, 3e. Bristol (UK): Wright. 34.

Robertson, V.J., Taylor, S.E., and Gage, T.W. (1984). Quantitative and qualitative analysis of the pressor effects of levonordefrin. *J. Cardiovasc. Pharmacol.* 6 (5): 929–935.

Ruffolo, R.R. Jr., Nichols, A.J., Stadel, J.M., and Hieble, J.P. (1991). Structure and function of α-adrenoceptors. *Pharmacol. Rev.* 43 (4): 475–505.

Rutherford, B., Zeller, J.R., and Thake, D. (2009). Local and systemic toxicity of intraoral submucosal injections of phentolamine mesylate (Oraverse). *Anesth. Prog.* 56 (4): 123–127.

Saunders, T.R., Psaltis, G., Weston, J.F. et al. (2011). In-practice evaluation of OraVerse® for the reversal of soft-tissue anesthesia after dental procedures. *Compend. Contin. Educ. Dent* 32 (5): 58–62.

Shanks, C.A. (1963). Intravenous octapressin during halothane anesthesia: a pilot study. *Br. J. Anaesth.* 35 (10): 640–643.

Smith, A.E. (1920). *Block Anesthesia and Allied Subjects. With Special Chapters on the Maxillary Sinus, the Tonsils, and Neuralgias of the Nervous Trigeminus for Oral Surgeons, Dentists, Laryngologists, Rhinologists, Otologists, and Students*. St. Louis (Mo): CV Mosby Co. 264, 266–267.

Stepke, M.T.H., Schwenzer, N., and Eichhorn, W. (1994). Vasoconstrictors during pregnancy – in vitro trial on pregnant and non pregnant mouse uterus. *Int. J. Oral Maxillofac. Surg.* 23 (6 Pt2): 440–442.

Sunada, K., Nakamura, K., Yamashiro, M. et al. (1996). Clinically safe dosage of felypressin for patients with essential hypertension. *Anesth. Prog.* 43 (4): 108–115.

Sung, C.-Y. and Truant, A.P. (1954). The physiological disposition of lidocaine and its comparison in some respects with procaine. *J. Pharmacol. Exp. Ther.* 112 (4): 432–443.

Sveen, K. (1979). Effect of the addition of a vasoconstrictor to local anesthetic solution on operative and postoperative bleeding, analgesia and wound healing. *Int. J. Oral Surg.* 8 (4): 301–306.

Tainter, M.L., Tuller, B.F., and Luduena, F.P. (1949). Levo-arterenol. *Science (Washington)* 107 (2767): 39–40.

Takamine, J. (1901). The blood-pressure-raising principle of the suprarenal glands – a preliminatry report. *Ther. Gaz.* 25 (4): 221–224.

Tavares, M., Goodson, J.M., Student-Pavlovich, D. et al. (2008). The Soft Tissue Anesthesia Recovery Group. Reversal of soft-tissue local anesthesia with phentolamine mesylate in pediatric patients. *J. Am. Dent. Assoc.* 139 (8): 1095–1104.

Tomlin, P.J. (1974). Death in outpatient dental anesthetic practice. *Anesthesia* 29 (5): 551–570.

Trendelenburg, U. (1988). The extraneuronal uptake and metabolism of catecholamines (Chapter 6). In: *Catecholamines I. Handbook of Experimental Pharmacology*, vol. 90/I (ed. U. Trendelenburg and N. Weiner). Berlin: Springer-Verlag. 279–319.

Tye, A., Patil, N., and Lapidus, J.B. (1967). Steric aspects of adrenergic drugs. III. Sensitization by cocaine to isomers of sympathomimetic amines. *J. Pharmacol. Exp. Ther.* 155 (1): 24–30.

Urech, E., Marxer, A., and Miescher, K. (1950). 182. 2-Aminoalkyl-imidazoline. *Helv. Chim. Acta* 33 (5): 1386–1407.

USP 38 (2015). *Farmacopea de los Estados Unidos de América*, 38e. Rockville, MD: The United States Pharmacopeial Convention 2488, 2694, 3584, 3586, 4474, 4490, 4658, 5011, 5414, 5427.

Van der Bijl, P. and Victor, A.M. (1992). Adverse reactions associated with norepinephrine in dental local anesthesia. *Anesth. Prog.* 39 (3): 87–89.

Volpato, M.C., Randi, J., Anard, J.M.G. et al. (1999). Acute toxicity ($LD_{50}$ and $CD_{50}$) of lidocaine and prilocaine in combination with adrenaline and felypressin. *Indian J. Dent. Res.* 10 (4): 138–144.

Von Euler, U.S. (1946a). A substance with sympathin E properties: spleen extracts. *Nature* 157 (3986): 369.

Von Euler, U.S. (1946b). A sympathomimetic ergone in adrenergic nerve fibers (sympathin) and its relations to adrenaline and noradrenaline. *Acta Physiol. Scand.* 12 (1): 73–97.

Von Fürth, O. (1900). Zur Kenntniss der brenzcatechinähulichen Substanz der Nebennieren. III. Mittheilung. *Hoppe-Seyler's Z. Physiol. Chem.* 29 (2): 105–123.

Weaver, J.M. (2008). New drugs on the horizon may improve the quality safety of anesthetic (Editorial). *Anesth. Prog.* 55 (2): 27–28.

Welsh, L.H. (1955). The analysis of solutions of epinephrine and norepinephrine. *J. Am. Pharm. Assoc.* 44 (8): 507–514.

Whitby, L.G., Axelrod, J., and Weil-Malherbe, H. (1961). The fate of $H^3$-norepinephrine in animals. *J. Pharmacol. Exp. Ther.* 132 (2): 193–201.

Wolfe, B.B. and Molinoff, P.B. (1988). Chatecolamine receptors (Chapter 7). In: *Catecholamines I. Handbook of Experimental Pharmacology*, vol. 90/I (ed. U. Trendelenburg and W. Weiner). Berlin: Springer-Verlag. 321–417.

Yagiela, J.A. (1985). Intravascular lidocaine toxicity: influence of epinephrine and route of administration. *Anesth. Analg.* 32 (2): 57–61.

Zurfluh, M.A., Daubländer, M., and Van Waes, H.J.M. (2015). Comparison of two epinephrine concentrations in an articaine solution for local anesthesia in children. *Swiss Dent. J.* 125 (6): 698–703.

# 7

# Injectable Anesthetic Solutions Used in Dentistry

This chapter describes the chemical and pharmaceutical composition of injectable anesthetic solutions in dental cartridges. It also analyzes procaine, which while rarely used today constitutes a reference against which the efficacy of all the others are compared.

## Solution Composition

Local anesthetic solutions available in cartridges have a number of components. In addition to the two most important, the local anesthetic and the vasoconstrictor, they contain other non-anesthetic constituents with specific functions that may have toxic or allergenic implications (Klein 1983).

### Local Anesthetic

This is the main drug and the one that induces the anesthetic effect. The five modern anesthetics used in dentistry today are all amides: lidocaine, articaine, mepivacaine, prilocaine, and bupivacaine.

With the exception of lidocaine, which is achiral, i.e. has no optical isomers (Tucker 1986; Calvey 1995; Mather and Chang 2001), the others are administered as a racemic mixture, i.e. equal parts of the two (levo or *S*- and dextro or *R*+) stereoisomers or asymmetric carbons (Tucker 1986; Strichartz et al. 1990; Calvey 1995; Mather and Chang 2001). In most, the two isomers have approximately the same anesthetic activity (Calvey 1995).

### Vasoconstrictor

This second most important component enhances the effect of the local anesthetic by promoting vasoconstriction of the blood vessels near the target tissue and inducing a mass-volume-time effect that heightens potency, lengthens the duration of the anesthetic effect, reduces hemorrhage where the solution is injected, and lowers the toxicity of the anesthetic by slowing its absorption into the bloodstream. There are two types of vasoconstrictors: one derived from vasopressin, namely felypressin (Octapressin®), which is less powerful and much less frequently used, and sympathomimetic vasoconstrictors such as epinephrine, norepinephrine, and levonordefrin, the three most powerful. Epinephrine is the one most commonly used worldwide.

These sympathomimetic vasoconstrictors are characterized by features with implications for dentistry.

- As they are highly sensitive to primarily oxidation-induced degradation, they determine the shelf life of local anesthetic solutions.
- They are combined with an antioxidant (sulfite) to increase shelf life (Milano et al. 1982; Klein 1983).
- They have an acidic pH, normally around 4 (Annex 14), but ranging from 2.7 to 5.5 (USP 38 2015), which also improves their stability and enhances their solubility in aqueous solutions.
- Their levo isomeric form is used, as it is 10–200 times more powerful than the dextro form (Table 6.5, Chapter 6).
- The bitartrate form of epinephrine is used because it is more stable than the base or hydrochloride forms and like those forms is water soluble (Smith 1920; Bonica 1959).

### Antioxidants (Sulfites)

These compounds lengthen the half-life of sympathomimetic vasoconstrictors such as epinephrine because they capture the oxygen penetrating the cartridge before it engages with and inactivates the vasoconstrictor (Milano et al. 1982; Klein 1983; Huang and Fraser 1984; Schwartz and Sher 1985; Seng and Gay 1986).

The sulfites most widely used are 0.5 mg/ml sodium bisulfite (Seng and Gay 1986), sodium or potassium

*Local Anesthesia in Dentistry: A Locoregional Approach*, First Edition. Jesús Calatayud and Mana Saraghi.
© 2024 John Wiley & Sons Ltd. Published 2024 by John Wiley & Sons Ltd.
Companion website: www.wiley.com/go/Calatayud/local

metabisulfite (Klein 1983; Seng and Gay 1986), and acetone sodium bisulfite 1 mg/ml (Seng and Gay 1986). Other characteristics associated with these compounds include their *bitter taste*, to which local anesthetics owe that same feature (Klein 1983), their contribution to maintaining an acid pH to preserve vasoconstrictors (Moorthy et al. 1984), and their efficacy *in protecting vasoconstrictors for the first 18 months* (American Dental Association 1983; Bennett 1984; Jastak et al. 1995). That capacity gradually declines with the amount of active antioxidant, lowering sympathomimetic vasoconstrictor activity and pH (Hondrum and Ezell 1996).

Although deemed to be safe (Bush et al. 1986; Seng and Gay 1986), low allergenic additives (Bush et al. 1986), the sulfites in local anesthetics used in dentistry have been known to trigger allergic reactions (Huang and Fraser 1984; Schwartz and Sher 1985; Schwartz et al. 1989; Dooms-Goossens et al. 1989; Campbell et al. 2001). For poorly understood reasons this intolerance is associated with severe, corticoid-treated asthma (Bush et al. 1986; Schwartz et al. 1989).

Seng and Gay (1986) proposed replacing sulfites with antioxidants suggested by Klein (1983), such as ascorbic acid and thioglycerol (only with Marcaine®), but they are less effective, more costly, and also pose health risks (Bush et al. 1986).

## Preservatives (Methylparaben)

Preservatives are used to keep dental cartridges containing local anesthesia sterile (i.e., bacterium-free) (Latronica et al. 1969; Larson 1977; Luebke and Walker 1978). These compounds are parabens (propyl-, butyl-, and methylparaben), the most widely used being methylparaben or methyl 4-hydroxy-benzoate (Larson 1977; Klein 1983) at concentrations of 1 mg/ml = 0.1% (Larson 1977).

Parabens are used for their bacteriostatic and fungistatic power (Schorr 1968; Latronica et al. 1969; Nagel et al. 1977; Larson 1977; Luebke and Walker 1978), low-dose efficacy (Larson 1977; Luebke and Walker 1978), and scant toxicity (Luebke and Walker 1978). Their primary drawback is that, like the alkyl-esters of aminobenzoic acid (Latronica et al. 1969; Nagel et al. 1977; Larson 1977; Luebke and Walker 1978; Giovannitti and Bennett 1979), they share a chemical structure with ester-type anesthetics. Allergic reactions to anesthetic solutions induced by these compounds and the cross-sensitivity to ester-type local anesthetics (Aldrete and Jonhson 1969; Latronica et al. 1969; Larson 1977; Luebke and Walker 1978) are consequently common (Aldrete and Jonhson 1969; Luebke and Walker 1978; Giovannitti and Bennett 1979). The US Food and Drug Administration (FDA) has therefore banned these compounds in dental cartridges and single (although not multi-dose) vials (Malamed 2004) because cartridge preparation and single-dose packaging with modern industrial techniques guarantee sterility and prevent infectious disease transmission. As a result, the use of parabens, the primary cause of allergic reactions, is no longer necessary. Since their prohibition this type of adverse reaction to local dental anesthesia has declined drastically (Malamed 2004).

Non-parabenic preservatives exist, but are seldom used. One, 0.25% (0.25 mg/ml) chlorobutanol (Klein 1983), is less effective (Luebke and Walker 1978) and edetate disodium calcium is only used in Marcaine, a brand name for bupivacaine (Klein 1983).

## pH Adjustment

Solutions with sympathomimetic vasoconstrictors such as epinephrine are the most acidic, around pH = 4, ranging from 3.5 to 4.5 (Annex 14), because a low (acid) pH is needed to preserve the vasoconstrictor, which breaks down in basic media (Tainter et al. 1939; Fyhr and Brodin 1987; Bowles et al. 1995). Epinephrine is most stable at pH = 3.4 (Hondrum et al. 1993) and breaks down in a matter of hours at pH > 6 (De Jong and Cullen 1963). Acidity poses problems, however.

1) Clinical trials have shown that injections are more painful, creating a burning or stinging sensation (Oikarinen et al. 1975; Moorthy et al. 1984; Kramp et al. 1999; Wahl et al. 2001).
2) The anesthetic effect may be delayed because at acidic pHs, most of the anesthetic molecules are cationic and unable to penetrate the cell membrane. Very few are free bases, the lipid-soluble form that crosses the membrane, establishing a new equilibrium with the cations in the axoplasm. That in turn activates the receptor that blocks the sodium channels, generating the anesthetic effect. The tissue is alkaline in pH (= 7.4) and buffers in the tissue mitigate the initial acidity of the solution (Tainter et al. 1939; Björn 1947b), however, although some studies (Björn 1947b) have shown that to take longer than initially believed. Today, it is known that cations can penetrate the membrane in other ways, crossing TRPV1 channels, for example (Butterworth and Oxford 2009) (see Chapter 4).
3) If the acidic solution comes into contact with a metal, such as in former hypodermic metal syringes, within a few hours the release of nickel, zinc, and especially copper ions begins to irritate the tissues, an effect that may last for several days (Lundqvist et al. 1948). Dental solutions fortunately come in glass cartridges that elude such problems.

For anesthetic solutions with sympathomimetic vasoconstrictors (epinephrine and levonordefrin) the USP has established pH ranges of 3.3–5.5 for solutions with lidocaine, mepivacaine, prilocaine, and bupivacaine, and of 2.7–5.2 for articaine with epinephrine (USP 38 2015). As these solutions age, their pH tends to decline further, with both the active antioxidant and vasoconstrictor content decreasing (Hondrum and Ezell 1996).

Solutions with non-sympathomimetic vasoconstrictors such as felypressin (Octapressin®), which is available in many European countries although not in the United States, have a pH of around 5 (Annex 14), more or less midway between solutions without vasoconstrictors and those with the sympathomimetic type.

The chemical compounds added to solutions to attempt to regulate their pH include hydrochloric acid (ClH) to lower it, and sodium hydroxide (NaOH) and sodium lactate ($C_3H_5NaO_3$) (only in Marcaine®, a brand name for bupivacaine) to raise it (Klein 1983).

### Other Compounds

Sterile water is used as a vehicle and salts, normally 3–6 mg/ml sodium chloride (NaCl), to render the solutions isotonic (Klein 1983). Clinical studies have shown that non-isotonic solutions do not raise anesthetic efficacy (Nordenram 1966) and irritate subcutaneous tissue, with concomitant pain (Lewis 1919; Nordenram 1966).

## Procaine (Novocaine)

Procaine, or Novocaine, is a derivative of para-amino benzoic acid, synthesized by German chemist Alfred Einhorn in 1904 (Farbwerke vorm 1904; Einhorn and Uhlfelder 1909). The first clinical trial of this anesthetic together with epinephrine was reported by Heinrich Braun (Braun 1905) under the name Novocaine. In 1910 German dentist Guido Fischer published the first book on local dental anesthesia featuring Novocaine as the primary anesthetic (Fischer 1910). It met with such success that it was translated into several languages and its second edition was translated into English (Fischer 1912). (The first German edition sold out in just a few months.) Around 1916, Novocaine began to be known among clinicians as procaine in the United States (Benedict et al. 1932; Link and Alfred Einhorn 1959).

In the first half of the twentieth century procaine was the prototypical local anesthetic and it is the standard used in this chapter for comparison of all others. Its most prominent characteristics are summarized in Table 7.1.

### Metabolism

When injected alone, procaine is retained in the injection site for 1.5 hours and in the presence of epinephrine for up to 3 h (Sung and Truant 1954). It has a short half-life, under 8 minutes (Seifen et al. 1979), because once in the bloodstream it is hydrolyzed by pseudocholinesterase (or plasma cholinesterase or butyrylcholinesterase). It scarcely penetrates the placenta. Its metabolites are eliminated in the urine, with only 2% eliminated in the free non-metabolized form (Brodie et al. 1948). Nonetheless, the pseudocholinesterase deficits or alterations found in one per 3000 people (Kalow and Gunn 1959) lengthen the half-life of procaine. Its possible biotransformation pathways are listed in Annex 12.

### Procaine with Epinephrine

Procaine is no longer marketed in dental cartridges, although 2% procaine ampoules and 1:1000 (1000 μg/ml) epinephrine ampoules are available. Therefore 50 ml of 2% procaine can be mixed with 1 ml of 1:1000 epinephrine to obtain 51 ml of 2% procaine with 1:50 000 (20 μ/ml) epinephrine.

The maximum absolute dose of this local anesthetic solution for adults weighing 70 kg or more is five and a half 1.8-ml cartridges. The limiting factor is the high epinephrine concentration, at 1:50 000. The maximum absolute dose established for procaine alone in dentistry is 400 mg (5.7 mg/kg) (American Dental Association 1984).

### Remarks

While procaine is less efficacious than other anesthetics (see anesthetic parameters and physical-chemical properties in Table 7.1), in the first half of the twentieth century it proved to be sufficiently effective and much safer than its predecessor cocaine, the first of the local anesthetics. Its primary drawback is the potential for hypersensitivity reactions (allergy reactions) and in particular its cross-sensitivity with all ester-type anesthetics (Aldrete and Johnson 1970).

Today procaine can be used in the event of multiple and severe allergies to several amide group anesthetics, although it has fallen into disuse and been replaced by modern amide-type anesthetic solutions that are less allergenic and exhibit an anesthetic parameter that attests to higher potency and efficacy.

## Lidocaine (Lignocaine)

Lidocaine was synthesized in 1943 by Swedish researchers Nils Löfgren (1913–1967) and Bengt Lundqvist (1922–1953) (Björn and Huldt IV 1947a; Löfgren 1948; Gordh

**Table 7.1** Procaine.

| Pharmacological factor | Reference |
|---|---|
| • Name and synonym: Procaine, Novocaine | |
| • First synthesized in 1904 by Alfred Einhorn | Farbwerke vorm (1904) |
| • Chemical name: 2-(diethylamino) ethyl 4-aminobenzoate | American Dental Association (1984) |
| • Formula: $C_{13}H_{20}N_2O_2$ | |
| $H_2N-\text{C}_6H_4-COO-CH_2-CH_2-N(C_2H_5)_2$ Procaine | |
| • Molecular weight: Base 236.3                Hydrochloride 272.8 | |
| • Clearance rate: 6.23 l/minute | Seifen et al. (1979) |
| • Volume of distribution: 58.7 l | Seifen et al. (1979) |
| • Half-life: <8 minutes | Seifen et al. (1979) |

| Physical–chemical property | |
|---|---|
| • pKa value or dissociation constant: 9.0    Denotes retarded onset | Annex 6 |
| • Lipid solubility or partition coefficient: *n*-heptane 0.02    *n*-octanol 2    Denotes low anesthetic potency and no topical anesthesia | Annex 7 |
| • Plasma protein binding: 5%    Denotes short duration of the anesthetic effect | Annex 9 |
| • Vasodilation: +++ (high)    Denotes need for a vasoconstrictor to be effective | Du Mesnil de Rochemont and Hensel (1960)<br>Lindorf et al. (1974) |

| Clinical factor | Reference |
|---|---|
| • Relative anesthetic potency: 1 | |
| • Relative toxicity: 1 | Annex 8 |
| • Maximum absolute dose in dentistry: 400 mg (5.7 mg/kg) | American Dental Association (1984) |
| • Usable during pregnancy: Yes (FDA category = C)    Denotes low risk | Haas et al. (2000) |
| • Usable during lactation: Yes    Denotes low risk | |
| • Usable with children: Yes    Denotes low risk | |

| Anesthetic parameter | Variable | 2% procaine + 1:50 000 epinephrine |
|---|---|---|
| Buccal infiltration | Successful pulpal anesthesia (%) | 80 |
| Superior lateral incisor | Duration, pulpal anesthesia (minutes) | 25 |
| 1 ml | Duration, anesthesia upper lip (minutes) | 95 |
| (Annex 21) | | |
| Mandibular block | Duration, anesthesia lower lip (minutes) | 110 |
| 1.8 ml | | |
| (Annex 27) | | |

Pharmacological, physical–chemical and clinical properties, and anesthetic parameter.
Summary: 2% procaine with 1:50 000 (20 µg/ml) epinephrine: 80%-25′/95′-110′.

et al. 2010), who first published their findings in 1946 (Löfgren and Lundqvist 1946). It was initially known as compound LL 30, the letters designating the two researchers' initials and the number the consecutive order of the compound of the many they studied (Gordh et al. 2010). After 1946 it was renamed Xylocaine® (Löfgren and Lundqvist 1946), a combination of the product from which it is derived, "xylidine," and the local anesthetic suffix "caine" (Gordh et al. 2010). In 1948 it was patented in Sweden and the United States (American Dental Association 1984; Gordh et al. 2010), where it quickly replaced procaine (American Dental Association 1984). In 1951 Xylocaine was adopted as the brand name and lidocaine as the generic name (McMahon and Woods 1951). It is presently known as lidocaine in the United States and most of the rest of the world and lignocaine in the United Kingdom. Lidocaine was the first amide-type local anesthetic to be successfully used and the only anesthetic discussed in this book, with the exception of tetracaine, that is achiral, i.e. with no levo/dextro stereoisomers (Calvey 1995).

Lidocaine has also been used since the 1960s as an antiarrhythmic drug in medical emergencies (Harrison et al. 1963; Katz and Epstein 1968). Its most prominent characteristics are summarized in Table 7.2.

## Metabolism

At a 2% concentration with 1:100 000 (10 µg/ml) epinephrine, lidocaine is removed from the injection site in around 4 hours and without epinephrine in less than 2 hours (Sung and Truant 1954). Once in the bloodstream it accumulates, in descending order, in the kidneys, lungs, brain, and heart (Sung and Truant 1954; Akerman et al. 1966). The hepatic microsomal system (Sung and Truant 1954; Akerman et al. 1966; Boyes et al. 1971; Stenson et al. 1971; Thomson et al. 1973), primarily isoform 3A of cytochrome P450 (Bargetzi et al. 1989), catabolizes 70% of the anesthetic (Boyes et al. 1971; Stenson et al. 1971). Around 80% is eliminated in the urine, although only 4% of it is excreted unchanged (Annex 12). Elimination is enhanced in acidic urine (Eriksson et al. 1966; Mihaly et al. 1978).

Lidocaine has a half-life of around 110 minutes (Annex 11). Severe liver and kidney disorders affect its catabolism, albeit in different manners (Thomson et al. 1973). Severe liver disease may raise its half-life by up to three times, whereas severe kidney conditions affect not half-life but the metabolites in the blood (Thomson et al. 1973), particularly monoethylglycinexylidide (MEGX) and glycinexylidide (GX), active agents involved in lidocaine toxicity (Blumer et al. 1973; Strong et al. 1973).

This drug diffuses passively across the placenta, reaching a concentration in the umbilical vein of 60% of that found in the maternal blood vessels (Covino 1971). Its possible biotransformation pathways are listed in Annex 12.

## Remarks

L-100 or 2% lidocaine with 1:100 000 (10 µg/ml) epinephrine and L-80, the same solution with 1:80 000 (12.5 µg/ml) epinephrine, are deemed to be the standard solutions in dentistry for several reasons (Cowan 1964):

1) Their efficacy in attaining pulpal anesthesia via buccal infiltration is only exceeded by potent solutions such as 4% articaine (double the anesthetic content) with 1:100 000 (10 µg/ml) epinephrine (A-100), or 2% lidocaine with 1:50 000 (20 µg/ml) epinephrine (L-50) (double the vasoconstrictor content) (Annex 21).
2) It is very safe, with a maximum absolute dose in dentistry of eight and a half cartridges in adults weighing 70 kg or over, more than most other solutions (Annex 10).
3) As an FDA pregnancy risk category B drug, it is very safe for pregnant or nursing women.

Lidocaine concentrations of 5% have shown to be highly toxic in animal experiments and are consequently not recommended (Lambert et al. 1994; Strichartz et al. 1994; Strichartz and Lambert 1995). Conversely, 2% lidocaine solutions with 1:200 000 (5 µg/ml) epinephrine (half the vasoconstrictor as in the standard solution) have proven to be scantly effective in clinical trials (Annex 21).

## Indications

Two local anesthetic solutions with epinephrine are presently available. Their characteristics and uses are discussed below.

**Standard 2% Lidocaine: L-100 with 1:100 000 (10 µg/ml) Epinephrine or L-80 with 1:80 000 (12.5 µg/ml) Epinephrine**

The epinephrine concentration used in the United States and many other countries is 1:100 000, although in some European countries, Japan, and India the standard is 1:80 000 (12.5 µg/ml). As in practice the two deliver similar results, they are indistinctly deemed to be the standard (Cowan 1964; Yamazaki et al. 2006). Nonetheless, while some authors eschew the 12.5 µg/ml dose where epinephrine is relative contraindicated, they find the 10 µg/ml concentration acceptable (Annex 17).

The maximum absolute dental dose in adults weighing 70 kg or more is 300 mg (4.3 mg/kg) of lidocaine, or *eight and a half 1.8-ml cartridges* (Annex 10). Its uses are as follows:

1) In mandibular blocks because:
    - Pulpal anesthetic efficacy in mandibular nerve blocks depends less on the potency of the local anesthetic solution (higher anesthetic or

**Table 7.2** Lidocaine.

| Pharmacological factor | Reference |
|---|---|
| • Name and synonyms: Lidocaine, lignocaine, LL 30, Xylocaine® | |
| • First synthesized in 1943 by Löfgren and Lundqvist | Löfgren (1948) |
| • Chemical name: alpha-diethylamino-2,6-acetoxylidide | American Dental Association (1984) |
| • Formula: $C_{14}H_{22}N_2O$ | Löfgren (1948) |
| • Molecular weight: Base 234.3 | Löfgren (1948) |
|                   Hydrochloride 270.8 | De Jong (1977) |
| | Strichartz (1990) |
| • Clearance rate: 0.83 l/min | Annex 11 |
| • Volume of distribution: 85 l | Annex 11 |
| • Half-life: 110 minutes | Annex 11 |

| Physical–chemical property | |
|---|---|
| • pKa value or dissociation constant: 7.9 | Annex 6 |
|         Denotes fast onset | |
| • Lipid solubility or partition coefficient: *n*-heptane 2.9 | Annex 7 |
|         *n*-octanol 45 | |
|         Denotes medium anesthetic potency and topical anesthesia | |
| • Plasma protein binding: 65% | Annex 9 |
|         Denotes medium duration of the anesthetic effect | |
| • Vasodilation: + (moderate) | Du Mesnil de Rochemont and Hensel (1960) |
|         Denotes need for a vasoconstrictor to be effective | Lindorf et al. (1974) |

| Clinical factor | Reference |
|---|---|
| • Relative anesthetic potency: 2 | |
| • Relative toxicity: 2 | Annex 8 |
| • Maximum absolute dose in dentistry: 300 mg (4.3 mg/kg) | American Dental Association (1984) |
| • Usable during pregnancy: Yes (FDA category = B) | Table 5.11 (Chapter 5) |
|         Denotes low risk | |
| • Usable during lactation: Yes | Table 5.11 (Chapter 5) |
|         Denotes low risk | |
| • Usable with children: Yes | |
|         Denotes low risk | |

| Anesthetic parameter | Variable | L-100 or L-80 | L-50 |
|---|---|---|---|
| Buccal infiltration | Successful pulpal anesthesia (%) | 95 | 100 |
| Superior lateral incisor | Duration, pulpal anesthesia (minutes) | 45 | 60 |
| 1 ml | Duration, anesthesia upper lip (minutes) | 190 | 165 |
| (Annex 21) | | | |
| Mandibular block | Duration, anesthesia lower lip (minutes) | 200 | 200 |
| 1.8 ml | | | |
| (Annex 27) | | | |

Pharmacological, physical–chemical, and clinical properties and anesthetic parameter.
Summary: (L-100) 2% lidocaine with 1:100 000 (10 µg/ml) epinephrine and (L-80) 2% lidocaine with 1:80 000 (12.5 µg/ml) epinephrine: 95%-45'/190'-200'.
(L-50) 2% lidocaine with 1:50 000 (20 µg/ml) epinephrine: 100%-60'/165'-200'.

vasoconstrictor concentration or both) (Annex 24) than on the proximity to the inferior alveolar nerve, the aponeuroses separating the anesthetic from the nerve, accessory innervation, or anatomical variations (see Chapter 19).
- Solutions with high concentrations of local anesthesia (4% articaine, 4% prilocaine) have not exhibited greater clinical efficacy in attaining pulpal anesthesia under normal circumstances (Annex 24), while inducing four to nine times more long-term paresthesia in the inferior alveolar and lingual nerves (Haas and Lennon 1995; Garisto et al. 2010) (see Chapter 22).

2) In children, for both mandibular blocks and maxillary and mandibular buccal infiltrations to achieve pulpal anesthesia because:
- The standard solution penetrates their smaller, more porous bones very well.
- A larger volume in milliliters per child kilogram can be administered because the maximum values are higher than with most other anesthetic solutions used in dentistry (Annex 10). The result is greater safety.

3) Where infiltrations need not achieve deep pulpal anesthesia, such as in gingivectomies, scaling and root planing, or gross debridement in patients with high dentinal sensitivity where only the gingival needs to be anesthetized because while it is as effective as other solutions a larger volume of anesthetic can be used at lower risk (before the maximum absolute dental dose is reached, therefore lowering the risk of toxicity) (Annex 10).

**L-50, 2% Lidocaine with 1:50 000 (20 μg/ml) Epinephrine**

As this solution has double the standard epinephrine concentration (20 μg/ml), it has a very beneficial hemostatic effect, raising the potency to achieve pulpal anesthesia more readily by keeping more local anesthetic in the infiltration area.

The maximum absolute dose of epinephrine in dentistry is 200 μg (2.8 μg/kg in adults >70 kg), the amount in *five and a half 1.8-ml cartridges* (Annex 10). Its uses are as follows:

1) Where *hemostasis* is required (Buckley et al. 1984) because abundant bleeding is expected, such as in oral surgery, scaling, and root planing (Chaikin 1977), the area to be treated (the gum during proximal or class V fillings or in the papillae when making impressions for fixed prosthesis) is infiltrated.
2) When pulpal anesthesia is not achieved with 2% lidocaine and 1:100 000 (10 μg/ml) epinephrine *L-50 can reinforce buccal infiltration* (Gruber 1950). As noted Chapter 5, two local anesthetics should not be used in the same site (see). The approach suggested here therefore calls for the same anesthetic, although the epinephrine concentration is doubled to make pulpal anesthesia more effective (Annex 21).

Interestingly, since the high epinephrine concentration in this solution delivers greater anesthetic potency by keeping more solution in the target site, the effect is shorter-lived (Klingenström and Westermar 1964) due to the significant vasodilatory reaction observed 2–3 hours later (Lindorf 1979). The result is a shorter duration of soft tissue anesthesia than with other less potent solutions (Annex 21).

## Articaine

Articaine was synthesized in 1969 (Frenkel 1989; Rahn and Ball 2001) by German pharmacologist Roman Muschaweck (1918–2007) for Farbwerke Hoechst AG at Frankfurt (Rahn and Ball 2001; Vogel 2007). In the first paper, published in 1972, it was given the experimental name Hoe 40 045 (Winther and Nathalang 1972). In 1974 it was renamed carticaine (Muschaweck and Rippel 1974; Winther and Patirupanusara 1974), acquiring its present name, articaine, in 1983 (Kirch et al. 1983; Mehta et al. 1983). It was first marketed in Germany and Switzerland in 1976 and afterwards very successfully in several countries (Table 7.3). Initially packaged in 1.7-ml cartridges under the brand name Ultracaín®, it is now available in 1.7- or 1.8-ml cartridges.

Articaine is an amide-type anesthetic but with two special characteristics. The first is that although the intermediate linkage is an amide, it also contains an ester linkage in the side chain of its aromatic ring. The other is that its aromatic ring is a thiophene rather than a benzene. Articaine's most prominent characteristics are summarized in Table 7.4.

Table 7.3 Articaine commercial availability: dates and countries.

| Year | Country | Reference |
|------|---------|-----------|
| 1976 | Germany, Switzerland | Isen (2000) |
| 1978 | Netherlands | Isen (2000) |
| 1980 | Austria, Spain | Isen (2000) |
| 1983 | Canada | Isen (2000) |
| 1998 | United Kingdom | Isen (2000) |
| 2000 | United States | Weaver (1999) |
|      | Denmark | Hillerup and Jensen (2006) |
| 2005 | Australia[a] | Yapp et al. (2012) |

[a] In Australia in 2.2-ml cartridges.

**Table 7.4** Articaine.

| Pharmacological factor | Reference |
|---|---|
| • Name and synonyms: Articaine, carticaine, Hoe 40 045 | |
| • First synthesized in 1969 by Roman Muschaweck | Rahn and Ball (2001) |
| | Vogel (2007) |
| • Chemical name: methyl 4-methyl-3-[2 (propylamino) propionamida]-2-thiophenecarboxylate | |
| • Formula: $C_{13}H_{20}N_2O_3S$ | |
| Articaine structural formula | |
| • Molecular weight: Base 284.4 | Muschaweck and Rippel (1974) |
|                   Hydrochloride 320.9 | Winther and Patirupanusara (1974) |
| • Clearance rate: 4.17 l/min | Annex 11 |
| • Volume of distribution: 120 l | Annex 11 |
| • Half-life: 25 minutes | Annex 11 |

| Physical–chemical property | |
|---|---|
| • pKa value or dissociation constant: 7.8 | Annex 6 |
|                   Denotes fast onset | |
| • Lipid solubility or partition coefficient: *n*-heptane 0.7 | Annex 7 |
|                   *n*-octanol 15 | |
| Denotes medium anesthetic potency and no topical anesthesia | |
| • Plasma protein binding: 60% | Annex 9 |
|                   Denotes medium duration of the anesthetic effect | |
| • Vasodilation: + (moderate) | Muschaweck and Rippel (1974) |
|                   Denotes need for a vasoconstrictor to be effective | |

| Clinical factor | Reference |
|---|---|
| • Relative anesthetic potency: 2 | |
| • Relative toxicity: 2 | Annex 8 |
| • Maximum absolute dose in dentistry: 500 mg (7 mg/kg) | Council on Clinical Affairs (2015) |
| | AAPD (2020) |
| • Usable during pregnancy: Yes (FDA category = C) | Table 5.11 (Chapter 5) |
|                   Denotes low risk | |
| • Usable during lactation: Yes | Table 5.11 (Chapter 5) |
|                   Denotes low risk | |
| • Usable with children: Yes, if over 4 years | Malamed et al. (2000) |
|                   Denotes low risk | Katyal (2010) |

Table 7.4 (Continued)

| Anesthetic parameter | Variable | A-100 | A-200 |
|---|---|---|---|
| Buccal infiltration | Successful pulpal anesthesia (%) | 98 | 92 |
| Superior lateral incisor 1.8 ml (Annex 21) | Duration, pulpal anesthesia (minutes) | 60 | 45 |
| | Duration, anesthesia upper lip (minutes) | 190 | 190 |
| Mandibular block 1.8 ml (Annex 27) | Duration, anesthesia lower lip (minutes) | 260 | 260 |

Pharmacological, physical-chemical, and clinical properties and anesthetic parameter.
Summary: (A-100) 2% articaine with 1:100 000 (10 µg/ml) epinephrine: 98%-60′/190′-260′.
(A-200) 2% articaine with 1:200 000 (5 µg/ml) epinephrine:92%-45′/190′-260′.

## Metabolism

Much less articaine (5–15%) than other amide anesthetics is metabolized in the liver by the P450 microsomal enzyme system (Isen 2000; Rahn and Ball 2001). Therein lies the advantage of this solution, as the ester side chain on its thiophene ring is rapidly hydrolyzed by plasma pseudocholinesterases (Becker and Reed 2006), which catabolize 85–95% of the drug. As articainic acid, the compound formed has no anesthetic activity or effect on the central nervous system (Müller et al. 1991; Oertel et al. 1997), the half-life of articaine is just 25 minutes. Nonetheless, in the 1 in 3000 individuals with deficient or altered plasma cholinesterases (Kalow and Gunn 1959) the drug is metabolized in the liver. Catabolism is a two-stage process (Vree et al. 1988; Van Oss et al. 1989) accelerated by alkaline pH (Oertel et al. 1996).

Articaine is classified as an amide-type local anesthetic, not an ester, and exhibits no cross-allergenic activity with para-aminobenzoic acid anesthetics, nor is allergic sensitization common (Becker and Reed 2006). The reason for the lack of allergic potential is that when articaine is metabolized to articanic acid, a metabolite with the structure similar to para-aminobenzoic acid (PABA) is not formed. The formation of a PABA metabolite is the reason for cross-allergenicity amongst ester anesthetics, not amides including articaine.

Articaine is eliminated primarily (85%) in the urine, 75% as articainic acid and only 3% as free and unaltered articaine (Annex 12). Two percent is also found in the feces (Hornke et al. 1984). This drug diffuses across the placenta passively, lodging in the umbilical vein at 32% of the concentration found in the maternal blood vessels (Strasser et al. 1977). Its possible biotransformation pathways are listed in Annex 12.

## Remarks

Several features of articaine merit comment.

### Maximum Dose and Toxicity

This issue was discussed in Chapter 5. By way of summary, its acute experimental toxicity is very similar to that of lidocaine (Annex 8; Albalawi et al. 2018), although the enormous advantage of articaine is its high clearance rate (4.17 l/minute) and short half-life (25 minutes) (Annex 11). The dose allowed in dentistry is therefore higher than for lidocaine (300 mg = 4.3 mg/kg). *The maximum absolute dose proposed for dentistry is 500 mg (7 mg/kg)* (Council on Clinical Affairs 2015; AAPD 2020), equivalent at 4% to seven 1.8-ml or seven and a half 1.7-ml cartridges. See Annex 10 of doses of dental local anesthetic solutions.

The use of articaine is *not recommended in children under 4 years of age* as there is little data to support its safety and efficacy, although a few trials have shown it to be safe (Wright et al. 1989), thus more data and clinical studies are needed to verify those findings (Malamed et al. 2000; Malamed et al. 2001; Katyal 2010; AAPD 2020).

### Anesthetic Potency

Articaine has been proven to carry higher anesthetic efficacy than lidocaine. Two recent meta-analyses comparing 4% articaine to 2% lidocaine solutions, both with 1:100 000 epinephrine, showed articaine to be more effective, particularly in pulpal anesthesia in buccal infiltrations (Katyal 2010; Brandt et al. 2011), while the adverse effects were observed to be similar (Katyal 2010). Clinical series have yielded the same results (Annexes 21 and 31). The reason for such greater efficacy may be attributed to two factors:

1) The slightly higher anesthetic potency in articaine, particularly "in vitro" (Den Hertog 1974; Borchard and Drouin 1980; Potocnik et al. 2006) but also in clinical trials using both solutions at the same concentration, with and without epinephrine (Winther and Nathalang 1972; Winther and Patirupanusara 1974). Some authors (Robertson et al. 2007) have associated higher potency with the thiophene ring in articaine, although research has shown the benzene ring to be more lipid soluble (Skjevik et al. 2011). The actual explanation appears to be that *articaine can form intramolecular hydrogen bonds* that raise its lipid solubility to levels above and beyond those observed in all local anesthetics, enhancing diffusion and tissue penetration (Skjevik et al. 2011).

2) *The concentration of articaine solutions is 4%, double that of lidocaine (2%)*, due precisely to the pharmacokinetic features discussed above. Consequently, a higher concentration yields greater anesthetic efficacy without adversely affecting safety due to the speed with which articaine is catabolized. In clinical studies 5% lidocaine exhibited better results than the 2% solution, both with epinephrine (Rood 1976; Eldridge and Rood 1977; Rood and Sowray 1980), although unfortunately they are not equally safe.

**Anesthetic Effect**

Although articaine has a short half-life in the plasma, its local effect is lengthy. The reason is that while in the blood it rarely exceeds 5 µg/ml, after infiltration it gathers in the dental alveolus, where it reaches a concentration of 120 µg/ml. The effect consequently persists due to the saturation of the local cholinesterases that catabolize the anesthetic (Oertel et al. 1993; Oertel et al. 1996).

Methylparaben, an allergenic-prone preservative, was withdrawn by the FDA in 1984 and removed from articaine in most European countries in the mid-1990s.

## Indications

Two local anesthetic solutions with epinephrine are presently available. Their characteristics and uses are discussed below.

**A-100, 4% Articaine with 1:100 000 (10 µg/ml) Epinephrine**

This effective anesthetic solution is designed to achieve pulpal anesthesia with buccal infiltration. As articaine efficacy is comparable to that of lidocaine, to enhance the effect double the concentration is used (4% vs. 2%) with the same epinephrine concentration. It therefore diffuses more readily across the periosteum and the cortical and spongy bone to reach the dental pulp (Schilly 1977). Clinical trials with maxillary infiltrations have proven its higher efficacy than the standard lidocaine solution (Kanna et al. 2006; Robertson et al. 2007; Abdulwahab et al. 2009; da Silva et al. 2010).

The maximum absolute dose in adults weighing 70 kg or over is 500 mg (7 mg/kg) or seven 1.8-ml or seven and a half 1.7-ml cartridges (Annex 10). The objective with this solution is to *achieve pulpal anesthesia with buccal infiltration* in:

- All adult teeth in the maxillary arch.
- Incisors, canines, and premolars in the mandibular arch.
- Post-mandibular block buccal reinforcement in molars and premolars to enhance mandibular block efficacy in achieving pulpal anesthesia (Haase et al. 2008).

It is neither advisable nor contraindicated in:

1) Buccal infiltrations, the sole technique (without mandibular block) to achieve pulpal anesthesia in mandibular molars. It only successfully anesthetizes the pulp in 65% of such cases (Annex 31) because the solution is deposited at a fair distance from the apices due to the presence of very thick barriers (cortical and spongy bone) (Arens et al. 1984; Denio et al. 1992; Poorni et al. 2011).

2) In mandibular block for two reasons:
   - Mandibular block efficacy in achieving pulpal anesthesia depends less on the potency of the anesthetic solution (higher anesthetic or vasoconstrictor concentration) (Annex 24) than on its proximity to the inferior alveolar nerve, the aponeuroses or fascias that separate the solution from the nerve, accessory innervation, and anatomical variations. Consequently, under normal conditions the standard L-100 solution delivers similar results.
   - In mandibular block, solutions with high local anesthetic concentrations, such as 4% articaine, may induce long-term paresthesia or persistent inoperable neuropathies due to anesthetic neurotoxicity. The incidence of that complication is fortunately very low, estimated to be 1 in 100 000 blocks, but the risk with 4% articaine is 22 times higher than with 2% lidocaine with epinephrine (L-100) (see Chapter 22).

Nonetheless, 4% articaine is indicated for acute pulpitis in the posterior mandibular teeth, in light of the difficulty involved in anesthetizing the area in such cases (Annex 35; Chapter 19).

3) It is not generally recommended in children because:
   - The standard 2% lidocaine solution with epinephrine is very successful in children, whose bones are smaller and more porous than adults', and can be administered at higher doses, depending on the child's weight, as the limits are higher (eight and a half cartridges in adults weighing >70 kg vs. seven for 4% articaine with epinephrine).
   - The anesthetic effects generated by articaine solutions last longer in the soft tissue, raising the risk of biting-induced self-injury to the tongue, lips, or buccal mucosa in children, especially those under 7 years of age (Adewuni et al. 2008).

This articaine solution would be indicated, however, to anesthetize the second primary mandibular molar with infiltration (e.g., in hemophilic children for whom mandibular blocks are contraindicated) because infiltration with the standard L-100 solution is less successful in that tooth (Wright et al. 1991; Sharaf 1997).

### A-200, 4% Articaine with 1:200 000 (5 µg/ml) Epinephrine

This solution has double the local anesthetic as the standard lidocaine solution (4% vs. 2%) but half the epinephrine (5 µg/ml vs. 10 µg/ml). As a result its efficacy in achieving pulpal anesthesia is similar to or slightly lower than in L-100 (Annex 21).

The maximum absolute dose in adults weighing 70 kg or over is 500 mg (7 mg/kg) or seven 1.8-ml or seven and a half 1.7-ml cartridges (Annex 10).

This solution would be indicated especially in patients for whom the epinephrine dose needs to be reduced (Mehta et al. 1983; American Dental Association 2003; Elad et al. 2008) but not eliminated altogether (see Chapter 10), such as:

- ASA III cardiovascular patients (with severe but not incapacitating illness, no symptoms during ordinary exercise such as fatigue, shortness of breath, dizziness, or chest pain) could be administered a maximum dose of 4.5 A-200 cartridges (40 µg of epinephrine). This includes patients with:
  - Uncontrolled high blood pressure: 95–115/160–200 mmHg.
  - Cardiac insufficiency and difficulty breathing on exertion or under stress but not when in repose.
  - Who have had a heart transplant.
  - Who more than 3 months prior had:
    - an acute heart attack
    - a stroke
    - a coronary bypass
    - stents in coronary artery disease.
- Patients who are on:
  - Non-selective beta-blockers (propanolol, carvedilol, nadolol, etc.) (Table 10.4, Chapter 10) could be administered a maximum dose of three A-200 cartridges (27 µg of epinephrine).
  - COMT (anti-Parkinson) inhibitors (tolcapone, entacapone) could be administered a maximum dose of three A-200 cartridges (27 µg of epinephrine).
  - Digoxin could be administered a maximum dose of four and a half A-200 cartridges (40 µg of epinephrine).
  - Amphetamines and psychostimulant derivatives (dextroamphetamine, methylphenidate, atomoxetine, etc.) could be administered a maximum dose of five and a half A-200 cartridges (50 µg of epinephrine).
  - Tri- and tetracyclic antidepressants (amitriptyline, nortriptyline, imipramine, mirtazapine, etc.) (Table 10.5, Chapter 10) could be administered a maximum dose of five and a half A-200 cartridges (50 µg of epinephrine).

In all these cases patients can be administered double the volume of the A-200 solution than with epinephrine 1:100 000 (10 µg/ml).

## Mepivacaine

Mepivacaine was synthesized in 1956 by Bo af Ekenstam et al. from piperidine carboxylic acid (Ekenstam et al. 1957). This anesthetic was the eighth of 35 compounds they produced. It was initially named Carbocaine® (Ekenstam et al. 1957) and renamed mepivacaine in 1960 (Luduena et al. 1960), retaining Carbocaine as the brand name. It was introduced in the United States in 1960 (Malamed 2004).

This anesthetic has two aromatic rings, the benzene typical of the amide group anesthetics, and piperidine in the amino terminus. Its most prominent characteristics are summarized in Table 7.5.

### Metabolism

Like all amide anesthetics, mepivacaine is metabolized in the liver and at least 50% is eliminated in the urine, with only 7% excreted unchanged (Annex 12). A higher proportion of unaltered mepivacaine is eliminated in acidic urine (Reynolds 1971; Meffin et al. 1973b). It crosses the placenta, with 70% of the maternal plasma found in the umbilical vein (Covino 1971). Its possible biotransformation pathways are listed in Annex 12.

**Table 7.5** Mepivacaine.

| Pharmacological factor | Reference |
|---|---|
| • Name and synonym: mepivacaine, Carbocaine® | |
| • First synthesized in 1956 by Ekenstam et al. | Ekenstam et al. (1957) |
| • Chemical name: 1-methyl-2,6-pipecoloxylidide | American Dental Association (1984) |
| • Formula: $C_{15}H_{22}N_2O$ | |
| Mepivacaine structure | |
| • Molecular weight: Base 246.16 Hydrochloride 282.8 | |
| • Clearance rate: 0.74 l/min | Annex 11 |
| • Volume of distribution: 85 l | Annex 11 |
| • Half-life: 120 minutes | Annex 11 |
| **Physical-chemical property** | |
| • pKa value or dissociation constant: 7.7<br>　　Denotes fast onset | Annex 6 |
| • Lipid solubility or partition coefficient: $n$-heptane 0.8<br>　　　　　　　　　　$n$-octanol 20<br>　　Denotes medium anesthetic potency and no topical anesthesia | Annex 7 |
| • Plasma protein binding: 75%<br>　　Denotes medium duration of the anesthetic effect | Annex 9 |
| • Vasodilation: − (weak vasoconstriction)<br>　　Denotes efficacy with no need for a vasoconstrictor | Du Mesnil de Rochemont and Hensel (1960)<br>Lindorf et al. (1974)<br>Lindorf (1979) |
| **Clinical factor** | **Reference** |
| • Relative anesthetic potency: 2 | |
| • Relative toxicity: 2 | Annex 8 |
| • Maximum absolute dose in dentistry: 300 mg (4.3 mg/kg) | American Dental Association (1984) |
| • Usable during pregnancy: Yes (FDA category = C)<br>　　Denotes low risk | Table 5.11 (Chapter 5) |
| • Usable during lactation: Yes<br>　　Denotes low risk | Table 5.11 (Chapter 5) |
| • Usable with children: Yes<br>　　Denotes low risk | |

Table 7.5 (Continued)

| Anesthetic parameter | Variable | M-3 | M-20 | M-100 |
|---|---|---|---|---|
| Buccal infiltration | Successful pulpal anesthesia (%) | 91 | 91 | 93 |
| Superior lateral incisor 1 ml (Annex 21) | Duration, pulpal anesthesia (minutes) | 15 | 45 | 35 |
|  | Duration, anesthesia upper lip (minutes) | 100 | 190 | 160 |
| Mandibular block 1.8 ml (Annex 27) | Duration, anesthesia lower lip (minutes) | 190 | 240 | 190 |

Pharmacological, physical-chemical, and clinical properties and anesthetic parameter.
Summary: (M-3) 3% with no vasoconstrictor: 91%-15′/100′-190′.
(M-20) 2% mepivacaine with 1:20 000 (50 µg/ml) levonordefrin: 91%-45′/190′-240′.
(M-100) 2% mepivacaine with 1:100 000 (10 µg/ml) epinephrine: 93%-35′/160′-190′.

## Remarks

Two features of mepivacaine merit comment: the recommended maximum doses and the solutions that can be used in dentistry.

### Maximum Doses

In the 1980s some European institutions proposed maximum mepivacaine doses of 500 mg with vasoconstrictor and 300 mg without (Die Arzneimittelkommission der Deutschen Ärzteschaft Informiert 1985). The FDA criterion is 400 mg with or without vasoconstrictor as the maximum absolute dose in dentistry (American Dental Association 2003). *The maximum absolute dental dose recommended here is 300 mg* with or without vasoconstrictor, further to the prudent recommendation published by the Council on Dental Therapeutics in 1984 (American Dental Association 1984).

### Mepivacaine Solutions

The three solutions of this local anesthetic presently available are discussed below.

- **M-3, 3% mepivacaine with no vasoconstrictor**
This solution is deemed here to pose a significant advantage because it performs better than any other vasoconstrictor-free local anesthetic for dentistry: 91%-15′/100′-190′ (Table 5.8, Chapter 5). While its results are modest compared to those of any other vasoconstrictor-enhanced solution, it is indisputably the best possible of those without such drugs, perhaps due to its own "inherent" vasoconstrictive effect, but very poor (Du Mesnil de Rochemont and Hensel 1960; Lindorf et al. 1974; Lindorf 1979). It is the most useful of the mepivacaine solutions because it constitutes a solution with the minimum requirements to attend to patients in whom vasoconstrictors are contraindicated for one reason or another.

- **M-20, 2% mepivacaine with 1:20 000 (50 µg/ml) levonordefrin**
This solution is marketed primarily in the United States and since 2004 has been difficult to find (Malamed 2004). Its two drawbacks are the small number of clinical studies and its lower anesthetic parameter (91%-45′/190′-240′) than observed for the standard lidocaine solution with epinephrine (95%-45′/190′-200′).

- **M-100, 2% mepivacaine with 1:100 000 (10 µg/ml) epinephrine**
This solution is marketed in some European countries, but has the same drawback as M-20: its anesthetic parameter (93%-35′/160′-200′) lower than in L-100, the standard lidocaine solution with the same epinephrine concentration.

## Indications

The only mepivacaine solution of interest is the one with *3% concentration and no vasoconstrictor*, for the reasons discussed above. This solution is indicated when vasoconstrictors are absolutely contraindicated (see Chapter 10), as listed below.

- Sympathomimetic vasoconstrictors (epinephrine, norepinephrine, and levonordefrin), in:
  1) Insulin-dependent, poorly controlled diabetes.
  2) Patients with sulfite sensitivity or intolerance.

3) Patients with severe, corticoid-controlled asthma because many are sulfite-intolerant.
4) Patients with pheochromocytoma, a tumor of the adrenal gland cromaffin tissue, which releases excess epinephrine and norepinephrine.
5) Patients who have consumed cocaine in the last 24 hours.
6) Cardiovascular patients simultaneously taking amphetamines or psychostimulants.
7) Exceptionally, patients allergic to artificial vasoconstrictors such as levonordefrin and the bitartrate or hydrochloride forms of natural vasoconstrictors such as epinephrine and norepinephrine (allergies to the base forms would be incompatible with life because they are natural hormones and neurotransmitters).

- Vasoconstrictors such as felypressin (Octapressin) are contraindicated during pregnancy due to the risk of provoking a premature birth or miscarriage. Felypressin (0.03 UL/ml = 0.54 µg/ml) is found in 3% prilocaine solutions.
Note: The contraindications for vasoconstrictors are discussed at length in Chapter 10.

The maximum absolute dose in adults weighing 70 kg or over is 300 mg (4.3 mg/kg) or five and a half 1.8-ml cartridges of M-3 (Annex 10).

## Prilocaine (Propitocaine)

Prilocaine was synthesized in 1953 by Nils Löfgren (1915–1967) and Claës Tegnér (Wielding 1960). A paper describing its synthesis was published in 1960 (Löfgren and Tegner 1960). Initially named L67 (Löfgren and Tegner 1960; Wielding 1960), in 1964 it was renamed propitocaine (Sadove et al. 1964) and prilocaine (Daly et al. 1964), and marketed under the name Citanest®. It was approved by the FDA for use in the United States in 1966 (Widman 1975). It is presently known as prilocaine the world over except in the United Kingdom, where the name propitocaine has prevailed (de Jong 1977). Prilocaine is an amide anesthetic derived from toluidine. Its most prominent characteristics are summarized in Table 7.6.

### Metabolism

Prilocaine concentrates, in descending order, in the lungs, kidneys, brain, and heart, more intensely than lidocaine (Akerman et al. 1966). It exits the bloodstream more rapidly than lidocaine, metabolized by amidase in the liver and to a lesser extent in the kidneys and lungs (Geddes 1965; Akerman et al. 1966). It is eliminated primarily in the urine, with less than 1% excreted unchanged (Akerman et al. 1966; Mather 1972), although that value is higher in acidic urine (Eriksson et al. 1966). Very little is eliminated in the feces (Akerman et al. 1966). Its possible biotransformation pathways are listed in Annex 12.

Prilocaine diffuses passively across the placenta, and although the concentration in the umbilical vein is the same as in the mother's plasma (Covino 1971; Poppers 1975), it is less toxic for the fetus than lidocaine or mepivacaine (Shnider and Gildea 1973).

Its main metabolite is ortho-toluidine (o-toluidine) or 2-methylalanine, the primary cause of toxic methemoglobinemia, which may be induced by this anesthetic (Onji and Tyuma 1965; Lund and Cwick 1965a; Spoerel et al. 1967). A second prilocaine metabolite, 4-hydroxy-o-toluidine, is also associated with methemoglobinemia, although to a lesser extent (Frayling et al. 1990).

### Remarks

The three most prominent factors meriting comment are toxicity and safety, clinical efficacy, and commercial solutions.

#### Toxicity and Safety

Prilocaine has a demonstrably lower toxicity than lidocaine in both laboratory animals (Annex 8) and human beings (Lund and Cwick 1965a; Lund et al. 1975). That may be because it is eliminated more quickly (Lund and Cwick 1965a), with blood levels declining more rapidly than in other anesthetics (Eriksson and Granberg 1965), in as much as it is metabolized not only in the liver but also in the lungs and kidneys, as noted.

Although its concentration in the fetal bloodstream is the same as in the mother's (Covino 1971; Poppers 1975), as it is less toxic than lidocaine and mepivacaine (Shnider and Gildea 1973), which are found in lower concentrations, it merits an FDA pregnancy risk category B (American Dental Association 2003).

The risk posed by prilocaine is that it causes *toxic methemoglobinemia*, an adverse effect directly related to the amount administered (Onji and Tyuma 1965; Hjelm and Holmdahl 1965; Lund and Cwick 1965b; Spoerel et al. 1967). Methemoglobinemia may be induced at doses of 400 mg (Daly et al. 1964; Lund and Cwick 1965b) and certainly at ≥900 mg (Scott et al. 1964; Lund and Cwick 1965b), although these values may vary depending on the individual (Spoerel et al. 1967). In 1984 the American Dental Association's Council on Dental Therapeutics consequently *recommended 400 mg as the maximum absolute dose* of prilocaine, with or without vasoconstrictor (American Dental Association 1984).

As discussed below, prilocaine comes in high concentrations (3–4%), raising the risk of long-term paresthesia or

Table 7.6  Prilocaine

| Pharmacological factor | Reference |
|---|---|
| • Name and synonyms: prilocaine, propitocaine, L 67 | |
| • First synthesized in 1953 by Löfgren and Tegnér | Wielding (1960) |
| • Chemical name: 2-propylamino-o-propionotoluidide | American Dental Association (1984) |
| • Formula: $C_{13}H_{20}N_2O$ | |
| Prilocaine structure | |
| • Molecular weight: Base 220.3<br>   Hydrochloride 256.8 | |
| • Clearance rate: 2.6 l/min | Annex 11 |
| • Volume of distribution: 190 l | Annex 11 |
| • Half-life: 95 minutes | Annex 11 |
| **Physical-chemical property** | |
| • pKa value or dissociation constant: 7.9<br>   Denotes fast onset | Annex 6 |
| • Lipid solubility or partition coefficient: $n$-heptane 0.9<br>   $n$-octanol 25<br>   Denotes medium anesthetic potency and no topical anesthesia | Annex 7 |
| • Plasma protein binding: 55%<br>   Denotes medium duration of the anesthetic effect | Annex 9 |
| • Vasodilation: ± (very weak vasodilation)<br>   Denotes efficacy with no need for a vasoconstrictor | Lindorf et al. (1974) Lindorf (1979)<br>Aström and Persson (1961) |
| **Clinical factor** | **Reference** |
| • Relative anesthetic potency: 1.5 | |
| • Relative toxicity: 1.5 | Annex 8 |
| • Maximum absolute dose in dentistry: 400 mg (5.7 mg/kg) | American Dental Association (1984) |
| • Usable during pregnancy: Yes (FDA category = B)<br>   Denotes low risk | Table 5.11 (Chapter 5) |
| • Usable during lactation: Yes<br>   Denotes low risk | Table 5.11 (Chapter 5) |
| • Usable with children: Yes<br>   Denotes low risk | |

(Continued)

**Table 7.6** (Continued)

| Anesthetic parameter | Variable | P-03 | P-200 | P-4 |
|---|---|---|---|---|
| Buccal infiltration | Successful pulpal anesthesia (%) | 88 | 85 | 87 |
| Superior lateral incisor 1 ml (Annex 21) | Duration, pulpal anesthesia (minutes) | 25 | 25 | 10 |
| | Duration, anesthesia upper lip (minutes) | 180 | 130 | 75 |
| Mandibular block 1.8 ml (Annex 27) | Duration, anesthesia lower lip (minutes) | 220 | 200 | 180 |

Pharmacological, physical-chemical and clinical properties and anesthetic parameter.
Summary: (P-03) 3% prilocaine with 0.03 IU/ml (0.54 µg/ml) felypressin: 88%-25'/180'-220'.
(P-200) 4% prilocaine with 1:200 000 (5 µg/ml) epinephrine: 85%-25'/130'-200'.
(P-4) 4% prilocaine with no vasoconstrictor: 87%-10'/75'-180'.

*persistent inoperable neuropathies* in the wake of mandibular block due to its neurotoxicity. The incidence of that complication is fortunately very low, estimated to be 1 in 100 000 blocks, but the risk with 4% prilocaine is 35 times higher than with 2% lidocaine with epinephrine (L-100) (see Chapter 22).

### Clinical Efficacy

As this anesthetic has been shown to be less potent in both laboratory animals (Aström and Persson 1961) and human beings (Annex 21), a higher concentration is needed for results comparable to those of lidocaine (3–4% vs. 2%).

In contrast, as it induces weaker vasodilation than lidocaine, likewise in laboratory animals (Aström and Persson 1961; Akerman et al. 1966) and humans (Lindorf et al. 1974; Lindorf 1979), it can be used without a vasoconstrictor, although such drugs enhance its efficacy (Annex 21).

### Prilocaine Solutions

All prilocaine solutions exhibit lower performance than other solutions.

- **P-4, 4% prilocaine with no vasoconstrictor**
  This solution would be indicated where vasoconstrictors are contraindicated, although as its anesthetic parameter (87%-10'/75'-180') is lower than in 3% mepivacaine with no vasoconstrictor (91%-15'/100'-190'), the latter is preferred in such situations.
- **P-200, 4% prilocaine with 1:200 000 (5 µg/ml) epinephrine**
  This solution would be indicated especially in patients in whom the epinephrine dose needs to be reduced but not eliminated altogether (see Chapter 10). As its anesthetic parameter (85%-25'/130'-190') is lower than in 4% articaine with 1:200 000 epinephrine (92%-45'/190'-260'), A-200 is preferred under these conditions.
- **P-03, 3% prilocaine with 0.03 IU/ml (0.54 µg/ml) felypressin**
  This solution would likewise be indicated where sympathomimetic vasoconstrictors are contraindicated. Although its anesthetic parameter is poor (88%-25'/180'-220'), as it induces longer-lasting pulpal and soft tissue anesthesia than vasoconstrictor-free 3% mepivacaine (91%-15'/100'-190'), it may be an alternative in such cases.

### Indications and Contraindications

The only prilocaine solution of interest is the one with a *3% concentration and 0.03 UI/ml (0.54 µg/ml) felypressin*, for the reasons discussed above.

The maximum absolute dose of prilocaine in dentistry for adults weighing 70 kg or more is 400 mg (5.7 mg/kg), which at 3% is equivalent to seven and a half 1.8-ml cartridges. The maximum dose of felypressin, however, is 7.02 µg (Oliver 1974; Roberts and Sowray 1987), *lowering the number of 1.8-ml cartridges to 7.2* at a concentration of 0.54 µg/ml (Annex 10).

### Indications

This solution is indicated when sympathomimetic vasoconstrictors (epinephrine, norepinephrine, and levonordefrin) are absolutely contraindicated (see Chapter 10), such as in:

1) Insulin-dependent, poorly controlled diabetes.
2) Patients with sulfite sensitivity or intolerance.
3) Patients with severe, corticoid-controlled asthma because many are sulfite-intolerant.
4) Patients with pheochromocytoma, a tumor of the adrenal gland cromaffin tissue, which releases excess epinephrine and norepinephrine.
5) Patients who have consumed cocaine in the last 24 hours.
6) Cardiovascular patients simultaneously taking amphetamines or psychostimulants.
7) Exceptionally, patients allergic to artificial vasoconstrictors such as levonordefrin and the bitartrate or hydrochloride forms of natural vasoconstrictors such as epinephrine and norepinephrine (allergies to the base forms would be incompatible with life because they are natural hormones and neurotransmitters).

**Contraindications**

This solution is also subject to contraindications, some deriving from its vasoconstrictor, felypressin, and others from the anesthetic.

- Felypressin-specific contraindications (see Chapters 6 and 10)
  1) It is *wholly contraindicated in pregnancy* due to the risk of miscarriage or premature birth because of the effect of its residual oxytoxicity (Anonymous 1970; Oliver 1974; Stepke et al. 1994).
  2) It is likewise contraindicated for heart attack (angina or myocardial infarction) patients. Although felypressin may cause the coronary vessels to contract, here the contraindication is not absolute. The maximum absolute dose in such cases is five 1.8-ml cartridges (Oliver 1974; Roberts and Sowray 1987).
- Prilocaine per se is contraindicated for patients in whom toxic methemoglobinemia may worsen their condition by further hampering oxygen transport to the tissues (see Chapter 9), such as in:
  1) Cardiovascular disease including
     - cardiac insufficiency, coronary insufficiency, arrhythmias
     - anemia and red blood cell alterations
     - insufficient cerebral or peripheral circulation
  2) Severe respiratory disease.
  3) Children under 1 year and in very old age.
  4) Rare cases of congenital methemoglobinemia.

Although in severe (ASA III) illness and congenital methemoglobinemia the solution is absolutely contraindicated, in all the others it may be administered, albeit at lower maximum doses.

# Bupivacaine

Like mepivacaine, bupivacaine was synthesized by Bo af Ekenstam et al. from piperidine carboxylic acid (Ekenstam et al. 1957). It was initially named LAC-43 (Ekenstam 1966) and subsequently bupivacaine. It was introduced for medical use under the brand name Marcaine (Moore 1984; Dunsky and Moore 1984) and approved by the FDA for use in dentistry in 1.8-ml cartridges in 1983 (Dean 1983).

This anesthetic is very similar to mepivacaine and like it has two aromatic rings, a benzene ring and a piperidine ring at the amino terminus which, rather than a single carbon atom (methyl, hence mepivacaine), has four (butyl, hence bupivacaine) (Lund et al. 1970; Pricco 1977; Moore 1984). The higher the number of terminal carbons the more potent and toxic is the anesthetic: termini with more than five carbons are too toxic and irritating to be used (Aberg et al. 1977). The most prominent characteristics of bupivacaine are summarized in Table 7.7.

## Metabolism

Large proportions of bupivacaine are observed at the injection site 1 hour later (Goehl et al. 1973), possibly because of its high lipid solubility. It is metabolized by cytochrome P450, primarily by the 3A4 isoform of the enzyme, although also by isoforms 2C19 and 2D6 (Gantebain et al. 2000). Around 80% is eliminated in the urine, only 5% as free unaltered bupivacaine (Annex 12). Elimination is enhanced by acid urine (Reynolds 1971) and 5% is also found in the feces (Goehl et al. 1973).

Bupivacaine crosses the placenta, with the umbilical vein containing 40% of the concentration found in the maternal plasma (Covino 1971). Its possible biotransformation pathways are listed in Annex 12.

## Remarks

Bupivacaine is a potent, long-lasting local anesthetic, but also more toxic than others (Annex 8) due to its high lipid solubility and high binding rate to plasma proteins. Like all local anesthetics it is toxic to the nervous and cardiovascular systems, although *bupivacaine is particularly toxic to the heart*, where it induces severe arrhythmia and fibrillation (Reiz and Nath 1986; Maxwell et al. 1994; Mather and Chang 2001) (see Chapter 9). As at concentrations of over 1% bupivacaine irritates the tissues (Henn and Brattsand 1966; Ekblom and Widman 1966), it is used at 0.25–0.75%, with the midway value, 0.5%, the most widely used.

It also has a very powerful vasodilatory effect, greater than in lidocaine (Aps and Reynolds 1976; Reynolds et al. 1976), and thus must be used with a vasoconstrictor. In light of its high pKa, its onset may be delayed.

**Table 7.7** Bupivacaine

| Pharmacological factor | Reference |
|---|---|
| • Name and synonym: bupivacaine, LAC 43 | |
| • First synthesized in 1957 by Ekenstam et al. | Ekenstam et al. (1957) |
| • Chemical name: 1-butyl-2′,6′-pipecoloxylide | American Dental Association (1984) |
| • Formula: $C_{18}H_{28}N_2O$ | |
| [Structural formula of Bupivacaine: 2,6-dimethylphenyl-NH–CO-piperidine with N-$C_4H_9$ substituent] | |
| • Molecular weight: Base 288.43    Hydrochloride 324.9 | |
| • Clearance rate: 0.52 l/min | Annex 11 |
| • Volume of distribution: 53 L | Annex 11 |
| • Half-life: 150 minutes | Annex 11 |

| Physical-chemical property | |
|---|---|
| • pKa value or dissociation constant: 8.1   Denotes slower onset | Annex 6 |
| • Lipid solubility or partition coefficient: $n$-heptane 27.5   $n$-octanol 350   Denotes high anesthetic potency and topical anesthesia | Annex 7 |
| • Plasma protein binding: 95%   Denotes long duration of the anesthetic effect | Annex 9 |
| • Vasodilation: ++ (high)   Denotes a need for a vasoconstrictor to be effective | Aps and Reynolds (1976) <br> Reynolds et al. (1976) |

| Clinical factor | Reference/s |
|---|---|
| • Relative anesthetic potency: 8 | |
| • Relative toxicity: 8 | Annex 8 |
| • Maximum absolute dose in dentistry: 90 mg (1.3 mg/kg) | Dean (1983) <br> American Dental Association (2003) |
| • Usable during pregnancy: Yes (FDA category = C)   Denotes low risk | Table 5.11 (Chapter 5) |
| • Usable during lactation: Yes   Denotes low risk | Table 5.11 (Chapter 5) |
| • Usable with children: Yes, if over 12 years | Laskin et al. (1977) <br> Jensen et al. (1981) |

| Anesthetic parameter | Variable | B-200 |
|---|---|---|
| Buccal infiltration <br> Superior lateral incisor <br> 1 ml <br> (Annex 21) | Successful pulpal anesthesia (%) | 80 |
| | Duration, pulpal anesthesia (minutes) | 35 |
| | Duration, anesthesia upper lip (minutes) | 410 |
| Mandibular block <br> 1.8 ml <br> (Annex 27) | Duration, anesthesia lower lip (minutes) | 490 |

Pharmacological, physical-chemical and clinical properties and anesthetic parameter.
Summary: (B-200) 0.5% bupivacaine with 1:200 000 (5 µg/ml) epinephrine: 80%-35′/410′-490′.

FDA authorization in dentistry is for 0.5% bupivacaine in 1.8-ml cartridges containing 1:200 000 (5 μg/ml) epinephrine (Dean 1983), with the maximum absolute dose set at 90 mg (American Dental Association 2003). *The main drawback to this solution is its low success rate in pulpal anesthesia when infiltrated* (anesthetic parameter 80%-35'/410'-500'), although its effect in soft tissues is long lasting. One of its advantages is that it retards the onset of initial post-operative pain after oral surgery (Table 7.8). A possible explanation for its scant infiltrative efficacy for pulpal anesthesia may be gleaned from experiments with ropivacaine (another long-lasting, high-potency local anesthetic with lipid solubility and plasma protein binding similar to bupivacaine). The former has been observed to bind to and concentrate in the soft tissues and nerves (hence its efficacy in mandibular blocks), but unfortunately to be unable to diffuse well across bone (Kimi et al. 2012), a highly mineralized tissue. That would explain the poor results when cortical and spongy bone must be penetrated to engage with the dental apex and reach the nerve and dental pulp.

*The wide gap between the 90 mg maximum authorized dose for dentistry* and the 225 mg allowed in medicine with and 175 mg without epinephrine (Lund et al. 1975; Moore et al. 1977; American Dental Association 1984, 2003) is striking. The medical dose is lower in some European countries: 150 mg with or without epinephrine (Die Arzneimittelkommission der Deutschen Ärzteschaft Informiert 1985; Wulf et al. 1988). Such a difference, much wider than in other anesthetics, may attest to health authorities' precautionary approach to the cardiotoxicity associated with bupivacaine.

Pulpal anesthesia is of cardinal importance in dentistry, however, and is a key concern in most solutions. Extensive oral surgery in soft tissue and bone may even entail tooth sectioning. An alternative is to use supplementary (intraligamental or intraosseous anesthetic techniques), although when tissue is surgically sectioned the results may not be optimal because of leakage from the opened flap (Yamazaki et al. 2006).

In light of the foregoing and based on the prudent 90 mg maximum dose, three lines of action are suggested to improve pulpal anesthesia.

1) Raise bupivacaine concentration to 0.75% with 1:200 000 (5 μg/ml) epinephrine. The results with this solution are promising: anesthetic parameter of 95%-25'/385' (Danielsson et al. 1985) at the maximum dose of 90 mg (1.3 mg/kg) for an adult weighing 70 kg or over, which is equivalent to six and a half 1.8-ml cartridges.
2) Raise epinephrine concentration in a 0.5% bupivacaine solution to 1:100 000 (10 μg/ml), the standard in dentistry (Annex 17). Experimental studies (Ohkado et al. 2000) and clinical trials (Oka et al. 1997) have yielded promising results. Onset time, retarded by the fairly high pKa value (8.1), can be shortened with this concentration (Nespeca 1976) and the higher epinephrine content improves hemostasis in surgery, offsetting the intense vasodilatory effect induced by bupivacaine.

With this solution, the maximum absolute dose, 90 mg (1.3 mg/kg) for a >70 kg adult, would translate into 10 1.8-ml cartridges.
3) Raise both concentrations, bupivacaine to 0.75% and epinephrine to 1:100 000. In that case, the maximum dose would be six and a half 1.8-ml cartridges. This alternative may be the cause for greatest concern because the heart may be sensitized by both bupivacaine and epinephrine.

### Indications and Contraindications

The sole bupivacaine solution commercially available in dental cartridges is 0.5% anesthetic with 1:200 000 (5 μg/ml) epinephrine (B-200). This solution provides for long-lasting anesthesia in soft tissue (Table 7.8), although its efficacy for pulpal anesthesia with buccal infiltration is

Table 7.8 Local anesthetic solutions: duration of lower lip anesthesia after mandibular block and onset of first pain after surgical extraction of mandibular wisdom teeth (data from Annex 27)

| | Duration, anesthesia lower lip | | Onset of first pain | |
|---|---|---|---|---|
| Local anesthetic solution | (minutes) | (hours) | (minutes) | (hours) |
| 0.5% bupivacaine with 1:100 000 epinephrine | 490 | 8 | 340 | 5.5 |
| 2% lidocaine with 1:100 000 epinephrine | 200 | 3.3 | 180 | 3 |
| 4% articaine with 1:100 000 epinephrine | 260 | 4.5 | 190 | 3.2 |
| 4% articaine with 1:200 000 epinephrine | 260 | 4.5 | 210 | 3.5 |
| 2% mepivacaine with 1:100 000 epinephrine | 190 | 3.2 | 150 | 2.5 |
| 3% mepivacaine, no vasoconstrictor | 190 | 3.2 | 150 | 2.5 |

low. It is consequently *recommended primarily for mandibular block. Patients must also be advised that anesthesia in the lower lip will last for 6–10 hours*, with the advantage that post-operative pain will be milder.

The maximum absolute dose of this local anesthesia for an adult weighing 70 kg or more is 90 mg (1.3 mg/kg) or 10 1.8-ml cartridges.

**Indications**

1) Bupivacaine prevents post-operative pain in extensive oral surgery (often surgical extraction of mandibular wisdom teeth) because it retards the onset of initial pain by prolonging anesthetic action in the soft tissue (Nespeca 1976; Laskin et al. 1977). Long-acting local anesthetics may also reduce the consumption of systemic analgesics such as nonsteroidal anti-inflammatory agents, acetaminophen, and/or opioids, which all have dose-dependent side effects (Chapman and Macleod 1985).
2) Bupivacaine prevents post-surgical pain in particularly painful endodontic therapy, such as in mandibular molars and premolars for the same reason as above (Moore and Dunsky 1983; Dunsky and Moore 1984; Parirokh et al. 2012).
3) Bupivacaine is used when long-lasting anesthesia is needed for the temporary relief of acute pain in soft tissues (not pulpal or osseous) in emergencies (Jensen et al. 1981).
4) Bupivacaine is used in chronic orofacial pain (such as causalgia, trigeminal neuralgia or post-herpetic neuralgia) to attempt to achieve permanent relief by blocking the Gasserian or the Stellate ganglion, sometimes repeatedly. In such cases it can be used with (Hanowell and Kennedy 1979) or without (Adler 1975; Hanowell and Kennedy 1979; Khoury et al. 1980) epinephrine.

**Contraindications**

Contraindications are associated primarily with the long duration of the anesthetic effect in soft tissue and concomitant discomfort in connection with drinking, eating, and speaking and the risk of self-injury to the tongue, lips, and buccal mucosa. Scantly effective pulpal anesthesia in infiltration, another major drawback, is reason not to use this solution in:

1) Short or medium duration routine procedures (Laskin et al. 1977; Jensen et al. 1981).
2) Children under 12 years, due to the high risk of self-injury to the soft tissues (Laskin et al. 1977; Jensen et al. 1981; Moore 1984).
3) Patients with special needs (Pricco 1977; Jensen et al. 1981) or psychiatric (Jensen et al. 1981) patients, for the above reason.

## References

AAPD (American Academy of Pediatric Dentistry) (2020). *Use of Local Anesthesia for Pediatric Dental Patients. The Reference Manual of Pediatric Dentistry*. Chicago, IL: American Academy of Pediatric Dentistry. 318–323.

Abdulwahab, M., Boynes, S., Moore, P. et al. (2009). The efficacy of six local anesthetic formulations used for posterior mandibular buccal infiltration anesthesia. *J. Am. Dent. Assoc.* 140 (8): 1018–1024.

Aberg, G., Dhuner, K.-G., and Sydnes, G. (1977). Studies on the duration of local anaesthesia: structures/activity relationships in a series of homologous local anesthetics. *Acta Pharmacol. Toxicol.* 41 (5): 432–443.

Adewuni, A., Hall, M., Guelmann, M., and Riley, J. (2008). The incidence of adverse reactions following 4% septocaine (articaine) in children. *Pediatr. Dent.* 30 (5): 424–428.

Adler, P. (1975). The use of bupivacaine for blocking the gasserian ganglion in major trigeminal neuralgia. *Int. J. Oral Sug.* 4 (6): 251–257.

Akerman, B., Aström, A., Ross, S., and Telc, A. (1966). Studies on the absorption, distribution and metabolism of labelled prilocaine and lidocaine in some animal species. *Acta Pharmacol. Toxicol.* 24 (4): 389–403.

Albalawi, F., Lim, J.C., DiRenzo, K.V. et al. (2018). Effects of lidocaine and articaine on neuronal survival and recovery. *Anesth. Prog.* 65 (2): 82–88.

Aldrete, J.A. and Johnson, D.A. (1970). Evaluation of intracutaneous testing for investigation of allergy to local anesthetic agents. *Anesth. Analg.* 49 (1): 173–183.

Aldrete, J.A. and Jonhson, D.A. (1969). Allergy to local anesthetics. *JAMA* 207 (2): 356–357.

American Dental Association (1983). *Dentists' desk reference: materials, instruments and equipment*, 2e. Chicago: American Dental Association. 355.

American Dental Association (1984). *Accepted Dental Therapeutics*, 40e. Chicago: Council on Dental Therapeutics, American Dental Association. 181–202.

American Dental Association (2003). *ADA Guide to Dental Therapeutics*, 3e. Chicago: American Dental Association. 2, 3.

Annex 6. Dissociation constant or pKa.

Annex 7. Partition coefficient or lipid solubility.

Annex 8. Acute experimental toxicity of local anesthetics.

Annex 9. Local anesthetic bonding to plasma proteins.

Annex 10. Maximum doses of dental local anesthetics solutions.

Annex 11. Pharmacokinetics of local anesthetics and vasoconstrictors.

Annex 12. Biotransformation of local anesthetics and vasoconstrictors.

Annex 14. Injectable anesthetic solutions pH.

Annex 17. Epinephrine III. Cardiovascular patients.

Annex 21. Maxillary pulpal anesthesia. Buccal infiltration.

Annex 24. Mandibular block I. Efficacy of standard solution L-100 or L-80.

Annex 27. Mandibular block IV. Anesthesia of the lower lip and time to first pain.

Annex 31. Mandibular pulpal anesthesia. Infiltrative.

Annex 35. Irreversible acute pulpitis (hot tooth). Efficacy of dental anesthesia.

Anonymous (1970). Felypressin – a new vasoconstrictor with prilocaine. *Drug Ther. Bull.* 8 (10): 38–40.

Aps, C. and Reynolds, F. (1976). The effect of concentration on vasoactivity of bupivacaine and lignocaine. *Br. J. Anaesth.* 48 (12): 1171–1174.

Arens, D.E., Adams, W.R., and de Castro, R.A. (1984). *Cirugía en endodoncia*. Barcelona: Ediciones Doyma SA. 38–50.

Aström, A. and Persson, N.H. (1961). Some pharmacological properties of o-methyl-propylaminopropionanilide, a new local anesthetic. *Br. J. Pharmacol.* 16 (1): 32–44.

Bargetzi, M.J., Aoyama, T., Gonzalez, F.J., and Meyer, U.A. (1989). Lidocaine metabolism in human liver microsomes by cytochrome P450 3A. *Clin. Pharmacol. Ther.* 46 (5): 512–527.

Becker, D.E. and Reed, K.L. (2006). Essentials of local anesthetic pharmacology. *Anesth. Prog.* 53 (3): 98–101.

Benedict, H.C., Clark, S.W., and Freeman, C.W. (1932). Studies in local anesthesia. *J. Am. Dent. Assoc.* 19 (12): 2087–2105.

Bennett, C.R. (1984). *Monheim's Local Anesthesia and Pain Control in Dental Practice*, 7e. St. Louis: The CV Mosby Co. 326.

Björn, H. (1947b). Studies on local anesthetics. V. The neutralization of acid local anesthetic solutions in the tissues. *Sven. Tandlak-Tidskr.* 40 (6): 853–867.

Björn, H. and Huldt, S. IV (1947a). The efficiency of xylocaine as a dental terminal anesthetic compared to that of procaine. *Sven. Tandlak-Tidskr.* 40 (6): 831–851.

Blumer, J., Strong, J.M., and Atkinson, A.J. Jr. (1973). The convulsant potency of lidocaine and its N-dealkylated metabolites. *J. Pharmacol. Exp. Ther.* 186 (1): 31–36.

Bonica, J.J. (1959). *Tratamiento del dolor, con estudio especial del empleo del bloqueo analgésico en el diagnóstico, pronóstico y terapéutica*. Barcelona (España): Salvat Editores SA. 159.

Borchard, U. and Drouin, H. (1980). Carticaine: action of the local anesthetic on myelinated nerve fibers. *Eur. J. Pharmacol.* 62 (1): 73–79.

Bowles, W.H., Frysh, H., and Emmons, R. (1995). Clinical evaluation of buffered local anesthetic. *Gen. Dent.* 43 (2): 182–184.

Boyes, R.N., Scott, D.B., Jebson, P.J. et al. (1971). Pharmacokinetics of lidocaine in man. *Clin. Pharmacol. Ther.* 12 (1): 105–116.

Brandt, R.G., Anderson, P.F., McDonald, N.J., Sohn, W., and Paters, M.C. (2011). The pulpal anesthetic efficacy of articaine versus lidocaine: a meta-analysis. *J. Am. Dent. Assoc.* 142 (5): 493–504.

Braun, H. (1905). Ueber einige neue örtliche Anaesthetica (Stovain, Alypin, Novocain). *Dtsch. Med. Wochenschr.* 31 (42): 1667–1671.

Brodie, B.B., Lief, P.A., and Poet, R. (1948). The fate of procaine in man following its intravenous administration and methods for the estimation of procaine and diethylaminoethanol. *J. Pharm. Exp. Ther.* 94 (4): 359–366.

Buckley, J.A., Ciancio, S.G., and McMullen, J.A. (1984). Efficacy of epinephrine concentration in local anesthesia during perioral surgery. *J. Periodontol.* 55 (11): 653–657.

Bush, R.K., Taylor, S.L., and Busse, W. (1986). A critical evaluation of clinical trials in reactions to sulfites. *J. Allergy Clin. Immunol.* 78 (1 Pt 2): 191–202.

Butterworth, J. and Oxford, G.S. (2009). Local anesthetics. A new hydrophilic pathway for the drug-receptor reaction (Editorial). *Anesthesiology* 111 (1): 12–14.

Calvey, T.N. (1995). Isomerism and anesthetic drugs. *Acta Anaesthsiol. Scand.* 39 (Suppl 106): 83–90.

Campbell, J.R., Maestrello, C.L., and Campbell, R.L. (2001). Allergy response to metabisulfite in lidocaine anesthetic solutions. *Anesth. Prog.* 48 (1): 21–26.

Chaikin, R.W. (1977). *Fundamentos clínicos prácticos del tratamiento periodontal*. Berlin: Quintessece Books. 35–39.

Chapman, P.J. and Macleod, A.W.G. (1985). A clinical study of bupivacaine for mandibular anesthesia in oral surgery. *Anesth. Prog.* 32 (2): 69–72.

Council on Clinical Affairs (2015). Guideline on use of local anesthesia for pediatric dental patients. *Pediatr. Dent.* 37 (Special issue): 199–205.

Covino, B.G. (1971). Comparative clinical pharmacology of local anesthetic agents. *Anesthesiology* 35 (2): 158–167.

Cowan, A. (1964). Minimun dosage in the clinical comparison of representative modern local anesthetic agents. *J. Dent. Res.* 43 (6): 1228–1249.

Da Silva, C.B., Berto, L.A., Volpato, M.C. et al. (2010). Anesthetic efficacy of articaine and lidocaine for incisive/mental nerve block. *J. Endod.* 36 (3): 438–441.

Daly, D.J., Davenport, J., and Newland, M.C. (1964). Methaemoglobinaemia following the use of prilocaine (Citanest). A preliminary report. *Br. J. Anaesth.* 36: 737–739.

Danielsson, K., Evers, H., and Nordenram, A. (1985). Long-acting local anesthetics in oral surgery: an experimental evaluation of bupivacaine and etidocaine for oral infiltration anesthesia. *Anesth. Prog.* 32 (2): 65–68.

De Jong, R.H. (1977). *Local Anesthetics*, 2e. Springfield (Illinois): Charles C Thomas Publisher. 279–282.

De Jong, R.H. and Cullen, S.C. (1963). Buffered-demand and pH of local anesthetic solutions containing epinephrine. *Anesthesiology* 24 (6): 801–807.

Dean, M. Cook-Waite Laboratories Inc. Comunication. In: Moorem P.A and Dunsky, J.L. (1983). Bupivacaine anesthesia – A clinical trial for endodontic therapy. *Oral Surg. Oral Med. Oral Pathol.* 55 (2): 176–179.

Den Hertog, A. (1974). The effect of carticain on mammalian non-myelinated nerve fibers. *Eur. J. Pharmacol.* 26 (2): 175–178.

Denio, D., Torabinejad, M., and Bakland, L.K. (1992). Anatomical relationship of the mandibular canal to its surrounding structures in mature mandibles. *J. Endod.* 18 (4): 161–165.

Die Arzneimittelkommission der Deutschen Ärzteschaft Informiert (1985). Lokalanästhetika: Bei Anwendung in der Praxis beachten. *Dtsch. Arztebl.* 82 (3): 100–101.

Dooms-Goossens, A., de Alam, A.G., Degreef, H., and Kochuyt, A. (1989). Local anesthetic intolerance due to metabisulfite. *Contact Dermatitis* 20 (2): 124–126.

Du Mesnil de Rochemont and Hensel, W., and Hensel, H. (1960). Messung der hautdurchblutung am menschen bei Einwirkung verscheidener lokalanasthetica. *Naunyn-Schmiedeberg Arch. Exp. Path. Pharmakol.* 239 (5): 464–474.

Dunsky, J.L. and Moore, P.A. (1984). Long-acting local anesthetics. A comparison of bupivacaine and etidocaine in endodontics. *J. Endod.* 10 (9): 457–460.

Einhorn, A. and Uhlfelder, E. (1909). Ueber den p-aminobenzoësäurdiäthyloamino – und – piperidoäthylester. *Justus Liebig's Ann. Chem.* 371 (2): 131–142.

Ekblom, L. and Widman, B. (1966). LAC-43 and tetracaine in spinal anaesthesia. A controlled clinical study. *Acta Anesthesiol. Scand. Suppl.* 23: 419–425.

Ekenstam, B. (1966). The effect of the structural variations on the local analgesic properties of the most commonly used groups of substances. *Acta Anaesth. Scand. Suppl.* 25: 10–18.

Ekenstam, B., Egner, B., Pettersson, G., and Local anesthetics, I. (1957). N-alkyl pyrrolidine and N-alkyl piperidine carboxylic acid amides. *Acta Chem. Scand.* 11 (7): 1183–1190.

Elad, S., Admon, D., Kedmi, M. et al. (2008). The cardiovascular effect of local anesthetic with articaine plus 1:200,000 adrenalin versus lidocaine plus 1:100,000 adrenalin in medically compromised cardiac patients: a prospective, randomized, double-blind study. *Oral Surg. Oral Med. Oral Pathol.* 105 (6): 725–730.

Eldridge, D.J. and Rood, J.P. (1977). A double blind trial of 5 per cent lignocaine solution. *Br. Dent. J.* 142 (4): 129–130.

Eriksson, E. and Granberg, P.-O. (1965). Studies on the renal excretion of Citanest® and Xylocaine®. *Acta Anaesth. Scand. Suppl.* 16: 79–85.

Eriksson, E., Granberg, P.-O., and Örtegren, B. (1966). Study of renal excretion of prilocaine and lidocaine. *Acta Chir. Scand.* Suppl 358: 55–69.

Farbwerke vorm (1904). Meister Lucius und Brüning in Höchst a. M. Verfahrenzur Darstellung von p-aminobenzoësäurealkaminestern. Kaiserliches Patentamt. Patentschrift nr 179627. Klasse 12q. Gruppe 6.

Fischer, G. (1910). *Di locale Anästhesie in der Zahanheilkunde. Mit spezieller Berück sichtingung der Schleimhaut und Leitungsanästhesie. Kurz gefaßtes lehrbuch für zahnärte, Ärzte und Studierende*. Berlin: Hermann Meusser.

Fischer, G. (1912). *Local Anesthesia in Dentistry. With Special Reference to Mucous and Conductive Methods. A Concise Guide for Dentists, Surgeons and Students*. Translated 2th German Ed. Philadelphia: Lea and Febiger.

Frayling, I.M., Addison, G.M., Chattergee, K., and Meakin, G. (1990). Methaemoglobinaemia in children treated with prilocaine-lignocaine cream. *Br. Med. J.* 301 (6744): 153–154.

Frenkel, G. (1989). Opening of the symposium (Foreword). En: Local anesthesia in dentistry today. Two decades of articaine. In: *Symposium 1–2 November 1989*. Bad Nauheim (Germany): Meducation Up-Date Hoechst. 5–6.

Fyhr, P. and Brodin, A. (1987). The effect of anaerobic conditions on epinephrine stability. *Acta Pharm. Suecica* 24 (3): 89–96.

Gantebain, M., Attolini, L., Bruguerolle, B. et al. (2000). Oxidative metabolism of bupivacaine into pipecolylxylidide in humans is mainly catalyzed by CYP3A. *Drug Metab. Dispos.* 28 (4): 383–385.

Garisto, G.A., Gaffen, A.S., Lawrence, H.P. et al. (2010). Ocurrence of parestesia after dental local anesthesia administration in the United States. *J. Am. Dent. Assoc.* 141 (7): 836–844.

Geddes, I.C. (1965). Studies of the metabolism of Citanest $C^{14}$. *Acta Anaesth. Scand. Suppl.* 16: 37–44.

Giovannitti, J.A. and Bennett, C.R. (1979). Assesment of allergy to local anesthetics. *J. Am. Dent. Assoc.* 98 (5): 701–706.

Goehl, T.J., Davenport, J.B., and Stanley, M.J. (1973). Distribution, biotransformation and excretion of bupivacaine in the rat and monkey. *Xenobiotica* 3 (12): 761–772.

Gordh, T., Gordh, T.E., and Lindqvist, K. (2010). Lidocaine: the origin of a modern local anesthetic. *Anesthesiology* 113 (6): 1433–1437.

Gruber, L.W. (1950). Preliminary report in the use of xylocaine as a local anesthetic in dentistry. *J. Dent. Res.* 29 (2): 137–142.

Haas, D.A. and Lennon, D. (1995). A 21 year retrospective study of reports of paresthesia following local anesthetic administration. *J. Can. Dent. Assoc.* 61 (4): 319–330.

Haas, D.A., Rynn, B.R., and Sands, T.D. (2000). Drug use for the pregnant or lactating patient. *Gen. Dent.* 48 (1): 54–60.

Haase, A., Reader, A., Nusstein, J. et al. (2008). Compare anesthetic efficacy of articaine versus lidocaine as a supplemental buccal infiltration on the mandibular first molar after an inferior alveolar nerve. *J. Am. Dent. Assoc.* 139 (9): 1228–1235.

Hanowell, S.T. and Kennedy, S.F. (1979). Phanton tonge pain and causalgia: case presentation and treatment. *Anesth. Analg.* 58 (5): 436–438.

Harrison, D.C., Sprouse, J.H., and Morrow, A.G. (1963). The antiarrhythmic properties of lidocaine and procaine amide. *Circulation* 28 (4): 486–491.

Henn, F. and Brattsand, R. (1966). Some pharmacological and toxicological properties of a new long-acting local analgesic, LAC-43 (Marcaine®), in comparison with mepivacaine and tetracaine. *Acta Anaesthesiol. Scand. Suppl.* 21: 9–30.

Hillerup, S. and Jensen, R. (2006). Nerve injury caused by mandibular block analgesia. *Int. J. Oral Maxillofac. Surg.* 35 (5): 437–443.

Hjelm, M. and Holmdahl, M.H. (1965). Methaemoglobinemia following lignocaine. *Lancet* 1 (7375): 53–54.

Hondrum, S.O. and Ezell, J.H. (1996). The relationship between pH and concentrations of antioxidants and vasoconstrictors in local anesthetic solutions. *Anesth. Prog.* 43 (4): 85–91.

Hondrum, S.O., Seng, G.F., and Rebert, N.W. (1993). Stability of local anesthetics in the dental cartridge. *Anesth. Pain Control Dent.* 2 (4): 198–202.

Hornke, I., Eckert, H.G., and Rupp, W. (1984). Pharmakokinetik und Metabolismus von Articain nach intramuskulärer Injection und männlichen Probanden. *Dtsch. Z. Mund. Kiefer Gesichts Chir.* 8 (1): 67–71.

Huang, A.S. and Fraser, W.M. (1984). Are sulfite additives really safe? *N. Engl. J. Med.* 311 (8): 542.

Isen, D.A. (2000). Articaine: pharmacology and clinical use of a recently approved local anesthetic. *Dent. Today* 19 (11): 72–77.

Jastak, J.T., Yagiela, J.A., and Donaldson, D. (1995). *Local Anesthesia of the Oral Cavity*. Philadelphia: WB Saunders Co. 161.

Jensen, O.T., Upton, L.G., Hayward, J.R., and Sweet, R.B. (1981). Advantages of long-acting local anesthetic using etidocaine hydrochloride. *J. Oral Surg.* 39 (5): 350–353.

Kalow, W. and Gunn, D.R. (1959). Some statistical data on atypical cholinesterase of human serum. *Ann. Hum. Genet.* 23 (3): 239–250.

Kanna, M.D., Whitworth, J.M., Corbett, I.P., and Meechan, J.G. (2006). Articaine and lidocaine mandibular buccal infiltration anesthesia: a prospective randomized double-blind cross-over study. *J. Endod.* 32 (4): 296–298.

Katyal, V. (2010). The efficacy and safety of articaine versus lidocaine in dental treatments: a meta-analysis. *J. Dent.* 38 (4): 307–317.

Katz, R.L. and Epstein, R.A. (1968). The interaction of anesthetic agents and adrenergic drugs to produce cardiac arrhythmias. *Anesthesiology* 29 (4): 763–784.

Khoury, R., Kennedy, S.F., and McNamara, R.E. (1980). Facial causalgia: report of a case. *J. Oral Surg.* 38 (10): 782–783.

Kimi, H., Yamashiro, M., and Hashimoto, S. (2012). The local pharmacokinetics of $^{3}$H-ropivacaine and $^{14}$C-lidocaine after maxillary infiltration anesthesia in rats. *Anesth. Prog.* 59 (2): 75–81.

Kirch, W., Kitteringham, N., Lambers, G. et al. (1983). Die klinische Pharmakokinetik von Articain nach intraoraler und intramuskuläres Application. *Schweiz. Mschr. Zahnheilk.* 93 (9): 714–719.

Klein, R.M. (1983). Components of local anesthetic solutions. *Gen. Dent.* 31 (6): 460–465.

Klingenström, P. and Westermar, K.L. (1964). Local tissue-oxygen tension after adrenaline, noradrenaline and octapressin® in local anaesthesia. *Acta Anaesth. Scand.* 8: 261–266.

Kramp, L.F., Eleazer, P.D., and Scheetz, J.P. (1999). Evaluation of prilocaine for the reduction of pain associated with transmucosal anesthetic administration. *Anesth. Prog.* 46 (2): 52–55.

Lambert, L.A., Lambert, D.H., and Strichartz, G.R. (1994). Irreversible conduction block in isolated nerve by high concentrations of local anesthetics. *Anesthesiology* 80 (5): 1082–1093.

Larson, C.E. (1977). Methylparaben – an overlooked cause of local anesthesia hypersensitivity. *Anesth. Prog.* 34 (3): 72–74.

Laskin, J.L., Wallace, W.R., and De Leo, B. (1977). Use of bupivacaine hydrochloride in oral surgery – a clinical study. *J. Oral Surg.* 35 (1): 25–29.

Latronica, R.J., Goldberg, A.F., and Wightman, J.R. (1969). Local anesthetic sensitivity. Report of a case. *Oral Surg. Oral Med. Oral Pathol.* 28 (3): 439–441.

Lewis, D.N. (1919). Pain following local anesthesia. *Dent. Cosmos.* 61: 407–408.

Lindorf, H.H. (1979). Investigation of the vascular effect of newer local anesthetics and vasoconstrictors. *Oral Surg. Oral Med. Oral Pathol.* 48 (4): 292–297.

Lindorf, H.H., Ganssen, A., and Mayer, P. (1974). Thermographic representation of vascular effects of local anaesthetics. *Electromedica* 42 (4): 106–110.

Link, W.J. and Alfred Einhorn, S.D. (1959). Inventor of novocaine. *Dent. Radiog. Photog.* 32 (1): 20.

Löfgren, N. (1948). *Studies on local anesthetics: xylocaine, a new synthetic drug*. Stockholm: Ivar Hoeggströms. 12.

Löfgren, N. and Lundqvist, B. (1946). Studies on local anaesthetics. II. *Svensk Kem Tidskr* 58 (8): 206–217.

Löfgren, N. and Tegner, C. (1960). Studies on local anesthetics XX. Synthesis of some α-monoalkylamino-methyl-2-methylpropionanilides. A new useful local anesthetic. *Acta Chem. Scand.* 14 (2): 486–490.

Luduena, F.P., Hoppe, J.O., Coulston, T., and Drobeck, H.P. (1960). The pharmacology and toxicology of mepivacaine, a new local anesthetic. *Toxicol. Appl. Pharmacol.* 2 (3): 295–315.

Luebke, N.H. and Walker, J.A. (1978). Discussion of sensitivity to preservatives in anesthetics. *J. Am. Dent. Assoc.* 97 (4): 656–657.

Lund, P.C. and Cwick, J.C. (1965a). Citanest®. . .a clinical and laboratory study. Part 1. *Anesth. Analg.* 44 (5): 623–631.

Lund, P.C. and Cwick, J.C. (1965b). Citanest®. . .a clinical and laboratory study. Part 2. *Anesth. Analg.* 44 (6): 712–721.

Lund, P.C., Cwick, J.C., and Vallesteros, F. (1970). Bupivacaine – A new long-acting local anesthetic agent. A preliminary clinical and laboratory report. *Anesth. Analg.* 49 (1): 103–114.

Lund, P.C., Cwick, J.C., and Cannon, R.T. (1975). Extradural anaesthesia: choice of local anaesthetic agents. *Br. J. Anaesth.* 47: 313–321.

Lundqvist, B., Löfgren, N., Persson, H., and Sjögren, B. (1948). Metal ion as a cause of swelling after local anesthesia in dental practice. *Acta Chir. Scand.* 97 (3): 239–258.

Malamed, S.F. (2004). *Handbook of Local Anesthesia*, 5e. St. Louis (Missouri): Elsevier-Mosby 65, 68, 71, 111–112.

Malamed, S.F., Gagnon, S., and Leblanc, D. (2000). A comparison between articaine HCl and lidocaine HCl in pediatric dental patients. *Pediatr. Dent.* 22 (4): 307–311.

Malamed, S.F., Cagnon, S., and Leblanc, D. (2001). Articain hydrochloride: a study of the safety of a new amide local anesthetic. *J. Am. Dent. Assoc.* 132 (2): 177–185.

Mather, L.E. (1972). *Studies in the Absorption, Distribution, Metabolism and Excretion of Drugs by Adult and Neonatal Humans* (Dissertation, Thesis). The University of Sydney. 216–229.

Mather, L.E. and Chang, D.H.-T. (2001). Cardiotoxicity with modern local anesthetics. Is there a safer choice? *Drugs* 61 (3): 333–342.

Maxwell, L.G., Martin, L.D., and Yaster, M. (1994). Bupivacaine-induced cardiac toxicity in neonates: successful treatment with intravenous phenytoin. *Anesthesiology* 80 (3): 682–686.

McMahon, F.G. and Woods, L.A. (1951). Further studies on the metabolism of lidocaine (xylocaine) in the dog. *J. Pharmacol. Exp. Ther.* 103 (4): 354. (abstract).

Meffin, P., Long, G.J., and Thomas, J. (1973b). Clearance and metabolism of mepivacaine in the human neonate. *Clin. Pharmacol. Ther.* 14 (2): 218–225.

Mehta, F.S., Daftary, D.K., Billimoria, R.B., and Trani, R.R. (1983). Carticaine in dentistry. *J. Indian Dent. Assoc.* 55 (12): 501–505.

Mihaly, G.W., Moore, G., Thomas, J. et al. (1978). The pharmacokinetics and metabolism of anilide local anaesthetics in neonates. I. Lignocaine. *Eur. J. Clin. Pharmacol.* 13 (2): 143–153.

Milano, E.A., Waraszkiewicz, S.M., and Dirubio, R. (1982). Aluminium catalysis of epinephrine degradation in lidocaine hydrochloride with epinephrine solutions. *J. Parent. Sci. Technol.* 36 (6): 232–236.

Moore, P.A. (1984). Bupivacaine: a long-acting local anesthetic for dentistry. *Oral Surg. Oral Med. Oral Pathol.* 58 (4): 369–374.

Moore, P.A. and Dunsky, J.L. (1983). Bupivacaine anesthesia – a clinical trial for endodontic therapy. *Oral Surg. Oral Med. Oral Pathol.* 55 (2): 176–179.

Moore, D.C., Bridenbaugh, L.D., Thompson, G.E. et al. (1977). Factors determining dosages of amide-type local anesthetic drugs. *Anesthesiology* 47 (3): 263–268.

Moorthy, A.P., Moorthy, S.P., and O'Neil, R. (1984). A study of pH of dental local anesthetic solutions. *Br. Dent. J.* 157 (11): 394–395.

Müller, W.P.E., Weiser, P., and Scholler, K.L. (1991). Pharmakokinetik vom Articain bei der Nervus mandibularis Blockade. *Reg. Anesth.* 14 (3): 52–55.

Muschaweck, R. and Rippel, R. (1974). Ein neues Lokalanästhetikum (Carticain) aus der Thiophenereihe. *Prakt. Anästh.* 9 (3): 135–146.

Nagel, J.E., Fuscaldo, J.T., and Fireman, P. (1977). Paraben allergy. *JAMA* 237 (15): 1594–1595.

Nespeca, J.A. (1976). Clinical trials with bupivacaine in oral surgery. *Oral Surg. Oral Med. Oral Pathol.* 42 (3): 301–307.

Nordenram, A. (1966). Influence of osmotic pressure on anaesthetic effect. A clinical, experiment comparison between different solutions of mepivacaine (Carbocaine®). *Odontol. Tidskr.* 74 (3): 217–222.

Oertel, R., Richter, K., Weile, K. et al. (1993). A simple method for the determination of articaine and its metabolite articainic acid in dentistry: application to a comparison of articaine and lidocaine concentrations in alveolus blood. *Methods Find Exp. Clin. Pharmacol.* 15 (8): 541–547.

Oertel, R., Berndt, A., and Kirch, W. (1996). Saturable in vitro metabolism of articaine by serum esterases. Does it contribute to the persistence of the local anesthetic effect? *Reg. Anesth.* 21 (6): 576–581.

Oertel, R., Rahn, R., and Kirch, W. (1997). Clinical pharmacokinetics of articaine. *Clin. Pharmacokinet.* 33 (6): 417–425.

Ohkado, S., Ichinohe, T., and Kaneko, Y. (2000). Comparative study on anesthetic potency depending on concentrations of lidocaine and epinephrine: assessment of dental local anesthetics using the jaw-opening reflex. *Anesth. Prog.* 48 (1): 16–20.

Oikarinen, V.J., Ylipaavalniemi, P., and Evers, H. (1975). Pain and temperature sensation related to local analgesia. *Int. J. Oral Surg.* 4 (4): 151–156.

Oka, S., Shimamoto, C., Kyoda, N., and Misaki, T. (1997). Comparison of lidocaine with and without bupivacaine for local dental anesthesia. *Anesth. Prog.* 44 (3): 83–86.

Oliver, L.P. (1974). Local anesthesia—a review of practice. *Aust. Dent. J.* 19 (5): 313–319.

Onji, Y. and Tyuma, I. (1965). Methemoglobin formation by local anesthetic and some related compounds. *Acta Anaesth. Scand. Suppl.* 16: 151–159.

Parirokh, M., Yosefi, M.H., Nakhaee, N. et al. (2012). Effect of bupivacaine on postoperative pain for inferior alveolar nerve block anesthesia after single-visit root canal treatment in teeth with irreversible pulpitis. *J. Endod.* 38 (8): 1035–1039.

Poorni, S., Veniashok, B., Senthilkumar, A.D. et al. (2011). Anesthetic efficacy of four percent articaine for pulpal anesthesia by using inferior alveolar nerve block and buccal infiltration techniques in patients with irreversible pulpitis: a prospective randomized double-blind clinical trial. *J. Endod.* 37 (12): 1603–1607.

Poppers, P.J. (1975). Evaluation of local anaesthetic agents for regional anaesthesia in obstetrics. *Br. J. Anaesth.* 47 (Suppl): 322–327.

Potocnik, I., Tomsic, M., Sketelj, J., and Bajrovic, F.F. (2006). Articaine is more effective than lidocaine or mepivacaine in rat sensory nerve conduction block in vitro. *J. Dent. Res.* 85 (2): 162–166.

Pricco, D.F. (1977). An evaluation of bupivacaine for regional nerve block in oral surgery. *J. Oral Surg.* 35 (2): 126–129.

Rahn, R. and Ball, B. (2001). Local anesthesia in dentistry. Articaine and epinephrine for dental anesthesia. In:. Seefeld (Germany): 3M ESPE AG. 6–13.

Reiz, S. and Nath, S. (1986). Cardiotoxicity of local anastetic agents. *Br. J. Anaesth.* 58 (7): 736–746.

Reynolds, F. (1971). Metabolism and excretion of bupivacaine in man: a comparison with mepivacaine. *Br. J. Anaesth.* 43 (1): 33–37.

Reynolds, F., Bryson, T.H.L., and Nicholas, A.D.G. (1976). Intradermal study of a new local anaesthetic agent: aptocaine. *Br. J. Anaesth.* 48 (4): 347–354.

Roberts, D.H. and Sowray, J.H. (1987). *Local Analgesia in Dentistry*, 3e. Bristol (UK): Wright. 34.

Robertson, D., Nusstein, J., Reader, A. et al. (2007). The anesthetic efficacy of articaine in buccal infiltration of mandibular posterior teeth. *J. Am. Dent. Assoc.* 138 (8): 1104–1112.

Rood, J.P. (1976). Inferior alveolar nerve block. The use of 5 per cent lignocaine. *Br. Dent. J.* 140 (12): 413–414.

Rood, J.P. and Sowray, J.H. (1980). Clinical experience with 5 per cent lignocaine solution. *J. Dent.* 8 (2): 128–131.

Sadove, M.S., Rosenberg, R., Heller, F.N. et al. (1964). Citanest®. A new local anesthetic agent. *Anesth. Analg.* 43 (5): 527–532.

Schilly, W. (1977). Vasoconstrictors in local anesthetics. *Quintessece Int.* 8 (12): 15–18.

Schorr, W.F. (1968). Paraben allergy. A case of intractable dermatitis. *JAMA* 204 (10): 859–866.

Schwartz, H.J. and Sher, T.H. (1985). Bisulfite sensitivity manifesting as allergy to local dental anesthesia. *J. Allergy Clin. Immunol.* 75 (4): 525–527.

Schwartz, H.J., Gilbert, I.A., Lenner, K.A. et al. (1989). Metabisulfite sensitivity and local dental anesthesia. *Ann. Allergy* 62 (2): 83–86.

Scott, D.B., Owen, J.A., and Richmond, J. (1964). Methaemoglobinaemia due to prilocaine. *Lancet* 2 (7362): 728–729.

Seifen, A.B., Ferrari, A.A., Seifen, E.E. et al. (1979). Pharmacokinetics of intravenous procaine infusion in humans. *Anesth. Analg.* 58 (5): 382–386.

Seng, G.F. and Gay, B.J. (1986). Dangers of sulfites in dental local anesthetic solutions: warning and recommendations. *J. Am. Dent. Assoc.* 113 (5): 769–770.

Sharaf, A.A.T. (1997). Evaluation of mandibular infiltration versus block anesthesia in pediatric dentistry. *J. Dent. Child.* 64 (4): 276–281.

Shnider, S.M. and Gildea, J. (1973). Paracervical block anesthesia in obstetrics. III. Choice of drug: fetal bradicardia following administration of lidocaine, mepivacaine, and prilocaine. *Am. J. Obstet. Gynecol.* 116 (3): 320–325.

Skjevik, A.A., Haug, B.E., Lygre, H., and Teigen, K. (2011). Intramolecular hydrogen bonding in articaine can be related to superior bone tissue penetration: a molecular dynamics study. *Biophys. Chem.* 154 (1): 18–25.

Smith, A.E. (1920). *Block Anesthesia and Allied Subjects. With Special Chapters on the Maxillary Sinus, the Tonsils, and Neuralgias of the Nervous Trigeminus for Oral Surgeons, Dentists, Laryngologists, Rhinologists, Otologists, and Students*. St Louis (Mo): CV Mosby Co. 266–267.

Spoerel, W.E., Adamson, D.H., and Eberhard, R.S. (1967). The significance of methaemoglobinaemia induced by prilocaine (Citanest). *Can. Anaesth. Soc. J.* 14 (1): 1–10.

Stenson, R.E., Constantino, R.T., and Harrison, D.C. (1971). Interrelationships of hepatic blood flow, cardiac output, and blood levels of lidocaine in man. *Circulation* 43 (2): 205–211.

Stepke, M.T.H., Schwenzer, N., and Eichhorn, W. (1994). Vasoconstrictors during pregnancy – in vitro trial on pregnant and non pregnant mouse uterus. *Int. J. Oral Maxillofac. Surg.* 23 (6 Pt2): 440–442.

Strasser, K., Huch, A., Huch, R., and Uihein, M. (1977). Plazenta-Passage von Carticain (Ultracain), einem neuen Lokalanästhetikum. *Z. Geburtshilfe Perinatol.* 181 (2): 118–120.

Strichartz, G.R. and Lambert, D.H. (1995). Neurotoxicity of 5% lignocaine. *Br. J. Anaesth.* 75 (3): 376.

Strichartz, G.R., Sanchez, V., Arthur, G.R. et al. (1990). Fundamental properties of local anesthetics. II. Measured octanol: buffer partition coefficients and pKa values of clinically used drugs. *Anesth. Analg.* 71 (2): 158–170.

Strichartz, G.R., Manning, T., and Datta, S. (1994). Irreversible conduction block in mammalian nerves by direct application of 2% and 5% lidocaine. *Reg. Anesth.* 19 (Suppl 2): 21. (Poster Discussion 2).

Strong, J.M., Parker, M., and Atkinson, A.J. Jr. (1973). Identification of glycinexylidide in patients treated with intravenous lidocaine. *Clin. Pharmacol. Ther.* 14 (1): 67–72.

Sung, C.-Y. and Truant, A.P. (1954). The physiological disposition of lidocaine and its comparison in some aspects with procaine. *J. Pharmacol. Exp. Ther.* 112 (4): 432–443.

Tainter, M.L., Throndson, A.H., and Moose, S.M. (1939). Alleged clinical importance of buffered local anesthetic solutions. *J. Am. Dent. Assoc.* 26: 920–927.

Thomson, P.D., Melmon, K.L., Richardson, J.A. et al. (1973). Lidocaine pharmacokinetics in advanced heart failure, liver disease, and renal failure in humans. *Ann. Intern. Med.* 78 (4): 499–508.

Tucker, G.T. (1986). Pharmacokinetics of local anesthetics. *Br. J. Anaesth.* 58 (7): 717–731.

USP 38 (2015). *Farmacopea de los Estados Unidos de América*, 38e. Rockville, MD: The United States Pharmacopeial Convention. 2488, 2694, 3584, 3586, 4474, 4490, 4658, 5011, 5414, 5427.

Van Oss, G.E.C.J.M., Vree, T.B., Baars, A.M. et al. (1989). Pharmacokinetics, metabolism, and renal excretion of articaine and its metabolite articainic acid in patients after epidural administration. *Eur. J. Anesthesiol.* 6 (1): 49–56.

Vogel, H.G. (2007). Nachruf für Dr. med. Roman Muschaweck. *BIOspektrum* 13 (5): 547. www.biospektrum.de/blatt/d_bs_pdf&_id=932179.

Vree, T.B., Baars, A.M., Van Oss, G.E.C.J.M., and Booij, L.H.D.J. (1988). High-perfomance liquid chromatography and preliminary pharmacokinetics of articaine and its 2-carboxy metabolite in human serum and urine. *J. Chromatogr.* 424 (2): 440–444.

Wahl, M.J., Overton, D., Howell, J. et al. (2001). Pain on injection of prilocaine plain vs lidocaine with epinephrine. A prospective double-blind study. *J. Am. Dent. Assoc.* 132 (10): 1396–1401.

Weaver, J.M. (1999). Articaine, a new local anesthetic for American dentists: will it supersede lidocaine (Editorial). *Anesth. Prog.* 49 (4): 111–112.

Widman, B. (1975). Plasma concentration of local anaesthetic agents in regard to absorption, distribution and elimination, with special reference to bupivacaine. *Br. J. Anaesth.* 47 (Suppl): 231–236.

Wielding, S. (1960). Studies on α-n-propylamino-2-methylpropionanilide – a new local anesthetic. *Acta Pharmacol. Toxicol.* 17 (3): 233–244.

Winther, J.E. and Nathalang, B. (1972). Effectivity of a new local analgesic Hoe 40 045. *Scand. J. Dent. Res.* 80 (4): 272–278.

Winther, J.E. and Patirupanusara, B. (1974). Evaluation of carticaine – a new local analgesic. *Int. J. Oral Surg.* 3 (6): 422–427.

Wright, G.Z., Weinberger, S.J., Friedman, C.S., and Plotzke, O.B. (1989). Use of articaine local anesthesia in children under 4 year age – a retrospective report. *Anesth. Prog.* 36 (6): 268–271.

Wright, G.Z., Weinberger, S.J., and Marti, R. (1991). The effectiveness of infiltration anesthesia in the mandibular primary molar region. *Pediatr. Dent.* 13 (3): 278–283.

Wulf, H., Winckler, K., Maier, C.H., and Heinzow, B. (1988). Pharmacokinetics and protein binding of bupivacaine in postoperative epidural analgesia. *Acta Anaesthesiol. Scand.* 32 (7): 530–534.

Yamazaki, S., Seino, H., Ozawa, S. et al. (2006). Elevation of a periosteal flap with irrigation of the bone for minor oral surgery reduces the duration of action of infiltration anesthesia. *Anesth. Prog.* 53 (1): 8–12.

Yapp, K.E., Hopcraft, M.S., and Parashos, P. (2012). Dentists' perceptions of a new local anesthetic drug – articaine. *Aust. Dent. J.* 57 (1): 18–22.

## Contraindications

# 8

# Contraindications for Local Anesthetic Techniques in Dentistry

In this chapter, we review cases and circumstances in which dental local anesthetic cannot be administered. These include the following:

- Lack of patient cooperation.
- Very poor health (ASA IV).
- Severe coagulopathies.
- Injection site infection.
- Severe restricted mouth opening (trismus, ankylosis of the temporomandibular joint).

In many situations where local anesthesia is contraindicated, we can turn to deep sedation or general anesthesia. In other cases, the patient's underlying condition must be treated first.

## Lack of Cooperation from the Patient

A lack of patient cooperation is a contraindication for dental local anesthetic, since it can entail very serious consequences for both the patient and the dentist, as follows:

- Pricks and injuries in the patient's mouth and face.
- Pricks on the dentist's hands.
- Breakage of the needle in the patient's mouth (Bacci et al. 2012).

### Predisposing Factors

Certain situations and types of patients are more likely to generate poor behavior, for example:

1) Preschool children under aged 5–6 years (pre-cooperators) (Wright et al. 1991; Sharaf 1997; Tyrer 1999; Lind-Strömberg 2001). Owing to their immaturity, they cannot understand the need to cooperate with the dentist (Pinkham and Schroeder 1975).
2) Patients with mental conditions, such as those with Down syndrome or cerebral palsy (Pinkham and Schroeder 1975; Tyrer 1999; Hulland and Sigal 2000), for the same reason as mentioned above, i.e., inability to cooperate, although this depends on the severity of the condition.
3) Patients with mental and psychiatric disorders (Berggren and Meynert 1984; Moore et al. 1993; Hulland and Sigal 2000), such as the following:
    - autism (Hulland and Sigal 2000; Lind-Strömberg 2001)
    - acute neurosis (Scott et al. 1984; Hägglin et al. 2001)
    - schizophrenia (Seeman and Molin 1976)
    - drug addiction and alcoholism (Pinkham and Schroeder 1975; Berggren and Meynert 1984)
    - psychotropic drug use (Berggren and Meynert 1984; Hulland and Sigal 2000)
    - phobias (Hägglin et al. 2001).
4) Patients with severe anxiety when receiving dental treatment. In these cases, we can highlight a series of characteristics:
    - Basic anxiety. Around 10% of people have high levels of anxiety with respect to dental treatment (Table 8.1), although they attend their appointments and try to cope with their anxiety to complete treatment (Molin and Seeman 1970; Kleinknecht and Bernstein 1978; Hall and Edmondson 1983; Scott et al. 1984). A further 5% have phobias or experience uncontrolled irrational and extreme fear (Table 8.1). Patients with phobias are not generally problematic with respect to dental work since their systematic avoidance behavior will result in many canceled or broken appointments. Often, these patients only attend the dentist's office when their neglected dental needs have mushroomed into a frank dental emergency such as an abscess, seeking acute dental treatment and possibly analgesics and antibiotics (Ayer et al. 1983; Sokol et al. 1985; Locker and Liddle 1991; Moore et al. 1993). To overcome their anxiety, these patients may benefit from psychological treatment or possibly sedation or general anesthesia (Moore et al. 1993).

*Local Anesthesia in Dentistry: A Locoregional Approach*, First Edition. Jesús Calatayud and Mana Saraghi.
© 2024 John Wiley & Sons Ltd. Published 2024 by John Wiley & Sons Ltd.
Companion website: www.wiley.com/go/Calatayud/local

Table 8.1 Patients who experience anxiety when undergoing dental treatment.

| Reference | Level of anxiety | | | |
|---|---|---|---|---|
| | Low | Medium | High | Phobia |
| Freidson and Feldman (1958) | — | — | — | 5% |
| SIFO (1962) | — | — | — | 9–14% |
| Gatchel et al. (1983) | 71% | 17% | 5% | 6% |
| Scott et al. (1984) | 44% | 25% | 21% | 10% |
| Rankin and Harris (1984) | 65% | 21% | 8% | 6% |
| Lindsay et al. (1987) | 63% | 22% | 10% | 5% |
| Milgrom et al. (1988) | 80% | 13% | 4% | 3% |
| Stouthard and Hoogstraten (1990) | 39% | 40% | 18% | 4% |
| Locker and Liddle (1991) | — | — | 8% | 4% |
| Hakeberg et al. (1992) | 59% | 25% | 11% | 5% |
| Moore et al. (1993) | 60% | 30% | 6% | 4% |
| Kaakko et al. (1998) | 39% | 41% | 17% | 4% |
| Ragnarsson (1998) | 72% | 19% | 10% | 0.3% |
| Hägglin et al. (2001) | — | — | 17% | — |
| Average | | | 11.2 | 5.7% |
| Rounded average | | | 10% | 5% |

Percentages rounded to whole units.

- Dental local anesthesia is the factor that causes the highest levels of anxiety in patients undergoing dental treatment (Lautch 1971; Gale 1972; Meldman 1972; Berggren and Meynert 1984; Scott et al. 1984; LeClaire et al. 1988). Seeing the syringe and needle, and feeling the prick of the needle are the most anxiety-inducing components of dental treatment.
- The behavior of anxious adults differs very little from that of those who are not anxious (McGimpsey 1977; Kleinknecht and Bernstein 1978; Ayer et al. 1983; Scott et al. 1984), therefore the health questionnaire should include a direct question on fear of dental treatment by category, for example five categories (no fear to very frightened) to identify patients with high degrees of anxiety (Kleinknecht and Bernstein 1978; Scott and Hirschman 1982; Ayer et al. 1983).
5) A history of behavioral problems and complications in previous situations, such as in dental treatment, vaccination, venipuncture for blood sampling, etc. Such behavior is thought to reoccur in around half of patients with such a history (Persson 1969; Hannington-Kiff 1969; McGimpsey 1977; Edmondson et al. 1978), therefore an appropriate question should be included on the health questionnaire.

## Evaluation of Risk

The best way of evaluating the risk of poor behavior is at the first visit, as follows:

- Review the patient's health questionnaire to obtain answers to the following questions:
  1) How anxious and fearful does dental treatment make you?
     Not at all ☐   A little ☐   Moderate ☐   Quite a lot ☐   A lot ☐
  2) Have you ever experienced an abnormal reaction, dizziness, or fainting at the dentist's office or with administration of local anesthetic, vaccinations, blood donations, etc.? Yes ☐   No ☐
  3) Are you being treated for any medical conditions? (Open answer)
  4) What medications are you taking, including prescription, over-the-counter, or herbal supplements? (Open answer)
  5) Do you use alcohol, tobacco, or any other substances? (Open answer)

The first two questions have already been commented on above, the last three provide us with information on the mental and psychiatric status of the patient, as well as about his/her medical problems and current medication to determine whether there are absolute or relative contraindications for administration of dental local anesthetic.

- The clinical examination at the first visit provides us with information on the risk of poor behavior, especially in the case of children since they are brought by their parents. Therefore, apart from age and physical appearance, there are two key moments for predicting disruptive behavior at future visits to the dentist:
  ○ During the oral examination.
  ○ During intraoral radiography.

Difficulty performing these two maneuvers points to a high risk for administration of local anesthesia at subsequent visits. In contrast, if the examination reveals that the patient has undergone major restoration work and complicated dental procedures and the parents report no special measures having been taken (sedation, medication, etc.), then the patient is likely to behave well since he/she has been able to undergo the above-mentioned treatments.

## Approach to Behavioral Problems

Patients with behavioral problems can be divided into two groups:

○ Patients who can receive local anesthetic but for whom this is very problematic (e.g., patients who experience

vasovagal syncope, etc.). In these cases, local anesthesia should be supplemented with methods to reduce anxiety, such as a good psychological strategy based on management of the personal relationship with the dentist (Gale et al. 1984; Maggirias and Locker 2002) and conscious sedation with short-acting benzodiazepines (triazolam) and/or nitrous oxide. However, such techniques are beyond the scope of this book.
- Patients who cannot receive local anesthetic. These patients require general anesthetic, and adults may require psychological or psychiatric care (Moore et al. 1993).

## ASA IV Physical Status

In 1963, the American Society of Anesthesiologists (ASA) developed a classification of physical status, which is now known as the ASA classification (Anonymous 1963; ASA 2019). This was initially designed to evaluate the threat to life of patients undergoing general anesthesia, although since it was introduced it has been extended to locoregional anesthesia and sedation, as is the case in dentistry (Malamed 2007, 2010). In this classification, we can observe the following:

- Some physicians consider patients with two or more conditions to have a higher ASA level than that of each of the conditions individually. For example, a patient with obesity and a stomach ulcer who is aged more than 65 years (all ASA II conditions) is classed as ASA III because of the fact that he/she has three conditions. ASA II means that the systemic illnesses are well-controlled. ASA III by definition means the conditions are not controlled. There is a degree of subjectivity among clinicians and some will consider a patient with multiple well-controlled comorbidities as ASA III, but the author adheres to the definition of ASA II as well-controlled systemic diseases.
- This classification of patients changes over time. For example, a patient who has had a myocardial infarction less than 3 months previously is classed as ASA IV, although if he/she has recovered after 3 months and subsequent progress is good, then he/she can be considered ASA III. If the condition continues to improve, the patient can be considered ASA II.

Below, we describe each of the ASA levels and provide examples, with emphasis on how local anesthesia is contraindicated in ASA IV cases.

### ASA I Patients

- Definition: healthy patients, no smoking, no or minimal alcohol use (ASA 2019).
- Consequences: good tolerance of physical stress (pain) and psychological stress (anxiety).
- Relevance in dentistry: can receive local anesthetics and standard dental treatment with no danger.

### ASA II Patients

- Definition: patients with well-controlled systemic disease that does not cause limitations.
- Consequences: minor limitations to tolerance of physical stress (pain) and psychological stress (anxiety).
- Relevance in dentistry: can receive local anesthetics and standard dental treatment.
- Examples include but not limited to:
  - Healthy patients with special circumstances, such as:
    - Pregnancy in a healthy woman (Malamed 2007, 2010; ASA 2019).
    - Healthy persons aged >65 years (Malamed 2007, 2010).
    - Obesity, body mass index (BMI) 30–40 (McCarthy 1982; Jastak et al. 1995; ASA 2019).
    - Patients who smoke tobacco (McCarthy and Malamed 1979; Abraham-Inpijn et al. 1988).
    - Social alcohol drinker (ASA 2019).
  - Cardiovascular disease:
    - Controlled arterial hypertension (90–95/140–160 mmHg) (Abraham-Inpijn et al. 1988; Malamed 2007; ASA 2019).
    - Congestive heart failure (caused by myocardial infarction, vascular disease, rheumatic disease, etc.) that is moderate and does not cause limitations. This is also said to be compensated congestive heart failure (Malamed 2007).
    - More than 6 months after a cerebrovascular accident that did not leave neurological sequelae.
    - Chronic orthostatic hypotension with vertigo or dizziness (Malamed 2007).
  - Endocrine-metabolic diseases:
    - Well-controlled diabetes (Malamed 2007, 2010; Wilson et al. 2008; ASA 2019).
    - Well-controlled hypo- or hyperthyroidism, i.e., normal function (euthyroid) (McCarthy 1982; Malamed 2007, 2010; Wilson et al. 2008).
    - Plasma pseudocholinesterase deficiency (Malamed 2003).
  - Respiratory disease:
    - Well-controlled asthma (Malamed 2007, 2010; Wilson et al. 2008).
    - Nonacute upper airway disease (common cold, influenza) (Malamed 2007).
    - Chronic sinusitis (McCarthy and Malamed 1979).

- Central nervous system (CNS) disease:
  - Well-controlled epilepsy with uncommon seizure episodes (less frequent than once every 3 months) (Malamed 2007; Wilson et al. 2008).
  - Psychiatric disorders such as controlled depression (Jastak et al. 1995).
  - Extreme fear of dental treatment (phobia) (McCarthy and Malamed 1979; Malamed 2007). These patients may require deep sedation or general anesthesia. Local anesthesia may be contraindicated.
- Other diseases:
  - Rheumatic diseases with chronic joint problems (arthritis, etc.) that do not require corticosteroids (Malamed 2007).
  - Stomach ulcer (McCarthy 1982; Malamed 2007).
  - Increased intraocular pressure (glaucoma) (McCarthy 1982; Malamed 2007).
  - Allergy to drugs, foods, or latex (McCarthy 1982; Malamed 2007).

## ASA III Patients

- Definition: patients with severe or uncontrolled systemic disease that limits activity but is not incapacitating (no symptoms at rest or with normal exercise).
- Consequences: reduced tolerance to physical stress (pain) and psychological stress (anxiety).
- Relevance for dentistry: patients can receive local anesthetic and standard dental treatment. However, it is important to take into account the following:
  - *If in doubt, the patient's doctor should be consulted.*
  - The patient may require additional measures such as sedation to reduce anxiety (oral, intravenous, intramuscular drugs, inhaled nitrous oxide, hypnosis), antibiotics, etc. Treatment of medically compromised patients is beyond the scope of this book. Excellent texts are available on this subject. Here, we only address the use of locoregional anesthetic in ASA III patients.
  - ASA III patients, especially those with cardiovascular disease, do not present further severe complications (arrhythmia, angina pectoris, myocardial infarction, etc.), although they do have increased minor complications such as tachycardia, dizziness, shaking, etc. *It is therefore recommended that appointments do not exceed 30 minutes*, where possible, since the number of complications can increase if the session is longer (Hughes et al. 1966; Daubländer et al. 1997).
  - Some authors suggest using vasoconstrictor-free anesthetic solutions. However, this is somewhat problematic because pain – a key factor in ASA III patients – is not well controlled. Anesthetic solutions with epinephrine should be used with caution (see Chapter 10).
- Examples include but are not limited to:
  - Patients with special circumstances, such as:
    - Morbid obesity (BMI > 40) (ASA 2019).
    - Alcohol dependence or abuse (ASA 2019).
    - Active hepatitis (ASA 2019).
  - Cardiovascular disease:
    - Uncontrolled arterial hypertension with moderate blood pressure values of around 95–115/160–200 mmHg (McCarthy 1982; Abraham-Inpijn et al. 1988; Malamed 2007, 2010).
    - Congestive heart failure (caused by myocardial infarction, vascular disease, rheumatic disease, etc.) with breathing difficulty (dyspnea) during exercise or with nervous tension, although not at rest. This is decompensated congestive heart failure (Malamed 2007).
    - Implanted pacemaker (ASA 2019).
    - More than 3 months after any of the following:
      - Cerebrovascular accident that has left neurological sequelae (McCarthy and Malamed 1979; Malamed 2007, 2010; Wilson et al. 2008).
      - Heart attack (angina pectoris or acute myocardial infarction) (McCarthy and Malamed 1979; Abraham-Inpijn et al. 1988; Malamed 2007, 2010; Wilson et al. 2008).
      - Coronary bypass surgery (Perusse et al. 1992a).
      - Stents in coronary artery disease (ASA 2019).
    - Heart transplant: surgical denervation resulting from removal of the nerve endings in the heart leaves the heart hypersensitive to the action of catecholamines (Carleton et al. 1969; Roca et al. 1993; Meechan et al. 2002).
    - Clotting disorders:
      - Platelet count >30 000–50 000 (Finucane et al. 2004; Scully and Cawson 2005).
      - Oral anticoagulants (warfarin, acenocoumarol) with international normalized ratio (INR) levels <3.5–4 (Table 8.3).
      - Hemophiliac patients with clotting factor >30–50% (we can assume that clotting factor has been added) (Evans and Aledort 1978; Segelman 1978; Katz and Terezhalmy 1988; Jastak et al. 1995).
  - Endocrine-metabolic diseases:
    - Poorly controlled diabetes (Malamed 2007, 2010; Wilson et al. 2008; ASA 2019).
    - Poorly controlled symptomatic hypo- or hyperthyroidism (Greenwood and Meechan 2003; Malamed 2007, 2010).

- Respiratory diseases:
  - Poorly controlled asthma (Malamed 2007: Wilson et al. 2008).
  - Poorly controlled chronic obstructive pulmonary disease (bronchitis, emphysema) with no breathing difficulty (dyspnea) in habitual daily activities (Malamed 2007; Wilson et al. 2008).
- CNS diseases:
  - Epilepsy controlled by drugs but with fewer than one seizure episode per month (Malamed 2007).
- Kidney diseases:
  - More than 3 months after a kidney transplant.
  - Chronic kidney failure requiring regular hemodialysis (Malamed 2007; ASA 2019).
- Other diseases:
  - Rheumatic disease with chronic joint problems (arthritis, etc.) requiring corticosteroids (Malamed 2007).
  - Cancer treated on an outpatient basis.
  - Myasthenia gravis (rare disease involving skeletal muscle weakness) that is stable and mild or moderate (Patil et al. 2012).
  - Malignant hyperthermia. Patients who have had this disease.
  - Patients who have received radiation on the maxillofacial area at risk of osteoradionecrosis.

## ASA IV Patients

- Definition: patients with severe systemic disease that is incapacitating and is constantly life-threatening. Patients present symptoms at rest, for example fatigue, dizziness, shortness of breath, or chest pain.
- Consequences: Poor tolerance of physical stress (pain) and psychological stress (anxiety).
- Relevance for dentistry:
  - *Local anesthesia and outpatient dental treatment are contraindicated in ASA IV patients. These patients are hospitalized.*
  - The only outpatient treatment is prescription of drugs such as analgesics, antibiotics, mouthwash, etc.
- Examples include but not limited to:
  - Cardiovascular disease:
    - Severe uncontrolled arterial hypertension, with(out) treatment, with pressures of >115/>200 mmHg, owing to the risk of heart attack or cerebrovascular accident (McCarthy 1982; Abraham-Inpijn et al. 1988; Malamed 2007).
    - Congestive heart failure (caused by myocardial infarction, vascular disease, rheumatic disease, etc.) that causes difficulty breathing (dyspnea) at rest (Perusse et al. 1992a; Malamed 2007; Wilson et al. 2008).
    - Unstable angina pectoris (Perusse et al. 1992a; Wilson et al. 2008).
    - Treatment-refractory arrhythmia (Perusse et al. 1992a).
    - Less than 3 months after:
      - A cerebrovascular accident (McCarthy and Malamed 1979; Malamed 2007; Wilson et al. 2008).
      - Heart attack (angina pectoris or acute myocardial infarction) (McCarthy and Malamed 1979; Perusse et al. 1992a; Malamed 2007; Wilson et al. 2008).
      - Coronary bypass surgery (Perusse et al. 1992a).
      - Stents in coronary artery disease (ASA 2019).
    - Clotting disorders:
      - Platelet count <30 000 (Finucane et al. 2004; Scully and Cawson 2005).
      - Oral anticoagulants (warfarin, acenocoumarol) with INR levels >3.5–4 (Table 8.3).
      - Hemophiliac patients with clotting factor lower than 5%, which is usual (Evans and Aledort 1978; Segelman 1978; Katz and Terezhalmy 1988; Jastak et al. 1995; Correa et al. 2006).
  - Endocrine-metabolic disease:
    - Poorly controlled or uncontrolled insulin-dependent diabetes (Perusse et al. 1992b; Malamed 2007; Wilson et al. 2008).
    - Poorly controlled hyperthyroidism, with frank signs and symptoms (thyroid storm) (Greenwood and Meechan 2003; Little 2006; Malamed 2007).
  - Respiratory disease:
    - Asthma with frequent attacks that is difficult to control and requires corticosteroids and admission to hospital (Perusse et al. 1992b; Steinbacher and Glick 2001; Malamed 2007).
    - Chronic obstructive pulmonary disease (bronchitis, emphysema) leading to difficulty breathing (dyspnea) at rest (Malamed 2007; Wilson et al. 2008).
    - Hereditary angioneurotic edema or angioedema (Barclay and Edwards 1971).
  - CNS disease:
    - Poorly controlled epilepsy with frequent seizures (more than one per week and/or a history of status epilepticus) (Malamed 2007; Wilson et al. 2008).
  - Kidney disease:
    - Within 3 months of a kidney transplant.
    - End state of renal disease not undergoing regularly scheduled dialysis (ASA 2019).
  - Other diseases:
    - Cancer with marked physical involvement, even if the disease is being treated on an outpatient basis.

- Myasthenia gravis (rare disease involving musculoskeletal weakness) that is severe and uncontrolled (Patil et al. 2012).

### ASA V Patients

- Definition: Dying patient who is unlikely to live more than 24 hours with or without surgery.
- Relevance for dentistry. This type of patient is outside the setting of dentistry, since he/she is hospitalized.

## Clotting Abnormalities

In cases of severe clotting abnormalities, truncal block with dental local anesthesia can damage vessels and cause unstoppable internal bleeding. This can occur if tissues are lax, leading to a dissecting hematoma that grows gradually in the parapharyngeal and submandibular space, with swelling of oral tissues, the face, and the neck as it advances toward the mediastinum. There may also be difficulty swallowing (dysphagia) and opening the mouth (trismus), appearance of bloody patches under the skin and oral mucosa (ecchymosis), and, finally, breathing difficulties resulting from compression of the airways by the hematoma (Archer and Zubrow 1954; Evans and Leake 1964; Evans and Aledort 1978; Mulligan and Weitzel 1988). Such a dramatic clinical picture is very unusual and was associated with mandibular block in hemophiliacs (Archer and Zubrow 1954: Evans and Leake 1964).

### High-risk Anesthetic Techniques

Not all dental local anesthetic techniques carry the same risk of dissecting hematoma in predisposed patients. High-risk techniques are characterized by specific factors. First, the needle is inserted deep into the tissue and the damaged vessel may be at some distance from the surface. Second, the tissues are very vascularized, with the result that it is easy to damage a vessel (Evans and Aledort 1978; Mulligan and Weitzel 1988). Third, as the surrounding tissue is lax and abundant, it cannot contain the hemorrhage owing to the absence of pressure (Evans and Aledort 1978; Mulligan and Weitzel 1988). *Truncal block techniques are the most problematic* (Jastak et al. 1995; Wilde 1998; Scully and Wolff 2002):

- Mandibular block (Sachs et al. 1978; Evans and Aledort 1978; Mulligan and Weitzel 1988; Johnson and Leary 1988; Brewer and Correa 2006; Zaliuniene et al. 2014).
- Maxillary block, both with the high-tuberosity or zygomatic approach and with the transpalatal approach or greater palatine canal approach (Evans and Aledort 1978; Johnson and Leary 1988).
- Lingual nerve block or even infiltration of terminal branches of the lingual nerve in the floor of the mouth (Brewer and Correa 2006; Zaliuniene et al. 2014).

Furthermore, while the risk of causing a hemorrhage is lower with these techniques than with extractions and oral surgery (Mulligan and Weitzel 1988; Dézsi et al. 2017), it is important to remember that bleeding in oral surgery is external and easier to contain with local measures (gelatin plugs, collagen, sutures, tranexamic acid, etc.). However, hemorrhages caused by truncal block are internal and deep and therefore not easily contained. In fact, there are almost no local methods other than compression, and even this is limited. Consequently, truncal block techniques carry a greater risk than initially thought.

### Systemic Causes of the Risk of Hemorrhage

Before commenting on the systemic causes of the risk of hemorrhage, we must make three observations:

1) *Patients generally arrive diagnosed and medicated*, as seen in the health questionnaire.
2) *In case of doubt, the patient's doctor or hematologist should be consulted* to determine the extent of the problem (Katz and Terezhalmy 1988; Brewer and Correa 2006; Zaliuniene et al. 2014).
3) Clotting analyses (INR) in patients taking vitamin K antagonists should be performed *on the same day as the dental procedure or no more than 48 hours later* in order to have reliable data on the situation at the time of the procedure (Rooney 1983; Blinder et al. 1999; Scully and Wolff 2002).

#### Antiplatelet Agents

Antiplatelet agents such as aspirin, clopidogrel, dipyridamole, ticlopidine, prasugrel, ticagrelor, etc. inhibit platelet aggregation (basic function during the initial phases of clotting). These drugs are prescribed to patients who have had a heart attack (ischemic heart disease) in the form of angina pectoris or myocardial infarction, or patients who have had a cerebrovascular accident (cerebral thrombosis) to ensure secondary prevention of thromboembolism.

If patients do not stop these medications, they may experience bleeding problems during oral surgery, although these are less serious than previously thought (Ardekian et al. 2000; Little et al. 2002; Becker 2008). However, they are not contraindicated for dental local anesthetics, not even for truncal block (Dézsi et al. 2017). A 2014 review advised not modifying antiplatelet medication during extractions or oral surgery since bleeding that is not controlled with local treatment is minimal (0.2%) and can be controlled in hospital without sequelae. Nevertheless, although the consequences of stopping treatment are very unusual (<1% of cases), they are very serious, with thromboembolic complications and myocardial infarction. Hence, we transmit the idea that the patient must "bleed or die" (Wahl 2014).

In conclusion, these patients can undergo truncal block or lingual infiltrations.

### Oral Vitamin K Antagonists: Anticoagulants

Oral vitamin K antagonists are coumarin derivatives such as warfarin and acenocoumarol. They inactivate vitamin K, thus reducing the action of clotting factors that depend on it, namely factors II, VII, IX, and X. They are prescribed to patients at risk of thromboembolism because of an underlying disease such as ischemic heart disease, a prosthetic heart valve, atrial fibrillation, deep vein thrombosis, etc. Consequently, they are not easily modified (Rooney 1983; Benoliel et al. 1986; Wahl 1998, 2000), and the current criterion is to maintain them during oral surgery and extractions (Wahl 1998, 2000).

The INR (International Normalized Ratio) is a clotting index based on prothrombin time (PT), which, as a coefficient between the PT of an anticoagulated patient and the PT of a control sample, represents a standardized value. This is subsequently corrected according to the International Sensitivity Index (ISI) and yields very stable and comparable values (ICSH/ICTH 1985; Steinberg and Moores 1995). The normal INR value is 1; the therapeutic value is 2–5 (Scully and Wolff 2002). Of note, the risk of bleeding increases with the INR because coagulability is reduced. As a guide, an INR of 3 may indicate that clotting time is three times longer than normal (while this is not exactly the case, it is approximate and easy to understand).

Clinical trials have shown that patients taking oral anticoagulants who underwent extractions or minor oral surgery did not experience serious bleeding problems because they were well controlled with local measures (Bailey and Fordyce 1983; Rooney 1983; Benoliel et al. 1986; Devani et al. 1998), even after mandibular block (Bailey and Fordyce 1983; Devani et al. 1998; Bajkin and Todorovic 2012). Table 8.2 shows mean INR values close to 3 and maximum values close to 4 recorded in clinical trials. Table 8.3 shows the maximum recommended INR levels at which we can perform extractions and oral surgery without stopping anticoagulant treatment. The absence of unanimity of criteria leads us to recommend a maximum INR value of 4 for truncal block.

Table 8.2 INR values in clinical trials involving patients who underwent oral surgery, with bleeding controlled using local measures.

| | INR | | |
|---|---|---|---|
| Reference | Number | Mean | Maximum |
| Ramström et al. (1993) | 45 | — | 4 |
| Borea et al. (1993) | 15 | 3.1 | — |
| Gaspar et al. (1997) | 32 | 2.5 | 3.5 |
| Devani et al. (1998) | 32 | 2.7 | 3.9 |
| Blinder et al. (1999) | 50 | 2.7 | 4 |
| Bajkin and Todorovic (2012) | 279 | 2.6 | 4 |
| Average | | 2.72 | 3.88 |
| Rounded average | | 3 | 4 |

Table 8.3 Maximum INR levels recommended by various authors for extractions and oral surgery.

| INR ≤ 3 | INR ≤ 3.5 | INR ≤ 4 |
|---|---|---|
| Weibert (1992) | Little et al. (2002) | Lippert and Gutschik (1994) |
| Greenwood (2008) | Scully and Wolff (2002) | Beirne and Koehler (1996) |
| | Rhodus and Little (2003) | Schardt-Sacco (2000) |
| | Dézsi et al. (2017) | Perry et al. (2007) |
| | | Becker (2008) |
| | | Renton et al. (2013) |
| | | Milla and Orlandi (2014) |

In conclusion, as a precautionary measure, *we do not recommend truncal block or lingual infiltrations in patients with INR values >4*.

### Direct Oral Anticoagulants

New oral anticoagulants, or direct oral anticoagulants, act by directly inhibiting activated factor II (thrombin) with dabigatran or activated factor X (Stuart-Power factor) with rivaroxaban, apixaban, and edoxaban. These new oral anticoagulants are more predictable and much easier to manage (González et al. 2016; Serrano-Sánchez et al. 2017; Hassona et al. 2018). To date, we do not have specific information on their involvement in locoregional anesthesia, although available data do seem to indicate that there are no contraindications to truncal block and lingual infiltration with current doses and regimens (Caliskan et al. 2017;

Serrano-Sánchez et al. 2017; Bensi et al. 2018; Hassona et al. 2018; Lababidi et al. 2018).

In conclusion, based on currently available data, which are in fact scarce, patients taking direct oral anticoagulants can undergo truncal block and lingual infiltrations.

**Low Platelet Counts**

Specific diseases such as idiopathic thrombocytopenic purpura, hypersplenism (excessive activity of the spleen), chronic liver disease, etc. can reduce the number of circulating platelets during the initial phase of clotting. Platelet counts are normally 150 000–400 000 platelets/mm$^3$, although counts above 50 000 platelets/mm$^3$, while low, involve no risk for extractions and oral surgery (Johnson and Leary 1988; Finucane et al. 2004; Renton et al. 2013; Bal et al. 2014). However, the limit for truncal block is established at counts lower than 30 000 platelets/mm$^3$ (Finucane et al. 2004; Scully and Cawson 2005).

In conclusion, *truncal block and lingual infiltration can be used in patients with platelet counts >30 000 platelets/mm$^3$*.

**Hemophilia**

Hemophilia is a congenital – generally inherited – clotting factor disorder caused by lack or poor functioning of clotting factors. The most frequent diseases are as follows:

o Factor VIII: hemophilia A or simply hemophilia.
o Factor IX: hemophilia B or Christmas disease.
o Factor XI: hemophilia C or Rosenthal syndrome.
o von Willebrand factor deficiency: pseudohemophilia or von Willebrand disease.
o Other, rarer deficiencies include those of factors II, V, VII, X, and XII. Even rarer deficiencies have been reported (Katz and Terezhalmy 1988).

It is interesting to remember that hemophilia C (Murphy et al. 1976; Sachs et al. 1978) and von Willebrand disease (Zakrzewska 1983; Wilde 1998) may occasionally go unnoticed and first manifest in the dentist's office after extractions or oral surgery.

These diseases cause the most severe clotting disorders and have led to the most dramatic cases of bleeding after mandibular block (Archer and Zubrow 1954; Evans and Leake 1964). Truncal block and extractions, and oral surgery can be performed when clotting factor levels are greater than 30–50% (Evans and Aledort 1978; Segelman 1978; Katz and Terezhalmy 1988) or greater than 50–75% (Renton et al. 2013), thus allowing us to assume that clotting factor has been added. It is important to remember that the normal level is 100% and that hemophiliacs have less than 5% (Mulkey 1976; Katz and Terezhalmy 1988; Correa et al. 2006). Furthermore, if clotting factor is added, the patient should not have autoantibodies against the clotting factor (Segelman 1978). Other authors directly advise against truncal block techniques (Mulkey 1976; Wilde 1998).

In conclusion, truncal block and lingual infiltration can only be used in hemophiliac patients when clotting factors have been added and levels are above 30–50%. It is important to remember that patients with hemophilia are considered ASA IV if their disease is not controlled.

**Alternatives and Recommendations**

- Alternatives to truncal block in cases of clotting disorders include the following:
  o Use of a supplementary technique such as the periodontal ligament technique (Mulkey 1976; Evans and Aledort 1978; Sachs et al. 1978; Pin 1987; Spuller 1988; Brewer and Correa 2006; Zaliuniene et al. 2014) or the intraosseous technique (Brewer and Correa 2006; Zaliuniene et al. 2014).
  o Periapical infiltration can be used instead of mandibular block in children with temporary molars (Dudkiewicz et al. 1987; Donohue et al. 1993). The same approach can be applied in permanent molars in adults, although treatment requires a potent solution, such as articaine 4% with epinephrine 1:100.000 (Annex 31; Brewer and Correa 2006; Zaliuniene et al. 2014).
  o Alternatively, we can use electronic dental anesthesia (EDA) (Savage 1982), although this has a less potent effect (see Chapter 20).
- The preferred approach in these patients is local anesthetic with a vasoconstrictor (mainly epinephrine), if there are no contraindications, because this helps to control bleeding (Mulkey 1976; Bisch et al. 1996; Devani et al. 1998; Scully and Wolff 2002; Zaliuniene et al. 2014) and increases the efficacy of anesthesia.

## Other Contraindications

### Injection Site Infection

Injections in areas of the mouth with acute infection are initially contraindicated for the following reasons:

1) The effect of the anesthetic is much less intense (Lewis 1919: Kramer and Mitton 1973):
   o Neurodegenerative changes in the axons of the inflamed area alter the thresholds of excitability and extend along the course of the nerve (Najjar 1977; Brown 1981; Wallace et al. 1985; Taylor and Byers 1990).

- Since tissue pH in the inflamed area can fall below 6 (Schade et al. 1921; De Jong and Cullen 1963) (normal pH is 7.4), there is little free base left for the anesthetic to penetrate the cell membranes (Bieter 1936; de Jong 1977).
- Vasodilation in the inflamed area favors rapid elimination of the anesthetic solution (Kramer and Mitton 1973; Meechan 1999).
- Other factors (see Chapter 19).

2) Injection can favor the diffusion and spread of the infection to neighboring tissue if the injection is into deep tissue and/or under pressure (Kramer and Mitton 1973). Furthermore, injection of epinephrine leads to hypoxia and reduced blood flow, thus reducing defenses in this area (Tran et al. 1985).

In these cases, an antibiotic is generally administered for a few days to control the acute phase. The dental procedure is then performed with anesthesia. In some cases, we can administer local infiltrative anesthetic gently in areas affected by abscesses to lance and drain them (Nordenram 1971). The contraindication is relative in these cases.

### Impossible Physical Access

It is sometimes impossible to reach the patient's mouth to administer local anesthetic, for example in patients with severe motor dysfunction caused by cerebral palsy (Hulland and Sigal 2000), advanced Parkinson disease, or with very severely restricted mouth opening (trismus) (Tyrer 1999). Intraoral local anesthetic techniques are absolutely contraindicated in these cases.

## Summary

- Lack of cooperation on the part of the patient → techniques involving dental local anesthesia are contraindicated.
- Patients in poor health classified as ASA IV → techniques involving dental local anesthesia are contraindicated.
- Severe clotting disorders:
    - Oral anticoagulants with INR >4 → truncal block and lingual infiltrations are contraindicated.
    - Platelet count <30 000 → truncal block and lingual infiltrations are contraindicated.
    - Hemophiliacs with clotting factor <30–50% → truncal block and lingual infiltrations contraindicated.
- Infection at the injection site → relative contraindication.
- Physically impossible access owing to severe motor dysfunction (advanced Parkinson disease, cerebral palsy, etc.) or very compromised ability to open the mouth (trismus) → intraoral dental local anesthesia is contraindicated.

## References

Abraham-inpijn, L., Borgmeijer-Hoelen, A., and Gortzak, R.A.T. (1988). Changes in blood pressure, heart rate, and electrocardiogram during dental treatment with use of local anesthetic. *J. Am. Dent. Assoc.* 116 (4): 531–536.

Anonymous (1963). New classification of physical status. *Anesthesiology* 24 (1): 111.

Annex 31. Mandibular pulpal anesthesia: infiltrative.

Archer, W.H. and Zubrow, H.J. (1954). Fatal hemorrhage following regional anesthesia for operative dentistry in a hemophiliac. *Oral Surg. Oral Med. Oral Pathol.* 7 (5): 464–470.

Ardekian, L., Gaspar, R., Peled, M. et al. (2000). Does low-dose aspirin therapy complicate oral surgical procedures? *J. Am. Dent. Assoc.* 131 (3): 331–335.

ASA House of Delegates (Executive Committee). ASA physical status classification system. Original approval October 15, 2014. Last amended October 23, 2019.

Ayer, A.A., Domoto, P.K., Gale, E.N. et al. (1983). Overcoming dental fear: strategies for its prevention and management. *J. Am. Dent. Assoc.* 107 (1): 18–27.

Bacci, C., Mariuzzi, M.L., Ghirotto, C., and Fustti, S. (2012). Local anesthesia needle breakage in a 5-year-old child during inferior alveolar nerve block with the Vazirani-Akinosi technique. *Minerva Stomatol.* 62 (7–8): 337–340.

Bailey, B.M.W. and Fordyce, A.M. (1983). Complications of dental extractions in patients receiving warfarin anticoagulant therapy. *Br. Dent. J.* 155 (9): 308–310.

Bajkin, B.V. and Todorovic, L.M. (2012). Safety of local anesthesia in dental patients taking oral anticoagulants: is it still controversial? *Br. J. Oral Maxillofac. Surg.* 50 (1): 65–68.

Bal, M.V., Koyuncuoglu, C.Z., and Saygun, I. (2014). Immune thrombocytopenic purpura presenting as unprovoked gingival hemorrhage: a case report. *Open Dent. J.* 8: 164–167.

Barclay, J.K. and Edwards, J.L. (1971). Angioneurotic edema. *Oral Surg. Oral Med. Oral Pathol.* 32 (4): 552–556.

Becker, D.E. (2008). Cardiovascular drugs: implications for dental practice. Part 2—Antihyperlipidemics and antithrombotics. *Anesth. Prog.* 55 (2): 49–56.

Beirne, O.R. and Koehler, J.R. (1996). Surgical management of patients on warfarin sodium. *J. Oral Maxillofac. Surg.* 54 (9): 1115–1118.

Benoliel, R., Leviner, E., Katz, J., and Tzukert, A. (1986). Dental treatment for the patient on anticoagulant therapy: prothrombin time value – what difference does it make? *Oral Surg. Oral Med. Oral Pathol.* 62 (2): 149–151.

Bensi, C., Belli, S., Paradiso, D., and Lomurno, G. (2018). Postoperative bleeding risk of direct anticoagulants after oral surgery procedures: a systematic review and meta-analysis. *Int. J. Oral Maxillofac. Surg.* 47 (7): 923–932.

Berggren, U. and Meynert, G. (1984). Dental fear and avoidance: causes, symptoms, and consequences. *J. Am. Dent. Assoc.* 109 (2): 247–251.

Bieter, R.N. (1936). Applied pharmacology of local anesthetics. *Am. J. Surg.* 34 (3): 500–510.

Bisch, F.C., Bowen, K.J., Hanson, B.S. et al. (1996). Dental considerations for a Glanzmann's thrombasthenia patient: case report. *J. Periodontol.* 67 (5): 536–540.

Blinder, D., Manor, Y., Martinowitz, V., and Taicher, S. (1999). Dental extractions in patients maintained on continued oral anticoagulant. Comparison of local hemostatic modalities. *Oral Surg. Oral Med. Oral Pathol.* 88 (2): 137–140.

Borea, G., Montebugnoli, L., Capuzzi, P., and Magelli, C. (1993). Tranexamic acid as a mouthwash in anticoagulant-treatment patients undergoing oral surgery. An alternative method to discontinuing anticoagulant therapy. *Oral Surg. Oral Med. Oral Pathol.* 75 (1): 29–31.

Brewer, A. and Correa, M.E. (2006). *Guidelines for Dental Treatment of Patients with Inherited Bleeding Disorders. Treatment of Hemophilia*, Monograph No 40. World Federation of Hemophilia (WFH). 4 (Open access).

Brown, R.D. (1981). The failure of local anaesthesia in acute inflammation. Some recent concepts. *Br. Dent. J.* 151 (2): 47–51.

Caliskan, M., Tückel, H.-C., Benlidayi, M.-E., and Deniz, A. (2017). Is it necessary to alter anticoagulant therapy for tooth extraction in patients taking direct oral anticoagulants? *Med. Oral Patol. Oral Cir. Bucal* 22 (6): e767–e773.

Carleton, R.A., Heller, S.J., Najafi, H., and Clark, J.G. (1969). Hemodynamic performance of a transplanted human heart. *Circulation* 40 (4): 447–452.

Correa, M.E.P., Annicchino-Bizzacchi, J.M., Jorge, J. Jr. et al. (2006). Clinical impact of oral health index in dental extraction of hemophilic patients. *J. Oral Maxillofac. Surg.* 64 (5): 785–788.

Daubländer, M., Müller, R., and Lipp, M.D.W. (1997). The incidence of complications associated with local anesthesia in dentistry. *Anesth. Prog.* 44 (4): 132–141.

De Jong, R.H. (1977). *Local Anesthetics*, 2e. Springfield (Illinois): Charles C Thomas Publisher. 43, 46.

De Jong, R.H. and Cullen, S.C. (1963). Buffer demand and pH of local anesthetic solutions containing epinephrine. *Anesthesiology* 24 (6): 801–807.

Devani, P., Lavery, K.M., and Howell, C.J.T. (1998). Dental extractions in patients on warfarin: is alteration of anticoagulant regime necessary? *Br. J. Oral Maxillofac. Surg.* 36 (2): 107–111.

Dézsi, C.A., Dézsi, B.B., and Dézsi, A.D. (2017). Management of dental patients receiving antiplatelet therapy or chronic oral anticoagulation: a review of the last evidence. *Eur. J. Gen. Pract.* 23 (1): 196–201.

Donohue, D., García-Godoy, F., King, D.L., and Barnwell, G.M. (1993). Evaluation of mandibular infiltration versus block anesthesia in pediatric patients. *J. Dent. Child* 60 (2): 104–106.

Dudkiewicz, A., Schwartz, S., and Laliberté, R. (1987). Effectiveness of mandibular infiltration in children using the local anesthetic Ultracaine® (articaine hydrochloride). *J. Can. Dent. Assoc.* 53 (1): 29–31.

Edmondson, H.D., Gordon, P.H., Lloyd, J.M. et al. (1978). Vasovagal episodes in the dental surgery. *J. Dent.* 6 (3): 189–195.

Evans, B.E. and Aledort, L.M. (1978). Hemophilia and dental treatment. *J. Am. Dent. Assoc.* 96 (5): 827–834.

Evans, R.E. and Leake, D. (1964). Bleeding in a hemophiliac after inferior alveolar nerve block. *J. Am. Dent. Assoc.* 6 (3): 352–355.

Finucane, D., Fleming, P., and Smith, O. (2004). Dentoalveolar trauma in patient with chronic idiopathic thrombocytopenic purpura: a case report. *Pediatr. Dent.* 26 (4): 352–354.

Freidson, E. and Feldman, J.J. (1958). The public looks at dental care. *J. Am. Dent. Assoc.* 57 (3): 325–335.

Gale, E.M. (1972). Fears of the dental situation. *J. Dent. Res.* 51 (4): 964–966.

Gale, E.N., Carlsson, S.G., and Jontell, M. (1984). Effects of dentists' behavior on patients' attitudes. *J. Am. Dent. Assoc.* 109 (3): 444–446.

Gaspar, R., Brenner, B., Ardekian, L. et al. (1997). Use of tranexamic acid mouthwash to prevent postoperative bleeding in oral surgical patients on oral anticoagulant medication. *Quintessene Int.* 28 (6): 375–379.

Gatchel, R.J., Ingersoll, B.D., Bowman, L. et al. (1983). The prevalence of dental fear and avoidance: a recent survey study. *J. Am. Dent. Assoc.* 107 (4): 609–610.

González, F., Álvarez, A., Torres, J., and Fernández-Tresguerres, I. (2016). New anticoagulants. Implications in odontology. *Cient. Dent. (Madrid)* 13 (Special Suppl): 4–15. Open access in www.cientificadental.es.

Greenwood, D.E. (2008). Medical emergencies in dental practice. *Periodontology 2000* (46): 27–41.

Greenwood, M. and Meechan, J.G. (2003). General medicine and surgery for dental practitioners. Part 6: The endocrine system. *Br. Dent. J.* 195 (3): 129–133.

Hägglin, C., Hakeberg, M., Hällström, T. et al. (2001). Dental anxiety in relation to mental health and personality factors. A longitudinal study of middle-aged and elderly women. *Eur. J. Oral Sci.* 109 (1): 27–33.

Hakeberg, M., Berggren, U., and Carlsson, S.G. (1992). Prevalence of dental anxiety in an adult population in major urban area in Sweden. *Commun. Dent. Oral Epidemiol.* 20 (2): 97–101.

Hall, N. and Edmondson, H.D. (1983). The etiology and psychology of dental fear. A five-year study of the use of intravenous diazepam in its management. *Br. Dent. J.* 154 (8): 247–252.

Hannington-Kiff, J.G. (1969). Fainting and collapse in dental practice. *Dent. Pract. Dent. Rec.* 20 (1): 2–7.

Hassona, Y., Malamos, D., Shaqman, M. et al. (2018). Management of dental patients taking direct oral anticoagulants: dabigatran. *Oral Dis.* 24 (1–2): 228–232.

Hughes, C.L., Leach, J.K., Allen, R.E., and Lambson, G.O. (1966). Cardiac arrhythmias during oral surgery with local anesthesia. *J. Am. Dent. Assoc.* 73 (5): 1095–1102.

Hulland, S. and Sigal, M.J. (2000). Hospital-based dental care for persons with disabilities: a study of patient sedation criteria. *Special Care Dent.* 20 (4): 131–138.

ICSH/ICTH (1985). ICSH/ICTH recommendations for reporting prothrombin time in oral anticoagulant control. *J. Clin. Pathol.* 38 (2): 133–134.

Jastak, J.T., Yagiela, J.A., and Donaldson, D. (1995). *Local Anesthesia of the Oral Cavity*. Philadelphia: WB Saunders Co. 128, 139.

Johnson, W.T. and Leary, J.M. (1988). Management of dental patients with bleeding disorders: review and update. *Oral Surg. Oral Med. Oral Pathol.* 66 (3): 297–303.

Kaakko, T., Milgrom, P., Coldwell, S.E. et al. (1998). Dental fear among university students: implications for pharmacological research. *Anesth. Prog.* 45 (2): 62–67.

Katz, J.O. and Terezhalmy, G.T. (1988). Dental management of the patient with hemophilia. *Oral Surg. Oral Med. Oral Pathol.* 66 (1): 139–144.

Kleinknecht, R.A. and Bernstein, D.A. (1978). The assessment of dental fear. *Behav. Ther.* 9 (4): 626–634.

Kramer, H.S. and Mitton, A.V. (1973). Complications of local anesthesia. *Dent. Clin. N. Am.* 17 (3): 443–460.

Lababidi, E., Breik, O., Savage, J. et al. (2018). Assessing an oral surgery specific protocol for patients on direct oral anticoagulants: a retrospective controlled cohort study. *Int. J. Oral Maxillofac. Surg.* 47 (7): 940–946.

Lautch, E. (1971). Dental phobia. *Br. J. Psychiatry* 119 (549): 151–158.

LeClaire, A.J., Skidmore, A.E., Griffin, J.A. Jr., and Balaban, F.S. (1988). Endodontic fear survey. *J. Endod.* 14 (11): 560–564.

Lewis, D.N. (1919). Pain following local anesthesia. *Dent. Cosmos* 61 (5): 407–408.

Lindsay, S.J.E., Humphris, G., and Barnby, G.J. (1987). Expectations and preferences for routine dentistry in anxious adult patients. *Br. Dent. J.* 163 (4): 120–124.

Lind-Strömberg, U. (2001). Rectal administration of midazolam for conscious sedation of uncooperative children in need of dental treatment. *Swed. Dent. J.* 25 (3): 105–111.

Lippert, S. and Gutschik, E. (1994). Views of cardiac-valve prosthesis patients and their dentists on anticoagulation therapy. *Scand. J. Dent. Res.* 102: 168.

Little, J.W. (2006). Thyroid disorders. Part I: Hyperthyroidism. *Oral Surg. Oral Med. Oral Pathol.* 101 (3): 276–284.

Little, J.W., Miller, C.S., Henry, R.G., and McIntosh, B.A. (2002). Antithrombotic agents: implications in dentistry. *Oral Surg. Oral Med. Oral Pathol.* 95 (5): 544–551.

Locker, D. and Liddle, A.M. (1991). Correlates of dental anxiety among older adults. *J. Dent. Res.* 70 (3): 198–203.

Maggirias, J. and Locker, D. (2002). Psychological factors and perception of pain associated with dental treatment. *Commun. Dent. Oral Epidemiol.* 30 (2): 151–159.

Malamed, S.F. (2003). *Sedation. A Guide to Patient Management*, 4e. St. Louis (Mi): Mosby. 575.

Malamed, S.F. (2007). *Medical Emergencies in the Dental Office*, 6e. St. Louis (Mi): Mosby-Elsevier. 23–28, 43, 50–52, 275, 292, 307, 332.

Malamed, S.F. (2010). Knowing your patient. *J. Am. Dent. Assoc.* 141 (Suppl 1): 3S–7S.

McCarthy, F.M. (1982). *Medical Emergencies in Dentistry. An Abridged Edition of Emergencies in Dental Practice*, 3e. Philadelphia: WB Saunders Co. 25, 49, 52, 54, 57.

McCarthy, F.M. and Malamed, S.F. (1979). Physical evaluation system to determine medical risk and indicated dental therapy modifications. *J. Am. Dent. Assoc.* 99 (2): 181–184.

McGimpsey, J.C. (1977). Fainting in the dental surgery. *Br. Dent. J.* 143 (2): 53–57.

Meechan, J.G. (1999). How to overcome failed local anesthesia. *Br. Dent. J.* 186 (1): 15–20.

Meechan, J.G., Parry, G., Rattray, D.T., and Thomason, J.M. (2002). Effects of dental local anesthetics in cardiac transplant recipients. *Br. Dent. J.* 192 (3): 161–163.

Meldman, M.J. (1972). The dental-phobia test. *Psychosomatic* 13 (6): 371–372.

Milgrom, P., Fiset, L., Melvick, S., and Weinstein, P. (1988). The prevalence and practice management consequences of dental fear in a major US city. *J. Am. Dent. Assoc.* 116 (6): 641–647.

Milla, J. and Orlandi, F.A. (2014). Manejo de los pacientes anticoagulados y/o antiagregados en odontología. Una revisión de la literatura. *RCOE (Madrid)* 19 (1): 29–33.

Molin, C. and Seeman, K. (1970). Disproportionate dental anxiety. Clinical and nosological considerations. *Acta Odontol. Scand.* 28 (2): 197–212.

Moore, R., Birn, H., Kirkegaard, E. et al. (1993). Prevalence and characteristics of dental anxiety in Danish adults. *Commun. Dent. Oral Epidemiol.* 21 (5): 292–296.

Mulkey, T.F. (1976). Outpatient treatment of hemophiliacs for dental extractions. *J. Oral Surg.* 34 (5): 428–434.

Mulligan, R. and Weitzel, K.G. (1988). Pretreatment management of the patient receiving anticoagulant drugs. *J. Am. Dent. Assoc.* 117 (3): 479–483.

Murphy, J.B., Robinson, K., and Segelman, A. (1976). PTA deficiency (factor XI deficiency). *Oral Surg. Oral Med. Oral Pathol.* 42 (1): 26–30.

Najjar, T.A. (1977). Why can't you achieve adequate regional anesthesia in the presence of infection? *Oral Surg. Oral Med. Oral Pathol.* 44 (1): 7–13.

Nordenram, A. (1971). *Manuel d'anesthesie locale enpractiquedentaire*. Möndal (Sweden): Lindgren and Söner. 37.

Patil, P.M., Singh, G., and Patil, S.P. (2012). Dentistry and the myasthenia gravis patient: a review of the current state of the art. *Oral Surg. Oral Med. Oral Pathol.* 114 (1): e1–e8.

Perry, D.J., Noakes, T.J.C., and Helliwell, P.S. (2007). Guidelines for the management of patients on oral anticoagulants requiring dental surgery. *Br. Dent. J.* 203 (7): 389–393.

Persson, G. (1969). General side effects of local anesthesia with special reference to catecholamines as vasoconstrictors and the effect of some premedications. *Acta Odontol. Scand.* 27 (Suppl 53): 1–141.

Perusse, R., Goulet, J.-P., and Turcotte, J.-Y. (1992a). Contraindications to vasoconstrictors in dentistry: Part I. Cardiovascular diseases. *Oral Surg. Oral Med. Oral Pathol.* 74 (5): 679–686.

Perusse, R., Goulet, J.-P., and Turcotte, J.-Y. (1992b). Contraindications to vasoconstrictors in dentistry: Part II. Hyperthyroidism, diabetes, sulfite sensitivity, cortico-dependent asthma, and pheochromocytoma. *Oral Surg. Oral Med. Oral Pathol.* 74 (5): 687–691.

Pin, P.J.A. (1987). The use of intraligamental injections in haemophiliacs. *Br. Dent. J.* 162 (4): 151–152.

Pinkham, J.R. and Schroeder, C.S. (1975). Dentist and psychologist: practical consideration for team approach to the intensely anxious patient. *J. Am. Dent. Assoc.* 90 (5): 1022–1026.

Ragnarsson, E. (1998). Dental fear and anxiety in an adult Icelandic population. *Acta Odontol. Scand.* 56 (2): 100–104.

Ramström, G., Sindet-Pedersen, S., Hall, G. et al. (1993). Prevention of postsurgical bleeding in oral surgery using tranexamic acid without dose modification of oral anticoagulants. *J. Oral Maxillofac. Surg.* 51 (11): 1211–1216.

Rankin, J.A. and Harris, M.B. (1984). Dental anxiety: the patient's point of view. *J. Am. Dent. Assoc.* 109 (1): 43–47.

Renton, T., Woolcombe, S., Taylor, T., and Hill, C.M. (2013). Oral surgery: Part I. Introduction and management of the medically compromised patient. *Br. Dent. J.* 215 (5): 213–223.

Rhodus, N.L. and Little, J.W. (2003). Dental management of the patient with cardiac arrhythmias: an update. *Oral Surg. Oral Med. Oral Pathol.* 96 (6): 659–668.

Roca, J., Caturla, M.C., Hjemdahl, P. et al. (1993). Effects of adrenaline on ventricular function and coronary haemodynamics in relation to catecholamine handling in transplanted human hearts. *Eur. Heart J.* 14 (4): 474–483.

Rooney, T.P. (1983). General dentistry during continuous anticoagulant therapy. *Oral Surg. Oral Med. Oral Pathol.* 56 (3): 252–255.

Sachs, S.A., Lipton, R., and Frank, R. (1978). Management of ambulatory oral surgical patients with hemophilia. *J. Oral Surg.* 36 (1): 25–29.

Savage, M. (1982). Clinical use of dental electro-analgesia. *Br. Dent. J.* 152 (7): 242–244.

Schade, H., Neukrich, P., and Halpert, A. (1921). Über locale Acidosen des Gewebes und die Methodik ihrer intravitalen Messung, zugleich ein Beitrag zur Lehre der Entzündung. *Z. Gesamte Exp. Med. (Berlin)* 24 (1-4): 11–56.

Schardt-Sacco, D. (2000). Update on coagulopathies. *Oral Surg. Oral Med. Oral Pathol.* 90 (5): 559–563.

Scott, D.S. and Hirschman, R. (1982). Psychological aspects of dental anxiety in adults. *J. Am. Dent. Assoc.* 104 (1): 27–31.

Scott, D.S., Hirschman, R., and Schroeder, K. (1984). Historical antecedents of dental anxiety. *J. Am. Dent. Assoc.* 108 (1): 42–45.

Scully, C. and Cawson, R.A. (2005). *Medical Problems in Dentistry*, 5e. Edinburgh: Elsevier Churchill Livingstone. 141.

Scully, C. and Wolff, A. (2002). Oral surgery in patients on anticoagulant therapy. *Oral Surg. Oral Med. Oral Pathol.* 94 (1): 57–64.

Seeman, K. and Molin, C. (1976). Psychopathology, feelings of confinement and helplessness in the dental chair, and relationship to the dentist in patients with disproportionate dental anxiety (DDA). *Acta Psychiatr. Scand.* 54 (2): 81–91.

Segelman, A.E. (1978). Protocol for the management of the hemophiliac having oral surgery (letter). *J. Oral Surg.* 36 (6): 423.

Serrano-Sánchez, V., Ripolles-de Ramón, J., Collado-Yurrita, L. et al. (2017). New horizons in anticoagulants and their implications in oral surgery. *Med. Oral Patol. Oral Cir. Bucal* 22 (5): e601–e608.

Sharaf, A.A.T. (1997). Evaluation of mandibular infiltration versus block anesthesia in pediatric dentistry. *J. Dent. Child* 64 (4): 276–281.

SIFO (1962). Cited by: Seeman K, Molin C. Psychopathology, feelings of confinement and helplessness in the dental chair, and relationship to the dentist in patients with disproportionate dental anxiety (DDA). *Acta Psychiatr. Scand. 1976* 54 (2): 81–91.

Sokol, D.J., Sokol, S., and Sokol, C.K. (1985). A review of nonintrusive therapies used to deal with anxiety and pain in the dental office. *J. Am. Dent. Assoc.* 110 (2): 217–222.

Spuller, R.L. (1988). Use of periodontal ligament injection in dental care of the patient with hemophilia: a clinical evaluation. *Special Care Dent.* 8 (1): 78–79.

Steinbacher, D.M. and Glick, M. (2001). The patient with asthma. An update and oral health considerations. *J. Am. Dent. Assoc.* 132 (9): 1229–1239.

Steinberg, M.J. and Moores, J.F. (1995). Use of INR to assess degree of anticoagulation in patients who have dental procedures. *Oral Surg. Oral Med. Oral Pathol.* 80 (2): 175–177.

Stouthard, M.E.A. and Hoogstraten, J. (1990). Prevalence of dental anxiety in the Netherlands. *Community Dent. Oral Epidemiol.* 18 (3): 139–142.

Taylor, P.E. and Byers, M.R. (1990). An immunocytochemical study of the morphological reaction of nerves containing calcitonin gene-related peptide to microabscess formation and healing in rat molars. *Arch. Oral Biol.* 35 (8): 629–638.

Tran, D.T., Miller, S.H., Buck, D. et al. (1985). Potentiation of infection by epinephrine. *Plast. Reconstr. Surg.* 76 (6): 933–934.

Tyrer, G.L. (1999). Referrals for dental general anaesthetics – how many really need GA? *Br. Dent. J.* 187 (8): 440–443.

Wahl, M.J. (1998). Dental surgery in anticoagulated patients. *Arch. Intern. Med.* 158 (15): 1610–1616.

Wahl, M.J. (2000). Myths of dental surgery in patients receiving anticoagulant therapy. *J. Am. Dent. Assoc.* 131 (1): 77–81.

Wahl, M.J. (2014). Dental surgery and antiplatelet agents: bleed or die. *Am. J. Med.* 127 (4): 260–267.

Wallace, J.A., Michanowicz, A.Z., Mundell, R.D., and Wilson, E.G. (1985). A pilot study of the clinical problem of regionally anesthetizing the pulp of an acutely inflamed mandibular molar. *Oral Surg. Oral Med. Oral Pathol.* 59 (5): 517–521.

Weibert, R.T. (1992). Oral anticoagulant therapy in patients undergoing dental surgery. *Clin. Pharm.* 11: 857.

Wilde, J.T. (1998). Von Willebrand disease and its management in oral and maxillofacial surgery. *Br. J. Oral Maxillofac. Surg.* 36 (2): 112–118.

Wilson, K.E., Dorman, M.L., Moore, P.A., and Girdler, N.M. (2008). Pain control and anxiety management for periodontal therapies. *Periodontology 2000* (46): 42–55.

Wright, G.Z., Weinberg, S.J., Martin, R., and Plotzke, O. (1991). The effectiveness of infiltration anesthesia in the mandibular primary molar region. *Pediatr. Dent.* 13 (5): 278–283.

Zakrzewska, J. (1983). Gingival bleeding as a manifestation of von Willebrand disease. *Br. Dent. J.* 155 (5): 157–160.

Zaliuniene, R., Peciuliene, V., Brukiene, V., and Aleksejuniene, J. (2014). Hemophilia and oral health. *Stomatologija* 16 (4): 127–131.

# 9

## Contraindications for Local Anesthetics

Not all anesthetic drugs have the same characteristics, therefore in this chapter we address those cases and circumstances where a specific anesthetic cannot be administered or where there may theoretically be an interaction. The chapter is divided into two parts: relevant contraindications, which may be absolute or relevant, and minor contraindications, most of which are not really contraindications but, on rare occasions, could become relative contraindications that require the dose of local anesthetic to be reduced.

## Relevant Contraindications

### Allergy to Local Anesthetics

Allergy is an adverse drug reaction triggered by immune mechanisms. Its duration is unlimited because of immunological memory (Seskin 1978), therefore *allergy is an absolute contraindication for this type of drug* and an alternative local anesthetic must be used.

Ester anesthetics undergo hydrolysis in the circulatory system and form metabolites such as para-aminobenzoic acid, which has considerable sensitizing power (Giovannitti and Bennett 1979). Consequently, allergic sensitization in this group is common, as is cross-sensitization (Adler and Simon 1949; Aldrete and Johnson 1970; Giovannitti and Bennett 1979; Schatz 1984; Adriani et al. 1986). The only drugs from this group used at present are tetracaine and benzocaine (very rarely procaine and cocaine), and these are used mainly as topical anesthetics.

Allergy to modern amide local anesthetics is very rare. At least 1% of adverse reactions attributed to local anesthetics are allergic (Verril 1975; Giovannitti and Bennett 1979) and rarely cross-reactions. However, cases of allergy to each of these drugs have been reported (Chapter 23).

There are no cases of cross-sensitization between amide and ester anesthetics since these have very different chemical structures, therefore in the case of multiple allergy to one group, we can use anesthetics from the other group (Incaudo et al. 1978; Schatz 1984).

### Long-acting Anesthetics

Long-acting anesthetics such as bupivacaine, which is available in 1.8-ml cartridges for dental use, are contraindicated in the following cases:

1) Routine short- or medium-duration procedures (Laskin et al. 1977; Jensen et al. 1981).
2) Children aged under 12 years, owing to the high risk of self-injury of soft tissues (Laskin et al. 1977; Jensen et al. 1981; Moore 1984).
3) Patients with developmental disabilities and special needs (Pricco 1977; Jensen et al. 1981) or patients with psychiatric diseases (Jensen et al. 1981), for the same reason as children aged under 12 years.

The main reason for these contraindications is to prevent discomfort on drinking, eating, and speaking, as well as the risk of self-injury of the soft tissues (tongue, lips, and buccal mucosa) owing to the long duration of anesthesia in these tissues. Furthermore, the absence of pulpal anesthesia in infiltrations is a major disadvantage in routine procedures (Chapter 7).

### Prilocaine, Benzocaine, and Methemoglobinemia

Hemoglobin is an iron transport protein in the red cells that transports oxygen to tissues. Through their metabolites, prilocaine and benzocaine can alter this protein to form methemoglobin (MHb), which does not fulfill its function of transporting oxygen. A review of 242 cases of local anesthetic-induced toxic MHb collected between 1947 and 2007 revealed that 65% were caused by benzocaine and 30% by prilocaine; both anesthetics were clearly the most frequently involved (Guay 2009).

*Local Anesthesia in Dentistry: A Locoregional Approach*, First Edition. Jesús Calatayud and Mana Saraghi.
© 2024 John Wiley & Sons Ltd. Published 2024 by John Wiley & Sons Ltd.
Companion website: www.wiley.com/go/Calatayud/local

Patients with diseases or disorders that hamper transport of oxygen to tissues are more vulnerable to the toxic methemoglobinemia caused by these local anesthetics. These diseases include the following:

1) Cardiovascular diseases:
   - Heart diseases (heart failure, coronary artery insufficiency, arrhythmia, etc.) because they reduce oxygen transport (Olson and McEvoy 1981; Duncan and Kobrinsky 1983; Rodriguez et al. 1994) and reduce the flow of blood to the liver, where the anesthetics are metabolized (Spoerel et al. 1967; Wilburn-Goo and Lloyd 1999).
   - Anemia and red cell disorders (Spoerel et al. 1967; Olson and McEvoy 1981; Duncan and Kobrinsky 1983; Rodriguez et al. 1994; Wilburn-Goo and Lloyd 1999).
   - Insufficient cerebral or peripheral irrigation (Spoerel et al. 1967).
2) Severe respiratory diseases, since oxygen exchange is reduced (Anonymous 1994; Wilburn-Goo and Lloyd 1999).
3) Extreme age groups:
   - Newborns and nursing infants have an immature enzyme system, therefore they have a larger proportion than normal of methemoglobinemia (Künzer von and Schneider 1953; Ross and Desforges 1959; Lo and Agar 1986). This situation continues, with some degree of risk, until the infant is 1 year old (Severinghaus et al. 1991; Kellet and Copeland 1983; Rodriguez et al. 1994).
   - Elderly people, given that they have diseases that reduce the oxygen supply to tissues (see points 1 and 2) and take drugs that can produce toxic methemoglobinemia (Wilburn-Goo and Lloyd 1999).
4) Congenital methemoglobinemia. A few hundred patients throughout the world have these diseases, which are diagnosed during the first year of life (Curry 1982):
   - Hemoglobin M.
   - Nicotinamide-adenine-dinucleotide-methemoglobin-reductase (NADH-MHb-reductase) system deficiency.
   - Nicotinamide-adenine-dinucleotide-phosphate-methemoglobin-reductase (NADPH-MHb-reductase) system deficiency.
   - Glucose-6-phosphatedehydrogenase deficiency.

Cases of congenital methemoglobinemia are considered *absolute contraindications* (Jastak et al. 1995; Coleman and Coleman 1996; Wilburn-Goo and Lloyd 1999). The first three causes are considered *relative contraindications*, therefore they can be administered with local anesthetics, albeit at reduced maximum doses, but the first three causes are considered *absolute contraindications* in ASA III patients. Other anesthetics, such as lidocaine and tetracaine, have been involved, although the association is much weaker. Chapter 23 contains a review of methemoglobinemia caused by dental local anesthetic.

## Cholinesterase Deficiency and Esther Anesthetics

Procaine and tetracaine are ester local anesthetics that are metabolized by the enzyme cholinesterase or pseudocholinesterase in blood (Kalow 1952). It is known that one in every 3000 people have a deficiency or abnormality of this enzyme (Kalow and Gunn 1959) and that the deficiency is hereditary (Kalow and Staron 1957; Foldes et al. 1963). Consequently, affected patients are at risk of intolerance and toxicity (Foldes et al. 1963).

At present, this problem is of little relevance, since procaine is rarely used as an injectable anesthetic (it has been replaced by more modern amide agents). In any case, the contraindication is absolute.

## Myasthenia Gravis and Esters

Myasthenia gravis is a rare autoimmune disease characterized by skeletal muscle weakness resulting from antibodies attacking acetylcholine receptors in the postsynaptic (motor) membrane. *In patients with myasthenia gravis, injected ester anesthetics (procaine and tetracaine) must be avoided* because they are hydrolyzed by plasma cholinesterases and the patients are treated with anticholinesterases (pyridostigmine, neostigmine), which inhibit the enzymes that metabolize these anesthetics, therefore there is a risk of poisoning by ester anesthetics (Patton and Howard 1997; Yarom et al. 2005; Patil et al. 2012). This is not the case, however, with benzocaine (also an ester anesthetic, although topical) (Yarom et al. 2005).

## Minor Contraindications

### Procaine and Sulfonamides

Procaine, or novocaine, is an ester anesthetic, like tetracaine. It inhibits the bacteriostatic effect of sulfonamides, which compete with para-aminobenzoic acid. This acid results from the metabolization of ester anesthetics (Woods 1940), which are a substrate of the acid for folic acid synthesis (De Jong 1977).

In conclusion, procaine and sulfonamides are not widely used today; in addition, this interaction between the doses and regimens used in dental local anesthetics is considered of minor relevance (Moore 1999).

### Lidocaine and Cimetidine

Cimetidine is a histamine $H_2$ receptor antagonist that inhibits secretion of hydrochloric acid in the stomach. It is therefore used in the treatment of stomach ulcers and in conditions requiring control of stomach acid secretion.

Clinical studies have shown that cimetidine diminishes the metabolism of lidocaine by 20–25% (Feely et al. 1982; Wing et al. 1984), thus increasing its plasma levels by 40–50% (Kishikava et al. 1990; Feely et al. 1982). This is because it reduces blood flow to the liver, which means that a smaller amount of lidocaine is metabolized (Feely et al. 1982) and the drug directly inhibits the oxidative mechanism for the biotransformation of lidocaine in the liver (Feely et al. 1982; Wing et al. 1984).

It is noteworthy that other $H_2$ receptor antagonists such as ranitidine (Feely and Guy 1983; Robson et al. 1985) and famotidine (Kishikava et al. 1990) are not subject to this interaction.

In conclusion, this interaction is considered to be of minor relevance in the doses and regimens used in the dental anesthetic lidocaine (Tucker 1986; Moore 1999).

### Lidocaine and Propranolol

Propranolol is a nonselective betablocker (it blocks adrenergic $\beta_1$ and $\beta_2$ receptors) that is used to treat patients with arterial hypertension, arrhythmia, angina pectoris, hyperthyroidism, etc. (Weiner 1988).

Clinical studies have shown how propranolol can reduce the metabolism of lidocaine by 20–40% (Svendsen et al. 1982; Bax et al. 1985) and thus increase its plasma levels by 20–30% (Ochs et al. 1980; Svendsen et al. 1982). This is because propranolol reduces blood flow in the liver by 20–30% (Price et al. 1967; Trap-Jensen et al. 1976; Westaby et al. 1984) – with the result that lower quantities of lidocaine are metabolized – and because of the direct action when enzyme activity against lidocaine is reduced in the liver (Bax et al. 1983, 1985).

Of note, other nonselective betablockers such as pindolol (Svendsen et al. 1982) do not present this interaction.

In conclusion, this interaction is considered to be of minor relevance in the doses and regimens used with lidocaine in dentistry (Tucker 1986; Moore 1999). However, it may prove important in medical practice during infusions for the treatment of arrhythmia (Moore 1999).

### Lidocaine and Succinylcholine

Succinylcholine is a potent muscle relaxant with rapid and short action (minutes). It is used for induction of general anesthesia to relax the muscles and thus facilitate intubation.

Clinical studies have shown that intravenous high-dose lidocaine prolongs the muscle block induced by succinylcholine (Usubiaga et al. 1967; Winkinski et al. 1970; Telivuo and Katz 1970). This effect has also been found, albeit less intensely, with other local anesthetics (mepivacaine, prilocaine, bupivacaine, etidocaine, procaine, and cocaine) (Telivuo and Katz 1970; Matsuo et al. 1978).

In conclusion, this interaction is considered to be of minor relevance in the doses and regimens used with lidocaine in dentistry.

### Bupivacaine and Cardiotoxicity

All local anesthetics are toxic for the central nervous system (CNS) and for the heart. However, bupivacaine is particularly toxic for the heart and can cause severe arrhythmia with tachycardia and ventricular fibrillation (Albright 1979; Reiz and Nath 1986; Maxwell et al. 1994; Mather and Chang 2001). Thus, when these conditions develop, resuscitation is more problematic and it may take 45 minutes to restore a normal heart rate (Albright 1979). Mortality has reached 40% (Reiz and Nath 1986). The toxic effect is caused directly through action on the myocardium (Moller and Covino 1988; Graf et al. 2002; Bozkurt et al. 2003) and indirectly via the CNS (Heavner 1986; Thomas et al. 1986).

Toxicity is disproportionately more pronounced with intravenous injection than with other routes of administration, for example intraoral administration (Albright 1979), owing to the high lipid solubility of this drug and marked binding to plasma proteins. In other words, after intraoral injection, the drug gradually enters the bloodstream and its free fraction (the truly toxic component) is low, although after intravenous injection a large amount enters the general circulation. The free fraction increases since increased concentrations of an anesthetic in blood are associated with lower levels of the fraction bound to plasma proteins (Shnider and Way 1968; Tucker et al. 1970; Mather et al. 1971).

The patients most predisposed to this type of adverse effect are as follows: (i) adults who receive high doses, above 50–360 mg (Reiz and Nath 1986) or above 90 mg (Moore et al. 1977; Albright 1979), which are generally associated with intravascular injections (Moore et al. 1977), and (ii) small children (aged under 12 months) owing their immature metabolism, which is unable to produce plasma proteins and transport high levels of bupivacaine as a free fraction (Mazoit et al. 1988; Luz et al. 1996; Knudsen et al. 1997; Meunier et al. 2001), and the immaturity of the liver, which prevents metabolism of the drug (Meunier et al. 2001). The risk is low in dentistry for the following reasons:

1) The maximum dose in dentistry is 90 mg (American Dental Association 2003).

2) Bupivacaine is contraindicated in children aged under 12 years (see above) to prevent the risk of self-injury of the soft tissues (tongue, lips, and buccal mucosa) owing to the long action of the anesthetic in these tissues (Pricco 1977; Jensen et al. 1981; Moore 1984).
3) It is important to remember that in dentistry, aspiration is mandatory to prevent intravascular injections.

In conclusion, cardiotoxicity is considered an extremely rare adverse effect with the doses and regimens of bupivacaine used in dentistry.

### Amide Anesthetics and Malignant Hyperthermia

Malignant hyperthermia (MH) or malignant hyperpyrexia is a rare and severe familial disease (Britt and Kalow 1970) that is triggered after administration of general anesthesia and with concomitant drugs, especially halothane and succinylcholine (Britt and Kalow 1970; Kalow et al. 1970; Adriani and Sundin 1984). The pathophysiology of MH is still not fully understood. During acute episode of MH, intracellular calcium increases in skeletal muscle, causing uncontrolled muscle contractions (Fukami and Ganzberg 2005). It appears that there may be a defect in the RYR1 gene for a calcium channel receptor in the sarcoplasmic reticulum. It is autosomally dominant with variable penetrance, but some patients without the genetic defect still can develop MH (Fukami and Ganzberg 2005).

Symptoms generally appear within 2 hours of onset of anesthesia, with increased exhaled carbon dioxide (hypercapnia), increased heart rate (tachycardia, which may progress to various types of arrhythmia), and increased body temperature (pyrexia) accompanied by sweating and muscle rigidity (including all muscles but notable masseter muscle rigidity and trimus is a presentation of MH), even if the patient has received a potent muscle relaxant such as succinylcholine (Britt and Kalow 1970; Kolb et al. 1982; Fukami and Ganzberg 2005). The condition is potentially fatal (Kolb et al. 1982; Ording 1985).

The problem arose when it was suggested that amide local anesthetics could trigger this clinical picture, given that sporadic cases had been described with lidocaine and bupivacaine (Britt 1972; Klimanek et al. 1976; Gibbs 1984). Furthermore, it has been suggested that stress (Gronert et al. 1980; Kolb et al. 1982) and infection (Adriani and Sundin 1984) – both of which circumstances arise in the dentist's office – could trigger MH. This concern was further reinforced with the publication of an important book on dental local anesthesia, where it was stated that these agents could act as triggers (Malamed 1986). Note: This point was corrected in subsequent editions.

Current data call into doubt this contraindication to the use of amide anesthetics in patients with MH, for various reasons:

1) Clinical cases of MH associated with amide anesthetics resolved spontaneously with no specific treatment (dantrolene and cooling) and did not present the mortality usually associated with these conditions (Britt 1972; Klimanek et al. 1976; Gibbs 1984). It is possible to think that some of these reactions were caused more by stress than by the anesthetics themselves (Minasian and Yagiela 1988; Dershwitz et al. 1989).
2) The disease has been reproduced in experimental porcine models with halothane and succinylcholine, although never with local anesthetics (only poisoning due to the excess dose administered) (Hall et al. 1972; Kerr et al. 1975; Wingard and Bobko 1979; Harrison and Morell 1980). The current body of evidence indicates that the triggering agents are succinylcholine and volatile inhalational anesthetics (sevoflurane, enflurane, isoflurane, desflurane, and halothane) (Morgan et al. 2013).
3) Patients diagnosed with MH who have received amide local anesthetics for muscle biopsy or dental treatment or epidural anesthesia during labor, etc. did not develop MH (Willatts 1979; Berkowitz and Rosenberg 1985; Adriani and Sundin 1984; Gielen and Viering 1986).
4) Similarly, no cases of MH were reported in the main reviews on adverse effects of local anesthetics: Danish Malignant Hyperthermia (Ording 1985), Malignant Hyperthermia Association of the United States (MHAUS) (Minasian and Yagiela 1988), and the reviews of the Massachusetts Society of Oral Maxillofacial Surgeons (MSOMS) (D'Eramo 1999; D'Eramo et al. 2003).

In conclusion, current data indicate that use of amide local anesthetics is not contraindicated in patients diagnosed with MH.

## References

Adler, P. and Simon, M. (1949). Contribution to the problem of allergy to local anesthetics. *Oral Surg. Oral Med. Oral Pathol.* 2 (8): 1029–1036.

Adriani, J. and Sundin, R. (1984). Malignant hyperthermia in dental patients. *J. Am. Dent. Assoc.* 108 (2): 180–184.

Adriani, J., Coffman, V.D., and Naraghi, M. (1986). The allergenicity of lidocaine and other amide and related local anesthetics. *Anesth. Rev.* 13 (6): 30–36.

Albright, G.A. (1979). Cardiac arrest following regional anesthesia with etidocaine or bupivacaine (editorial). *Anesthesiology* 51 (4): 285–286.

Aldrete, J.A. and Johnson, D.A. (1970). Evaluation of intracutaneous testing for investigation of allergy to local anesthetic agents. *Anesth. Analg.* 49 (1): 173–183.

American Dental Association (2003). *ADA Guide to Dental Therapeutics*, 3e. Chicago: American Dental Association. 2.

Anonymous (1994). Prilocaine-induced methemoglobinemia – Wisconsin, 1993. *Morb. Mortal. Wkly. Rep.* 43 (35): 655–657.

Bax, N.D.S., Lennard, M.S., Al-Asay, S. et al. (1983). Inhibition of drug metabolism by B-adrenoceptor antagonists. *Drugs* 25 (Suppl 2): 121–126.

Bax, N.D.S., Tucker, G.T., Lennard, M.S., and Woods, H.F. (1985). The impairment of lignocaine clearance by propanolol—major contribution from enzyme inhibition. *Br. J. Clin. Pharmacol.* 19 (5): 597–603.

Berkowitz, A. and Rosenberg, H. (1985). Femoral block with mepivacaine for muscle biopsy in malignant hyperthermia patients. *Anesthesiology* 62 (5): 651–652.

Bozkurt, P., Süzer, Ö., Ekici, E. et al. (2003). Effects of bupivacaine used with sevoflurane on the rhythm and contractility in isolated rat heart. *Eur. J. Anaesthesiol.* 20 (3): 199–204.

Britt, B.A. (1972). Recent advances in malignant hyperthermia. *Anesth. Analg.* 51 (5): 841–849.

Britt, B.A. and Kalow, W. (1970). Malignant hyperthermia: a statistical review. *Can. Anaesth. Soc. J.* 17 (4): 293–315.

Coleman, M.D. and Coleman, N.A. (1996). Drug-induced methaemoglobinaemia. Treatment issues. *Drug Saf.* 14 (6): 394–405.

Curry, S. (1982). Methemoglobinemia. *Ann. Emerg. Med.* 11 (4): 214–221.

De Jong, R.H. (1977). *Local Anesthetics*, 2e. Springfield (IL): Charles C. Thomas Publisher. 228, 229.

D'Eramo, E.M. (1999). Mortality and morbidity with outpatient anesthesia: the Massachusetts experience. *J. Oral Maxillofac. Surg.* 57 (5): 531–536.

D'Eramo, E.M., Bookless, S.J., and Howard, J.B. (2003). Adverse events with outpatient anesthesia in Massachusetts. *J. Oral Maxillofac. Surg.* 61 (7): 793–800.

Dershwitz, M., Ryan, J.F., and Guralnick, W. (1989). Safety of amide local anesthetics in patients susceptible to malignant hyperthermia. *J. Am. Dent. Assoc.* 118 (3): 276–280.

Duncan, P.G. and Kobrinsky, N. (1983). Prilocaine-induced methemoglobinemia in a newborn infant. *Anesthesiology* 59 (1): 75–76.

Feely, J. and Guy, E. (1983). Lack of effect of ranitidine on the disposition of lignocaine. *Br. J. Clin. Pharmacol.* 15 (3): 378–379.

Feely, J., Wilkinson, G.R., McAllister, C.B., and Wood, A.J.J. (1982). Increased toxicity and reduced clearance of lidocaine by cimetidine. *Ann. Intern. Med.* 96 (5): 592–594.

Foldes, F.F., Foldes, V.M., Smith, J.C., and Zsigmond, E.K. (1963). The relation between plasma cholinesterase and prolonged apnea caused by succinylcholine. *Anesthesiology* 24 (2): 208–216.

Fukami, M.C. and Ganzberg, S.I. (2005). A case report of malignant hyperthermia in a dental clinic operation room. *Anesth. Prog.* 52 (1): 24–28.

Gibbs, J.M. (1984). Unexplained hyperpyrexia during labour. *Anaesth. Intensive Care* 12 (4): 375.

Gielen, M. and Viering, W. (1986). 3-in-1 lumbar plexus block for muscle biopsy in malignant hyperthermia patients. Amide local anaesthetics may be used safely. *Acta Anaesthesiol. Scand.* 30 (7): 581–583.

Giovannitti, J.A. and Bennett, C.R. (1979). Assessment of allergy to local anesthetics. *J. Am. Dent. Assoc.* 98 (5): 701–706.

Graf, B.M., Abraham, I., Eberbach, N. et al. (2002). Differences in cardiotoxicity of bupivacaine and ropivacaine are the result of the physicochemical and stereoselective properties. *Anesthesiology* 96 (6): 1427–1434.

Gronert, G.A., Thompson, R.L., and Onofrio, B.M. (1980). Human malignant hyperthermia: awake episodes and correction by dantrolene. *Anesth. Analg.* 59 (5): 377–378.

Guay, J. (2009). Methemoglobinemia related to local anesthetics: a summary of 242 episodes. *Anesth. Analg.* 108 (3): 837–845.

Hall, L.W., Trim, C.M., and Wolf, N. (1972). Further studies of porcine malignant hyperthermia. *Br. Med. J.* 2 (5806): 145–148.

Harrison, G.G. and Morell, D.F. (1980). Response of MHS swine to i.v. infusion of lignocaine. *Br. J. Anaesth.* 52 (4): 385–387.

Heavner, J.E. (1986). Cardiac dysrhythmias induced by infusion of local anesthetics into the lateral cerebral ventricle of cats. *Anesth. Analg.* 65 (2): 133–138.

Incaudo, G., Schatz, M., Patterson, R. et al. (1978). Administration of local anesthetics to patients with history of prior adverse reaction. *J. Allergy Clin. Immunol.* 61 (5): 339–345.

Jastak, J.T., Yagiela, J.A., and Donaldson, D. (1995). *Local Anesthesia of the Oral Cavity*. Philadelphia: WB Saunders Co. 143.

Jensen, O.T., Upton, L.G., Hayward, J.R., and Sweet, R.B. (1981). Advantages of long-acting local anesthetic using etidocaine hydrochloride. *J. Oral Surg.* 39 (5): 350–353.

Kalow, W. (1952). Hydrolysis of local anesthetics by human serum cholinesterase. *J. Pharmacol. Exp. Ther.* 104 (2): 122–134.

Kalow, W. and Gunn, D.R. (1959). Some statistical data on atypical cholinesterase of human serum. *Ann. Hum. Genet.* 23 (3): 239–250.

Kalow, W. and Staron, N. (1957). On distribution and inheritance of atypical forms of human serum cholinesterase as indicated by dibucaine numbers. *Can. J. Biochem. Physiol.* 35 (12): 1305–1317.

Kalow, W., Britt, B.A., Terran, M.E., and Haist, C. (1970). Metabolic error of muscle metabolism after recovery from malignant hyperthermia. *Lancet* 2 (7679): 895–898.

Kellet, P.B. and Copeland, C.S. (1983). Methemoglobinemia associated with benzocaine-containing lubricant. *Anesthesiology* 59 (5): 463–464.

Kerr, D.D., Wingard, D.W., and Gatz, E.E. (1975). Prevention of porcine malignant hyperthermia by epidural block. *Anesthesiology* 42 (3): 307–311.

Kishikava, K., Namiki, A., Miyashita, K., and Saitoh, K. (1990). Effects of famotidine and cimetidine on the plasma levels of epidurally administered lignocaine. *Anaesthesia* 45 (9): 719–721.

Klimanek, J., Majewski, W., and Walencik, K. (1976). A case of malignant hyperthermia during epidural analgesia. *Anaesth. Resusc. Intensive Ther.* 4 (2): 143–145.

Knudsen, K., Suurküla, M.B., Blomberg, S. et al. (1997). Central nervous and cardiovascular effects of i.v. infusions of ropivacaine, bupivacaine and placebo in volunteers. *Br. J. Anaesth.* 78 (5): 507–514.

Kolb, M.E., Horne, M.L., and Martz, R. (1982). Dantrolene in human malignant hyperthermia. *Anesthesiology* 56 (4): 254–262.

Künzer, W. von and Schneider, D. (1953). Zur Aktivität der reduzierenden Fermetsysteme in der Erythrozyten junger Säuglinge. *Acta Haematol.* 9 (6): 346–353.

Laskin, J.L., Wallace, W.R., and De Leo, B. (1977). Use of bupivacaine hydrochloride in oral surgery – a clinical study. *J. Oral Surg.* 35 (1): 25–29.

Lo, S.C.-L. and Agar, N.S. (1986). NADH-methemoglobin reductase activity in the erythrocytes of newborn and adult mammals. *Experientia* 42 (11–12): 1264–1265.

Luz, G., Innerhofer, P., Bachmann, B. et al. (1996). Bupivacaine plasma concentrations during continuous epidural anesthesia in infants and children. *Anesth. Analg.* 82 (2): 231–234.

Malamed, S.F. (1986). *Handbook of Local Anesthesia*, 2e. St. Louis (IL): Mosby Co. 112.

Mather, L.E. and Chang, D.H.-T. (2001). Cardiotoxicity with modern local anesthetics. Is there a safer choice? *Drugs* 61 (3): 333–342.

Mather, L.E., Long, G.J., and Thomas, J. (1971). The intravenous toxicity and clearance of bupivacaine in man. *Clin. Pharmacol. Ther.* 12 (6): 935–943.

Matsuo, S., Rao, D.B., Chandry, I., and Foldes, F.F. (1978). Interaction of muscle relaxants and local anesthetics at the neuromuscular junction. *Anesth. Analg.* 57 (5): 580–587.

Maxwell, L.G., Martin, L.D., and Yaster, M. (1994). Bupivacaine-induced cardiac toxicity in neonates: successful treatment with intravenous phenytoin. *Anesthesiology* 80 (3): 682–686.

Mazoit, J.-X., Denson, D.D., and Samii, K. (1988). Pharmacokinetics of bupivacaine following caudal anesthesia in infants. *Anesthesiology* 68 (3): 387–391.

Meunier, J.-F., Goujard, E., Dubonsset, A.-M. et al. (2001). Pharmacokinetics of bupivacaine after continuous epidural infusion in infants with and without biliary atresia. *Anesthesiology* 95 (1): 87–95.

Minasian, A. and Yagiela, J.A. (1988). The use of amide local anesthetics in patients susceptible to malignant hyperthermia. *Oral Surg. Oral Med. Oral Pathol.* 66 (4): 405–415.

Moller, R.A. and Covino, B.G. (1988). Cardiac electrophysiologic effects of lidocaine and bupivacaine. *Anesth. Analg.* 67 (2): 107–114.

Moore, P.A. (1984). Bupivacaine: a long-acting local anesthetic for dentistry. *Oral Surg. Oral Med. Oral Pathol.* 58 (4): 369–374.

Moore, P.A. (1999). Adverse drug interactions in dental practice: interactions associated with local anesthetics, sedatives and anxiolytics. Part IV of a series. *J. Am. Dent. Assoc.* 130 (4): 541–554.

Moore, D.C., Mather, L.E., Bridenbaugh, L.D. et al. (1977). Bupivacaine (Marcaine®): an evaluation of its tissue and systematic toxicity in humans. *Acta Anaesth. Scand.* 21 (2): 109–121.

Morgan, G.E., Mikhail, M.S., and Murray, M.J. (ed.) (2013). *Clinical Anesthesiology*, 5e. New York: McGraw-Hill Companies. 167–172.

Ochs, H.R., Carstens, G., and Greenblatt, D.J. (1980). Reduction in lidocaine clearance during continuous infusion and by coadministration of propranolol. *N. Engl. J. Med.* 303 (7): 373–377.

Olson, M.L. and McEvoy, G.K. (1981). Methemoglobinemia induced by local anesthetics. *Am. J. Hosp. Pharm.* 38 (1): 89–93.

Ording, H. (1985). Incidence of malignant hyperthermia in Denmark. *Anesth. Analg.* 64 (7): 700–704.

Patil, P.M., Singh, G., and Patil, S.P. (2012). Dentistry and the myasthenia gravis patient: a review of the current state of the art. *Oral Surg. Oral Med. Oral Pathol.* 114 (1): e1–e8.

Patton, L.L. and Howard, J.F. (1997). Myasthenia gravis: dental treatment considerations. *Spec. Care Dent.* 17 (1): 25–32.

Pricco, D.F. (1977). An evaluation of bupivacaine for regional nerve block in oral surgery. *J. Oral Surg.* 35 (2): 126–129.

Price, H.L., Cooperman, L.H., and Warden, J.C. (1967). Control of the splanchnic circulation in man. Role of Beta-adrenergic receptors. *Circ. Res.* 21 (3): 333–340.

Reiz, S. and Nath, S. (1986). Cardiotoxicity of local anaesthetic agents. *Br. J. Anaesth.* 58 (7): 736–746.

Robson, R.A., Wing, L.M.H., Miners, J.O. et al. (1985). The effect of ranitidine on the disposition of lignocaine. *Br.J. Clin. Pharmacol.* 20 (2): 170–173.

Rodriguez, L.F., Smolik, L.M., and Zbehlik, A.J. (1994). Benzocaine-induced methemoglobinemia: report of a severe reaction and review of the literature. *Ann. Pharmacother.* 28 (5): 643–649.

Ross, J.D. and Desforges, J.F. (1959). Reduction of methemoglobin by erythrocytes from cord blood. Further evidence of deficient enzyme activity in the newborn period. *Pediatrics* 23 (4): 718–726.

Schatz, M. (1984). Skin testing and incremental challenge in the evaluation of adverse reactions to local anesthetics. *J. Allergy Clin. Immunol.* 74 (4-part 2): 606–616.

Seskin, L. (1978). Anaphylaxis due to local anesthetic hypersensitivity: report of case. *J. Am. Dent. Assoc.* 96 (5): 841–843.

Severinghaus, J.W., Xu, F.-D., and Spellman, M.J. Jr. (1991). Benzocaine and methemoglobin: recommended actions. *Anesthesiology* 74 (2): 385–386.

Shnider, S.M. and Way, E.L. (1968). The kinetics of transfer of lidocaine (xylocaine®) across the human placenta. *Anesthesiology* 29 (5): 944–950.

Spoerel, W.E., Adamson, D.H., and Eberhard, R.S. (1967). The significance of methaemoglobinemia induced by prilocaine (Citanest). *Can. Anaesth. Soc. J.* 14 (1): 1–10.

Svendsen, T.L., Tango, M., Waldorff, S. et al. (1982). Effects of propanolol and pindolol on the plasma lignocaine clearance in man. *Br. J. Clin. Pharmacol.* 13 (Suppl): 223s–226s.

Telivuo, L. and Katz, R.L. (1970). The effects of modern intravenous local analgesic on respiration during partial neuromuscular blockade in man. *Anesthesia* 25 (1): 30–35.

Thomas, R.D., Behbehani, M.M., Coyke, D.E., and Denson, D.D. (1986). Cardiovascular toxicity of local anesthetics: an alternative hypothesis. *Anesth. Analg.* 65 (5): 444–450.

Trap-Jensen, J., Clansen, J.P., Noer, I. et al. (1976). The effects of beta-adrenoceptor blockers on cardiac output, liver blood flow and skeletal muscle blood flow in hypertensive patients. *Acta Physiol. Scand.* 30 (Suppl 440): 30. (abstract n° 27).

Tucker, G.T. (1986). Pharmacokinetics of local anesthetics. *Br. J. Anaesth.* 58 (7): 717–731.

Tucker, G.T., Noyes, R.N., Bridenbaugh, P.O., and More, D.C. (1970). Binding of anilide-type local anesthetics in human plasma. I. Relation-ships between binding, physicochemical properties, and anesthetic activity. *Anesthesiology* 33 (3): 287–303.

Usubiaga, J.E., Wikinski, J.A., Morales, R.L., and Usubiaga, L.E. (1967). Interaction of intravenous administered procaine, lidocaine and succinylcholine in anesthetized subjects. *Anesth. Analg.* 46 (1): 39–45.

Verril, P.J. (1975). Adverse reactions to local anesthetics and vasoconstrictor drugs. *Practitioner* 214 (1281): 380–387.

Weiner, N. (1988). Drogas que inhiben los nervios adrenérgicos y bloquean los receptores adrenérgicos. In: *Goodman and Gilman. Las bases farmacológicas de la terapéutica*, 7e. Madrid: Editorial Medica panamericana. 186–217.

Westaby, D., Bihari, D.J., Gimson, A.E.S. et al. (1984). Selective and non-selective beta receptor blockade in the reduction of portal pressure in patients with cirrhosis and portal hypertension. *Gut* 25 (2): 121–124.

Wilburn-Goo, D. and Lloyd, L.M. (1999). When patients become cyanotic: acquired methemoglobinemia. *J. Am. Dent. Assoc.* 130 (6): 826–831.

Willatts, S. (1979). Malignant hyperthermia susceptibility. Management during pregnancy and labour. *Anaesthesia* 34 (1): 41–46.

Wing, L.M.H., Miners, J.O., Birkett, D.J. et al. (1984). Lidocaine disposition-sex differences and effects of cimetidine. *Clin. Pharmacol. Ther.* 35 (5): 695–701.

Wingard, D.W. and Bobko, S. (1979). Failure of lidocaine to trigger porcine malignant hyperthermia. *Anesth. Analg.* 58 (2): 99–103.

Winkinski, J.A., Usubiaga, J.E., Morales, R.L. et al. (1970). Mechanism of convulsions elicited by local anesthetic agents: I. Local anesthetic depression of electrically induced seizures in man. *Anesth. Analg.* 49 (3): 504–510.

Woods, D.D. (1940). The relation of p-aminobenzoic acid to the mechanism of action of sulphanilamide. *Br. J. Exp. Pathol.* 21 (2): 74–90.

Yarom, N., Barnea, E., Nissan, J., and Gorsky, M. (2005). Dental management of patients with myasthenia gravis: a literature review. *Oral Surg. Oral Med. Oral Pathol.* 100 (2): 158–163.

# 10

## Contraindications for Vasoconstrictors

Below, we review the contraindications for sympathomimetic vasoconstrictors (epinephrine, norepinephrine, and levonordefrin) in three sections: absolute contraindications, relative contraindications, and contraindications of little relevance. In the last part, we examine the contraindications to felypressin. We also explain that, although there is potential for further research, including well-designed studies on the effects of local anesthetics with vasoconstrictors, most clinical studies on the doses and regimens used in dentistry have shown that these solutions are very safe and that relatively few cases of adverse effects have been reported (Brown and Rhodus 2005).

## Absolute Contraindications

Below, we analyze some situations in which sympathomimetic vasoconstrictors, especially epinephrine, are absolutely contraindicated and cannot be used (Table 10.1).

### Uncontrolled Insulin-dependent Diabetes Mellitus

Administration of epinephrine in healthy patients increases plasma levels of the drug, therefore when levels of 150–200 pg/ml are reached (as with administration of two cartridges of a 1:100 000 solution [10 μg/ml]) (Annex 16), the blood sugar level increases (Clutter et al. 1980) as glucose is released by the liver as a result of increased neoglycogenesis (Christensen 1979; Hamburg et al. 1980). Furthermore, when blood epinephrine levels greater than 400 pg/ml are reached (as with administration of five cartridges of a 1:100 000 solution [10 μg/ml]) (Annex 16), release of insulin is inhibited through the direct action of epinephrine on the cells of the pancreas (Christensen 1979; Hamburg et al. 1980), thus aggravating the increase in plasma glucose (Clutter et al. 1980).

Studies on intraoral injection of anesthetic solutions with epinephrine confirm this data (Meechan et al. 1991a; Meechan 1996). In addition, the anxiety felt by the patient (as is often the case in the dentist's office) worsens the situation by activating the sympathetic nervous system and increasing the release of glucose to the bloodstream (Christensen 1979; Hamburg et al. 1980; Berk et al. 1985). Increased blood glucose (glycemia) for 20–30 minutes is well tolerated by healthy persons (Meechan et al. 1991a; Meechan 1991b, 1996).

Such situations are very serious in diabetic patients (Christensen 1979) and are worse for patients with insulin-dependent diabetes mellitus (Berk et al. 1985). Nevertheless, both types of patients can be treated at the dentist's office and receive anesthetic solutions with epinephrine, provided they are carefully monitored (Dos Santos-Paul et al. 2015). It is important to remember that these patients, and any patients with uncontrolled systemic disease, are considered ASA (American Society of Anesthesiologists) III (Wilson et al. 2008). However, most insulin-dependent diabetic patients are young and need considerable discipline to administer insulin, maintain a balanced diet, and take regular and well-planned physical exercise. These requirements are often difficult to meet owing to the fact that young people participate in sports, group activities, and activities that do not facilitate the necessary discipline for appropriate insulin treatment (Munroe 1983). In these circumstances, there is an increased risk of diabetic ketoacidosis or hyperglycemic reaction or worsening of an ongoing one (onset of these reactions is slow, usually hours or days) (Munroe 1983; Perusse et al. 1992b).

In conclusion, in patients with poorly controlled or uncontrolled insulin-dependent diabetes, dental local anesthetic solutions with epinephrine are absolutely contraindicated (Munroe 1983; Perusse et al. 1992b). Furthermore, since these patients are considered ASA IV (Malamed 2007; Wilson et al. 2008), only emergency dental treatment (analgesics, antibiotics, etc.) is indicated for control of pain and infection (Munroe 1983).

*Local Anesthesia in Dentistry: A Locoregional Approach*, First Edition. Jesús Calatayud and Mana Saraghi.
© 2024 John Wiley & Sons Ltd. Published 2024 by John Wiley & Sons Ltd.
Companion website: www.wiley.com/go/Calatayud/local

**Table 10.1** Summary of absolute contraindications for sympathomimetic vasoconstrictors.

1) Poorly controlled or uncontrolled insulin-dependent diabetes mellitus.
2) Intolerance to sulfites.
3) Severe asthma controlled by corticosteroids.
4) Arterial hypertension due to pheochromocytoma.
5) Consumption of cocaine in the previous 24 hours.
6) Consumption of psychostimulants by patients with cardiovascular disease
7) Allergy to vasoconstrictors.

## Intolerance to Sulfites

Sulfites (sulfite, bisulfite, sodium/potassium metabisulfite, and sulfur dioxide) are used as antimicrobial drugs, reducing agents, and antibrowning agents in foods such as fruit, vegetables, salads, mushrooms, potatoes, shellfish, wine, beer, and juices; in addition, they are used in foods that do not contain thiamine, such as red meat (Bush et al. 1986; Simon 1986; Seng and Gay 1986). Sulfites are also used as antioxidants in various medicines, including local anesthetic solutions containing sympathomimetic vasoconstrictors (Huang and Fraser 1984; Schwartz and Sher 1985; Bush et al. 1986; Simon 1986; Seng and Gay 1986), therefore all dental local anesthetic solutions with epinephrine, norepinephrine, and levonordefrin contain sulfites (Huang and Fraser 1984; Schwartz and Sher 1985; Seng and Gay 1986). The United States Food and Drug Administration (FDA) includes sulfites in the Generally Recognized As Safe category (Bush et al. 1986; Simon 1986; Seng and Gay 1986).

Little is known about the mechanism of sensitization to sulfites (Schwartz and Sher 1985; Bush et al. 1986; Simon 1986). It is thought to result from the following: (i) release of histamine via a nonimmune pathway, (ii) action of the parasympathetic nervous system and gastrin, and (iii) deficiency of the enzyme sulfite oxidase (responsible for oxidizing sulfite to inactive sulfate). It is therefore more appropriate to talk of intolerance or reactions to sulfites than allergy until we can better determine to what extent these reactions are immunological.

The prevalence of intolerance to sulfites in the general population is unknown, although the condition is considered extremely rare (except in the case of asthmatic patients [see below]) (Bush et al. 1986). Furthermore, although it has been demonstrated that subcutaneous sensitization to sulfites is very difficult (the oral route and, even more so, the inhaled route are the most common routes of sensitization) (Goldfarb and Simon 1984; Bush et al. 1986), there have been reports of reactions (urticaria, angioedema, inflammation, dyspnea, etc.) after administration of dental local anesthesia with epinephrine solutions caused by the sulfites they contain (Huang and Fraser 1984; Schwartz and Sher 1985; Schwartz et al. 1989; Dooms-Goossens et al. 1989; Campbell et al. 2001).

In conclusion, anesthetic solutions containing adrenergic vasoconstrictors are absolutely contraindicated in patients who do not tolerate sulfites, since these solutions contain sulfites as antioxidants.

## Asthma Controlled with Corticosteroids

For reasons that remain unknown, asthmatic patients are particularly sensitive to sulfites, and it has been estimated that around 5% of asthmatics could be very sensitive to these drugs (Seng and Gay 1986; Simon 1986). Although other authors have reported this figure to be excessive (Bush et al. 1986), a more selective study has shown that not all asthmatics are the same. Thus, *8% of patients with severe asthma controlled by corticosteroids are sensitized to sulfites, whereas fewer than 1% of asthmatics who do not need corticosteroids are sensitized* (Bush et al. 1986). In addition, the literature shows that most asthmatics who experience bronchospasms and reactions to sulfites are patients who need corticosteroids (Bush et al. 1986; Schwartz et al. 1989).

In conclusion, in patients with severe asthma whose disease is controlled with corticosteroids, local anesthetic solutions containing adrenergic vasoconstrictors are absolutely contraindicated, since 8% do not tolerate the sulfites used as antioxidants in these solutions. Furthermore, asthma patients whose disease is difficult to control and have frequent attacks that require admission to hospital and corticosteroids are classed as ASA IV, therefore only immediate dental treatment is indicated (analgesics, antibiotics, etc.) for control of pain and infection (Perusse et al. 1992b; Steinbacher and Glick 2001; Malamed 2007).

## Pheochromocytoma-induced Arterial Hypertension

Pheochromocytoma is an unusual tumor of the medulla of the adrenal gland that is generally benign and produces epinephrine and norepinephrine (Hickler and Thorn 1977; Cryer 2001; Keiser 2001). The most typical symptom in most cases is arterial hypertension, and the tumor is thought to cause fewer than 0.1–0.5% of diagnosed cases of hypertension (Sutton et al. 1981; Plouin et al. 1981).

The arterial hypertension produced by this tumor is permanent in 50–60% of cases, although 25–50% of cases involve paroxysmal hypertension (Hickler and Thorn 1977; Keiser 2001), that is, hypertension that takes the form of crises lasting minutes or even hours that are usually spontaneous or caused by physical effort, emotional tension, or abdominal palpation. Attacks of paroxysmal hypertension, which result from release of catecholamines, can lead to death from myocardial infarction (even in the absence of heart disease), from arrhythmias, or from brain hemorrhage (Hickler and Thorn 1977; Keiser 2001).

In conclusion, sympathomimetic vasoconstrictors are contraindicated in patients with pheochromocytoma owing to the risk of fatal heart abnormalities or cerebrovascular accidents (Perusse et al. 1992b). In addition, these patients can be considered ASA III or IV depending on the degree of severity.

### Recent Consumption of Cocaine

Cocaine was addressed in Chapter 1, since it was the first local anesthetic, and in Chapter 12, since it is a topical anesthetic that is still in use. Illegal consumption of and addiction to cocaine in developed countries cause serious medical and social problems (Friedlander and Gorelick 1988; Goulet et al. 1992).

Cocaine taken intranasally is quickly inactivated on entering the bloodstream by plasma pseudocholinesterase. However, it remains in blood for more than 6 hours, with a peak at 60 minutes and a half-life of 1.5 hours (Annex 11). This is because the drug remains in the mucosa for more than 3 hours owing to its vasoconstrictive effect (Van Dyke et al. 1976). Consumption stimulates the central nervous system (CNS) and peripheral sympathetic nervous system (Benchimol et al. 1978; Pasternack et al. 1985) with *generalized sensitization of the body to the action of catecholamines* (Tainter et al. 1949; Tye et al. 1967; Benchimol et al. 1978; Kossowosky and Lyon 1984; Nanji and Filipenko 1984; Howard et al. 1985; Goulet et al. 1992). Therefore, high doses can produce a direct toxic effect on the heart, with possible coronary spasm (Benchimol et al. 1978; Kossowosky and Lyon 1984; Schachne et al. 1984; Friedlander and Gorelick 1988). Ingestion results in increased arterial blood pressure and heart rate, with increased oxygen consumption by the heart that can in turn lead to the following:

- Hypertensive crises with a risk of cerebrovascular accidents (Friedlander and Gorelick 1988).
- Arrhythmias (Benchimol et al. 1978; Nanji and Filipenko 1984; Friedlander and Gorelick 1988).
- Angina pectoris (Pasternack et al. 1985) or acute myocardial infarction, even in young patients with no previous history of heart disease (Kossowosky and Lyon 1984; Schachne et al. 1984; Cregler and Mark 1985; Howard et al. 1985; Pasternack et al. 1985; Weiss 1986).

The dentist should try to identify recent consumption of cocaine based on suspicious behavior (mania, restlessness, irritability, or depression, dilated pupils, red eyes, runny, or bloody nose, frequent intakes of breath through the nose without allergy or having a cold, etc.), careless appearance (Friedlander and Gorelick 1988), or as part of taking a medical history and asking about recreational drug use (Goulet et al. 1992), although patients may not disclose their consumption.

In conclusion, anesthetic solutions containing sympathomimetic vasoconstrictors, especially epinephrine, are contraindicated in patients who have consumed cocaine during the *previous 24 hours* (Goulet et al. 1992), given that plasma levels of the drug are maintained for more than 6 hours (Van Dyke et al. 1976).

### Patients with Cardiovascular Diseases Who Take Amphetamines and Psychostimulants

Children with psychological disorders, such as attention-deficit hyperactivity disorder, are generally treated with amphetamine and other psychostimulants (atomoxetine, dexamfetamine, modafinil, etc.) (Table 10.2) (Moore and Hersh 2006). If these patients also have cardiovascular problems such as arrhythmia or arterial hypertension, then local anesthetic solutions with sympathomimetic vasoconstrictors (mainly epinephrine and levonordefrin) are contraindicated (Moore and Hersh 2006; Hersh and Moore 2008).

Note: For some authors, *selegiline*, an antiparkinson and antidepressant monoamine oxidase inhibitor (MAOI), is absolutely contraindicated in patients receiving sympathomimetic amines such as epinephrine. Selegiline can cause increases in arterial pressure since it produces amphetamine compounds (L-metamfetamine and L-amfetamine) during metabolism in the liver (Friedlander et al. 2009).

### Allergy to Vasoconstrictors

We generally think of vasoconstrictors as epinephrine and norepinephrine. Given that these drugs are natural neurotransmitters and hormones, there are no cases of allergy to their base forms, as this would not be compatible with human life. However, exogenous forms administered in local anesthetics include bitartrates and hydrochlorides,

Table 10.2 Amphetamines and psychostimulants.

| Amphetamine | Atomoxetine |
| --- | --- |
| Dexamphetamine | Dexmethylphenidate |
| Methamphetamine | Methylphenidate |
| Modafinil | Pemoline |

and two cases of allergy to epinephrine have been reported (Kohase and Umino 2004).

Felypressin (Octapressin®), which is used in many countries in the European Union, and levonordefrin (synthetic vasoconstrictor), which is used in the United States, are artificial drugs, therefore they can cause allergic sensitization. In fact, one case of allergy to levonordefrin has been reported (Germishuys and Anderson 1982). Allergy is an absolute contraindication for these drugs.

Of note, these situations are exceptional since, despite years of experience with these drugs, only three cases of allergy have been reported.

## Relative Contraindications

Below, we present those situations (mainly drug interactions) where sympathomimetic vasoconstrictors such as norepinephrine and levonordefrin are absolutely contraindicated, *but where epinephrine can be administered, albeit with important restrictions*. In such situations, we have two alternatives:

1) Solutions with epinephrine where limitations are applied, as follows:
   - The maximum concentration is 1:100000 (10 μg/ml), therefore higher concentrations are contraindicated (1:80000 [12.5 μg/ml] and 1:50000 [20 μg/ml]), but not lower concentrations (1:200000 [5 μg/ml]) (McCarthy 1982; American Dental Association 2003; Malamed 2004).
   - The current maximum dose of epinephrine is no longer 200 μg, although much lower doses of 27–50 μg can be administered depending on the case.
     A suitable alternative in these cases is articaine 4% with epinephrine 1:200000 (5 μg/ml) and an anesthetic parameter of 92%-45′/190′-260′.
2) Solutions that do not contain epinephrine or any other sympathomimetic vasoconstrictor, such as the following (see Chapter 7):
   - Solutions that do not contain a vasoconstrictor, such as mepivacaine 3% with an anesthetic parameter of 91%-15′/100′-190′ or prilocaine 4% with an anesthetic parameter of 87%-10′/75′-180′.
   - Prilocaine 3% with felypressin 0.03 IU (0.54 μg/ml) and an anesthetic parameter of 88%-25′/180′-220′.

The problem with an epinephrine-free alternative is that the anesthetic parameter is not very potent (see Chapter 7), and we must remember that onset of pain owing to deficient anesthesia leads to a more marked reaction of the sympathetic nervous system, with an increased risk for the patient (Annex 17).

The maximum number of 1.8-ml cartridges that can be administered with epinephrine in these circumstances is summarized in Table 10.3.

### Nonselective Beta-blockers

Beta-blockers, also known as beta-adrenergic antagonists and beta-adrenergic receptor blockers, are classified into two types (Table 10.4): (i) cardioselective beta-blockers, which only act on $\beta_1$ receptors, mainly in the heart, and (ii) nonselective beta-blockers, which act by blocking both cardioselective $\beta_1$ receptors and $\beta_2$ vasodilators in the arterioles of skeletal muscle and via many other actions (Table 6.7, Chapter 6). These drugs are used in patients with disease such as arterial hypertension, angina pectoris or myocardial infarction, arrhythmias, vascular headaches (migraine), hyperthyroidism, pheochromocytoma, etc. (Foster and Aston 1983; Goulet et al. 1992; Yagiela 1999).

Clinical trials in hypertensive patients (Houben et al. 1982) and with healthy volunteers (Hjemdahl et al. 1983; Reeves et al. 1984; Dzubow 1986; Rehling et al. 1986; Sugimura et al. 1995; Niwa et al. 1996) have demonstrated the following:

- Administration of epinephrine in patients who take cardioselective beta-blockers produces very moderate hemodynamic effects (Houben et al. 1982; Hjemdahl et al. 1983; Rehling et al. 1986); the same can be said of norepinephrine (Hjemdahl et al. 1983). The selective beta blockers block $\beta_1$ effects, leaving the alpha effects and $\beta_2$ effects, namely vasoconstriction and vasodilatation, respectively, and therefore there is less of a hypertensive response to epinephrine.
- Administration of epinephrine in patients taking nonselective beta-blockers produces *severe hemodynamic effects*, with increased arterial pressure and a reflex decrease in heart rate (bradycardia) (Houben et al. 1982; Hjemdahl et al. 1983; Reeves et al. 1984; Dzubow 1986; Rehling et al. 1986; Sugimura et al. 1995; Niwa et al. 1996). The same is true of norepinephrine (Hjemdahl et al. 1983; Reeves et al. 1984), although with lesser intensity, given that the vasodilatory $\beta_2$ effect of norepinephrine is much less pronounced than that of epinephrine (Reeves et al. 1984). The same is true of levonordefrin (Mito and Yagiela 1988). The nonselective beta blockers block all $\beta_1$ and $\beta_2$ effects, leaving the alpha effects, namely vasoconstriction, unopposed, and therefore there is a risk for a hypertensive response to epinephrine.

The mechanism underlying the interaction between sympathomimetic vasoconstrictors (epinephrine and norepinephrine) and nonselective beta-blockers is based on

Table 10.3 Summary of the maximum doses of epinephrine and maximum number of cartridges in situations of relative contraindication.

| Maximum doses of epinephrine | Number of 1.8-ml cartridges | | Clinical situations |
|---|---|---|---|
| | 1:100 000 (10 µg/ml) | 1:200 000 (5 µg/ml) | |
| 27 µg | 1.5 | 3 | Nonselective beta-blockers<br>Antiparkinson COMTi |
| 40 µg | 2.2 | 4.5 | ASA III cardiovascular<br>Digoxin |
| 50 µg | 2.7 | 5.5 | Amphetamines and psychostimulants<br>Tricyclic antidepressants<br>Older antihypertensive<br>Halothane and thiopental |
| Example LAS[a] | Lidocaine 2% + epinephrine 1:100 000 | Articaine 4% + epinephrine 1:200 000 | |
| Anesthetic parameter | 95%-45'/190'-200' | 92%-45'/190'-260' | |
| Example LAS | Articaine 4% + epinephrine 1:100 000 | Bupivacaine 0.5% + epinephrine 1:200 000 | |
| Anesthetic parameter | 98%-60'/190'-260' | 80%-35'/410'-490' | |

Epinephrine can be used, albeit at lower doses (lower number of cartridges). Articaine 4% with epinephrine 1:200 000 (5 µg/ml) is very useful in these cases since, as it contains half the amount of epinephrine as the 1:100 000 solution (10 µg/ml), we can administer double the amount of solution with similar potency and efficacy, although this is somewhat lower than the standard solution of lidocaine 2% with epinephrine 1:100 000, as indicated in its anesthetic parameter.

[a] LAS, local anesthetic solution.

Table 10.4 Beta-blockers.

| Cardioselective | Nonselective |
|---|---|
| **Atenolol** | Carteolol |
| **Bisoprolol** | **Carvedilol** |
| Celiprolol | Labetalol |
| Esmolol | Nadolol |
| **Metoprolol** | Oxprenolol |
| Nebivolol | Pindolol |
| | **Propranolol** |
| | Sotalol |
| | Timolol |

The most common drugs are shown in bold.

blockade of the vasodilatory $β_2$ receptors of the arterioles of skeletal muscle by the beta-blocker, which increases arterial pressure (systolic and diastolic). Given that only the vasoconstrictor α effect remains, there is a risk of cerebrovascular accidents (Hansbrough and Near 1980) and a reflex decrease in heart rate (bradycardia) resulting from blockade of the cardioselective $β_1$ receptors, thus increasing the risk of cardiac arrest (Foster and Aston 1983). Furthermore, this effect is more intense, given that nonselective beta-blockers reduce clearance of epinephrine and, to a lesser extent, norepinephrine, thus extending the duration of action of the exogenous catecholamines (Hjemdahl et al. 1983). It is interesting that, even though these reactions are thought to be dose-dependent, there may be idiopathic cases in which specific sensitivity to these adrenergic receptors aggravates the reaction (Dzubow 1986). A curious effect is that by blocking the vasodilatory $β_2$ effect, nonselective beta-blockers indirectly increase the vasoconstrictor α affect, thus increasing the anesthetic potency of local anesthetic solutions with epinephrine and the duration of soft tissue and pulpal anesthesia (Zhang et al. 1999).

A review of the literature reveals case reports of patients treated with propranolol (nonselective beta-blocker) who were given epinephrine at 40–320 µg (Kram et al. 1974; Hansbrough and Near 1980; Foster and Aston 1983) or levonordefrin at 75 µg (Mito and Yagiela 1988). After a few minutes, the patients experienced an episode of arterial hypertension accompanied by bradycardia lasting 10–15 minutes, which, in some cases, was complicated by a cerebrovascular accident (Hansbrough and Near 1980) or cardiac arrest (Foster and Aston 1983).

The measure proposed in these cases was not to use local anesthetic solutions containing epinephrine (Goulet et al. 1992) or if they did contain epinephrine, then the dose had to be very low (Dzubow 1986), namely, the equivalent of 1.5 cartridges of epinephrine 1:100 000 (10 μg/ml), which represents 27 μg (Yagiela 1999; Naftalin and Yagiela 2002). In addition, arterial pressure and heart rate had to be monitored after 5 minutes (Yagiela 1999; Naftalin and Yagiela 2002; Malamed 2004).

In conclusion, in these patients, local anesthetic solutions containing epinephrine can be used, although at a maximum concentration of 1:100 000 (10 μg/ml) and an *absolute maximum dose of 27 μg* (1.5 × 1.8-ml cartridges). Heart rate and arterial pressure should be monitored before administration of local anesthetic containing vasopressor as well as 5 minutes following administration.

### COMT Inhibitor-type Antiparkinson Drugs

The new antiparkinson medicines tolcapone (Tasmar®) and entacapone produce reversible blockade of catechol-O-methyltransferase (COMT), an enzyme that inactivates peripheral levodopa, therefore these drugs are dopaminergics since they increase dopamine levels. However, they also inhibit inactivation of exogenously administered catecholamines (e.g., epinephrine, norepinephrine, and levonordefrin) by COMT, leading to increased arterial pressure, increased heart rate, and risk of arrhythmias (Illi et al. 1995; Ganzberg 2003; Friedlander et al. 2009). There have been no reports of this interaction to date, probably because the drugs are new and little experience is available.

In conclusion, epinephrine should be reduced to 1.5–3 cartridges of epinephrine 1:100 000 (10 μg/ml), that is, an *absolute maximum dose of 27–50 μg* (Hersh and Moore 2008; Friedlander et al. 2009).

### ASA III Patients with Cardiovascular Conditions

ASA III patients have severe systemic disease that limits activity but is not disabling (no symptoms at rest or with standard exercise). They have reduced tolerance to physical stress (pain) and psychological stress (anxiety). Cardiovascular disorders affecting this group include the following:

- Uncontrolled arterial hypertension with moderate blood pressure (95–115/160–200 mmHg) (McCarthy 1982; Abraham-Inpijn et al. 1988; Malamed 2007).
- Congestive heart failure (caused by myocardial infarction, vascular disease, rheumatic disease, etc.) that leads to difficulty breathing (dyspnea) with exercise or nervous tension, but not at rest (Malamed 2007).
- Implanted pacemaker (ASA 2019).
- Conditions occurring more than 3 months after the following:
  - Cerebrovascular accident that has left neurological sequelae (McCarthy and Malamed 1979; Malamed 2007; Wilson et al. 2008).
  - Heart attack (angina pectoris or acute myocardial infarction) (McCarthy and Malamed 1979; Abraham-Inpijn et al. 1988; Malamed 2007; Wilson et al. 2008).
  - Coronary bypass surgery (Perusse et al. 1992a).
  - Stents in coronary artery disease (ASA 2019).
- Heart transplant. Surgical denervation: the transplanted heart has been denervated, meaning that the vagus nerve has been transected, losing parasympathetic input and leaving the heart hypersensitive to the action of catecholamines (Carleton et al. 1969; Roca et al. 1993; Meechan et al. 2002).

Special attention should be given to the good tolerance of hypertensive patients (controlled and uncontrolled) to dental local anesthetic solutions with epinephrine reported in a systematic review (Bader et al. 2002) and of patients with cardiovascular disease in general, albeit within certain limits (Annex 17). Of note, it is important to control pain in these patients, and, as epinephrine in local anesthetic solutions plays a key role in pain control (Annex 17), patients should receive local anesthetic solutions with epinephrine, although not exceeding the maximum concentration of 1:100 000 (10 μg/ml) and not exceeding the *absolute maximum dose of 40 μg* (McCarthy 1982; Campbell et al. 1996; Rahn and Ball 2001; American Dental Association 2003; Malamed 2004, 2007; Herman and Ferguson 2010; Anderson and Bosack 2014), that is, 2.2–2.5 cartridges of epinephrine 1:100 000.

Note: See ASA classification in Chapter 8.

### Digitalis Glycosides (Digoxin)

Digoxin and digitoxin are digitalis glycosides used as cardiotonic agents for heart failure and arrhythmias. These drugs have a low therapeutic index, that is, the difference between therapeutic and toxic levels is small. Small dose modifications can easily lead to toxic levels (Hersh and Moore 2008).

Intravenous infusion of epinephrine (Fellows et al. 1985) and intraoral injection (Meechan and Rawlins 1987, 1988; Meechan et al. 1991a) reduce plasma potassium levels on entering the cells (Fellows et al. 1985). Infusion reaches maximum levels at 10–20 minutes and then tends to normalize (Meechan and Rawlins 1987, 1988; Meechan et al. 1991a). This is of no relevance in healthy persons. However, in patients with cardiovascular disease who take digitalis glycosides, epinephrine can cause arrhythmias (Kunin et al. 1962; Meechan et al. 1991a; Naftalin and Yagiela 2002; Hersh and Moore 2008), since reduction of plasma potassium levels worsens these situations (Meechan and Rawlins 1988).

Although there is no recommended regimen in these cases, some authors recommend an *absolute maximum dose of 40 μg* of epinephrine until more information becomes available (Hersh and Moore 2008). The dose is equivalent to 2.2 cartridges of epinephrine 1:00 000.

## Amphetamines and Psychostimulants

Amphetamines and psychostimulant derivatives (Table 10.2) are used in children with attention-deficit and hyperactivity disorder (see above) (Nissen 2006; Moore and Hersh 2006; Hersh and Moore 2008). These diseases can persist into adolescence and even into adulthood (Hersh and Moore 2008).

The drugs act by releasing norepinephrine and other catecholamines or by blocking their uptake (Hersh and Moore 2008), with the result that they increase heart rate and blood pressure (Nissen 2006; Moore and Hersh 2006). There have been reports of children with acute myocardial infarction and cerebrovascular accidents after receiving these drugs (Nissen 2006; Hersh and Moore 2008). In these conditions, exogenous administration of catecholamines in local anesthetic solutions can increase the risks (Hersh and Moore 2008).

While no definitive criterion has been established, some authors recommend reducing the maximum doses of epinephrine in line with the recommendations for tricyclic antidepressants, that is, an *absolute maximum dose of 50 μg* of epinephrine (Hersh and Moore 2008), which is equivalent to 2.7 cartridges of epinephrine 1:100 000 (10 μg/ml).

## Tricyclic Antidepressants

Antidepressive drugs are grouped into four major categories (Table 10.5) according to their mechanism of action and chemical structure. For our purposes, the most important are tricyclic and tetracyclic or heterocyclic antidepressants, since these inhibit uptake of norepinephrine in adrenergic nerve endings, thus increasing their concentration at receptor sites (Boakes et al. 1973; Hollister 1978; Yagiela et al. 1983; Yagiela 1999; Naftalin and Yagiela 2002), including heart muscle (Fowler et al. 1976; Yagiela 1999), and boosting the effect of

**Table 10.5** Different types of antidepressants and their mechanism of action.

| Tricyclic: Norepinephrine and serotonin uptake inhibitors | |
|---|---|
| Amitriptyline | Clomipramine |
| Desipramine | Doxepin |
| Imipramine | Nortriptyline |
| Protriptyline | Venlafaxine[a] |
| Duloxetine[a] | |
| Tetracyclic: Norepinephrine uptake inhibitors | |
| Amoxapine | Lofepramine |
| Maprotiline | Mianserin |
| Mirtazapine | Reboxetine[b] |
| MAOIs: Monoamine oxidase (MAO) inhibitors | |
| Phenelzine | Isocarboxazid |
| Moclobemide | Nialamide |
| Tranylcypromine | Selegiline |
| SSRIs: Selective serotonin reuptake inhibitors | |
| Citalopram | Escitalopram |
| Fluoxetine | Fluvoxamine |
| Paroxetine | Sertraline |
| Trazodone | |

Table adapted from Rodríguez and Reneses (2002). Inhibit the reuptake of norepinephrine and serotonin.
[a] Venlafaxine and duloxetine are not tricyclics but inhibit the reuptake of norepinephrine and serotonin.
[b] Reboxetine is not a tetracyclic but inhibits the reuptake of norepinephrine.

sympathomimetic vasoconstrictors. Tricyclic antidepressants are used to treat depression, neuropathic pain (atypical orofacial pain, chronic pain, etc.), severe abnormalities caused by anxiety, nocturnal enuresis in children etc. (Goulet et al. 1992; Yagiela 1999; Naftalin and Yagiela 2002).

Experimental animal studies (Goldman 1971a; Goldman et al. 1971b; Yagiela et al. 1983, 1985) and clinical trials in healthy volunteers (Svedmyr 1968; Boakes et al. 1973) and in patients with depression (Persson and Siwers 1975) have shown that administration of catecholamines such as epinephrine, norepinephrine, and levonordefrin in patients taking tricyclic or tetracyclic antidepressants produces hypertensive reactions and alterations of heart rhythm (arrhythmias) by boosting the effect of epinephrine two- to fourfold and that of norepinephrine and levonordefrin four- to ninefold (Svedmyr 1968; Boakes et al. 1973; Yagiela et al. 1985). It is interesting to point out that long-term administration of this type of antidepressant (more than 2–3 weeks) can lead to desensitization to sympathomimetic vasoconstrictors and therefore a reduced effect of the interaction (Moyer et al. 1979; Weiss et al. 1980; Brown and Rhodus 2005).

MAOI (Monoamine Oxidase Inhibitors) antidepressants are still associates with this interaction in many books on dental local anesthesia (Bennett 1984; Roberts and Sowray 1987; Gaudi and Arreto 2005). However, experimental animal studies (Yagiela et al. 1983, 1985) and clinical trials (Elis et al. 1967; Boakes et al. 1973) have been unable to demonstrate this type of interaction. This is logical, given that the main enzyme responsible for inactivation of adrenergic vasoconstrictors (epinephrine, norepinephrine, and levonordefrin) is COMT and not the monoamine oxidase (MAO) inhibited by MAOI drugs (Boakes et al. 1973; Yagiela et al. 1985). Phenylephrine, a vasoconstrictor that is no longer in use, is the only drug that is metabolized by MAO and can be boosted by MAOIs (Yagiela et al. 1985).

Modern selective serotonin reuptake inhibitors (SSRIs), such as those derived from fluoxetine (Prozac®), are not subject to this type of interaction because they do not inhibit the reuptake of norepinephrine, only serotonin (De Jonghe and Swinkles 1992). These antidepressants are rapidly replacing tricyclic antidepressants.

In conclusion, in the case of patients who take tricyclic and tetracyclic antidepressants, many authors have agreed that local anesthetic solutions with epinephrine can be used, although at a maximum concentration of 1:100 000 (10 μg/ml) and an *absolute maximum dose of 50 μg* (Yagiela et al. 1985; Goulet et al. 1992; Naftalin and Yagiela 2002; Malamed 2004), which is equivalent to 2.7 cartridges.

## Interactions Involving Drugs that are No Longer in Use

Below, we analyze potential drug interactions involving drugs that are no longer or very rarely in use; however, the provider should be aware of the interactions.

### Older Antihypertensive Agents (Anti-adrenergic Drugs)

Guanethidine and reserpine (alkaloid of rauwolfia) are neuro-adrenergic blockers that are used in the treatment of arterial hypertension (Jastak and Yagiela 1983; Jastak et al. 1995; Yagiela 1999). The drugs have almost been replaced by new antihypertensive agents, which are much more efficacious and safer.

Guanethidine and reserpine act by impairing the release of neurotransmitters (norepinephrine) in the sympathetic nerve endings and leading to depletion of catecholamines in many organs (Boura and Green 1965; Mitchell and Oates 1970), therefore prolonged use causes hypersensitivity of the adrenergic receptors to the direct action of sympathomimetic vasoconstrictors (Emmelin and Engström 1961; Fleming 1962; Boura and Green 1965; Katz and Epstein 1968), thus generating a risk of exaggerated response to exogenous catecholamines and increased arterial pressure and arrhythmias (Fleming 1962; Katz and Epstein 1968; Jastak et al. 1995). The effect is more pronounced with norepinephrine (Fleming 1962; Boura and Green 1965).

In conclusion, patients treated with older antihypertensive agents can receive local anesthetic solutions with epinephrine, although at a maximum concentration of 1:100 000 (10 μg/ml) and an *absolute maximum concentration of 50 μg*, that is, equivalent to 2.7 cartridges.

### General Anesthesia (Halothane and Thiopental)

Halothane is a potent inhaled general anesthetic that sensitizes the heart to the action of epinephrine (Joas and Stevens 1971; Munson and Tucker 1975; Johnston et al. 1976; Hayashi et al. 1993) and, probably, levonordefrin (Yagiela 1999). Sodium thiopental is an ultrashort-acting barbiturate that is administered intravenously for induction of general anesthesia. It also sensitizes the heart to the action of epinephrine (Hayashi et al. 1993; Christensen et al. 1993). However, in the presence of exogenous epinephrine, both halothane and thiopental can alter heart rhythm, thus leading to severe arrhythmia (Hilley et al. 1984). Of note, the action of norepinephrine is more intense than that of epinephrine when altering heart rate in these cases (Deterling et al. 1954; Katz and Katz 1966).

In the case of general anesthesia in patients undergoing oral surgery, sympathomimetic vasoconstrictors can be used as hemostatic agents to reduce bleeding and thus make it easier for the surgeon to visualize the field. In these circumstances – general anesthesia with halothane and complementary local anesthesia – a paradoxical finding is that the likelihood of arrhythmias is reduced (Kaufman 1965; Plowman et al. 1974; Johnston et al. 1976). In addition, concomitant administration of local anesthesia and general anesthesia reduce post-operative pain and is safer than general anesthesia alone (Kaufman et al. 2005). This observation seems to result from the fact that local anesthetic interrupts the painful stimulus reaching the brain and prevents the adrenal sympathetic response (Alexander et al. 1972; Plowman et al. 1974). The new general anesthetics (isoflurane, desflurane, and sevoflurane) are not subject to these interactions. Consequently, halothane has fallen into disuse.

In conclusion, patients placed under general anesthesia can receive local anesthetic solutions with epinephrine, albeit at a maximum concentration of 1:100 000 (10 μg/ml) and an *absolute maximum dose of 100 μg* (Katz et al. 1962; Katz and Epstein 1968; Buhrow and Bastron 1981). Similarly, patients receiving sodium thiopental can receive the same solutions of local anesthetic with epinephrine at the same concentrations with an *absolute maximum dose of 1 μg/kg if used in combination with halothane and 2 μg/kg if used with another general anesthetic gas* (Christensen et al. 1993; Yagiela 1999).

## Contraindications of Little Relevance

Below, we describe those situations where sympathomimetic vasoconstrictors have traditionally been contraindicated and that are no longer considered contraindications or that are of little relevance, but in which it may be prudent not to use high concentrations of epinephrine (e.g., 1:50000 [20 µg/ml]) or administer large quantities of epinephrine, even when not contraindicated.

### Uncontrolled Hyperthyroidism

The most dramatic change in how the danger of catecholamines such as epinephrine is perceived can be seen in patients with hyperthyroidism (uncontrolled or poorly controlled), Graves–Basedow disease, Hashimoto thyroiditis, toxic thyroid adenoma, etc. Until recently, there was broad consensus on the absolute contraindication of sympathomimetic vasoconstrictors in these patients (Allen 1979; Jastak and Yagiela 1983; Cawson et al. 1983; Bennett 1984; Malamed 1986; Roberts and Sowray 1987; Perusse et al. 1992b). This criterion of maximum prudence is based on the "sympathetic component of hyperthyroidism," which caused 0.5–20% of these patients to experience episodes of angina pectoris (Kotler et al. 1973) and led to – fortunately very few – cases of myocardial infarction in patients with hyperthyroidism and no previous coronary disease (Kotler et al. 1973; Proskey et al. 1977; Symmes et al. 1977).

However, the literature contains no cases of toxic reactions to the administration of epinephrine in patients with hyperthyroidism (Cawson et al. 1983), and the so-called sympathetic component is a direct effect of excess thyroid hormone, but not of catecholamines. Furthermore, experiments with animals (Cravey and Gravenstein 1965; Schoot van der and Moran 1965; Margolius and Caffney 1965; Cairoli and Crout 1967) and humans in which hyperthyroidism was provoked by exogenous hormone (Wilson et al. 1966; Aoki et al. 1967), such as in clinical trials involving patients with hyperthyroidism (Aoki et al. 1972; Varma et al. 1976; McDevitt et al. 1978), were unable to demonstrate hypersensitivity to catecholamines in the cardiovascular system. Therefore, during the last 20–30 years, authors who considered uncontrolled hyperthyroidism an absolute contraindication for epinephrine (Jastak and Yagiela 1983; Malamed 1986) no longer do so (Yagiela 1999; Malamed 2004).

Nevertheless, in the case of patients with poorly controlled hyperthyroidism, which some authors class as ASA III (Malamed 2007), we must remember that if they present clear signs and symptoms, then they could be ASA IV. Therefore, they are subject to the limitations and precautions of this group, since they run the risk of developing a medical emergency known as thyroid storm or thyrotoxic crisis (nervousness, fever, sweating, palpitations, etc.), which can progress to loss of consciousness and coma (Little 2006). In the latter case, the patient is classified as ASA IV, which means that the systemic disease poses a threat to the patient's life (Greenwood and Meechan 2003).

In conclusion, at present there is no absolute contraindication for epinephrine and the other sympathomimetic vasoconstrictors in symptomatic patients with uncontrolled or poorly controlled hyperthyroidism (ASA III), although it is important to remember that, given their physical status, they may be ASA IV, patients experiencing a thyroid storm (Chapter 8).

### Phenothiazines and Antipsychotic Drugs

The phenothiazine family shares many common aspects, although it can be divided into two large groups (Table 10.6):

- Antipsychotic or neuroleptic drugs, also known as major tranquilizers such as chlorpromazine, which are used to treat severe mental disorders such as schizophrenia, manic-depressive psychosis or bipolar disease, severe paranoia and mania, delirium, etc. (Hollister and Kosek 1965; Giles and Modlin 1968; Fowler et al. 1976; Friedlander and Brill 1986).
- Antihistamines such as promethazine, which are used as antiallergic drugs, sedatives, and antiemetics.

These drugs can interact with sympathomimetic vasoconstrictors to produce, in theory, alterations of heart rate (Alvarez-Mena and Frank 1973) and dizziness on standing up (orthostatic hypotension) caused by the blockade of α adrenergic receptors produced by these drugs (Jastak and Yagiela 1983; Yagiela et al. 1985; Yagiela 1999). The latter effect can be much less obvious with norepinephrine and levonordefrin, given that these agents act poorly against vasodilatory $\beta_2$ receptors, in contrast with epinephrine.

Table 10.6 Phenothiazines: two main groups.

| Phenothiazine antipsychotics | |
| --- | --- |
| Chlorpromazine | Fluphenazine |
| Levomepromazine | Perphenazine |
| Pericyazine | Pipotiazine |
| Trifluoperazine | Thioproperazine |
| **Phenothiazine antihistamines** | |
| Alimemazine or trimeprazine | Mequitazine |
| Promethazine | Thiethylperazine |

All antipsychotic phenothiazines have a certain tendency to cause these effects in a very moderate way. However, they were seen to be problematic when a former antipsychotic phenothiazine, *thioridazine*, which produces severe alterations of heart rate, proved fatal as a result of adverse effects (Hollister and Kosek 1965; Giles and Modlin 1968; Fowler et al. 1976). It was therefore withdrawn from the market in 2005 (Agencia Española de Medicamentos y Productos Sanitarios 2005; Australian Health Department 2007). Animal experiments have shown these interactions to be of little relevance with current drugs (Yagiela et al. 1983, 1985) and, to date, there has been no evidence of a significant clinical interaction between the two drugs groups in healthy normotensive patients (Jastak and Yagiela 1983; Jastak et al. 1995; Goulet et al. 1992; Yagiela 1999).

In conclusion, there is no contraindication for phenothiazines at the doses and concentrations used in dental local anesthesia, although every precaution should be taken owing to the theoretical possibility of a reaction. The ASA status of psychiatric patients should be evaluated by assessing the patient and reviewing their medical history.

### Vasoconstrictors and Osteoradionecrosis

Radiotherapy used to treat head and neck cancer causes a series of complications, such as mucositis, xerostomia, caries, trismus, etc. (Rothwell 1987; Carl 1993; Scully and Epstein 1996). Osteoradionecrosis, a less frequent complication (Rothwell 1987; Scully and Epstein 1996), is defined as mucosal or cutaneous ulceration (loss of soft tissue integrity) lasting more than 3 weeks, with the irradiated bone exposed (maxilla or mandible) in the absence of cancer (Wong et al. 1997).

Current knowledge of the physiology of this condition is much improved. Radiotherapy affects all irradiated tissues, especially bone, leaving tissue that is hypoxic, poorly vascularized, and hypocellular. In the case of trauma, such as that resulting from tooth extraction, surgery, rubbing against a prosthesis, etc., it is not possible to provide the resources necessary to cure the lesion, leaving a chronic wound that does not heal (Marx 1983; Scully and Epstein 1996). In such circumstances, trauma and bacterial invasion are lesser factors. Spontaneous necrosis, i.e. with no previous trauma, can appear (Marx 1983; Scully and Epstein 1996; Wong et al. 1997; Clayman 1997).

Some authors recommend using vasoconstrictor-free local anesthetic solutions in the irradiated areas as a coadjuvant measure to avoid increasing the risk of osteoradionecrosis (Narang and Wells 1970; Roberts and Sowray 1987), although we do not know if this measure actually has a positive effect (Clayman 1997). However, most reviews on management of irradiated patients do not comment on whether the local anesthetic should contain vasoconstrictors (Topazian 1959; Bottomley and Ebsersole 1966; Rahn and Drone 1967; Rothwell 1987; Carl 1993; Scully and Epstein 1996; Wong et al. 1997), and there are even authors who perform extractions with epinephrine-containing anesthetic solutions in these patients (Marx et al. 1985).

In conclusion, according to currently available information, we believe that there is no evidence for contraindicating vasoconstrictors in irradiated patients at risk of osteoradionecrosis.

## Contraindications of Felypressin

Felypressin is a vasoconstrictor derived from the hormones of the posterior lobe of the hypophysis (vasopressin and oxytocin). It is marketed under the name Octapressin with prilocaine 3% at a concentration of 0.03 IU/ml (0.54 µg/ml). Felypressin is subject to two main contraindications in dentistry (see Chapter 6):

1) Patients who have experienced a *heart attack* (angina pectoris or myocardial infarction). The *contraindication is relative*, since felypressin can be administered at lower doses:
   - The reason is that the vasoconstrictor effect on the coronary vessels decreases blood flow and oxygen supply to the heart (ischemia) (Light et al. 1965; Miyachi et al. 2003). However, it is interesting to note that administration of doses equivalent to 14 cartridges of 0.03 IU/ml to hypertensive patients scarcely affects ischemia in the heart (Sunada et al. 1996).
   - The United Kingdom Dunlop Committee on Safety of Drugs recommends a *maximum dose of 5 × 1.8-ml cartridges* of felypressin at 0.03 IU/ml (Oliver 1974; Roberts and Sowray 1987). Experimental data from dogs suggest that similar doses should be applied (Miyachi et al. 2003).

2) *Pregnancy is an absolute contraindication* (Anonymous 1970; Oliver 1974). The residual oxytocic effect of felypressin stimulates the $v_1$ receptors, which cause uterine contractions, thus reducing blood flow to the placenta and increasing the risk of contractions with premature labor or miscarriage (Anonymous 1970; Oliver 1974; Stepke et al. 1994). In addition, felypressin is used with prilocaine, a local anesthetic that can produce fetal methemoglobinemia and worsen the situation (Anonymous 1970; Oliver 1974).

# References

Abraham-Inpijn, L., Borgmeijer-Hoelen, A., and Gortzak, R.A.T. (1988). Changes in blood pressure, heart rate, and electrocardiogram during dental treatment with use of local anesthetic. *J. Am. Dent. Assoc.* 116 (4): 531–536.

Agencia Española de Medicamentos y Productos Sanitarios (2005). *Suspensión de comercialización de la especialidad farmacéutica Meleril (Tioridazina)*. Subdirección General de Medicamentos de uso Humano. Agencia Española de Medicamentos y Productos Sanitarios. Ref: 2005/01. Madrid, 18 de enero de 2005.

Alexander, J.P., Bekheit, S., and Fletcher, E. (1972). Dysrhythmia and oral surgery. II: Junctional rhythms. *Br. J. Anaesth.* 44 (11): 1179–1182.

Allen, G.D. (1979). *Dental Anesthesia and Analgesia (Local and General)*, 2e. Baltimore: Williams and Wilkins. 76, 77.

Alvarez-Mena, S.C. and Frank, M.J. (1973). Phenothiazine-induced T-wave abnormalities. Effects of overnight fasting. *JAMA* 224 (13): 1730–1733.

American Dental Association (2003). *ADA Guide to Dental Therapeutics*, 3e. Chicago: American Dental Association. 4.

Anderson, E. and Bosack, R. (2014). Anesthetic considerations for patients with cardiovascular disease (Chapter 5). In: *Anesthesia Complications in the Dental Office* (ed. R. Bosack and S. Lieblich). Ames (Iowa): Wiley Blackwell. 25–48.

Annex 11. Pharmacokinetics of local anesthetics and vasoconstrictors.

Annex 16. Epinephrine II. Dose administered and plasma levels.

Annex 17. Epinephrine III. Cardiovascular patients.

Anonymous (1970). Felypressin – a new vasoconstrictor with prilocaine. *Drug Ther. Bull.* 8 (10): 38–40.

Aoki, V.S., Wilson, W.R., Theilen, E.O. et al. (1967). The effects of triiodothyronine on hemodynamic responses to epinephrine and norepinephrine in man. *J. Clin. Pharmacol. Exp. Ther.* 157 (1): 62–68.

Aoki, V.S., Wilson, W.R., and Theilen, E.O. (1972). Studies of the reputed augmentation of the cardiovascular effects of catecholamines in patients with spontaneous hyperthyroidism. *J. Clin. Pharamacol. Exp. Ther.* 181 (2): 362–368.

ASA House of Delegates (Executive Committee) (2019). ASA physical status classification system. Original approval October 15, 2014. Last amended October 23,

Australian Health Department (2007). Withdrawal of thioridazine. *Aust. Prescr.* 30 (3): 82.

Bader, J.D., Bonito, A.J., and Shugars, D.A. (2002). A systematic review of cardiovascular effects of epinephrine on hypertensive dental patients. *Oral Surg. Oral Med. Oral Pathol.* 93 (6): 647–653.

Benchimol, A., Bartall, H., and Desser, K.H. (1978). Accelerated ventricular rhythm and cocaine abuse. *Ann. Intern. Med.* 88 (4): 519–120.

Bennett, C.R. (1984). *Monheim's Local Anesthesia and Pain Control in Dental Practice*, 7e. St. Louis: The CV Mosby Co. 180, 206, 255.

Berk, M.A., Clutter, W.E., Skor, D. et al. (1985). Enhanced glycemia responsiveness to epinephrine in insulin-dependent diabetes mellitus is the result of the inability to secreta insulin. Augmented insulin secretion normally limits the glycemic, but not the lipolytic or ketogenic, response to epinephrine in humans. *J. Clin. Invest.* 75 (6): 1842–1851.

Boakes, A.J., Laurence, D.R., Teoh, P.C. et al. (1973). Interactions between sympathomimetic amines and antidepressant agents in man. *Br. Med. J.* 1 (5849): 311–315.

Bottomley, W.K. and Ebsersole, J.H. (1966). Guidelines for dental care when patients receive radiation therapy to the head and neck. *Oral Surg. Oral Med. Oral Pathol.* 22 (2): 252–256.

Boura, A.L.A. and Green, A.F. (1965). Adrenergic neurone blocking agents. *Ann. Rev. Pharmacol.* 5: 183–212.

Brown, R.S. and Rhodus, N.L. (2005). Epinephrine and local anesthesia revised. *Oral Surg. Oral Med. Oral Pathol.* 100 (4): 401–408.

Buhrow, J.A. and Bastron, R.D. (1981). A comparative study of vasoconstrictors and determination of their safe dose under halothane anesthesia. *J. Oral Surg.* 39 (12): 934–937.

Bush, R.K., Taylor, S.L., and Busse, W. (1986). A critical evaluation of clinical trials in reactions to sulfites. *J. Allergy Clin. Immunol.* 78 (1 Pt 2): 191–202.

Cairoli, V.J. and Crout, R. (1967). Role of the autonomic nervous system in the resting tachycardia of experimental hyperthyroidism. *J. Pharmacol. Exp. Ther.* 158 (1): 55–65.

Campbell, J.H., Huizinga, P.J., Das, S.K. et al. (1996). Incidence and significance of cardiac arrhythmia in geriatric oral surgery patients. *Oral Surg. Oral Med. Oral Pathol.* 82 (1): 42–46.

Campbell, J.R., Maestrello, C.L., and Campbell, R.L. (2001). Allergic response to metabisulfite in lidocaine anesthetic solution. *Anesth. Prog.* 48 (1): 21–26.

Carl, W. (1993). Local radiation and systemic chemotherapy: preventing and managing the oral complications. *J. Am. Dent. Assoc.* 124 (3): 119–123.

Carleton, R.A., Heller, S.J., Najafi, H., and Clark, J.G. (1969). Hemodynamic performance of a transplanted human heart. *Circulation* 40 (4): 447–452.

Cawson, R.A., Curson, I., and Whittington, D.R. (1983). The hazards of dental local anaesthetics. *Br. Dent. J.* 154 (8): 253–258.

Christensen, N.J. (1979). Catecholamines and diabetes mellitus. *Diabetologia* 16 (4): 211–224.

Christensen, L.Q., Bonde, J., and Kampmann, J.P. (1993). Drug interactions with inhalation anesthetics. *Acta Anaesthesiol. Scand.* 37 (3): 231–244.

Clayman, L. (1997). Management of dental extractions in irradiated jaws: a protocol without hyperbaric oxygen therapy. *J. Oral Maxillofac. Surg.* 55 (3): 275–281.

Clutter, W.E., Bier, D.M., Shah, S.D., and Cryer, P.E. (1980). Epinephrine plasma metabolic clearance rates and physiologic thresholds for metabolic and hemodynamic action in man. *J. Clin. Invest.* 66 (1): 94–101.

Cravey, G.M. and Gravenstein, J.S. (1965). The effect of thyroxin, corticosteroids, and epinephrine on atrial rate. *J. Pharmacol. Exp. Ther.* 148 (1): 75–79.

Cregler, L.L. and Mark, H. (1985). Relation of acute myocardial infarction to cocaine abuse. *Am. J. Cardiol.* 56 (12): 794.

Cryer, P.E. (2001). Diseases on the sympathochromaffin system (Chapter 12). In: *Endocrinology and Metabolism*, 4e (ed. P. Felig and L.A. Frohman). New York: McGraw-Hill Inc., Medical Publishing Division. 525–551.

De Jonghe, F. and Swinkles, J.A. (1992). The safety of antidepressants. *Drugs* 43 (Suppl 2): 40–47.

Deterling, R.A., Ngai, S.H., Laragh, J.H., and Papper, C.M. (1954). The cardiovascular effects of continuous intravenous infusion of norepinephrine, epinephrine and neosynephrine during cyclopropane and ether anesthesia in the dog. *Anesthesiology* 15 (1): 11–18.

Dooms-Goossens, A., de Alam, A.G., Degreef, H., and Kochyt, A. (1989). Local anesthetic intolerance due to metabisulfite. *Contact Dermat.* 20 (2): 124–126.

Dos Santos-Paul, M.A., Neves, I.L.I., Neves, E.S., and Ramires, J.A.F. (2015). Local anesthesia with epinephrine is safe and effective for oral surgery in patients with type 2 diabetes mellitus and coronary disease: a prospective randomized study. *Clinics (Sao Paulo)* 70 (3): 185–189.

Dzubow, L.M. (1986). The interaction between propranolol and epinephrine as observed in patients undergoing Mohs' surgery. *J. Am. Acad. Dermatol.* 15 (1): 71–75.

Elis, J., Laurence, D.R., Mattie, H., and Prichard, B.N.C. (1967). Modification by monoamine oxidase inhibitors of the effect of some sympathomimetics on blood pressure. *Br. Med. J.* 2 (5544): 75–78.

Emmelin, N. and Engström, J. (1961). Supersensitivity of salivary glands following treatment with bretylium or guanethidine. *Br. J. Pharmacol. Chemother.* 16 (3): 315–319.

Fellows, I.W., Bennett, T., and Macdonald, I.A. (1985). The effect of adrenaline upon cardiovascular and metabolic functions in man. *Clin. Sci. (London)* 69 (2): 215–222.

Fleming, W.W. (1962). Supersensitivity of the cat heart to catecholamine-induced arrhythmias following reserpine pretreatment (27830). *Proc. Soc. Exp. Biol. Med.* 111 (2): 484–486.

Foster, C.A. and Aston, S.J. (1983). Propranolol–epinephrine interaction: a potential disaster. *Plast. Reconstr. Surg.* 72 (1): 74–78.

Fowler, N.O., McCall, D., Chou, T.-C. et al. (1976). Electrocardiographic changes and cardiac arrhythmias in patients receiving psychotropic drugs. *Am. J. Cardiol.* 3 (2): 223–230.

Friedlander, A.A. and Brill, N.Q. (1986). The dental management of patients with bipolar disorder. *Oral Surg. Oral Med. Oral Pathol.* 61 (6): 579–581.

Friedlander, A.H. and Gorelick, D.A. (1988). Dental management of the cocaine addict. *Oral Surg. Oral Med. Oral Pathol.* 65 (1): 45–48.

Friedlander, A.H., Mahler, M., Norman, K.M., and Ettinger, R.L. (2009). Parkinson disease. Systemic and orofacial manifestations, medical and dental management. *J. Am. Dent. Assoc.* 140 (6): 658–669.

Ganzberg, S. (2003). Neurological drugs (Chapter 20). In: *ADA Guide to Dental Therapeutics*, 3e. Chicago: American Dental Association. 366–381.

Gaudi, J.F. and Arreto, C.D. (2005). *Manual de anestesia en odontoestomatología*. Barcelona: Ed Masson/Elsevier. 165.

Germishuys, P.J. and Anderson, R. (1982). Allergy to vasoconstrictor in a local anaesthetic solution: a case report. *J. Dent. Assoc. S. Afr.* 37 (4): 233–235.

Giles, T.D. and Modlin, R.K. (1968). Death associated with ventricular arrhythmia and thioridazine hydrochloride. *JAMA* 205 (2): 98–100.

Goldfarb, G. and Simon, R. (1984). Provocation of sulfite sensitive asthma. *J. Allergy Clin. Immunol.* 73: 135. (Abstract no 107).

Goldman, V. (1971a). Local anaesthetics containing vasoconstrictors. *Br. Med. J.* 1 (5741): 175.

Goldman, V., Astrom, A., and Evers, H. (1971b). The effect of tricyclic antidepressant on the cardiovascular effects of local anaesthetic solutions containing different vasoconstrictors. *Anaesthesia* 26 (1): 91.

Goulet, J.-P., Perusse, R., and Turcotte, J.-Y. (1992). Contraindications to vasoconstrictors in dentistry: Part III. Pharmacological interactions. *Oral Surg. Oral Med. Oral Pathol.* 74 (5): 692–697.

Greenwood, M. and Meechan, J.G. (2003). General medicine and surgery for dental practitioners. Part 6: The endocrine system. *Br. Dent. J.* 195 (3): 129–133.

Hamburg, S., Hendler, R., and Sherwin, R.S. (1980). Influence of small increments of epinephrine on glucose tolerance in normal humans. *Ann. Intern. Med.* 93 (4): 566–568.

Hansbrough, J.F. and Near, A. (1980). Propranolol–epinephrine antagonism with hypertension and stroke. *Ann. Intern. Med.* 92 (5): 717.

Hayashi, Y., Kamibayashi, T., Sumikawa, K. et al. (1993). Adrenoceptor mechanism involved in thiopental-epinephrine-induced arrhythmias in dogs. *Am. J. Physiol.* 265 (4): H 1380–H 1385.

Herman, W.W. and Ferguson, H.W. (2010). Dental care for patients with heart failure. An update. *J. Am. Dent. Assoc.* 141 (7): 845–853.

Hersh, E.V. and Moore, P.A. (2008). Adverse drug interactions in dentistry. *Periodontol 2000* 46: 109–142.

Hickler, R.B. and Thorn, G.W. (1977). Pheochromocytoma (94). In: *Harrison's Principles of Internal Medicine*, 8e. Tokyo: McGraw-Hill Kogakusha Ltd. 557–563.

Hilley, M.D., Milam, S.B., Gieske, A.H. Jr., and Giovannitti, J.A. (1984). Fatality associated with the combined use of halothane and gingival retraction cord. *Anesthesiology* 60 (6): 587–588.

Hjemdahl, O., Akerstedt, T., Pollare, T., and Gillberg, M. (1983). Influence of B-adrenoceptor blockade by metoprolol and propanolol on plasma concentrations and effects of noradrenaline and adrenaline during i.v. infusion. *Acta Physiol. Scand.* (Suppl 515): 45–53.

Hollister, L.E. (1978). Tricyclic antidepressants (second of two parts). *N. Engl. J. Med.* 229 (21): 1168–1172.

Hollister, L.E. and Kosek, J.C. (1965). Sudden death during treatment with phenothiazine derivatives. *JAMA* 192 (12): 1035–1038.

Houben, H., Thien, T., and Van't Laar, A. (1982). Effect of low-dose epinephrine infusion on hemodynamics after selective and non selective B-blockade in hypertension. *Clin. Pharmacol. Ther.* 31 (6): 685–690.

Howard, R.E., Hueter, D.C., and Davis, G.J. (1985). Acute myocardial infarction following cocaine abuse in a young woman with normal coronary arteries. *JAMA* 254 (1): 95–96.

Huang, A.S. and Fraser, W.M. (1984). Are sulfite additives really safe? *N. Engl. J. Med.* 311 (8): 542.

Illi, A., Sunderberg, S., Ojala-karlsson, P. et al. (1995). The effect of entacapone on the disposition and hemodynamic effects of intravenous isoproterenol and epinephrine. *Clin. Pharmacol. Ther.* 58 (2): 221–227.

Jastak, J.T. and Yagiela, J.A. (1983). Vasoconstrictors and local anesthesia: a review and rationale for use. *J. Am. Dent. Assoc.* 107 (4): 623–629.

Jastak, J.T., Yagiela, J.A., and Donaldson, D. (1995). *Local Anesthesia of the Oral Cavity*. Philadelphia: WB Saunders Co. 131–133.

Joas, T.A. and Stevens, W.C. (1971). Comparison of the arrhythmic doses of epinephrine during Forane, halothane, and fluroxene anesthesia in dogs. *Anesthesiology* 35 (1): 48–53.

Johnston, R.R., Eger, E.I., and Wilson, C. (1976). A comparative interaction of epinephrine with enflurane, isoflurane, and halothane in man. *Anesth. Analg.* 55 (5): 709–712.

Katz, R.L. and Epstein, R.E. (1968). The interaction of anesthetic agents and adrenergic drugs to produce cardiac arrhythmias. *Anesthesiology* 29 (4): 763–784.

Katz, R.L. and Katz, G.J. (1966). Surgical infiltration of pressor drugs and their interaction with volatile anaesthetics. *Br. J. Anaesth.* 38 (9): 712–718.

Katz, R.L., Matteo, R.S., and Papper, E.M. (1962). The injection of epinephrine during general anesthesia with halogenated hydrocarbons and cyclopropane in man. *Anesthesiology* 23 (5): 597–600.

Kaufman, L. (1965). Cardiac arrhythmias in dentistry (letter). *Lancet* 2 (7406): 287.

Kaufman, E., Epstein, J.B., Gorsky, M. et al. (2005). Preemptive analgesia and local anesthesia as a supplement to general anesthesia: a review. *Anesth. Prog.* 52 (1): 29–38.

Keiser, H.R. (2001). Pheochromocytoma and other diseases of the sympathetic nervous system (Chapter 86). In: *Principles and Practice of Endocrinology and Metabolism* (ed. K.L. Becker). Philadelphia: Lippincott Williams and Wilkins. 827–834.

Kohase, H. and Umino, M. (2004). Allergic reaction to epinephrine preparation in 2% lidocaine. Two reports. *Anesth. Prog.* 51 (4): 134–137.

Kossowosky, W.A. and Lyon, A.T. (1984). Cocaine and acute myocardial infarction. A probable connection. *Chest* 86 (5): 729–731.

Kotler, M.N., Michaelides, K.M., Bouchard, R.J., and Warbasse, J.R. (1973). Myocardial infarction associated with thyrotoxicosis. *Arch. Intern. Med.* 132 (5): 723–728.

Kram, J., Bourne, H.R., Melmon, K.L., and Maibach, H. (1974). Propranolol (letter). *Ann. Intern. Med.* 80 (2): 282.

Kunin, A.S., Surawicz, B., and Sims, E.A.H. (1962). Decrease in serum potassium concentrations and appearance of cardiac arrhythmias during infusion of potassium with glucose in potassium-depleted patients. *N. Engl. Med. J.* 266 (5): 228–233.

Light, G.A., Rattenborg, C., and Holaday, D.A. (1965). A new vasoconstrictor: preliminary studies of phelypressin. *Anesth. Analg.* 44 (3): 280–287.

Little, J.W. (2006). Thyroid disorders. Part I: Hyperthyroidism. *Oral Surg. Oral Med. Oral Pathol.* 101 (3): 276–284.

Malamed, S.F. (1986). *Handbook of Local Anesthesia*, 2e. St. Louis (Missouri): The CV Mosby Co. 40, 49.

Malamed, S.F. (2004). *Handbook of Local Anesthesia*, 5e. St. Louis (Missouri): Elsevier-Mosby. 150, 151, 364.

Malamed, S.F. (2007). *Medical Emergencies in the Dental Office*, 6e. St. Louis (Missouri): Mosby-Elsevier. 24–26, 43–47, 292, 458–459.

Margolius, H.S. and Caffney, T.E. (1965). The effects of injected norepinephrine and sympathetic nerve stimulation in hypothyroid and hyperthyroid dogs. *J. Pharmacol. Exp. Ther.* 149 (3): 329–335.

Marx, R.E. (1983). Osteoradionecrosis: a new concept of its pathophysiology. *J. Oral Maxillofac. Surg.* 41 (5): 283–288.

Marx, R.E., Johnson, R.P., and Kline, S.N. (1985). Prevention of osteoradionecrosis: a randomized prospective clinical trial of hyperbaric oxygen versus penicillin. *J. Am. Dent. Assoc.* 111 (1): 49–54.

McCarthy, F.M. (1982). *Medical Emergencies in Dentistry. An Abridged Edition of Emergencies in Dental Practice*, 3e. Philadelphia: WB Saunders Co 39.

McCarthy, F.M. and Malamed, S.F. (1979). Physical evaluation system to determine medical risk and indicated dental therapy modifications. *J. Am. Dent. Assoc.* 99 (2): 181–184.

McDevitt, D.G., Riddel, J.G., Hadden, D.R., and Montgomery, D.A.D. (1978). Catecholamine sensitivity in hyperthyroidism and hypothyroidism. *Br. J. Clin. Pharmacol.* 6 (4): 297–301.

Meechan, J.G. (1991b). The effects of dental local anaesthetics on blood glucose concentration in healthy volunteers and in patients having third molar surgery. *Br. Dent. J.* 170 (10): 373–376.

Meechan, J.G. (1996). Epinephrine, magnesium, and dental local anesthetic solutions. *Anesth. Prog.* 43 (4): 99–102.

Meechan, J.G. and Rawlins, M.D. (1987). A comparison of the effect of two different dental local anaesthetic solutions on plasma potassium concentration. *Br. Dent. J.* 163 (6): 191–193.

Meechan, J.G. and Rawlins, M.D. (1988). The effects of two different dental local anaesthetic solutions on plasma potassium levels during third molar surgery. *Oral Surg. Oral Med. Oral Pathol.* 66 (6): 650–653.

Meechan, J.G., Thomson, C.W., Blair, G.S., and Rawlins, M.D. (1991a). The biochemical and haemodynamic effects of adrenalin in lignocaine local anaesthetic solutions in patients having third molar surgery under general anaesthesia. *Br. J. Oral Maxillofac. Surg.* 29 (4): 263–268.

Meechan, J.G., Parry, G., Rattray, D.T., and Thomason, J.M. (2002). Effects of dental local anesthetics in cardiac transplant recipients. *Br. Dent. J.* 192 (3): 161–163.

Mitchell, J.R. and Oates, J.A. (1970). Guanethidine and related agents. I. Mechanism of the selective blockade of adrenergic neurons and its antagonism by drugs. *J. Pharmacol. Exp. Ther.* 172 (1): 100–107.

Mito, R.S. and Yagiela, J.A. (1988). Hypertensive response to levonordefrin in a patient receiving propranopol: report of case. *J. Am. Dent. Assoc.* 116 (1): 55–57.

Miyachi, K., Ichinohe, T., and Kaneko, Y. (2003). Effects of local injection of prilocaine-felypressin on the myocardial oxygen balance in dogs. *Eur. J. Oral Sci.* 111 (4): 339–345.

Moore, P.A. and Hersh, E.V. (2006). Common medications prescribed for adolescent dental patients. *Dent. Clin. N. Am.* 50 (1): 139–149.

Moyer, J.A., Greenberg, L.H., Frazer, A. et al. (1979). Opposite effects of acute and repeated administration of desmethylimipramine on adrenergic responsiveness in rat pineal gland. *Life Sci.* 24 (24): 2237–2244.

Munroe, C.O. (1983). The dental patient and diabetes mellitus. *Dent. Clin. N. Am.* 27 (2): 329–340.

Munson, E.S. and Tucker, W.K. (1975). Doses of epinephrine causing arrhythmia during enflurane, methoxyflurane and halothane anaesthesia in dogs. *Can. Anaesth. Soc. J.* 22 (4): 495–501.

Naftalin, L.W. and Yagiela, J.A. (2002). Vasoconstrictors: indications and precautions. *Dent. Clin. N. Am.* 46 (4): 733–746.

Nanji, A.A. and Filipenko, J.D. (1984). Asystole and ventricular fibrillation associated with cocaine intoxication. *Chest* 85 (1): 132–133.

Narang, R. and Wells, H. (1970). The avoidance of osteoradionecrosis of the mandible after of a number of teeth in a patient given radiotherapy for oral carcinoma. *Oral Surg. Oral Med. Oral Pathol.* 29 (5): 656–659.

Nissen, S.E. (2006). ADHD drugs and cardiovascular risk. *N. Engl. J. Med.* 354 (14): 1445–1448.

Niwa, H., Shibutani, T., Hori, T. et al. (1996). The interaction between pindolol and epinephrine contained in local anesthetic solution to the left ventricular diastolic filling velocity in normal subjects. *Anesth. Prog.* 43 (3): 78–84.

Oliver, L.P. (1974). Local anesthesia—a review of practice. *Aust. Dent. J.* 19 (5): 313–319.

Pasternack, P.F., Colvin, S.B., and Baumann, F.G. (1985). Cocaine-induced angina pectoris and acute myocardial infarction in patients younger than 40 years. *Am. J. Cardiol.* 55 (6): 847.

Persson, G. and Siwers, B. (1975). The risk of potentiating effect of local anaesthesia with adrenalin in patients treated with tricyclic antidepressants. *Swed. Dent. J.* 68 (1): 9–18.

Perusse, R., Goulet, J.-P., and Turcotte, J.-Y. (1992a). Contraindications to vasoconstrictors in dentistry: part I. Cardiovascular diseases. *Oral Surg. Oral Med. Oral Pathol.* 74 (5): 679–686.

Perusse, R., Goulet, J.-P., and Turcotte, J.-Y. (1992b). Contraindications to vasoconstrictors in dentistry: Part II. Hyperthyroidism, diabetes, sulfite sensitivity, cortico-dependent asthma, and pheochromocytoma. *Oral Surg. Oral Med. Oral Pathol.* 74 (5): 687–691.

Plouin, P.F., Degoulet, P., Tugaye, A. et al. (1981). Le dépistage du phéochromocytoma: chez quels hypertension?: etude sémiologique chez 2585 hypertensos don't 11 ayant un phéochromocytoma. *Nouv Presse Med.* 10 (11): 869–872.

Plowman, P.E., Thomas, W.J.W., and Thurlow, A.C. (1974). Cardiac dysrhythmias during anaesthesia for oral surgery. The effect of local blockade. *Anaesthesia* 29 (5): 571–575.

Proskey, A.J., Saksena, F., and Towne, W.D. (1977). Myocardial infarction associated with thyrotoxicosis. *Chest* 72 (1): 109–111.

Rahn, R. and Ball, B. (2001). Articaine and epinephrine for dental anesthesia. In: *Local Anesthesia in Dentistry*. Seefeld (Germany): 3M ESPE AG. 29–33.

Rahn, A.O. and Drone, J.B. (1967). Dental aspects of the problems, care, and treatment of the irradiated oral cancer patient. *J. Am. Dent. Assoc.* 74 (5): 957–966.

Reeves, R.A., Boer, W.H., DeLeve, L., and Leenen, F.H.H. (1984). Non selective beta-blockade enhances pressor responsiveness to epinephrine, norepinephrine, and angiotensin II in normal man. *Clin. Pharmacol. Ther.* 35 (4): 461–466.

Rehling, M., Svendsen, T.L., Maltbaek, N. et al. (1986). Haemodynamic effects of atenolol, pindolol and propranolol during adrenaline infusion in man. *Eur. J. Clin. Pharmacol.* 30 (6): 659–663.

Roberts, D.H. and Sowray, J.H. (1987). *Local Analgesia in Dentistry*, 3e. Bristol (UK): Wright. 34, 70–72.

Roca, J., Caturla, M.C., Hjemdahl, P. et al. (1993). Effects of adrenaline on ventricular function and coronary haemodynamics in relation to catecholamine handling in transplanted human hearts. *Eur. Heart J.* 14 (4): 474–483.

Rodríguez, A.L. and Reneses, A. (2002). Manejo de los fármacos en el tratamiento de la depresión. *Infor. Terap. SS (Madrid)* 26 (1): 1–8.

Rothwell, B.R. (1987). Prevention and treatment of the orofacial complications of radiotherapy. *J. Am. Dent. Assoc.* 114 (3): 316–322.

Schachne, J.S., Roberts, B.H., and Thompson, P.D. (1984). Coronary-artery spasm and myocardial infarction associated with cocaine use (letter). *N. Engl. J. Med.* 310 (25): 1665–1666.

Schoot van der, J.B. and Moran, N.C. (1965). An experimental evaluation of the reputed influence of thyroxine on the cardiovascular effects of catecholamines. *J. Pharmacol. Exp. Ther.* 149 (3): 336–345.

Schwartz, H.J. and Sher, T.H. (1985). Bisulfite sensitivity manifesting as allergy to local dental anesthesia. *J. Allergy Clin. Immunol.* 75 (4): 525–527.

Schwartz, H.J., Gilbert, I.A., Lenner, K.A. et al. (1989). Metabisulfite sensitivity and local dental anesthesia. *Ann. Allergy* 62 (2): 83–86.

Scully, C. and Epstein, J.B. (1996). Oral health care for the cancer patient. *Eur. J. Cancer B Oral. Oncol.* 32B (5): 281–292.

Seng, G.F. and Gay, B.J. (1986). Dangers of sulfites in dental local anesthetic solutions: warning and recommendations. *J. Am. Dent. Assoc.* 113 (5): 769–770.

Simon, R.A. (1986). Sulfite sensitivity. *Ann. Allergy* 56 (4): 281–291.

Steinbacher, D.M. and Glick, M. (2001). The patient with asthma. An update and oral health considerations. *J. Am. Dent. Assoc.* 132 (9): 1229–1239.

Stepke, M.T.H., Schwenzer, N., and Eichhorn, W. (1994). Vasoconstrictors during pregnancy – in vitro trial on pregnant and nonpregnant mouse uterus. *Int. J. Oral Maxillofac. Surg.* 23 (6 Pt 2): 440–442.

Sugimura, M., Hirota, Y., Shibutani, T. et al. (1995). An echocardiographic study of interactions between pindolol and epinephrine contained in local anesthetic solutions. *Anesth. Prog.* 42 (2): 29–35.

Sunada, K., Nakamura, K., Yamashiro, M. et al. (1996). Clinically safe dosage of felypressin for patients with essential hypertension. *Anesth. Prog.* 43 (4): 108–115.

Sutton, M.G., Sheps, S.G., and Lie, J.T. (1981). Prevalence of clinically unsuspected pheochromocytoma. Review of a 50 year autopsy series. *Mayo Clin. Proc.* 56 (6): 354–369.

Svedmyr, N. (1968). The influence of tricyclic antidepressive agent (protriptyline) on some of circulatory effects of noradrenaline and adrenaline in man. *Life Sci.* 7 (1): 77–84.

Symmes, J.C., Lenkei, S.C.M., and Berman, N.D. (1977). Myocardial infarction, hyperthyroidism and normal coronary arteries: report of two cases. *Can. Med. Assoc. J.* 117 (5): 489–491.

Tainter, M.L., Tullar, B.F., and Luduena, F.P. (1949). Levo-arterenol. *Science (Washington)* 107 (2767): 39–40.

Topazian, D.S. (1959). Prevention of osteoradionecrosis of the jaws. *Oral Surg. Oral Med. Oral Pathol.* 12 (5): 530–538.

Tye, A., Patil, P.N., and LaPidus, J.B. (1967). Steric aspects of adrenergic drugs. III. Sensitization by cocaine to isomers of sympathomimetic amines. *J. Pharmacol. Exp. Ther.* 155 (1): 24–30.

Van Dyke, C., Barash, P.G., Jatlow, P., and Byck, R. (1976). Cocaine: plasma concentrations after intranasal application in man. *Science (Washington)* 191 (4229): 859–861.

Varma, D.R., Sharma, K.K., and Arora, R.C. (1976). Response to adrenaline and propranolol in hyperthyroidism (letter). *Lancet* 1 (7953): 260.

Weiss, R.J. (1986). Recurrent myocardial infarction caused by cocaine abuse. *Am. Heart J.* 111 (4): 793.

Weiss, B., Prozialeck, W., and Cimino, M. (1980). Acute and chronic effects of psychoactive drugs on adrenergic receptors and calmodulin. *Adv. Cyclic Nucleotide Res.* 12: 213–215.

Wilson, W.R., Theilen, E.O., Hege, J.H., and Valenca, M.R. (1966). Effects of beta-adrenergic receptor blockade in normal subjects before, during and after triiodothyronine-induced hypermetabolism. *J. Clin. Invest.* 45 (7): 1159–1169.

Wilson, K.E., Dorman, M.L., Moore, P.A., and Girdler, N.M. (2008). Pain control and anxiety management for periodontal therapies. *Periodontol 2000* 46: 42–55.

Wong, J.K., Wood, R.E., and McLean, M. (1997). Conservative management of osteoradionecrosis. *Oral Surg. Oral Med. Oral Pathol.* 84 (1): 16–21.

Yagiela, J.A. (1999). Adverse drug interactions in dental practice: interactions associated with vasoconstrictors. Part V of a series. *J. Am. Dent. Assoc.* 130 (5): 701–709.

Yagiela, J.A., Duffin, S.R., and Hunt, L.M. (1983). Drugs interactions involving vasoconstrictors in local anesthetic solutions. *J. Dent. Res.* 62 (Special issue: AADR abstracts): 231. (Abstract no 562).

Yagiela, J.A., Duffin, S.R., and Hunt, L.M. (1985). Drug interactions and vasoconstrictors used in local anesthetic solutions. *Oral Surg. Oral Med. Oral Pathol.* 59 (6): 565–571.

Zhang, C., Banting, D.W., Gelb, A.W., and Hamilton, J.T. (1999). Effect of β-adrenoreceptor blockade with nadolol on the duration of local anesthesia. *J. Am. Dent. Assoc.* 130 (12): 1773–1780.

# Instruments and Topical Anesthesia

## 11

## Instrument Set and Equipment

In this chapter, we examine the armamentarium for dental local anesthesia, mainly needles, cartridges, syringes, and other instruments.

## Needles

Needles enable the local anesthetic solution to pass from the cartridge to the tissues surrounding the tip. Current dental needles are disposable (single-use) and double-tipped for use in cartridge-type syringes (ISO 7885: 2010). They were introduced in 1959 (Dobbs 1965) and the early 1960s (Bedrock et al. 1999; Pogrel 2009), and are recommended for use in dentistry by the Council on Dental Materials and Devices of the American Dental Association (ADA) (Alling and Christopher 1974). This type of needle has the advantage that it resolves some of the older problems (Alling and Christopher 1974), namely, loss of sharpness and barbing owing to repeated use, breakage of the needle owing to metal fatigue, and cross-infection resulting from the needle being used in more than one patient.

Needles come in individual wrappers and are sealed with protective caps that maintain the sterility ensured during manufacture using ethylene oxide or gamma irradiation (Oikarinen and Perkki 1975a; Council on Dental Materials 1986).

Needles are made of *flexible stainless steel* (18/8 type) to prevent them from breaking if bent. According to the manufacturer, the metal contains up to 17 compounds, the most important being iron, chrome, and nickel (Oikarinen and Perkki 1975a). It is important to note that the manufacturing technique and the composition can affect the characteristics of rigidity and deflection (Robinson et al. 1984; Van der Bijl and Rossouw 1996).

Modern disposable dental needles of all lengths and gauges are *very resistant to breakage* resulting from traction or bending and easily exceed safety standards (Oikarinen and Perkki 1975a; Cooley and Robinson 1979; Robinson et al. 1984; Van der Bijl and Rossouw 1996; Tomas et al. 2000). Nonetheless, it is important to note the following: (i) the finest 30G needles are weaker than thicker gauges (27 and 25G) (Oikarinen and Perkki 1975a; Robinson et al. 1984; Tomas et al. 2000; Pietruszka et al. 1986; Bhatia and Bounds 1998; Zelster et al. 2002) and (ii) the hub is the weakest part of the needle and the point where most break (Pietruszka et al. 1986; Bhatia and Bounds 1998; Zelster et al. 2002).

### Parts of a Needle

Modern double-tipped disposable needles comprise the following parts (Figure 11.1).

**Anterior Part**

This is the active part of the needle, which penetrates the tissues and is in turn made up of the following:

- The shaft, or shank. This is the external part, which is characterized by being very polished and smooth (Van der Bijl 1995), as well as being covered by a thin layer of silicone to ensure that the shaft passes easily through the tissue with the least resistance, thus making the insertion less painful (Winther and Petersen 1979; Van der Bijl 1995). The silicone layer also helps to prevent oxidation of the metallic surface (Van der Bijl 1995).
- Tip. Current needle tips are tribevel with an eccentric bevel on one side, a main bevel, and two secondary bevels on the beveled surface of the main bevel (Figure 11.2). This modern concept is based on multibevel tips or scalpel points ensure the best possible edge and reduce the force of penetration, thus decreasing pain and injury in the mucosa and tissues (Winther and Petersen 1979; Lehtinen and Oksala 1979). The bevel angles are also shallow (9–12°) to reduce deflection as the needle crosses the tissues (Aldous 1968; Robinson et al. 1984; Stacy and Hajjar 1994; Meechan 2002).

---

*Local Anesthesia in Dentistry: A Locoregional Approach*, First Edition. Jesús Calatayud and Mana Saraghi.
© 2024 John Wiley & Sons Ltd. Published 2024 by John Wiley & Sons Ltd.
Companion website: www.wiley.com/go/Calatayud/local

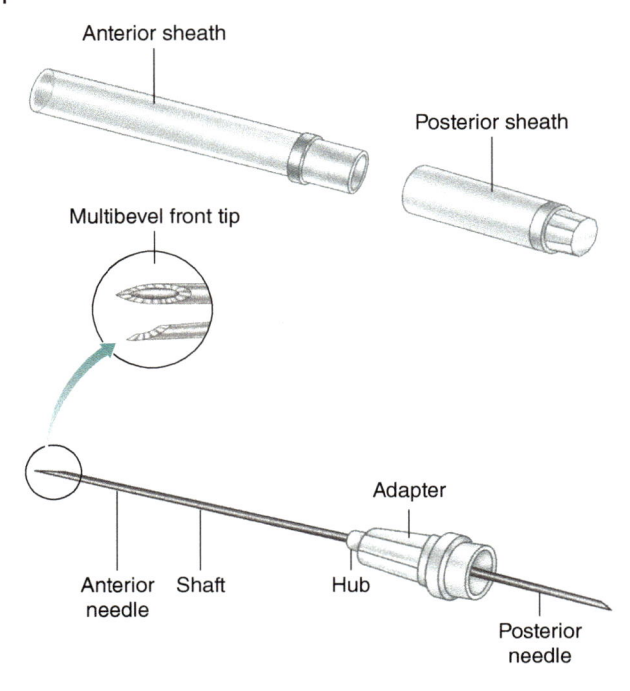

**Figure 11.1** Parts of a disposable double-tip needle. *Source:* Redrawn with modifications from Jastak et al. (1995).

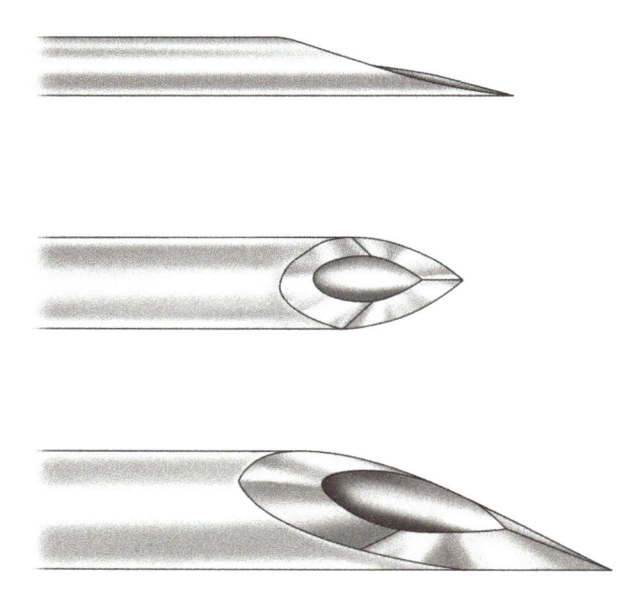

**Figure 11.2** Multibevel tip of double-tip disposable needles.

It is interesting to observe that once injected, the anesthetic solution spreads around the tip of the needle in an oval, with approximately equal quantities on both sides of the bevel.

### Middle Part
This part is in turn composed of two parts, the hub and the socket (adapter).

- The hub separates the anterior part of the needle from the posterior part. It is the weakest part and the point where the needle usually breaks, therefore the needle must never be completely inserted into the tissues up to the hub (Pietruszka et al. 1986; Bhatia and Bounds 1998; Zelster et al. 2002).
- The socket, or adapter, is the point where the needle is attached to the mouth of a cartridge-type syringe. Plastic sockets lack an internal thread. The thread is created by screwing the socket onto the threaded mouth of the syringe. Metallic sockets are already threaded. Many manufacturers place a triangle or arrow or some other mark on the socket to help the dentist align the needle with the bevel.

### Posterior Part
This is a shorter needle (17–25 mm) that perforates the diaphragm of the cartridge and is located inside the syringe. Its tip is beveled at a steeper angle (15–55°) (Meechan 2002). Manufacturers sometimes make the back part of the needle too short, in which case it does not perforate the diaphragm of the cartridge, or too long, thus leaving anesthetic solution inside the cartridge because the plunger cannot reach the final stage owing to its contact with the posterior part of the excessively long needle.

Of note, the lumen of the needle has a rough surface (Oikarinen and Perkki 1975a) (Figure 11.3) and a larger lumen does not make injections less painful (McPherson et al. 2015).

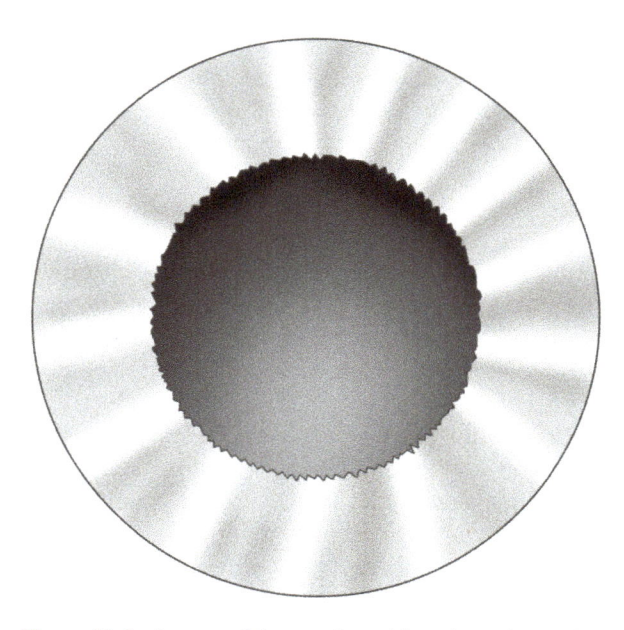

**Figure 11.3** Lumen of the needles with an irregular surface. *Source:* Drawn from Oikarinen and Perkki (1975a).

## Protective Sheath

This is the sheath that keeps the needle sterile and sealed. It is formed by two protective caps:

- The anterior cap, which covers the front, or active, part of the needle and is fitted to the socket or adapter.
- The posterior cap, which covers the short posterior needle and is fitted to the socket or adapter. At the same time, it overlies the anterior cap so that it is the first part to be removed when the seal is broken. The needle can be screwed into the anterior part or needle adapter of the syringe, while the anterior part of the needle remains covered and is protected.

Where the protective caps join, at the level of the adapter, there is a label showing the gauge, length, manufacturer, and expiry date of the needle (Meechan 2002).

## Lengths and Gauges

As we shall see, length and gauge (G) play a key role in the selection of needles for the various anesthetic techniques.

Table 11.1 shows the different lengths of needle in the active (anterior) part, which is that running from the hub to the tip. As we can see, there are three lengths – long, short, and extrashort – although each varies depending on the manufacturer. However, the most widely used lengths at present are shown.

The gauges used during the first half of the twentieth century were thick (20 or 23G), although after the Second World War new needles appeared. These were made of stainless steel and were much more resistant and flexible, therefore the gauge could be reduced to 25G (Harrison 1948). Each gauge has an external diameter (gauge) and an internal diameter (lumen): the smaller the gauge number, the thicker the external and internal diameters of the needle (Table 11.2). The main gauges used at present are 25, 27, and 30G. However, by far the most widely used is 27G (Alling and Christopher 1974).

## Needles: Critical Aspects

Needles are subject to limitations that should be clarified to facilitate appropriate choice and use.

Table 11.1 Lengths of needles.

| Type | Length Millimeters | Inches |
|---|---|---|
| Long | 41 | 1 5/8 |
|  | 38 | 1 1/2 |
|  | **35** | **1 3/8** |
|  | 30 | 1 1/8 |
| Short | **25** | **1** |
|  | 20 | 3/4 |
| Extra-short | **12** | **1/2** |
|  | 10 | — |
|  | 8 | 1/3 |

The most common gauges used in dentistry are shown in bold.

Table 11.2 Needle gauges.

| International gauge | Gauge France | External diameter Millimeters | Inches | Internal diameter Millimeters | Inches |
|---|---|---|---|---|---|
| 20G | 90/100 | 0.90 | 0.360 | — | — |
| 22G | 70/100 | 0.70 | 0.280 | — | — |
| 23G | 60/100 | 0.60 | 0.024 | 0.30 | 0.012 |
| **25G** | 50/100 | 0.50 | 0.020 | 0.25 | 0.010 |
| 26G | 45/100 | 0.45 | 0.018 | 0.25 | 0.010 |
| **27G** | 40/100 | 0.40 | 0.016 | 0.20 | 0.008 |
| 28G | 35/100 | 0.35 | 0.014 | 0.20 | 0.008 |
| **30G** | 30/100 | 0.30 | 0.012 | 0.15 | 0.006 |
| 32G | 26/100 | 0.26 | 0.010 | — | — |

The most common gauges used in dentistry are shown in bold.
*Source:* Data from Oikarinen and Perkki (1975a), Council on Dental Materials and Devices (1978), Trapp and Davies (1980), Lehtinen (1983), Jastak et al. (1995), Meechan (2002), Malamed (2004), Gaudy and Arreto (2005), and ISO 7885 (2010).

## Aspiration and Gauge

Poiseuille's law describes the relationship between diameter and resistance to flow of a liquid in a tube, intravenous catheter, or needle. The resistance to flow is inversely related to the radius to the fourth power. For example, if the internal diameter of the needle (lumen) is halved, the resistance to the flow of liquid inside the needle increases 16-fold (Wittrock and Fischer 1968). Furthermore, as blood transports formed elements (red cells, lipoproteins, etc.) (Guyton 1976), it is three to four times more viscous and dense than water, with the result that resistance is greater.

Both *in vitro* studies (Smith 1968a, 1968b; Wittrock and Fischer 1968; Cooley and Robinson 1979; Piesold et al. 1998) and clinical studies (Cohen et al. 1969; Watson and Colman 1976; Trapp and Davies 1980; Brownbill et al. 1987) have shown that blood can be aspirated with fine, narrow gauges (30G) and thick gauges (25G). However, the narrowest gauges (30G) have a slow and reduced aspiration flow rate, since they must overcome higher flow pressure (Smith 1968a, 1968b; Cooley and Robinson 1979; Piesold et al. 1998). In addition, the evaluation of a true positive aspiration requires a sufficient volume of aspirated blood such that a color change is noted in the cartridge (Watson and Colman 1976). For this reason, it is not advisable to use 30G needles and *we should use 27 and 25G needles to ensure that aspirated blood is present in sufficient quantities when a positive aspiration does indeed occur and can therefore be seen by the provider* (Cooley and Robinson 1979; Piesold et al. 1998).

## Pain and Gauge

Most dentists think that smaller calibers (30 and 27G) cause less pain during insertion and injection (Smith 1968a; Cooley and Robinson 1979; Mollen et al. 1981; Van der Bijl 1995). However, clinical studies indicate that there is little difference in the perception of pain; six clinical trials revealed no statistically significant differences in the pain produced by different gauges of needle (30, 27, and 25G) and a further two trials show that the finest 30G needle produces less pain than a 27G needle (Table 11.3). In any case, the differences are negligible (even if they are statistically significant, as in the latter two trials they were of minimal clinical relevance). With respect to needles, the truly important factors involved in injection pain are as follows:

1) Design of the tip. This is possibly the most important factor (Lehtinen and Oksala 1979) and the reason why modern needles are multibevel (Lehtinen and Oksala 1979; Winther and Petersen 1979).
2) The fine layer of silicone covering the surface of the shaft of the needle reduces resistance during insertion into tissue (Winther and Petersen 1979; Van der Bijl 1995).

**Table 11.3** Clinical trials that compare the pain caused by dental injection with needles of various gauges.

| Nonsignificant results | | Statistically significant results | |
|---|---|---|---|
| Reference | Gauge | Reference | Gauge |
| Fuller et al. (1979) | 30G, 27G, 25G | Ram et al. (2007) | **30G**, 27G |
| Mollen et al. (1981) | 27G, 25G | Ghasemi et al. (2014) | **30G**, 27G |
| Lehtinen (1983) | 30G, 27G | | |
| Brownbill et al. (1987) | 30G, 25G | | |
| Carr and Horton (2001) | 27G, 25G | | |
| Flanagan et al. (2007) | 30G, 27G, 25G | | |

The gauges that produce the least pain are shown in bold.

As we shall see in Chapter 13, possibly the most important individual factor involved in pain during insertion and injection is the skill/technique of the dentist (Mollen et al. 1981; Saloum et al. 2000; Goodell et al. 2000; Ram and Peretz 2003; Nusstein and Beck 2003).

## Deflection of the Needle and Gauge

Deep linear insertions (e.g. regional block, such as mandibular block) with cartridge-type syringes and the palm-thumb grasp (e.g. traditional technique) cause the needle to deflect as it advances owing to the quantity of tissue taken up by the lumen (Jeske and Boshart 1985). This *deflection is toward the tip*, that is, the side opposite the bevel (Cooley and Robinson 1979; Hochman and Friedman 2000). The factors affecting this deflection are as follows:

1) Gauge. The thicker the gauge, the more rigid the needle is and the less likely it is to deflect (Aldous 1968; Robinson et al. 1984; Jeske and Boshart 1985; Van der Bijl and Rossouw 1996; Hochman and Friedman 2000), therefore *25G needles (the thickest) are recommended for regional block* by specification no. 54 of the Council on Dental Materials, Instruments and Equipment of the ADA (Council on Dental Materials 1986), since these are the needles that are least likely to deflect.
2) Length. The longer the needle is, the more likely it is to deflect (Aldous 1968; Van der Bijl 1995).
3) Bevel. The greater the angle is, the more likely it is to deflect (Aldous 1968); this is why current bevels have shallow angles (9–18°) and the steep angles of previous versions are no longer used.

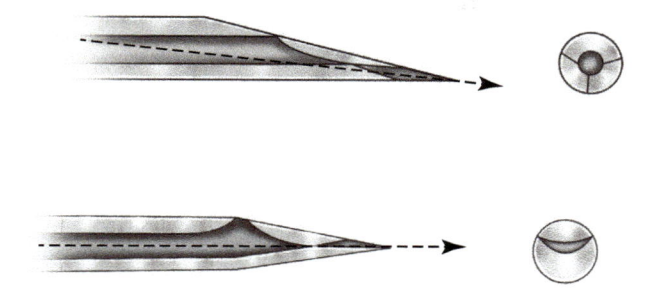

**Figure 11.4** Tip of nondeflecting needles (Truject®) vs. conventional needles.

4) Characteristics of the metal used and manufacturing techniques. Needles of the same gauge and length from different manufacturers deflect to different degrees (Robinson et al. 1984; Van der Bijl and Rossouw 1996).

The currently marketed fine 28G Truject® needle is almost nondeflective during deep linear insertions owing to the design of the tip, which is centered on the longitudinal axis of the needle (Figure 11.4). This decreases the central area by 75%, thus reducing the amount of tissue taken up in the lumen as the needle advances (Jeske and Boshart 1985). The point of traditional needles is situated eccentrically; if it is placed more centrally, the needle is less likely to deflect (Aldous 1968).

### Lesions Caused by a Barbed Needle

Repeated use in the same patient leads to loss of the edge at the tip in 80% of needles, thus causing tip of the needle to bend or barb (Oikarinen and Perkki 1975a). Barbing can be caused accidentally during preparation of the syringe (Jastak et al. 1995) – the most unusual cause – and during injection, when the needle meets the bone (Dentists' Desk 1983; Jastak et al. 1995; Malamed 2004).

When a barbed needle is removed and/or inserted at another site (especially if the tip of the needle is deflected outwards), it can damage the muscles (causing trismus), the nerve stems (causing long-lasting paresthesia), and the vessels (causing hemorrhage) (Stacy and Hajjar 1994).

It is difficult to see a barbed needle, although it is easily observed by wiping a sterile gauze across the tip, which catches in the material (Dentists' Desk 1983; Jastak et al. 1995). A barbed needle should be discarded and a new one selected; hence the recommendation to change the needle after two to four injections (Dentists' Desk 1983; Jastak et al. 1995; Malamed 2004).

### Breakage of Needles

One of the main causes of needle breakage is the use of unsuitable needles in truncal block, owing to the depth of the insertion. It is important to note the following causes:

1) The use of short needles that are inserted deep into the soft tissues as far as the hub, which is the weakest part, where the needle usually breaks (Pietruszka et al. 1986; Bhatia and Bounds 1998; Zelster et al. 2002). Around 50% of breakages in the dentist's office occur in this situation (Annex 37).
2) The use of fine-gauge needles (30G), which are the weakest and have proven to be more fragile *in vitro* (Oikarinen and Perkki 1975a; Robinson et al. 1984). Around 60% of breakages in mandibular block involve needles of this gauge (Annex 37).

In conclusion, in regional block techniques such as mandibular block, it is not recommended to use short needles, fine-gauge needles (e.g. 30G), or short and fine-gauge needles, *all of which account for more than 75% of cases of breakage* (Annex 37).

### Criteria for the Selection of Needles

Given the above, we can list practical criteria for selecting needles, depending on the technique and specific needs, as follows:

- Long 25G needles (the thickest) should be used for deep insertions in regional block, e.g. mandibular block, for several reasons:
  - This is the gauge that is least likely to deflect during deep insertions.
  - Aspiration is successful with 25G needles and in deep insertions positive aspirations are common.
  - The injection is no more painful than with smaller gauges (27G or 30G), as shown in clinical trials.
- Short 27G needles should be used for infiltrative techniques that require little depth but successful aspiration, for two reasons:
  - In these cases, a short needle is more comfortable than a long one.
  - Aspiration is successful if a vessel is punctured.
- Short or extra-short 30G needles are recommended in the following cases:
  - When it is not necessary to aspirate, since their ability to reveal truly positive aspirations is very poor (see Chapter 13).
  - When it is not necessary to inject deep into the tissue, since the needle deflects considerably more than with other gauges and is at greater risk of breakage.

## Cartridges

The cartridge is a cylindrical tube that encloses the anesthetic solution between an opening sealed by a rubber diaphragm at the anterior part and a plunger, or plug, at the

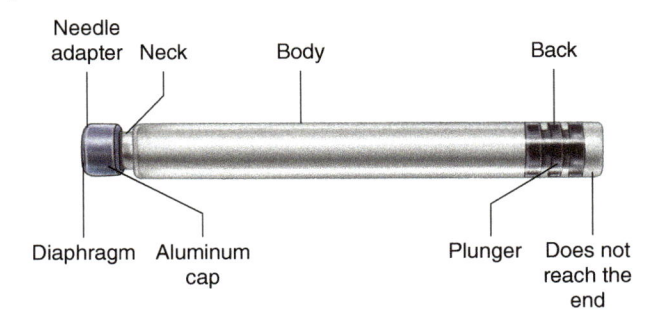

**Figure 11.5** Parts of a cartridge.

posterior part (Figure 11.5). Cartridges are disposable (a cartridge can only be used for one patient) and have several advantages:

1) They guarantee the sterility of the anesthetic solution.
2) They are easy and quick to load and clean. Modern cartridges do not require the dentist to break the ampule, draw up local anesthetic, and expel the air, therefore the dentist's skin does not come into contact with the solution, which may spill during these maneuvers.
3) They prevent contact with the metal of the syringe. Acidic solutions with epinephrine and other sympathomimetic vasoconstrictors interact with metals to release metal ions (nickel, zinc, copper) that irritate tissues and cause pain on injection, especially copper ions (Lundqvist et al. 1948).

Cartridges were introduced in 1920 by the army surgeon Harvey S. Cook, who compared them to a rifle cartridge, in the sense that one cartridge per patient is loaded and "fired" (Dobbs 1965). The Cook-Waite company subsequently introduced the cartridge with the commercial name "Carpule", which became so popular that many professionals today use the term "carpule" for all cartridges (Nevin and Putterbaugh 1949).

Cartridge volume is worthy of comment. Initially, cartridges contained 1, 2, and 2.5 ml (Nevin and Putterbaugh 1949). The 2-ml cartridges contained 1.8 ml of anesthetic solution, with 0.2 ml taken up by the plunger. From 1950 onward, the standard 1.8-ml cartridge became widely used (Gruber 1950). At present, use of these cartridges is standard practice throughout the world (Dentists' Desk 1983; Malamed 2004). They measure 63–65 mm in length and 8–9 mm in diameter (Meechan 2002). The cartridges make it possible to inject up to 1.7 ml of anesthetic solution since the other 0.1 ml is trapped in the neck of the cartridge between the diaphragm and the plunger (Cannell et al. 1975).

Cartridges containing 2 and 2.2 ml are currently available, but only in certain countries, such as the United Kingdom and Australia. They are used less frequently because, being longer, holding the syringe is difficult when the dentist has small hands, thus hampering the aspiration maneuver.

The tube is made of one of two materials: (i) glass, which is better quality, with the result that most anesthetic solutions come in this type of container, and (ii) plastic, which is only used in some countries and is worse, for the following reasons:

1) The plunger does not move as easily or as smoothly against plastic as against glass (Jastak et al. 1995; Malamed 2004).
2) Plastic is less transparent, thus making it more difficult to evaluate positive aspirations (Jastak et al. 1995).
3) Spills and leaks of solution are more common during injection than with glass cartridges (Malamed 2004).
4) Resistance to pressure is half that of glass cartridges, therefore they are not recommended for the periodontal ligament technique (Table 18.2, Chapter 18). Plastic cartridges have the advantage that they do not break under pressure, but the tube becomes deformed and the anesthetic solution leaks out (Meechan et al. 1990).

Of particular interest is the fact that the diaphragm and the plunger contain small quantities of latex, therefore latex allergens may be present in the solution (Brown et al. 2002). However, to date there have been no reports of allergy to latex via local anesthetic cartridges (Shojaei and Haas 2002).

## Parts of a Cartridge

### Anterior Part or Needle Adapter

This part comprises the diaphragm, a fine latex membrane through which the needle penetrates, and the aluminum cap, which is generally silver in color and surrounds and holds the diaphragm to the needle adapter (Figure 11.5). The aluminum must not come into contact with the local anesthetic solution, since this can speed up the degradation of sympathomimetic vasoconstrictors such as epinephrine (Milano et al. 1982).

### Neck

The needle adapter is joined to the body by a narrowing of the glass tube, where 0.1 ml of anesthetic solution is trapped and therefore cannot be injected (Cannell et al. 1975).

### Cylindrical Body

The body is made of transparent glass in order to see blood clearly in positive aspirations and the volume injected via the movement of the plunger. The cylinder is the body of the syringe. As the plunger advances down the syringe pushed by the piston of the syringe, it can inject the solution via the needle.

**Posterior Part**

The posterior part contains the plunger or rubber stopper that is inside the cylindrical tube. This rubber stopper does not reach the end of the tube; if it does reach the end, then this could indicate that the solution is contaminated. The harpoon of the piston is attached to the rubber stopper and thus enables aspiration. Its main function is to move along the cylindrical tube pushed by the piston to inject the anesthetic solution.

The plunger may be solid, which is the most usual case, so that it can attach to the harpoon or the plunger support system. Less often, it is hollow to house a special system such as the blades of the Uniject® syringe (Meechan 2002).

**Other Elements**

- Silicone lubricant on the interior surface of the cylinder enables the plunger to slide smoothly along the glass tube. This lubricant was previously paraffin (wax) or glycerin. Both compounds could harden with time or with low ambient temperatures, thus creating resistance to the movement of the plunger or making it move along in fits and starts, especially at the beginning of the maneuver (blocked or sticky stopper).
- There is a transparent security foil on the surface of the cylinder. The foil serves the following purposes:
  o To prevent pieces of glass falling into the patient's mouth by limiting uncontrolled shattering of the cartridge if it breaks owing to excessive pressure during injection (e.g. during the periodontal ligament technique) (Rawson and Orr III 1985) or if it is cracked/split because of damage during transport (see Chapter 21).
  o To facilitate administration of the exact volume of anesthesia by means of a line along the axis of the cartridge that acts as a volume indicator (graduated scale).
  o To provide information on the name of the anesthetic solution and vasoconstrictor, concentrations, commercial name, lot number, and date of expiry.
- Content color code. This code may be a colored ring around the cylinder or the color of the rubber stopper or the aluminum cap at the needle adapter. A ring code system is used in the United States but not in Europe, where manufacturers have their own codes, therefore different brands can use the same colors on cartridges with different contents.

## Storage of Cartridges

To ensure optimal performance with good preservation of the active ingredients, cartridges should be stored following a series of norms that can be divided in two groups: those that apply to all cartridges and those that also apply to cartridges containing sympathomimetic vasoconstrictors.

**Norms for All Cartridges**

1) *Store in their original packaging* (Passon et al. 1992). Cartridges are not airtight compartments and may be contaminated by chemical vapors (Chasteen et al. 1988; Passon et al. 1992) via penetration of the rubber part of the diaphragm or the plunger (Passon et al. 1992); however, the package is completely closed and sealed.

   Packages come in two formats: vacuum packed cans with 50 cartridges, which are rarely used today, and, more frequently, packages with five blister packs each containing 10 perfectly sealed and closed cartridges (the packages may also contain 10 blister packs).

2) Store in a *dry place*, since humidity tends to deteriorate both the packages and the cartridges.

3) Return damaged or deteriorated packages because the cartridges may be cracked or split and thus carry a risk of breakage during injection and/or loss of stability of the anesthetic solution (Meechan 2002; Malamed 2004). Cartridges should also be returned if the aluminum cap of the diaphragm in the needle adapter is dented or damaged, since the underlying glass may also be broken (Malamed 2004).

Cartridges should never be stored in the following ways:

- Submerged in disinfectant, since this can penetrate the cartridge and contaminate the anesthetic solution, leading to painful injections and long-term paresthesia (Shannon and Feller 1972; Shannon and Wescottt 1974).
- Together with products that release chemical vapors, such as resin solvents, since these too can penetrate the cartridge (Chasteen et al. 1988; Passon et al. 1992).

**Norms for Cartridges Containing Catecholamines**

Sympathomimetic vasoconstrictors such as epinephrine, norepinephrine, and levonordefrin are all very sensitive to degradation, therefore the expiry date appears on the cartridge (Hondrum et al. 1993). In addition to the abovementioned norms, these cartridges are subject to additional storage conditions:

1) *Darkness*, given that light speeds up oxidation of the vasoconstrictors, especially epinephrine. By light, we mean daylight (Gerke et al. 1977; Thoma and Struve 1986), fluorescent light in rooms (Hondrun and Ezell 1996), and ultraviolet light (Ciarlone and Fry 1980).

2) The recommended storage temperature is 20–22 °C (68–72 °F), which is equivalent to ambient temperature,

with minimum and maximum values of *15–30 °C (59–86 °F)* (Hondrum et al. 1993). High temperatures speed up oxidation of the catecholamines and therefore their degradation (Fry and Ciarlone 1980; Kelly and Dalm 1985; Thoma and Struve 1986), thus cartridges should never be kept in cartridge warmers for long periods.

3) *Packages indicating that more than half of the lifetime of the drug has passed, that is 18 months, should be rejected before the expiry date* (Dentists' Desk 1983; Jastak et al. 1995), since the duration of the solution is 3 years. Solutions previously lasted for a shorter period when they were in good condition (Gerke et al. 1977), although with new manufacturing and packaging techniques, we can extend the optimal time point until 18 months.

Studies of stored samples that have not yet reached their expiry date show that the drugs are well preserved and adhere to the minimum levels set by the United States Pharmacopeia (USP) (Kirchhoefer et al. 1986a, 1986b; Smith 1991). Nevertheless, as time passes, it is important to bear in mind the following:

- Anesthetics become more painful as their pH decreases (Oikarinen et al. 1975b; Moorthy et al. 1984; Crose 1991), since the sulfites become sulfates and release protons (Hondrun and Ezell 1996).
- Solutions lose potency as a result of the decrease in the concentration of sympathomimetic vasoconstrictor (epinephrine): as time passes, the solution will contain lower quantities of antioxidant (sulfite), which protects it (Smith 1991; Hondrun and Ezell 1996), even if minimum levels are maintained (Smith 1991).

## Problems Affecting Cartridges

Dental local anesthetic cartridges may be subject to some of the following problems:

1) Small bubbles (<1–2 mm). These are the remnants of nitrogen used during manufacture to eliminate air and oxygen from anesthetic solutions containing sympathomimetic vasoconstrictors and thus extend the half-life of the catecholamines (Milano et al. 1982; Thoma and Struve 1986). These bubbles are harmless, and the cartridges can be used without risk for the patient (Dentists' Desk 1983; Jastak et al. 1995; Malamed 2004).
2) Signs indicating that the cartridge has been frozen, namely, large bubbles (>2 mm, the main sign), extruded plunger, and suspended particles. When a cartridge has been frozen and then thawed, suspended particles may remain inside (Hondrum et al. 1993). These are formed by the residue of lubricants such as silicone or paraffin (Cooley and Lubow 1981). Furthermore, the extruded plunger may compromise sterilization of the solution, therefore these cartridges must be withdrawn (Dentists' Desk 1983; Jastak et al. 1995; Malamed 2004). Of interest, lidocaine with epinephrine solution freezes at −3 °C (Hondrum et al. 1993).
3) Extruded plunger. This situation is the result of a plunger being frozen (see above) or of contamination of the anesthetic solution. The contamination may have been caused by chemical vapors (Chasteen et al. 1988) or by submerging the cartridge in disinfectant solution (Shannon and Feller 1972; Shannon and Wescottt 1974). In both cases, the contaminant enters the cartridge via the semipermeable membranes, that is, the diaphragm of the needle adapter or, even more likely, via the rubber stopper (Fyhr and Brodin 1987; Passon et al. 1992). In any case, the cartridges should not be used owing to the risk of injecting the patient with solution contaminated by chemical products.
4) Corroded/rusted aluminum cap. When the corrosion is white in color, it usually means that the cartridge has been placed in a quaternary ammonium disinfectant, which tends to cause an electrolytic reaction (Dentists' Desk 1983; Jastak et al. 1995; Malamed 2004). When the corrosion is red in color, it means that in the box where cartridge was stored another cartridge has broken and its liquids have rusted the metal of the cap (Dentists' Desk 1983; Malamed 2004). The cartridge should be disposed of in both cases.
5) Abnormal appearance of the anesthetic solution inside the cartridge (Jastak et al. 1995). The cartridge should be disposed of in the following cases:
   - Yellow, brown, or dark-brown color. This is caused by oxidation of epinephrine resulting from the formation of melanins and other inactive compounds. While not toxic, the solution lacks vasoconstrictive activity (Smith 1920).
   - Particles and sediments from lubricant residue on the plunger (silicone, paraffin, glycerin) after freezing (Cooley and Lubow 1981).
   - Milky color due to contamination by chemical vapors (Chasteen et al. 1988; Passon et al. 1992) or bacterial contamination (Meechan 2002).

## Degradation of Drugs in the Cartridge

The half-life of a drug is the time between its manufacture (manufacture and packaging) and the point where its biological activity falls below 90%. The physical and safety properties of the drug are maintained throughout this period (Hondrum et al. 1993). The life of local anesthetic solutions is determined by sympathomimetic vasoconstrictors since local anesthetic is very resistant to degradation (Hondrum et al. 1993). Below, we discuss the degradation of various compounds of local anesthetic solutions inside cartridges.

**Local Anesthesia**

Local anesthetics undergo hydrolysis, although they are very resistant to degradation and can last up to 6 years in storage at extreme temperatures without deteriorating (Hondrum et al. 1993).

**Sympathomimetic Vasoconstrictors (Epinephrine)**

Unlike local anesthetics, catecholamines are very vulnerable to degradation, therefore the active half-life and expiry date of the solutions are marked on the cartridges (Hondrum et al. 1993). These drugs degrade in three ways:

- Oxidation (the main route). Oxidation is the loss of electrons by an atom with addition of oxygen or removal of hydrogen in the organic molecules (Hondrum et al. 1993). The oxidative pathway of epinephrine in aqueous solutions is shown in Table 11.4. Oxidation has various causes: oxygen (Milano et al. 1982: Hondrum et al. 1993), increases in pH (Fyhr and Brodin 1987), given that above pH 6 the solution degrades in a few hours (de Jong and Cullen 1963), increases in temperature (Gerke et al. 1977; Fry and Ciarlone 1980; Thoma and Struve 1986), and sunlight or fluorescent/ultraviolet light (Gerke et al. 1977; Ciarlone and Fry 1980; Thoma and Struve 1986; Hondrum et al. 1993).
- Racemization. Racemization is the conversion from the levo/levoisomer form, which is 15–20 times more potent, to the dextro/dextroisomer form to create a mixture of the two (racemic mixture) that has half the vasoconstrictive potency (see Chapter 6). The main cause of this transformation is the fall in pH below pH 2 (Milano et al. 1982). Other, less important causes are increases in temperature and light (Hondrum et al. 1993).

**Table 11.4** Oxidative pathway of epinephrine in aqueous solutions.

Epinephrine
↓
Leucoadrenochrome
↓
Adrenochrome (red)
↓
Adrenolutin (yellow or brown)
↓
Melanins (Brown) nonvasoactive

*Source:* Data from: Milano et al. (1982), Kirchhoefer et al. (1986b).

- Degradation by sulfites (sulfonation). Sulfites protect epinephrine and vasoconstrictive catecholamines from oxidation, but they also produce anaerobic degradation of these substances (Hajratwala 1975; Fyhr and Brodin 1987). However, fortunately, the process is very slow (Milano et al. 1982; Fyhr and Brodin 1987; Hondrum et al. 1993). Epinephrine becomes epinephrine sulfonic acid via this pathway. The main causes of this process are time and, to a much lesser extent, soluble aluminum, which speeds up the reaction (Milano et al. 1982).

To better preserve sympathomimetic vasoconstrictors inside the cartridge, the options available are as follows: (i) degasification with nitrogen to eliminate oxygen during the manufacture of anesthetic solutions (Milano et al. 1982; Thoma and Struve 1986), (ii) maintaining an acid pH (2.7–5.5) (USP 38 2015), because this helps to keep vasoconstrictive amines stable, and (iii) adding sulfites as antioxidants, since this extends the active life of these vasoconstrictors by preventing the oxygen that enters the cartridge from inactivating the amine through oxidation (Milano et al. 1982; Klein 1983; Hondrum et al. 1993) and helps to maintain an acidic pH.

**Sulfites**

On oxidation, sulfites become sulfates and release two protons that tend to reduce the pH of local anesthetic solutions. This transformation is caused by oxygen entering the cartridge and increased temperature and light (Hondrum and Ezell 1991, 1996).

## Syringes

The syringe is the instrument that contains the cartridge. The needle through which the anesthetic is injected is also screwed to the syringe. Today, standard dental syringes are made of metal (chrome or stainless steel), thus making them robust, long-lasting, and sterilizable. They vary according to the manufacturer and enable use of local anesthetic cartridges and aspiration before injection. They are used with one hand and are designed for a thumb-palm or palm-thumb grasp (Figure 11.6) and linear insertion (Council on Dental Materials and Devices 1974, 1978). This is the most widely used dental syringe today, therefore we call it the conventional cartridge-type syringe.

### Parts of a Cartridge-type Syringe

#### Anterior Part or Needle Adapter

This is the part where the disposable double-tipped needle is screwed onto the adapter (Figure 11.7).

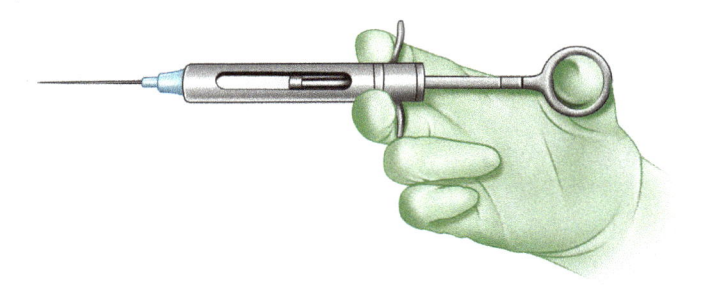

**Figure 11.6** Palm-thumb grasp.

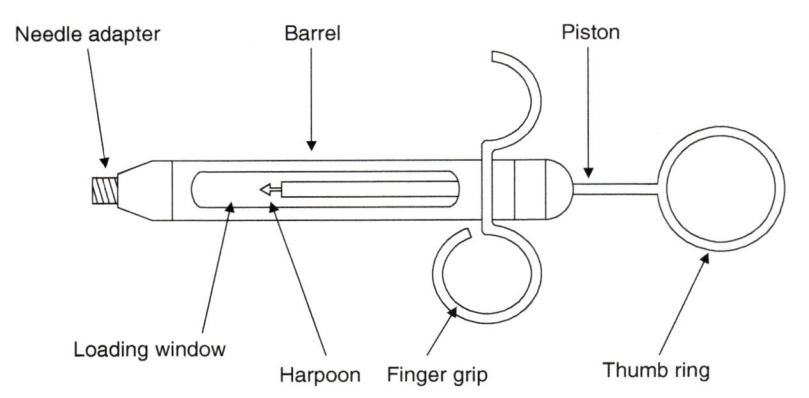

**Figure 11.7** Parts of a cartridge-type syringe.

There are two types of thread: the European thread and the American thread.

### Syringe Barrel or Body of the Syringe
The barrel is cylindrical and houses the cartridge. It has the advantage of a longitudinal loading window for insertion of the cartridge and a window on the opposite side so that the cartridge is visible in any position. We can then determine whether or not there has been a positive aspiration or know the amount of anesthetic that is injected at a given time.

### Posterior Part (Back)
The posterior part has a finger support on the external part of the body of the syringe. The dentist uses this to support the index and middle finger and thus hold the syringe. The internal part contains a spring to better adjust the cartridge to the barrel so that it does not come out.

### Piston
The piston is a cylindrical barrel that enters the posterior part of the syringe. Its functions are to perform aspiration by pulling the plunger or rubber stopper backwards and to do the opposite, namely, push the rubber stopper forward to inject the solution across the needle.

The piston comprises two parts. The anterior part is composed of the system for holding the cartridge by means of a harpoon or spiral that enables the piston to attach to the plunger and thus pull the plunger backward and perform the aspiration (Council on Dental Materials and Devices 1978; Council on Dental Materials 1982). The posterior part comprises the thumb ring (Figure 11.7), where the thumb is placed to pull the piston back, perform the aspiration, and push forward to inject the anesthetic solution across the needle.

## Using the Syringe

### Set-up
1) Retract the piston so that the spring of the posterior part of the barrel moves backward and leaves free space for the cartridge in the body of the syringe.
2) Load the cartridge by the lateral loading window so that the anterior part faces the anterior part of the syringe and with the posterior part toward the posterior part of the syringe (Figure 11.8).
3) Attach the piston support system to the plunger or rubber stopper of the cartridge by pressing firmly while avoiding force that can break the cartridge. Remember that if the plunger is not attached firmly when aspirating, then the piston will become unattached.
4) Remove the posterior cap of the double-tipped needle to leave the adapter and the posterior needle open (Figure 11.9).
5) Screw the needle to the anterior part of the needle adapter of the syringe with the anterior cap still in place and place a protective disk over the cap (Figure 11.10).
6) Hold the syringe with the palm-thumb grasp (Figure 11.6).

### Dismantling
1) Replace, using one hand only, the anterior cap with the protective disk over the needle (anterior or active

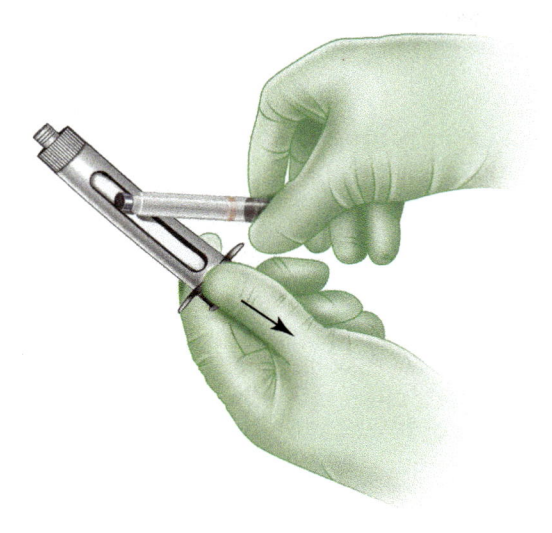

**Figure 11.8** Loading the cartridge by the lateral window after pulling the piston backwards to leave space for the cartridge.

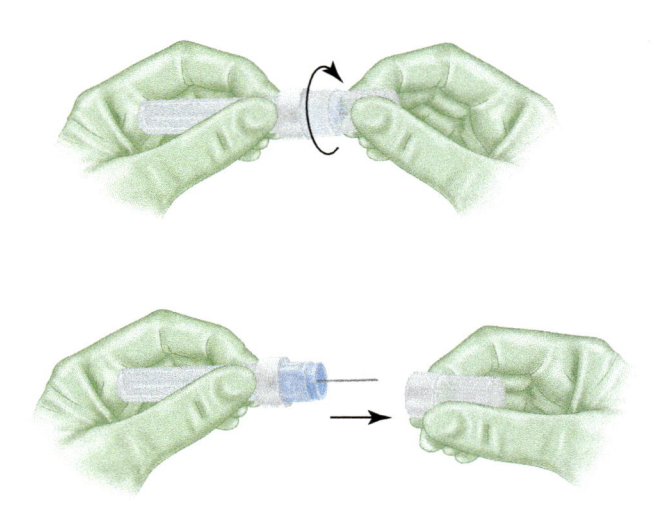

**Figure 11.9** Removal of the back cap of the needle.

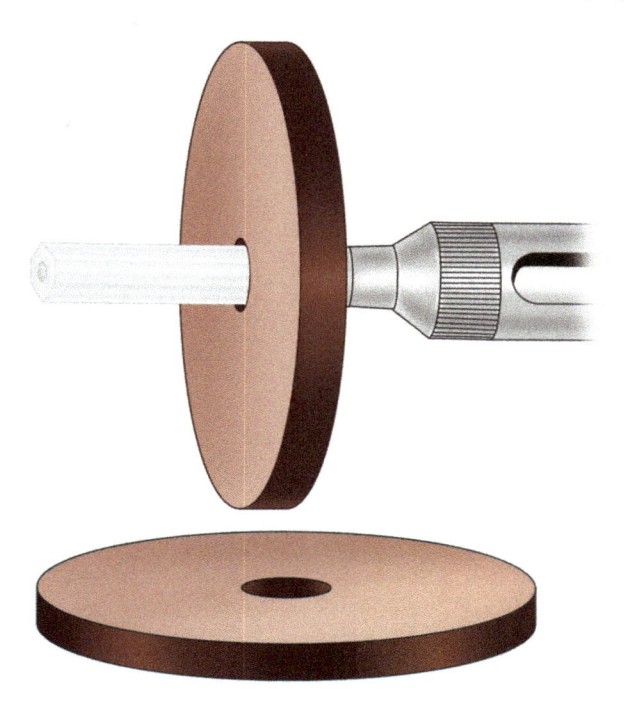

**Figure 11.10** Protective disk.

needle). Recapping with two hands has a higher risk of a needle stick injury.

2) Unscrew the needle of the adapter of the syringe and place it in the sharps container, always holding the needle by the cap of the anterior part and the protective disk so as to avoid needle stick injury.
3) Disconnect the piston of the plunger from the cartridge.
4) Pull the piston backwards until it is disconnected from the body of the empty cartridge and loosen the spring from the back part of the barrel of the cartridge to release it.
5) Pull the empty cartridge out through the loading window.
6) Another cartridge can be loaded using the maneuvers described above.

### Cleaning and Sterilization

- Clean the syringe after use with cold water to remove any remaining anesthetic solution, saliva, or disinfectant, which may form deposits over time and must then be removed using brushes and ultrasound baths.
- Sterilize the syringe before use on another patient (Council on Dental Materials and Devices 1974, 1978).

## Self-aspirating Syringes

Self-aspirating syringes are a variant of the conventional metal cartridge-type syringes, although they take advantage of the elasticity of the diaphragm of the needle adapter to perform aspiration.

### Characteristics

The inside of the anterior part of the syringe, or needle adaptor, contains a type of metal stud, or aspirating nipple, around the opening of the posterior needle. This projects outward and presses on the diaphragm of the cartridge (Figure 11.11).

The piston differs somewhat from that of a conventional syringe. First, its anterior part is *flat*, and it does not have a device for holding the plunger; it is only prepared for pushing the plunger and not pulling it back. The Astra® system is a variant of this approach in which the anterior part of the piston finishes in a type of projection that penetrates a hollow plunger to deform it, making this the passive

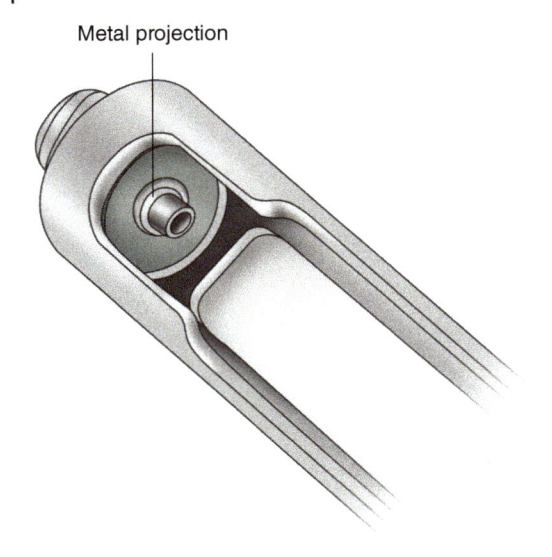

Figure 11.11 Metal projection or aspirating nipple of the self-aspirating syringe.

aspiration mechanism (Meechan and McCabe 1992). Furthermore, the posterior part of the piston of the syringe has a *flat thumb rest*, but no ring, since it does not need to pull backwards. In the middle, near the finger grip of the syringe, there is a metal disk to help with aspiration.

### Mechanism of Action

When the piston is pushed, the cartridge causes the diaphragm to become deformed on contact with the metal aspirating nipple. When the piston is released, the diaphragm recovers its initial shape by producing gentle negative pressure within the cartridge, thus causing the aspiration.

A variant of this mechanism is as follows: once the piston is pressed, the thumb is released and the metal disk is relaxed with the thumb immediately under the finger grip. This maneuver makes for a more intense deformation of the diaphragm and enables an aspiration that is twice as strong as that of the previous system.

We have already mentioned a variant known as the Astra system, in which the posterior part of the plunger deforms instead of the diaphragm (Meechan and McCabe 1992). This system is problematic in that it requires special cartridges in which the plunger or posterior stopper of the cartridge is hollow.

### Advantages and Disadvantages

The advantages of self-aspirating syringes are as follows:

1) The syringe can be set up and dismantled more quickly, with the cartridge in place, since there is no need to connect or disconnect the plunger of the cartridge to or from the piston aspiration system (Williams and Simm 1975).
2) The plunger is not at risk of becoming disconnected from the piston support system (Cowan 1972; Williams and Simm 1975).
3) The movement of the thumb needed to pull backwards to perform the aspiration in conventional syringes can momentarily displace the tip of the needle and lead to false positives or negatives (Cowan 1972; Williams and Simm 1975; Lloyd 1992). An *in vitro* study carried out in 2016 revealed that the tip of the needle was deflected by about 2 mm during this maneuver with self-aspirating syringes and about 2.5 mm with conventional cartridge-type syringes, in which the plunger is pulled with the thumb in the ring (Kämmerer et al. 2016).
4) They are ideal for dentists with small hands, for whom the pull of the piston backwards could surpass the reach of their hand.

The main disadvantage of this type of syringe is that it feels less stable and safe in aspiration in the case of dentists accustomed to using conventional syringes, which are heavier and feel more substantial.

### Variants of Cartridge-type Syringes

#### Plastic Syringes

These syringes are identical to conventional syringes, although the fact that they are made of plastic means that they have specific characteristics. They are less resistant to sterilization in the long term, they are lighter and feel less stable for dentists who are accustomed to metal syringes, and they should be used with needles with a plastic adapter (not metal), since a metal adapter quickly wears out the anterior part of the syringe. Furthermore, when the plunger is pulled back with the thumb to perform the aspiration, the tip of the needle moves about 3 mm (Kämmerer et al. 2016).

#### Uniject-type Syringes

These syringes are designed for Ultracain® brand cartridges, which take articaine with epinephrine. The cartridge is loaded through the posterior part instead of through the lateral window (Figure 11.12), and the system for holding the cartridge for aspiration includes a piston with blades in the front part that open after the piston enters a special hollow in the posterior part of the plunger. These syringes are only useful for this cartridge system.

#### Disposable Antineedle Stick Syringes

These are also known as "safety syringes", and the whole system – needle, cartridge, and syringe – comes as an

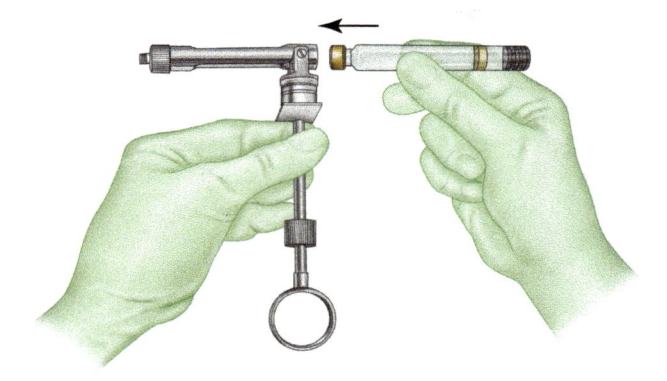

**Figure 11.12** Loading the cartridge into the back end of the Uniject® syringe.

integrated block. They are made of disposable plastic and come sterilized. They comprise a cylindrical protective sheath around the needle to prevent accidental needlestick injury. This is removed before injecting the patient. There are two basic models: the fully disposable model (all plastic) and the model that retains the posterior part (piston and finger grip), which is generally made of metal and is recyclable and sterilizable. The anterior part, the injection unit (needle, cartridge, and body of the syringe) is disposable (Meechan 2002; Gaudy and Arreto 2005).

The advantage of this system is that it reduces the risk of accidental needlestick injury for health professionals (Meechan 2002; Gaudy and Arreto 2005). Its disadvantages are its cost, the storage space it requires before use and for disposal, its poorer maneuverability in the case of dentists accustomed to more comfortable and effective conventional syringes, and the fact that, in many models, the quality of the safety lock is imperfect (Gaudy and Arreto 2005). In addition, the cartridge replacement system is complicated in those models that retain the posterior part.

In any case, new models of this syringe come onto the market every so often, and after some time in fashion, they disappear to make way for other models (Table 11.5), and in some case tests indicate that the devices tested

**Table 11.5** Safety dental syringes used in the United States.

Hypo Safety syringe[a]
RevVac safety syringe
Safe-Mate needle system
Safety Plus XL syringe[a]
SafetyWand
UltraSafe syringe[a]
Ultra Safety Plus XL syringe

[a] Tests indicate that the devices tested were no safer than traditional anesthetic needles (Cuny et al. 2000). Source: Data from Cuny et al. (2000) and Saxena et al. (2013).

did not confer a significant additional margin of safety when compared traditional anesthetic syringes (Cuny et al. 2000).

### Power-operated Syringes

In power-operated syringes, the piston is moved by means of a power source, which may be gas (e.g. freon) or springs and not by movement of the thumb (Roberts and Sowray 1987; Jastak et al. 1995). Every so often, models go out of fashion and are no longer manufactured. The main disadvantages of these syringes compared with conventional syringes include their greater cost, the fact that they are less manageable owing to their size and weight, and the absence of an aspiration system in some models.

### Other Injection Devices

Other devices are available. These are addressed in their corresponding sections, since they have specific methodologies and techniques.

1) High-pressure syringes for the periodontal ligament technique. These are addressed in Chapter 18 on supplementary techniques in the case of failure.
2) High-pressure jet injectors. These are addressed in Chapter 20 on alternatives to traditional techniques.
3) Computer-controlled injection techniques. These are also addressed in Chapter 20.

## Additional Instruments

### Complementary Devices

In addition to needles, cartridges, and syringes, other devices are necessary for correct administration of dental local anesthesia.

1) A protective disk, to protect against needle stick injury, is a needle-recapping device (Cleveland et al. 2007). The need to leave the syringe on the tray for further injections increases the risk of accidental needle stick injury when replacing the cap on the needle in the syringe. While several systems have been developed (Jastak et al. 1995), the simplest, cheapest, and most effective method is to place a disk over the anterior cap of a double-tipped needle (Figure 11.10).
2) Timer. The timer is very useful for setting the time until the anesthetic takes effect after injection. This obviates the need to watch the clock and the possibility of forgetting how much time has passed owing to distraction. Furthermore, the timer tells us exactly when the time set has passed, thus enabling us to forget about it and do

other things during the interval, from chatting to the patient to preparing the material necessary for the procedure.
3) Rigid recipient for disposal of waste (sharps container) (Cleveland et al. 2007). This recipient is mandatory for disposal of sharps such as needles, scalpels, suture material, etc. after use. In some countries, dentists use electrofusion needle destroyers based on an electric arc, although there is always a small portion of the needle that is not destroyed (near the hub and adapter) (Gaudy and Arreto 2005).
4) Scale for weighing patients. This can be kept in the patients' toilet, restroom or the reception area. Determining the patient's weight is very important when estimating the maximum dose to be administered, especially in the case of children (Annex 10).
5) Small utensils such as cotton swabs for application of topical anesthetic or cotton rolls or gauze for cleaning the injection site and/or covering the areas once the topical anesthetic has been applied (Figure 11.13).

### Alkalinization System (pH Onset System®)

The pH Onset System® is a commercial system for automated alkalinization of 1.8-ml dental local anesthetic cartridges that contain sympathomimetic vasoconstrictors, such as epinephrine, which have an acid pH of around 4 (Annex 14). Thus, we can reduce the sensation of burning, stinging, and pain of the initial injection caused by anesthetic solutions. The system also reduces the latency time of the anesthetic. The device was developed by Dr. Mic Falkel and was first applied in the field of dentistry in 2012 by Onpharma in the United States (Reed et al. 2012; Logothetis 2013).

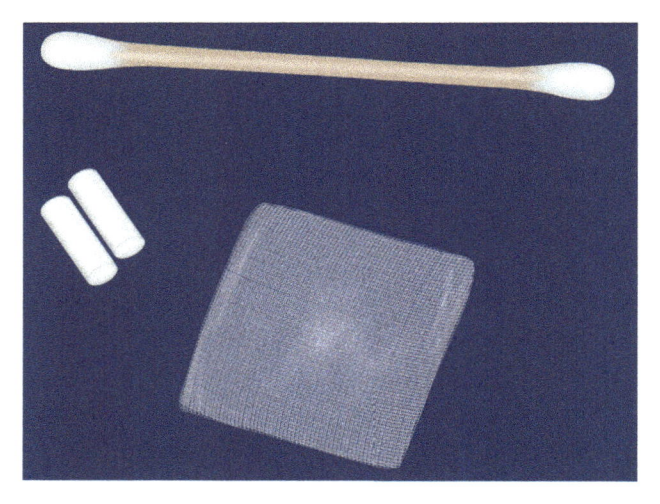

**Figure 11.13** Complementary devices for local anesthetic such as cotton swabs, cotton rolls, and gauze.

**Advantages**

Alkalinization of local anesthetic solutions can achieve the following:

1) Reduced injection pain (Annex 39). Clinical trials have shown that acidic dental local anesthetic solutions can cause a sensation of burning, stinging, or pain during injection, the "bee sting effect" (Oikarinen et al. 1975b; Moorthy et al. 1984; Kramp et al. 1999; Wahl et al. 2001). In medicine, alkalinization has been used for decades to alkalinize acid local anesthetic solutions before intradermal and subcutaneous injection to avoid this sensation (Primosch and Robinson 1996; Cepeda et al. 2010; Malamed and Falkel 2013a). In addition, the results of several systematic reviews with meta-analyses have demonstrated its efficacy (Davies 2003; Cepeda et al. 2010). In addition, given that dental anesthetics come prepared in ready-to-use manufactured cartridges, it is not necessary to add the bicarbonate ampule to the syringe, only to fill the cartridge with alkali, which is more difficult.
2) Reduced latency time (Annex 39). This approach has been proven in clinical trials in dentistry using the pH Onset System (Malamed et al. 2013b). It seems that it is made possible because the new automated system achieves optimal efficacy in the alkalinization process by taking full advantage of the base form of the local anesthetic and the formation of carbon dioxide ($CO_2$). There is no loss of these elements to the air or through absorption in the plastic of the mixing pen (Takamura et al. 2000), since the complete operation is carried out very quickly (less than 15 seconds) inside the glass cartridges of the anesthetic itself and with stainless-steel connecting tubes (Malamed et al. 2013b). Further clinical trials are necessary to verify this observation. If shown to be true, it would save the dentist precious time (Malamed et al. 2013b).
3) Increased anesthetic potency. To date, this is more a theoretical than proven advantage (Annex 39), but a meta-analysis with five select clinical trials reported better results with buffered solutions (statistically significant differences) (Kattan et al. 2019). A possible explanation is that there may be other mechanisms that introduce the anesthetic in cationic form within the axoplasm, such as transient receptor potential vanilloide 1 (TRPV1) channels (Butterworth and Oxford 2009) (see Chapter 4).

**Mechanism of Action**

The new system has advantages because it has direct actions (known for some time) and indirect actions that improve its efficacy.

Table 11.6 Percentage of lidocaine molecules in the form of B and BH$^+$ according to pH in the medium and considering its pKa = 7.9.

| pH | Ratio of B:BH$^+$ | %B | %BH$^+$ |
|---|---|---|---|
| 3.5 | 1:15 000 | 0.006% | 99.994% |
| 6.5 | 1:25 | 3.83% | 96.17% |
| 7.1 | 1:8 | 13% | 87% |
| 7.4 | 1:4 | 25% | 75% |

- Direct actions:
  1) Alkalinization of the medium. Local anesthetic solutions with sympathomimetic vasoconstrictors, such as epinephrine, have an acid pH, generally around 4 (Annex 14). Under these conditions, the local anesthetic molecules are mainly cationic (BH$^+$), with few in their free base form (B), which, as it is liposoluble, spreads across the axon membrane to the cytoplasm, where it re-establishes a new BH$^+$ ↔ B balance, with BH$^+$ able to bind to the sodium channel receptor and block nerve conduction. Table 11.6 shows the base form proportion of lidocaine for different levels of pH, starting from a base of pKa = 7.9. However, the real results are a little less dramatic, given that the pKa value of local anesthetics is calculated under standard laboratory conditions and at a temperature of 25 °C, whereas body temperature is 37 °C and the pKa of lidocaine is 7.6 under these conditions (Kamaya et al. 1983). Therefore, the level of base form anesthetic increases slightly, so that at pH = 7.4, the real B percentage is 40%.
  2) Release of carbon dioxide ($CO_2$). The interaction between sodium bicarbonate ($NaHCO_3$) and hydrochloric acid (HCl) of the local anesthetic solution produces water ($H_2O$) and carbon dioxide ($CO_2$) (Malamed et al. 2013b). $CO_2$ spreads much more quickly than the anesthetic and therefore reaches the axons earlier (Catchlove 1972) to act directly on the membrane by depressing its activity (Condouris and Shakalis 1964; Catchlove 1972) and thus boosting the anesthetic effect.

- Indirect actions:
  1) Retention of the base form of the anesthetic in the glass cartridge. It is important to remember that the base form tends to adhere to plastics, silicones, and synthetic resins (Takamura et al. 2000; Mizogami et al. 2004; Malamed et al. 2013b), although not to Teflon or glass (Malamed et al. 2013b).
  2) Retention of $CO_2$ in the glass cartridge. $CO_2$ is volatile, and plastic materials are permeable to it and absorb it (DeLuca and Kowalsky 1972), therefore the mixture inside the glass cartridge prevents its immediate leakage. However, given that after the first 90 seconds it tends to form microbubbles that move toward the glass walls and grow over time, the mixture is made in less than 15 seconds once the pieces are assembled (Reed et al. 2012). Consequently, the cartridge should be used as soon as it is prepared by loading it into a cartridge-type syringe.

  Of note, as the mixture is inside the glass cartridge itself, the loss of base form anesthetic and $CO_2$ is minimized. In addition, as this process occurs quickly and the mixture is available almost immediately, maximum use can be made of its possibilities. Since the mixture is not prepared in a separate plastic syringe, some of these components are lost; in addition, the process is time-consuming and cumbersome.

### Cartridges for the Device

1) A conventional 1.8-ml cartridge containing the local anesthetic solution (now mainly lidocaine) with epinephrine. This cartridge is inserted into the component known as the cartridge connector through the end of the mixing pen.
2) A 3-ml cartridge with sodium bicarbonate ($NaHCO_3$) 8.4% and an osmolar concentration of 2 mOsmol/ml, 1 mEq/1 ml, and pH 7–8.5 in sterile, nonpyrogenic solution (USP 38 2015). The cartridge contains the component that neutralizes acid pH and is inserted into the chamber of the mixing pen, where it has a lateral window enabling the dentist to observe how it gradually empties with use.

### Mixing Pen

The mixing pen consists of three independent components that are assembled to form a unit (Figure 11.14).

- Body. This is found at the end of the pen and consists of several parts:
  - The body itself, which houses the piston that pushes the plunger the back of the 3-ml cartridge of bicarbonate to mix it with the 1.8 ml of local anesthetic solution.
  - The display, which is situated near the end and shows the amount of bicarbonate that is to be transferred to the anesthetic cartridge, generally 10% (ratio 1:10), which is equivalent to 0.18 ml, or 11.1% (ratio 1:9), which is equivalent to 0.2 ml.
  - Regulating dial. We use this to select the amount of bicarbonate we wish to enter the anesthetic cartridge (marked on the display).

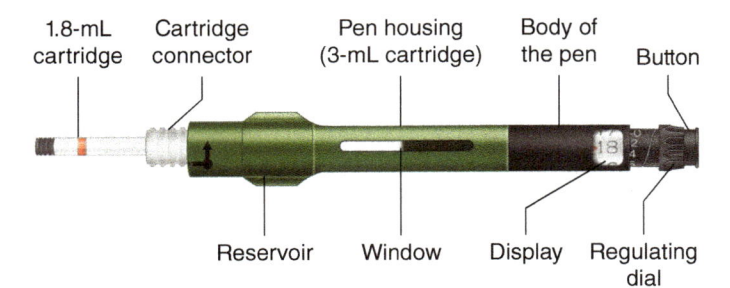

**Figure 11.14** Parts of the mixing pen once assembled.

Labels: 1.8-mL cartridge, Cartridge connector, Pen housing (3-mL cartridge), Body of the pen, Button, Reservoir, Window, Display, Regulating dial

- Mixing button. The final part of the body of the pen once assembled and prepared. Once pressed, the mix is prepared in two seconds.
- Pen housing. Housing for 3-ml bicarbonate cartridges, where the bicarbonate cartridge is loaded. A lateral window makes it possible to see the cartridge emptying as anesthetic cartridges are reloaded (1.8 ml) with a small quantity of bicarbonate (0.18–0.2 ml).
- Cartridge connector. This sterile tube is used to enable passage of fluids between cartridges. It is inserted into the other end of the mixing pen, and a cartridge of local anesthetic (1.8 ml) is adjusted at the end. This component has a reservoir to store anesthetic solution that leaves the cartridge to make room for the bicarbonate solution that enters it. The whole unit is connected with metal tubes that join the two cartridges and the outlet of the reservoir.

**Mixing**

Once the mixing pen is assembled and set up, the end button is pressed (Figure 11.15). The piston pushes the plunger of the bicarbonate cartridge (3 ml) so that the 0.18 ml that flows through the connecting tube toward the local anesthetic cartridge (1.8 ml) at the same time as the other 0.18 ml of anesthetic solution flows out to make room for the bicarbonate and is deposited in the reservoir of the cartridge connector. The whole assembly and mixing maneuver takes 15 seconds (Reed et al. 2012) and should be performed immediately after using the anesthetic cartridge to optimize performance, as we have seen.

**pH**

The ideal pH is 7–7.4 (Malamed and Falkel 2013a). A pH value above 7.9 is irritant for tissues and causes cellulitis and tissue damage (Whitcomb et al. 2010). Furthermore, at different levels of alkaline pH, local anesthetics precipitate. Thus, lidocaine precipitates at levels higher than 7.6 (Reed et al. 2012; Malamed and Falkel 2013a), mepivacaine at levels greater than 7.83, and bupivacaine at levels over 7.2 (Schwab and Watson 1996). Therefore, bupivacaine cannot be used in these alkalinization systems. Articaine at pH 7.6 has not yielded the results expected, although more clinical trials are necessary (Shurtz et al. 2015).

## Vibrating Devices

These devices act as vibrators (counter stimulating effect) applied before and/or during injection of local anesthetic *to reduce the pain of the needle prick and the injection*. They operate based on the gate control theory. While several devices are available, the two most commonly used today are VibraJect® and DentalVibe®. The two advantages of these devices are as follows:

1) Use of the devices does not require the traditional dental local anesthesia protocol to be modified.
2) As they do not involve administration of drugs, there is no risk of toxicity or allergy to the components of drugs.

Annex 40 shows clinical trial findings from the various types of vibrating devices used in dentistry.

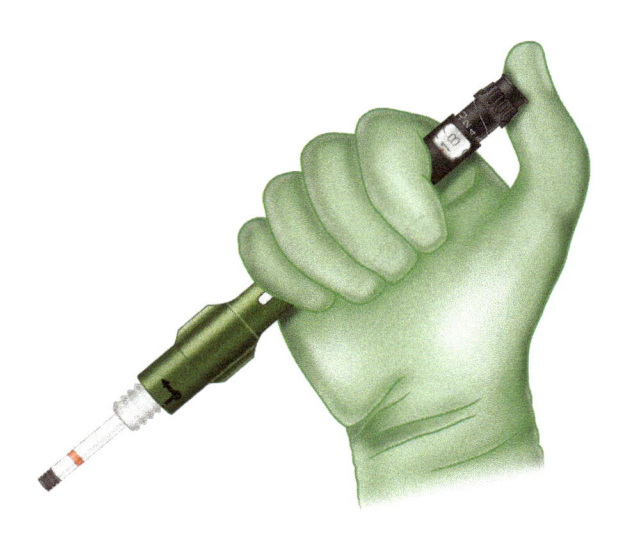

**Figure 11.15** Activation of the mixture of bicarbonate by pressing the button at the end of the mixing pen.

## Gate Control Theory

This theory was formulated by Melzack and Wall (1965). As an example of the theory, we can imagine a situation where we accidentally hit a finger while hammering a nail. The immediate result is intense pain. Our natural reflex is to hold the finger with the other hand and press tightly. This maneuver partly relieves the pain we feel in our finger.

The mechanism underlying this reaction is much more complex, although it can be summarized as follows: each metamer of the spinal cord (in this case the caudate nucleus of the trigeminal nerve) is penetrated by thick fibers (non-nociceptive A and B fibers), which transmit impulses generated by vibrations, pressure, or scratching and transport very fast nerve impulses, and by thin fibers (delta A and polymodal C fiber nociceptors), which transmit painful impulses much more slowly (Table 4.1, Chapter 4). When they reach the spinal cord, both types of fiber transmit their impulses to the central transmission neurons so that they can be sent to higher centers. However, the thickest fibers also stimulate the small neurons of the Substantia Gelatinosa of Rolando in the spinal cord, which tend to reduce the action of the fine pain fibers (Figure 11.16).

Since tactile stimuli reaching the cerebral cortex can modulate pain (Inui et al. 2006), modulation of pain can occur at various levels, and these levels may even interact with each other (Inui et al. 2006).

## VibraJect

VibraJect is a small device that first came onto the market in the United States in 2003. It temporarily attaches at an angle by means of a clip to the barrel of traditional cartridge type syringe (Figure 11.17). VibraJect transfers high-frequency microvibrations to the needle (3000 Hz)

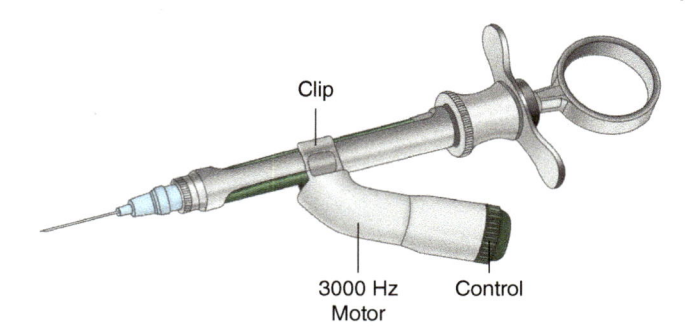

**Figure 11.17** VibraJect, with its clip, 3000-Hz motor, and control.

(Yoshikawa et al. 2003). The device weighs 18 g, measures 59 mm in length, and is 16–26 mm wide at its largest part (Yoshikawa et al. 2003). Its 2019 cost is $299, and it uses 1.5-V batteries. The disadvantages are as follows:

1) It can occasionally jump off the syringe if the clip comes loose.
2) The dentist should ensure that the tip of the needle does not make contact with a tooth, because the resulting sensation is unpleasant.
3) Its effectiveness is questionable because of the ambiguous results reported; data from several clinical trials reveal that it was not effective in half of the cases studied (Annex 40). One possible explanation for these poor results is that the vibration is too small to activate the thick A and B fibers (Roeber et al. 2011).

A currently available variant is the Syringe Micro Vibrator (SMV), which is mounted in parallel on the barrel of the syringe and held with four flexible clips. The device transmits an ultrahigh-frequency, low-amplitude vibration (Bonjar 2011).

## DentalVibe

This device was invented by Dr. Steven G. Goldberg and came onto the market in the United States in 2010 (Fa et al. 2016). It comprises a rechargeable cordless handpiece. The active part is the two-pronged U-shaped vibrating tip (micro-oscillations), which is disposable and latex-free (Figure 11.18) and serves as a soft tissue retractor. It also has a light between the two prongs to illuminate the area where the injection is to be placed. When the device is activated, it emits a sound that helps to distract the patient. The 2019 cost of DentalVibe is $995, and each disposable tip costs $2.

DentalVibe is used by placing the tip over the area to be injected, as if it was a dental mirror, and separating the soft tissues. The device is activated for 5–10 seconds before inserting the needle. The device remains active throughout the injection and even for 5–10 seconds after the needle is

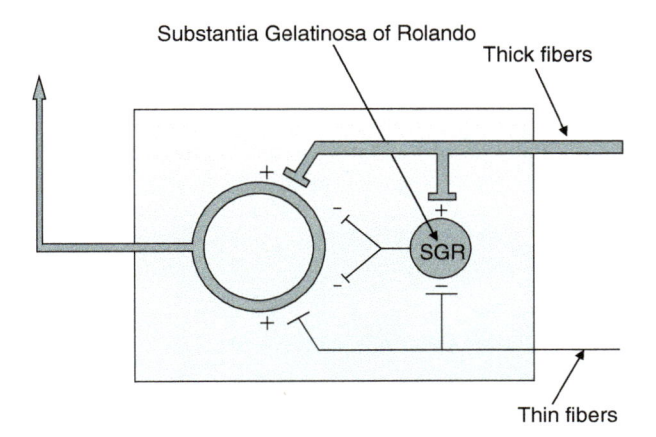

**Figure 11.16** Schematic representation of the gate control theory. Thick axon with non-nociceptive A and B fibers; fine axon with nociceptive fibers. When the faster thick fibers are activated, the substantia gelatinosa of Rolando (SGR) tends to deactivate the pain impulses.

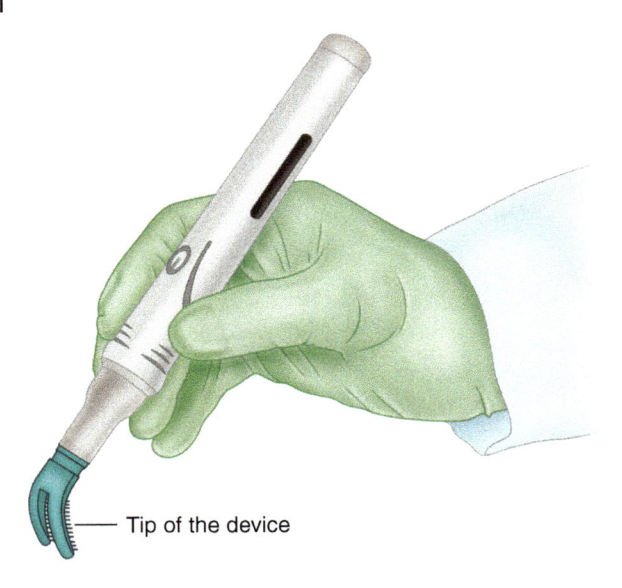

**Figure 11.18** DentalVibe.

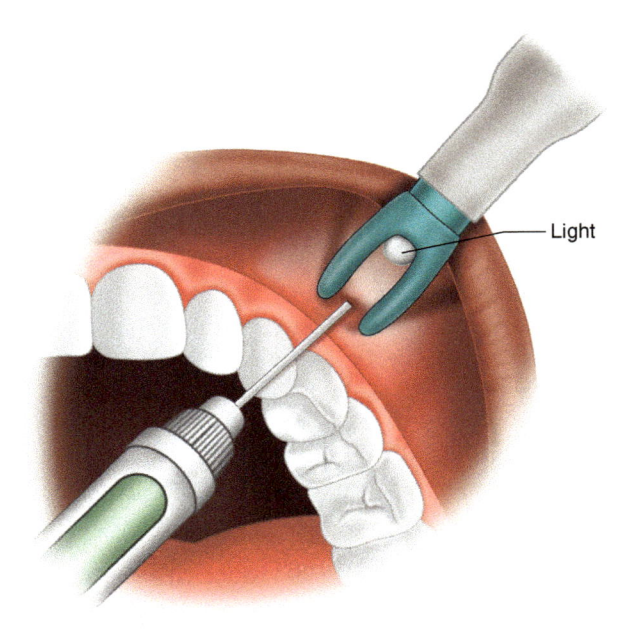

**Figure 11.19** Tip of DentalVibe. The cheek is separated from the gums to enable injection in maxillary buccal infiltration. Note the light between the two prongs of the tip.

withdrawn (Shaefer et al. 2017) (Figure 11.19). The disadvantages of the device are as follows:

1) It should not be applied to alveolar bone, since this produces an unpleasant sensation.
2) Given that the soft tissues are not separated with the fingers, the anatomical structures are not palpated as easily. But this is a clear advantage for some authors, as it removes the need for the dentist to introduce his/her fingers into the patient's mouth during administration of the anesthetic, thus preventing needle stick accidents (David et al. 2007; Fa et al. 2016).

The effectiveness of the technique is addressed in Annex 40. In almost all clinical trials, injection of dental local anesthetic using DentalVibe was less painful than using standard techniques.

### Cartridge Heaters

These are used very little today. Storage of cartridges with sympathomimetic vasoconstrictors such as epinephrine in these heaters for long periods degrades the vasoconstrictor through the action of high temperatures (Fry and Ciarlone 1980).

Experiments that studied the temperature of the cartridge from the point where it leaves the heater until it is placed in the cold metal cartridge-type syringe and the anesthetic solution flows out of the tip of the needle show that the temperature falls considerably until it reaches room temperature (Malamed 2004). This problem could be resolved using modern heaters, which simultaneously heat cartridges, syringes, and needles (Volk and Gargiulo 1984). However, clinical trials show that patients are not able to distinguish an injection at 20–21 °C (room temperature) from one at 35–37 °C (Oikarinen et al. 1975b; Rood 1977; Ram et al. 2002), but they are able to feel less pain when the temperature is higher, 42 °C (107.6 °F) (Aravena et al. 2015, 2018).

## References

Aldous, J.A. (1968). Needle deflection: a factor in the administration of local anesthetics. *J. Am. Dent. Assoc.* 77 (3): 602–604.

Alling, C.C. and Christopher, A. (1974). Status report on dental anesthetic needles and syringes. *J. Am. Dent. Assoc.* 89 (5): 1171–1176.

Annex 10. Maximum doses of local anesthetics in dentistry.

Annex 14. Injectable anesthetic solutions pH.

Annex 37. Needle breakage.

Annex 39. Alkalinized (buffered) local anesthetic solutions.

Annex 40. Vibration devices.

Aravena, P.C., Barrientos, C., and Troncoso, C. (2015). Effect of warming anaesthetic solutions on pain during dental injection. A randomized clinical trial. *J. Oral Res.* 4 (5): 306–312.

Aravena, P.C., Barrientos, C., Troncoso, C. et al. (2018). Effect of warming anesthetic on pain perception during dental injection: a split-mouth randomized clinical trial. *Local Reg. Anesth.* 11: 9–13.

Bedrock, R.D., Skigen, A., and Dolwick, M.F. (1999). Retrieval of a broken needle in the pterygomandibular space. *J. Am. Dent. Assoc.* 130 (5): 685–687.

Bhatia, S. and Bounds, G. (1998). A broken needle in the pterygomandibular space: report of a case and review of the literature. *Dent. Update* 25 (1): 35–37.

Bonjar, A.H.S. (2011). Syringe micro vibrator (SMV) a new device being introduced in dentistry to alleviate pain and anxiety of intraoral injections, and a comparative study with a similar device. *Ann. Surg. Innov. Res.* 5 (1): 1. https://doi.org/10.1186/1750-1164-5-1.

Brown, R.S., Paluvoi, S., Choksi, S. et al. (2002). Evaluating a dental patient for local anesthesia allergy. *Compend. Contin. Edu. Dent.* 23 (2): 125–138.

Brownbill, J.W., Walker, P.O., Bourcy, B.D., and Keenan, K.M. (1987). Comparison of inferior dental nerve block injections in child patients using 30-gauge and 25-gauge short needles. *Anesth. Prog.* 34 (6): 215–219.

Butterworth, J. and Oxford, G.S. (2009). Local anesthetics. A new hydrophilic pathway for the drug-receptor reaction (Editorial). *Anesthesiology* 111 (1): 12–14.

Cannell, H., Walters, H., and Beckett, A.H. (1975). Circulating levels of lignocaine after peri-oral injections. *Br. Dent. J.* 138 (3): 87–93.

Carr, M.P. and Horton, J.E. (2001). Evaluation of a transoral delivery system for topical anesthesia. *J. Am. Dent. Assoc.* 132 (12): 1714–1719.

Catchlove, R.F.H. (1972). The influence of $CO_2$ and pH on local anesthetic action. *J. Pharmacol. Exp. Ther.* 181 (2): 298–309.

Cepeda, M.S., Tzortzopoulou, A., Thackrey, M. et al. (2010). Adjusting the pH of lidocaine for reducing pain on injection. *Cochrane Database Syst. Rev.* (12): Art. No: CD006581. DOI: https://doi.org/10.1002/14651858.CD006581.pub2.

Chasteen, J.E., Hatch, R.A., and Passon, J.C. (1988). Contamination of local anesthetic cartridges with acrylic monomers. *J. Am. Dent. Assoc.* 116 (3): 375–379.

Ciarlone, A.E. and Fry, B.W. (1980). Decreased vasoconstrictor content in local anesthetic cartridges exposed to ultraviolet irradiation. *J. Dent. Res.* 59 (4): 724.

Cleveland, J.L., Barker, L.K., Cuny, E.J., and Panlilio, A.L., NaSH Group(2007). Preventing percutaneous injuries among dental health care personnel. *J. Am. Dent. Assoc.* 138 (2): 169–178.

Cohen, M.B., Gravitz, L.A., and Knappe, T.A. (1969). Twenty-five versus twenty-seven-gauge needles. *J. Am. Dent. Assoc.* 78 (6): 1312–1314.

Condouris, G.A. and Shakalis, A. (1964). Potentiation of the nerve-depressant effect of local anaesthetic by carbon dioxide. *Nature* 204 (4953): 57–59.

Cooley, R.L. and Lubow, R.M. (1981). Particulate contamination of local anesthetic solutions. *Oral Surg. Oral Med. Oral Pathol.* 51 (5): 481–483.

Cooley, R.L. and Robinson, S.F. (1979). Comparative evaluation of the 30-gauge dental needle. *Oral Surg. Oral Med. Oral Pathol.* 48 (5): 400–404.

Council on Dental Materials (1982). Instruments and Equipment. Addendum to American National Standards Institute/American Dental Association specification no. 34 for dental aspirating syringes. *J. Am. Dent. Assoc.* 104 (1): 69–70.

Council on Dental Materials (1986). Instruments and Equipment. ANSI/ADA specification no. 54* for double-pointed, parenteral, single use needles for dentistry. *J. Am. Dent. Assoc.* 113 (6): 952.

Council on Dental Materials and Devices (1974). Acceptance program for dental anesthetic syringe devices. *J. Am. Dent. Assoc.* 89 (5): 1177.

Council on Dental Materials and Devices (1978). New American National Standards Institute/American Dental Association specification no. 34* for dental aspirating syringes. *J. Am. Dent. Assoc.* 97 (2): 236–238.

Cowan, A. (1972). A new aspirating syringe. *Br. Dent. J.* 133 (12): 547–548.

Crose, V.W. (1991). Pain reduction in local anesthetic administration through pH buffering. *J. Indiana Dent. Assoc.* 70 (2): 24–27.

Cuny, E., Fredekind, R.E., and Budenz, A.W. (2000). Dental safety needles' effectiveness: results of a one-year evaluation. *J. Am. Dent. Assoc.* 131 (10): 1443–1448.

David, H.T., Aminzadeh, K.K., Kae, A.H., and Radomsky, S.C. (2007). Instrument retraction to avoid needle-stick injuries during intraoral local anesthesia. *Oral Surg. Oral Med. Oral Pathol.* 103 (3): e11–e13.

Davies, R.J. (2003). Buffering the pain of local anaesthetics: a systematic review. *Emerg. Med. (Fremantle)* 15 (1): 81–88.

De Jong, R.H. and Cullen, S.C. (1963). Buffer demand and pH of local anesthetic solutions containing epinephrine. *Anesthesiology* 24 (6): 801–807.

DeLuca, P.P. and Kowalsky, R.J. (1972). Problems arising from the transfer of sodium bicarbonate injection from ampuls to plastic disposable syringes. *Am. J. Hosp. Pharm.* 29 (3): 217–222.

Dentists' Desk (1983). *Dentists' Desk Reference: Materials, Instruments and Equipment*, 2e. Chicago: American Dental Association. 351–356.

Dobbs, E.C. (1965). A chronological history of local anesthesia in dentistry. *J. Oral Ther. Pharmacol.* 1 (5): 546–549.

Fa, B.A., Gupta, S., and Bhattacharyya, M. (2016). Operator reference of retraction method during anesthesia delivery. *Stomatol. Edu. J.* 3 (1): 10–15.

Flanagan, T., Wahl, M.J., Schmitt, M.M., and Wahl, J.A. (2007). Size doesn´t matter: needle gauge and injection pain. *Gen. Dent.* 55 (3): 216–217.

Fry, B.W. and Ciarlone, A.E. (1980). Concentrations of vasoconstrictor in local anesthetics. Change during storage in cartridge heaters. *J. Dent. Res.* 59 (7): 1163.

Fuller, N.P., Menke, R.A., and Meyers, W.J. (1979). Perception of pain to three different intraoral penetrations of needles. *J. Am. Dent. Assoc.* 99 (5): 822–824.

Fyhr, P. and Brodin, A. (1987). The effect of anaerobic conditions on epinephrine stability. *Acta Pharm. Suec.* 24 (3): 89–96.

Gaudy, J.-F. and Arreto, C.D. (2005). *Manuel d´analgesie en odontoestomatologie*, 2e. Paris: Masson. 68–69, 73, 79.

Gerke, D.C., Crabb, G.A., Frewin, D.B., and Frost, B.R. (1977). The effect of storage on the activity of adrenaline in local anaestheticsolutions: an evaluation using bioassay and fluorometric techniques. *Aust. Dent. J.* 32 (6): 423–427.

Ghasemi, D., Rajaei, S., and Aghasizadeh, E. (2014). Comparison of inferior dental nerve block injections in child patients using 30-gauge and 27-gauge short needles. *J. Dent. Mater. Tech.* 3 (2): 71–76.

Goodell, G.G., Gallager, F.J., and Nicoll, B.K. (2000). Comparison of controlled injection pressure system with a conventional technique. *Oral Surg. Oral Med. Oral Pathol.* 90 (1): 88–94.

Gruber, L.W. (1950). Preliminary report in the use of xylocaine as a local anesthetic in dentistry. *J. Dent. Res.* 29 (2): 137–142.

Guyton, A.C. (1976). *Textbook of Medical Physiology*, 5e. Philadelphia: WB Saunders Co. 223.

Hajratwala, B.R. (1975). Kinetics of sulfite-induced anaerobic degradation of epinephrine. *J. Pharm. Sci.* 64 (1): 45–48.

Harrison, S.M. (1948). Regional anesthesia for children. *Dent. Record* 68: 146–155.

Hochman, M.N. and Friedman, M.J. (2000). In vitro study of needle deflection: a linear insertion technique versus a bidirectional rotation insertion technique. *Quintessence Int.* 31 (1): 33–39.

Hondrum, S.O. and Ezell, J.H. (1991). Changes in the acidity of local anesthetics over time. *J. Dent. Res.* 70 (Special Issue): 516 (abstract no. 2002).

Hondrum, S.O., Seng, G.T., and Rebert, N.W. (1993). Stability of local anesthetics in the dental cartridge. *Anesth. Pain Control Dent.* 2 (4): 198–202.

Hondrun, S.O. and Ezell, J.H. (1996). The relationship between pH and concentrations of oxidants and vasoconstrictors in local anesthetic solutions. *Anesth. Prog.* 43 (4): 85–91.

Inui, K., Tsuji, T., and Kakgi, R. (2006). Temporal analysis of cortical mechanisms for pain relief by tactile stimuli in humans. *Cereb. Cortex* 16 (3): 355–365.

ISO 7885: 2010 (2010). *Dentistry – Sterile injection needles for single use*. Geneve: International Organization for Standardization.

Jastak, J.T., Yagiela, J.A., and Donaldson, D. (1995). *Local Anesthesia of the Oral Cavity*. Philadelphia: WB Saunders Co. 145–168.

Jeske, A.H. and Boshart, B.F. (1985). Deflection of conventional versus nondeflecting dental needles in vitro. *Anesth. Prog.* 32 (2): 62–64.

Kamaya, H., Hayes, J.J. Jr., and Ueda, I. (1983). Dissociation constants of local anesthetics and their temperature dependence. *Anesth. Analg.* 62 (11): 1025–1030.

Kämmerer, P.W., Schneider, D., Pacyna, A.A., and Daubländer, M. (2016). Movement control during aspiration with different injection systems via video monitoring – an in vitro model. *Clin. Oral Invest.* 21 (1): 105–110.

Kattan, S., Lee, S.-M., Hersh, E.V., and Karabucack, B. (2019). Do buffered local anesthetics provide more successful anesthesia than nonbuffered solutions in patients with pulpally involved teeth requiring dental therapy? A systematic review. *J. Am. Dent. Assoc.* 150 (3): 165–177.

Kelly, J.R. and Dalm, G.W. (1985). Stability of epinephrine in dental anesthetic solutions: implications for autoclave sterilization and elevated temperature storage. *Mil. Med.* 150 (2): 112–114.

Kirchhoefer, R.D., Allgire, J.F., and Juenge, E.C. (1986a). Stability of sterile aqueous lidocaine hydrochloride and epinephrine injections submitted by US hospitals. *Am. J. Hosp. Pharm.* 43 (7): 1736–1741.

Kirchhoefer, R.D., Thornton, L.K., and Allgiere, J.F. (1986b). Stability of sterile aqueous epinephrine injections submitted by US hospitals. *Am. J. Hosp. Pharm.* 43 (7): 1741–1746.

Klein, R.M. (1983). Components of local anesthetic solutions. *Gen. Dent.* 31 (6): 460–465.

Kramp, L.F., Eleazer, P.D., and Scheetz, J.P. (1999). Evaluation of prilocaine for the reduction of pain associated with transmucosal anesthetic administration. *Anesth. Prog.* 56 (2): 52–55.

Lehtinen, R. (1983). Penetration of 27- and 30-gauge dental needles. *Int. J. Oral Surg.* 12 (6): 444–445.

Lehtinen, R. and Oksala, E. (1979). Penetration of disposable needles. *Int. J. Oral Surg.* 8 (2): 145–148.

Lloyd, J.M. (1992). Aspiration in dental local anesthesia (letter). *Br. Dent. J.* 172 (4): 136.

Logothetis, D.D. (2013). Anesthetic buffering: new advances for use in dentistry. *RDH* (January): 61–66.

Lundqvist, B., Löfgren, N., Persson, H., and Sjögren, B. (1948). Metal ion as a cause of swelling after local anesthesia in dental practice. *Acta Chir. Scand.* 97 (3): 239–258.

Malamed, S.F. (2004). *Handbook of Local Anesthesia*, 5e. St. Louis (Missouri): Elsevier-Mosby. 99–117.

Malamed, S.F. and Falkel, M. (2013a). Buffered local anaesthetics: the importance of pH and $CO_2$. *SAAD Dig.* 29 (January): 9–17.

Malamed, S.F., Tavana, S., and Falkel, M. (2013b). Faster onset and more comfortable injection with alkalinized 2% lidocaine with epinephrine 1:100,000. *Compend. Contin. Edu. Dent.* 34 (Special 1): 10–20.

McPherson, J.S., Dixon, S.A., Townsend, R., and Vanderwalle, K.S. (2015). Effect of needle design on pain from dental local anesthetic injections. *Anesth. Prog.* 62 (1): 2–7.

Meechan, J.G. (2002). *Practical Dental Local Anaesthesia*. London: Quintessence Publishing Co. Ltd. 14–17, 22.

Meechan, J.G. and McCabe, J.F. (1992). Effect of different storage methods on the performance of dental local anaesthetic cartridges. *J. Dent.* 20 (1): 38–43.

Meechan, J.G., McCabe, J.F., and Carrick, T.E. (1990). Plastic dental local anaesthetic cartridges: a laboratory investigation. *Br. Dent. J.* 169 (2): 54–56.

Melzack, R. and Wall, P.D. (1965). Pain mechanism: a new theory. *Science* 150 (3699): 971–979.

Milano, E.A., Waraskiewicz, S.M., and Dirubio, R. (1982). Aluminium catalysis of epinephrine degradation in lidocaine hydrochloride with epinephrine solutions. *J. Parent. Sci. Technol.* 36 (6): 232–236.

Mizogami, M., Tsuchiya, H., and Takakura, K. (2004). Local anesthetics adsorbed onto infusion balloon. *Anesth. Analg.* 99 (3): 764–768.

Mollen, A.J., Ficara, A.J., and Provant, D.R. (1981). Needles – 25 gauge versus 27 gauge – can patients really tell? *Gen. Dent.* 29 (5): 417–418.

Moorthy, A.P., Moorthy, S.P., and O'Neil, R. (1984). A study of pH of dental local anaesthetic solutions. *Br. Dent. J.* 157 (11): 394–395.

Nevin, M. and Putterbaugh, P.G. (1949). *Conduction, Infiltration and General Anesthesia in Dentistry*, 5e. New York: Dental Items of Interest Publishing Co Inc. 296–297.

Nusstein, J.M. and Beck, M. (2003). Effectiveness of 20% benzocaine as a topical anesthetic for intraoral injections. *Anesth. Prog.* 50 (4): 159–163.

Oikarinen, V.J. and Perkki, K. (1975a). A metallurgic and bacteriological study of disposable injection needles in dental and oral surgery practice. *Proc. Finn. Dent. Soc.* 71 (5): 147–161.

Oikarinen, V.J., Ylipaavalniemi, P., and Evers, H. (1975b). Pain and temperature sensations related to local analgesia. *Int. J. Oral Surg.* 4 (4): 151–156.

Passon, C., Hatch, R.A., and Chasteen, J.E. (1992). Route of entry of vapors into anesthetic cartridges. *Gen. Dent.* 40 (4): 293–297.

Piesold, J., Müller, W., and Dreissig, J. (1998). An experimental study on the aspirating reliability of different types of injection syringes with regard to the formation of punch cylinders. *Br. J. Oral Maxillofac. Surg.* 36 (1): 39–43.

Pietruszka, J.F., Hoffman, D., and McGivern, B.E. Jr. (1986). A broken needle and its surgical removal: a case report. *N. Y. State Dent. J.* 52 (7): 28–31.

Pogrel, M.A. (2009). Broken local anesthetic needles. A case series of 16 patients, with recommendations. *J. Am. Dent. Assoc.* 140 (12): 1517–1522.

Primosch, R.E. and Robinson, L. (1996). Pain during intraoral infiltration with buffered lidocaine. *Am. J. Dent.* 9 (1): 5–10.

Ram, D. and Peretz, B. (2003). The assessment of pain sensation during local anesthesia using a computerized local anesthesia (Wand) and a conventional syringe. *J. Dent. Child* 70 (2): 130–133.

Ram, D., Hermida, L.B., and Peretz, B. (2002). A comparison of warmed and room-temperature anesthetic for local anesthesia in children. *Pediatr. Dent.* 24 (4): 333–336.

Ram, D., Hermida, D., and Amir, E. (2007). Reaction of children to dental injection with 27- or 30 gauge needles. *Int. J. Paediatr. Dent.* 17 (5): 383–387.

Rawson, R.D. and Orr, D.L. III (1985). Vascular penetration following intraligamental injection. *J. Oral Maxillofac. Surg.* 43 (8): 600–604.

Reed, K.L., Malamed, S.F., and Fonner, A.M. (2012). Local anesthesia part 2: technical considerations. *Anesth. Prog.* 59 (3): 127–137.

Roberts, D.H. and Sowray, J.H. (1987). *Local Analgesia in Dentistry*, 3e. Bristol (UK): Wright. 44–45.

Robinson, S.F., Mayhew, R.B., Cowan, R.D., and Hawley, R.J. (1984). Comparative study of deflection characteristics and fragility of 25-, 27-, and 30-gauge short dental needles. *J. Am. Dent. Assoc.* 109 (6): 920–924.

Roeber, B., Wallace, D.P., Rothe, V. et al. (2011). Evaluation of the effects of the VibraJect attachment on pain in children receiving local anesthesia. *Pediatr. Dent.* 33 (1): 46–50.

Rood, J.P. (1977). The temperature of local anesthetic solutions. *J. Dent.* 5 (3): 213–214.

Saloum, F.S., Baumgartner, J.C., Marshall, G., and Tinkle, J. (2000). A clinical comparison of pain perception to the Wand and a traditional syringe. *Oral Surg. Oral Med. Oral Pathol.* 89 (6): 691–695.

Saxena, R., Gupta, S.K., Newaskar, V., and Chandra, A. (2013). Advances in dental local anesthesia techniques and devices: an update. *Natl. J. Maxillofac. Surg.* 4 (1): 19–24.

Schwab, R.A. and Watson, W.A. (1996). Bicarbonate buffering of local anesthetics. *Ann. J. Emerg. Med.* 14 (3): 339.

Shaefer, J.R., Lee, S.J., and Anderson, N.K. (2017). A vibration device to control injection discomfort. *Comp. Cont. Edu. Dent.* 38 (6): e5–e8.

Shannon, I.L. and Feller, R.P. (1972). Contamination of local anesthetic carpules by storage in alcohol. *Anesth. Prog.* 19 (1): 6–8.

Shannon, I.L. and Wescottt, W.B. (1974). Alcohol contamination of local anesthetic cartridges. *J. Acad. Gen. Dent.* 22 (11): 20–21.

Shojaei, A.R. and Haas, D.A. (2002). Local anesthetic cartridges and latex allergy: a literature review. *J. Can. Dent. Assoc.* 68 (10): 622–626.

Shurtz, R., Nusstein, J., Reader, A. et al. (2015). Buffered 4% articaine as a primary buccal infiltration of the mandibular first molar: a prospective, ramdomized, double-blind study. *J. Endod.* 41 (9): 1403–1407.

Smith, A.E. (1920). *Block Anesthesia and Allied Subjects. With Special Chapters on the Maxillary Sinus, the Tonsils, and Neuralgias of the Nervous Trigeminus for Oral Surgeons, Dentists, Laryngologists, Rhinologists, Otologists, and Students*. St Louis (Mo): CV Mosby Co. 267–268.

Smith, N. (1968a). An investigation of the influence of gauge on some physical properties of hypodermic needles. Part I. The relation between gauge and flexibility of the needle. *Aust. Dent. J.* 13 (2): 158–161.

Smith, N. (1968b). An investigation of the influence of gauge on some physical properties of hypodermic needles. Part II. The relation between needle gauge and time taken to aspirate blood. *Aust. Dent. J.* 13 (2): 161–163.

Smith, J.R. (1991). Stability of epinephrine in local anesthetic cartridges. *Gen. Dent.* 39 (4): 261–263.

Stacy, G.C. and Hajjar, G. (1994). Barbed needle and inexplicable paresthesias and trismus after dental regional anesthesia. *Oral Surg. Oral Med. Oral Pathol.* 77 (6): 585–588.

Takamura, K., Muramatsu, I., and Miyamoto, E. (2000). Absorption of lidocaine into a plastic infusion balloon. *Anesth. Analg.* 91 (1): 192–194.

Thoma, K. and Struve, M. (1986). Untersuchungenzur Photo- Thermostabilität von Adrenalin-Lösungen .1. MitteilungzurStabilität von Adrenalin-Lösungen. *Pharm. Acta Helv.* 61 (1): 2–9.

Tomas, M., Hubbard, R., Shah, T., and Reilly, J. (2000). Anesthetic needle breakage subsequent bending. *J. Dent. Res.* 79 (Special issue): 441 (abstract no. 2380).

Trapp, L.D. and Davies, R.O. (1980). Aspiration as a function of hypodermic needle internal diameter in the in-vivo human upper limbs. *Anesth. Prog.* 27 (2): 49–51.

USP 38 (2015). *Farmacopea de los Estados Unidos de America*, 38e. Rockville, MD: The United States Pharmacopeial Convention 2488, 2694, 4490, 4658, 5414.

Van der Bijl, P. (1995). Injection needles for dental local anesthesia. *Compend. Contin. Edu. Dent.* 16 (11): 1106–1115.

Van der Bijl, P. and Rossouw, R.J. (1996). Rigidity of dental local anaesthetic injection needles. *J. Dent. Assoc. S. Afr.* 51 (3): 149–151.

Volk, R.J. and Gargiulo, A.V. (1984). Local anesthetic cartridge warmer – first in, first out fresh. *Ill Dent. J.* 53 (2): 92–94.

Wahl, M.J., Overton, D., Howell, J. et al. (2001). Pain on injection of prilocaine plain vs lidocaine with epinephrine. A prospective double-blind study. *J. Am. Dent. Assoc.* 132 (10): 1396–1401.

Watson, J.E. and Colman, R.S. (1976). Interpretation of aspiration tests in local anesthetic injections. *J. Oral Surg.* 34 (12): 1069–1074.

Whitcomb, M., Drum, M., Reader, A. et al. (2010). A prospective, randomized, double-blind study of the anesthetic efficacy of sodium bicarbonate buffered 2% lidocaine with 1:100,000 epinephrine in inferior alveolar nerve blocks. *Anesth. Prog.* 57 (2): 59–66.

Williams, M.J.R. and Simm, W. (1975). Practical aspiration for local anaesthesia. *Dent. Update* 2 (1): 23–27.

Winther, J.E. and Petersen, J.K. (1979). Penetration resistance of dental injection needles. *Int. J. Oral Surg.* 8 (5): 363–369.

Wittrock, J.W. and Fischer, W.E. (1968). The aspiration of blood through small-gauge needles. *J. Am. Dent. Assoc.* 76 (1): 79–81.

Yoshikawa, F., Ushito, D., Ohe, C. et al. (2003). Vibrating dental local anesthesia attachment to reduce injection pain. *J. Jpn. Dent. Soc. Anesthesiol.* 31 (2): 194–195. (Japanese).

Zelster, R., Cohen, C., and Casap, N. (2002). The implications of a broken needle in the pterygomandibular space: clinical guidelines for prevention and retrieval. *Pediatr. Dent.* 24 (2): 153–156.

# 12

# Topical Anesthesia

Topical or surface anesthetic is applied to the oral mucosa without injection. This is possible because some local anesthetics have the ability to superficially anesthetize the mucosa. In contrast, the skin is anesthetized poorly because of the barrier effect of the stratum corneum, with only base forms proving somewhat efficacious (Dalili and Adriani 1971). However, non-intact skin (i.e. affected by wounds, abrasions, or burns), as well as the oral mucosa, can be anesthetized with cationic and base forms (Campbell and Adriani 1958; Wehner and Hamilton 1984).

## Factors Affecting Topical Anesthesia with Local Anesthetics

A series of factors affect the efficacy of this approach and must be taken into account.

### Local Anesthetic

For a local anesthetic to be effective, it must have a high partition coefficient (*highly liposolubility*) if it is to act as a clinically useful topical anesthetic (Gangorosa 1981). It must also have *higher concentrations* than those used in infiltrative techniques. However, the *absolute maximum doses are lower*. This is because in the 1950s, tetracaine (an ester anesthetic) was very used as a topical anesthetic. The drug was very easily absorbed with higher peak plasma levels as compared to peak plasma levels achieved after subcutaneous administration (Adriani and Campbell 1956), thus leading to poisoning due to overdose, more frequently when administered topically than parenterally (Adriani and Campbell 1956; Campbell and Adriani 1958). The peaks observed in currently used topical anesthetic preparations are not as high as initially suspected (Table 12.1).

The hydrochloride forms (salt) must have an optimal pH of 6.1–6.6, since more acidic levels (pH < 6.1) have the disadvantage that their efficacy and duration is decreased. This is because the free base form is better absorbed in the mucosa (Campbell and Adriani 1958), and although acid salt is more stable, it must be alkalinized to become the base form on coming into contact with the mucosa. In addition, the buffering capacity of the mucosa is very limited, in contrast with subcutaneous administration, where tissue fluid is an effective buffer against acids (Campbell and Adriani 1958; Adriani et al. 1964; Adriani and Zepernick 1964). Base form preparations have the disadvantage that they are not very stable and are easily inactivated.

### Application Time

Application time is very important because some anesthetics or anesthetic formulations require shorter application times to be effective, e.g. benzocaine 20% or lidocaine 5%, both in gel or ointment or paste. Others need longer times, e.g. EMLA 5% cream (eutectic mixture of local anesthetic consisting of 2.5% lidocaine and 2.5% prilocaine) and lidocaine adhesive strips (Dentipatch®) (Annexes 19 and 20).

It is important to remember that the considerable moisture of the oral cavity tends to inhibit adhesion to the mucosal surface, therefore maximum absorption is achieved in the first 30 seconds (Carr and Horton 2001a). Furthermore, the longer the anesthetic remains in contact with the mucosa, the better it will penetrate (Meechan 2000).

### Method of Application

As mentioned above, the high degree of moisture in the mouth disperses topical local anesthetics easily by diluting them in saliva and preventing them from reaching suitable concentrations at a specific site, thus causing them to lose their efficacy (Carr and Horton 2001a). Formulations in solution, i.e. liquids, are those that most easily disperse in the mouth, with the result that they lose much of their efficacy and are more likely to fail (Annex 19) and anesthetize

*Local Anesthesia in Dentistry: A Locoregional Approach*, First Edition. Jesús Calatayud and Mana Saraghi.
© 2024 John Wiley & Sons Ltd. Published 2024 by John Wiley & Sons Ltd.
Companion website: www.wiley.com/go/Calatayud/local

Table 12.1 Peak blood levels after administration of topical anesthetic to the oral mucosa.

| Commercial formulation | Amount (mg) | Anesthetic administered | | | Peak | | Reference |
| --- | --- | --- | --- | --- | --- | --- | --- |
| | | Anesthetic | Amount (mg) | Time (min) | Concentration (ng/ml) | Time (min) | |
| Lidocaine 10% aerosol | 2000 | Lidocaine | 200 | 4 | 350 | 30 | Haasio (1990) |
| Lidocaine patch | 50 | Lidocaine | 50 | 30 | 95 | 45 | Brook (1989) |
| Dentipatch 20% | 46 | Lidocaine | 46 | 2.5–15 | 22 | 15 | Hersh (1996) |
| Dentipatch 20% | 46 | Lidocaine | 46 | 5–15 | 22.5 | 45 | Houpt (1997) |
| Dentipatch 20% | 46 | Lidocaine | 46 | 5 | 64 | 10 | Leopold (2002) |
| EMLA 5% cream | 4000 | Lidocaine | 100 | 4 | 200 | 5 | Haasio (1990) |
| | | Prilocaine | 100 | | 100 | 15 | |
| EMLA 5% cream | 4000 | Lidocaine | 100 | 5 | 210 | 30 | Pere (1992) |
| | | Prilocaine | 100 | | 50 | 30 | |
| EMLA 5% cream | 8000 | Lidocaine | 200 | 30 | 221 | 40 | Vickers (1997) |
| | | Prilocaine | 200 | | 131 | 40 | |
| Oraqix 5% | 3500 | Lidocaine | 175 | 20–27 | 99–266 | 20–40 | Huledal and Friskopp (2000) |
| | | Prilocaine | 175 | | 46–118 | 20–40 | |
| Oraqix 5% | 2000 | Lidocaine | 50 | 6–9 | 172 | 30 | Friskopp and Huledal (2001) |
| | | Prilocaine | 50 | | 76 | 30 | |
| Oraqix 5% | 8500 | Lidocaine | 212.5 | 6 | 280 | 189 | Herdevall (2003) |
| | | Prilocaine | 212.5 | | 110 | 189 | |

The dose becomes toxic from 5 μg/ml (= 5000 ng/ml) in the case of lidocaine and from 4 μg/ml (= 4000 ng/ml) in the case of prilocaine (Annex13).

distal parts of the mouth such as the pharynx, thus hampering swallowing (Haasio et al. 1990). They can also cause a bad taste, which often leads to increased salivation to counter it, thus further increasing dilution and reducing efficacy (Evers and Haegerstam 1981).

Aerosol formulations are subject to the same problems as liquid formulations. In addition, the doses administered are difficult to control (Campbell and Adriani 1958) and the drug is sometimes inhaled on application (Roberts and Sowray 1987). Aerosols are not recommended in children because the noise they make and their bad taste (which spreads through the mouth) can lead to uncontrollable bad behavior (Frasier 1967; Evers and Haegerstam 1981).

We can therefore deduce that *topical anesthetics in a liquid formulation and aerosol should not be recommended owing to their low efficacy* (Annex 19) and the abovementioned problems, therefore gel, ointment, cream, and paste formulations are preferred.

### Amount Administered

The amount may have some impact, although we do not know the optimal amounts to ensure maximum efficacy.

It is important to distinguish between the amount of formulation and the amount of anesthetic, for example 100 mg of benzocaine 20% in cream = 20 mg of benzocaine and 1 g of lidocaine (1000 mg) 5% in gel = 50 mg of lidocaine.

We must remember that in many cases, *anesthetic is also administered by injection and that this amount must be added to the amount of the topical agent to avoid problems with toxicity due to excessive dosing* (Cannel 1996; Meechan et al. 1998). If a patient were to receive the maximum recommended dose of a topical anesthetic, the patient could not receive any other topical or injected local anesthetic.

### Types of Pain

Some clinical trials have shown that needle prick is a painful stimulus that can be anesthetized better than contact with bone or an injection (Annex 19). In addition, electrical stimuli or pressure can be more intense and therefore more useful for evaluating the efficacy of topical anesthesia (Adriani et al. 1964; Adriani and Zepernick 1964).

### Area of the Mouth

Topical anesthesia is not as effective in all areas of the mouth. The mucosa and the buccal, maxillary, and *mandibular gingiva are anesthetized easier than the palate*, as shown in clinical trials (Annex 19). This observation is logical, given that the palatal mucosa is much thicker and keratinized, therefore its permeability is lower than in any other part of the oral mucosa (Lesch et al. 1989). Furthermore, as it has less subcutaneous tissue, the fibromucosa, which is formed by denser fibers, adheres tightly to the periosteum, thus leading to a more painful injection resulting from stretching of the tissue (Gill and Orr II 1979; Keller 1985; Kreider et al. 2001; Bhalla et al. 2009).

*Topical anesthesia is not effective at reducing the discomfort or pain caused by mandibular block* (Annex 19), since the needle penetrates about 20–25 mm into the pterygomandibular space and topical anesthetic cannot reach this depth (Meechan et al. 1998).

### Effect of Topical Anesthesia

Topical anesthesia has a series of effects, which can be summarized as follows:

1) Anesthesia of the fibromucosa is the main function, since it penetrates 1–3 mm, at which point most of the nerve endings can detect pain. In infiltrative techniques, penetration of the needle into the subcutaneous tissues and muscle fascia by a few millimeters is less painful because sensitivity to pain is reduced at this level (Meadows 1970).
2) It has an important placebo effect that boosts the action of the anesthetic and calms the patient (Kincheloe et al. 1991; Martin et al. 1994; Roghani et al. 1999), therefore it is very important to inform the patient that you are going to use topical anesthesia before the injection in order to reduce the pain (Martin et al. 1994).
3) Anesthetic solutions containing disinfectant can also help to disinfect the surface of the mucosa (Winther and Khan 1971). Topical anesthetics (lidocaine, tetracaine, cocaine, EMLA), in addition to their anesthetic properties, also possess antimicrobial effects (Mullin and Rubinfeld 1997; Aldous et al. 1998; Aydin et al. 2001; Berg et al. 2006; Gocmen et al. 2008; Reynolds et al. 2016), but the rate of onset of antimicrobial activity as well as whether the activity is bactericidal or bacteriostatic is still unknown (Kaewjiaranai et al. 2018).

### Topical Anesthetics in Dentistry

Below, we set out the topical anesthetics that are currently used in dentistry. However, it is clear that the most widely used are benzocaine 20% and lidocaine 5%, both of which can be applied in ointment or gel.

### Benzocaine

Benzocaine, or ethyl aminobenzoate, is an ester-type anesthetic that was synthesized by Eduard Ritser (1859–1946) in 1890 and initially called Anesthesin (Neue Arzneimittel und pharmaceutische Spezialitäten 1902). It has been used exclusively as a topical anesthetic since 1903 (Sveen et al. 1982). Since benzocaine lacks the hydrophilic cationic amino terminus (Ritchie and Ritchie 1968; de Jong 1977), it is practically free of any charge, and is only a neutral free base (pKa 3.2) at physiological pH. It is therefore not water soluble (Adriani and Campbell 1956; Anonymous 1964; Takman 1975; de Jong 1977) and its action is pH-independent (Ritchie and Ritchie 1968) and very fast. As very little is absorbed, benzocaine scarcely causes toxic systemic reactions (it is considered to be very safe) (Adriani and Campbell 1956) and cannot be injected because it is very irritant and is only used as a topical anesthetic. Table 12.2 summarizes its main characteristics.

**Maximum Dose**

While no official dose has been established by the United States Food and Drug Administration (US FDA) (Beutlich 1991; American Dental Association 2003), some researchers, based on cases of toxic methemoglobinemia, have estimated that it is not recommended to exceed 15–25 mg/kg (Potter and Hillman 1979; Rodriguez et al. 1994). This criterion is followed by a number of authors (Klein et al. 1983; Severinghaus et al. 1991; Wilburn-Goo and Lloyd 1999). Therefore, as a guide, the absolute maximum dose in a 70-kg adult could be set at 1050 mg (15 mg/kg), which, at 20%, represents 5.5 ml of gel or ointment. Figure 12.1 shows different doses in gel for use in dentistry.

**Advantages and Disadvantages**

The main advantages of benzocaine are that its action is very quick, 20–30 seconds, it is cheap, it adheres to the oral mucosa better than EMLA cream, and its taste is more agreeable than that of EMLA (Tulga and Mutlu 1999; Primosch and Rolland-Assensi 2001; Al-Melh et al. 2005). In addition, it is almost not absorbed because it is not water-soluble (see above), therefore it is considered safe.

**Table 12.2** Benzocaine.

| Pharmacological factors | Reference |
|---|---|
| • Name and synonyms: benzocaine, Anesthesin, Americaine | |
| • First synthetized in 1890 by Eduard Ritsert | Neue Arzneimittel und pharmaceutische Spezialitäten (1902) |
| • Chemical name: Ethyl aminobenzoate | Anonymous (1964) |
| • Formula: $C_9H_{11}NO_2$ $$H_2N-\text{C}_6H_4-COO-C_2H_5$$ Benzocaine | |
| Molecular weight: Base 165.2     Hydrochloride | Martindale (1982) |
| **Physicochemical properties** | |
| • pKa value or dissociation constant: 3.2 | Annex 6 |
| • Lipid solubility or partition coefficient: N-heptane 3.1     n-octanol 80     Indicating capacity for topical anesthesia | Annex 7 |
| • Binding to plasma proteins: ? | |
| • Vasodilation:? | |
| **Clinical factors** | |
| • Relative anesthetic potency: 1 | |
| • Relative toxicity: ? | |
| • Absolute maximum dose in dentistry: 1050 mg (15 mg/kg)     This is only a guide. Equivalent to 5.5 ml of gel or ointment at 20% | Potter and Hillman (1979) Rodriguez (1994) |
| • Use during pregnancy: Yes (FDA category = C)     Indicating that it is safe | Haas (2000) (Table 5.11) |
| • Use during breastfeeding: Yes (indicating that it is safe) | Haas (2000) Singh and Al (2019) |
| • Use in children: Yes (indicating that it is safe)     Contraindicated in children aged under 2 years | Singh and Al (2019) |
| **Clinical efficacy (mouth)** | |
| Benzocaine 20% in gel, ointment, or paste | |
| • Onset of action: 20–30 s (very fast) | Annex 20 |
| • Maximum effect: ? | |
| • Duration of effect of topical anesthesia: 5 min | |

Main pharmacological factors, physicochemical properties, clinical factors, and clinical efficacy.
Benzocaine has a pKa = 3.2 because it lacks the hydrophilic N-terminus, therefore it is not absorbed (safer than topical anesthetic). It is very irritating when injected. In addition, pharmacokinetic data (clearance, volume of distribution, and plasma half-life) are lacking. Similarly, it does not bind to plasma proteins.

Its main disadvantages are the short duration of the anesthetic effect (5 minutes) and its low potency, although it is better than placebo (Annex 19).

### Specific Adverse Effects

There are two specific adverse effects: sensitization and allergic reactions, which can appear in 3–6% of cases owing to continued exposure (Martindale 1982) and which occur as cross-reactions with sulfonamide allergy (Anonymous 1964).

Benzocaine can also lead to toxic methemoglobinemia when administered at doses greater than the recommended dose, especially in children aged under 1 year owing to the immaturity of their enzyme system (Anonymous 1964; Rodriguez et al. 1994) (see Chapter 23). In a few

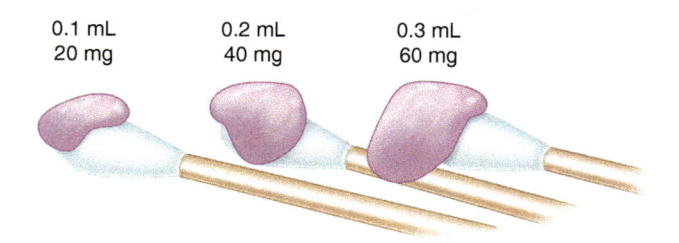

**Figure 12.1** Example of different amounts and doses of topical anesthetic benzocaine 20% gel on a cotton swab.
*Source:* Redrawn from Künisch et al. (2017).

0.1 mL / 20 mg
0.2 mL / 40 mg
0.3 mL / 60 mg

susceptible individuals, there is no "therapeutic window" between the doses required to produce a therapeutic effect and that producing toxic methemoglobinemia (Guay 2009). Benzocaine is contraindicated in patients with history of methemoglobinemia and should not be used in children younger than 2 years old (American Academy of Pediatric Dentistry 2020).

## Lidocaine

Lidocaine is an amide-type anesthetic that can be injected and applied topically. It is one of the most commonly used anesthetics throughout the world in both of its formulations. Its main pharmacological factors, physicochemical properties, and clinical factors were discussed in Chapter 7 (Table 7.2).

In this section, we examine the gel, ointment, and paste 5% formulations because the liquid and aerosol formulations are very poor (see Annex 19).

### Maximum Dose

The absolute maximum dose for a ≥70-kg adult has been set at 250 mg (Adriani et al. 1964; American Dental Association 2003) (3.6 mg/kg), which in gel or ointment 5% is equivalent to 5 ml. The maximum dose for topical anesthetic is lower than the maximum dose for injectable solution (300 mg) (Table 7.2, Chapter 7).

### Advantages and Disadvantages

The main advantages are that onset is rapid, the drug is inexpensive, and its action lasts longer than that of benzocaine (12 minutes) (Annex 20) (Table 12.3).

### Specific Adverse Effects

The main adverse effect is that of toxicity due to overdosing, therefore the recommended maximum dose should not be exceeded. In addition, some formulations of lidocaine contain methylparaben as a preservative, which can cause allergic sensitization (see Chapters 7 and 23).

## Lidocaine Adhesive Patches (DentiPatch®)

These patches measure 8×26×2 or 10×20×2 mm in a bioadhesive matrix that is stuck directly onto the oral mucosa (Houpt et al. 1997; Kreider et al. 2001; Carr and Horton 2001b; Stecker et al. 2002). The patches contain lidocaine 20%, which is equivalent to 46 mg per patch (Stecker et al. 2002). This method enables the anesthetic to spread in the mucosa without becoming diluted in the mouth or dispersing in the saliva owing to the fact that it is confined to the mouth. Consequently, the patch has an advantage over gels, ointments, creams, liquid solutions, and aerosols.

The patch formulation was approved by the US FDA in 1996 (Hersh et al. 1996; Houpt et al. 1997), although the first study with adhesive strips appeared in 1968 (Giddon et al. 1968).

### Maximum Dose

As we have already seen, the absolute maximum dose for lidocaine as a topical anesthetic for a ≥70-kg adult has been set at 250 mg (Adriani et al. 1964; American Dental Association 2003) (3.6 mg/kg), which in 20% lidocaine patches with 46 mg per patch represents a maximum of 5.5 patches.

### Advantages and Disadvantages

Lidocaine adhesive strips have several advantages. They prevent spread of the anesthetic in the mouth, as they are confined (Howitt and Lowell 1972; Hersh et al. 1996), therefore the anesthetic does not spread and anesthetize the tongue or pharynx (Nakamura et al. 2013). The dose administered is well controlled and the anesthetized area is easily seen (Howitt and Lowell 1972). In addition, as the patch has a relatively potent effect (Table 12.4), the dental hygienist can use it for dental procedures such as scaling and root planing

**Table 12.3** Lidocaine.

| Clinical efficacy (mouth) | Reference |
|---|---|
| • Onset of action: 1–2 min | Annexes 19 and 20 |
| • Maximum effect: 5 min | |
| • Duration of the effect of topical anesthesia: 12 min | |

5% formulation in gel, ointment, or paste.

**Table 12.4** Lidocaine.

| Clinical efficacy (mouth) | Reference |
|---|---|
| • Onset of action: 2–5 min | Annexes 19 and 20 |
| • Maximum effect: 15 min | |
| • Duration of the effect of topical anesthetic: 25 min | |

Adhesive strips or patches (DentiPatch).

(Carr and Horton 2001b) or to fit the clamps for rubber dams (Stecker et al. 2002) and the dentist can take small superficial biopsy specimens (Roller and Ship 1975).

The disadvantages are that onset of action is slow, 2–5 minutes, and it is four times more expensive than benzocaine (Stecker et al. 2002). Occasionally, adhesion fails owing to a fault in the system (Stecker et al. 2002), insufficient depth of the buccal area, and excessively viscous saliva (Taware et al. 1997). Of note, it has not been declared safe in patients aged under 12 years (American Dental Association 2003).

**Specific Adverse Effects**
Specific adverse effects include mild irritation of the mucosa the patch adheres to in 10–20% of cases owing to the long periods of time it remains in the same place (Brook et al. 1989; Hersh et al. 1996; Houpt et al. 1997), its unpleasant – generally bitter – taste (Brook et al. 1989; Houpt et al. 1997; Taware et al. 1997), and the fact that it sometimes increases salivation and the sensation of retching or nausea (Stern and Giddon 1975).

## EMLA Cream

EMLA (Eutectic Mixture of Local Anesthetic). Eutexia is a physical phenomenon by which the mixture of two correctly dosed substances has a lower melting point than either of the two separately or mixed at any other proportion. In this case, the two substances are the anesthetics lidocaine and prilocaine.

The mixture was first proven to be effective on the skin in 1980 (Juhlin et al. 1980). In 1981, the patent was registered in Europe (Broberg and Evers 1981). The FDA authorized the drug in the United States in 1993 (Primosch and Rolland-Assensi 2001). Currently, the manufacturer (Astra) and the FDA do not recommend application of EMLA on the oral mucosa (Oraqix®, an oral variant is recommended [see below]), restricting it to the skin, since the safe doses remain unknown (Primosch and Rolland-Assensi 2001; Lim and Julliard 2004; Al-Melh and Anderson 2007; Franz-Montan et al. 2008). However, EMLA cream has been used in dentistry in clinical trials, from which we provide data.

**Advantages of the Structure and Composition of EMLA**
The oil–water emulsion of lidocaine normally forms drops with an anesthetic concentration of 20% (Reiz and Reiz 1982). In addition, lidocaine and prilocaine have melting points of 96 and 37 °C, respectively (Vickers and Punnia-Moorthy 1993; Munshi et al. 2001). When lidocaine and prilocaine are mixed 1:1 in an oil–water emulsion with ester ethoxylate surfactant of neutralized fatty acids such as Carboner 934P, the resulting emulsion does not contain lipophilic solvent (Nyqvist-Mayer et al. 1986), and a cream is obtained with the following characteristics:

1) Emulsion drops with a high concentration of anesthetic (80%) (Juhlin et al. 1980; Reiz and Reiz 1982) and a lower size (1 µ) (Nyqvist-Mayer et al. 1986).
2) The melting point of both anesthetics falls to 18 °C (Brodin et al. 1984), that is lower than for each separately. The mixture behaves as a pure solid (eutectic), thus enabling it to be absorbed at body temperature.
3) The high water concentration facilitates penetration via the skin and mucosa.

In theory, the above-mentioned factors make it possible to create a more powerful anesthetic compound than each separately at the same concentration. The complete composition of EMLA is set out in Table 12.5.

**Maximum Dose**
There is no established maximum dose, although the results from a clinical trial showed that it was possible to administer 8000 mg of EMLA 5% cream (400 mg of local anesthetic: 200 mg of lidocaine and 200 mg of prilocaine) with no risk of toxicity, since it generated peak levels that were far from toxic (Vickers et al. 1997) (Table 12.1). In addition, Oraqix (variant of EMLA cream [see below]) has an established maximum dose of 8500 mg (Herdevall et al. 2003).

In conclusion, we can propose an absolute maximum dose for a ≥70-kg adult of 8000 mg (115 mg/kg), which is equivalent to 5.7 mg/kg of anesthesia (2.85 mg/kg of lidocaine and 2.85 mg/kg of prilocaine).

**Advantages and Disadvantages**
The main advantage is that it makes it possible to achieve a relatively potent anesthetic effect, therefore the dental hygienist can carry out small dental tasks such as scaling and root planing or measuring periodontal pocket depth

**Table 12.5** Composition per 1 ml = 1 g = 1000 mg of EMLA 5% cream.

| Component | Function | Milligrams (mmol/l) |
| --- | --- | --- |
| Lidocaine | Local anesthetic | 25 (107) |
| Prilocaine | Local anesthetic | 25 (117) |
| Arlatone 289 | Surfactant/emulsifier | 19 |
| Carbopol 934 | Thickener | 10 |
| Sodium hydroxide | Up to pH = 9.6 | — |
| Purified water | Up to 1 ml | ±921 |

Arlatone 289 is hydrogenated and ethoxylated castor oil. Carbopol 934 or Carbomer 934P is carboxypolymethylene.
*Source:* Data from Reiz and Reiz (1982), Nyqvist-Mayer et al. (1986), Engberg (1987), Haasio (1990), Munshi et al. (2001).

**Table 12.6** EMLA.

| Clinical efficacy (mouth) | Reference |
|---|---|
| • Onset of action: 3 min (2–5)<br>• Maximum effect: 5 min<br>• Duration of the effect of topical anesthetic: 20 min | Annexes 19 and 20 |

5% cream.

(Donaldson and Meechan 1995) and removing orthodontic arch bars (Pere et al. 1992). In addition, the dentist can remove small fibromas from the palate (Meechan 2001). Table 12.6 shows data on their clinical efficacy.

The disadvantages include the slow onset of action (2–5 minutes, mean 3 minutes), the fact that it is more expensive than benzocaine (Meechan and Donaldson 1994), and the low viscosity of EMLA cream (Meechan and Donaldson 1994; Donaldson and Meechan 1995; Tulga and Mutlu 1999; Primosch and Rolland-Assensi 2001), which reduces its power of absorption through dispersion in the mouth and dilution in saliva, and means that a large amount of cream remains on the cotton swab or roll (Holst and Evers 1985; Lim and Julliard 2004). EMLA cream is not recommended in children owing to the lack of data or for application in the oral cavity in adults. However, we do have an equivalent for oral use, namely, Oraqix (see below).

### Specific Adverse Effects

A burning sensation occurs in the oral mucosa after long applications (30–40 minutes) (Vickers and Punnia-Moorthy 1993; Franz-Montan et al. 2008) owing to the high pH (9.6) (Vickers and Punnia-Moorthy 1993) and, very rarely, ulcers on the superficial mucosa for the same reason (Franz-Montan et al. 2008). Patients also complain of the bitter taste (Svensson and Petersen 1992; Meechan and Donaldson 1994; Tulga and Mutlu 1999; Primosch and Rolland-Assensi 2001). Prilocaine can induce toxic methemoglobinemia in children aged under 6 years (Frayling et al. 1990). This is also the case for children aged under 1 year (Engberg et al. 1987), whose enzymes are not sufficiently mature to metabolize high doses of EMLA (see Chapter 23).

### Tetracaine (Amethocaine)

Tetracaine is an ester-type anesthetic that was first synthesized in 1928 by the German chemist Otto Eisleb (1887–1948) in IG Farben (Hoechst). It was patented in the United States in 1932 (Eisleb 1932) and marketed under the name of Pantocaine (Eisleb 1934).

Tetracaine is known as Amethocaine in the British pharmacopeia. As it has a pKa of 8.5, onset of action can sometimes be delayed. In addition, as with lidocaine, it is one of the few local anesthetics that is achiral, that it, it does not have optic isomers (Calvey 1995). The main characteristics of tetracaine are summarized in Table 12.7.

### Maximum Dose

Tetracaine is an old topical anesthetic, which, when applied to the mucosa, is absorbed rapidly owing to its potent vasodilator effect. The resulting anesthesia is deeper and more potent, although there is also a greater risk of the drug passing to the bloodstream (Bonica 1950; Adriani and Campbell 1956). Given that the maximum dose as a topical anesthetic has been set at 20 mg (Carabelli 1952; American Dental Association 2003), the absolute maximum dose in a ≥70-kg adult is 20 mg (0.3 mg/kg), which is equivalent to 2000 mg (=2 ml) in 1% creams.

When tetracaine is applied as an aerosol, it is easy to lose control of the dose administered, therefore it is recommended not to apply the drug for more than 1–2 seconds to avoid administering a toxic dose or, preferably, the drug should be administered using a fixed-dose applicator so as not to exceed the maximum dose.

### Advantages and Disadvantages

The main advantage of tetracaine is that it is a potent topical anesthetic, as seen in its clinical effect in 1% formulations, which lasts 50 minutes (Table 12.7). Its main disadvantage is the ease with which it produces toxic reactions when absorbed after application on the mucosa and the dose is greater than de 20 mg (Weisel and Tella 1951; Carabelli 1952).

### Specific Adverse Effects

Key adverse effects include allergic and hypersensitivity reactions caused by the fact that tetracaine is an ester anesthetic. The other main problem is toxic reactions resulting from overdose when the drug is applied to the mucosa (it is barely absorbed by intact skin; Mazumdar et al. 1991). Tetracaine is a topical anesthetic that not only anesthetizes the surface but also reaches a certain depth. Consequently, its potent vasodilator effect passes to the systemic circulation in such a way that it is the only anesthetic that can reach higher levels in blood after topical application on the mucosa than after parenteral injection (Adriani and Campbell 1956). In the 1940s and 1950s, tetracaine was the anesthetic that caused the highest number of toxic reactions when the doses administered were greater than 30–40 mg (Weisel and Tella 1951; Carabelli 1952; Adriani and Campbell 1956) (see Chapter 23).

**Table 12.7** Tetracaine.

| Pharmacological factors | Reference |
|---|---|
| • Name and synonyms: Tetracaine, Amethocaine, Pontocaine<br>• First synthesized in 1928 by Otto Eisleb<br>• Chemical name: 2-dimethylaminoethyl 4-butylaminobenzoate<br>• Formula: $C_{15}H_{24}N_2O_2$<br><br>$C_4H_9\text{—HN—}\bigcirc\text{—COO—CH}_2\text{—CH}_2\text{—N}\begin{smallmatrix}CH_3\\CH_3\end{smallmatrix}$<br>Tetracaine | Council on Dental Therapeutics (1984) |
| • Molecular weight: Base 264.4<br>        Hydrochloride 300.8 | Martindale (1982) |
| • Clearance: ? | Annex 11 |
| • Volume of distribution: ? | Annex 11 |
| • Half-life: ? | Annex 11 |
| **Physicochemical properties** | |
| • pKa value or dissociation constant: 8.5 | Annex 6 |
| • Lipid solubility or partition coefficient: N-heptane 4.1<br>        n-octanol 220<br>  Indicates high anesthetic potency and topical anesthetic capability | Annex 7 |
| • Binding to plasma proteins: 85%<br>        Indicating long duration of anesthesia | Annex 9 |
| • Vasodilation: ++ (high) | Martindale (1982) |
| **Clinical properties** | |
| • Relative anesthetic potency: 8 | |
| • Relative toxicity: 8 | Annex 8 |
| • Absolute maximum dental dose: 20 mg (0.3 mg/kg) | Carabelli (1952)<br>ADA guide (2003) |
| • Use during pregnancy: Yes (FDA category = C)<br>        Indicating that it is safe | Haas (2000)<br>(Table 5.11) |
| • Use during breastfeeding: Yes<br>        Indicating that it is safe | Haas (2000)<br>(Table 5.11) |
| • Use in children: NOT in children aged <12 years<br>        Not established in the USA | ADA guide (2003) |
| **Clinical efficacy (mouth)** | |
| Formulations of tetracaine 1%<br>• Onset of action: 1–2 min<br>• Maximum effect: ?<br>• Duration of effect of topical anesthetic: 50 min | Annexes 19 and 20 |

Main pharmacological factors, physicochemical properties, clinical factors, and clinical efficacy.
Surprisingly for an anesthetic as old as tetracaine, data on pharmacokinetics are lacking (clearance, volume of distribution, and half-life) (Annex 11).

## Cocaine

Cocaine is an ester anesthetic that appears naturally as an alkaloid in the coca leaf (*Erythroxylum coca*), which grows in South America, mainly in Bolivia and Peru. The drug accounts for 0.7–1.8% of the weight of the leaf (Caldwell and Sever 1974; Van Dyke and Byck 1982). Cocaine was isolated in 1860 by Albert Niemann, who also gave it the name "cocaine" (Niemann 1860). The drug was artificially synthesized in 1923 by Richard Willstätter (Willstätter et al. 1923).

Cocaine has a pKa of 8.8 (Annex 6), therefore its onset of action should be late. However, in practice, this latency period is very short and its action manifests itself very quickly for various reasons: (i) the high concentration (it is generally used at ≥20%) (Adriani 1963; Adriani et al. 1964; Adriani and Zepernick 1964) and (ii) its vasoconstrictor effect, which becomes apparent when it blocks the monoaminoxidase enzyme and prevents reuptake of norepinephrine from the nerve endings (Muscholl 1961; Covino and Giddon 1981).

It is worth highlighting that plasma pseudocholinesterases rapidly inactivate cocaine in blood. However, the drug persists in the mucosa (especially the nasal mucosa) for 4–6 hours, with a peak at 60 minutes and a half-life of 95 minutes (Annex 11). This is due to the slow passage to the bloodstream resulting from the vasoconstrictor effect (Van Dyke et al. 1976). Also interesting is the fact that in addition to catabolism by plasma cholinesterases, cocaine, like all ester anesthetics, is metabolized slowly in the liver (McLure and Rubin 2005). Table 12.8 summarizes the main characteristics of cocaine.

### Maximum Dose

Cocaine is a safer topical anesthetic than originally thought because its vasoconstrictor effect reduces its systemic toxicity, with the result that, paradoxically, the drug is less toxic at higher concentration, since it increases vasoconstriction in the affected mucosa (Campbell and Adriani 1958; Adriani et al. 1964; Van Dyke et al. 1976). The maximum dose for injectable anesthetic was set at 50 mg at the beginning of the twentieth century (Fischer 1912; Bieter 1936). The American Dental Association (ADA) guidelines recommend a maximum topical dose of 400 mg, although in a 1–4% solution (American Dental Association 2003). We favor using higher concentrations (≥20%), therefore we suggest a smaller maximum dose than that recommended by other authors, that is, *a maximum absolute dose of 100 mg* (1.5 mg/kg) for an adult weighing ≥70 kg (DiFazio 1981; Martindale 1982). As the most widely used concentration is 20%, this would be equal to 0.5 ml of solution, gel, or ointment, therefore it should be applied in small dabs.

### Advantages and Disadvantages

The main advantage is its potent and rapid effect (30 seconds), which is long-lasting (55 minutes) (Table 12.8). Its disadvantages are drug trafficking and illegal recreational use (Anonymous 1979) and its ability to create dependence with repeated use, especially in the case of recreational inhalation (Caldwell and Sever 1974; Van Dyke and Byck 1982). Due to reuptake inhibition of norepinephrine, cocaine may not be well tolerated in patients with cardiovascular disease.

### Specific Adverse Effects

Allergy and sensitization, since this is an ester anesthetic, as well as the problems of trafficking, illegal recreational use, and drug addiction through repeated use (see above) (Caldwell and Sever 1974; Van Dyke and Byck 1982).

### Formulations for Use in Dentistry

There are no commercial formulations (except for compounded formulas such as TAC gel; Kravitz 2007), only the generic form, although it can be obtained in pharmacies with special prescriptions for controlled substances. The most popular formulation in Europe is a solution that has been used in ear, nose, and throat medicine since 1898 known as BONAIN, which comprises one-third cocaine (anesthetic), one-third phenol (disinfectant), and one-third menthol to improve the taste (Martindale 1982; Jyväkorpi 1996; Tainmont 2007).

## Topical Anesthetic Compounds

These are compounded formulas obtained by mixing various topical anesthetics and a vasoconstrictor (Table 12.9). They are very popular in the United States, although their main drawback is that they carry very high doses (see below). *They are mainly used in orthodontic surgery for the placement of intraosseous anchors* (microscrews or orthodontic mini-implants).

### Composition

The formulations are very diverse. The most popular for dentistry are shown in Table 12.9. Their components include the following (Kravitz et al. 2015):

1) Local anesthetics that are generally a mixture of several components and may be amide- and ester-type.
2) Vasoconstrictor. The vasoconstrictor in this case is phenylephrine, which has fallen into disuse in injectable solutions and whose vasoconstrictive potency is 5% of that of epinephrine (Furchgott 1972). Furthermore, when the formulation contains this vasoconstrictor, its expiry date is 90 days after the preparation (Kravitz et al. 2015).

**Table 12.8** Cocaine.

| Pharmacological factors | Reference |
|---|---|
| • Name and synonyms: Cocaine | |
| • First synthesized in 1923 by Richard Willstätter<br>　First isolated in 1860 by Albert Niemann | Niemann (1860)<br>Willstätter (1923) |
| • Chemical name: Benzoylmethylecgonine | Caldwell and Sever (1974)<br>Council on Dental Therapeutics (1984) |
| • Formula: $C_{17}H_{21}NO_4$ | Martindale (1982) |
| • Molecular weight: Base 303.4<br>　　　　　　　　Hydrochloride 339.8 | Martindale (1982)<br>Council on Dental Therapeutics (1984) |
| • Clearance: 1.83 l/min | Annex 11 |
| • Volume of distribution: 207 l (intranasal) | Javaid (1983) |
| • Half-life: 95 min (intranasal) | Annex 11 |
| **Physicochemical properties** | |
| • pKa value or dissociation constant: 8.8 | Annex 6 |
| • Lipid solubility or partition coefficient: ? | |
| • Binding to plasma proteins: 98% | McLure and Rubin (2005) |
| • Vasodilation: − (marked vasoconstriction) | Muscholl (1961) |
| **Clinical factors** | |
| • Relative anesthetic potency: ? | |
| • Relative toxicity: 3? | Annex 8 |
| • Absolute maximum dose in dentistry: 100 mg (1.5 mg/kg) | DiFazio (1981)<br>Martindale (1982) |
| • Use during pregnancy: ? (FDA category = C) | ADA guide (2003) |
| • Use during breastfeeding: ? | |
| • Use in children: NOT in children aged <6 years<br>• Not established in the USA | ADA guide (2003) |
| **Clinical efficacy (mouth)** | |
| Formulations at 20% or higher | Annex 20 |
| • Onset of action: 30 s (very fast) | |
| • Maximum effect: ? | |
| • Duration of effect of topical anesthesia: 55 min | |

Main pharmacological factors, physicochemical properties, clinical factors, and clinical efficacy.

Table 12.9 Popular topical anesthetic compounds used on the mucosa in the USA: mixtures and high concentrations (Kravitz 2007; Kravitz et al. 2015).

| Topical compound | Drug | % | Amount per milliliter | Absolute maximum dose |
|---|---|---|---|---|
| TAC 20% Alternative | Tetracaine | 4 | 40 mg | [a]20 mg[b] |
| | Lidocaine | 20 | 200 mg | 250 mg[c] |
| | Phenylephrine | 2 | 2000 μg | 4000 μg[d] |
| Profound PET gel | Tetracaine | 4 | 40 mg | [a]20 mg[b] |
| | Lidocaine | 10 | 100 mg | 250 mg[c] |
| | Prilocaine | 10 | 100 mg | 250 mg[d] |
| | Phenylephrine | 2 | 2000 μg | 4000 μg[d] |
| Baddest Topical in Town (BTT) | Tetracaine | 12.5 | 125 mg | [a]20 mg[b] |
| | Lidocaine | 3 | 30 mg | 250 mg[c] |
| | Prilocaine | 12.5 | 125 mg | 250 mg[e] |
| | Phenylephrine | 2 | 3000 μg | 4000 μg[d] |
| Best Topical Ever | Tetracaine | 12.5 | 125 mg | [a]20 mg[b] |
| | Lidocaine | 12.5 | 125 mg | 250 mg[c] |
| | Prilocaine | 3 | 30 mg | 250 mg[e] |
| | Phenylephrine | 3 | 3000 μg | 4000 μg[d] |

[a] Indicates values that already exceed the maximum recommended doses in the milliliter amount, without taking into account the cumulative effect of other drugs.
[b] Carabelli (1952), ADA guide (2003).
[c] Adriani et al. (1964), ADA guide (2003).
[d] Jastak and Yagiela (1983), Malamed (2004).
[e] Estimated to be equal to lidocaine in topical anesthetic.

3) Wetting agent. This is usually alcohol, propylene glycol, or ethoxydiglycol. It serves as a base for the mixture of the drugs mentioned above, displaces air, and enhances penetration of the active ingredients into the mucosa.
4) Base for drug transport, to formulate creams, gels, and ointments. This has a soft, creamy consistency.
5) Favoring and colorant to sweeten and suppress the bitterness of these products.

**Advantages and Application**

The main advantage for orthodontists is that they do not have to administer local anesthetic injections to place mini-implants. In addition, the compounds are very easy to apply.

The compounds are applied on clean mucosa at a volume of 0.2–0.4 ml (Kwong et al. 2011; Lamberton et al. 2016), although some authors consider that up to 2 ml can be applied (Kravitz 2007; Kravitz et al. 2015). This amount is excessive (see Table 12.9). It is left to act for 2–4 minutes, reaching its maximum effect in 5 minutes, and lasts 25–30 minutes (Kravitz 2007; Kravitz et al. 2015).

**Adverse Effects**

The main drawback of these compounds is that they have a low therapeutic margin, that is, a very narrow margin between the effective dose and a toxic dose. In addition, their formulation (cream, ointment, or gel) makes it difficult to calculate and monitor the dose administered (Kravitz 2007). Two cases of severe reactions to the formulations and two deaths (caused by application of the compound on the skin for depilation) have been reported in the United States, therefore, in 2006, the FDA published an alert on the potential risks of these compounds (Kravitz 2007; Baumgaertel 2009).

Other drawbacks include irritation of the mucosa (probably because of the high concentrations of active ingredient) and the bad – generally bitter – taste, which is managed with sweeteners and flavorings (Kravitz 2007; Kravitz et al. 2015).

**Clinical Efficacy**

Clinical trials have shown that these formulations are efficacious (Kravitz and Kusnoto 2006; Reznik et al. 2009), even more so than benzocaine 20% (Reznik et al. 2009) and Oraqix (Kwong et al. 2011), although they are less effective than the traditional 0.45-ml injection (one-quarter of a 1.8-ml cartridge) of the standard solution of lidocaine 2% with epinephrine 1:100 000 (Lamberton et al. 2016).

### Other Experimental Formulations

Over time, variants or new methods have been sought to achieve a potent, rapid, efficacious, and safe topical anesthetic, although the results have ranged from poor to encouraging in some cases, as follows:

- Mixtures of topical anesthetics with detergents, cations, diffusion agents (Hyaluronidase) (Adriani and Zepernick 1964), and vasoconstrictors (Adriani and Campbell 1956; Campbell and Adriani 1958; Adriani 1964; Nakamura et al. 2013) have not improved topical anesthesia or diminished its systemic absorption.
- Similarly, alkalization and acidification of topical anesthesia formulations have been unable to improve the results (Adriani et al. 1964; Adriani and Zepernick 1964).
- Mixtures of two or more topical anesthetics have not shown a cumulative anesthetic effect (Adriani and Zepernick 1964), although they have – unfortunately – led to cumulative systemic toxic effects (Adriani 1963; Adriani et al. 1964). Compound topical anesthetics have become popular in the United States. These compounded

formulas are composed of a mixture of several topical anesthetics and a vasoconstrictor (see above). The exception to the lack of recommendations in favor of mixtures is EMLA cream (or its oral variant, Oraqix), which, as we have seen, is not included in this section owing to its pharmaceutical peculiarities and its low doses (5%, that is, 2.5% of lidocaine and 2.5% of prilocaine).

- Iontophoresis. This process involves placing a positively charged topical anesthetic on the oral mucosa (e.g. lidocaine 2% with epinephrine, both drugs are positively charged) and placing an electrode on top of the anesthetic to enable current to flow for about 10 minutes (5–15 minutes) (Gangorosa 1974; Won et al. 1995). Iontophoresis has proven successful in mobile primary tooth extraction, and the local anesthetic is not painful (Gangorosa 1974). This is a promising proposal, although it is time-consuming and cumbersome.
- Liposomes. Liposomes are small empty spheres (0.03–10 μm) with a double-phospholipid wall that act as vehicles by encapsulating the topical anesthetic before transport and helping them to penetrate the oral mucosa (McLure and Rubin 2005; Franz-Montan et al. 2007, 2012). They have been used with tetracaine 5% (Zed et al. 1996) and with ropivacaine 1–2% (Franz-Montan et al. 2007, 2010); outcome has been standard to promising.
- Sonophoresis. This technique involves using ultrasonic energy to generate microchannels across lipids between the keratinized cells of the stratum corneum and thus facilitate penetration of topical anesthetic. The results are no different from those of standard techniques (Packer et al. 2013).

Finally, Table 12.10 summarizes data on all recommended topical anesthetics, with all their clinical characteristics and maximum recommended doses.

## Topical Cooling

Cold reduces the velocity of nerve conduction, which ceases when the temperature falls from 10 to 0 °C (Harbert 1989), thus inducing anesthesia. Topical cooling techniques are *only used before injection of local anesthesia* to ensure that the procedure is as painless as possible. The only contraindication would be in patients who cannot tolerate cold (Harbert 1989).

## Cold Aerosols

Cold aerosols are the old, traditional method. The aerosols contain ethyl chloride, which is a highly volatile component. On evaporation, the aerosol quickly reduces the temperature of the mucous membrane at the application site. Ethyl chloride is the model on which newer aerosols are based and exits the container at −10 or −16 °C (Cohen et al. 1993; Nusstein et al. 1998).

The main advantage of these aerosols is their rapid action, which is almost instantaneous. Moreover, there is no maximum dose since they do not enter the bloodstream and their action is limited to cooling the surface of the mucous membrane. When the surface of the membrane is covered with white frosting, the solution can be injected.

The main drawback is the short duration of effect, which lasts only a few seconds (Roberts and Sowray 1987). The other drawbacks of these formulations are as follows:

- They can be inhaled, especially when applied to the back of the mouth. In addition, given that they are derived from ethyl chloride, they have a general anesthetic effect and thus carry a risk of loss of consciousness (Roberts and Sowray 1987).

**Table 12.10** Summary of topical anesthetics in their most widely used formulations: clinical effect, absolute maximum dose, and use in pregnancy (FDA, risk of pregnancy), breastfeeding, and children.

| Topical anesthetic | | Clinical effect (minutes) | | | Maximum dose | | | Clinical factors | | | |
|---|---|---|---|---|---|---|---|---|---|---|---|
| Anesthetic | Formulation | Onset minutes | Maximum effect | Duration | mg total | mg/kg | ml | FDA risk | Pregnancy | Breast-feeding | Children |
| Benzocaine | 20% gel/ointment | 0.3–0.5 | — | 5 | 1050 | 15 | 5.5 | C | Yes | Yes | Yes |
| Lidocaine | 5% gel/ointment | 1–2 | 5 | 12 | 250 | 3.6 | 5 | B | Yes | Yes | Yes |
| Lidocaine | 20% patch | 2–5 | 15 | 25 | 250 | 3.6 | $5.5^a$ | B | Yes | Yes | Not <12 years |
| EMLA | 5% cream | 3 | 5 | 20 | 400 | 5.7 | 8 | B | Yes | Yes | Not <12 years |
| Tetracaine | 1% | 1–2 | — | 50 | 20 | 0.3 | 2 | C | Yes | Yes | Not <12 years |
| Cocaine | 20% | 0.5 | — | 55 | 100 | 1.5 | 0.5 | C | ? | ? | Not <12 years |

[a] In the case of lidocaine adhesive patches, the maximum dose is in the number of 20% patches, with 46 mg per patch, so 5.5 patches.

- They are not recommended in children because the noise of the aerosol and the bad taste resulting from their dispersion in the mouth could lead the child to behave badly (Frasier 1967; Evers and Haegerstam 1981).
- They can cause sensitization to cold in sensitive teeth since it is difficult to control the area of application (Roberts and Sowray 1987)

### Refrigerants

Even colder compounds can also be used in dentistry. Initially, the substance used was dichlorodifluoromethane (DDN) (Fuss et al. 1986; Duncan et al. 1992), which exits the container at −50 °C (Fuss et al. 1986; Cohen et al. 1993; Nusstein et al. 1998; Hsiao-Wu et al. 2007) and which was initially used in vitality testing. It has been replaced by 1,1,1,2 tetrafluoroethane spray (TFE) (Green Ice or Endo-Ice), which exits the container at −26 °C (Nusstein et al. 1998; Hsiao-Wu et al. 2007), has a weaker ozone-depleting effect (Nusstein et al. 1998; Kennedy et al. 2003; Lathwal et al. 2015), and is not flammable. It was approved by the US FDA in 2004 (Lathwal et al. 2015).

The main advantage of these refrigerants is their rapid action, which is almost instantaneous (a few seconds). In addition, they are not subject to maximum doses, since they do not enter the bloodstream, and act only by cooling the surface of the mucous membranes, as is the case with cold aerosols. Furthermore, they are not toxic when inhaled (Kosaraju and Vandewalle 2009) and have proven superior to benzocaine 20% for 2 minutes (Kosaraju and Vandewalle 2009).

However, refrigerants do have a drawback, namely, *they can only be used on the palate* (Duncan et al. 1992; Kosaraju and Vandewalle 2009; Wiswall et al. 2014) owing to the nature of the palatal epithelium, which can resist low temperatures (Duncan et al. 1992). Nevertheless, they can cause frostbite of the palatal mucosa in 80% of cases, with erythema and soreness, which appear after 2–48 hours and last 1–10 days (Wiswall et al. 2014). Carbon dioxide ($CO_2$) snow, or dry ice, is not used for this purpose since its temperature is excessively low (−78 °C) (Fuss et al. 1986; Loetscher et al. 1988) and it can severely damage the mucosa.

The technique involves soaking the tip of a cotton swab (Kosaraju and Vandewalle 2009; Wiswall et al. 2014) or a cotton pellet held in tweezers (Duncan et al. 1992) in 1,1,1,2-tetrafluoroethane (Green Ice or Endo Ice). The solution is then applied for only 5–10 seconds (never more, owing to the low temperature) by pressing it against the area of the palate that is to be injected. After this short period, the tip of the needle is inserted in the immediate area of the swab (pressed against the surface of the palate), which is withdrawn. The anesthetic solution is then injected (Kosaraju and Vandewalle 2009).

### Topical Ice

The use of ice was proposed by Henry Harbert (Harbert 1989). This approach has several advantages:

- Since the temperature of the ice is −4 to 0 °C, the mucous membrane is not damaged by frostbite (Hindocha et al. 2019).
- It can be used throughout the mouth, not only in the palate.
- As the ice contains no drugs, it does not cause allergic or toxic reactions (Hindocha et al. 2019).
- It is inexpensive, since it is composed of tap water (Lathwal et al. 2015; Hindocha et al. 2019).
- In clinical trials, it has proven superior to benzocaine 20% gel for 1 minute (Harbert 1989; Aminabadi and Farahani 2009; Ghaderi et al. 2013; Lathwal et al. 2015), lidocaine 2% gel for 1 minute (Mohiuddin et al. 2015), and refrigerants for 5 seconds (Lathwal et al. 2015). It is equally effective as lidocaine 5% gel for 1 minute (Hindocha et al. 2019).
- It can be used in both children and adults.

The only problem with this approach is that it requires the device to be prepared. The various systems available are as follows:

- The empty glass cartridge is filled with water and stored upright in the freezer at −4° (Ghaderi et al. 2013).
- An ice cube, tube, or cone is made by cutting and filling the little finger of a latex glove with water. The latex finger is closed and placing it in the freezer (Aminabadi and Farahani 2009; Mohiuddin et al. 2015).

The main problem with these systems is that the ice is contained in glass or latex and is not in direct contact with the mucous membrane. Therefore, the surface of the ice melts and surrounds the covered ice, thus reducing its effect on the oral mucosa in a very short time (Hindocha et al. 2019). Furthermore, the dentist has to hold the frozen device with his/her fingers.

- The tip of a cotton bud can be soaked in water and the whole bud frozen (Jayasuriya et al. 2017). However, this technique generates very little ice, which melts very quickly. Consequently, contact between the ice and the mucosa ceases after a short time (Hindocha et al. 2019).

All three methods are simple and relatively easy to prepare, although they are subject to the drawbacks we have mentioned. In our opinion, the two best methods are as follows:

- A bar of ice is prepared with an empty glass anesthetic cartridge or the protective sheath of a needle. The empty sheath or empty cartridge is filled with water and a toothpick is inserted through the silicone stopper (as this is thinner, the toothpick can penetrate more easily in the plunger), thus leaving an active part (the anterior part of the frozen water) measuring around 25 mm. The sheath is then stored upright in the freezer at −4 °C) (Harbert 1989). Before use, the bar of ice is removed from the sheath using the handle (toothpick) (Figure 12.2).
- A bar of ice is prepared with a small plastic syringe. A 2.5-ml syringe is filled with water and placed in the freezer at −4 °C. When this is frozen, the tip of the syringe is cut with a scalpel (Figure 12.3) and the plunger is pressed so that the tip of the ice appears (Figure 12.4) (Hindocha et al. 2019).

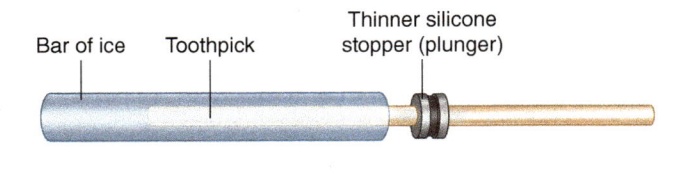

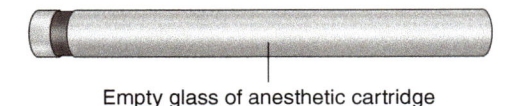

**Figure 12.2** Bar of ice with a toothpick get from an empty glass of anesthetic cartridge.

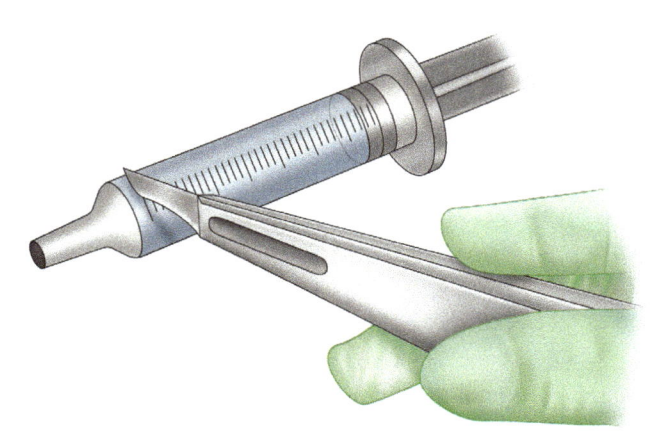

**Figure 12.3** A scalpel is used to cut the anterior part of the syringe containing frozen water. *Source:* Redrawn from Hindocha (2019).

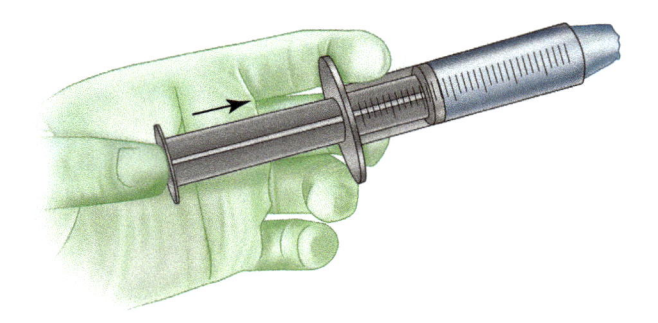

**Figure 12.4** The plunger is pressed to force the ice through the tip of the syringe. *Source:* Redrawn from Hindocha (2019).

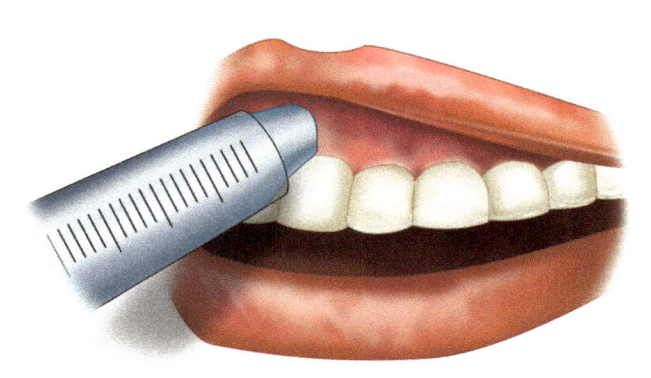

**Figure 12.5** The bar of ice in the syringe is pressed against the area of the oral mucosa to be injected. *Source:* Redrawn from Hindocha (2019).

Application is simple. The bar of ice is applied directly to the mucous membrane, with the ice held by the toothpick (Harbert 1989) or via the plastic syringe (Hindocha et al. 2019) (note that we do not touch the ice directly with our fingers) and *pressing firmly against the mucous membrane for 45–60 seconds*. The ice gradually melts (Figure 12.5) and the mucous membrane quickly changes color from pink to white owing to the blanching produced by the pressure and cold. After the recommended time, the bar of ice is slightly withdrawn and the anesthetic solution is injected at the point where the ice was applied. The ice continues to melt, and the pressure is maintained.

## Indications for Topical Anesthetic

The two main indications of topical anesthetic are preparation for injection of local anesthetic and use during periodontal treatments administered by the hygienist. We examine these indications in more detail below, the first in Chapter 13 and the second at the end of the present chapter, with Oraqix. Other indications are as follows.

### For Symptomatic Relief of Pain

Topical anesthetic is indicated for symptomatic relief of pain in the following situations.

#### Pain Resulting from Tooth Decay

Benzocaine has been used since 1926 (Sveen et al. 1982) as a topical anesthetic for relief of pain resulting from tooth decay, loss of a filling, or a broken/cracked tooth. Clinical studies have shown the efficacy of this agent at concentrations of 7.5% (Sveen et al. 1982) and 10–20% (Hersh et al. 2005; Hersh et al. 2013) – both in the gel formulation – and report promising data for the 12% patches (Hersh et al. 2003). In order for it to function, the gel must be placed on the gum surrounding the tooth.

#### Painful Ulcers and Lesions on the Mucosa

Clinical studies have also demonstrated the efficacy of applying lidocaine 5% on painful lesions caused by recurrent aphthous ulcers, acute herpetic gingivostomatitis, or mouth ulcers (Ship et al. 1960). The anesthetic is applied directly on the lesion using cotton swabs. Benzocaine 10–20% (three times daily) has also proven efficacious on mucosa damaged by friction from removable prostheses (Graser 1984).

### Indication as Anesthetic

*Topical anesthetics cannot replace injectable solutions when pulpal anesthesia is required* (Annex 20), although, in some cases, they can replace injections in minor procedures and can help in specific interventions, as follows.

#### Minor Surgical Interventions

Topical anesthetic can be used for various minor interventions: superficial biopsies of the oral mucosa with lidocaine adhesive strips applied for 5 minutes (DentiPatch) (Roller and Ship 1975), removal of small soft tissue tumors, such as palatal fibromas, with EMLA 5% cream for 15 minutes (Meechan 2001), lancing a dental abscess (Roberts and Sowray 1987), and placement of temporary orthodontic mini-implants (Reznik et al. 2009; Kwong et al. 2011). However, the results are poorer than with standard injectable anesthetics (Lamberton et al. 2016) (as seen with topical anesthetic compounds).

#### Clinical Procedures

These include placement of retraction clamps that function apically in children with budding teeth in whom the midpoint of the crown is still below the gum line. In these cases, the anesthetic used is benzocaine 20% for 1 minute (Stecker et al. 2002), DentiPatch for 5 minutes (Stecker et al. 2002), EMLA 5% cream for 5 minutes (Lim and Julliard 2004), or Oraqix for 2 minutes (Yoon and Chussid 2009). All of these methods relieve discomfort and pain, although they do not eliminate them completely. Topical anesthetic in the form of EMLA 5% cream for 5 minutes can also be used to relieve discomfort during removal of orthodontic bars (Pere et al. 1992).

#### Management of the Gag Reflex

Topical anesthetics can be used to reduce gagging, which can affect patients when taking impressions or periapical radiographs (in the upper posterior part) (Ship et al. 1960; Graser 1984; Roberts and Sowray 1987). In such cases, it is better to administer topical anesthetics in the form of aerosols on the soft palate, including the uvula and tonsillar pillars (Roberts and Sowray 1987).

## Periodontal Oraqix® Gel

As mentioned above, Oraqix is EMLA cream adapted for the oral mucosa, although it has been designed more specifically for periodontal work, therefore it is suitable for regular periodontal examination and scaling and root planning. In addition, as these procedures are painful, they require local anesthetic injections in 92% of cases (Van Steenberghe et al. 2004). The disadvantages of such injections are as follows:

1) Many patients are afraid of the needle and the injection (Donaldson et al. 2003; Jeffcoat et al. 2001; Magnusson et al. 2003). The local anesthetic injection is estimated to cause moderate or intense pain in 35% of patients undergoing periodontal procedures (Van Steenberghe et al. 2004).
2) The long duration of the anesthetic effect, with swelling of the soft tissues (Donaldson et al. 2003; Jeffcoat et al. 2001; Magnusson et al. 2003), is considered a disadvantage by more than 25% of patients undergoing periodontal procedures (Van Steenberghe et al. 2004).
3) Hygienists who usually perform tartar removal and scaling and root planing are not authorized to administer local anesthetic injections in many countries of the European Union (Stern and Giddon 1975; Svensson et al. 1994). In the United States, most states allow the hygienist to administer local anesthetic injections under the supervision of the dentist, although some states do not authorize this practice (Boynes et al. 2010).

It was therefore necessary to find alternatives to local anesthetic injections. In 1975 (Stern and Giddon 1975) and in 2001 (Carr and Horton 2001a), lidocaine patches applied to specific quadrants for 5–15 minutes yielded promising results. In addition, in 1994 and 1995 (Svensson et al. 1994; Donaldson and Meechan 1995), EMLA 5% cream applied to a specific quadrant with an intraoral splint for 5 minutes also yielded promising results.

## Oraqix System (Needle-free Anesthesia)

The Oraqix periodontal gel system came onto the market in 2005. This formulation, which is derived from EMLA cream, contains 5% topical anesthetic in a 1:1 eutectic mixture of 2.5% lidocaine and 2.5% prilocaine. It is designed specifically for use in the oral cavity. Since Oraqix is a thermosetting noninjectable anesthetic gel, it has low viscosity at ambient temperature (fluid-like), although when it is applied to periodontal pockets the heat of the body converts it into an elastic gel that remains at the application site to produce anesthesia and reduce the risk of dispersion to other areas of the mouth (Friskopp and Huledal 2001; Friskopp et al. 2001; Herdevall et al. 2003; Magnusson et al. 2003).

Oraqix comes in cartridges containing 1.7 ml or 1.7 g, with 5% anesthetic (Herdevall et al. 2003; Kwong et al. 2011), therefore it contains 2.5% lidocaine (42.5 mg) and 2.5% prilocaine (42.5 mg), i.e. a total of 85 mg of anesthetic per cartridge. The maximum dose has been set at five cartridges, i.e. 8.5 ml or 8.5 g (425 mg of anesthetic, thus 212.5 mg of lidocaine and 212.5 mg of prilocaine) (Herdevall et al. 2003; Kwong et al. 2011). Studies on peak levels in blood show that these amounts are far from toxic (Table 12.1) and that methemoglobinemia caused by prilocaine also remains below 2% (i.e. normal levels) (Herdevall et al. 2003) (see Chapter 23).

Oraqix can be applied using a cartridge-type syringe or, even better, a specially designed applicator (Figure 12.6), in such a way that each click administers 0.07–0.08 ml (Kwong et al. 2011). The anesthetic is paced on a specific tooth, semiarch, or the whole mouth, with a dose of 0.2 ml per tooth (three clicks) or one-eighth of a cartridge (Donaldson et al. 2003). In a specific quadrant, it is administered at a dose of one to two cartridges (1.7–3.4 ml) (Magnusson et al. 2003; Van Steenberghe et al. 2004). It is only authorized for adults. The absence of data for children (age <12 years), means that it is not indicated in this population.

The system has special 23G blunt applicators (0.6 mm external diameter) with a lateral outlet (Friskopp and Huledal 2001; Friskopp et al. 2001; Jeffcoat et al. 2001); hence the term "needle-free anesthetic" (Van Steenberghe et al. 2004).

**Method of Application**

Below we provide a step-by-step explanation of how this anesthetic is prepared before use in scaling and root planing:

- The Oraqix is loaded into the applicator (Figure 12.7) or a cartridge-type syringe and the 23G blunt applicator is put into position.
- The quadrant is isolated with cotton roll (Donaldson et al. 2003).
- Saliva is aspirated to keep the mouth dry (Herdevall et al. 2003).
- The applicator is inserted into the periodontal pockets, which are filled with Oraqix up to the gingival margin until it begins to overflow (Friskopp and Huledal 2001; Friskopp et al. 2001). The patient may experience minor discomfort during this maneuver (5–20% of cases) (Friskopp and Huledal 2001; Friskopp et al. 2001).
- If the procedure is to be performed by quadrants, the best approach is to fill the most distal pockets and gradually fill the remainder while moving forward (Jeffcoat et al. 2001).
- The gel should be applied as quickly as possible to maximize its extension and absorption (Friskopp and Huledal 2001).
- The dentist can begin to work 0.5–2 minutes after application (Friskopp et al. 2001; Jeffcoat et al. 2001; Donaldson et al. 2003; Van Steenberghe et al. 2004), therefore the effect is very quick.
- The anesthetic effect lasts for 17–20 minutes (Friskopp et al. 2001).

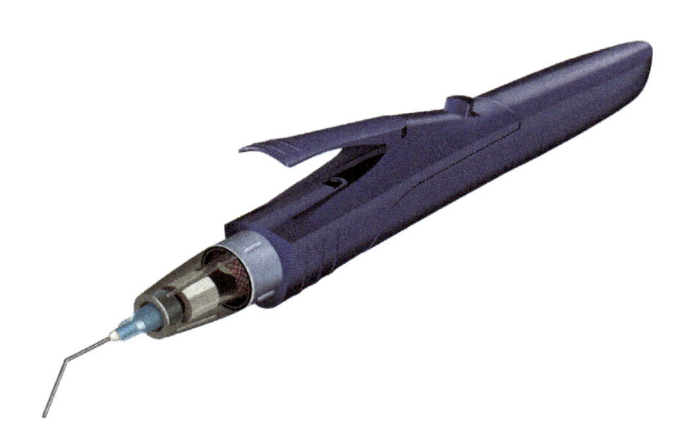

**Figure 12.6** Oraqix device set up and ready for use.

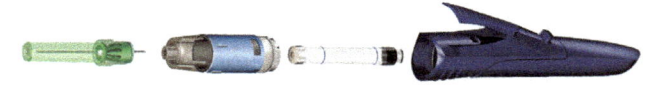

**Figure 12.7** Different elements during the set-up of the Oraqix device and order of assembly.

- If the scaling process continues to hurt, then we can apply the following measures:
  - Reinforcement, by re-administering Oraqix to the tooth in question. This occurs in 30% of cases (Magnusson et al. 2003).
  - If the tooth continues to hurt despite reinforcement with Oraqix, then a rescue strategy based on infiltration with standard anesthetic can be adopted. This situation may arise in 5–10% of cases (Jeffcoat et al. 2001; Donaldson et al. 2003; Magnusson et al. 2003).
- During treatment, the patient can expectorate/spit, but not rinse (Herdevall et al. 2003). If the patient's mouth is very dry and uncomfortable, then it can be moistened with the air-water aerosol of the device (Herdevall et al. 2003).
- Once treatment is complete, the patient can rinse with water to remove any remaining Oraqix (Friskopp and Huledal 2001).

**Efficacy**

Application of the above-mentioned method in scaling and root planing has revealed the following:

- Oraqix is better than placebo (Friskopp and Huledal 2001; Jeffcoat et al. 2001; Donaldson et al. 2003; Magnusson et al. 2003).
- Oraqix is more effective in deeper pockets (Jeffcoat et al. 2001; Donaldson et al. 2003; Magnusson et al. 2003).
- Seventy percent of patients prefer Oraqix, even though it is not as effective against pain as standard local anesthetic injections (Van Steenberghe et al. 2004).

**Specific Adverse Effects**

1) Between 10% and 30% of patients complain of the bad taste of this anesthetic (Friskopp and Huledal 2001; Friskopp et al. 2001).
2) The anesthetic extends to the throat and tongue in 20% of cases, since the gel flows out of an over-filled periodontal pocket (Friskopp and Huledal 2001; Herdevall et al. 2003).
3) In theory, there is a risk of toxic methemoglobinemia induced by prilocaine in predisposed patients (see Chapter 23).

# References

Adriani, J. (1963). Comparative potency and duration of action of topical anesthetic drugs in man (Abstract). *Anesthesiology* 24 (1): 120–121.

Adriani, J. and Campbell, D. (1956). Fatalities following topical application of local anesthetics to mucous membranes. *JAMA* 162 (17): 1527–1530.

Adriani, J. and Zepernick, R. (1964). Clinical effectiveness of drugs used for topical anesthesia. *JAMA* 188 (8): 711–716.

Adriani, J., Zepernick, R., Arens, J., and Authement, E. (1964). The comparative potency and effectiveness of topical anesthetics in man. *Clin. Pharmacol. Ther.* 5 (1): 49–62.

Aldous, W.K., Jensen, R., and Sieck, B.M. (1998). Cocaine and lidocaine with phenylephrine as topical anesthetics: antimicrobial activity against common nasal pathogens. *Ear Nose Throat J.* 77 (7): 554–557.

Al-Melh, M.A. and Anderson, L. (2007). Comparison of topical anesthetics (EMLA/Oraqix vs benzocaine) on pain experience during palatal needle injection. *Oral Surg. Oral Med. Oral Pathol.* 103 (5): e16–e20.

Al-Melh, M.A., Anderson, L., and Behbehani, E. (2005). Reduction of pain from needle stick in the oral mucosa by topical anesthetics: a comparative study between lidocaine/prilocaine and benzocaine. *J. Clin. Dent.* 16 (2): 53–56.

American Academy of Pediatric Dentistry (2020). *Use of Local Anesthesia for Pediatric Dental Patients. The Reference Manual of Pediatric Dentistry*. Chicago IL: American Academy of Pediatric Dentistry. 318–323.

American Dental Association (2003). *ADA Guide to Dental Therapeutics*, 3e. Chicago: American Dental Association. 1–16.

Aminabadi, N.A. and Farahani, R.M.Z. (2009). The effect of pre-cooling the injection site on pediatric pain perception during the administration of local anesthesia. *J. Contemp. Dent. Pract.* 10 (3): 43–50.

Annex 6. Dissociation constant or pKa.

Annex 7. Partition coefficient or lipid solubility.

Annex 8. Acute experimental toxicity of local anesthetics.

Annex 9. Local anesthetic bonding to plasmatic proteins.

Annex 11. Pharmacokinetics of local anesthetics and vasoconstrictors.

Annex 13. Toxic plasma levels of local anesthetics.

Annex 19. Topical anesthesia I. Results of clinical trials.

Annex 20. Topical anesthesia II. Clinical efficacy.

Anonymous (1964). Benzocaine. *Med. Lett. Drugs Ther.* 6: 86–87.

Anonymous (1979). Cocaine. *Br. Med. J.* 1 (6169): 971–972.

Aydin, O.N., Eyigor, M., and Aydin, N. (2001). Antimicrobial activity of ropivacaine and other local anesthetics. *Eur. J. Anaesthesiol.* 18 (10): 687–694.

Baumgaertel, S. (2009). Compound topical anesthetics in orthodontics: putting the facts into perspective. *Am. J. Orthod. Dentofacial. Orthop.* 135 (5): 556–557.

Berg, J.O., Mössner, B.K., Skow, M.N. et al. (2006). Antibacterial properties of EMLA and lidocaine in wound tissue biopsies for culturing. *Wound Repair Regen.* 14 (5): 581–585.

Beutlich, F.W. (1991). *Letter. Anesthesiology* 74 (2): 387.

Bhalla, J., Meechan, J.G., Lawrence, H.P. et al. (2009). Effect of time on clinical efficacy of topical anesthesia. *Anesth. Prog.* 56 (2): 36–41.

Bieter, R.N. (1936). Applied pharmacology of local anesthetics. *Am. J. Surg.* 34: 500–510.

Bonica, J.J. (1950). Regional anesthesia with tetracaine. *Anesthesiology* 11 (5): 606–622.

Boynes, S.G., Zovko, J., and Peskin, R.M. (2010). Local anesthesia administration by dental hygienists. *Dent. Clin. N. Am.* 54 (4): 769–778.

Broberg, B.F.J and Evers, H.CA. (1981). Local anesthetic mixture for topical application, and process for its preparation. European Patent 0002425 A1.

Brodin, A., Nyqvist-Mayer, A., Wadsten, T. et al. (1984). Phase diagram and aqueous solubility of the lidocaine–prilocaine binary system. *J. Pharm. Sci.* 73 (4): 481–484.

Brook, L.M., Tucker, G.T., Tuckley, E.C., and Boynes, R.N. (1989). A lignocaine patch for dental analgesia safety and early pharmacology. *J. Controlled Release* 10 (2): 183–188.

Caldwell, J. and Sever, P.S. (1974). The biochemical pharmacology of abused drugs. I. Amphetamines, cocaine, and LSD. *Clin. Pharmacol. Ther.* 16 (4): 625–638.

Calvey, T.N. (1995). Isomerism and anesthetic drugs. *Acta Anaesthesiol. Scand.* 39 (Suppl 106): 83–90.

Campbell, D. and Adriani, J. (1958). Absorption of local anesthetics. *JAMA* 168 (7): 873–877.

Cannel, H. (1996). Evidence of safety margins of lignocaine local anesthetics for perioral use. *Br. Dent. J.* 181 (7): 243–249.

Carabelli, A.A. (1952). Use of pantocaine in subposologic quantities for bronchoscopy and bronchography. *Anesthesiology* 13 (2): 169–183.

Carr, M.P. and Horton, J.E. (2001a). Clinical evaluation and comparison of 2 topical anesthetics for pain caused by needle sticks and scaling and root planning. *J. Periodontol.* 72 (4): 479–484.

Carr, M.P. and Horton, J.E. (2001b). Evaluation of a transoral delivery system for topical anesthesia. *J. Am. Dent. Assoc.* 132 (12): 1714–1719.

Cohen, H.P., Cha, B.Y., and Spångberg, L.S.W. (1993). Endodontic anesthesia in mandibular molars. A clinical study. *J. Endod.* 19 (7): 370–373.

Council on Dental Therapeutics (1984). *Accepted Dental Therapeutics*, 40e. Chicago (IL): American Dental Association. 181–202.

Covino, B. and Giddon, D.B. (1981). Pharmacology of local anesthetic agents. *J. Dent. Res.* 60 (8): 1454–1459.

Dalili, H. and Adriani, J. (1971). The efficacy of local anesthetics in blocking the sensation of itch, burning, and pain in normal and "sunburned" skin. *Clin. Pharmacol. Ther.* 12 (6): 913–919.

De Jong, R.H. (1977). *Local Anesthetics*, 2e. Springfield (IL): Charles C Thomas Publisher. 230.

DiFazio, C. (1981). Local anesthetics: action, metabolism and toxicity. *Otolaryngol. Clin. N. Am.* 14 (3): 515–519.

Donaldson, D. and Meechan, J.G. (1995). A comparison of the effects of EMLA® cream and topical 5% lidocaine on discomfort during gingival probing. *Anesth. Prog.* 42 (1): 7–10.

Donaldson, D., Gelskey, S.C., Landry, R.G. et al. (2003). A placebo-controlled multi-center evaluation of an anesthetic gel (Oraqix®) for periodontal therapy. *J. Clin. Periodontol.* 30 (3): 171–175.

Duncan, J.D., Reeves, G.W., and Fitchie, J.G. (1992). Technique to diminish discomfort from the palatal injection. *J. Prosth. Dent.* 67 (6): 901–902.

Eisleb O. (1932). Of Hofheim-on-Taunus, Germany, assignor to Winthrop Chemical Company, Inc., of New York, NY, a corporation of New York. Beta-dimethylaminoethyl ester of para-butylamino-benzoic acid. US Patent 1,889,645. Patented Nov. 29.

Eisleb, O. (1934). Vom Cocain zum Pantocain. Der Werdegang der örtlichen Betäubung. *Med. Chem. (Leverkusen)* 2: 364–376.

Engberg, G., Danielson, K., Henneberg, S., and Nilsson, A. (1987). Plasma concentrations of prilocaine and lidocaine and methaemoglobin formation in infants after epicutaneous application of a 5% lidocaine-prilocaine cream (EMLA). *Acta Anaesthsiol. Scand.* 31 (7): 624–628.

Evers, H. and Haegerstam, G. (1981). *Handbook of Dental Local Anesthesia*. Copenhagen: Schultz Medical International. 65, 171.

Fischer, G. (1912). *Local Anesthesia in Dentistry. With Special Reference to the Mucous and Conductive Methods. A Concise Guide for Dentists, Surgeons and Students*. Philadelphia: Lea and Febiger. 37.

Franz-Montan, M., Silva, A.L.R., Cogo, K. et al. (2007). Liposome-encapsulated ropivacaine for topical anesthesia of human oral mucosa. *Anesth. Analg.* 104 (6): 1528–1531.

Franz-Montan, M., Ranali, J., Ramacciato, J.C. et al. (2008). Ulceration of gingival mucosa after topical application of EMLA: report of four cases. *Br. Dent. J.* 204 (3): 133–134.

Franz-Montan, M., de Paula, E., Groppo, F.C. et al. (2010). Liposome-encapsulated ropivacaine for intraoral topical anesthesia. *Oral Surg. Oral Med. Oral Pathol.* 110 (6): 800–804.

Franz-Montan, M., de Paula, E., Groppo, F.C. et al. (2012). Liposomal delivery system for topical anaesthesia of the palatal mucosa. *Br. J. Oral Maxillofac. Surg.* 50 (1): 60–64.

Frasier, I.M. (1967). Local anesthetics. In: *Premedication, Local and General Anesthesia in Dentistry* (ed. A.B. Jorgensen and J. Hayden). Philadelphia: Lea and Febiger. 89–96.

Frayling, I.M., Addison, G.M., Chattergee, K., and Meakin, G. (1990). Metahaemoglobinemia in children treated with prilocaine-lignocaine cream. *Br. Med. J.* 301 (6744): 153–154.

Friskopp, J. and Huledal, G. (2001). Plasma level of lidocaine and prilocaine after application of Oraqix®, a new intrapocket anesthetic, in patients with advanced periodontitis. *J. Clin. Periodontol.* 28 (5): 425–429.

Friskopp, J., Nilsson, M., and Isacsson, G. (2001). The anesthetic onset and duration of a new lidocaine/prilocaine gel intra-pocket anesthetic (Oraqix®) for periodontal scaling/root planing. *J. Clin. Periodontol.* 28 (5): 453–458.

Furchgott, R.F. (1972). *The classification of adrenoceptors (adrenergic receptors). An evaluation from the standpoint of receptor theory (Chapter 9)* Catecholamines. Handbook of experimental pharmacology (New series), vol. 33 (ed. H. Blaschko and E. Muscholl). Berlin: Springer-Verlag. 283–335.

Fuss, Z., Trowbridge, H., Bender, I.B. et al. (1986). Assessment of reliability of electrical and thermal pulp testing agents. *J. Endod.* 12 (7): 301–305.

Gangorosa, L.P. (1974). Iontophoresis for surface local anesthesia. *J. Am. Dent. Assoc.* 88 (1): 125–128.

Gangorosa, L.P. (1981). Newer local anesthetics and techniques for administration. *J. Dent. Res.* 60 (8): 1471–1480.

Ghaderi, F., Banakar, S., and Rostami, S. (2013). Effect of pre-cooling injection site on pain perception in pediatric dentistry: a randomized clinical trial. *Dent. Res. J.* 10 (6): 790–794.

Giddon, D.B., Quadland, M., Rachwall, P.C. et al. (1968). Development of a method for comparing topical anesthetics in different application and dosage forms. *J. Oral Ther. Pharmacol.* 4 (4): 270–274.

Gill, C.J. and Orr, D.L. II (1979). A double-blind crossover comparison of topical anesthetics. *J. Am. Dent. Assoc.* 98 (2): 213–214.

Gocmen, J.S., Buyukkocak, U., Caglayan, O., and Aksoy, A. (2008). In vitro antibacterial effects of topical local anesthetics. *J. Dermatol. Treat.* 19 (6): 351–353.

Graser, G.N. (1984). The efficacy of topical anesthetics in reducing intraoral discomfort. *Oral Surg. Oral Med. Oral Pathol.* 58 (1): 42–46.

Guay, J. (2009). Methemoglobinemia related to local anesthetics: a summary of 242 episodes. *Anesth. Analg.* 108 (3): 837–845.

Haas, D.A., Rynn, B.R., and Sands, T.D. (2000). Drug use for the pregnant or lactating patient. *Gen. Dent.* 48 (1): 54–60.

Haasio, J., Jokinen, T., Numminen, M., and Rosenberg, P.H. (1990). Topical anaesthesia of gingival mucosa by 5% eutectic mixture of lignocaine and prilocaine or by 10% lignocaine spray. *Br. J. Oral Maxillofac. Surg.* 28 (2): 99–101.

Harbert, H. (1989). Topical ice: a precursor to palatal injections. *J. Endod.* 15 (1): 27–28.

Herdevall, B.-M., Klinge, B., Persson, L. et al. (2003). Plasma levels of lidocaine, o-toluidine, and prilocaine after application of 8.5 g Oraqix® in patients with generalized periodontitis: effect on blood methemoglobin and tolerability. *Acta Odontol. Scand.* 61 (4): 230–234.

Hersh, E.V., Houpt, M.I., Cooper, S.A. et al. (1996). Analgesic efficacy and safety on an intraoral lidocaine patch. *J. Am. Dent. Assoc.* 127 (11): 1626–1634.

Hersh, E.V., DeRossi, S.S., Ciarrocca, K.N. et al. (2003). Efficacy and tolerability of an intraoral benzocaine patch in the relief of spontaneous toothache pain. *J. Clin. Dent.* 14 (1): 1–6.

Hersh, E.V., Stoopler, E.T., Secreto, S.A., and DeRossi, S.S. (2005). A study of benzocaine gel dosing for toothache. *J. Clin. Dent.* 16 (4): 103–108.

Hersh, E.V., Ciancio, S.G., Kuperstein, A.S. et al. (2013). An evaluation of 10 percent and 20 percent benzocaine gels in patients with acute toothaches: efficacy, tolerability and compliance with label dose administration directions. *J. Am. Dent. Assoc.* 144 (5): 517–526.

Hindocha, N., Manhem, F., Bäckyrd, E., and Bagesund, M. (2019). Ice versus lidocaine 5% for topical anaesthesia of oral mucosa – a randomized cross-over study. *BMC Anesthesiol.* 19 (1): 227.

Holst, A. and Evers, H. (1985). Experimental studies of new topical anaesthetics on the oral mucosa. *Swed. Dent. J.* 9 (5): 185–191.

Houpt, M.I., Heins, P., Lamster, I. et al. (1997). An evaluation of intraoral lidocaine patches in reducing needle-insertion pain. *Compend. Contin. Edu. Dent.* 18 (4): 309–316.

Howitt, J.W. and Lowell, C. (1972). Topical anesthetic effectiveness. An old and new product evaluated. *N. Y. State Dent. J.* 38 (9): 549–550.

Hsiao-Wu, G.W., Susarla, S.M., and White, P.P. (2007). Use of the cold test as a measure of pulpal anesthesia during endodontic therapy: a randomized, blinded, placebo-controlled clinical trial. *J. Endod.* 33 (4): 406–410.

Huledal, G. and Friskopp, J. (2000). A new anesthetic gel for periodontal use; plasma levels of lidocaine and prilocaine. *J. Clin. Periodontol.* 27 (Suppl 1): 52. (Abstract no. 136).

Jastak, J.T. and Yagiela, J.A. (1983). Vasoconstrictors and local anesthesia: a review and rationale for use. *J. Am. Dent. Assoc.* 107 (4): 623–630.

Javaid, J.I., Musa, M.N., Fischman, M. et al. (1983). Kinetics of cocaine in humans after intravenous and intranasal administration. *Biopharm. Drug Dispos.* 4 (1): 9–18.

Jayasuriya, N.S.S., Weerapperuma, I.D., and Amarasinghe, M.G.C.K. (2017). The use of an iced cotton bud as an effective pre-cooling method for palatal anaesthesia: a technical note. *Sing. Dent. J.* 38: 17–19.

Jeffcoat, M.K., Geurs, N.C., Magnusson, I. et al. (2001). Intrapocket anesthesia for scaling and root planing: results of a double-blind multicenter trial using lidocaine prilocaine dental gel. *J. Periodontol.* 72 (7): 895–900.

Juhlin, L., Evers, H., and Broberg, F. (1980). A lidocaine-prilocaine cream for superficial skin surgery and painful lesions. *Acta Derm. Veneorol. (Stockholm)* 60 (6): 544–546.

Jyväkorpi, M. (1996). A comparison of topical Emla cream with Bonain's solution for anesthesia of the tympanic membrane during tympanocentesis. *Eur. Arch. Otorhinolaryngol.* 253 (4): 234–236.

Kaewjiaranai, T., Srisatjaluk, R.L., Sakdajeyont, W. et al. (2018). The efficiency of topical anesthetics as antimicrobial agents: a review of use in dentistry. *J. Dent. Anesth. Pain Med.* 18 (4): 223–233.

Keller, B.J. (1985). Comparison of the effectiveness of two topical anesthetics and a placebo in reducing injection pain. *Hawaii Dent. J.* 16 (12): 10–11.

Kennedy, S., Reader, A., Nusstein, J. et al. (2003). The significance of needle deflection in success of the inferior alveolar nerve block in patients with irreversible pulpitis. *J. Endod.* 29 (10): 630–633.

Kincheloe, J.E., Mealiea, W.L. Jr., Mattison, G.D., and Seib, K. (1991). Psychophysical measurement on pain perception after administration of a topical anesthetic. *Quintessence Int.* 22 (4): 311–315.

Klein, S.L., Nustad, R.A., Feinberg, S.E., and Fonseca, R.J. (1983). Acute toxic methemoglobinemia caused by a topical anesthetic. *Pediatr. Dent.* 5 (2): 107–108.

Kosaraju, A. and Vandewalle, K.S. (2009). A comparison of a refrigerant and topical anesthetic gel as preinjection anesthetics. A clinical evaluation. *J. Am. Dent. Assoc.* 140 (6): 68–72.

Kravitz, N.D. (2007). The use of compound topical anesthetics. A review. *J. Am. Dent. Assoc.* 138 (10): 1333–1339.

Kravitz, N.D. and Kusnoto, B. (2006). Placement of mini-implants with topical anesthetic. *J. Clin. Orthod.* 40 (10): 602–604.

Kravitz, N.D., Graham, J.W., and Nicozisis, J.L. (2015). Compound topical anesthetics in orthodontics. *J. Clin. Orthod.* 49 (6): 371–377.

Kreider, K.A., Stratmann, R.G., Milano, M. et al. (2001). Reducing children's injection pain: lidocaine patches versus topical benzocaine gel. *Pediatr. Dent.* 23 (1): 19–23.

Künisch, J., Daunbländer, M., Klingberg, G. et al. (2017). Best clinical practice guidance for local analgesia in pediatric dentistry: an EAPD policy document. *Eur. Arch. Paediatr. Dent.* 18 (5): 313–321.

Kwong, T.S., Kusnoto, B., Viana, G. et al. (2011). The effectiveness of Oraqix versus TAC(a) for placement of orthodontic temporary anchorage devices. *Angle Orthod.* 81 (5): 754–759.

Lamberton, J.A., Oesterle, L.J., Shellhart, W.C. et al. (2016). Comparison of pain perception during miniscrew placement in orthodontic patients with a visual analog scale survey between compound topical and needle-injected anesthetic: a crossover, prospective, randomized clinical trial. *Am. J. Orthod. Dentofac. Orthop.* 149 (1): 15–23.

Lathwal, G., Pandit, I.K., Gugnani, N., and Gupta, M. (2015). Efficacy of different precooling agents and topical anesthetics on the pain perception during intraoral injection: a comparative clinical study. *Int. J. Clin. Pediatr. Dent.* 8 (2): 119–122.

Leopold, A., Wilson, S., Weaver, J.S., and Mori, A.M. (2002). Pharmacokinetics of lidocaine delivered from a transmucosal patch in children. *Anesth. Prog.* 49 (3): 82–87.

Lesch, C.A., Squier, C.A., Cruchley, A. et al. (1989). The impermeability of human oral mucosa and skin to water. *J. Dent. Res.* 68 (9): 1345–1349.

Lim, S. and Julliard, K. (2004). Evaluating the efficacy of EMLA topical anesthetic in sealant placement with rubber dam. *Pediatr. Dent.* 26 (6): 497–500.

Loetscher, C.A., Melton, D.C., and Walton, R.E. (1988). Injection regimen for anesthesia of the maxillary first molar. *J. Am. Dent. Assoc.* 117 (2): 337–340.

Magnusson, I., Geurs, N.C., Harris, P.A. et al. (2003). Intrapocket anesthesia for scaling and root planing in pain-sensitive patients. *J. Periodontol.* 74 (5): 597–602.

Malamed, S.F. (2004). *Handbook of Local Anesthesia*, 5e. St. Louis (MO): Elsevier-Mosby. 50.

Martin, M.D., Ramsay, D.S., Whitney, C. et al. (1994). Topical anesthesia: differentiating the pharmacological and psychological contribution to efficacy. *Anesth. Prog.* 41(2): 40–47.

Martindale (1982). *The Extra Pharmacopoeia*, 28e. London: Reynolds JEF Editor. 899–923.

Mazumdar, B., Tomlinson, A.A., and Faulder, G.C. (1991). Preliminary study to assay plasma amethocaine concentrations after topical application of a new local anaesthetic cream containing amethocaine. *Br. J. Anaesth.* 67 (4): 432–436.

McLure, H.A. and Rubin, A.P. (2005). Review of local anaesthetic agents. *Minerva Anesthesiol.* 71 (3): 59–74.

Meadows, J.C. (1970). Observations on muscle pain in man, with particular reference to pain during needle electromyography. *J. Neural Neurosurg. Psychiatry* 33 (4): 519–523.

Meechan, J.G. (2000). Intraoral topical anaesthetics: a review. *J. Dent.* 28 (1): 3–14.

Meechan, J.G. (2001). The use of EMLA® for oral soft-tissue biopsy in a needle phobic: a case report. *Anesth. Prog.* 48 (1): 32–34.

Meechan, J.G. and Donaldson, D. (1994). The intraoral use of EMLA cream in children: a clinical investigation. *J. Dent. Child* 61 (4): 260–262.

Meechan, J.G., Gowans, A.J., and Welbury, R.R. (1998). The use of patient-controlled transcutaneous electronic nerve stimulation (TENS) to decrease the discomfort of regional anaesthesia in dentistry: a randomized controlled clinical trial. *J. Dent.* 26 (5–6): 417–420.

Mohiuddin, I., Setty, J.V., Srinivasan, I., and Desai, J.A. (2015). Topical application of local anaesthetic gel vs ice in pediatric patients for infiltration anaesthesia. *J. Evol. Med. Dent. Sci.* 4 (74): 12,934–12,940.

Mullin, G.S. and Rubinfeld, R.S. (1997). The antibacterial activity of topical anesthetics. *Cornea* 16 (6): 662–665.

Munshi, A.K., Hegde, A.M., and Latha, R. (2001). Use of EMLA®: is it an injection free alternative? *J. Clin. Pediatr. Dent.* 25 (3): 215–219.

Muscholl, E. (1961). Effect of cocaine and related drugs on the uptake of noradrenaline by heart and spleen. *Br. J. Pharmacol. Chemother.* 16 (3): 352–359.

Nakamura, S., Matsuura, N., and Ichinohe, T. (2013). A new method of topical anesthesia by using anesthetic solution in a patch. *J. Endod.* 39 (11): 1369–1373.

Neue Arzneimittel und pharmaceutische Spezialitäten (1902). Dr Ritsert's Anästhesin. *Pharm. Ztg.* 47: 356.

Niemann, A. (1860). Ueber eine neue organische Base in den Cocablättern. *Arch. Pharm.* 153: 129–155 and 291–308.

Nusstein, J., Reader, A., Nist, R. et al. (1998). Anesthetic efficacy of the supplemental intraosseous injection of 2% lidocaine with 1:100,000 epinephrine in irreversible pulpitis. *J. Endon.* 24 (7): 487–491.

Nyqvist-Mayer, A.A., Brodin, A.F., and Frank, S.G. (1986). Drug release studies on an oil-water emulsion on a eutectic mixture of lidocaine and prilocaine as the dispersed phase. *J. Pharm. Sci.* 75 (4): 365–373.

Packer, J.I., Krall, B., Makki, A., and Torabinejad, M. (2013). The effect of sonophoresis on topical anesthesia: a pilot project. *Anesth. Prog.* 60 (2): 37–41.

Pere, P., Iizuka, T., Rosenberg, P.H., and Lindqvist, C. (1992). Topical application of 5% eutectic mixture of lignocaine and prilocaine (EMLA®) before removal of arch bars. *Br. J. Oral Maxillofac. Surg.* 30 (3): 153–156.

Potter, J.L. and Hillman, J.V. (1979). Benzocaine-induced methemoglobinemia. *J. Am. Coll. Emerg. Physicians (JACEP)* 8 (1): 26–27.

Primosch, R.E. and Rolland-Assensi, G. (2001). Comparison of topical EMLA 5% oral adhesive to benzocaine 20% on the pain experienced during palatal anesthetic infiltration in children. *Pediatr. Dent.* 23 (1): 11–14.

Reiz, G.M.E.E. and Reiz, S.L.A. (1982). EMLA – a eutectic mixture of local anaesthetics for topical anaesthesia. *Acta Anaesthsiol. Scand.* 26 (6): 596–598.

Reynolds, M.M., Greenwood-Quaintance, K.E., Patel, R., and Pulido, J.S. (2016). Selected antimicrobial activity of topical ophthalmic anesthetics. *Transf. Vis. Sci. Technol.* 5 (4): 2.

Reznik, D.S., Jeske, A.H., Chen, J.-W., and English, J. (2009). Comparative efficacy of 2 topical anesthetics for the placement of orthodontic temporary anchorage devices. *Anesth. Prog.* 56 (3): 81–85.

Ritchie, J.M. and Ritchie, B.R. (1968). Local anesthetics: effect of the pH on activity. *Science* 162 (3860): 1394–1395.

Roberts, D.H. and Sowray, J.H. (1987). *Local Analgesia in Dentistry*, 3e. Bristol (UK): Wright. 34, 74–77.

Rodriguez, L.F., Smolik, L.M., and Zbehlik, A.J. (1994). Benzocaine-induced methemoglobinemia: report of a severe reaction and review of the literature. *Ann. Pharmacother.* 28 (5): 643–649.

Roghani, S., Duperon, D.F., and Barcohana, N. (1999). Evaluating the efficacy of commonly used topical anesthetics. *Pediatr. Dent.* 21 (3): 197–200.

Roller, N.W. and Ship, I.I. (1975). Lidocaine topical film strip for oral mucosa biopsies. *J. Oral Med.* 30 (2): 55–58.

Severinghaus, J.W., Xu, F.-D., and Spellman, M.J. Jr. (1991). Benzocaine and methemoglobin: recommended actions (Letter). *Anesthesiology* 74 (2): 385–386.

Ship, I.I., Williams, A.F., and Osheroff, B.J. (1960). Development and clinical investigation of a new oral surface anesthetic for acute and chronic oral lesions. *Oral Surg. Oral Med. Oral Pathol.* 13 (5): 630–636.

Singh, R. and Al Khalili, Y. (2019). *Benzocaine. StatPearls [Internet]*. Treasure Island (FL): StatPearls Publishing.

Stecker, S.S., Swift, J.Q., Hodges, J.S., and Erickson, P.R. (2002). Should a mucoadhesive patch (DentiPatch) be used for gingival anesthesia in children? *Anesth. Prog.* 49 (1): 3–8.

Stern, I. and Giddon, D.B. (1975). Topical anesthesia for periodontal procedures. *Anesth. Prog.* 22 (4): 105–108.

Sveen, O.B., Yaekel, M., and Adair, S.M. (1982). Efficacy of using benzocaine for temporary relief of toothache. *Oral Surg. Oral Med. Oral Pathol.* 53 (6): 574–576.

Svensson, P. and Petersen, J.K. (1992). Anesthetic effect of EMLA occluded with orahesive oral bandages on oral mucosa. A placebo—controlled study. *Anesth. Prog.* 39 (3): 79–82.

Svensson, P., Petersen, J.K., and Svensson, H. (1994). Efficacy of topical anesthetic on pain and unpleasantness during scaling of gingival pockets. *Anesth. Prog.* 41 (2): 35–39.

Tainmont, J. (2007). Dr Bonain, an ENT surgeon with an ocean background. *B-ENT* 3 (4): 217–230.

Takman, B.H. (1975). The chemistry of local anaesthetic agents: classification of blocking agents. *Br. J. Anesth.* 47 (Suppl): 183–190.

Taware, C.P., Mazumdar, S., Pendharkar, M. et al. (1997). A bioadhesive delivery system as an alternative to infiltration anesthesia. *Oral Surg. Oral Med. Oral Pathol.* 84 (6): 609–615.

Tulga, F. and Mutlu, Z. (1999). Four types of topical anaesthetic agents: evaluation of clinical effectiveness. *J. Clin. Padiatr. Dent.* 23 83): 217–220.

Van Dyke, C. and Byck, R. (1982). Cocaine. *Sci. Am.* 246 (3): 128–141.

Van Dyke, C., Barash, P.G., Jatlow, P., and Byck, R. (1976). Cocaine: plasma concentrations after intranasal application in man. *Science* 191 (4229): 859–861.

Van Steenberghe, D., Bercy, P., De Boever, J. et al. (2004). Patient evaluation of a novel non-injectable anesthetic gel: a multicenter crossover study comparing the gel to infiltration anesthesia during scaling and root planing. *J. Periodontol.* 75 (11): 1471–1478.

Vickers, E.R. and Punnia-Moorthy, A. (1993). Pulpal anesthesia from an application of a eutectic topical anesthetic. *Quintessence Int.* 24 (8): 547–551.

Vickers, E.R., Marzbani, N., Gerzina, T.M. et al. (1997). Pharmacokinetics of EMLA cream 5% application to oral mucosa. *Anesth. Prog.* 44 (1): 32–37.

Wehner, D. and Hamilton, G.C. (1984). Seizures following topical application of local anesthetics to burn patients. *Ann. Emerg. Med.* 13 (6): 456–458.

Weisel, E. and Tella, R.A. (1951). Reactions to tetracaine (Pontocaine) used as topical anesthetic in bronchoscopy: study of 1,000 cases. *JAMA* 147 (3): 218–222.

Wilburn-Goo, D. and Lloyd, L.M. (1999). When patients become cyanotic: acquired methemoglobinemia. *J. Am. Dent. Assoc.* 130 (6): 826–831.

Willstätter, R., Wolfes, D., and Mäder, H. (1923). Synthese des natürlichen Cocaïns. *Justus Liebig's Ann. Chem.* 434 (2): 111–139.

Winther, J.E. and Khan, M.W. (1971). Antimicrobial effect of topical anesthetics. *Acta Odontol. Scand.* 29 (3): 337–347.

Wiswall, A.T., Bowles, W.R., Lunos, S. et al. (2014). Palatal anesthesia: comparison of four techniques for decreasing injection discomfort. *Northwest. Dent.* 93 (4): 25–29.

Won, S.H., Lee, S.W., and Kho, H.S. (1995). Penetration of lidocaine into oral mucosa by iontophoresis and its clinical application. *J. Dent. Res.* 74 (Special issue): 576. (abstract no. 1404).

Yoon, R.K. and Chussid, S. (2009). Topical anesthesia for rubber dam clamp placement in sealant placement: comparison of lidocaine/prilocaine gel and benzocaine. *Pediatr. Dent.* 31 (5): 377–381.

Zed, C.M., Epstein, J., and Donaldson, D. (1996). Topical liposome encapsulated tetracaine versus benzocaine – a clinical investigation. *J. Dent. Res.* 75 (Special issue): 247. (abstract no. 1840).

**Local Anesthetic Techniques in Dentistry**

# 13

# Basic Injection Technique

In this chapter, we review the basic technique for injecting local anesthetic intraorally. We present the various phases in order and with all the relevant steps (even though these often overlap in clinical practice), placing emphasis on those aspects that make dental injections safer and more comfortable, given that injections are the main reason people fear dental treatment (Kleinknecht et al. 1973; Messer 1977; Berggren and Meynert 1984; Milgrom et al. 1997). Furthermore, following the approach we present here helps to reduce the stress experienced by almost 20% of dentists themselves with respect to administration of local anesthetic (Simon et al. 1994).

In the second part of the chapter, we address the components of the injection technique that lead to pain by separating them into those that directly produce pain and those that are much less significant but are popularly considered to be closely associated with pain. The final part of the chapter will address the terminology of the different anesthetic techniques. We have divided the basic technique into 10 phases (sections "Initial Preparation" to "Post-treatment Phase").

## Comment on Retraction

With the aim of preventing accidental needle-stick injury and the resulting risk of transmission of HIV, hepatitis B, or hepatitis C infection to the health professional (Cleveland et al. 2007; David et al. 2007), dentists now tend to avoid placing their fingers into the patient's mouth during administration of local anesthetic to retract the soft tissues and palpate dental structures (Cleveland et al. 2007; David et al. 2007; Fa et al. 2016). Alternatives include a dental mirror (David et al. 2007; Fa et al. 2016), a Minnesota retractor, a tongue depressor (David et al. 2007), or even devices such as the vibrating device DentalVibe® (Fa et al. 2016) (Chapter 11).

Nevertheless, a study based on information collected from 1995 to 2004 in the United States that provides a wide-ranging review of previous studies found that, since 1987, the frequency of accidental needle-stick injury in dentistry had decreased, and that of the 59 recorded cases of transmission of HIV infection to healthcare personnel, none involved dental professionals (Cleveland et al. 2007). Furthermore, of the 360 accidental needle-stick cases recorded in dental health personnel, 88 were caused by dental needles (25%), with 70% affecting dentists and oral surgeons and 25% affecting dental assistants and hygienists (Cleveland et al. 2007).

In this book, dental local anesthetic techniques are addressed by inserting the fingers of the supporting hand into the patient's mouth (left hand in right-handed dentists) to separate the soft tissues and thus stabilize the area to facilitate injection. This is the approach recommended in all of the texts in this specialty, although emphasis is placed on methods to prevent accidental needle-stick injuries.

## Phases of the Injection

### Initial Preparation

Before the patient enters the dental office, we should evaluate and anticipate a series of concerns.

1) Assess how well the patient will cooperate.
   The previous visit (generally the first visit), especially in children, gives an idea of how the patient will behave. It is important to remember that children are brought to the dentist by their parents. Thus, aside from age, demeanor, and physical appearance, two specific situations enable us to predict disruptive behavior in future visits to the dentist:
   - Examination of the mouth.
   - Intraoral radiographs.
   
   Any difficulty observed while these maneuvers are being performed points to a high risk of disruptive

---

*Local Anesthesia in Dentistry: A Locoregional Approach*, First Edition. Jesús Calatayud and Mana Saraghi.
© 2024 John Wiley & Sons Ltd. Published 2024 by John Wiley & Sons Ltd.
Companion website: www.wiley.com/go/Calatayud/local

behavior during administration of oral anesthesia at the following visits.

In contrast, if the examination reveals the patient to have undergone considerable restorative work and complicated dental procedures and the parents report that no specific measures were taken (sedation, medication), then the patient's behavior should be acceptable for the administration of local anesthesia.

2) Review the health questionnaire and dental history.
   We can review the following questions:

   1) What level of anxiety and fear does dental treatment cause you?
      None ☐   A little ☐   Moderate ☐   Quite a lot ☐   A lot ☐

   2) Have you ever experienced abnormal reactions, fainting, dizziness when receiving local anesthetic or vaccinations or when giving blood?
      Yes ☐   No ☐

   These two questions enable us to better evaluate disruptive behavior. Other questions on health status, medical problems, and medications taken will enable us to determine whether there are absolute or relative contraindications for administration of dental local anesthetic or whether there are limitations for the use of anesthetics or vasoconstrictors (see Chapters 8, 9, and 10 on contraindications for the techniques, anesthetics, and vasoconstrictors).

3) Review body weight in small patients and children.
   The basic purpose of reviewing body weight is to avoid overdose, which can have serious consequences (Goodson and Moore 1983; Hersh et al. 1991; Moore 1992; Virts 1999; Council on Clinical Affairs 2015). Surveys among dentists show that around half believe (erroneously) that the maximum dose should not be based on the patient's weight but that the same dose should be administered to all patients, therefore in patients weighing less than 40 kg there may be a risk of overdose (Linscott et al. 1978; Cheatham et al. 1992; Daubländer et al. 1997). Annex 10 shows the maximum absolute doses by body weight in dentistry.

4) Organize all local anesthetic equipment.
   Before the patient comes into the dental office, the dental equipment should be prepared and covered so as not to increase the anxiety generally felt by the patient (Mink and Spedding 1966). Some authors recommend having tweezers or mosquito clamp to prepare for the unfortunate case where a needle breaks in the patient's mouth, so that the end protruding from the soft tissue can be removed before it disappears completely into the tissue (Armbrecht and Schwetz 1962; Orr 1983; McDonogh 1996).

## Preparation Phase

Once the patient is in the office, we can proceed as follows:

1) Position of the dentist and patient.
   - The dentist should be seated at between 8 and 10 o'clock (maximum 7–11 o'clock) with respect to the patient's mouth, depending on the technique and approach used, and on the patient's right (for right-handed dentists). Being seated ensures better accuracy and control.
   - The patient should be in a semi-recumbent position so that the dentist can work from a seated position, thus improving accuracy and reducing risk for the patient: having the patient in a semi-recumbent position reduces the risk of a vasovagal reaction caused by the lack of blood flow to the brain resulting from anxiety. Consequently, the risk of serious complications is reduced (Bourne 1957, 1970).

2) Assistant beside the dentist.
   Having the assistant seated at 2–4 o'clock can make it easier to pass the syringe and hold the patient to prevent sudden movements (especially in children) and help where necessary, such as in cases of needle breakage, when he/she can pass the dentist tweezers or a mosquito clamp to remove the protruding end of the needle (Orr 1983).

3) Where possible, remove prosthesis and braces from the patient's mouth. Where possible orthodontic braces in children and dentures in adults should be removed, since these hamper administration of anesthetic and increase the risk of lesions in uncooperative patients.

4) Preparation of the syringe by the assistant.
   - Insert the cartridge into the syringe. Some dentists prefer to disinfect the mouth of the cartridge by wiping it with gauze soaked in alcohol immediately before loading the syringe. This maneuver is not necessary with modern packaging (blister packs). Cartridges should never be placed in disinfectant since this can reach the interior of the cartridge and contaminate the solution (Shannon and Feller 1972; Shannon and Wescott 1974).
   - Place the needle over the mouth of the syringe loaded with the cartridge by removing the posterior cap of the needle and screwing the posterior part of the needle into the mouth of the syringe. Note that the anterior cap covering the front part of the needle, the active part, is not removed. The needle should not be bent for intraoral injections (Dentists' Desk 1983). In cases where it is necessary to bend the needle to reach a difficult area, then it should be bent half-way down the shaft of the needle and not at the hub-adapter, since this is the weakest area and thus increases the risk of breakage (Burgess 1988).

- Finally, place a protective disk on the front cap of the needle to prevent needle-stick injury when the syringe containing the cartridge and needle is passed to the dentist (needle-stick protector) (Figure 11.10, Chapter 11).

5) Do not use words with a high emotional content.
   Try to avoid these terms and use more pleasant euphemisms:
   - Do not use the terms "syringe," "injection," or "prick"; instead use "anesthesia," which is more general and less aggressive.
   - Do not use the words "pain" or "harm"; instead use "notice" or "discomfort."
   - Do not use the term "soft tissue anesthesia," as it is too technical; instead use "numbness," "dullness," "tingling," "tickling," or "swelling" (Table 13.1).
   
   Using words with a high emotional content in explanations increases anxiety and makes more predisposed patients consider low levels of stimulus as pain (Jackson 1974; Firestein 1976; Wepman 1978).

6) With children, use the tell-show-do technique (Addelston 1959), which is actually the tell-do technique (McClure 1968), since in this case neither the needle nor the syringe should be shown: seeing these objects increases anxiety in children (Spedding and Mink 1964; Majstorovic and Veerkamp 2004) (Figure 13.1). The approach should be as follows (Spedding and Mink 1964: Mink and Spedding 1966):
   - Provide brief explanations with positive sentences and continuous specific references in a level of language that is suited to the patient's age. Prolonged explanations lead the child to stop listening and begin to feel anxious.
   - The dentist can tell the child that only his/her "teeth are going to sleep" and that these are small (show using the fingers), unlike him/her, who is big (show using the arms). This strategy is aimed at reassuring the child by showing him/her that he/she is big in comparison with the teeth, which are small and that, therefore, the maneuver will be "a little one."

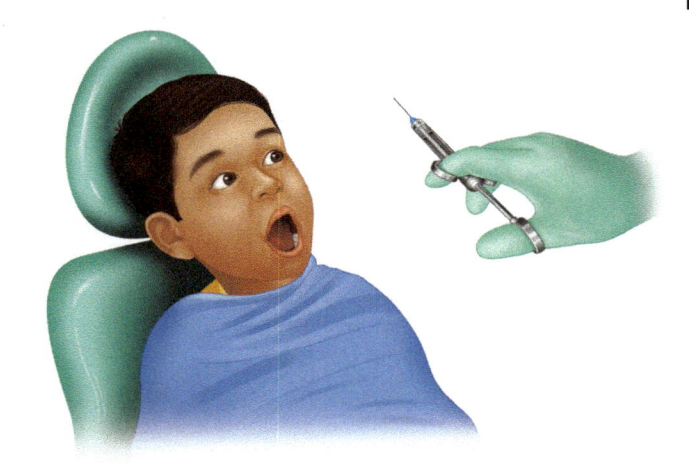

**Figure 13.1** Do not show children the syringe with the needle in place. *Source:* Drawn with modifications according to Snawder (1987).

- The dentist explains that he/she is going to use "anesthetic" on the gum near the teeth and touches the area to be injected with a finger (this should be clearly visible). Thus, the patient becomes familiar with the touch and pressure on this area of the mouth. The dentist can tell the child that when the anesthetic goes in, "it will feel just as it does now."
- The dentist then explains how the anesthetized lips and mouth will feel "fat" or that they will feel "ticklish" or that the "lip will feel swollen." These terms are nicer than those used with adults, such as "tickling sensation," "tingling," "numbness," or "dullness" (Table 13.1).
- The dentist should ensure that the patient does not confuse the sensation of "pressure" at the injection site with "discomfort," therefore the dentist carefully takes the child's wrist (without hurting) and presses it so that the patient notices the sensation of pressure without pain and moves the patient's arm.
- It is important to use a calm, soft, gentle, and monotone voice to ensure an atmosphere of normality where everything is known, understood, and accepted (Addelston 1959).
- Finally, tell the patient that he/she will feel like they have a "fat lip" or "swollen lip" and that this will last for some time and then go away. You can even give the patient a mirror so that he/she can see that the lip is not swollen even if it feels like it is.

Questions commonly asked by children:

- Will it be painful? Will it hurt? Simply tell the patient that he/she will feel the same "discomfort" as when you put your finger in his/her mouth.
- Are you going to stick a needle in me? Are you going to give me an injection? Tell the patient that "you give

**Table 13.1** The most common terms used with patients in dentistry to explain the feeling of soft tissue anesthetized (lips, tongue, and mouth).

| Children | Adults |
| --- | --- |
| - Fat → feeling a "fat lip" sensation<br>- Tickling<br>- Swollen | - Tingling<br>- Numbness<br>- Dullness<br>- Itching<br>- Pins and needles<br>- Frozen → getting frozen |

injections in the backside, in the mouth you use anesthesia." This way, we separate the two parts of the body and the two concepts.
- The patient may ask to see the syringe and needle. In this case, you say "No, because it's clean and doesn't have germs, so I can't show it to you." This explanation is generally sufficient. Some dentists tell children that they'll show it to them at the end (only if the child remembers; if not, do nothing) and if they do, they do so with only the syringe (not the needle), or if they do show the needle it has the cap on.

7) Similarly, with adults, it is a good idea to explain what you are about to do, how you are going to anesthetize them, and how comfortable they will feel. Something like this: "Just let me anesthetize you and you'll see that it's much less than you expect." Or inject a dose of humor: "After I inject the anesthetic you'll get addicted and be back every day for more." Or "It's not worth worrying about the anesthetic. You'll see that it's much easier than you think. Just let me show you."

Remember, studies show that patients are anxious and have expectations of pain caused by the anesthetic and dental treatment that are more negative than necessary (Rousseau et al. 2002; Nanitsos et al. 2009). Giving the patient positive information allays and reduces the fear and anxiety (Van Wijk and Hoogstraten 2006).

## Application of Topical Anesthetic

Approximately 95% of dentists in the United States (Kohli et al. 2001) and UK (Meechan 2008) administer topical anesthetic before intraoral injections to reduce pain and fear.

The time between applying the topical agent and the injection is very important. Many dentists wait less than 30 seconds (Gill and Orr 1979), and a survey in the United States showed that 70% wait less than a minute (Kohli et al. 2001). Holst and Evers estimated that the maximum time tolerated in clinical practice for topical anesthetic to take effect should not exceed 5 minutes (Holst and Evers 1985). In addition, moisture in the mouth tends to inhibit adhesion of gels, ointments, pastes, creams, and solutions to the mucosal surface, thus hampering absorption of the anesthetic, therefore maximum absorption is achieved during the first 30 seconds (Carr and Horton 2001b). For all the above reasons, we need topical anesthetics that have a short onset of action, generally under 1–2 minutes, therefore the most commonly used agents in clinical practice are *benzocaine 20% and lidocaine 5% in gels, ointments, and creams* (Kohli et al. 2001; Meechan 2008).

As seen in the chapter on topical anesthetic (Chapter 12), aerosols and liquid solutions yield the worst results, therefore the preferred form is gel, ointment, cream, or paste (Annex 19). In addition, topical anesthetic has little efficacy on the palate, which has a thicker and more keratinized mucous membrane, thus making it the least permeable part of the oral mucosa (Lesch et al. 1989). Similarly, its efficacy is poor for reducing the discomfort/pain produced by mandibular block, since the needle is inserted approximately 20–25 mm into the pterygomandibular space. As reported in clinical trials (Annex 19), topical anesthetic cannot reach this level (Meechan et al. 1998). Remember that in truncal injections the most painful part is the advance of the needle into the soft tissue (Annex 23). In any case, the placebo effect of the topical anesthetic is observed.

**Method of Application**

1) Tell the patient that topical anesthetic is going to be used to reduce the "discomfort" associated with administration of local anesthetic. This measure has been shown to reduce anxiety and increase tolerance to pain (Martin et al. 1994).
2) Clean and dry the puncture site with gauze or air pressure to remove saliva and soft debris (Figure 13.2). If this is not sufficient, the amount of saliva in the mouth can be reduced by placing cotton roll in the vestibule, at the orifice of the Stenon duct, or under the tongue at the orifice of the Wharton duct.
3) Aspirate saliva to ensure that it does not dilute the topical anesthetic which is about to be applied.
4) Apply the ointment or gel by rubbing a cotton swab directly over the injection site (Figure 13.3). Apply a small amount; it is important to remember that the

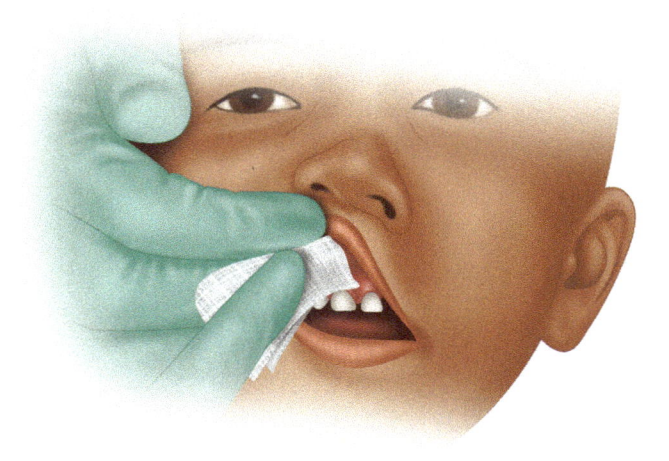

**Figure 13.2** Using gauze to clean the area where the topical anesthetic is to be applied.

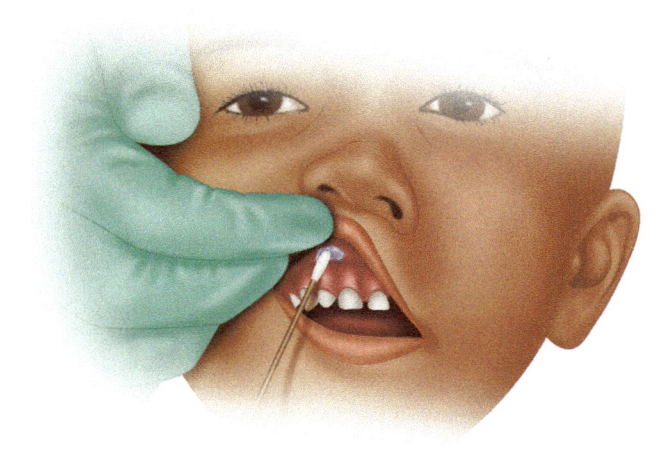

**Figure 13.3** Application of topical anesthesia with a cotton swab.

cotton bud will absorb part of the gel or ointment (Holst and Evers 1985).
5) Cover the area with gauze or a cotton roll so that the anesthetic remains in place and is not dispersed throughout the mouth or diluted in saliva (or at least as little as possible) (Roghani et al. 1999; Munshi et al. 2001). Here, again, some of the gel or ointment will be absorbed by the gauze or cotton roll (Lim and Julliard 2004).
6) Wait sufficient time for the anesthetic to take effect, generally 30 seconds to 1 minute for benzocaine and 1–2 minutes for lidocaine. Remember that one of the reasons for failure of topical anesthetic is that not enough time is left for it to take effect (Gill and Orr 1979).
7) Clean the area before injection to remove the topical anesthetic and leave the area clean. Owing to continuous stimulation with saliva, the injection site is always being contaminated, therefore it is more important to keep it clean than disinfected (Mink and Spedding 1966).
8) Prevent contact between the anesthetic and skin, since many anesthetics are ester agents (benzocaine, tetracaine, cocaine) and can lead to allergic sensitization (Roberts and Sowray 1987).

*Note*: Owing to diffusion of the topical anesthetic, the mucosa of the tongue or pharynx often becomes anesthetized at some distance from where the topical anesthetic was applied. This is a common complaint (Nakamura et al. 2013).

**Observations on Aerosols**

As we have seen, topical anesthetic in the form of aerosols is not recommended owing to the low efficacy resulting from dispersion in the mouth and dilution in saliva (Annex 19), although when they are used, it is important to take into account the following:

1) A cannula should be used to prevent – as much as possible – the aerosol solution from extending and dispersing.
2) Advise the patient to hold his/her breath when the agent is applied so that the drug is not inhaled. This would lead to anesthesia of the pharynx and an uncomfortable sensation of anxiety (Roberts and Sowray 1987).
3) Press the aerosol for 1 second, no more than 2 seconds, especially if it contains tetracaine, since it is easy to administer a toxic dose (Bennett 1984; Roberts and Sowray 1987).

Finally, aerosols are not recommended in children because they may lead to sudden uncooperative behavior owing to the noise they make and bad taste as the anesthetic spreads through the mouth (Frasier 1967; Evers and Haegerstam 1981).

**Transfer of the Syringe**

1) The assistant finishes preparing the syringe (continuation of section "Preparation Phase", point 4).
   Once the syringe is prepared with the cartridge, needle, and protective disk, the assistant separates the anterior cap to break the seal and replaces it using the protective disk. The risk of a needle-stick injury is minimized because of the protective disk (Figure 11.10, Chapter 11).
2) The dentist's supporting hand, i.e. the hand not holding the syringe (the left hand for right-handed dentists) must carry out the following operations simultaneously (Figure 13.4):
   - Stabilize the patient's head by holding it with the hand and fingers. The objective is to prevent sudden movements by the patient during insertion of the needle (Marks et al. 1984).
   - Separate the soft tissue to ensure that the injection site is clearly visible.
   - Block the view of the syringe (especially in children) with the fingers extended over the face or the wrist. There may also be cases where the upper lip can be raised.
3) Children. *The dentist must look the child directly in the eye throughout the transfer maneuver* to ensure the following:
   - The child is prevented from seeing the syringe, given that he/she tends to follow all the dentist's actions and movements. Look directly at the child throughout, especially if he/she is nervous.
   - By looking directly at the child's face, the dentist can observe whether he/she is feeling pain or notices the

prick of the needle by gestures such as frowning, raising the eyebrows, blinking, or moving the nose. On the other hand, the patient may not modify his/her expression, thus indicating that the insertion has been asymptomatic or well-tolerated.
- The child should not close his/her eyes (almost no children do it, on the contrary, they look at everything the dentist is doing) (Mink and Spedding 1966), since the disappearance of one sense increases the sensitivity of the others, with the result that sensations such as touch and pressure are more easily perceived as pain. Furthermore, with the eyes closed, the patient can imagine horrible threats that are not seen when the eyes are open (Mink and Spedding 1966).
- The dentist can also ask the patient to place his/her hands under his/her bottom, that is, away from the mouth and supported by his/her own body (Figure 13.4). In addition, since children see the word "bottom" as a nice word, even a little naughty, they accept it very well.

4) The dentist extends and opens his/her right hand (right-handed dentist) to receive the syringe from the assistant without looking (he/she is looking at the child) and outside the child's field of vision (behind the head rest or under the chin and near the left ear).

5) The assistant places the syringe in the dentist's hand:
   - The syringe is presented with the needle cap and protective disk pointing toward the assistant (Figure 13.5).
   - The assistant takes the syringe with his/her right hand by the body of the syringe, or barrel (Figure 13.5).

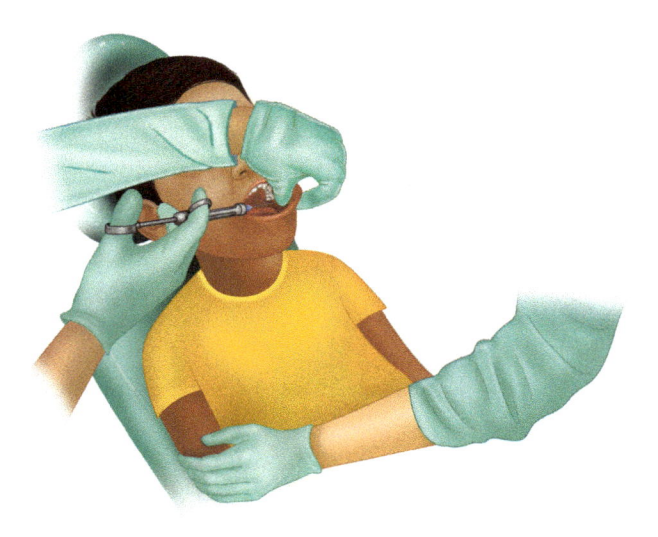

**Figure 13.4** Note the following: (1) the position and function of the dentist's supporting hand, and (2) the assistant's arm extended across the child's body. *Source:* Redrawn with modifications from Snawder (1987).

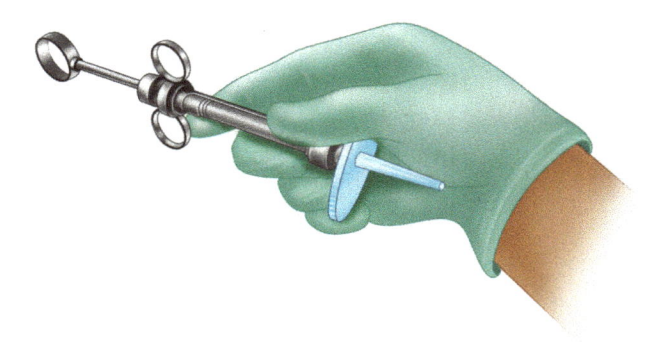

**Figure 13.5** The assistant holds the syringe before passing it to the dentist with the right hand on the body or barrel of the syringe. Note the protective disk over the cap of the needle.

- The syringe is passed across out of the view of the patient, that is, behind the headrest or under the patient's chin.
- The syringe is placed correctly in the dentist's hand with a slight tap on the dentist's open hand (so that the dentist is aware of receiving the syringe).
- The assistant removes the anterior sheath or cap of the needle so that it is exposed. Remember that the seal of the cap has already been broken (section "Transfer of the Syringe", point 1), therefore it is easy to remove the cap.

6) With the syringe in his/her hand, the dentist pushes the plunger slightly to:
   - Purge the syringe (one or two drops) to eliminate silicone and aluminum powder residue that have entered the lumen of the needle when it pierces the silicone diaphragm of the mouth of the cartridge with the posterior needle (Kelly and Cohen 1984; Piesold et al. 1998). This residue is found in around 10% of cases and can measure as much as 0.3–0.5 mm and carries a risk of entering a vessel or muscle and causing pain or trismus (Kelly and Cohen 1984).
   - Eliminate the initial sudden pushing and shaking movement (Tzafalia and Sixou 2011) caused by the fact that the plunger is usually blocked or sticks to the glass of the cartridge. This will ensure that it moves smoothly down the barrel (Figure 13.6). The plunger used to be lubricated with paraffin or glycerine wax that became hard over time and at low ambient temperatures. Lubricants are currently made of silicone and are much better than the previous ones. However, even though the problem has been somewhat resolved, it has not disappeared (Jastak et al. 1995; Malamed 2004). The problem is worse with plastic cartridges than with glass cartridges (Malamed 2004).

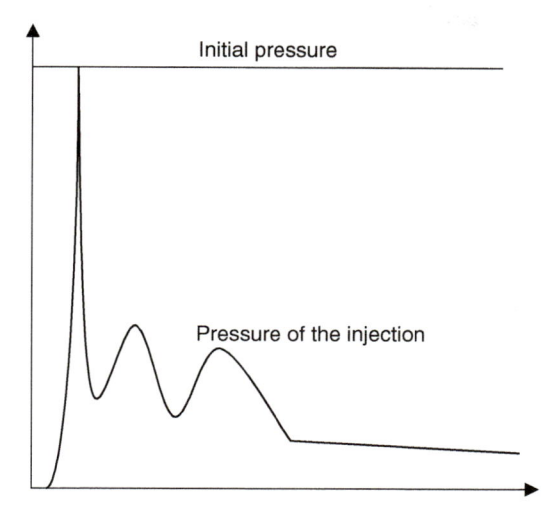

**Figure 13.6** Control the sudden shaky initial movement to ensure that the solution is injected smoothly.

The way the hand moves and the use of cartridge-type metal syringes make these initial brusque movements difficult to control. This is one of the advantages of computerized injection techniques, which solve this problem almost perfectly (Tzafalia and Sixou 2011).

7) With the syringe now purged in his/her right hand, the dentist can direct it toward the patient's mouth.

### Insertion of the Needle

1) Children. The assistant extends his/her left arm over the child's body to hold the arms in place gently but firmly and remains alert to possible disruptive movements (Mink and Spedding 1966; Ram and Peretz 2002) (Figure 13.4).
2) The dentist warns the patient when pain is unavoidable. Our body does not react well to surprises and reactions are often uncontrollable.
  For example, injections into the palate or using the intrapulpal technique can be painful, therefore we must tell the patient that the pain will last only a second and show interest and concern for the fact.
  For the same reason, when we say "this won't hurt," we should be sure that this is in fact the case. If the injection actually does hurt, then the patient may become counter-conditioned, with the result that every time we say something similar, the patient will expect to feel pain (Jackson 1974) and not relax. This defective approach to providing information is disliked by 75% of patients (Rankin and Harris 1985).
3) The dentist always holds the syringe stable to maintain control and prevent unexpected movements of the needle (Ram and Peretz 2002). This is done by supporting the body of the syringe on the patient's teeth or lips or with the dentist's fingers placing the syringe on the patient's mouth or face.
  Do not rest on the patient's arms or shoulders, since he/she can move them unexpectedly while keeping the mouth still.
4) *The dentist should perform counter-irritant/counter-stimulant measures immediately before inserting the needle.*
  Traction and stretching of the soft tissue can be applied with the fingers in the area near the injection site to leave the area tense. This enables the needle to penetrate the mucous membrane with minimum resistance and discomfort. If the soft tissue remains lax and soft, the needle will push against it before being inserted, therefore insertion will be more difficult and painful.
  Pressure or vibratory stimulus can also be applied by making rapid movements with the fingers or a cotton-tip applicator. These maneuvers enable the following:
    - The patient's attention is diverted from the "prick," thus ensuring that the pain threshold does not decrease (anxiety reduces the pain threshold) and the stimulus of the penetration of the needle (which is at its limit) falls below the pain threshold (Woolgrove 1983; Sokol et al. 1985).
    - Activation of the gate control system at the level of the trigeminal caudate nucleus, which partially inhibits the passage of painful stimuli upwards, thus helping to maintain the stimulus below the pain threshold (Melzack and Wall 1965; Dubner 1978) (see Chapter 11).
5) During the insertion of the needle, the dentist can distract the patient further with a continuous monolog, for example, "I hope everything is OK...now open your mouth, a little more,... that's it, a little more,... that's it, perfect, just like that,..."
6) Depending on whether the injection is an infiltration or mandibular block, we can make a few suggestions:
    - Buccal infiltration. *We recommend the minimum intervention* (minimum volume/minimum injection time), which consists of injecting a single drop at the injection site in 1–2 seconds and waiting a minute; we then inject again at the same site (the appearance of a blood spot is common), one or two drops in 1–2 seconds and waiting half a minute. We inject at the same site again, although this time ±0.25 ml (an eighth of a 1.8-ml cartridge) in 7–10 seconds after aspirating; we now wait another half minute. Finally, we inject, slowly at the same site, the quantity we intended to administer (again, after aspirating). This method enables anesthesia of the soft tissues and prevents the discomfort resulting from distension of the tissues by injecting most of the solution.

- Mandibular block. *We recommend a light but firm tap followed by quick insertion.* This approach involves giving a light but firm tap with the supporting hand (generally the left in right-handed persons) at the same time as the hand holding the syringe (generally the right) inserts the needle quickly to reach the bone immediately. This is a very important maneuver, since the traumatic stimulus limits the pain threshold (in this case, the passage of the needle across the soft tissue), which lasts some time, so that the initial threshold can be overcome and pain appears (Fuller et al. 1979). A slower advance reduces the threshold considerably, and, if some drops of anesthetic are injected as the needle advances, then the situation worsens (Appendix), in addition, the anesthetic does not act immediately (Nusstein et al. 2006; McCarney et al. 2007). It is important to remember that passage of the needle is the factor that produces most pain in truncal blocks (Annex 23).

7) Avoid injuring the periosteum. The periosteum is rich in nerve endings and any injury to it causes pain at the time of the lesion and in the post-operative period. In order to avoid this injury, we recommend the following:
    - Place the bevel of the needle facing toward the bone (Figure 13.7) since if it comes into contact with the periosteum, it will tend to slide across without damaging it. This classic concept is currently under discussion since evidence from clinical trials indicates that the direction of the bevel does not affect the onset of pain (Carr and Horton 2001b) or the efficacy of the anesthetic in achieving pulpal anesthesia (Steinkruger et al. 2006).
    - If the tip of the needle touches the bone, we withdraw it 1–2 mm before injecting (we do not exert pressure by pressing it against the bone) for the following reasons: (i) so as not to leave anesthetic solution below the periosteum and (ii) so as not to blunt the needle, especially if the tip barbed outwards, since this can damage muscles, nerves, and vessels on withdrawal (Stacy et al. 1994) (Figure 22.2, Chapter 22).

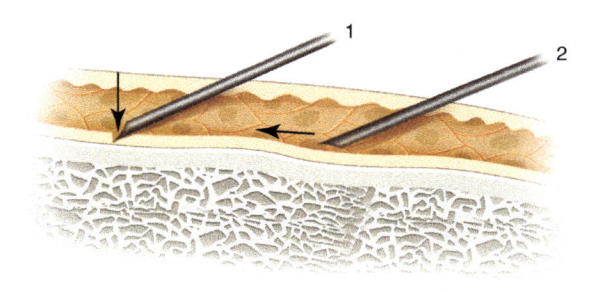

**Figure 13.7** Prevent the tip of the needle from damaging the periosteum (1) by placing the bevel parallel to it (2).

8) Never insert the needle up to the hub. This is the weakest and most vulnerable part and the level at which needles always break (Orr 1983; Marks et al. 1984; Burgess 1988; McDonogh 1996; Zelster et al. 2002). Therefore, in the case of a breakage, the end part of the needle will remain outside the soft tissue and can be withdrawn before it disappears fully into the tissue.
   Long needles should be used in techniques where it is necessary to insert the needle deep into the soft tissue, for example mandibular block (Dentists' Desk 1983).
9) In children, voice control should be used if the patient complains, cries, or tries to move when the needle is inserted.

    In principle, the syringe should not be withdrawn, since this would reinforce the child's disruptive behavior and hamper subsequent administration of local anesthesia (Mink and Spedding 1966).

    Voice control accompanied by strict facial expression (nonverbal communication) gives us an authoritarian air. We can then move close to the child's ear and tell him/her in a soft voice that it is time to stop behaving badly. If the child's behavior continues to be disruptive, we raise our voice suddenly and considerably, and use expressions such as "Open your mouth!", "Don't move!" Once we have the child's attention, we change our tone of voice, thanking him/her for stopping behaving badly and gently explaining that "You'll hardly feel a thing."

## Aspiration

In 1957, the Council on Dental Therapeutics of the American Dental Association highlighted the need for systematic aspiration before injecting dental local anesthetic (Council on Dental Therapeutics 1957). Today, there are still many dentists who do not routinely use aspiration in the belief that intravascular injection is very uncommon or that if it does occur, it has few adverse effects (Bartlett 1972; Meechan and Rood 1992). Some surveys show that more than 20% of dentists do not routinely aspirate (Malamed 2004).

The aim of aspiration before injection is to prevent intravascular injection and therefore systemic toxic effects resulting from the sudden passage of the solution into the bloodstream (Forrest 1959; Shira 1962; Bos et al. 1971), which can sometimes increase toxicity 200-fold (Meechan and Rood 1992).

### False Positives and Negatives

Matters may be further complicated by false positives and false negatives:

- False positives, when the cartridge fills with blood without a vessel having been injected (Alling and Christopher 1974;

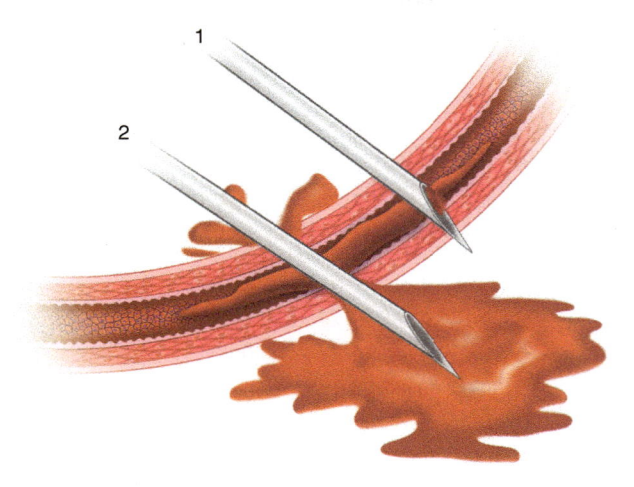

**Figure 13.8** False positives in aspirations due to residual blood on crossing a vessel (1) or by aspirating blood extravasated from the tissue spaces (2). *Source:* Redrawn from Alling and Christopher (1974).

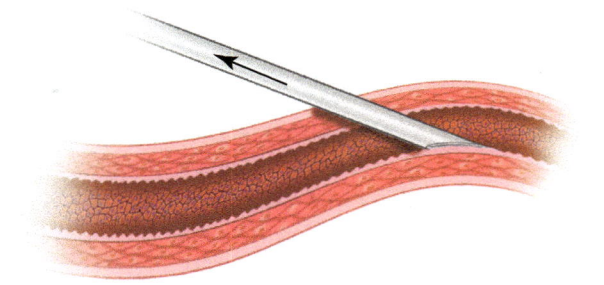

**Figure 13.9** False negative caused by the bevel being on the internal layer of the vessel (adventitia or endothelium). *Source:* Redrawn and modified from Watson and Colman (1976).

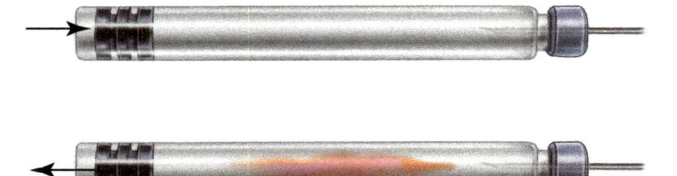

**Figure 13.10** Genuinely positive aspiration, shown by the fact that the cartridge is colored by an intense stream of blood.

Watson and Colman 1976) as a result of the following (Figure 13.8):

1) Aspiration of extravasated blood from tissue spaces caused by the trauma resulting from passage of the needle.
2) Residual blood remaining in the lumen of the needle as it crosses a vessel.

- False negatives, when the cartridge does not fill with blood despite the fact that the tip of the needle is in a vessel as a result of:
   1) Excess negative pressure when the plunger is pulled backward to aspirate, thus leading to collapse of the vessels, especially vessels measuring less than 1.5 mm (Alling and Christopher 1974; Watson and Colman 1976).
   2) If the angle of insertion of the needle has the misfortune to lie parallel to the inner layer (adventitia) of the vessel, then the endothelium (adventitia) occludes the lumen of the needle on aspiration, especially in small vessels (Figure 13.9).
   3) Formation of a punch cylinder of epithelial mucosal cells in a little more than 1% of cases, leading to obstruction of the lumen (Piesold et al. 1998).

**How to Interpret a Positive Aspiration**

While it is impossible to make an infallible interpretation, we suggest the following (Watson and Colman 1976; Cooley and Robinson 1979):

- A cartridge colored lightly or more intensely but in a diffuse fashion usually indicates a false positive.
- An intensely colored cartridge with blood return entering it is usually a true positive (Figure 13.10). If the return reaches halfway up the syringe, it usually indicates a small vein (<1.5 mm); if it is very intense and fills the cartridge, it usually indicates an artery or a large vein (>1.5 mm). it is therefore important to use 25G or 27G needles (25G is better) since these make it possible to evaluate the characteristics of the blood return that colors the cartridge. This is not possible with 30G needles because the return is always weak (see Chapter 11).

**Aspiration Technique**

According to the criteria of Forrest, we can indicate the following steps to ensure correct aspiration (Forrest 1959):

1) Move the tip of the needle to the target area.
2) Inject a few drops to clear the lumen of punch cylinder (thus avoiding false negatives) and any blood remaining in the interior after crossing tissues or a vessel (thus avoiding false positives).
3) Aspiration is performed by dragging the plunger smoothly back by pulling the support ring of the syringe 1–2 mm with the thumb (without moving the tip of the needle) for 2–3 seconds to create a "soft" negative pressure. This prevents a false negative through collapse of the small veins owing to excessive traction.
4) If the result is negative (the cartridge does not fill with blood), we turn the needle a few degrees and re-inject a few drops before softly aspirating again. We thus

prevent a false negative that would have occurred if we had initially placed the bevel parallel to the adventitia. If the result had been a positive aspiration (the cartridge fills with blood), the needle is withdrawn 1–2 mm and we aspirate again, as indicated above. If the result is negative again, we proceed with the injection; however, if it is positive again, we recommend removing the cartridge, changing it for a new one, and starting again, since it is difficult to evaluate a new aspiration with the syringe reddened by blood (Forrest 1959; Allen 1979).

5) If the result is finally negative, we proceed with the injection, but we aspirate every 0.25–0.5 ml to slow the injection and prevent false negatives, given that in conventional aspiration syringes (where it is necessary to pull back), the tip of the needle can be moved a little during the maneuver, therefore some authors prefer self-aspirating syringes (Lloyd 1992).

**Remarks**

- In positive aspirations, it is impossible to know whether we have reached an artery or a vein (Bartlett 1972).
- For reasons that are not clear, there is considerable individual variability in the percentages of positive aspirations (Bos et al. 1971; Persson et al. 1974; Meechan and Blair 1989; Lopez and Rosello 1995).
- Even if the aspiration is negative, a new cartridge should be used for each patient, since blood or tissue liquid is detected in 10–25% of cartridges (Trapp and Davies 1980; Lipp et al. 1993), with the risk of transfer of organic materials and fluids and, therefore, infection.
- There is little correlation between adverse effects (vasovagal reactions, palpitations, pallor) and positive aspirations (Forrest 1959; Goldman and Gray 1963; Persson et al. 1974; Blair and Meechan 1985; Lipp et al. 1988), possibly owing to the following:
  ○ Other factors that can contribute to adverse effects, such as anxiety and fear, pain, vascular irritation when the needle comes in contact with a vessel.
  ○ During aspiration, traction of the plunger with the thumb in the ring leads the tip of the needle to move involuntarily for a second (Cowan 1972; Williams and Simm 1975; Lloyd 1992) and in such a way that it is practically imperceptible (Kämmerer et al. 2016). An in vitro study performed in 2016 found that this movement of the needle was around 2.5 mm with syringes that took a conventional cartridge and some 2 mm with self-aspirating syringes (Kämmerer et al. 2016). Aspiration should therefore be repeated at each stage to ensure that it is successful (McClure 1968; Lloyd 1992), bearing in mind that there is general agreement that the risk of intravascular injection increases if the syringe is not aspirated first (Horowitz et al. 2005). Partial intravascular injection has been reported in around 25% of cases despite previous negative aspiration (Eickbohm et al. 1991).
- After a second or third injection at the same site, the probability of a positive aspiration increases as a result of aspiration of extravasated blood from injured vessels (Lopez and Rosello 1995; Lustig and Zusman 1999).
- Finally, Table 13.2 shows the mean prevalence of positive aspirations in the various dental intraoral anesthetic techniques. Truncal block is the technique that most frequently leads to positive aspirations.

**Table 13.2** Percentage of positive aspirations in anesthetic techniques

| Arch | Technique | Percentage (%) |
|---|---|---|
| Maxillary | Periapical infiltration (buccal infiltration) | 2 |
| | Periapical infiltration – molars | 4 |
| | Posterior superior alveolar nerve block | 5 |
| | High tuberosity technique[a] | 13 |
| | Transpalatal technique | 5 |
| | Infraorbital nerve technique[b] | 1 |
| | Palate | 1 |
| Mandible | Mandibular block: | |
| | – Standard technique | 10 |
| | – Gow–Gates technique | 5–10 |
| | – Laguardia–Akinosi technique | 5 |
| | Periapical infiltration (buccal infiltration) | <1 |
| | Infiltration mental area | 5 |
| | Buccal nerve block | 1 |
| | Lingual nerve block | 1 |

[a] Data from Goldman and Gray (1963).
[b] Data from Karkut et al. (2010).
*Source:* data from Annex 22.

### Injection

1) *Inject the solution slowly by pushing the plunger at a rate of 1.8 ml in 40–60 seconds.* This maneuver enables us to avoid the following:
   - Pain during the injection caused by tissue expansion with an excessively rapid entry of the solution and the resulting increase in pressure (Mamiya et al. 2001; Primosch and Brooks 2002; Kudo 2005; Kanaa et al. 2006; Whitworth et al. 2007; Aggarwal et al. 2012). This pain is even greater than that caused

by the prick of the needle during insertion (Carr and Horton 2001a; Annex 19).
- Toxicity of the anesthetic solution, since there may be rapid increases in plasma levels, especially with unnoticed intravascular injections (Adriani and Campbell 1956; Campbell and Adriani 1958; Adriani et al. 1959; Scott 1986). Slow injections enable dilution of the anesthetic solution in the systemic circulation (Adriani and Campbell 1956; Campbell and Adriani 1958), thus enabling the lungs to retain the drug and attenuate the toxic effect (Tucker and Mather 1979; Scott 1986). Some authors consider slow injections to be the key to prevention of adverse reactions in dental anesthesia, even more so than aspiration (Malamed 2004).
- Ineffectiveness of the anesthetic. Rapid injection under pressure leads to turbulent diffusion of the solution to areas that are distant from the tip of the needle, thus reducing the amount of drug at the target area, with the corresponding loss of effectiveness (McClure 1968; Jorgensen and Hayden 1970; Mamiya et al. 2001). Furthermore, clinical trials show that slow injections increase the percentage of success in pulpal anesthesia (Kanaa et al. 2006).

Table 13.3 shows the injection rates recommended by several authors, as well as real values from surveys. Most dentists inject a 1.8-ml cartridge in under 20–30 seconds. The conventional recommendation was to inject 1 ml per minute to avoid injection pain and prevent toxicity. Clinical trials have shown that injections administered in more than 36 seconds are not painful in children (Maragakis and Musselman 1996) and that there is no difference between administering injections in 60 or 100 seconds (de Souza Melo et al. 2015). Furthermore, in the case of a child, the longer the injection takes, the more nervous the patient becomes and the more he/she associates the injection with pain (Jones et al. 1995). Therefore, modern convention suggests injecting a 1.8-ml cartridge in 40–60 seconds.

2) Aspirate every 0.25–0.5 ml of solution injected (McClure 1968; Lloyd 1992) to confirm the safety of the injection, with multiple negative aspirations (remember the problem of movement of the tip of the needle), and to help slow the injection by blocking the natural tendency to inject quickly, as shown by surveys.

3) Keep the patient distracted with a monolog to ensure that his/her attention is drawn away from the injection. Thus, "… hold your mouth open, that's it, like that, …don't move, keep it like that, perfect,… you can feel my fingers touching your lip,… raise your hand if it hurts,…"

**Final Phase**

1) Remove the needle slowly and smoothly from the injection site when the injection is complete. The direction of insertion and withdrawal should not be changed because of the risk of needle breakage (Orr 1983; Marks et al. 1984; Zelster et al. 2002). If it is necessary to change the direction of the needle, then this should be done just below the mucous membrane, when the needle is almost completely out. We do so by reinserting the needle in the new direction (Orr 1983; Marks et al. 1984).

2) The assistant will place the cap on the needle. Remember the importance of the protective disk on the cap to prevent needle-stick injury during the maneuver. The needle should remain covered to prevent contamination and needle stick accidents (Dentists' Desk 1983).
The assistant also takes the syringe from the dentist's hands (once the cap has been replaced) out of the patient's line of vision, generally under the chin.

3) The injection site should not be massaged or rubbed. Massaging forces the anesthetic solution to spread throughout the more lax tissues along the least path of resistance and at some distance from the injection site, thus reducing its concentration and ability to cross the periosteum, cortical bone, and cancellous bone, and, paradoxically, increasing the area of superficially anesthetized soft tissue.

Table 13.3 Rate of injection of a 1.8-ml cartridge in seconds, as recommended by various authors and surveys

| Reference | Seconds | Remarks |
|---|---|---|
| **Recommendations** | | |
| Fischer (1912) | 108 | Classic 1 ml/min |
| Nordenram (1971) | 108 | |
| Bennett (1984) | 108 | |
| National Heath Foundation Australia (Oliver 1974) | 60 | Currently, most common criterion |
| Malamed (1986) | 60 | |
| Roberts and Sowray (1987) | 60 | |
| Linscott et al. (1978) | 60 | |
| Kanaa et al. (2006) | 60 | |
| Meechan (1998) | 30 | |
| **Survey** | | |
| Malamed (1986) | 20 | 80% of dentists |
| Kohli et al. (2001) | <30 | 56% of dentists |
| | 30–60 | 33% of dentists |

We may occasionally massage the area gently to reduce the burning sensation (beesting effect) caused by the acid pH of solutions containing sympathomimetic vasoconstrictors, such as epinephrine.

4) If anesthetic solution enters the mouth, the patient usually complains of a bitter taste resulting from sulfites in solutions with vasoconstrictors such as epinephrine (Klein 1983).

   We can reassure adults that swallowing the solution is not toxic and we can use the aerosol of the syringe to force air and water into the mouth and use the aspirator to remove the bad taste.

   Moreover, in children, we can gain their confidence by telling them that the "medicine" (the anesthesia) tastes bad and that it would be a good idea if it tasted of chocolate, strawberry, or ice cream and asking them what they thought, if we should invent it, and what flavor would they prefer.

   Solution can enter the mouth for several reasons: (i) a few drops may be released when the needle is withdrawn from the tissue as a result of the remaining pressure in the plunger (the most frequent cause); (ii) if it occurs during the injection, it is caused by the fact that the needle pierced the diaphragm of the mouth of the cartridge off-center, thus forming an oval hole around the needle between the diaphragm and needle through which some of the solution escapes (Dentists' Desk 1983; Malamed 1986; Jastak et al. 1995), but this problem can be resolved by removing the needle and reinserting it appropriately into the mouth of the syringe; and (iii) breakage of the cartridge, although this is very rare (see Chapter 22).

5) Children. The dentist continues to support the head with his/her hand and looking directly at the child to monitor the situation. When the cap is placed on the syringe and the syringe is removed from the dentist's hands, both the dentist and the assistant should *keep the needle and syringe out of the child's line of vision* (Mink and Spedding 1966; McClure 1968). Very often, it is during this phase that we drop our guard and the child sees the needle and syringe, thus removing any benefit gained with the maneuvers made to reassure him/her (Mink and Spedding 1966) (Figure 13.1).

6) We must warn the patient that he/she will start to feel the effect of the anesthesia on the lips and tongue. As the term "soft tissue anesthesia" is somewhat technical, the words "numbness," "tingling," "dullness," "itching," and feeling "pins and needles," can be used; in children, we should use words like "tickling" or tell them that they'll feel like they have a "fat lip" or a "fat tongue" (Table 13.1).

7) The dentist, hygienist, or the assistant should remain near the patient while the anesthesia takes effect (Nordenram 1971; Evers and Haegerstam 1981; Council on Clinical Affairs 2015; AAPD 2020). Remember, most adverse reactions occur during the first 15–30 minutes (Nordenram 1971; Kelly and Patterson 1974). Clinical studies have found that around 50% of complications occur during the first 30 minutes and that a further 20–30% occur before 2–6 hours (Kaufman et al. 2000; Batinac et al. 2013).

8) Children who are more difficult to control. An available option just after administering the anesthetic, and one which many pediatric dentists recommend, is to rinse the mouth to prevent the child from crying (if they are about to cry). This helps to take the child's mind off the recent injection (Mink and Spedding 1966).

### Evaluation of Anesthesia

1) Subjective response. When the patient tells us that he/she is experiencing soft tissue anesthesia (sensation described as numbness, tingling, dullness, tickling, or fat lip) (Table 13.1), we know that the anesthetic is having an effect at least on the soft tissues. Phases of soft tissue anesthesia have been reported as follows (Lindsay 1929): first, sensation of heat followed by a sensation of numbness; when the numbness is more advanced, it is more marked and eventually very marked and accompanied by sensation of swelling.

2) Objective response in the soft tissue. We can check by pinching the gingival papilla to the canine with a sickle probe and observing that it is in fact insensitive (Ellis et al. 1990). However, this does not guarantee pulpal anesthesia (Vreeland et al. 1989; Cohen et al. 1993; Childers et al. 1996; Certosimo and Archer 1996).

3) Objective pulpal response. This occurs later (Figure 5.3, Chapter 5) and can be evaluated in two ways:
   - With an electric pulp tester. The electric stimulus is very reliable in permanent teeth and only presents false negatives (the electric stimulus is negative, although there is still pain during the procedure) in 0–5% of cases (Dreven et al. 1987; Certosimo and Archer 1996). Owing to the lack of complete innervation in the odontoblast layer, the electric stimulus not very reliable in primary teeth (Fuss et al. 1986). It is also important to bear in mind that in permanent teeth with acute pulpitis, false negatives occur in 20–40% of cases (Table 13.4).
   - With cold stimulus. Initially dichlorodifluoromethane (DDN) was used. This is at −50 °C when it leaves the container (Fuss et al. 1986; Cohen et al. 1993; Hsiao-Wu et al. 2007) and is reliable not only in permanent teeth, but also in primary teeth (Fuss et al. 1986), although this has now been replaced by

Table 13.4 Percentage of failure of pulpectomy with pain after anesthesia and lack of response of the pulp to the stimulus of the electric pulp meter in teeth (mainly molars) with acute irreversible pulpitis (hot tooth)

| Reference | ml/LAS/time (min) | Percentage (%) with pain (proportion) |
|---|---|---|
| *After mandibular block* | | |
| Dreven et al. (1987) | 3.6/L-100/10′ | 38 (6/16) |
| Nusstein et al. (1998) | 1.8/L-100/5′ | 80 (8/10) |
| Allegretti et al. (2016) | 3.6/*/15′ | 14 (6/43) |
| Visconti et al. (2016) | 3.6/L-100/20′ | 36 (5/14) |
| Ghoddusi et al. (2018) | 3.6/L-100/15′ | 45 (13/29) |
| | | 42.6 ≈ **40** |
| *After infiltration in the maxillary buccal space* | | |
| Dreven et al. (1987) | 3.6/L-100/10′ | 14 (2/14) |
| Nusstein et al. (1998) | 3.6/L-100/3′ | 26 (6/23) |
| | | **20** |

LAS, local anesthetic solution; ml, milliliters injected.
Times are given in minutes: 5′ = 5 minutes.
L-100 = lidocaine 2% with epinephrine 1:100 000.
*Solutions of L-100, A-100, and M-100.
A-100 = articaine 4% with epinephrine 1:100 000.
M-100 = mepivacaine 2% with epinephrine 1:100 000.

1,1,1,2-tetrafluoroethane (TFE) (Green Endo-Ice), which is more ozone-friendly (Kennedy et al. 2003) and leaves the container at −26 °C (Nusstein et al. 1998; Miller et al. 2004; Hsiao-Wu et al. 2007). It is applied in 10–25 seconds, even in vital teeth with crowns (Miller et al. 2004). This method can also produce false negatives in teeth with acute pulpitis (Reader et al. 2011; Chavarria-Bolaños et al. 2017). The cold test has advantages over electric stimulus, in that it is easier and faster and does not require special equipment (Reader et al. 2011).

In cases of acute pulpitis, these methods are always helpful even if they fail, since in the case of a negative response we always run the risk of a false negative. However, if there is already pain when the electrical or cold stimulus is applied, then this indicates that the tooth has not been anesthetized and that anesthesia should be reinforced (Reader et al. 2011; Chavarria-Bolaños et al. 2017).

Finally, it is important to note that in clinical practice, *systems of objective evaluation are not common* (except in acute pulpitis); we wait for standard periods after the patient reports a subjective response, except in special cases.

4) Wait for the standard periods to ensure pulpal anesthesia.

- We wait 5 minutes in maxillary buccal infiltrations, once the infiltration has finished, to guarantee pulpal anesthesia in most cases.
- In mandibular block, the criterion is to wait 5 minutes for the onset of soft tissue anesthesia of the lower lip and from there, a further 5–10 minutes to guarantee pulpal anesthesia, which takes longer (10–15 minutes in total) (see Chapter 16).

5) The definitive proof is treatment itself, therefore the patient should be warned at the start of the procedure that he/she may feel a sensation of touch, pressure, or temperature (cold or heat), but not pain, since the anesthetic solution is very effective at suppressing pain, but not other stimuli (de Jong 1977). We can also tell the patient that he/she can raise his/her hand in the case of discomfort and we will stop immediately (this gives the patient a sensation of control and thus reduces anxiety).

We also insist on the need to avoid sudden movements since this could lead us to hurt the patient.

We proceed cautiously with drilling instruments and the scalpel, monitoring constantly to see if the patient complains and/or raises a hand.

We also follow a progressive system in children. We place the head of the drilling instrument over the tooth to observe the child's response to the vibration. If this is appropriate, we place the drill over the enamel, and if the response is suitable, we continue with the procedure.

## Post-treatment Phase

1) Inform the patient how long the sensation of numbness will last in the soft tissues when dental treatment has been completed. As a guide, *it can last around 200 minutes (3–4 hours) with the standard solution of lidocaine 2% and epinephrine 1:100000 (10 μg/ml) or 1:80000 (12.5 μg/ml)* and more than 5 hours in a little over 5% of cases (Hersh et al. 2008). These times may vary with other solutions (see Chapter 7).

A degree of residual local anesthesia is desirable as it prevents the onset of pain. However, patients should be informed about the prolonged duration of soft tissue anesthesia, especially as it may impact their ability to speak, sing, drink, and eat, which may be a concern if the patient plans on going to a meeting or event following the appointment where they may be participating in aforementioned activities.

2) Warn against chewing while the soft tissues remain anesthetized, since this can lead the patient to bite his/her lips, tongue, and buccal mucosa (self-injury), which are numb, and cause injury and pain. Although many patients say that they can chew with "the other side," it is wise to insist because it is difficult to control the

subconscious use of both sides during chewing. It is also important to be careful with very hot drinks and cigarettes (risk of burn).
3) Children. Stress both to them and their parents or guardians that they must not bite their tongue, lips, or buccal mucosa while they are anesthetized, since it will hurt and they could injure themselves. Little children tend to bite themselves repeatedly when they see that it does not hurt. A trick used by many pediatric dentists is to place a cotton roll between the lips or between the cheek and the gum for as long as the anesthetic lasts to remind children not to bite themselves (Mink and Spedding 1966).
4) With respect to the dose of anesthetic, it is important to remember the following:
   - Topical anesthesia also contributes to the total dose administered (Cannell 1996; Meechan 1998).
   - When it is necessary to inject a large quantity of anesthetic solution, try to reserve 20–25% of the absolute maximum dose to address unexpected events (Meechan 1998).
   - *Do not dispose of the empty cartridges after administration.* Keep them until the procedure is complete in order to know exactly how much anesthetic has been administered, especially in cases where it is necessary to administer new injections halfway through treatment (Meechan 1998).
   - Remember the patient's height and weight, especially in the case of children and small adults (often elderly persons) to minimize the risk of overdose (Goodson and Moore 1983; Hersh et al. 1991; Virts 1999). See Annex 10 on maximum doses.
5) Used needles should be disposed of in a safe container for sharps and contaminated instruments (Dentists' Desk 1983).

## Causes of Pain During the Injection

Below, we analyze the real causes of pain, factors that play a role in pain, and factors that are of almost no importance but that many dentists still believe to be relevant.

### Factors That Cause Pain

1) The injection. Insertion/penetration of the needle into the mucosa is the main cause of pain during the injection (Annex 19). It can be mitigated by the following: (i) using topical anesthetic before the injection and (ii) distracting the patient with counter-stimulus maneuvers (traction, stretching, pressure) and a continuous monolog.
2) The advance of the needle across the soft tissue until it reaches its target in truncal block (Annex 23 and Appendix). The pain can be relieved with a continuous monolog and the rapid advance of the needle toward its objective with counter-stimulus maneuvers.
3) Injection of acidic solutions (low pH). Solutions containing sympathomimetic vasoconstrictors, such as epinephrine also contain antioxidants (sulfites), which reduce the pH (Annex 14). This leads to an initial sensation of stinging and burning, as shown in clinical trials (Oikarinen et al. 1975; Moorthy et al. 1984; Kramp et al. 1999; Wahl et al. 2001). Fortunately, this effect disappears quickly, since tissue fluids contain buffers which neutralize the pH. A smooth and short massage can help to relieve this sensation.
4) The speed of the injection. This factor has been considered important since the early years of dental local anesthesia (Lewis 1919), and this remains the case today (Malamed 1986; Roberts and Sowray 1987; Linscott et al. 1978). Clinical trials have clearly proven this impression (Mamiya et al. 2001; Primosch and Brooks 2002; Kudo 2005; Kanaa et al. 2006; Whitworth et al. 2007), especially in buccal infiltrations (Annex 23). The explanation is that a rapid injection leads to a sudden distension of the tissues, which increases pressure and is painful. This specific factor is more painful than the needle insertion (Nist et al. 1992; Quarnstrom and Libed 1994; Carr and Horton 2001a; Kennedy et al. 2001; Wiswall et al. 2014). It can be mitigated by slow injection and a continuous monolog.

### Factors That Play a Role in Pain

Regardless of the objective causes of pain, a series of factors contribute to the perception that pain is more intense.

1) The part of the mouth where the injection is performed. The clinical impression is that the palate is the part where most pain is felt (Kramp et al. 1999; Wahl et al. 2001; Primosch and Brooks 2002); this impression is confirmed in the literature (Annexes 19 and 23). Furthermore, it is known that pain is most intense in the anterior part of the hard palate than in the posterior part (Meechan et al. 2005; Ozec et al. 2010). Other sites where pain is more intense include buccal periapical infiltrations in the anterior teeth of the maxilla; in contrast, buccal periapical infiltrations in the posterior teeth of the maxilla are the least painful (Annex 23).
2) The patient's age and sex. Most anxiety and sensitivity to pain during injection of local anesthetic and dental treatment in general is observed with women (LeClaire et al. 1988; Liddell and Locker 1997; Baht et al. 2000;

Van Wijk and Hoogstraten 2006; Meechan et al. 2005), and adolescents and young adults (Kleinknecht and Berstein 1978; LeClaire et al. 1988; Liddell and Locker 1997; Wahl et al. 2001; Maggirias and Locker 2002; Gazal 2015).

3) Intense anxiety reduces the pain tolerance threshold and makes it more likely that nonpainful stimuli (e.g. pressure) are interpreted as painful, therefore anxious patients overestimate the degree of pain that dental treatment causes (Wepman 1978; Corah et al. 1979; Woolgrove 1983; Sokol et al. 1985; LeClaire et al. 1988; Maggirias and Locker 2002; Van Wijk and Makkes 2008) and can enter a vicious cycle of overestimating pain and increasing anxiety.

4) The dentist. Many physicians agree that the main factor in reducing pain during the administration of anesthesia is the dentist him/herself (Mollen et al. 1981; Goodell et al. 2000; Saloum et al. 2000; Nusstein and Beck 2003; Ram and Peretz 2003), for two key reasons:
   - The dentist's touch, skill, and ability when administering local anesthetic. Many of these small details have been addressed in this chapter during the 10 phases of injection, where emphasis was placed on safety, psychology, careful management of oral tissues, and the ways pain can be reduced during the injection. It is of critical importance that the that clinician maintains an optimistic demeanor before, during, and after the injection process (Kravitz 2006).
   - The dentist's management of the interpersonal relationship, improved communication, and use of psychological strategies that increase patient satisfaction (Gale et al. 1984; Maggirias and Locker 2002). Patient satisfaction may even be high in treatments that are painful (Lindemann et al. 2008) owing to the dentist's positive and professional approach (i.e. not appearing indifferent or being on the defensive) and the fact that he/she gives the patient encouragement, especially at difficult points during the procedure. While not within the scope of this book, some aspects are worthy of mention (Gale et al. 1984):
     – Welcome the patient and ask him/her to sit in the dental chair.
     – Explain what is going to be done.
     – Approach the patient carefully.
     – Talk about things in general when administering the anesthetic.
     – Explain to the patient during the treatment that everything is going well. Even if a problem arises, we can say something like "This is interesting, but we'll have it fixed in second." Note the use of the euphemism "interesting" and not words such as "problem" and "difficulty."
     – Converse with the patient on completion of treatment and say goodbye.

   Patient expectations of pain and anxiety are not modified by a simple pain-free procedure; however, repeated exposures to pain-free treatment attenuate expectations of anxiety and pain (Maggirias and Locker 2002).

Finally, it is important to remember that the two principal factors by which patients judge dentists are whether they administer the injection without pain and whether there is pain during the procedure (St Georges 2004).

## Unimportant Causes (Myths)

There are two myths that, unfortunately, are widespread among dentists with respect to the cause of pain during injection. They are of little relevance.

1) The needle caliber myth. Most dentists think that smaller calibers (30G and 27G) cause less pain during the insertion and the injection (Smith 1968; Cooley and Robinson 1979; Mollen et al. 1981; Van der Bijl 1995). However, clinical studies seem to indicate that there is little difference with respect to perception of pain (see Chapter 11). Six clinical trials found no statistically significant differences in pain with the different calibers of needle (30G, 27G, and 25G), and a further two trials showed that the finest-gauge needle (30G) caused less pain than the 27G needle. The clinical differences were very small but statistically significant (Table 11.3, Chapter 11).

   To verify differences between the calibers, we must use thicker needles (20G or 22G), such as those used in intramuscular injections or those that were once used in dental injections (Smith 1920).

2) The cartridge temperature myth. Even in the earliest texts on dental local anesthesia, authors insisted that solutions be at body temperature (around 36 °C) to prevent pain during the injection (Fischer 1912; Lewis 1919).

   Clinical trials have shown that patients cannot distinguish between ambient temperature (20–21 °C) and injections at body temperature (35–37 °C) (Oikarinen et al. 1975; Rood 1977; Ram et al. 2002).

   Furthermore, heating the cartridges for a short time is harmless, although storing them at body temperature for long periods deteriorates sympathomimetic vasoconstrictors such as epinephrine (Gerke et al. 1977; Fry and Ciarlone 1980; Thoma and Struve 1986; Hondrum et al. 1993).

   If the cartridge is cold (less than 20 °C = 68 °F), it can be heated up before placing it in the syringe by holding it in the hand for 30 seconds (Malamed 2004).

## Terminology

Below, we classify dental anesthesia and comment on the terms used to define the different anesthetic techniques (Jorgensen and Hayden 1970; Allen 1979; Jastak et al. 1995).

- Classification of anesthesia with respect to the *periosteum*:
  - Infraperiosteal or subperiosteal. When the needle goes below the periosteum to deliver the anesthetic solution at this level. The technique was used many years ago, when anesthetic solutions were weak, so that they could cross a barrier (the periosteum), penetrate more deeply, and thus cross the cortical bone to reach the cancellous bone. The approach is complicated by pain during penetration of the periosteum and postoperative pain.
  - Supraperiosteal or paraperiosteal. When the needle remains above the periosteum and does not cross it. *Today, all techniques are supraperiosteal* because modern anesthetic solutions cross the periosteum well.
- *Classification of anesthesia according to basic techniques* (Figure 13.11):
  - Topical or surface anesthesia, which results from application of the anesthetic on the oral mucosa without administering an injection.
  - Infiltrative anesthesia, which involves injection of anesthetic solution into the tissues to be treated. Several nerve endings (many of which are microscopic) are anesthetized. Anesthesia is limited to the area reached by the solution.
  - Nerve or truncal block, which involves anesthesia of a whole nerve or nerve trunk (macroscopic), such as the inferior alveolar nerve (mandibular block). The advantage of this approach is that it anesthetizes at some distance and thus covers a large anatomical area.

Note: Nerve blocks can be of smaller secondary trunks; some authors call these blocks "field blocks" or "regional blocks." We refer to them all as nerve blocks, for example maxillary nerve block ($V_2$) via the high tuberosity (main nerve trunk) and anterior superior alveolar nerve block via the infraorbital nerve (secondary trunk) (see Chapter 14).

- Variants of infiltrative techniques:
  - Periapical or para-apical anesthesia. The filtration placed at the apex of the teeth (buccal infiltration).
  - Intrapapillary anesthesia. Infiltration in the interdental papilla (Figure 13.12).
  - Plexus anesthesia. Anesthetic administered by infiltration of the superior dental plexus or superior alveolar nervous plexus in the maxilla at the level of or above the apexes of the teeth at the junction of the posterior, medial, and anterior alveolar nerves, and even the nasopalatine nerve in the anterior part (see Chapter 2).
  - Transpapillary technique. Infiltration of the interdental papilla to anesthetize the palate through the buccal part.
  - Intrapulpal anesthesia. Injection directly into the open dental pulp.
  - Intraosseous anesthesia. Penetration of the needle into the cancellous bone after crossing the periosteum and cortical bone to inject directly into the trabecular or cancellous bone.

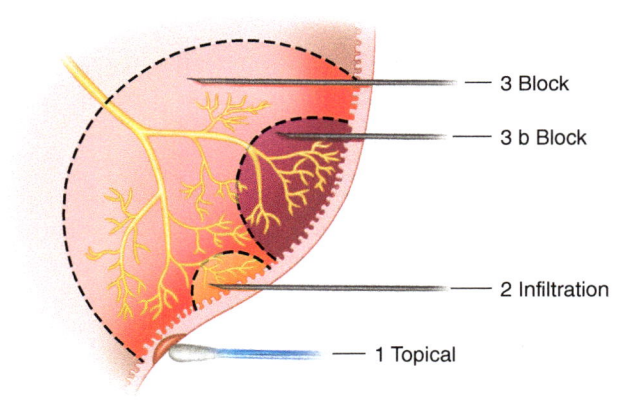

**Figure 13.11** Basic techniques in dental local anesthesia: (1) topical anesthesia; (2) infiltrative anesthesia; (3) nerve trunk block; and (3b) smaller, secondary nerve trunk block (field or regional anesthesia or field block). *Source:* Redrawn from Allen (1979) and Jastak et al. (1995).

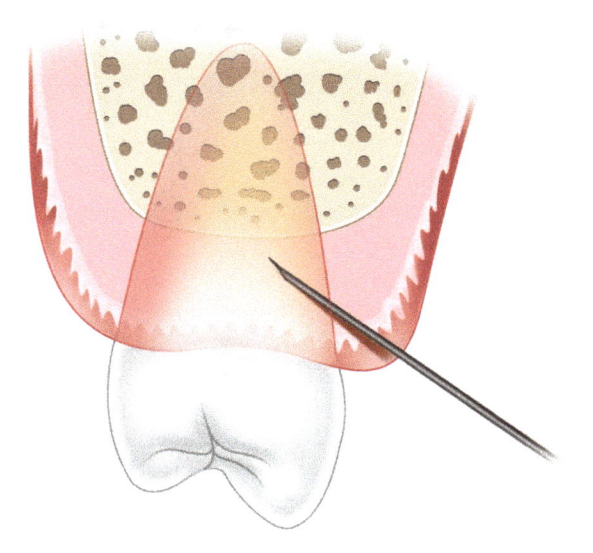

**Figure 13.12** Intrapapillary infiltrative anesthesia.

- Intraligamentous anesthesia or anesthesia of the periodontal ligament. A pressure injection across the periodontal ligament.
- Intraseptal anesthesia. Penetration of the needle into the interdental papilla to perforate the interdental bone crest and inject the anesthetic solution into the cancellous bone. This is a variant of the intraosseous and intraligamentous techniques.

## Appendix

Data from McCarney et al. (2007).

Mandibular block. Pain in scale of none, mild, moderate, and severe. Pain during advance of the needle (needle placement) in a group with deposition of anesthetic solution (anesthetic given) and a group without deposition (no anesthetic given).

|  | Severe pain | None, mild, moderate pain | Total |
|---|---|---|---|
| Anesthetic given | 20 (35%) | 38 | 58 |
| No anesthetic given | 5 (11%) | 39 | 44 |
|  | 25 | 77 | 102 |

The worse pain is experienced during deposition of the anesthetic solution during the advance of the needle (anesthetic given). Fisher exact test $= 0.0099$ (two sides $P$ value).

Molar with irreversible acute pulpitis.

## References

Addelston, H.K. (1959). Child patient training. *Fortn. Rev. Chic. Dent. Soc.* 38 (2): 7–9, 27–29.

Adriani, J. and Campbell, D. (1956). Fatalities following topical application of local anesthetics to mucous membranes. *JAMA* 162 (17): 1527–1530.

Adriani, J., Campbell, D., and Yarberry, D.H. Jr. (1959). Influence of absorption on systemic toxicity of local anesthetic agents. *Anesth. Analg.* 38 (5): 370–377.

Aggarwal, V., Singla, M., Miglani, S. et al. (2012). A prospective randomized single-blind evaluation of effect of injection speed on anesthetic efficacy of inferior alveolar nerve block in patients with symptomatic irreversible pulpitis. *J. Endod.* 38 (12): 1578–1580.

Allegretti, C.E., Sampaio, R.M., Horliana, A.C.R.T. et al. (2016). Anesthetic efficacy in irreversible pulpitis: a randomized clinical trial. *Braz. Dent. J.* 27 (4): 381–386.

Allen, G.D. (1979). *Dental Anesthesia and Analgesia (Local and General)*, 2e. Baltimore: Williams and Wilkins. 86–89, 95–96.

Alling, C.C. and Christopher, A. (1974). Status report on dental anesthetic needles and syringes. Council on dental materials and devices and council on dental therapeutics. *J. Am. Dent. Assoc.* 89 (5): 1171–1176.

American Academy of Pediatric Dentistry (AAPD) (2020). *Use of Local Anesthesia for Pediatric Dental Patients. The Reference Manual of Pediatric Dentistry*. Chicago IL: American Academy of Pediatric Dentistry. 318–323.

Annex 10. Maximum doses of dental local anesthetics solutions.

Annex 14. Injectable anesthetic solutions pH.

Annex 19. Topical anesthesia I. Results of clinical trials.

Annex 22. Positive aspirations.

Annex 23. Pain resulting from injection techniques.

Armbrecht, E.C. and Schwetz, W.S. (1962). A case report. Recovery of a broken needle. *West Virginia Dent. J.* 36: 120–121.

Baht, E.I., Baht, R., Kozlovsky, A., and Simon, H. (2000). Effect of gender on acute pain prediction and memory in periodontal surgery. *Eur. J. Oral Sci.* 108 (2): 99–103.

Bartlett, S.Z. (1972). Clinical observations on the effects of injections of local anesthetic preceded by aspiration. *Oral Surg. Oral Med. Oral Pathol.* 33 (4): 520–526.

Batinac, T., Tokmadzic, V.S., Peharda, V., and Brajac, I. (2013). Adverse reactions and alleged allergy to local anesthetics: analysis of 331 patients. *J. Dermatol.* 40 (7): 522–527.

Bennett, C.R. (1984). *Monheim's Local Anesthesia and Pain Control in Dental Practice*, 7e. St Louis (Missouri): The CV Mosby Co. 106, 165.

Berggren, U. and Meynert, G. (1984). Dental fear and avoidance: causes, symptoms, and consequences. *J. Am. Dent. Assoc.* 109 (2): 247–251.

Blair, G.S. and Meechan, J.G. (1985). Local anesthesia in dental practice I. A clinical study of self-aspirating system. *Br. Dent. J.* 159 (3): 75–77.

Bos, A.L., Coppes, L., Determann, E.J. et al. (1971). Aspiration control in the administration of local anesthesia in dentistry. *Ned. Tijdschr. Tandheelkd.* (Suppl 6): 24–38.

Bourne, J.G. (1957). Fainting and cerebral damage. Dosage in patients kept upright during dental gas anesthesia and after surgical operations. *Lancet* 273 (6994): 499–505.

Bourne, J.G. (1970). Deaths with dental anesthetics. *Anaesthesia* 25 (4): 473–481.

Burgess, J.O. (1988). The broken dental needle – a hazard. *Special Care Dent.* 8 (2): 71–73.

Campbell, D. and Adriani, J. (1958). Absorption of local anesthetics. *JAMA* 168 (7): 873–877.

Cannell, H. (1996). Evidence of safety margins of lignocaine local anaesthetics for perioral use. *Br. Dent. J.* 181 (7): 243–249.

Carr, M.P. and Horton, J.E. (2001a). Evaluation of transoral delivery system for topical anesthesia. *J. Am. Dent. Assoc.* 132 (12): 1714–1719.

Carr, M.P. and Horton, J.E. (2001b). Clinical evaluation and comparison of 2 topical anesthetics for pain caused by needle sticks and scaling and rootplaning. *J. Periodontol.* 72 (4): 479–484.

Certosimo, A.J. and Archer, R.D. (1996). A clinical evaluation of the electric pulp tester as an indicator of local anesthesia. *Oper. Dent.* 21 (1): 25–30.

Chavarria-Bolaños, D., Rodríguez-Wong, I., Noguera-Gonález, D. et al. (2017). Sensitivity, specificity, predictive values, and accuracy of three diagnostic tests to predict inferior alveolar nerve blockade failure in symptomatic irreversible pulpitis. *Pain Res. Mange.* 2017: 3108940.

Cheatham, B.D., Primosch, R.E., and Courts, F.J. (1992). A survey of local anesthetic usage in pediatric patients by Florida dentists. *J. Dent. Child.* 59 (6): 401–407.

Childers, M., Reader, A., Nist, R. et al. (1996). Anesthesia efficacy of the periodontal ligament injection after an inferior alveolar nerve block. *J. Endod.* 22 (6): 317–320.

Cleveland, J.L., Barker, L.K., Cuny, E.J. et al. (2007). Preventing percutaneous injuries among dental health care personnel. *J. Am. Dent. Assoc.* 138 (2): 169–178.

Cohen, H.P., Cha, B.Y., and Spangberg, L.S.W. (1993). Endodontic anesthesia in mandibular molars: a clinical study. *J. Endod.* 19 (7): 370–373.

Cooley, R.L. and Robinson, S.F. (1979). Comparative evaluation of the 30-gauge dental needle. *Oral Surg. Oral Med. Oral Pathol.* 48 (5): 400–404.

Corah, N.L., Gale, E.N., and Illig, S.J. (1979). Psychological stress reduction during dental procedures. *J. Dent. Res.* 58 (4): 1347–1351.

Council on Clinical Affairs (2015). Guideline on use of local anesthesia for pediatric dental patients. *Pediatr. Dent.* 37 (Special issue): 199–205.

Council on Dental Therapeutics. Chicago: American Dental Association. 1957: 109.

Cowan, A. (1972). A new aspirating syringe. *Br. Dent. J.* 133 (12): 547–548.

Daubländer, M., Müller, R., and Lipp, M.D.W. (1997). The incidence of complications associated with local anesthesia in dentistry. *Anesth. Prog.* 44 (4): 132–144.

David, H.T., Aminzadeh, K.K., Kae, A.H., and Radomsky, S.C. (2007). Instrument retraction to avoid needle-stick injuries during intraoral local anesthesia. *Oral Surg. Oral Med. Oral Pathol.* 103 (3): e11–e13.

De Jong, R.H. (1977). *Local Anesthetics*, 2e. Springfield (IL): Charles C Thomas Publisher. 61.

De Souza Melo, M.R., Sabey, M.J.S., Lima, C.J. et al. (2015). The effect of 2 injection speeds on local anesthetic discomfort during inferior alveolar nerve blocks. *Anesth. Prog.* 62 (3): 106–109.

Dentists' Desk (1983). *Reference: Materials, Instruments and Equipment*, 2e. Chicago: American Dental Association. 351–356.

Dreven, L.J., Reader, A., Beck, M. et al. (1987). An evaluation of an electric pulp tester as a measure of analgesia in human vital teeth. *J. Endod.* 13 (5): 233–238.

Dubner, R. (1978). Neurophysiology of pain. *Dent. Clin. N. Am.* 22 (1): 11–30.

Eickbohm, J.E., Wulf, H., Hoffmann, C., and Becker, C.H. (1991). Klinische Pharmakokinetik von Lidocain nach intraoraler Leitungsanästhesie. *Dtsch. Zahnärztl. Z.* 46 (12): 812–814.

Ellis, R.K., Berg, J.H., and Raj, P.P. (1990). Subjective signs of efficacious inferior alveolar nerve block in children. *J. Dent. Child.* 57 (5): 361–365.

Evers, H. and Haegerstam, G. (1981). *Handbook of Dental Local Anesthesia*. Copenhagen: Schultz Medical International. 65, 75, 171.

Fa, B.A., Gupta, S., and Bhattacharyya, M. (2016). Operator preference of retraction method during anesthesia delivery. *Stomatol. EDU J.* 3 (1): 10–15.

Firestein, S.K. (1976). Patient anxiety and dental practice. *J. Am. Dent. Assoc.* 93 (6): 1180–1187.

Fischer, G. (1912). *Local Anesthesia in Dentistry. With Special Reference to the Mucous and Conductive Methods. A Concise Guide for Dentists, Surgeons and Students*. Philadelphia: Lea and Febiger. 51, 135.

Forrest, J.O. (1959). Notes on aspiration before injection of local anesthetics using dental cartridges. *Br. Dent. J.* 107 (3): 259–262.

Frasier, I.M. (1967). Local anesthetics. In: *Premedication, Local and General Anesthesia in Dentistry* (ed. A.B. Jorgensen and J. Hayden). Philadelphia: Lea and Febiger. 89–96.

Fry, B.W. and Ciarlone, A.C. (1980). Concentrations of vasoconstrictor in local anesthetics during storage in cartridges heaters. *J. Dent. Res.* 59 (7): 1136.

Fuller, N.P., Menke, R.A., and Meyers, W.S. (1979). Perception of pain to three different intraoral penetrations of needles. *J. Am. Dent. Assoc.* 99 (5): 822–824.

Fuss, Z., Towbridge, H., Bender, I.B. et al. (1986). Assessment of reliability of electrical and thermal pulp testing agents. *J. Endod.* 12 (7): 301–305.

Gale, E.N., Carlsson, S.G., and Jontell, M. (1984). Effects of dentists' behavior on patients' attitudes. *J. Am. Dent. Assoc.* 109 (3): 444–446.

Gazal, G. (2015). Comparison of speed of action and injection discomfort of 4% articaine and 2% mepivacaine for pulpal anesthesia in mandibular teeth: a randomized, double-blind cross-over trial. *Eur. J. Dent.* 9 (2): 201–206.

Gerke, D.C., Crabb, G.A., Frewin, D.B., and Frost, B.R. (1977). The effect of storage on the activity of adrenaline in local anesthetic solutions: an evaluation using bioassay and fluorometric techniques. *Aust. Dent. J.* 22 (6): 423–427.

Ghoddusi, J., Zarrabi, M.H., Daneshvar, F., and Naghavi, N. (2018). Efficacy of IANB and Gow-Gates techniques in madibular molars with symptomatic irreversible pulpitis: a prospective randomized double blind clinical study. *Iran. Endod. J.* 13 (2): 143–148.

Gill, C.J. and Orr, D.L. II. (1979). A double-blind crossover comparison of topical anesthetics. *J. Am. Dent. Assoc.* 98 (2): 213–214.

Goldman, V. and Gray, W. (1963). A clinical trial of a new local analgesic agent. *Br. Dent. J.* 115 (2): 59–65.

Goodell, G.G., Gallager, F.J., and Nicoll, B.K. (2000). Comparison of controlled injection pressure system with a conventional technique. *Oral Surg. Oral Med. Oral Pathol.* 90 (1): 88–94.

Goodson, J.M. and Moore, P.A. (1983). Life-threatening reactions after pedodontic sedation: an assessment of narcotic, local anesthetic, and antiemetic drug interaction. *J. Am. Dent. Assoc.* 107 (2): 239–245.

Hersh, E.V., Helpin, M.L., and Evans, O.B. (1991). Local anesthetic mortality: report of case. *J. Dent. Child.* 58 (6): 489–491.

Hersh, E.V., Moore, P.A., Papas, A.S. et al. (2008). Reversal of soft-tissue local anesthesia with phentolamine mesylate in adolescents and adults. *J. Am. Dent. Assoc.* 139 (8): 1080–1093.

Holst, A. and Evers, H. (1985). Experimental studies of new topical anaesthetics on the oral mucosa. *Swed. Dent. J.* 9 (5): 185–191.

Hondrum, S.O., Seng, G.F., and Rebert, N.W. (1993). Stability of local anesthetics in the dental cartridge. *Anesth. Pain Control Dent.* 2 (4): 198–202.

Horowitz, J., Almong, Y., Wolf, A. et al. (2005). Ophthalmic complications of dental anesthesia: three new cases. *J. Neuroophthalmol.* 25 (2): 95–100.

Hsiao-Wu, G.W., Susarla, S.M., and White, P.P. (2007). Use of the cold test as a measure of pulpal anesthesia during endodontic therapy: a randomized, blinded, placebo-controlled clinical trial. *J. Endod.* 33 (4): 406–410.

Jackson, E. (1974). Managing dental fear's: a tentative code of practice. *J. Oral Med.* 29 (4): 96–101.

Jastak, J.T., Yagiela, J.A., and Donaldson, D. (1995). *Local Anesthesia of the Oral Cavity*. Philadelphia: WB Saunders Co. 161–162, 185–186.

Jones, C.M., Heidmann, J., and Gerrish, A.C. (1995). Children's ratings of dental injection and treatment pain, and influence of the time taken to administer the injection. *Int. J. Paediatr. Dent.* 5 (2): 81–85.

Jorgensen, N.B. and Hayden, J. Jr. (1970). *Anestesia odontológica*. Mexico, DF: Editorial Interamericana SA. (Spanish translation of: Jorgensen, N.B. and Hayden, J. Jr. (1967). Premedication, Local and General Anesthesia in Dentistry. Philadephia: Lea and Febiger). 24, 33.

Kämmerer, P.W., Schneider, D., Pacyna, A.A., and Daubländer, M. (2016). Movement control during aspiration with different injection systems via video monitoring – an in vitro model. *Clin. Oral Investig.* 21 (1): 105–110.

Kanaa, M.D., Meechan, J.G., Corbett, I.P., and Whitworth, J.M. (2006). Speed of injection influences efficacy for inferior alveolar nerve blocks: a double-blind randomized controlled trial in volunteers. *J. Endod.* 32 (10): 919–923.

Karkut, B., Reader, A., Drum, M. et al. (2010). A comparison of the local anesthetic efficacy of the extraoral versus intraoral infraorbital nerve block. *J. Am. Dent. Assoc.* 141 (2): 185–192.

Kaufman, E., Gaharian, S., and Katz, Y. (2000). Adverse reactions triggered by dental local anesthetics: a clinical survey. *Anesth. Prog.* 47 (4): 134–138.

Kelly, J.R. and Cohen, M.E. (1984). Injectable debris associated with dental anesthetic delivery. *J. Am. Dent. Assoc.* 108 (4): 621–624.

Kelly, J.F. and Patterson, R. (1974). Anaphylaxis. Course, mechanisms and treatment. *J. Am. Med. Assoc.* 227 (12): 1431–1436.

Kennedy, M., Reader, A., Beck, M., and Weaver, J. (2001). Anesthetic efficacy of ropivacaine in maxillary anterior infiltration. *Oral Surg. Oral Med. Oral Pathol.* 91 (4): 406–412.

Kennedy, S., Reader, A., Nusstein, J. et al. (2003). The significance of needle deflection in success of the inferior alveolar nerve block in patients with irreversible pulpitis. *J. Endod.* 29 (10): 630–633.

Klein, R.M. (1983). Components of local anesthetic solutions. *Gen. Dent.* 31 (6): 460–465.

Kleinknecht, R.A. and Berstein, D.A. (1978). The assessment of dental fear. *Behav. Ther.* 9 (4): 626–634.

Kleinknecht, R.A., Klepac, R.K., and Alexander, L.D. (1973). Origins and characteristic of fear of dentistry. *J. Am. Dent. Assoc.* 86 (4): 842–948.

Kohli, N., Ngan, O., Crout, R., and Lindscott, C.C. (2001). A survey of local and topical anesthesia use by pediatric dentists in the United States. *Pediatr. Dent.* 23 (3): 265–269.

Kramp, L.F., Eleazer, P.D., and Acheetz, J.P. (1999). Evaluation of prilocaine for the reduction of pain associated with transmucosal anesthetic administration. *Anesth. Analg.* 46 (2): 52–55.

Kravitz, J. (2006). The palatal press and roll anesthesia technique. *Pract. Proced. Aesthet. Dent.* 18 (4): 242–245.

Kudo, M. (2005). Initial injection pressure for dental local anesthesia: effects on pain and anxiety. *Anesth. Prog.* 52 (3): 95–101.

LeClaire, A.J., Skidmore, A.E., Griffin, J.A. Jr., and Balaban, F.S. (1988). Endodontic fear survey. *J. Endod.* 14 (11): 560–564.

Lesch, C.A., Squier, C.A., Cruchley, A. et al. (1989). The impermeability of human oral mucosa and skin to water. *J. Dent. Res.* 68 (9): 1345–1349.

Lewis, D.N. (1919). Pain following local anesthesia. *Dent. Cosmos* 61 (5): 407–408.

Liddell, A. and Locker, D. (1997). Gender and age differences in attitudes to dental pain and dental control. *Community Dent. Oral Epidemiol.* 25 (4): 314–318.

Lim, S. and Julliard, K. (2004). Evaluating the efficacy of EMLA topical anesthetic in sealant placement with rubber dam. *Pediatr. Dent.* 26 (6): 497–500.

Lindemann, M., Reader, A., Nusstein, J. et al. (2008). Effect of sublingual triazolam on the success of inferior alveolar nerve block in patients with irreversible pulpitis. *J. Endod.* 34 (10): 1167–1170.

Lindsay AW. The direct approach technique in mandibular block anesthesia. Thesis. Faculty of Dentistry, University of Toronto. 1929; 34–35.

Linscott, C., Kohli, K., Ngan, P., and Crout, R. (1978). Local anesthesia practices among United States pediatric dentists. *J. Dent. Res.* 77 (Special Issue A): 290. (abstract no 1479).

Lipp, M.D.W., Dick, W.F., Daubländer, M. et al. (1988). Examination of the central-nervous epinephrine level during local dental infiltration and block anesthesia using tritium-marked epinephrine as vasoconstrictor. *Anesthesiology* 69 (3A-Suppl): A371.

Lipp, M., Dick, W., Daubländer, M. et al. (1993). Exogenous and endogenous plasma levels of epinephrine during dental treatment and local anesthesia. *Reg. Anesth.* 18 (1): 6–12.

Lloyd, J.M. (1992). Aspiration in dental local anaesthesia (letter). *Br. Dent. J.* 172 (4): 136.

Lopez, J. and Rosello, X. (1995). Anestesiatroncular del nerviodentario inferior. Porcentaje de aspiracionespositivas. *Rev. Eur. Odontoestomatol. (Barcelona)* 7 (6): 353–356.

Lustig, J.P. and Zusman, S.P. (1999). Immediate complications of local anesthetic administered to 1,007 consecutive patients. *J. Am. Dent. Assoc.* 130 (4): 496–499.

Maggirias, J. and Locker, D. (2002). Psychological factors and perception of pain associated with dental treatment. *Community Dent. Oral Epidemiol.* 30 (2): 151–159.

Majstorovic, M. and Veerkamp, J.S.J. (2004). Relationship between needle phobia and dental anxiety. *J. Dent. Child.* 71 (3): 201–205.

Malamed, S.F. (1986). *Handbook of Local Anesthesia*, 2e. St. Louis (Missouri): The CV Mosby Co. 116–127.

Malamed, S.F. (2004). *Handbook of Local Anesthesia*, 5e. St. Louis (Missouri): Elsevier-Mosby. 115, 160, 166–167, 309–311.

Mamiya, H., Katagiri, N., Ichinohe, T., and Kaneko, Y. (2001). The effects of the injection speed of local anesthesia. *J. Dent. Res.* 80 (Special Issue): 667. (abstract no 1122).

Maragakis, G.M. and Musselman, R.J. (1996). The time used to administer local anesthesia to 5 and 6 year olds. *J. Clin. Pediatr. Dent.* 20 (4): 321–323.

Marks, R.B., Carlton, D.M., and McDonald, J. (1984). Management of a broken needle in the pterygomandibular space: report a case. *J. Am. Dent. Assoc.* 109 (2): 263–264.

Martin, M.D., Ramsay, D.S., Whitney, C. et al. (1994). Topical anesthesia: differentiating the pharmacological and psychological contribution to efficacy. *Anesth. Prog.* 41 (2): 40–47.

McCarney, M., Reader, A., and Beck, M. (2007). Injection pain of the inferior alveolar nerve block in patients with irreversible pulpitis. *Oral Surg. Oral Med. Oral Pathol.* 104 (4): 571–575.

McClure, D.B. (1968). Local anesthesia for the preschool child. *J. Dent. Child.* 35 (6): 441–448.

McDonogh, T. (1996). An unusual case of trismus and dysphagia. *Br. Dent. J.* 180 (12): 465–466.

Meechan, J. (1998). How to avoid local anaesthesia toxicity. *Br. Dent. J.* 184 (7): 334–335.

Meechan, J.G. (2008). Intra oral topical anesthesia. *Periodontology* 46: 56–79.

Meechan, J.G. and Blair, G.S. (1989). Clinical experience in oral surgery with 2 different automatic aspirating syringes. *Int. J. Oral Maxillofac. Surg.* 18 (2): 87–89.

Meechan, J.G. and Rood, J.P. (1992). Aspiration in dental local anesthesia. *Br. Dent. J.* 172 (2): 40.

Meechan, J.G., Gowans, A.J., and Welbury, R.R. (1998). The use of patient-controlled transcutaneous electronic nerve stimulation (TENS) to decrease the discomfort of regional anaesthesia in dentistry: a randomized controlled clinical trial. *J. Dent.* 26 (5–6): 417–420.

Meechan, J.G., Howlett, P.C., and Smith, B.D. (2005). Factors influencing the discomfort of intraoral needle penetration. *Anesth. Prog.* 52 (3): 91–94.

Melzack, R. and Wall, P.D. (1965). Pain mechanism: a new theory. *Science* 150 (3699): 971–979.

Messer, J.G. (1977). Stress in dental patients undergoing routine procedures. *J. Dent. Res.* 56 (4): 362–367.

Milgrom, P., Coldwell, S.E., Getz, T. et al. (1997). Four dimensions of fear of dental injections. *J. Am. Dent. Assoc.* 128 (6): 756–762.

Miller, S.O., Johnson, J.D., Allemang, J.D., and Strother, J.M. (2004). Cold testing through full-coverage restorations. *J. Endod.* 30 (10): 695–700.

Mink, J.R. and Spedding, R.H. (1966). An injection procedure for the child dental patient. *Dent. Clin. N. Am.* 10: 309–325.

Mollen, A.J., Ficara, A.J., and Provant, D.R. (1981). Needles – 25 gauge versus 27-gauge – can patients really tell? *Gen. Dent.* 29 (5): 417–418.

Moore, P. (1992). Preventing local anesthetic toxicity. *J. Am. Dent. Assoc.* 123 (9): 60–64.

Moorthy, A.P., Moorthy, S.P., and O'Neil, R. (1984). A study of pH of dental local anesthetic solutions. *Br. Dent. J.* 157 (11): 394–395.

Munshi, A.K., Hegde, A.M., and Latha, R. (2001). Use of EMLA®: is it an injection free alternative? *J. Clin. Pediatr. Dent.* 25 (3): 215–219.

Nakamura, S., Matsuura, N., and Ichinohe, T. (2013). A new method of topical anesthesia by using anesthetic solution in a patch. *J. Endod.* 39 (11): 1369–1373.

Nanitsos, E., Vartuli, R., Forte, A. et al. (2009). The effect of vibration on pain during local anaesthesia injections. *Aust. Dent. J.* 54 (2): 94–100.

Nist, R.A., Reader, A., Beck, M., and Meyers, W.J. (1992). An evaluation of the incisive nerve block and combination inferior alveolar and incisive nerve blocks in mandibula anesthesia. *J. Endod.* 18 (9): 455–459.

Nordenram, A. (1971). *Manuel d'anesthésie locale enpractiquedentaire*. Mölndal (Sweden): Lindgren and Söner. Bofors Nobel-Pharma. 24, 39.

Nusstein, J.M. and Beck, M. (2003). Effectiveness of 20% benzocaine as a topical anesthetic for intraoral injections. *Anesth. Prog.* 50 (4): 159–163.

Nusstein, J., Reader, A., Nist, R. et al. (1998). Anesthetic efficacy of the supplemental intraosseous injection of 2% lidocaine with 1:100,000 epinephrine in irreversible pulpitis. *J. Endod.* 24 (7): 487–491.

Nusstein, J., Steinkruger, G., Reader, A. et al. (2006). The effects of a 2-stage technique on inferior alveolar nerve block injection pain. *Anesth. Prog.* 53 (4): 126–130.

Oikarinen, V.J., Ylipaavalniemi, P., and Evers, H. (1975). Pain and temperature sensations related to local analgesia. *Int. J. Oral Surg.* 4 (4): 151–156.

Oliver, L.P. (1974). Local anesthesia –a review of practice. *Aust. Dent. J.* 19 (5): 313–319.

Orr, D.L. II. (1983). The broken needle: report of case. *J. Am. Dent. Assoc.* 107 (4): 603–604.

Ozec, I., Tasdemir, U., Gümüs, C., and Solak, O. (2010). Is it possible to anesthetize palatal tissues with buccal 4% articaine injection? *J. Oral Maxillofac. Surg.* 68 (5): 1032–1037.

Persson, G., Keskitalo, E., and Evers, H. (1974). Clinical experiences in oral surgery using a new self-aspirating injection system. *Int. J. Oral Surg.* 3 (6): 428–434.

Piesold, J., Müller, W., and Dreiβig, J. (1998). An experimental study on the aspirating reliability of different types of injection syringes with regard to formation of punch cylinders. *Br. J. Oral Maxillofac. Surg.* 36 (1): 39–43.

Primosch, R.E. and Brooks, R. (2002). Influence of anesthetic flow rate delivered by the wand local anesthetic system on pain response to palatal injections. *Am. J. Dent.* 15 (1): 15–20.

Quarnstrom, F. and Libed, E.N. (1994). Electronic anesthesia versus topical anesthesia for the control of injection pain. *Quintessence Int.* 25 (10): 713–716.

Ram, D. and Peretz, B. (2002). Administering local anesthesia to paediatric dental patients – current status and prospects for future. *Int. J. Paediatr. Dent.* 12 (2): 80–89.

Ram, D. and Peretz, B. (2003). The assessment of pain sensation during local anesthesia using a computerized local anesthesia (wand) and a conventional syringe. *J. Dent. Child.* 70 (2): 130–133.

Ram, D., Hermida, L.B., and Peretz, B. (2002). A comparison of warmed and room-temperature anesthetic for local anesthesia in children. *Pediatr. Dent.* 24 (4): 333–336.

Rankin, J.A. and Harris, M.B. (1985). Patient's preferences for dentists' behaviors. *J. Am. Dent. Assoc.* 110 (3): 323–327.

Reader, A., Nusstein, J., and Drum, M. (2011). *Successful Local Anesthesia. For Restorative Dentistry and Endodontics*. Chicago: Quintessence Publishing Co, Inc. 132.

Roberts, D.H. and Sowray, J.H. (1987). *Local Analgesia in Dentistry*, 3e. Bristol (UK): Wright. 74–77, 87.

Roghani, S., Duperon, D.F., and Barcohana, N. (1999). Evaluating the efficacy of commonly used topical anesthetics. *Pediatr. Dent.* 21 (3): 197–200.

Rood, J.P. (1977). The temperature of local anesthetic solutions. *J. Dent.* 5 (3): 213–214.

Rousseau, W.H., Clark, S.J., Newcomb, B.E. et al. (2002). A comparison of pain levels during pulpectomy, extractions, and restorative procedures. *J. Endod.* 28 (2): 108–110.

Saloum, F.S., Baumgartner, J.C., Marshall, G., and Tinkle, J. (2000). A clinical comparison of pain perception to the wand and a traditional syringe. *Oral Surg. Oral Med. Oral Pathol.* 89 (6): 691–695.

Scott, D.B. (1986). Toxic effects of local anesthetic agents on the central nervous system. *Br. J. Anaesth.* 58 (7): 732–735.

Shannon, I.L. and Feller, R.P. (1972). Contamination of local anesthetic carpules by storage in alcohol. *Anesth. Prog.* 19 (1): 6–8.

Shannon, I.L. and Wescott, W.B. (1974). Alcohol contamination of local anesthetic cartridges. *J. Acad. Gen. Dent.* 22 (11): 20–21.

Shira, R.B. (1962). Changing concepts in the practice of exodontic and oral surgery. *J. Ontario Dent. Assoc.* 39 (1): 8–13.

Simon, J.F., Peltier, B., Chambers, D., and Dower, I. (1994). Dentist troubled by the administration of anesthetic injections: long-term stresses and effects. *Quintessence Int.* 25 (9): 641–646.

Smith, A.E. (1920). *Block Anesthesia and Allied Subjects. With Special Chapters on the Maxillary Sinus, the Tonsils, and Neuralgias of the Nervous Trigeminus for Oral Surgeons, Dentists, Laryngologists, Rhinologists, Otologists, and Students.* St Louis (MO): CV Mosby Company. 380–524.

Smith, N. (1968). An investigation of the influence of gauge on some physical properties of hypodermic needles. Part I. The relation between gauge and flexibility of the needle. *Aust. Dent. J.* 13 (2): 158–161.

Snawder, K.D. (1987). *Manual de Odontopediatría clínica.* Barcelona: Editorial Labor SA (Spanish translation of: Handbook of clinical pedodontics. St. Louis: The CV Mosby Co. 1982). 81–82.

Sokol, D.J., Sokol, S., and Sokol, C.K. (1985). A review of nonintrusive therapies used to deal with anxiety and pain in the dental office. *J. Am. Dent. Assoc.* 110 (2): 217–222.

Spedding, R.H. and Mink, J.R. (1964). An approach to the injection procedure for the child patient. *J. N. J. State Dent. Soc.* 35: 161–168.

St Georges, J. (2004). How dentists are judged by patients. *Dent. Today* 23 (8): 96–99.

Stacy, G.C., Orth, D., and Hajjar, G. (1994). Barbed needle and inexplicable paresthesias and trismus after dental regional anesthesia. *Oral Surg. Oral Med. Oral Pathol.* 77 (6): 585–588.

Steinkruger, G., Nusstein, J., Reader, A. et al. (2006). The significance of needle bevel orientation in achieving a successful inferior alveolar nerve block. *J. Am. Dent. Assoc.* 137 (12): 1685–1691.

Thoma, K. and Struve, M. (1986). Untersuchungerzur Photon und Thermostabilität von Adrenlin-Lösungen. 1. MitteilungzurStabilität von Adrenalin-Lösungen. *Pharm. Acta Helv.* 61 (1): 2–9.

Trapp, L.D. and Davies, R.O. (1980). Aspiration as a function of hypodermic needle internal diameter in the in vivo human upper limb. *Anesth. Prog.* 49 (2): 49–51.

Tucker, G.T. and Mather, L.E. (1979). Clinical pharmacokinetics of local anesthetics. *Clin. Pharmacokinet.* 4 (4): 241–278.

Tzafalia, M. and Sixou, J.-L. (2011). Administration of anesthetics using metal syringes. An ex vivo study. *Anesth. Prog.* 58 (2): 61–65.

Van der Bijl, P. (1995). Injection needles for dental local anesthesia. *Compend. Contin. Educ Dent.* 16 (11): 1106–1115.

Van Wijk, A.J. and Hoogstraten, J. (2006). Reducing fear of pain associated with endodontic therapy. *Int. Endod. J.* 39 (5): 384–388.

Van Wijk, A.J. and Makkes, P.C. (2008). Highly anxious dental patients report more pain during dental injections. *Br. Dent. J.* 205 (3): 142–143.

Virts, B.E. (1999). Local anesthesia toxicity review. *Pediatr. Dent.* 21 (6): 375.

Visconti, R.P., Tortamano, I.P., and Buscariolo, I.P. (2016). Comparison of the anesthetic efficacy of mepivacaine and lidocaine in patients with irreversible pulpitis: a double-blind randomized clinical trial. *J. Endod.* 42 (9): 1314–1319.

Vreeland, D.L., Reader, A., Beck, M. et al. (1989). An evaluation of volumes and concentrations of lidocaine in human inferior alveolar nerve block. *J. Endod.* 15 (1): 6–12.

Wahl, M., Overton, D., Howell, J. et al. (2001). Pain on injection of prilocaine with epinephrine. A prospective double-blind study. *J. Am. Dent. Assoc.* 132 (10): 1396–1401.

Watson, J.E. and Colman, R.J. (1976). Interpretation of aspirating test in local anesthetic injections. *J. Oral Surg.* 34 (12): 1069–1074.

Wepman, B.J. (1978). Psychological components of pain perception. *Dent. Clin. N. Am.* 22 (1): 101–113.

Whitworth, J.M., Kanaa, M.D., Corbett, I.P., and Meechan, J.G. (2007). Influence of injection speed on the effectiveness of incisive/mental nerve block: a randomized, controlled, double-blind study in adult volunteers. *J. Endod.* 33 (10): 1149–1154.

Williams, M.J.R. and Simm, W. (1975). Practical aspiration for local anaesthesia. *Dent. Update* 2 (1): 23–27.

Wiswall, A.T., Bowles, W.R., Lunos, S. et al. (2014). Palatal anesthesia: comparison of four techniques for decreasing injection discomfort. *Northwest Dent.* 93 (4): 25–29.

Woolgrove, J. (1983). Pain perception and patient management. *Br. Dent. J.* 154 (8): 243–246.

Zelster, R., Cohen, C., and Casap, N. (2002). The implications of a broken needle in the pterygomandibular space: clinical guidelines for prevention and retrieval. *Pediatr. Dent.* 24 (2): 153–156.

# 14

# Maxillary Anesthesia I: Pulpal Anesthesia

## Introduction

This chapter on pulpal anesthetic methods for the upper arch (maxillary) teeth addresses the following procedures.

- Buccal infiltration anesthesia and the variation known as the modified cotton roll approach.
- Intra- and extraoral infraorbital nerve block as an approach to block the anterior superior alveolar nerve.
- Posterior superior alveolar nerve block (PSA) and the variation known as the modified Adatia technique.
- High tuberosity approach to block the maxillary nerve ($V_2$) through the mucobuccal fold.
- Transpalatal approach (also known as the greater palatine canal technique) to block the maxillary nerve ($V_2$).

The chapter also reviews certain aspects affecting the anesthesia of maxillary teeth to provide a fuller understanding of the anesthetics used.

## Maxilla

The thin layer of porous cortical bone in the maxilla is perforated by many small foramina through which the anesthetic solution can diffuse (DuBrul 1988). As the tooth apices are very close to the cortical surface (Table 2.7, Chapter 2), the technique of choice in most cases is buccal infiltration, in light of its efficacy, simplicity, and safety. Another advantage to the technique is that more than one tooth can be anesthetized with more infiltration.

## Maxillary Nerve ($V_2$)

The second division of the trigeminal (cranial nerve V), the maxillary nerve, distributes to three superior alveolar nerves (anterior, middle, and posterior) that innervate the dental pulp. In over 80% of individuals these branches intermingle in a superior dental plexus at the dental apices (Table 2.3, Chapter 2), although the middle superior alveolar nerve is missing in just under 50% (Table 2.2, Chapter 2). As those circumstances render independent block of each branch very difficult, the procedure actually used is buccal infiltration near the apex of the teeth, which affects all three.

### Buccal Anesthesia of the Upper Molars

Inserting the needle in the buccal cavity around the upper molars may involve three types of anesthetic techniques, depending on needle depth and angle (Figure 14.1): the deeper the penetration and the wider the angle, the greater the number of teeth affected, although the risk of causing hematomas by penetrating pterygoid plexus vessels is also greater.

- Buccal infiltration of the molars is the simplest and most effective technique for anesthetizing molar pulp. As the needle need not be inserted very deeply, the risk of hematoma is minimal.
- PSA (Posterior superior alveolar nerve block) or the tuberosity approach is a more complex technique because the needle is inserted higher and at a wider angle to skirt around the posterior wall of the maxilla (tuberosity) and reach the foramina through which the one to four branches forming this nerve trunk transmit. This technique anesthetizes molars as well as premolars, albeit less effectively. The likelihood of causing hematoma is logically greater with this method and part of its clinical efficacy is due to the buccal infiltrative effect, for the solution diffuses across the molars.
- The high tuberosity approach is designed to block the maxillary nerve ($V_2$) in the pterygopalatine fossa. This technique is even more difficult and arbitrary than the tuberosity approach due to the lack of osseous references to guide the needle during injection. The needle is

---

*Local Anesthesia in Dentistry: A Locoregional Approach*, First Edition. Jesús Calatayud and Mana Saraghi.
© 2024 John Wiley & Sons Ltd. Published 2024 by John Wiley & Sons Ltd.
Companion website: www.wiley.com/go/Calatayud/local

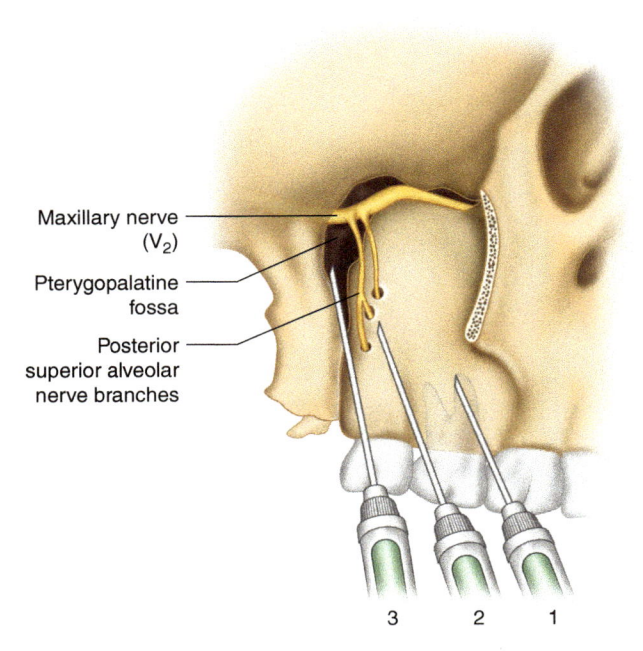

**Figure 14.1** Needle 1, short, buccal infiltrations (4% positive aspirations); needle 2, longer, posterior superior alveolar nerve branch blocks (5% positive aspirations); needle 3, longest, maxillary nerve ($V_2$) block in pterygopalatine fossa (13% positive aspirations).

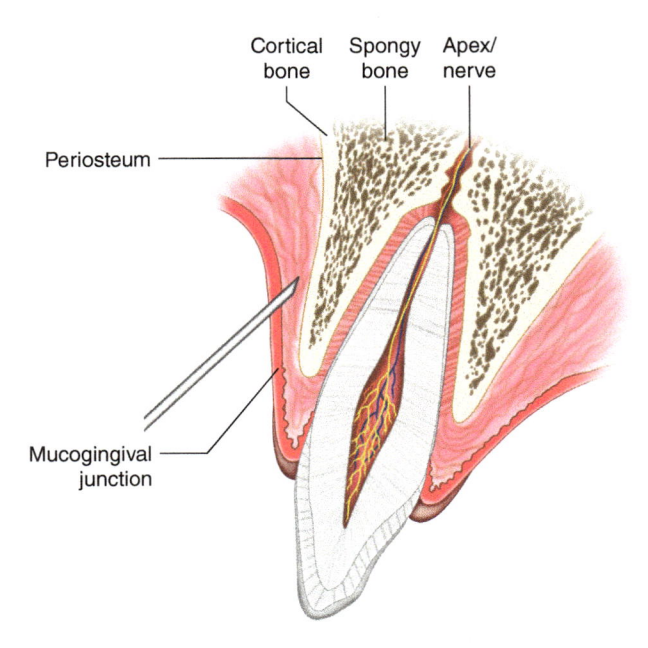

**Figure 14.2** Insertion of needle immediately below the mucogingival junction with the solution crossing the periosteum, cortical, and spongy bone to reach the nerve at the entrance to the dental apex.

inserted at a much greater height and wider angle to reach the pterygopalatine fossa, greatly raising the risk of hematoma and other adverse effects. This method anesthetizes molars, premolars, and the palate on the side injected.

## Buccal Infiltration

This technique has a number of synonyms: supraperiosteal buccal infiltration (all modern techniques are supraperiosteal), buccal infiltration, and anesthesia of the plexus.

*This is by far the technique most commonly used to anesthetize maxillary tooth pulp*, given its simplicity, efficacy, and safety. It consists essentially of administering the local anesthesia around the teeth to be treated, crossing the periosteum, the cortical bone, and the trabecular or spongy bone to reach the dental apex and anesthetize the pulp and adjacent tissues (Figure 14.2).

### Zones Anesthetized

- Tooth (pulp and periodontal ligament) injected, often extending to the adjacent mesial and distal teeth.
- Buccal cavity, including fibromucosa (alveolar mucosa, gingiva, and interdental papillae), bone, and periosteum.

### Technique

- Short (20–25 mm), 25G or 27G needle.
- Dentist's and patient's positions.
  - Dentist at 9:00 to 10:00 o'clock.
  - Patient in supine position with head slightly hyperextended to enable the dentist to administer the anesthesia to the anterior and posterior teeth on the right side and turn the patient's head as required if the anesthesia is to be administered to the posterior teeth on the left side.
- Bring the roof of the buccal cavity in the area to be anesthetized into view with the non-injection hand.
  - For anterior teeth (incisors and canines), pull the upper lip upward and ask the patient to open their mouth (Figure 14.3).
  - For posterior teeth (premolars and molars), pull the cheek and labial commissure outward and slightly upward to firmly stretch the jugal mucosa (Figure 14.4). Ask the patient to half-close their mouth to prevent the coronoid apophysis of the mandible from shifting forward (and getting in the way) as it does when the mouth is wide open (Figure 14.5).
- Needle insertion.
  - With the non-injection hand *stretch and tense* the (lax, mobile, dark) buccal alveolar mucosa and then insert the needle; a tense buccal cavity is readily visible, facilitating painless penetration. Insert the needle *as*

Buccal Infiltration | 243

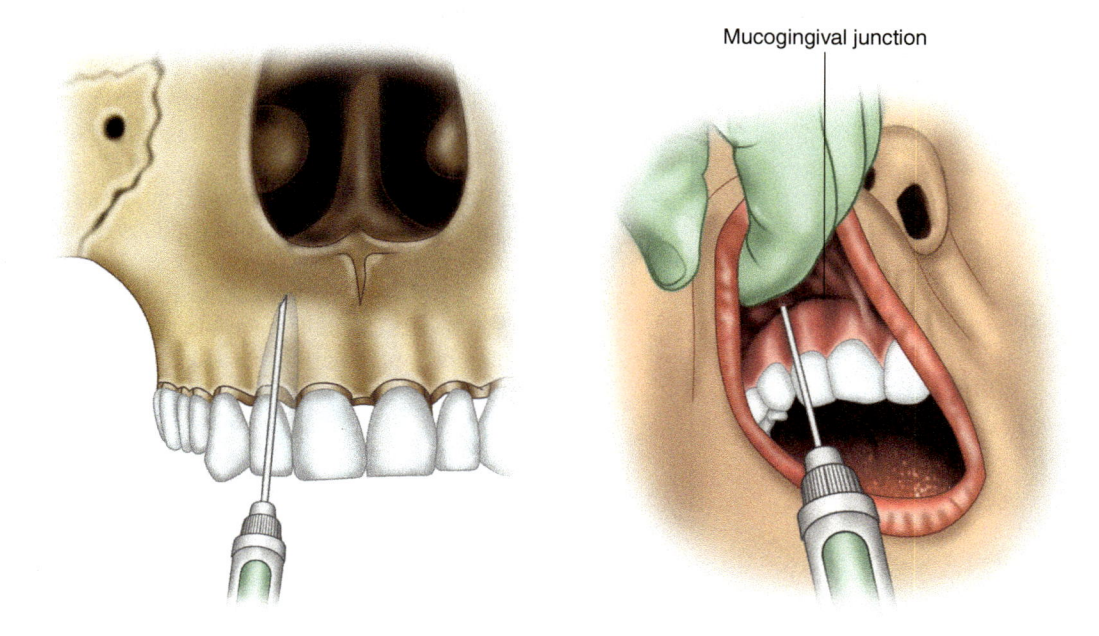

**Figure 14.3** Insertion of needle alongside the mucogingival junction in anterior teeth, with the patient's mouth wide open, pulling the upper lip upward.

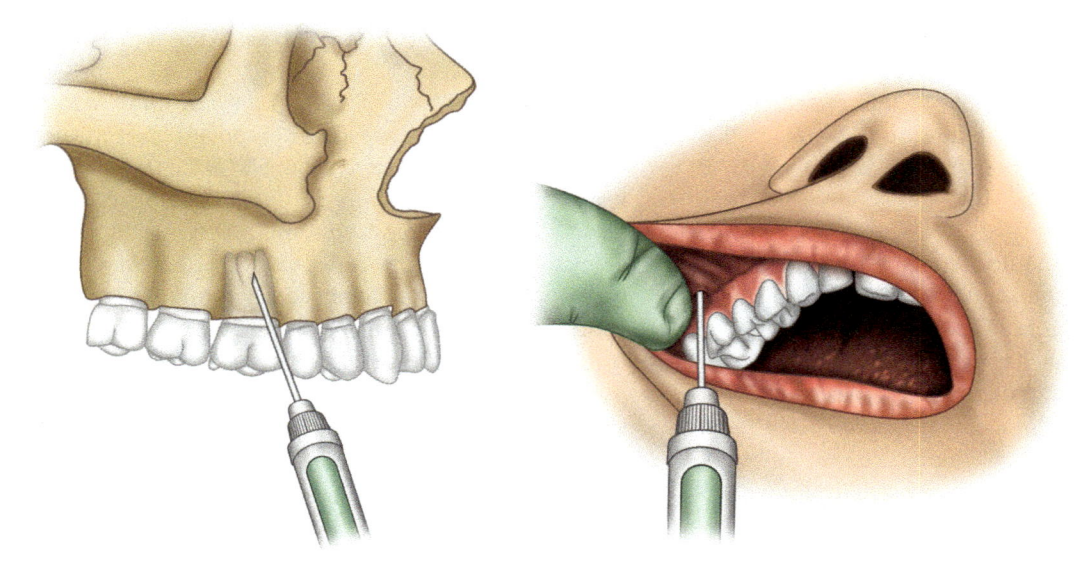

**Figure 14.4** Insertion of needle alongside the mucogingival junction in molars, pulling the labial commissure outward and upward, and asking the patient to partially close their mouth.

*close to the apex of the tooth to be treated as possible* (key to success), introducing the *tip of the needle only 2–3 mm underneath the mucosa.*

- The periosteum and bone are rarely touched with this technique but if that happens draw the needle back slightly to avoid impact.
- *Inject immediately above the mucogingival junction* (line between the attached gingiva and the alveolar mucosa) for the following reasons.

- As the surface of the maxilla is buccally concave, the surface of the bone is farther from the root in the apical direction, in the central incisors due to the position of the anterior nasal spine and in the molars to the position of the zygomatic apophysis of the malar bone.
- As the submucosa is less lax than the roof of the buccal cavity due to the proximity of the attached gingiva, when the needle is inserted immediately

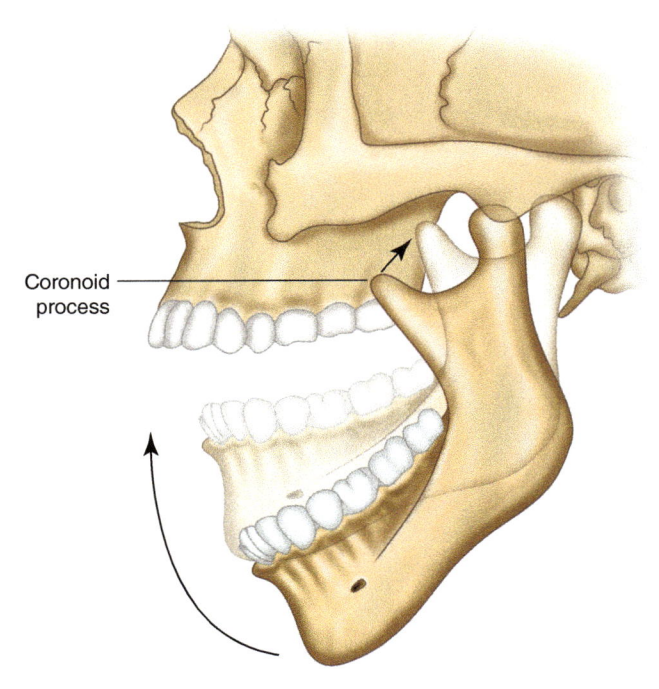

**Figure 14.5** Partially closed mouth in which the coronoid process rises, leaving room to reach the molars buccally.

above the mucogingival junction the anesthetic solution is kept in a smaller area in closer contact with the bone, tending to diffuse to the apex. If it were injected at the roof of the buccal cavity, it would tend to diffuse to softer tissues and away from the bone.

- Since the injected liquid is stored a little beyond the tip of the needle, *the insertion site should always be slightly mesial relative to the tooth.*
- Aspire before injecting. Aspiration is positive in 2% of anterior teeth and 4% of molars (Annex 22).
- *Injection proceeds to minimal intervention* (minimum volume/minimum injection time) criterion. Injection pain is greatly reduced with this four-step technique.
  1) First inject only one or two drops of anesthetic solution within 1–2 seconds and wait 60 seconds after withdrawing the needle to anesthetize the soft tissue around the injection zone.
  2) Inject another one or two drops at the same site (normally identifiable by tiny blood droplets caused by the first insertion) during 1–2 seconds and wait 30 seconds after withdrawing the needle.
  3) Inject a larger amount of anesthetic (about an eighth of a cartridge or 0.25 ml) slowly within 7–10 seconds and, after aspirating, wait 30 seconds after withdrawing the needle. Note that just a small amount is injected to reinforce the preceding injections and begin pulpal anesthesia.
  4) After aspirating, slowly inject the full amount of anesthesia envisaged at the same site, after aspiration. *Note*: Clinical studies have shown that anterior maxillary (incisor) infiltrations are painful, only slightly less than palatal infiltrations (hence heeding the importance of minimal intervention criterion), whereas infiltration in the maxillary molars is one of the least painful techniques (Annex 23; Bataineh and Al-Sabri 2017). Another advantage is that anesthetizing the soft tissues (happily) fails to confirm patients' expectation of a more painful second than first injection (Martin et al. 1994; Meechan and Day 2002; Paschos et al. 2006; Badcock et al. 2007; Kuscu et al. 2014).
- Amount of anesthetic to be used. Clinical studies today recommend slightly larger amounts than classical texts to ensure good pulpal anesthesia (Mikesell et al. 1987; Premdas and Pitt Ford 1995; Brunetto et al. 2008; Guglielmo et al. 2011; Sreekumar and Bhargava 2011).
  o In anterior teeth: a little less than a full 1.8-ml cartridge, 1.5 ml, for instance.
  o In posterior teeth: a full cartridge or slightly more, 1.8–2.5 ml.
  *Note*: In children under 6–8 years, the dose should be halved.
- *The submucosa lump or blister forming must not be touched* to enable the anesthetic to spread across the periosteum, cortical, and spongy bone to reach the apex and from there the nerve fibers in the teeth (Figure 14.2). Massaging the blister forces the anesthetic to spread along the pathway of least resistance, the lax soft tissues, carrying it away from the injection site and lowering the concentration at the target zone and hence the capacity to diffuse toward the dental apex.
- Subjective symptoms of anesthesia. Soft tissue anesthesia, defined by patients as dullness, numbing, tingling, itching, pins and needles feeling, or fattening in the lip (Table 13.1, Chapter 13) varies depending on the injection site.
  o In anterior teeth. Soft tissue anesthesia begins in the upper lip, labial commissure, and even the *ala nasi* within 2 minutes.
  o In posterior teeth. As labial anesthesia is scant, especially where molars are concerned, a waiting period of at least 5 minutes must be allowed. Alternatively, some clinicians insert a probe in the mucosa to determine soft tissue anesthesia.
- Time needed for pulpal anesthesia. In 70% of individuals anesthesia is effective in less than 2 minutes (Annex 21), although *the recommended waiting period is 5 minutes from the time of injection*. Where the minimal intervention criterion is followed, a minute or more may be necessary.

- Soft tissue anesthesia usually lasts 3–4 hours (200 minutes) (Annex 21), a fact which the patient should be notified of after treatment.

### Efficacy of this Technique

Clinical studies have proven the efficacy of this technique to be high (Table 14.1), with success rates of 95% in posterior and 98% in anterior teeth in adults with a powerful solution such as 4% articaine, 1:100 000 epinephrine (10 μg/ml) (A-100), and around 87% and 95% of a standard lidocaine solution (L-100). Palatal reinforcement with a small amount of anesthetic solution (±0.25–0.3 ml) raises pulpal anesthetic efficacy and duration, particularly in posterior teeth with palatal roots (Aggarwal et al. 2011; Guglielmo et al. 2011; Ulusoy and Alacam 2014).

### Complications Specific to this Technique

The most common of the very few complications associated are listed below.

1) Appearance of small, asymptomatic intraoral hematomas in the submucosa that disappear spontaneously in a few days and that are attributable to repeated needle insertion in the same site as recommended for minimal intervention.
2) Injection site inflammation in 2% of cases (Moore et al. 2006), which also subsides spontaneously in a few days.
3) Failure to anesthetize the pulp is uncommon with this technique, as noted. In some individuals failure in the central incisors may be due to thickening of the anterior nasal spine and in molars to thickening of the zygomatic arch of the malar bone.

### Factors That Lead to Success

1) The tooth. Poorer results are obtained with molars than with anterior teeth (Cowan 1964; Certosimo and Archer 1996) for two reasons: (i) cortical thickening at the zygomatic crest and (ii) separation of the palatal roots.
2) The anesthetic solution. While 2% lidocaine, 1:100 000 epinephrine (L-100) delivers good results, success rates are higher with powerful solutions such as 4% articaine, 1:100 000 epinephrine (A-100) or 2% lidocaine, 1:50 000 epinephrine (L-50) (Annex 21). The use of powerful solutions such as A-100 is therefore preferred in adults, given that in such cases *the potency of the solution enhances penetration* and the capacity to cross the periosteum, cortical, and spongy or trabecular bone to reach the dental apex and bathe the nerve fibers, intensifying the effect and lengthening the duration of pulpal anesthesia (Annex 21).
3) The volume of solution injected. As clinical tests have shown that overly small volumes lead to a higher number of failures (Mikesell et al. 1987; Premdas and Pitt Ford 1995; Brunetto et al. 2008), the volumes specified above are preferred.
4) The waiting time. The recommended waiting time is 5 minutes after completing injection (Mikesell et al. 1987; Certosimo and Archer 1996) (Annex 21).

### Modified Cotton Roll Approach

Jorgensen and Hayden recommended using a cotton roll to raise the success rate (Jorgensen and Hayden 1970).

The technique is the same as specified above except that a small cotton roll is placed at the roof of the buccal cavity before injecting the solution and held firmly against the mucosa with the non-injection index finger or thumb. The needle is inserted between the roll and the mucogingival junction, maintaining the pressure on the roll during and for a few minutes after injection (Figure 14.6).

The aim is to create a nearly closed deposition area in the lax alveolar soft tissue to hinder diffusion along that initially easier route (carrying it away from the injection site) and force the solution to diffuse across the cortical layer of the bone to the apices.

## Infraorbital Nerve Block

*Infraorbital nerve block is not recommended for routine dental treatment* (Kleier et al. 1983; Roberts and Sowray 1987; Jastak et al. 1995) and is consequently seldom used because (i) the buccal infiltration alternative is simpler, safer, and more effective and (ii) many patients reject the approach psychologically for fear of injury to the eye (Jastak et al. 1995; Malamed 2004).

Table 14.1 Successful (%) pulpal anesthesia in anterior and posterior teeth with buccal infiltration (electrical pulp tester assessment).

| Anesthetic solution | Successful pulpal anesthesia (%) | |
| --- | --- | --- |
| | Anterior teeth 1 ml | First molar 1.8 ml |
| 2% lidocaine + 1:100 000 epinephrine (L-100) | 95 | 87 |
| 4% articaine + 1:100 000 epinephrine (A-100) | 98 | 95 |

*Source:* Data from Annex 21.

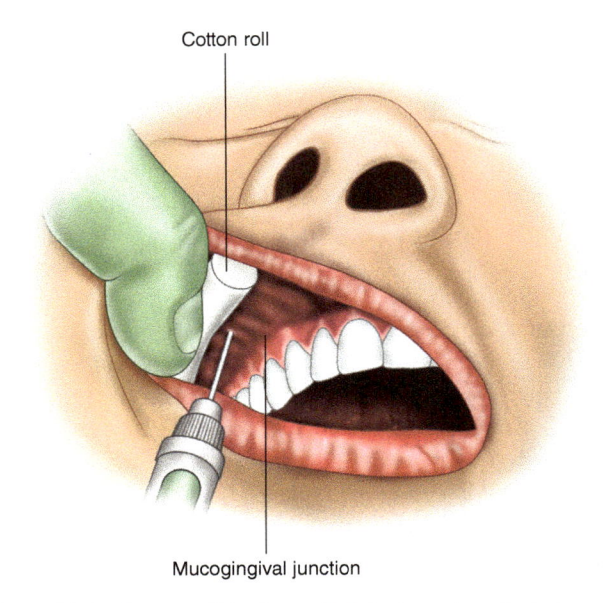

**Figure 14.6** Cotton roll in the roof of the buccal cavity to trap the anesthetic solution between it and the mucogingival junction, forcing diffusion toward the periosteum, cortical, and spongy bone.

The technique theoretically aims to fully block the anterior and partially anesthetize the middle alveolar nerve by diffusing the anesthetic solution across the infraorbital foramen to anesthetize the incisors, canines, and premolars on the side injected.

The technique has two variations, intraoral (the most common) and extraoral or transcutaneous, normally used by oral and maxillofacial surgeons. The drawback to the extraoral approach is that it is more painful (Karkut et al. 2010) and poses more local complications (Kleier et al. 1983; Karkut et al. 2010), although as it does not involve the canine fossa, it is useful in infectious or inflammatory processes affecting the roof of the buccal cavity in the zone (Jastak et al. 1995; Malamed 2004).

## Uses

- Circumstances for using either the intraoral or the extraoral approach.
  1) Surgical operations on the anterior aspect of the maxilla on the side injected, such as surgical extraction of impacted canines, apicoectomies, epulis extractions, and maxillary sinus surgery (Kleier et al. 1983; Roberts and Sowray 1987).
  2) Multiple tooth treatments, for theoretically it calls for a smaller volume of anesthesia, avoiding the need for multiple injections in restorations and extractions (Kleier et al. 1983; Jastak et al. 1995; Malamed 2004).
  3) After buccal infiltration failure in anterior teeth (Kleier et al. 1983; Roberts and Sowray 1987; Jastak et al. 1995; Malamed 2004).
- Additional circumstances for use of the extraoral approach only.
  1) *Inflammation and infection of the canine fossa* and surroundings in which buccal infiltration is not appropriate (Jastak et al. 1995; Malamed 2004).
  2) *Trauma to anterior teeth* where the alveolar bone must be repositioned and the soft tissue sutured (Kleier et al. 1983).

## Zones Anesthetized

- Anesthesia of the anterior and middle superior alveolar nerves.
  - Teeth, including pulp and periodontium of the canine, first premolar and second premolar on the side injected. The central and lateral incisors and the first molar on the side injected are likewise anesthetized, albeit only partially.
  - Buccal cavity, including fibromucosa (alveolar mucosa, gingiva, and interdental papillae), bone and periosteum around incisors, canines and premolars on the side injected.
  - Maxillary sinus, anterior and lateral walls and floor.
- Anesthesia of the peripheral branches of the infraorbital nerve affects the skin on the upper lip, *ala nasi*, and lower eyelid on the side injected.

## Intraoral Technique

- Long (35–38 mm), 27G or 25G needle.
- Dentist's and patient's positions:
  - Dentist at 8:00–10:00 o'clock.
  - Patient in supine position with their neck slightly extended. Mouth moderately open. If the neck is bent rather than extended, the patient's chest interferes with the syringe.
- Location of the infraorbital foramen.
  - Ask the patient to look straight ahead. In 85% of individuals, the foramen lies on the imaginary line joining the pupil and the longitudinal axis of the second premolar (Annex 2). The line also runs very close to the labial commissure on the side injected (Figure 14.7).
  - With the non-injection index finger, feel the slight depression on the rim of the orbit at the point crossed by the imaginary line running from the pupil. That is the zygomaticomaxillary suture, normally found at a point two-fifths inward on the lower orbital rim (Figure 14.8).

○ Run the finger downward from there along the lower infraorbital rim for 5–10 mm until it reaches the infraorbital depression (infraorbital nocht, which is where the infraorbital foramen lies) (Annex 2). Hold the finger in that position, pressing gently (Kleier et al. 1983; Karkut et al. 2010).

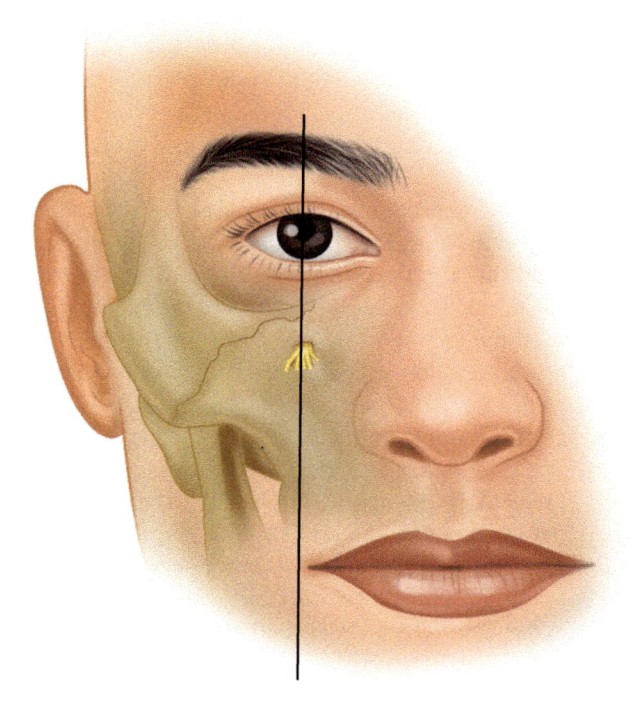

- Retract the upper lip with the non-injection thumb to view the anterior maxillary teeth and the plexus on the buccal aspect of incisors, canines, and premolars, while tensing the roof of the buccal cavity (Figure 14.9).
- There are two possible approaches to the infraorbital foramen.
  1) The vertical or direct or second premolar approach, deemed here to be the better of the two, for in 85% of individuals the infraorbital foramen lies on or near the extended second maxillary premolar axis (Annex 2) (Figure 14.8).
     ○ Insert the needle at the roof of the buccal cavity over the second premolar with the bevel facing the bone (so that when the anesthetic solution is injected it diffuses toward the infraorbital foramen) and *separated from the alveolar bone by around 5 mm* to prevent premature contact with the roof of the canine fossa as the needle travels toward the infraorbital foramen (Bennett 1984; Jastak et al. 1995) (Figure 14.9).
     ○ Place the needle parallel to the longitudinal axis of the second premolar and guide it gently toward the infraorbital foramen underneath the tip of the non-injection index finger. The needle courses along the second premolar cementoenamel junction (CEJ) to the infraorbital foramen for about 30–35 mm (Annex 2) or, if measured from the roof of the buccal cavity, for around 15 mm (Jastak et al. 1995; Malamed 2004).

     *Note*: Remember that injection around premolars and molars is much less painful than around anterior maxillary teeth (Annex 23).

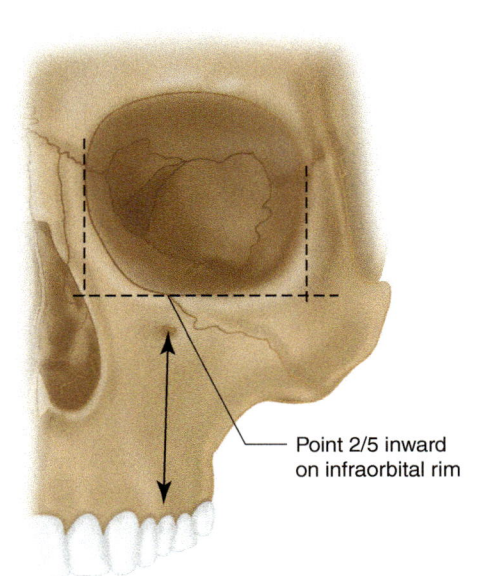

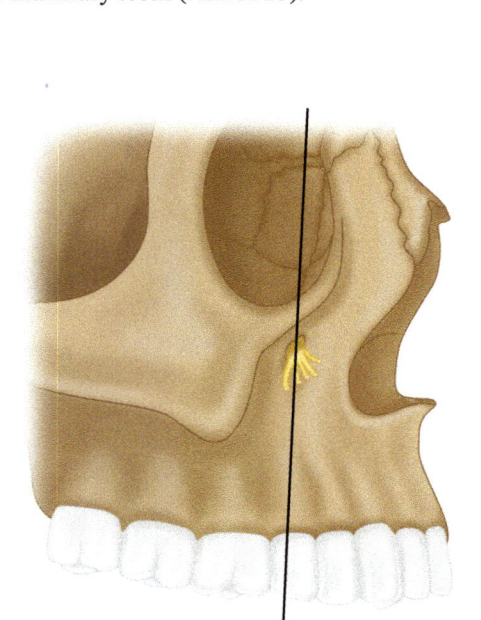

**Figure 14.7** Infraorbital foramen on the imaginary line joining the pupil (looking straight ahead) and the labial commissure.

**Figure 14.8** Infraorbital foramen on the axis extending upward from the second maxillary premolar at a point two-fifths inward on the lower orbital rim.

Point 2/5 inward on infraorbital rim

**Figure 14.9** Non-injection index finger over the skin on the infraorbital foramen as the thumb lifts the upper lip, keeping the needle a few millimeters away from the alveolar process and running it parallel to the axis of the second premolar (direct or vertical approach).

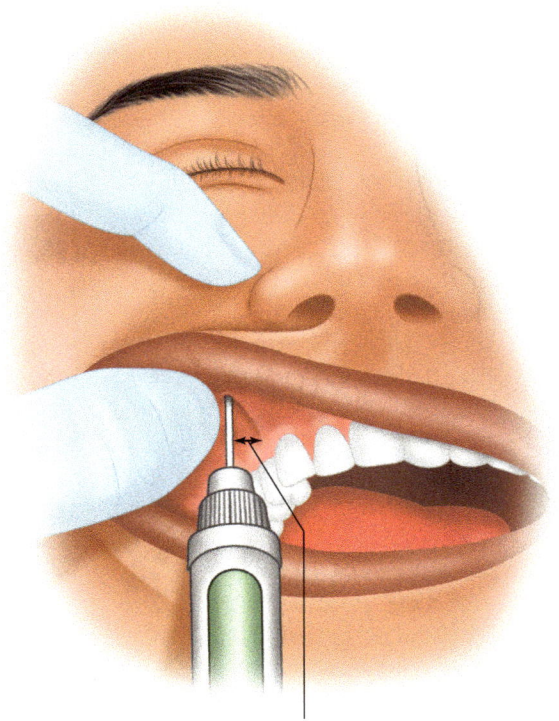

Separation from alveolar process

In a variation on this approach, which is nearly direct, the reference is the first rather than the second premolar (Malamed 2004).
2) Oblique or from the midline or from the lateral incisor.
   ○ Insert the needle at the roof of the buccal surface in alongside the lateral incisor, obliquely, i.e. on the imaginary line running from the mesial incisal angle to the gingival distal angle, with the bevel facing the bone (so that when the anesthetic solution is injected it diffuses toward the infraorbital foramen) and *separated from the alveolar bone by around 5 mm* to prevent premature contact with the roof of the canine fossa as the needle travels toward the infraorbital foramen.
   ○ Advance the needle obliquely and gently toward the infraorbital foramen underneath the tip of the index finger. This route is less direct and somewhat longer, with the needle running along 20 mm of soft tissue (Bennett 1984; Roberts and Sowray 1987).

*Note*: Remember that injections around the anterior maxillary teeth are among the most painful, nearly as painful as palatal injections (Annex 23).

Another variation is from the canine, a less oblique and slightly shorter approach.
- The tip of the needle reaches the infraorbital foramen underneath the tip of the non-injection index finger. It impacts the roof of the infraorbital foramen (lower rim of the orbit), preventing penetration in the orbit. The infraorbital foramen runs downward and medially (toward the nose) in nearly 60% of individuals and downward only in 20% (Annex 2).
- Aspire before injecting: 1% of cases are positive (Karkut et al. 2010).
- Inject a 1.8-ml cartridge over the course of 40–60 seconds (Berberich et al. 2009; Karkut et al. 2010). The index finger should feel the deposition. As the bevel faces the bone, the anesthesia is distributed toward the entrance to the infraorbital foramen.
- Massage the area after injection, pressing gently with the index finger for a few seconds (Karkut et al. 2010) to enhance diffusion of the solution inside the foramen.
- Subjective symptoms of anesthesia (numbness, tingling, etc.) (Table 13.1, Chapter 13) appear in 1–3 minutes in the upper lip, *nasi ala*, and lower eyelid. Pulpal anesthesia is reached in 5–10 minutes (Berberich et al. 2009; Karkut et al. 2010) and the soft tissue remains anesthetized for 3–4 hours (Feige 1978; Corbett et al. 2010).

### Extraoral Technique

- Needle. Either (i) short (20–25 mm) double-tip, cartridge-like, caliber 27G or 25G, or (ii) short, strong insulin syringe. Remember that the route is shorter and the needle has to penetrate the skin and firm subcutaneous tissue.
- Dentist's and patient's positions as in the intraoral approach.
- Location of the infraorbital foramen. As in the intraoral approach.
- Ask the patient to close their eyes for protection while disinfecting the skin in the suborbital area and for psychological reasons because extraoral injection of the infraorbital foramen is not a pleasant sight.
- Insert the needle in the skin below the non-injection index finger rests, marking the location of the infraorbital foramen.
  ○ Hold the needle with the bevel toward the skin so that when injected the anesthetic solution diffuses toward the infraorbital foramen (Kleier et al. 1983).
  ○ As the foramen follows a downward and inward course (Annex 2), place the needle at a site slightly inward of

and lower than the mark on the skin at an angle of around 45° and tilted slightly outward.
- Insert the needle in the skin and continue until touching bone. Inject around 0.2 ml to anesthetize the soft tissues and wait 30 seconds before removing the needle (Kleier et al. 1983; Roberts and Sowray 1987).
- When re-inserting, use the needle as a probe to locate the entrance to the infraorbital foramen or a site near it (Karkut et al. 2010). Push the needle in no more than 10 mm (Kleier et al. 1983; Karkut et al. 2010). Remember that the soft tissue over the foramen is around 7 mm thick and the needle must not penetrate into the foramen more than 1–3 mm (Kleier et al. 1983; Karkut et al. 2010). Do not try to penetrate the foramen, but merely to reach a nearby site to prevent the risk of penetrating the orbit and affecting the eye (Saeedi et al. 2011).
- Aspire before injecting. Aspiration is positive in 1% of cases (Karkut et al. 2010).
- Inject the rest of the cartridge (1.6–1.7 ml) over the course of 40–60 seconds. During this operation, the non-injection index finger should feel the deposition of the solution underneath the skin. As the bevel faces the bone the anesthesia is distributed toward the infraorbital foramen.
- After injection massage and gently press the area with the index finger for a few seconds (Karkut et al. 2010) to enhance diffusion of the solution toward the inside the foramen.
- The subjective symptoms of anesthesia are as described for the intraoral approach.

### Efficacy of this Technique

As Table 14.2 shows, according to clinical trials pulpal anesthesia is successful, on the side injected, in 25% of maxillary incisors, in around 90% in canine and premolars, and 60% in the first maxillary molar (Figure 14.10) after injecting 1.8 ml of standard lidocaine solution (L-100). The pulp is anesthetized in around 3 minutes on average (Corbett et al. 2010). The effect is most intense after 5–10 minutes.

Table 14.2 also shows that the results with the intra- and extraoral approaches are very similar, although poorer tooth-by-tooth than obtained with buccal infiltration anesthesia.

### Complications Specific to this Technique

1) A facial hematoma may appear under the lower eyelid in 2% of cases due to injury to the inferior facial vein or some vascular nervous package in the infraorbital foramen (Phillips 1943; Berberich et al. 2009; Karkut et al. 2010). It disappears spontaneously in 10–14 days (Berberich et al. 2009; Karkut et al. 2010).
2) Moderate to severe postoperative pain in the area in 1% of cases, lasting normally 1–3 days (Berberich et al. 2009).
3) Temporary double vision (diplopia) in nearly 3% of patients with the extraoral technique (Kleier et al. 1983; Karkut et al. 2010), even one case with intraoral technique (Ceylan et al. 2010), disappearing with the effect of the anesthesia.

Table 14.2 Successful (%) pulpal anesthesia with the infraorbital nerve technique (electrical pulp tester assessment and standard anesthetic solutions L-80 or L-100).

| Tooth | Intraoral | | | | Extraoral |
|---|---|---|---|---|---|
| | Feige (1978) $n = 62$ | Berberich et al. (2009) $n = 40$ | Karkut et al. (2010) $n = 40$ | Corbett et al. (2010)[a] $n = 28$ | Karkut et al. (2010) $n = 40$ |
| Central incisor (%) | 40 | 15 | 15 | 11 | 15 |
| Lateral incisor (%) | 50 | 28 | 22 | 18 | 22 |
| Canine (%) | 100 | 85 | 92 | 93 | 92 |
| First premolar (%) | 100 | 82 | 90 | 89 | 87 |
| Second premolar (%) | 100 | 75 | 80 | 96 | 82 |
| First molar (%) | — | 52 | 70 | — | 65 |
| Amount injected (ml) | 0.5 | 1.8 | 1.8 | 1.0 | 1.8 |
| Solution injected | L-80 | L-100 | L-100 | L-80 | L-100 |

L-80 → 2% lidocaine + 1:80 000 (12.5 µg/ml) epinephrine.
L-100 → 2% lidocaine + 1:100 000 (10 µg/ml) epinephrine.
[a] Using "the wand" (computer-controlled local anesthetic).

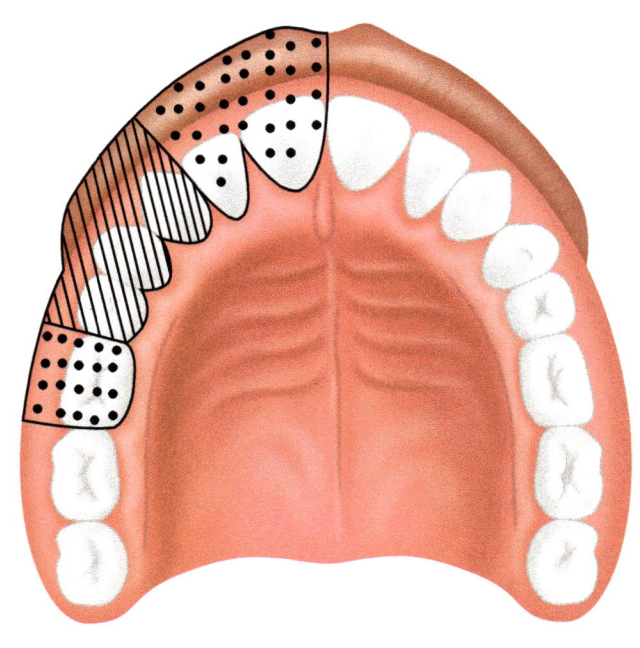

**Figure 14.10** Efficacy of anesthesia: greatest in ruled area and only partial in dotted area.

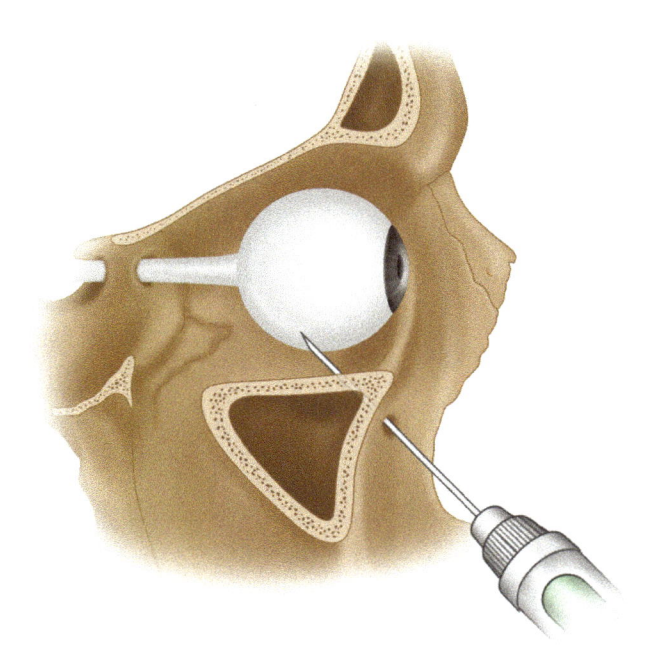

**Figure 14.11** Needle penetration through the infraorbital foramen at the posterior part of the eyeball. *Source:* Redrawn from Saeedi (2011).

4) Needle penetration in the eyeball (Weinand et al. 1997; Chan et al. 2011; Saeedi et al. 2011) (Figure 14.11). This is very unusual because the needle normally impacts the roof of the infraorbital foramen. Nonetheless, if the needle crosses the roof of the foramen or if the roof is missing, it may impact the posterior side of the globe and injure the retina, causing the following harm.

- *Acute and immediate ocular pain* (Weinand et al. 1997; Chan et al. 2011). In some cases pain is absent but other symptoms appear several minutes later (Saeedi et al. 2011).
- *Dilated (mydriasis)* or immobile pupil or failure to react to light (Chan et al. 2011; Saeedi et al. 2011).
- Loss of visual acuity and vision impaired by floating spots (Chan et al. 2011).
- Blood extravasation to the conjunctiva (ecchymosis) (Saeedi et al. 2011) or avulsed or extruded orbit (exophthalmos) (Chan et al. 2011).
- Ocular infection (endophthalmitis) (Weinand et al. 1997).

All such cases require the intervention of an ophthalmologist. This rare complication may be more frequent in the extraoral approach because the needle may be inserted too horizontally, thereby entering the infraorbital canal more deeply (Saeedi et al. 2011).

### Remarks

Infraorbital nerve block aims to anesthetize the one to four branches of the anterior superior alveolar nerve that innervate incisors, canines, and occasionally the first premolar (Chapter 2). It is scantly effective for a number of reasons.

1) In the infraorbital foramen, the anterior superior alveolar nerve branches lie at a distance of around 10–15 mm from the infraorbital foramen (Table 2.3, Chapter 2) and in some series 20% of individuals at over 20 mm (FitzGerald and Scott 1958; Heasman et al. 1984). They are therefore normally at a considerable depth and difficult to reach.

2) If the needle penetrates the infraorbital canal the risks include (i) damaging the neurovascular bundle, sufficient reason to avoid this maneuver and confide in diffusion of the solution in the area around the infraorbital foramen (Haglund and Evers 1985; Evers and Haegerstam 1981) and (ii) penetrating the orbit and affecting the eye (Weinand et al. 1997; Saeedi et al. 2011).

3) Accessory foramina appear in 15% of individuals, and in 15% of those they may be multiple (Annex 2). These accessory foramina may be located at a considerable distance from the main infraorbital foramen (Kadanoff et al. 1970; Leo et al. 1995) in up to 40% of individuals in some series (Kadanoff et al. 1970). These are important findings because they explain why anesthetic block may not be successful in the infraorbital foramen (Leo et al. 1995; Canan et al. 1999).

4) Anterior superior alveolar nerve block via the infraorbital foramen is insufficient to anesthetize incisor and canine pulp because these teeth may be cross-innervated contralaterally or even by the nasopalatine nerve (Hoffer 1922a; Phillips 1943; Phillips and Maxmen 1941; Cook 1949; Roda and Blanton 1994). Supplementary buccal infiltration is therefore required.

In practice much of the efficacy of this technique depends on the buccal diffusion of the anesthetic solution, since the anterior wall of the maxilla (along which the anterior superior alveolar nerve branches course) is very thin (Cook 1950a). For that reason the teeth actually anesthetized are the canine and premolars and surrounding tissue (Figure 14.10). Generally speaking, then, the advantages of this technique over simple buccal infiltration are nearly negligible.

## Posterior Superior Alveolar Nerve Block

Posterior superior alveolar nerve block (PSA) is also known as zygomatic or tuberosity anesthesia because the idea is to carry the anesthetic solution to the maxillary tuberosity.

This method is somewhat more complex than buccal infiltration in molars because the needle must be inserted a little higher and at an angle to skirt over the buccinator muscle insertion, avoid the posterior wall of the maxilla (tuberosity), and reach the foramina through which the one to four branches of this nerve trunk transmit (Figure 14.12). The risk of hematomas due to injury to the vessels in the zone is also higher. Recent clinical tests have questioned its efficacy and utility, as the success rate for anesthetizing maxillary molars is no higher than in simple buccal infiltration (Padhye et al. 2011; Al-Delayme 2014).

### Zones Anesthetized

- Teeth, including pulp and periodontium of the molars and less frequently the premolars on the side injected.
- Buccal cavity, including fibromucosa (alveolar mucosa, gingiva, and interdental papillae), bone and periosteum in the buccal area around the molars as well as the premolars, although less effectively.

### Technique

- Short (25 mm), 27G needle.
- Dentist's and patient's positions.
   - Dentist at 9:00–10:00 o'clock.
   - Patient in supine position with head slightly hyperextended to enable the dentist to turn it slightly to the left to anesthetize the right side or to the right to anesthetize the left side.
- *Examine the entire roof of the upper molar buccal cavity with the non-injection index finger* to locate the osseous bridge that protrudes from the zygomatic crest on the malar bone (normally alongside the first maxillary molar).
- *Retract the labial commissure outward and upward* with the non-injection hand to firmly stretch the jugal mucosa (Figure 4.12).
   - Stretch the tissue intraorally with the index finger on the right side and the thumb on the left.
   - The aim is to (i) bring the concavity of the buccal cavity around the molars into view and (i) reduce any injection-induced pain by inserting the needle in a tense mucosa.
- Increase the space for maneuvering by asking the patient to partially close their mouth (Figure 14.5). The result is (i) greater labial commissure width and (ii) rearward shift of the coronoid process of the mandible to keep it from obstructing the operation.
- Insert the needle in the roof of the buccal cavity.
   - *Behind the zygomatic crest of the malar bone*, which is usually the same as saying behind the second molar (Figure 14.1).
   - *Orient the needle upward* and as perpendicularly as possible to the occlusal plane of the maxillary molars. As a full 90° angle is not possible due to the presence of the jugal mucosa, the needle should be posteriorly oblique, which is also desirable.
   - *Avoid the osseous wall* to prevent the needle from impacting or catching in the surface of the maxillary tuberosity (outer and posterior wall of the maxilla).
   - Push the needle a few millimeters into the buccal cavity.

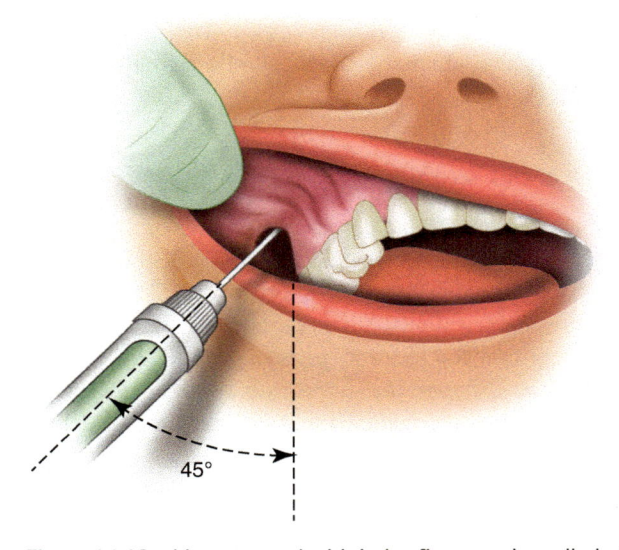

**Figure 14.12** Lip separated with index finger and needle held at 45° relative to the sagittal plane.

- Needle orientation and course.
  - *Tilt the tip of the needle inward* (the syringe tilts outward), theoretically forming an angle of around 30–45° relative to the sagittal or medial plane to keep it flush against the posterior wall of the maxilla (Figure 14.12). The tilt angle must be wider, up to 70°, in children (Hayden 1965).
  - *Advance the needle upward, inward, and slightly rearward*, trying to keep as close as possible to the bone without tearing the periosteum. That precaution normally (but not always) protects the pterygoid plexus vessels and the posterior superior alveolar artery from puncture (DuBrul 1988).
  - If resistance is encountered (because the needle hits bone), draw the needle back slightly, narrow the angle of the inward tilt, and continue.
- Insertion length (Figure 14.13).
  - *Insert the needle 15–20 mm on average* (Loetscher et al. 1988; Pfeil et al. 2010). Remember that the deeper the needle, the greater the risk of injuring a vessel and causing hematomas. In children with mixed dentition, insert the needle 10–15 mm (Maljaei et al. 2017).
  - Remember as well that the posterior superior alveolar nerve has one to four branches (Jones 1939; McDaniel 1956; Heasman 1984) that in most individuals lie less than 30 mm from the lower part of the maxillary tuberosity and only rarely higher (maximum 40 mm) (Heasman 1984). Subtracting from that distance the 3–12 mm between the roof of the buccal cavity and the gingival margin in molars (Jorgensen 1948) and given that the anesthetic diffuses there, an insertion 15–20 mm (15–20 mm plus the 3–12 mm for the roof, total 18–32 mm) deep should ensure an effective block.
- Aspire before injecting. Aspiration is positive in 5% of cases (Annex 22).
- Inject 1.8 ml (one full cartridge) slowly, over the course of 40–60 seconds. Injecting two cartridges (3.6 ml) yields better results and increases the duration of pulpal anesthesia (Pfeil et al. 2010). Inject 1 ml in children with mixed dentition (Hayden 1965: Maljaei et al. 2017).
- Subjective symptoms of anesthesia. Soft tissue anesthesia, defined by patients as dullness, numbing, tingling, tickling or "fattening" sensation in the lip (Table 13.1, Chapter 13), appears after 2–3 minutes.
  - Tests with a 15–20-minute wait (Loetscher et al. 1988; Pfeil et al. 2010) report better results than those with a 5-minute wait (Padhye et al. 2011). A compromise might be *a waiting period of 5–10 minutes after injection* to enable the anesthetic solution to take full effect.
  - Optionally some clinicians insert a probe in the buccal mucosa around the molars to determine soft tissue anesthesia.
  - The definitive sign of efficacy is obtained by working on the molars (i.e. prepping into dentin), initially cautiously and then proceeding normally if the patient expresses no discomfort.
- Soft tissue anesthesia usually lasts 3–4 hours (200 minutes), a fact of which the patient should be notified after treatment.

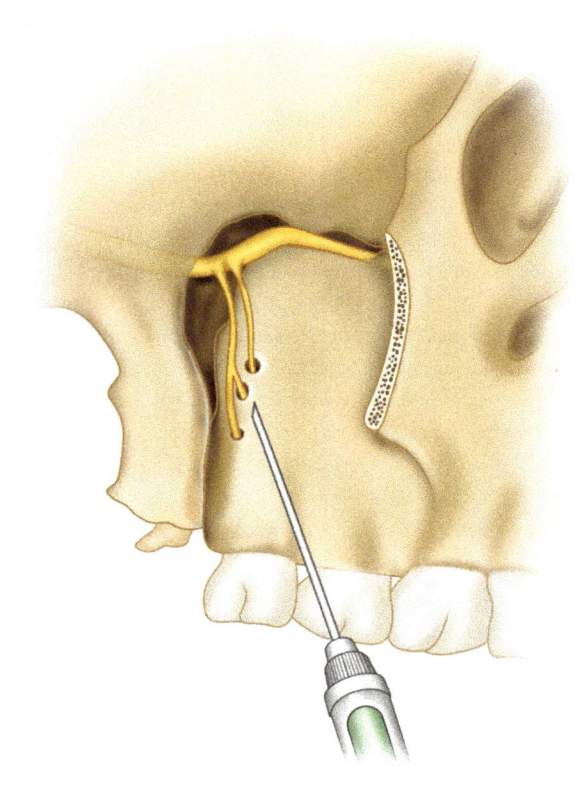

**Figure 14.13** Needle height necessary to block the posterior superior alveolar nerve.

### Efficacy of this Technique

When assessed with an electrical pulp tester or dry ice (at −78 °C), pulpal anesthesia is successful in 90% of maxillary molars, but in only 25–50% of premolars (Table 14.3). Similar results (around 90%) are reported for children with mixed dentition for the first permanent and second primary molars, although the success rate drops to 65% in the first primary molar (Hayden 1965) (assessed with the less rigorous extraction method). As the preceding values are referred to the standard local anesthetic, 2% lidocaine, 1:100 000 (10 μg/ml) epinephrine (L-100), use of a more powerful solution such as articaine (A-100) would be expected to improve the results.

Table 14.3 Successful (%) pulpal anesthesia with posterior superior alveolar nerve block (−78 °C dry ice or electrical pulp tester assessment and standard solution L-100)

| Variable | | Loetscher et al. (1988) n = 45–56 | Pfeil (2010) n = 31 | Pfeil (2010) n = 31 |
|---|---|---|---|---|
| Tooth | Second molar (%) | 96 | 97 | 100 |
| | First molar (%) | 88 | 77 | 84 |
| | Second premolar (%) | 31 | 45 | 68 |
| | First premolar (%) | 10 | 10 | 32 |
| Amount injected (ml) | | 1.2 | 1.8 | 3.6 |
| Stimulus | | Cold (−78 °C) | Electrical | Electrical |

L-100 → 2% lidocaine + 1:100 000 (10 μg/ml) epinephrine.

### Complications Specific to this Technique

1) Extraoral hematomas may appear on the face in less than 0.5% of cases (further to the Kuster and Udin 1984; Loetscher et al. 1988; Pfeil et al. 2010; Padhye et al. 2011 series). They occur when the needle pierces a vein in the pterygoid plexus or the buccogingival branches of the posterior superior alveolar artery that course somewhat erratically near the maxillary tuberosity (Harn et al. 2002; Padhye et al. 2011). They may present with *swelling in the malar or superior masseteric region.* Swelling appears earlier if an artery rather than a venous plexus vein is injured. In both cases the symptom is a dark brown spot on the skin due to blood extravasation (ecchymosis) that in the next few days spreads forward and downward along the muscular planes of the cheek, while changing to a purple-yellowish hue. The process is painless, causing no discomfort through the 10–15 days it takes to reabsorb the spot.
2) *Acute trismus*, with the inability to open the mouth partially or wholly, normally a painful process sensitive to exploration at the insertion site. The cause is needle penetration in the lateral (external) pterygoid muscle, inducing irritation and spasms (Kramer and Mitton 1973; Stone and Kaban 1979). This complication, which may appear in less than 0.5% of cases (further to the Kuster and Udin 1984; Loetscher et al. 1988; Pfeil et al. 2010; Padhye et al. 2011 series), can be treated as described in Chapter 22.

### Modified Adatia Technique

In 1968, Adatia (1968) introduced a simple method that prevents the risk of hematomas and swelling (Adatia 1974, 1976).

- It is identical to buccal infiltration at the second maxillary molar behind the zygomatic osseous crest of the malar bone except that the needle runs a distance of *around 10 mm* instead of 2–3 mm to pass over the buccinator muscle insertion.
- A 1.8-ml cartridge is injected, forming a sort of subcutaneous blister immediately over the buccinator muscle in the molar buccal cavity. *The blister should be pushed backward, upward, and inward with the fingertip.* This operation is easier if the patient's mouth is completely closed (Figure 14.5).

This procedure facilitates diffusion of the anesthetic solution toward the molar apices as well as toward the upper posterior part of the maxilla, i.e. toward the posterior superior alveolar nerve branches before they course into the foramina in the tuberosity.

The success rate, assessed in extractions only (rather than with the more rigorous electrical pulp tester), comes to nearly 100% in molars and nearly 90% in premolars with the standard lidocaine solution (L-80) (Adatia 1976).

## High Tuberosity Approach

This technique aims to block the maxillary nerve ($V_2$), the second division of the trigeminal nerve, within the pterygopalatine fossa, numbing a wide area by anesthetizing all its branches at once.

It is known as high tuberosity because the tuberosity approach (without "high") is a synonym for PSA nerve block. Here the needle must travel further (higher) into the pterygopalatine fossa, hence the name. Other synonyms for this approach are posterior infraorbital approach because it is like infraorbital block but posterior, or Smith's technique because it was developed by Dr. Arthur Ervin Smith of Chicago around 1913 (Smith 1920).

*This is a difficult technique* because it is highly arbitrary because of the lack of osseous references to guide the needle during injection. It calls for introducing the needle higher and at a wider angle to avoid the posterior wall of the maxilla (tuberosity) and reach the pterygopalatine fossa (Figure 14.1). That raises the risk of hematomas due to puncture of pterygoid plexus veins or branches of the posterior superior alveolar artery. *It is also one of the most painful techniques* (Annex 23).

### Uses

As noted earlier, the most common technique in the upper arch is buccal infiltration anesthesia, although on occasion a more powerful anesthetic effect is required, as in the following examples.

1) Lengthy oral surgery in the maxillary zone because the high tuberosity approach covers a larger area with less anesthetic and fewer injections.
2) After buccal infiltration failure, particularly in the molar zone.

## Zone Anesthetized

Theoretically the technique would affect the entire area innervated by the second division of the trigeminal nerve, the maxillary nerve ($V_2$), including the following.

- Teeth, including pulp and periodontium of molars and premolars on the side injected. Whilst incisors and canines may be anesthetized, as they are contralaterally cross-innervated, they may require reinforcement via buccal infiltration.
- Buccal cavity, including fibromucosa (alveolar mucosa, gingiva, and interdental papillae), bone, and periosteum around molars and premolars. As discussed earlier, the anterior teeth are often contralaterally cross-innervated. On occasion the upper area in the roof of the buccal cavity at the first maxillary molar may require supplementary infiltration, as it may be innervated by a branch of the ophthalmic nerve (first division of the trigeminal nerve) (Saborido 1977).
- Palate, including the fibromucosa, bone, and periosteum of the entire hemi-arch except the anterior part, which is contralaterally cross-innervated by the nasopalatine nerve (Saborido 1977).
- Maxillary sinus on the side injected.
- Terminal branches of the infraorbital nerve that innervate the upper half-lip, the *nasi ala*, and the lower eyelid on the side injected.

## Technique

- Long (42 mm), 27G or (preferably) 25G needle. In patients with small mouths or where a high angle is needed (see below), the needle should be bent at a 30–45° angle several millimeters ahead of the cone or hub to facilitate needle progress along the posterior wall of the maxilla. Note that the needle is not bent at the hub itself because as this is the weakest part it might readily break.
- Dentist's and patient's positions.
  - Dentist at 9:00–10:00 o'clock.
  - Patient in supine position with head slightly hyperextended to enable the dentist to turn it slightly to the left to anesthetize the right side or to the right to anesthetize the left side.
- Advise the patient that during injection they may experience (i) heart palpitations (up to 30% of individuals in some series; Forloine et al. 2010) due to the use of epinephrine solutions and (ii) temporary ocular and visual alterations (up to 10–15% of individuals) (Table 14.4).
- Determine the depth of the needle (Jorgensen 1948; Hayden 1965).
  - The height of the posterior maxilla or distance the needle should travel may vary from 30 to 50 mm (Jorgensen 1948), and although the normal range is 30–40 mm with a *mean of around 35 mm* (Broering et al. 2009; Forloine et al. 2010), the distance must be individually estimated. One fairly reliable procedure is to measure the height of the anterior maxilla from the first maxillary premolar gingival margin to the edge of the inferior orbit because in 90% of individuals this is practically the same distance as the height of the posterior maxilla. The latter is 4–6 mm higher in only 5% of

Table 14.4 Successful (%) pulpal anesthesia after the high tuberosity approach (electrical pulp tester assessment and 3.6 ml of standard solution L-100): percentage of ocular complications and lower lip anesthesia

| Variable | | Broering et al. (1991) $n = 40$ | Broering et al. (2009) $n = 40$ | Forloine et al. (2010) $n = 50$ |
|---|---|---|---|---|
| Tooth | Second molar (%) | 100 | 100 | 98 |
| | First molar (%) | 78 | 95 | 92 |
| | Second premolar (%) | 52 | 73 | 76 |
| | First premolar (%) | 30 | 52 | 58 |
| | Canine (%) | 22 | 32 | 54 |
| | Lateral incisor (%) | 4 | 18 | 8 |
| | Central incisor (%) | 4 | 5 | 10 |
| Lower lip anesthesia (%) | | — | 2 | 32 |
| Ocular complications | Diplopia (%) | — | 10 | 12–16 |
| | Blurred vision (%) | — | 5 | 0 |
| | Mydriasis (%) | — | 2 | 0 |

individuals, in which case the needle may not be inserted high enough, and 1–3 mm lower in the other 5%, leading to an overly high insertion site (Jorgensen 1948). Only in the presence of open anterior bite is the height of the posterior maxilla 2–9 mm lower than the anterior (90% of individuals affected), raising the risk of overestimating the desired height (Jorgensen 1948).
- The height of the anterior maxilla is measured along the face with a dental caliper from the first premolar gingival margin to immediately below the infraorbital bone margin, taking care not to accidentally injure the eye and marking the distance with a rubber stop on the needle to prevent over-insertion (Hayden 1965).

- *Examine the entire roof of the buccal cavity over the maxillary molars with the non-injection index finger* to locate the osseous bridge that protrudes from the zygomatic crest on the malar bone (normally alongside the first maxillary molar).
- *Pull the labial commissure outward and upward* with the non-injection hand to firmly stretch the jugal mucosa (Figure 4.12).
  - Stretch the tissue intraorally with the index finger on the right side and the thumb on the left.
  - The aim is to (i) bring the concavity of the buccal cavity around the molars into view and (ii) reduce any injection-induced pain by inserting the needle in a tense mucosa.
- Increase the space for maneuvering in the mouth.
  - Ask the patient to partially close their mouth to enlarge the workspace, which (i) broadens the labial commissure and (ii) shifts the coronoid apophysis of the mandible rearward to prevent it from taking up space and getting in the way (Figure 14.5).
  - If despite the foregoing the space is insufficient, ask the patient to shift their mandible toward the side to be injected to increase the separation between the ascending ramus of the mandible and the posterior maxilla (Sicher 1950).
- Insert the needle in the roof of the buccal cavity.
  - *Behind the zygomatic crest of the malar bone*, which is usually the same as saying behind the second or third molar.
  - Point the needle upward and as perpendicularly as possible to the molar occlusal plane. As a full 90° angle is not possible due to the presence of the jugal mucosa, the needle should be rearwardly oblique, which is also desirable.
  - *Avoid the osseous wall* to prevent the needle from hitting or catching in the surface of the maxillary tuberosity (outer and posterior wall of the maxilla).
  - Push the needle a few millimeters into the buccal cavity.

- Needle re-orientation and course.
  - *Tilt the tip of the needle inward* (the syringe tilts outward), theoretically forming an angle of around 30–45° relative to the sagittal or medial plane to keep it flush against the posterior wall of the maxilla (Figure 14.12).
  - *Push the needle upward, inward, and slightly rearward*, trying to keep as close as possible to the bone without tearing the periosteum. That protects the pterygoid plexus veins, the posterior superior alveolar artery, Bichat's fat pads, and the lateral (external) pterygoid muscle from puncture. Note that it is not always possible to avoid impacting the vessels in this zone (Sicher 1950).
  - If resistance is met (because the needle hits bone), withdraw the needle slightly, re-enter at a less inward angle, and continue.
  - Needle progress is interrupted when the rubber stop (used to mark the insertion length) reaches the second and third molar CEJ or gingival margin. Remember that the mucosa at the roof of the buccal cavity is not a good reference because its depth may vary from 3 to 12 mm (Jorgensen 1948).
- Aspire before injecting. Aspiration is positive in 13% of cases (Goldman and Gray 1963).
- Inject the full 1.8-ml cartridge over the course of 40–60 seconds, after which the entire operation is repeated to inject a second cartridge, *for a total of 3.6 ml*. Many authors deem a single cartridge to be insufficient because as the tip of the needle does not reach but merely comes close to the pterygopalatine fossa (where the maxillary nerve lies), the anesthetic solution must diffuse across a longer distance to bathe the nerve (Smith 1920; Collon 1946; Jorgensen 1948; Forloine et al. 2010).
- Subjective symptoms of soft tissue anesthesia appear in 3–5 minutes with patients describing tickling, tingling, or numbing (Table 13.1, Chapter 13) at the injection site and (i) the lower eyelid, *nasi ala* and half of the upper lip and (ii) the half of the palate on the side injected.
  - *Wait 5–10 minutes after injection to allow the anesthetic to take effect* and anesthetize the pulp of maxillary molars and premolars. Note that this approach takes a little more time.
  - Optionally some clinicians insert a probe in the buccal mucosa around the molars to determine soft tissue anesthesia.
  - The definitive sign of efficacy is obtained by working on the molars (i.e. prepping into dentin), initially cautiously and then proceeding normally if the patient expresses no discomfort.
- Soft tissue anesthesia usually lasts 3–4 hours (200 minutes), a fact which the patient should be notified of after treatment.

### Efficacy of this Technique

As Table 14.4 shows, according to several clinical tests pulpal anesthesia is successful in nearly 95% of molars, but just 60% of premolars. The success rate drops even lower in the anterior teeth. Surprisingly, although this is an upper arch approach, it anesthetizes the lower lip in a small percentage of cases. As these findings are referred to a standard 2% lidocaine, 1:100 000 (10 μg/ml) epinephrine solution (L-100), a more powerful solution such as 4% articaine, 1:100 000 (10 μg/ml) epinephrine (A-100) would be expected to deliver somewhat better results.

### Complications Specific to this Technique

1) Anesthetic failure is fairly common due to the difficulty and arbitrary nature of this approach.
    - If the needle is not close enough to the pterygopalatine fossa, rather than the entire maxillary nerve ($V_2$), its posterior superior alveolar nerve branches are blocked, anesthetizing the molars only.
    - If the solution is injected too outwardly, in the infratemporal fossa (formerly the zygomatic fossa), it is too far away from the pterygopalatine fossa to anesthetize the whole nerve. This can be corrected by tilting the needle more medially, closer to the posterior side of the maxilla (Collon 1946).
    - If only one instead of two 1.8-ml cartridges (3.6 ml) is injected, the amount of the solution diffusing is insufficient to anesthetize the maxillary nerve ($V_2$) (Collon 1946).
2) *An extraoral hematoma on the face is the most common complication.* This dark-brown purplish, normally swollen spot in the malar or superior masseteric area is generally painless. Its cause is blood extravasation (ecchymosis) due to puncture of a vein in the pterygoid plexus or the buccogingival branches of the posterior superior alveolar artery that course somewhat erratically near the maxillary tuberosity (Harn et al. 2002). In either case in the next few days the lesion spreads forward and downward along the muscular planes of the cheek, while changing to a purple-yellowish hue. It is wholly reabsorbed in 10–15 days.
3) Ocular and visual alterations in the eye on the side injected appear in 10–15% of cases. The most common symptom is double vision (dipoplia), although others such as blurred vision, dilated pupil (mydriasis), and drooping eyelid (ptosis) may also appear. When the anesthetic solution is deposited too high in the pterygopalatine fossa (rather uncommon in this approach), the solution diffuses across the inferior orbital fissure to the interior of the orbit, anesthetizing ocular nerves, and muscles with the concomitant loss of motor coordination (Collon 1946; Forloine et al. 2010). In such situations, (i) reassure the patient that the effect will disappear spontaneously with the effect of the anesthesia, (ii) protect the eye with a patch until the effect subsides, and (iii) advise the patient that they may neither drive nor operate hazardous machinery while the effect lasts.
4) Acute trismus, with the inability to open the mouth partially or wholly, is normally a painful process sensitive to exploration at the insertion site. The cause is needle penetration in the lateral (external) pterygoid muscle, inducing irritation and spasms (Kramer and Mitton 1973; Stone and Kaban 1979). Permanent trismus may appear more rarely (Stone and Kaban 1979) (see Chapter 22).
5) Pain is inherent in this technique, one of the most painful.
    - Needle progression may induce moderate to severe pain in 50% of patients (Annex 23).
    - Moderate to severe post-operative pain around the injection site may last 1–3 days in 25% of individuals (Broering et al. 2009; Forloine et al. 2010), subsiding spontaneously with no sequelae.

### Remarks

The high tuberosity approach is not recommended for routine dentistry practice because it is difficult, entails more complications, and delivers results only marginally better than simple buccal infiltration anesthesia. The most important factors for success with this approach are as follows:

1) The tip of the needle must be placed at the right height.
2) The tip of the needle must be oriented at the angle that brings it closest to the pterygopalatine fossa.
3) Two 1.8-ml (3.6-ml) cartridges must be injected to provide sufficient volume for the solution to diffuse to the pterygopalatine fossa and reach the maxillary nerve ($V_2$).

## Transpalatal Technique

As in the high tuberosity approach, this technique aims to block the maxillary nerve ($V_2$), the second division of the trigeminal nerve, within the pterygopalatine fossa, rendering a wide area numb by anesthetizing all its branches at once.

It is also known as the *greater palatine canal technique*. The term "transpalatal," coined by Dr. Gerardo Saborido (1977), seems to be much more illustrative of what the technique actually involves. It was first described in 1921 by Juan Ubaldo Carrea of Buenos Aires, who recommended it in molars and premolars (Carrea 1921a,b), and subsequently applied in 1922 by Otto Hofer of Vienna (Hofer 1922b). It was also described in 1922 by Mendel Nevin of New York, who claimed to have developed it in 1917, but did not recommend it due to the high frequency of obstructions in the canal and the risk of injury to the vascular nervous package (Nevin 1922). The following year Samuel Silverman of Atlanta (Silverman 1923), apparently unaware of Carrea's work, described it as his own.

*Note*: In the 1921 paper the surname "Carrea" is misspelled as "Carrba."

In this relatively simple technique (an enormous advantage over the high tuberosity approach) the needle penetrates the greater palatine foramen through the greater palatine canal to reach the pterygopalatine fossa, where the second division of the trigeminal nerve (maxillary nerve, $V_2$) transmits before entering the infraorbital canal.

## Uses

As noted earlier, buccal infiltration is the most common technique to anesthetize the upper arch, although on occasion a more powerful anesthetic is required, such as in the following examples.

1) Lengthy oral surgery in the maxillary zone, as the transpalatal approach covers a larger area with less anesthetic and fewer injections.
2) After buccal infiltration failure, particularly in the molar zone.
3) *In acute buccal cavity infection around molars and premolars.* Under such circumstances the buccal infiltration, superior alveolar nerve block, and high tuberosity procedures are contraindicated since the needle must be inserted in this area (Szerlip and Morristown 1950; Sved et al. 1992). Today, in 95% of the cases where the transpalatal technique is chosen it is for this reason (Sved et al. 1992).

## Zone Anesthetized

Theoretically the technique would affect the entire area innervated by the second division of the trigeminal nerve, the maxillary nerve ($V_2$).

- Teeth, including pulp and periodontium of the molars and premolars on the side injected. Whilst incisors and canines may be anesthetized, as they are contralaterally cross-innervated, they may require reinforcement via buccal infiltration.
- Buccal cavity, including fibromucosa (alveolar mucosa, gingiva, and interdental papillae), bone, and periosteum around molars and premolars. As discussed earlier, the anterior teeth are often contralaterally cross-innervated.
- On occasion the upper area in the roof of the buccal cavity at the first maxillary molar may require supplementary infiltration, as it may be innervated by a branch of the ophthalmic nerve (first division of the trigeminal nerve) (Saborido 1977).
- Palate, including the fibromucosa, bone, and periosteum of the entire hemi-arch except the anterior part, which is contralaterally cross-innervated by the nasopalatine nerve (Saborido 1977).
- Maxillary sinus on the side injected.
- Terminal branches of the infraorbital nerve that innervate the upper half-lip, the *nasi ala*, and the lower eyelid on the side injected.

## Technique

- *Very long (42 mm), 27G needle* (preferred over 25G as it is more flexible and less prone to jamming as it progresses; Cohn 1986). In patients with small mouths or where a sharp angle is needed (see below), the needle should be bent at a 30–45° angle, several millimeters ahead of the cone or hub to facilitate needle progress along the greater palatine canal (Cook 1950b; Mercuri 1979; Lepere 1993; Douglas and Wormald 2006). Note that the needle is not bent at the hub itself because as this is the weakest part it could break.
- Dentist's and patient's positions.
  - Dentist at 9:00–10:00 o'clock.
  - Patient in supine position with head slightly hyperextended to enable the dentist to turn it slightly to the left to anesthetize the right side or to the right to anesthetize the left side.
- Anesthetize the greater palatine nerve where it exits from the greater palatine foramen and wait 2 minutes before continuing (Chapter 15). This measure aims to minimize possible discomfort during the rest of the procedure.
- Advise the patient that during the injection they may feel (i) pressure below the maxillary facial tissues on the side injected and (ii) temporary ocular and visual alterations such as double vision (diplopia), drooping eyelid (ptosis), or blurred vision (10% of cases) (Table 14.5).
- Determine the depth (length) of the insertion.
  - In dry skulls, the mean length along the greater palatine canal between the greater palatine foramen and the roof of the pterygopalatine fossa is around 35 mm, normally ranging from 20 to 45 mm (Table A 42.6, Annex 42). As the 4–6 mm (3–7 mm) thickness of the fibromucosa over the greater palatine foramen (Table 14.6) must be added to that dimension, and take away 1–2 mm of soft tissues overlaying the alveolar crest in bicuspids

**Table 14.5** Percentage of visual/ocular alterations and their relationship to needle length and amount (ml) of solution injected with the transpalatal technique

| Reference | Sample size | Percentage of visual/ocular alterations (%) | Needle length (mm) | Amount injected (ml) |
|---|---|---|---|---|
| Dickson and Coates (1945) | 80 | 6 | 42 | 2.0 |
| Malamed and Trieger (1983) | 150 | 1 | 35 | 1.8 |
| Sved et al. (1992) | 101 | 39 | 42 | 4.4 |
| Schwartz-Arad et al. (2004)[a] | 76 | 0 | 30 | 3, 2 |
| Broering et al. (2009) | 40 | 18 | — | 3.6 |
| Torres et al. (2011) | 82 | 7 | 41 | 1.2–1.8 |
| Mean | | 11, 8 | | |
| Rounded mean | | **10** | | |

[a] Computer-controlled device (the wand).

**Table 14.6** Depth of soft tissue overlaying the grater palatine foramen

| Reference | Sample | Depth (mm) |
|---|---|---|
| Dickson and Coates (1945) | Patients | 3–4 |
| Cook (1950b) | Patients | 4–7 |
| Canter et al. (1964) | Patients | 2–7 |
| Viegas and Hemphill (1961) | Patients | 2–5 |
| Malamed and Trieger (1983) | Patients | 3–4 |
| Methathrathip et al. (2005) | Cadavers | 6.7 ± 2.3 (2–13) |
| Douglas and Wormald (2006) | Cadavers | 6.9 |
| Nimigean et al. (2013) | Patients | 6 (4–8) |
| Shalaby et al. (2015) | Cadavers | 4, 9 ± 1, 9 |
| Mean | | 4.7 |
| Rounded mean | | 4–6 |

(Malamed and Trieger 1983), the total may come to around 37–39 mm on average. Clinical trials yield lower heights, however, *around 33 mm (29–35 mm)*, because the needle need not reach the roof of the pterygopalatine fossa (Broering et al. 2009).

o Two methods for a more personalized estimate, particularly for children or adults with very small or large faces, are in place and closely correlated to the posterior part of the maxilla.

  1) Measurement of the low anterior height. This consists of measuring the distance between the infraorbital foramen and the alveolar crest of the second maxillary premolar. The mean is 30–35 mm (Table A 2.5, Annex 2).

  2) Measurement of the high anterior or orbit height. This consists of measuring the distance between the upper rim of the orbit and the lower rim at the infraorbital foramen. The mean is 33–34 mm (Canter et al. 1964; Slavkin et al. 1966).

o The measurement as estimated with one method or the other should be increased by 5 mm to accommodate the fibromucosa over the greater palatine foramen. A stop is placed on the needle to prevent over-insertion (silicone or rubber stop) (Figure 14.14).

- Ask the patient to open their mouth as widely as possible for full vision and to insert the needle in the greater palatine canal. A mouth-opener (bite block or mouth prop) may be optionally placed on the non-injection side (Mercuri 1979; Malamed and Trieger 1983).
- Locate the greater palatine foramen.
  o This formation lies on the horizontal hard palate at the abutment with the vertical alveolar process: *in nearly 90% of individuals it is located around the third maxillary molar* (Annex 42) (Figure 14.15). The third molar zone refers to the area ranging from a point slightly forward of the third molar (between it and the second molar) to a point slightly backward of the third molar and including the third molar zone.
  o It also helps to know that it lies around 15 mm, laterally, from the midline of the palate (Szerlip and Morristown 1950; Annex 42).
  o It is around 4 mm forward of the posterior edge of the hard palate (Annex 42). This is important when the maxillary arch is edentulous (Mercuri 1979; Wong and Sved 1991). One way of distinguishing the hard and soft palate is by locating the line where the color of the palatal mucosa changes.
- Insert the needle in the greater palatine foramen.
  o The approach is from the opposite side of the mouth to more readily locate and insert the needle into the greater palatine canal (Figure 14.14).
  o Insert the needle slightly forward of where the foramen is presumed to be (Figure 14.15). Remember that the foramen is covered by around 4–6 mm of fibromucosa (Cook et al. 1950b) (Table 14.6).
  o If the needle does not go in after the first puncture, *repeat the operation several times until the foramen is reached* (Hofer 1922b; Peckham 1938; Wong and Sved 1991). Contrary to what some authors contend, the foramen is not readily found by touch and must be located by trial and error (Wong and Sved 1991). It is nearly impossible to detect the foramen if the diameter is too small (it varies from 3 to 4 mm; Annex 42) and/or the fibromucosa is thick.

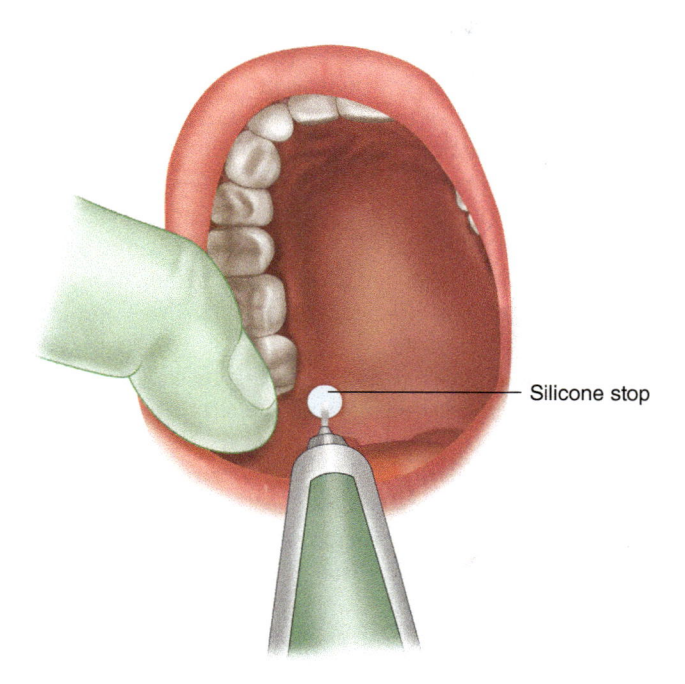

**Figure 14.14** Silicone stop or rubber stop to mark the needle insertion limit; maneuver facilitated by non-injection side approach.

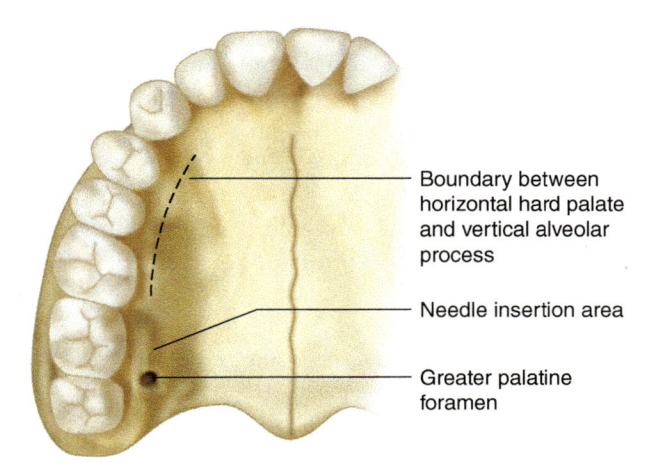

**Figure 14.15** Location of greater palatine foramen and needle insertion area.

**Table 14.7** Angulation to occlusal plane and mid-sagittal plane (°) in the transpalatal technique

| Reference | Sample | Angle occlusal plane (°) | Angle sagittal plane (°) |
|---|---|---|---|
| Carrea (1921a) | Patients | — | 5–10 |
| Dickson and Coates (1945) | Patients | 45 | 5–10 |
| Cook (1950b) | Patients | 60–70 | |
| Ries Centeno (1979) | Dry skulls | 60 | |
| Malamed and Trieger (1983) | Dry skulls | 46 (20–70) | — |
| Chentanez et al. (1985) | Dry skulls | 60 ± 9 | — |
| Austin (1987) | Dry skulls | 60 ± 8 (51–76) | 7 ± 5 (−3 to 20) |
| Wong and Sved (1991) | Patients | 60 | 5–8 |
| Methathrathip et al. (2005) | Dry skulls | 58 ± 6 | 7 ± 5 |
| Douglas and Wormald (2006) | Cadavers | 60 | — |
| Howard-Swirzinski et al. (2010) | CBCT | 63 | — |
| Shalaby et al. (2015) | Dry skulls | 50 | — |
| | Mean | 57.7 | 7.1 |
| | Rounded mean | **50–60** | **5–10** |

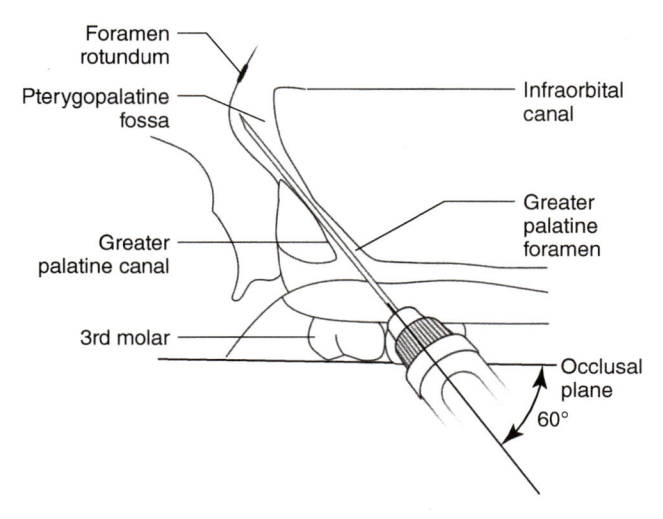

**Figure 14.16** Needle angle relative to the occlusal plane of the maxillary molars. Schematic representation in saggital section.

- Push the needle slowly and gently across the greater palatine canal.
  - Direct the needle rearward and upward at an *angle of around 50–60°* relative to the occlusal plane of the upper molars (Table 14.7 and Figure 14.16) (sagittal section: antero-posterior direction). It is frequent that the needle has to be bent in the shaft but not in the hub, the weakest part.
  - Needle movement relative to the medial plane should be *5–10° outward* (Table 14.7 and Figure 14.17) (coronal section: medial-lateral direction).

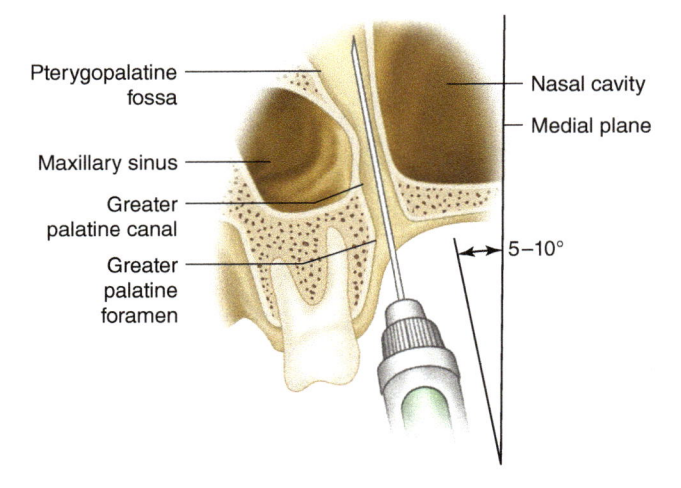

**Figure 14.17** Needle angle relative to the medial plane (coronal section).

- *Never force the needle.* Any resistance is an indication that it is not running parallel to the canal walls. This minor angle deviation can be corrected by drawing the needle back by 1–3 mm to free it of any contact with the bone and readjusting the orientation with minor movements (Peckham 1938; Dickson and Coates 1945; Saborido 1977; Malamed and Trieger 1983; Wong and Sved 1991). Note that the scant space available in a greater palatine canal with a narrow diameter (1.5 mm) severely limits any possible redirection of the needle (Cook 1950b). This circumstance is fortunately not very common.
- The clinical impression is that maneuvering inside the canal causes patients little discomfort (Silverman 1923; Malamed and Trieger 1983) and clinical tests show that this technique is less painful than the tuberosity approach (Annex 23).
- Advance the needle until the rubber stop used to mark the insertion depth is reached. Allow at least 2–3 mm of the needle to protrude outside the mucosa over the greater palatine foramen so it can be withdrawn in the event of breakage (Dickson and Coates 1945; Mercuri 1979; Wong and Sved 1991).
- Aspire before injecting. Aspiration is positive in 5% of cases (Annex 22).
- Slowly inject a 1.8-ml cartridge of solution over the course of 40–60 seconds and then a second cartridge for *a total of 3.6 ml*. Some authors deem 1.8 ml to be too little and therefore recommend two (Wong and Sved 1991; Sved et al. 1992). Either repeat the entire operation or, where the patient is highly cooperative, unscrew the needle from the syringe while still in the mouth, load another cartridge and re-screw the syringe onto the needle for the second injection (Wong and Sved 1991).

- Subjective symptoms of anesthesia appear in 3–5 minutes, with patients describing soft tissue anesthesia as tickling, tingling, or numbing (Table 13.1, Chapter 13) at the injection site and (i) the lower eyelid, *nasi ala* and half of the upper lip; and (ii) the half of the palate on the side injected.
  - *Wait 5–10 minutes* after injection to allow the anesthetic to take effect and anesthetize the pulp of maxillary molars and premolars. Note that this approach takes a little more time.
  - Optionally some clinicians insert a probe in the buccal mucosa around the molars to determine soft tissue anesthesia.
  - The definitive sign of efficacy is obtained by working on the molars, initially cautiously and then proceeding normally if the patient expresses no discomfort.
- Soft tissue anesthesia usually lasts 2–3 hours (Sved et al. 1992; Lepere 1993), a fact of which the patient should be notified after treatment.

### Efficacy of this Technique

As Table 14.8 shows, according to several clinical tests pulpal anesthesia is successful in nearly 95% of molars, but just 65% of premolars. The success rate drops even lower in the anterior teeth. Surprisingly, although this is an upper arch approach, it anesthetizes the lower lip in a small percentage of cases. The clinical success rate in maxillary molars and premolars determined via extractions, oral surgery, and dental treatment (less rigorous method) is in the order of 80% (Table 14.9). As these findings are referred to a standard 2% lidocaine, 1:100 000 (10 µg/ml) epinephrine solution (L-100), a more powerful anesthetic

**Table 14.8** Successful (%) pulpal anesthesia with the transpalatal technique (electrical pulp tester assessment and 3.6 ml of standard solution L-100) and percentage of lower lip anesthesia

| Variable | | Broering et al. (1991) n = 40 | Broering et al. (2009) n = 40 |
|---|---|---|---|
| Tooth | Second molar (%) | 96 | 100 |
| | First molar (%) | 83 | 95 |
| | Second premolar (%) | 65 | 80 |
| | First premolar (%) | 35 | 68 |
| | Canine (%) | 26 | 60 |
| | Lateral incisor (%) | 17 | 43 |
| | Central incisor (%) | 4 | 23 |
| Lower lip anesthesia (%) | | — | 12 |

Table 14.9 Clinical successful (%) in molars and premolars with the transpalatal technique

| Reference | Sample size | Success rate (%) |
|---|---|---|
| Dickson and Coates (1945) | 80 | 80 |
| Corbett and Helmore (1948) | — | 78 |
| Malamed and Trieger (1983) | 150 | 90 |
| Sved et al. (1992) | 101 | 89 |
| Schwartz-Arad et al. (2002) | 66 | 91 |
| Torres et al. (2011) | 82 | 60 |
| Mean | | 81.3 |
| Rounded mean | | 80 |

such as 4% articaine, 1:100 000 (10 μg/ml) epinephrine (A-100) would be expected to deliver somewhat better results.

## Complications Specific to This Technique

1) Full or partial anesthetic failure for the following reasons.
   - The greater palatine foramen cannot be located (Mercuri 1979; Schwartz-Arad et al. 2004), especially in edentulous patients. In such cases, review the anatomy (Mercuri 1979).
   - The needle continuously catches on the posterior wall of the canal, a common occurrence in canals highly angled relative to the occlusal plane. Bending the needle is very useful in such cases, as noted earlier (Mercuri 1979; Cohn 1986).
   - The needle is not inserted far enough and the tip fails to reach the pterygopalatine fossa, so the gravity-driven anesthetic solution flows downward (Wong and Sved 1991). In such cases, repeat the technique with a longer needle (Mercuri 1979).
   - The amount of anesthetic administered is insufficient. The solution is to inject another cartridge (Wong and Sved 1991).
2) Anatomical variations may induce failure.
   - Canal obstructed because it is contorted or irregular, with osseous protrusions that hinder passage of the needle, a situation found in 5% of individuals (Table 14.10). In such cases desist and seek alternative techniques such as the high tuberosity approach (Dickson and Coates 1945; Mercuri 1979; Cohn 1986; Wong and Sved 1991). Nonetheless, when the obstacle is less than 15 mm from the total length envisaged the injection may often be successful (Sved et al. 1992).
   - Excessive rearward slant on the greater palatine canal at a very small angle relative to the occlusal plane of the maxillary molars. This anatomic variation may result in the dose being delivered anterior to the pterygoid process, preventing the needle from reaching the pterygopalatine fossa (Cook 1950b). This circumstance is uncommon.
   - Excessive lateral slant on the greater palatine canal, which empties into the lateral side the pterygoid process without reaching the pterygopalatine fossa (Cook 1950b). This circumstance is also uncommon.

Table 14.10 Percentage of obstructed greater palatine canal in dry skulls and clinical trials

| Dry skulls | | | Clinical trials | | |
|---|---|---|---|---|---|
| Reference | n | Obstructed (%) | Reference | n | Obstructed (%) |
| Canter et al. (1964) | 205 | 39 | Dickson and Coates (1945) | 80 | 2.5 |
| Slavkin et al. (1966) | 58 | 37 | Mercuri (1979) | — | 5 |
| Jorgensen and Hayden (1970) | 200 | 15 | Cohn (1986) | — | 10 |
| Ries Centeno (1979) | 50 | 6 | Sved et al. (1992) | 101 | 6 |
| Malamed and Trieger (1983) | 204 | 3 | Schwartz-Arad et al. (2002 and 2004) | 66–76 | 0 |
| Chentanez et al. (1985) | 120 | 54 | Broering et al. (2009) | 40 | 8 |
| Austin (1987) | 42 | 5 | | | |
| Ferreira et al. (1990) | 100 | 10 | | | |
| Sharma and Garud (2013) | 100 | 4 | | | |
| Mean | | 19.2 | | | 5.2 |
| Rounded mean | | 20 | | | 5 |

The values used are from clinical trials; dry skull values are not representative of clinical reality.

3) Needle protrusion outside the greater palatine canal, which also induces anesthetic failure for the following reasons.
   - The needle penetrates the greater palatine foramen too far rearward, reaching the soft (nasal-pharyngeal) palate. The clinician's perception is an overly smooth injection and the patient's a bitter taste in their throat because the liquid drips behind the soft palate and ultimately into the esophagus (Szerlip and Morristown 1950; Saborido 1977; Sved et al. 1992).
   - The needle penetrates the anterior wall of the greater palatine canal and the anesthetic solution is deposited in the maxillary sinus (Mercuri 1979).
   - The needle penetrates the posterior wall of the greater palatine canal and the anesthetic solution is deposited in the infratemporal fossa (formerly zygomatic fossa), to no anesthetic effect (Mercuri 1979; Wong and Sved 1991).
- The needle penetrates the lateral/medial wall of the canal and the tip enters the nasal-pharynx and nasal cavity. In such cases, aspiration prior to injection may draw bubbles into the cartridge (a sign that the needle is in the nasal pharynx) and the patient begins to cough, with a bitter taste in their throat, and may bleed through the nose on the side injected (epistaxis) when the needle penetrates the highly vascularized nasal mucosa (Saborido 1977; Mercuri 1979; Wong and Sved 1991).

   *Note*: As the osseous walls of the greater palatine canal tend to be very thin, they may be readily perforated if the clinician forces the needle (Malamed and Trieger 1983; Wong and Sved 1991).
4) *Visual and ocular alterations in the eye on the side injected in around 10% of cases* (Table 14.5).
   - The cause of these complications is the use of very long needles and/or the injection of large amounts of anesthetic solution, some of which reaches the upper area of the pterygopalatine fossa and may seep across the inferior orbital fissure, entering the eye socket and anesthetizing ocular nerves and muscles (Table 14.5). For some authors these symptoms confirm that the anesthetic has reached the maxillary nerve ($V_2$) (Sved et al. 1992).
   - The possible complications are as follows.
     - Double vision (diplopia) due to ocular muscle anesthesia. This is the most common complication and in 90% of cases appears alone or with strabismus or a drooping eyelid (Sved et al. 1992; Torres et al. 2011).
     - Inability to coordinate and synchronize the movements of the two eyes (strabismus) due to paralysis of the eye muscles (the lateral rectus muscle is the one most severely affected). It is usually attendant on diplopia, seldom appearing alone (Sved et al. 1992).
     - Drooping upper eyelid (ptosis) due to anesthesia of the branches of the oculomotor nerve in the upper eyelid. It is likewise usually attendant on diplopia, seldom appearing alone (Sved et al. 1992).
     - Other rare complications include dilated pupil (mydriasis), corneal anesthesia, blurred vision (Broering et al. 2009), and, very exceptionally, temporary blindness due to optical nerve (cranial nerve II) anesthesia.
   - These complications generally disappear spontaneously with the effect of the anesthesia without any sequelae (Dickson and Coates 1945; Saborido 1977; Mercuri 1979).
   - Treatment in such cases consists of the following:
     1) Reassure the patient that the effect will disappear spontaneously with the effect of the anesthesia.
     2) Place a protective patch over the eye for the duration.
     3) Advise the patient that they may not drive nor operate hazardous machinery while the effect lasts.
5) The side of the face affected may also be pale and exhibit blanching (ischemic paling). This is usually because the needle punctures or rubs against the internal maxillary artery that transmits through the upper part of the pterygopalatine fossa, causing spasm/contraction in all its branches and paling in the entire area of the face covered by the artery. It is more readily visible in people with lighter skin (Mercuri 1979). The patient may occasionally also feel a sudden burning sensation in the whole area. Note that the area covered by the internal maxillary artery is nearly parallel to the facial area innervated by the maxillary nerve ($V_2$). Treatment in these cases consists of reassuring the patient that the effect is temporary and will disappear spontaneously in a few minutes.
6) *In 1% of cases the needle punctures the nerve inducing a kind of electric shock, cramp, or intense burning sensation in the posterior and medial half of the palate on the side injected*, with no sequelae (Sved et al. 1992). No chronic or long-lasting lesions of this nature have been reported in clinical practice, despite their theoretical likelihood (Silverman 1923; Dickson and Coates 1945; Mercuri 1979; Wong and Sved 1991), perhaps because the technique is seldom used.
7) With this technique:
   - Pain is less severe, especially during needle travel, than in the alternative high tuberosity approach (Annex 23).
   - Moderate to severe post-operative pain around the injection site may last 1–3 days in only 2% of individuals (Broering et al. 2009), subsiding spontaneously with no sequelae.

### Factors That Lead to Success

Three major factors determine the success of this technique (Wong and Sved 1991).

1) The greater palatine foramen on the posterior palate must be located, which is not always a simple task.
2) The needle must travel a long enough distance to reach the pterygopalatine fossa. If the needle is too short, as is often the case, the anesthetic solution fails to bathe the maxillary nerve ($V_2$), remaining rather in the canal. Long needles measuring 42 mm are therefore needed.
3) A sufficient amount of anesthetic must be injected to diffuse satisfactorily across the roof of the pterygopalatine fossa. Clinicians tend not to use enough (Hofer 1922b; Wong and Sved 1991), despite the recommended two 1.8-ml cartridges or 3.6 ml.

### Final Remarks

Buccal infiltration is by far the most common of the techniques used for pulpal anesthesia in the maxilla for its simplicity, safety, and efficacy. None of the other techniques is routinely used.

Of the two maxillary nerve ($V_2$) block techniques, the transpalatal or greater palatine canal technique, which can be applied when the buccal cavity around molars and premolars is affected by acute infection (because the approach is from the palate), is deemed here to be more useful than the alternative high tuberosity approach. Moreover, it is simpler and less painful both during injection and in the post-operative period.

## References

Adatia, A.K. (1968). Posterior superior alveolar nerve block. *Dent. Pract.* 18 (9): 321–322.

Adatia, A.K. (1974). Local analgesia of maxillary first molars (letter). *Br. Dent. J.* 137 (12): 459.

Adatia, A.K. (1976). Regional nerve block for maxillary permanent molars. *Br. Dent. J.* 140 (3): 87–92.

Aggarwal, V., Singla, M., Miglani, S. et al. (2011). A prospective, randomized, single-blind comparative evaluation of anesthetic efficacy of posterior superior alveolar nerve blocks, buccal infiltration, and buccal plus palatal infiltrations in patients with irreversible pulpitis. *J. Endod.* 37 (11): 1491–1494.

Al-Delayme, R.-M.-A. (2014). A comparison of two anesthesia methods for surgical removal of maxillary third molars: PSA nerve block technique vs. local infiltration technique. *J. Clin. Exp. Dent.* 6 (1): e12–e16.

Annex 2. Infraorbital foramen.

Annex 21. Maxillary pulpal anesthesia: buccal infiltration.

Annex 22. Positive aspirations.

Annex 23. Pain resulting from injection techniques.

Annex 42. Grater palatine canal and foramen.

Austin, B.W. (1987). *Maxillary Nerve Block Anaesthesia (Thesis)*. Sydney (Australia): The University of Sydney. 279, 282.

Badcock, M.E., Gordon, I., and McCullough, M.J. (2007). A blinded randomized controlled trial comparing lignocaine and placebo administration to the palate for removal of maxillary third molars. *Int. J. Oral Maxillofac. Surg.* 36 (12): 1177–1182.

Bataineh, A.B. and Al-Sabri, G.A. (2017). Extraction of maxillary teeth using articaine without a palatal injection: a comparison between the anterior and posterior regions of the maxilla. *J. Oral Maxillofac. Surg.* 75 (1): 87–91.

Bennett, C.R. (1984). *Monheim's Local Anesthesia and Pain Control in Dental Practice*, 7e. St Louis (MI): The CV Mosby Company. 77, 81.

Berberich, G., Reader, A., Drum, M. et al. (2009). A prospective, ramdomized, double-blind comparison of the anesthetic efficacy of two percent lidocaine with 1:100,000 and 1:50,000 epinephrine and tree percent mepivacaine in intraoral, infraorbital nerve block. *J. Endod.* 35 (11): 1598–1504.

Broering, R., Reader, A., Beck, M., and Meyers, W. (1991). Evaluation of the second division nerve blocks in human maxillary anesthesia. *J. Endod.* 17 (4): 194 (Abstract no. 29).

Broering, R., Reader, A., Drum, M. et al. (2009). A prospective, randomized comparison of the anesthetic efficacy of the greater palatine and high tuberosity second division nerve blocks. *J. Endod.* 35 (10): 1337–1342.

Brunetto, P.C., Ranali, J., Ambrosano, G.M.B. et al. (2008). Anesthesia efficacy of 3 volumes of lidocaine with epinephrine in maxillary infiltration anesthesia. *Anesth. Prog.* 55 (2): 29–34.

Canan, S., Asim, O.M., Okan, B. et al. (1999). Anatomic variations of the infraorbital foramen. *Ann. Plast. Surg.* 43 (6): 613–617.

Canter, S.R., Slavkin, H.C., and Canter, M.R. (1964). Anatomical study of pterygopalatine fossa and canal: considerations applicable to the anesthetization of the second division of the fifth cranial nerve. *J. Oral Surg. Anesth. Hosp. Dent. Serv.* 22 (4): 318–323.

Carrea, J.U. (1921a). Anestesia troncular del nervio maxilar superior por el conducto palatino posterior. *La Odontología (Madrid)* 30 (6): 266–271.

Carrea, J.U. (1921b). Procedimientos de anestesias tronculares de los nervios maxilares. *La Odontología (Madrid)* 30 (9): 393–405.

Certosimo, A.J. and Archer, R.D. (1996). A clinical evaluation of the electric pulp tester as a indicator of local anesthesia. *Oper. Dent.* 21 (1): 25–30.

Ceylan, O.M., Mutlu, F.M., and Altinsoy, H.I. (2010). Transient binocular diplopia as a rare complication of local anesthesia (letter). *J. Pediatr. Ophthalmol. Strabismus* 47 (6): 381–382.

Chan, B.J., Koushan, K., Liszauer, A., and Martin, J. (2011). Iatrogenic globe penetration in a case of infraorbital nerve block (letter). *Can. J. Opthalmol.* 46 (3): 290–291.

Chentanez, V., Kaweewongprasert, S., Thunvarachorn, P., and Punrut, N. (1985). Position of greater palatine foramens, length and direction of greater palatine canals: anatomic study of 120 adult human skulls. *Chula. Med. J.* 29 (11): 1187–1197.

Cohn, S.A. (1986). The advantages of the greater palatine foramen block technique. *J. Endod.* 12 (6): 268–269.

Collon, D. (1946). Maxillary block anesthesia. *J. Am. Dent. Assoc.* 33 (15): 989–992.

Cook, W.A. (1949). The nerve supply to the maxillary incisors. *J. Oral. Surg. (Chicago)* 7 (2): 149–154.

Cook, W.A. (1950a). The anterior superior alveolar nerve and its control with local anesthetics. *Dent. Items Interest* 72 (10): 1021–1028.

Cook, W.A. (1950b). The second division block via the pterygopalatine canal. *Dent. Items Interest* 72 (12): 1270–1278.

Corbett, T.R. and Helmore, F.E. (1948). Block anaesthesia of the maxillary nerve via the greaterpalatine foramen. In: *Proceedings of the 11th Australian Dental Congress* (ed. K.F. Henderson and J.L. Prichard). Perth (WA). 137–145.

Corbett, I.P., Jaber, A.A., Whitworth, J.M., and Meechan, J.G. (2010). A comparison of the anterior middle superior alveolar nerve block and infraorbital nerve block for anesthesia of maxillary anterior teeth. *J. Am. Dent. Assoc.* 141 ((12): 1442–1448.

Cowan, A. (1964). Minimun dosage technique in clinical comparison of representative modern local anesthetic agents. *J. Dent. Res.* 43 (6): 1228–1249.

Dickson, G.C. and Coates, R.H. (1945). Regional anaesthesia of the maxillary nerve by the palatal method. *Br. Dent. J.* 79: 242–244.

Douglas, R. and Wormald, P.J. (2006). Pterygopalatine fossa infiltration through the greater palatine foramen; where to bend the needle. *Laryngoscope* 116 (7): 1255–1257.

DuBrul, E.L. (1988). *Sicher and Dubrul's Oral Anatomy*, 8e. St. Louis (MI): Ishiyaku EuroAmerica Inc. 269–284.

Evers, H. and Haegerstam, G. (1981). *Handbook of Dental Local Anesthesia*. Copenhagen: Schultz Medical Information. 74.

Feige, I. (1978). Technik und Erfolgsbewertung der Infraorbitalanästhesie be idem Zugangsweg entlang der Achse des 2, Prämolaren. *Stomatol. DDR* 28 (9): 649–653.

Ferreira, S.S., Reis, L.R., Gomes, J.C., and Ferreira, S.S. Jr. (1990). Analise do foramen palatinum majus e canalis palatinus major no esplancnocranio humano, para acesso ao bloqueio do nervus maxilaris. *Acta Biol. Paran* 19 (1–4): 1–19.

FitzGerald, M.J.T. and Scott, J.H. (1958). Observations on the anatomy of the superior dental nerves. *Br. Dent. J.* 104 (6): 205–208.

Forloine, A., Drum, M., Reader, A. et al. (2010). A prospective, randomized, double-blind comparison of the anesthetic efficacy two percent lidocaine 1:100,000 epinephrine and tree percent mepivacaine in the maxillary high tuberosity second division nerve block. *J. Endod.* 36 (11): 1770–1777.

Goldman, V. and Gray, W. (1963). A clinical trial of a new local analgesic agent. *Br. Dent. J.* 115 (2): 59–65.

Guglielmo, A., Drum, M., Reader, A., and Nusstein, J. (2011). Anesthetic efficacy a combination palatal and buccal infiltration of the maxillary first molar. *J. Endod.* 37 (4): 460–462.

Haglund, J. and Evers, H. (1985). *Local Anaesthesia in Dentistry*, 6e. Södertälje (Sweden): Astra Läkemedel AB. 31.

Harn, S.D., Durham, T.M., Callahan, B.P., and Kent, D.K. (2002). The triangle of safety: a modified posterior superior alveolar injection technique based on the anatomy of the PSA artery. *Gen. Dent.* 50 (6): 554–557.

Hayden, J. Jr. (1965). The innervation of the maxillary first permanent and primary molars a determinate by the deposition of local anesthetic solutions. A preliminary report. *Acta Odontol. Scand.* 23 (2): 147–162.

Heasman, P.A. (1984). Clinical anatomy of the superior alveolar nerves. *Br. J. Oral Maxillofac. Surg.* 22 (6): 439–447.

Hofer, O. (1922a). Die Leitungsästhesie des Nervus nasopalinus Scarpae bei stomatologischen Eingriffen. *Z. Stomatol.* 20: 411–416.

Hofer, O. (1922b). Die punktion des II. Trigeminusstammes vom gaumen aus. *Z. Stomatol.* 20 (6): 337–340.

Howard-Swirzinski, K., Edwards, P.C., Saini, T.S., and Norton, N.S. (2010). Length and geometric patterns of the greater palatine canal observed in cone beam computed tomography. *Int. J. Dent.* 292753. https://doi.org/10.1155/2010/292753.

Jastak, J.T., Yagiela, J.A., and Donaldson, D. (1995). *Local Anesthesia of the Oral Cavity*. Philadelphia: WB Saunders Co. 214, 216.

Jones, F.W. (1939). The anterior superior alveolar nerve and vessels. *J. Anat. (London)* 73 (Pt 4): 583–591.

Jorgensen, N.B. (1948). Measurements for intra-oral block of the maxillary nerve. *J. Oral Surg.* 6 (1): 1–8.

Jorgensen, N.B. and Hayden, J. Jr. (1970). *Anestesia odontológica*. Mexico DF: Editorial Interamericana SA. 34, 49. (Spanish translation of: Jorgensen, N.B and Hayden, J. Jr. (1967). *Premedication, Local and General Anesthesia in Dentistry*. Philadephia: Lea and Febiger).

Kadanoff, D., Mutafov, S.T., and Jordanov, J. (1970). Über die Hauptöffunngen resp. Incisurae des Gesichtsschädels (Incisurae frontalis seu Foramen frontale, Foramen supraorbitale seu Incisurae supraorbitalis, Foramen infraorbitale, foramen mentale). *Gegenbaurs Morphol. Jahrb.* 115 (1): 102–118.

Karkut, B., Reader, A., Drum, M. et al. (2010). A comparison of the local anesthetic efficacy of the extraoral versus the intraoral infraorbital nerve block. *J. Am. Dent. Assoc.* 141 (2): 185–192.

Kleier, D.J., Deeg, D.K., and Averbach, R.E. (1983). The extraoral approach to the infraorbital nerve block. *J. Am. Dent. Assoc.* 107 (5): 758–760.

Kramer, H.S. and Mitton, V.A. (1973). Complications of local anesthesia. *Dent. Clin. N. Am.* 17 (3): 443–460.

Kuscu, O.O., Scandalli, N., Calgar, E., and Meechan, J.G. (2014). Use of pre-injection diffusion of local anesthesia as a means of reducing needle penetration discomfort. *Acta Stomatol. Croat.* 48 (3): 193–198.

Kuster, C.G. and Udin, R.D. (1984). Frequency of hematoma formation subsequent to injection of dental local anesthetics in children. *Anesth. Prog.* 31 (3): 130–132.

Leo, J.T., Cassell, M.D., and Bergman, R.A. (1995). Variation in human infraorbital nerve, canal and foramen. *Ann. Anat.* 177 (1): 93–95.

Lepere, A.J. (1993). Maxillary nerve block via the greater palatine canal: new look at an old technique. *Anesth. Pain Control Dent.* 2 (4): 195–197.

Loetscher, C.A., Melton, D.C., and Walton, R.E. (1988). Injection regimen for anesthesia of the maxillary first molar. *J. Am. Dent. Assoc.* 117 (2): 337–340.

Malamed, S.F. (2004). *Handbook of Local Anesthesia*, 5e. St. Louis (Missouri): Elsevier-Mosby. 192–199.

Malamed, S.F. and Trieger, N. (1983). Intraoral maxillary nerve block: an anatomical and clinical study. *Anesth. Prog.* 30 (2): 44–48.

Maljaei, E., Pourkazemi, M., Ghanizadeh, M., and Ranjbar, R. (2017). The efficacy of buccal infiltration of 4% articaine and PSA injection of 2% lidocaine on anesthesia of maxillary second molars. *Iran Endod. J.* 12 (3): 276–281.

Martin, M.D., Ramsay, D.S., Whitney, C. et al. (1994). Topical anesthesia: differentiating the pharmacological and psychological contribution to efficacy. *Anesth. Prog.* 41 (2): 40–47.

McDaniel, V.M.L. (1956). Variations in nerve distributions of the maxillary teeth. *J. Dent. Res.* 35 (6): 916–921.

Meechan, J.G. and Day, P.F. (2002). A comparison of intraoral injection discomfort produced by plain and epinephrine-containinig lidocaine local anesthetic solutions: a randomized, double-blind, split-mouth, volunteer investigation. *Anesth. Prog.* 49 (2): 44–48.

Mercuri, L.G. (1979). Intraoral second division nerve block. *Oral Surg. Oral Med. Oral Pathol.* 47 (2): 109–113.

Methathrathip, D., Apinhasmit, W., Chompoopong, S. et al. (2005). Anatomy of greater palatine foramen and canal and pterygopalatine fossa in Thais: considerations for maxillary nerve block. *Surg. Radiol. Anat.* 27 (6): 511–516.

Mikesell, A., Reader, A., Beck, M., and Meyers, W. (1987). Analgesic efficacy of volumes of lidocaine in human maxillary infiltration. *J. Endod.* 13 (3): 128 (Abstract no. 3).

Moore, P.A., Boynes, S.G., Hersh, E.V. et al. (2006). The anesthetic efficacy of 4% articaine 1:200,000 epinephrine: two controlled clinical trials. *J. Am. Dent. Assoc.* 137 (11): 1572–1581.

Nevin, M. (1922). Blocking the superior maxillary nerve and its branches. *Dent. Items Interest* 44 (10): 740–749.

Nimigean, V., Nimigean, V.R., Buincu, L. et al. (2013). Anatomical and clinical considerations regarding the greater palatine foramen. *Romanian J. Morphol. Embryol.* 54 (3 Suppl): 779–783.

Padhye, M., Gupta, S., Chandiramani, G., and Bali, R. (2011). PSA block for maxillary molar's anesthesia – an obsolete technique? *Oral Surg. Oral Med. Oral Pathol.* 112 (6): e39–e43.

Paschos, E., Huth, K.C., Benz, C. et al. (2006). Efficacy of intraoral anesthetics in children. *J. Dent.* 34 (6): 398–404.

Peckham, R.N. (1938). Block anesthesia of the maxilla. *Am. J. Orthod. Oral Surg.* 24: 683–686.

Pfeil, L., Drum, M., Reader, A. et al. (2010). Anesthetic efficacy of 1.8 milliliters and 3.6 milliliters of 2% lidocaine with 1:100.000 epinephrine for posterior superior alveolar nerve blocks. *J. Endod.* 36 (4): 598–601.

Phillips, W.H. (1943). Anatomical considerations in local anesthesia in dental surgery. *Anesth. Analg.* 22 (1): 5–14.

Phillips, W.H. and Maxmen, H.A. (1941). The nasopalatine block injection as an aid in operative procedures for maxillary incisors. *Am. J. Orthod. Oral Surg.* 27 (8): 426–434.

Premdas, C.E. and Pitt Ford, T.R. (1995). Effect of palatal injections on pulpal blood flow in premolars. *Endod. Dent. Traumatol.* 11 (6): 274–278.

Ries Centeno, G.A. (1979). *Cirugía bucal*, 8e. Buenos Aires: Ed El Ateneo. 122.

Roberts, D.H. and Sowray, J.H. (1987). *Local Analgesia in Dentistry*, 3e. Bristol (UK): Wright. 105, 106.

Roda, R.S. and Blanton, P.L. (1994). The anatomy of the local anesthesia. *Quintessence Int.* 25 (1): 27–38.

Saborido, G. (1977). Anestesia troncular del nervio maxilar superior por vía transpalatina. *Bol. Inf. Dent. (Madrid)* 37 (287): 37–47.

Saeedi, O.J., Wang, H., and Blomquist, P.H. (2011). Penetrating globe injury during infraorbital nerve block. *Arch. Otolaryngol. Head Neck Surg.* 137 (4): 396–397.

Schwartz-Arad, E., Dolev, E., and Williams, W.P. (2002). Greater palatine nerve block – a new approach using a computer-controlled anesthetic delivery for maxillary sinus elevation procedures. *J. Dent. Res.* 81 (Special issue B): B-310. (Abstract no. 54).

Schwartz-Arad, E., Dolev, E., and Williams, W.P. (2004). Maxillary nerve block – a new approach using a computer-controlled anesthetic delivery system for maxillary sinus elevation procedure. A prospective study. *Quintessence Int.* 35 (6): 477–480.

Shalaby, S.A., Eid, E.M., Sarg, N.A.S., and Sewilam, A.M.A. (2015). Morphometric analysis of hard palate in Egyptian skulls. *Benha. Med. J.* 32 (1): 59–72.

Sharma, N.A. and Garud, R.S. (2013). Greater palatine foramen – key to successful hemimaxillary anaesthesia: a morphometric study and report of a rare aberration. *Singap. Med. J.* 54 (3): 152–159.

Sicher, H. (1950). Aspects in the applied anatomy of local anesthesia. *Int. Dent. J.* 1 (1): 70–82.

Silverman, S.L. (1923). Advances in block anesthesia, including an original technique of injecting the superior maxillary nerve. *Dent. Cosmos.* 65 (9): 974–977.

Slavkin, H.C., Canter, M.R., and Canter, S.R. (1966). An anatomic study of the pterygomaxillary region in the craneous of infants and children. *Oral Sug. Oral. Med. Oral Pathol.* 21 (2): 225–235.

Smith, A.E. (1920). *Block Anesthesia and Allied Subjects. With Special Chapters on the Maxillary Sinus, the Tonsils, and Neuralgias of the Nervous Trigeminus for Oral Surgeons, Dentists, Laryngologists, Rhinologists, Otologists, and Students.* St Louis (MO): CV Mosby Co. 380–386.

Sreekumar, K. and Bhargava, D. (2011). Comparison of onset and duration of action of soft tissue and pulpal anesthesia with three volumes of 4% articaine with 1:100,000 epinephrine maxillary infiltration anesthesia. *Oral Maxillofac. Sug.* 15 (4): 195–199.

Stone, J. and Kaban, L.B. (1979). Trismus after injection of local anesthetic. *Oral Surg. Oral Med. Oral Pathol.* 48 (1): 29–32.

Sved, A.M., Wong, J.D., Donkor, P. et al. (1992). Complications associated with maxillary nerve block anaesthesia via the greater palatine canal. *Aust. Dent. J.* 37 (5): 340–345.

Szerlip, L. and Morristown, N.J. (1950). A roentgenographic study of the pterygopalatine injection for blocking the maxillary nerve. *J. Oral Surg.* 8 (4): 327–330.

Torres, P.A., Sinning, N.C., Sagredo, K.B. et al. (2011). Relationship between of pterygopalatine fossa and block anesthesia of maxillary nerve. A pilot study. *Int. J. Morphol.* 29 (3): 857–861.

Ulusoy, Ö.I.A. and Alacam, T. (2014). Efficacy of single buccal infiltrations for maxillary first molars in patients with irreversible pulpitis: a randomized controlled trial. *Int. Endod. J.* 47 (3): 222–227.

Viegas, A.R. and Hemphill, F.M. (1961). Predicting depth of insertion of needle required to anesthetize the maxillary nerve by way of the pterygopalatine canal. *J. Oral Surg. Anesth. Hosp. Dent. Serv.* 19 (2): 105–109.

Weinand, F.S., Pavlovic, S., and Dick, B. (1997). Endophthalmitis nach enoraler Blockade des Nervus infraorbitalis. *Klin. Monatsbl. Augenheilkd.* 210 (5): 402–404.

Wong, J.D. and Sved, A.M. (1991). Maxillary nerve block anaesthesia via the greater palatine canal: a modified technique and case reports. *Aust. Dent. J.* 36 (1): 15–21.

# 15

# Maxillary Anesthesia II: Complementary Anesthesia of the Palate

## Introduction

Clinical experience shows that the buccal infiltrative technique applied via the buccal area does not usually anesthetize the palate, therefore some interventions must be completed with anesthesia of the palate, hence the concept of complementary anesthesia of the palate. In any case it is important to remember that the palate is innervated and that the fibromucosa, periosteum, and bone are innervated by two nerve trunks:

- The nasopalatine nerve, which emerges from the incisive foramen, supplies the area of the palate at the incisive papilla and the areas close to the central and lateral incisors.
- The greater palatine nerve, which emerges at the back part of the palate via the greater palatine foramen, supplies the palate in the canine, premolar, and molar areas on each side as far as the raphe.

This chapter reviews three techniques for anesthetizing the nerve trunks of the palate:

- Nasopalatine nerve block and its intranasal variant.
- Greater palatine nerve block and its variant in the area of cross-innervation extending from the first premolar to the lateral incisor.
- Transpapillary technique for children.

Some of the characteristics of the techniques used to anesthetize the palate are now reviewed.

## The Nasopalatine Nerve Innervates Less than Previously Thought

Many texts continue to attribute a much greater area of innervation to the nasopalatine nerve than it actually has (Bennett 1984; Jastak et al. 1995; Malamed 2004). Clinical research has shown that the area between the lateral incisor and the first premolar is an area of cross-innervation where the main supply is from the greater palatine nerve. Thus, the greater palatine nerve supplies the first premolar in 95% of cases, the canine in 75% of cases, and the lateral incisor in 50% (see Table 2.1, Chapter 2).

### The Potency of the Anesthetic is not Important

The potency of the anesthetic solution, according to the type and concentration of the anesthetic and/or vasoconstrictor, is not important for ensuring anesthesia of these nerves via the palate because they are superficial and not covered by periosteum or cortical bone, therefore little anesthetic is required to anesthetize the area.

### Anesthesia of the Palate Without Complementary Palatal Anesthesia

Clinical studies show that use of potent solutions such as articaine 4% with epinephrine 1:100 000 (10 µg/ml) (A-100) in extractions in the area of the molars and premolars principally is successful in 94% of cases with the buccal infiltrative technique. This approach does not require complementary palatal anesthetic, although patients may complain of mild discomfort in the palate. However, when the standard solution is used (lidocaine 2% with epinephrine 1:100 000) (L-100), the success rate falls to 55% (Table 15.1). Some authors recommend waiting longer (7–9 minutes) for the solution to reach the palate. In addition, this approach is more effective in anterior teeth than in posterior teeth (Kumaresan et al. 2015).

Studies based on magnetic resonance imaging do not reveal diffusion of the anesthetic solution from the buccal area to the palate (Özec et al. 2010); however, experimental

---

*Local Anesthesia in Dentistry: A Locoregional Approach*, First Edition. Jesús Calatayud and Mana Saraghi.
© 2024 John Wiley & Sons Ltd. Published 2024 by John Wiley & Sons Ltd.
Companion website: www.wiley.com/go/Calatayud/local

**Table 15.1** Success (%) of extraction of maxillary molars (M) and premolars (PM) after buccal infiltration with a potent anesthetic solution (A-100) or standard solution (L-100 or L-80) and no complementary palatal anesthetic.

| Reference | Sample size | Tooth | Solution ml/LAS/time (min) | Palatal anesthetic ml/LAS | Success (%) (proportion) |
|---|---|---|---|---|---|
| **No complementary anesthesia with A-100** | | | | | |
| Uckan et al. (2006) | 53 | — | 2.0/A-100/5′ | No | 96% (51/53) |
| Fan et al. (2009) | 71 | — | 1.7/A-100/5′ | No | 90% (64/71) |
| Lima-Junior et al. (2009) | 50 | 3rdM | 1.8/A-100/10′ | No | 94% (47/50) |
| Lima-Junior et al. (2013) | 15 | 3rdM | 1.8/A-100/5′ | No | 100% (15/15) |
| Somuri et al. (2013) | 30 | PM | 1.7/A-100/—— | No | 90% (27/30) |
| Darawade et al. (2014) | 50 | PM | 0.8/A-100/— | No | 100% (50/50) |
| Sharma et al. (2014) | 80 | M, PM | 0.9/A-100/— | No | 94% (75/80) |
| Kandasamy et al. (2015) | 116 | — | 1.7/A-100/10′ | No | 93% (106/116) |
| Bataineh and Al-Sabri (2017) | 48 | M, PM | 1.8/A-100/5′ | No | 92% (44/48) |
| Majid and Ahmed (2018) | 28 | M | 1.8/A-100/10′ | No | 86% (24/28) |
| Bataineh et al. (2019) | 50 | I, PM, M | 1.3/A-87/12′ | No | 94% (47/50) |
| | | | | Mean | **94%** |
| **No complementary anesthesia with L-100** | | | | | |
| Badcock et al. (2007) | 51 | 3rdM | 2.2/L-80/5′ | No | 86% (44/51) |
| Lassemi et al. (2008) | 30 | IC | 1.8/L-80/6′ | No | 77% (23/30) |
| Darawade et al. (2014) | 50 | PM | 1.3/L-100/— | No | 2% (1/50) |
| Kandasamy et al. (2015) | 111 | — | 1.7/L-80/10′ | No | 1% (1/111) |
| Kumaresan et al. (2015) | 25 | M | 1.5/L-80/7–9′ | No | 52% (13/25) |
| Majid and Ahmed (2018) | 28 | M | 3.6/L-100/10′ | No | 86% (24/28) |
| Bataineh et al. (2019) | 50 | I, PM, M | 1.3/L-75/10′ | No | 96% (48/50) |
| | | | | Mean | **55%** |

N, sample size; ml, milliliters injected; LAS, local anesthetic solution; A-100, articaine 4% + epinephrine 1:100 000 (10 μg/ml); A-87, articaine 4% + epinephrine 1:87 000 (11.5 μg/ml); L-100, lidocaine 2% + epinephrine 1:100 000 (10 μg/ml); L-80, lidocaine 2% + epinephrine 1:80 000 (12.5 μg/ml); L-75, lidocaine 2% + epinephrine 1:75 000 (13.3 μg/ml); 5 is 5 minutes waiting time after administering the anesthetic.

animal studies did find concentrations of anesthetic solution in the bone and the mucous membrane of the palate. These are greater with A-100 than with L-100 (Al-Mahalawy et al. 2018). Reported findings are contradictory.

Nevertheless, when complementary palatal anesthetic is used, irrespective of whether it is with A-100 or L-100, the success rate is practically 100% (Table 15.2).These successes in the third maxillary molars may be due to the fact that extraction at this level is relatively simple and rapid (less than 1 minute in most cases) and that the depth of anesthesia necessary for these extractions is lower than that needed in other procedures, such as endodontic procedures (Badcock et al. 2007). However, extraction of first molars may take longer (around 4 minutes) and be more complicated, although it is also successful, and extractions with complementary palatal anesthetic are more comfortable for the patient (Majid and Ahmed 2018).

## Indications

These techniques are not aimed at achieving pulpal anesthesia (Hicks et al. 1995), but rather at providing complementary anesthesia of the palate in the following cases:

1) Dental surgery and extractions (Roberts and Sowray 1987; Evers and Haegerstam 1981).
2) Reinforcing pulpal anesthesia after a buccal infiltration in healthy teeth (Guglielmo et al. 2011) or in the case of irreversible acute pulpitis (Aggarwal et al. 2011;

Table 15.2 Success (%) of extraction of maxillary molars (M) and premolars (PM) after buccal infiltration, based on a potent anesthetic (A-100) or the standard solution (L-100 or L-80) with complementary palatal anesthesia.

| Reference | Sample size | Tooth | Solution ml/LAS/time (min) | Palatal anesthetic ml/LAS | Success (%) (proportion) |
|---|---|---|---|---|---|
| **Complementary anesthesia with L-100** | | | | | |
| Uckan et al. (2006) | 53 | — | 1.8/L-100/5' | 0.5/L-100 | 98% (52/53) |
| Lassemi et al. (2008) | 30 | IC | —/L-80/6' | —/L80 | 100% (30/30) |
| Somuri et al. (2013) | 30 | PM | 1.8/L-100/— | 0.25/L-100 | 100% (30/30) |
| Sharma et al. (2014) | 80 | M, PM | 1.8/L-100/— | —/L-100 | 100% (80/80) |
| Kumaresan et al. (2015) | 25 | M | 1.5/L-80/2' | 0.3/L-80 | 100% (25/25) |
| Bataineh et al. (2019) | 55 | I, PM, M | 0.9/L-75/7' | 0.2/L-75 | 100% (55/55) |
| | | | | Mean | 99.6% ≈ **100%** |
| **Complementary anesthesia with A-100** | | | | | |
| Fan et al. (2009) | 71 | — | 1.7/A-100/5' | 0.4/A-100 | 95% (67/71) |
| Lima-Junior et al. (2009) | 100 | 3M | 1.8/A-100/5–10' | —/A-100 | 100% (100/100) |
| Majid and Ahmed (2018) | 28 | M | 1.8/A-100/10' | 0.2/A-100 | 100% (28/28) |
| | | | | Mean | 98.3 ≈ **100%** |

N, sample size; ml, milliliters injected; LAS, local anesthetic solution; A-100, articaine 4% + epinephrine 1:100 000 (10 μg/ml); L-100, lidocaine 2% + epinephrine 1:100 000 (10 μg/ml); L-80, lidocaine 2% + epinephrine 1:80 000 (12.5 μg/ml); L-75, lidocaine 2% + epinephrine 1:75 000 (13.3 μg/ml); 5 is 5 minutes waiting time after administering the anesthetic.

Ulusoy and Alacam 2014; Askari et al. 2016), given that in teeth with palatal roots the percentage of pulpal anesthesia increases.

3) Scaling and root planing.
4) Subgingival preparations in the palate:
   o Restorations.
   o Restorations by cervical caries.
   o Placement of a retraction cord.
   o Gingival retraction in the palate.
5) Insertion of subgingival matrix bands at the level of the palate (Malamed 2004).
6) Placement of clamps for a dental dam that penetrate or pinch the mucous membrane of the palate.

## Methods for Reducing Pain in Palatal Techniques

Clinical observation tells us that injections into the palate are the most painful (Kramp et al. 1999; Wahl et al. 2001; Primosch and Brooks 2002). Clinical studies confirm this observation (Annexes 19 and 23). This is because the palatal fibromucosa is formed by dense fibers, with little subcutaneous tissue, and is firmly attached to the periosteum. Consequently, elasticity is minimal, the ability to spread after administration is limited, and the technique is painful (Gill and Orr II 1979; Keller 1985; Kreider et al. 2001; Bhalla et al. 2009). In addition, the anterior part of the palate is known to be somewhat more painful than the posterior part, precisely because the fibromucosa is more firmly attached (Meechan et al. 2005; Özec et al. 2010).

Several methods are used to prevent or at least minimize the pain induced by injection into the palate. However, as expected, when several methods are available and no consensus has been reached on which is best, this is because neither is completely satisfactory.

### Topical Anesthesia

Topical anesthesia is poorly effective in the palate, as shown in clinical trials (Annex 19). These poor results are due not only to previous comments (fibromucosa firmly attached to the periosteum), but also to the fact that because the mucous membrane of the palate is more keratinized, its permeability is lower than that of the rest of the oral mucous membrane (Lesch et al. 1989), leading to reduced penetration of topical anesthetic.

In any case, topical anesthesia reduces the average perception of pain compared with placebo, although the differences are not significant.

## Pressure Techniques

**Conventional methods** (Malamed 2004)

These techniques involve applying firm and continuous pressure with a cotton swab (e.g. those used for application of topical anesthesia) on the surface of the mucous membrane of the palate to be injected for 20–30 seconds before insertion. The pressure should be sufficiently firm for the mucous membrane to change from its usual pink color to a white or pale color owing to the blanching caused by the pressure applied. The injection should be made very close to the head of the swab, and pressure should be maintained throughout the injection.

**"Press and roll" technique** (Kravitz 2006)

Inform the patient that you are about to place topical anesthetic on the palate (optional, although it does reassure the patient) and that he/she will feel considerable pressure on the palate during the maneuver.

- Dry the mucous membrane with a gauze.
- Cover the area with topical anesthesia and leave it for about 1–2 minutes (optional).
- Apply pressure on the area of the palate to be injected with the end of the shaft of a dental mirror.
- Insert the needle while pressing it against the shaft of the mirror, almost pushing it below the shaft and at the same time press with the shaft.
- Inject a few drops of anesthetic and then turn the shaft of the mirror toward the needle. Inject for only 3–5 seconds. This maneuver leaves the mucous membrane white or pale owing to the blanching induced by the pressure (Figure 15.1).
- Remove the needle, remove the shaft of the mirror, and wait a minute for the few drops of anesthetic solution to take effect and the soft tissues at the injection site to become anesthetized.
- After aspirating, reinsert the needle at the same site to inject a larger quantity of anesthesia ($\pm 1/8$ of a cartridge or 0.25 ml) slowly (7–10 seconds) and wait a further 30 seconds. A small amount of anesthetic is preferred to a large amount to reinforce the previous amount and ensure that the palate starts to become anesthetized.

This technique is fairly fast without topical anesthetic.

Pressure maneuvers act by activating the gate control system in the trigeminal nerve nuclei. This partially inhibits the passage of pain stimuli to higher pathways, thus helping the stimulus to remain below the pain threshold (Melzack and Wall 1965; Dubner 1978) (see Chapter 11).

## Topical Cooling

Cold reduces the velocity of nerve conduction, which ceases when the temperature falls from 10 to 0 °C (Harbert 1989), thus inducing anesthesia. Topical cooling techniques are used before injection of palatal local anesthesia to ensure that the procedure is as painless as possible. The only contraindication would be in patients who cannot tolerate cold (Harbert 1989).

There are three different approaches: (i) old cold aerosols, like ethyl chloride; (ii) refrigerants, only used on the palate (Duncan et al. 1992; Kosaraju and Vandewalle 2009; Wiswall et al. 2014); and (iii) topical ice. All these methods are explained in Chapter 12.

## Periodontal Ligament Technique

This technique was first proposed by Dr. Barry McArdle as being almost painless (McArdle 1997; Aslin 2001).

- In the first stage, buccal infiltration is used to anesthetize the buccal gingiva and the buccal part of the papillae of the tooth at the point on the palate to be anesthetized. This maneuver may take some time since, as the anesthesia begins to take effect, it is necessary to inject into the attached gingiva while moving gradually toward the interdental papilla.
- A high-pressure pistol-grip syringe for the periodontal ligament technique is prepared with an extrashort needle (8–12 mm, 27 G or 30 G). In posterior teeth, it may be necessary to deflect the needle halfway up the shaft, but never at the hub, which is where the needle can break.

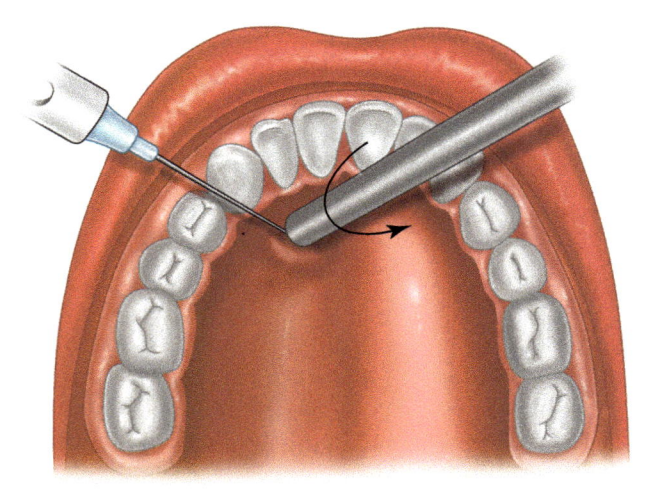

**Figure 15.1** Needle inserted under the tip of the shaft. The exact point at which a few drops are injected and the shaft turns toward the needle while applying pressure. *Source:* Redrawn from Kravitz (2006).

- The needle is inserted carefully into the papilla, in the anesthetized mesiobuccal area, and the injection is performed slowly with careful application of pressure. The papilla will blanche and the pale area will gradually extend toward the palatal part of the papilla. As the pressure builds up, the blanching extends toward the neighboring palatal area.
- The maneuver can be repeated in the distal-buccal papilla. If a greater area of the palate is to be covered, then the needle can be inserted into the area of the palate affected by blanching to slowly inject while gradually applying pressure and thus extending the anesthetized blanched area.

This method rarely leads to palatal ulceration induced by ischemia. If this does occur, it resolves spontaneously in a few days.

### Minimal Intervention Technique

The minimum technique, or minimum intervention technique (minimum volume/minimum injection time), has already been examined in the buccal infiltration technique (Chapter 14). Its advantages are that it is fast, does not require special equipment, and can be carried out in combination with other techniques such as pressure or cold (if so desired) to enhance its efficacy. The technique involves the following steps:

1) Warn the patient that he/she "will feel some discomfort" in the palate when the anesthetic is administered. Stress that this "will be very quick." This prepares the patient psychologically, since unexpected events are perceived as being more painful; in addition, during the painless part of administration, the patient relaxes, reassured by the explanation (Jackson 1974; Wepman 1978).
2) insert the needle 2–4 mm into the palate in the area to be treated and inject only one or two drops of solution over 1–2 seconds. Wait 60 seconds after removing the needle. This ensures that the soft tissue at the injection site is anesthetized.
3) Once again, inject one or two drops at the same site (this is usually the same blood spot from the first injection) over 1–2 seconds, only this time wait 30 seconds.
4) After aspirating, inject a greater quantity of anesthetic (±1/8 of a cartridge, 0.25 ml) slowly over 7–10 seconds at the same site and wait a further 30 seconds. Do not inject a large quantity, but rather small quantities to complement the previous injections and begin anesthesia of the palate.

*Notes*

- With respect to perception of pain, patients expect the second injection to be more painful than the first (Martin et al. 1994; Paschos et al. 2006; Badcock et al. 2007; Kuscu et al. 2014). Injecting the initial drops induces anesthesia in the soft tissue and thus largely resolves the problem.
- It is important to remember that pain is felt somewhat less intensely in the posterior part of the hard palate than in the anterior part (Meechan et al. 2005; Özec et al. 2010) because the fibromucosa is less dense and less attached to the periosteum, therefore this technique is particularly successful in the posterior part.
- In practice, many clinicians use their own methods, which involve a mix of those described above.

## Nasopalatine Nerve Block

In older books, this technique is also known as Scarpa's nasopalatine nerve or long sphenopalatine nerve block technique or the incisive or retroincisive canal injection technique.

In fact, the technique involves double anesthesia, since both nasopalatine nerves (right and left), which emerge together via a single incisive foramen, are anesthetized simultaneously (Phillips and Maxmen 1941).

### Anesthetized Area

This area corresponds to the fibromucosa, periosteum, and palatine bone (Table 2.1 and Figure 2.7, Chapter 2). The areas anesthetized are as follows:

- 100% of the interincisive papilla.
- 100% of the palate behind the central incisors.
- 50% of the palate behind the lateral incisors.
- 25% of the palate behind the canines on both sides.
- 5% of the palate, together with the first premolar on both sides.

### Technique

- Short 27 G needle (20–25 mm).
- Position of the dentist and patient:
  - The dentist is at 11:00 o'clock.
  - The patient is reclines with his/her head back and neck extended (hyperextension). The patient's mouth is open as wide as possible so that the dentist can see the palate directly.

The patient's head can turn slightly to the right or left, depending on the needs of the dentist.

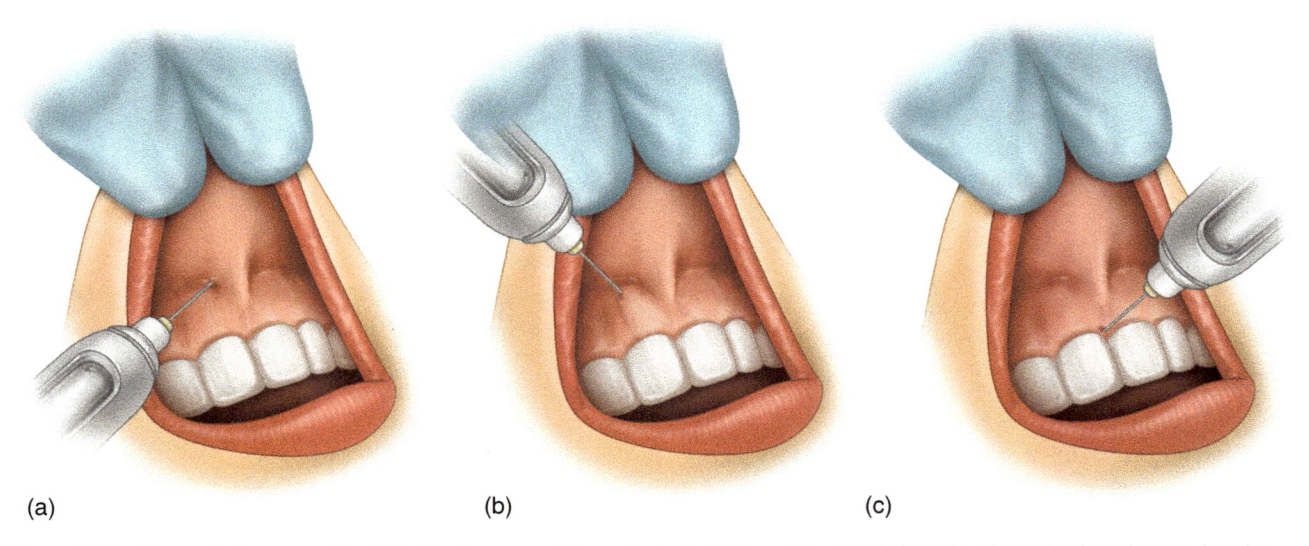

**Figure 15.2** Nasopalatine nerve block. Indirect approach from the buccal area: (a) buccal infiltration from the frenulum and under the maxillary central incisors, (b) insertion and infiltration in the gingiva oriented toward the interdental papilla, and (c) perpendicular insertion that crosses the interdental papilla toward the palatine nerve.

- Approach the interincisive papilla, which is situated on the palate, immediately behind and between the central incisors along the midline. There are two methods, as follows:

1) **Indirect approach from the buccal area**
   Since the papilla is in one of the most sensitive and painful areas of the mouth, many authors prefer an indirect approach before injecting directly into the papilla (Salagaray and Salagaray 1982; Bennett 1984; Malamed 1986), therefore they infiltrate via the buccal area. It is also important to remember that pain is also felt more intensely in the anterior part of the buccal area at the maxilla, although less so than the palate (Annex 23), therefore the technique should be performed very carefully.
   - Buccal infiltration technique applied via the buccal area between the central incisors at the level of the frenulum using the minimum intervention technique (see Chapter 14) (Figure 15.2a). Remember that while in this stage, the patient's position must be modified in order to approach the anterior buccal area of the maxilla and not the palate. Then wait 30–60 seconds for the anesthetic to take effect in the soft tissue.
   - The submucosal bulge can be gently massaged for a short time in order to extend the anesthetic solution throughout the soft tissue. Excessive massage will hamper successful pulpal anesthesia.
   - From the area of the oral mucous membrane of the anesthetized frenulum, one can gradually infiltrate along the attached gingiva close to the interdental papilla of the central incisors. Gingival blanching is an indicator of the extent of the anesthetized area (Figure 15.2b). Then, wait 30 seconds.
   - Insert the needle perpendicularly into the interdental papilla of the central incisors from the buccal area, immediately above what is estimated to be the top of the alveolar ridge (if the needle comes into contact with the bone, raise it a little more to pass over it), thus ensuring that the needle crosses from the buccal area to the palate (Figure 15.2c).
   - The needle initially penetrates the palate to a small degree. Inject a few drops under some pressure and observe the blanching of the interincisive papilla or of the part that is closest to the buccal area. Wait some 15–30 seconds before withdrawing the needle to prevent reflux of the anesthetic solution as a result of the pressure (remember that the fibromucosa is attached).
   - Repeat the maneuver by inserting the needle perpendicularly via the buccal area (the position is generally indicated by a blood spot), thus penetrating more deeply into the palate in the interincisive papilla, and inject a few additional drops. Once again, blanching of the interincisve papilla can be observed.

   There are several problems associated with the indirect approach.

- Since this method is time-consuming, many clinicians use it when nasopalatine nerve block is applied as a complement to buccal infiltration of the anterior maxilla.
- When the needle is inserted perpendicularly from the buccal area, it falls just within the patient's field of vision and may prove somewhat uncomfortable in psychological terms (Malamed 1986).

2) **Direct approach**
   - Press the interincisive papilla firmly with the tip of a cotton swab, a little bar of ice, or the end of the shaft of the mirror (see Methods for making palatal anesthesia less painful).
   - The papilla should be injected laterally from the palate in the area where pressure is being applied (lateral groove of the papilla that separates the papilla from the palate) to 1–2 mm (Figure 15.3). Inject one or two drops in 1–2 seconds (minimum intervention technique) and wait 30 seconds.
   - The maneuver should be repeated to inject a further one to two drops in 1–2 seconds so that the whole papilla can be anesthetized.
- Anesthesia of the maxillary incisive canal, which is immediately below the papilla. The procedure is as follows:
  - Insert the needle perpendicularly into the interincisive papilla along the axis of the buccal plate of the central incisors (Phillips and Maxmen 1941; Annex 41) (Figure 15.4).
  - Advance the needle to a depth of 5–10 mm (Figure 15.4). Remember that the foramen is 2–4 mm below the papilla.
  - Aspirate before injecting. Positive aspirations are observed in approximately 1% of cases (Annex 22).

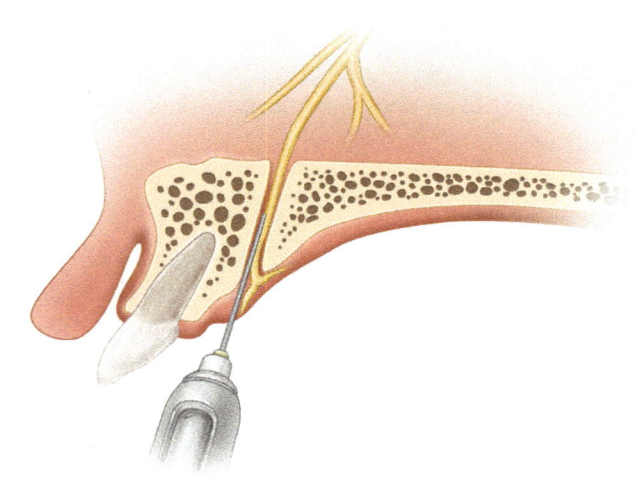

**Figure 15.4** Insert the needle following the axis of the central incisors and advance 5–10 mm in the maxillary incisive canal.

  - Slowly inject a few drops of anesthetic (<1/8 of a cartridge, <0.2 ml), and the papilla will begin to blanch.
- The subjective symptoms of anesthesia, i.e. the soft tissue anesthesia that patients define as dullness, numbness, or tingling (Table 13.1, Chapter 13), appear in 1 minute in the anterior part of the palate. This is more obvious when the patient touches the area with his/her tongue.
- Anesthesia is complete in 2–3 minutes and lasts 1–2 hours (80 minutes). The patient should be informed about this.

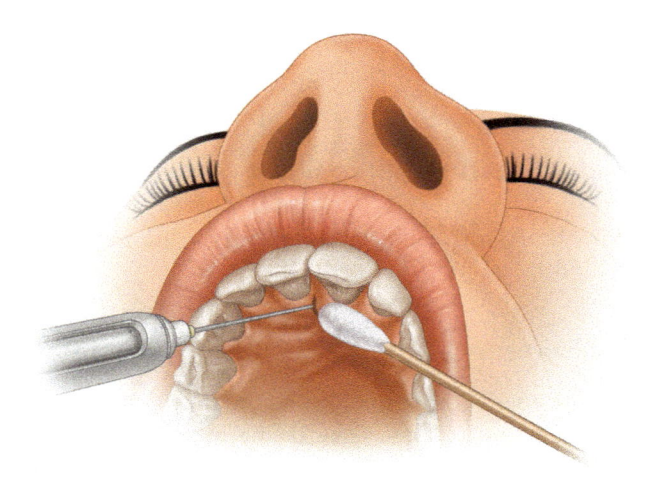

**Figure 15.3** With the papilla under pressure from the cotton swab, the needle is inserted laterally into the papilla.

### Specific Complications of This Technique

The technique has few complications and the most relevant are the following:

1) Inflammation and reddening (erythema) of the interincisive papilla after the procedure. Hematoma appears more rarely and sterile abscess caused by mucosal necrosis is even more exceptional. The complications are usually caused by the high volume of anesthetic injected or the anesthetic being injected too quickly, since the capacity of the palatal fibromucosa to distend is very limited at this level. The lesions resolve spontaneously in a few days.
2) Trophic ulcer is a possible complication, although very rare (Hartenian and Stenger 1976) (see Chapter 22 on local complications).

3) Overpenetration of the needle by more than 10 mm in the incisive canal can cause the anesthetic solution to enter the nostril and cross the choanae to the pharynx, thus leaving the patient with a sensation of liquid in his/her throat.

### Intranasal Variant

The nasopalatine nerve cannot be anesthetized via the interincisive papilla when this is infected, therefore the nerve is blocked at the level of the nasal septum, immediately before entering the interincisive canal, since at this level it is immediately below the nasal mucosa of the septum (Birn and Winther 1977; Evers and Haegerstam 1981; Haglund and Evers 1985). This method has the disadvantage of being less efficacious than the previous method since it requires the diffusion of a topical anesthetic, which is weaker.

### Technique

- The patient's nose must be perfectly clean and the mouth must remain open to enable breathing.
- With the cotton tip soaked in topical anesthetic (generally benzocaine 20% or lidocaine 5% gel, ointment, cream, or paste), the swabs should be inserted via the nostrils first on one side and then on the other using the following method:
  - Insert the swab upwards and backwards so that it enters the nostril (Figure 15.5).
  - Once the swab is inside the nostril, adjust the position by placing it horizontally to the floor of the nose.
  - Insert the swab approximately 15–20 mm into the nostril while maintaining contact with the floor of the nose and septum (Figure 15.6).

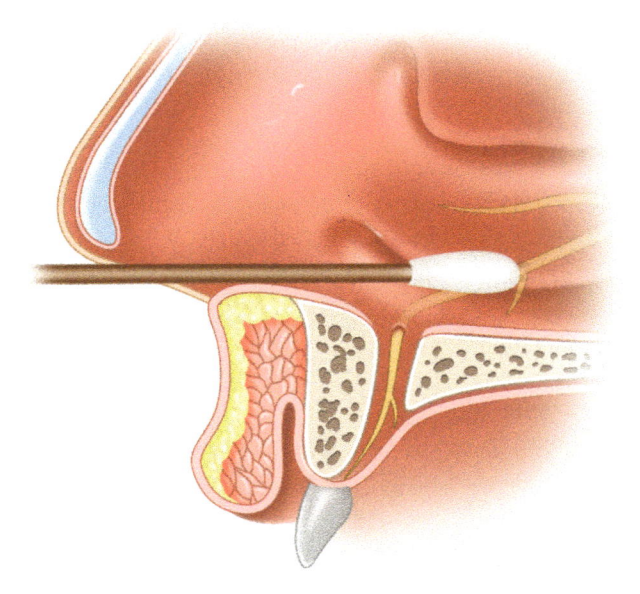

**Figure 15.6** Swabs in contact with the nasal septum and floor. Note how far they extend into the nasal cavity. *Source:* Redrawn from Birn and Winther (1977).

- With the swab in position, wait 1–3 minutes for the anesthetic to take effect (Figure 15.5).
- The subjective symptoms of anesthesia may appear after 1–3 minutes in the anterior part of the palate and become more obvious when the patient touches the interincisive papilla with the tip of the tongue.
- Before starting the procedure, it is necessary to do the following:
  - Remove the swabs from the nostrils to facilitate work on the mouth.
  - Allow the patient to blow his/her nose to remove any remaining topical anesthetic and to relieve nasal discomfort (mucus and itching).

## Greater Palatine Nerve Block

In older books, this technique is known as anterior palatine nerve block.

### Area Anesthetized

The area anesthetized corresponds to the fibromucosa, periosteum, and palatine bone in the part to be treated (Table 2.1 and Figure 2.7, Chapter 2), as follows:

- 100% of the molars on the respective side.
- 100% of the second premolars on the respective side.
- 95% of the first premolars on the respective side.

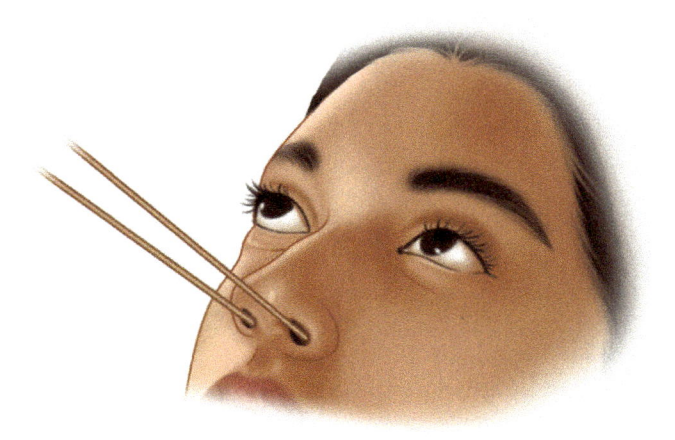

**Figure 15.5** Placement of the cotton swabs inside the nostrils. *Source:* Redrawn from Birn and Winther (1977).

- 75% of the canines on the respective side.
- 50% of the palate behind the lateral incisor on the respective side.

## Technique

- Short 27 G needle (20–25 mm).
- Position of the dentist and patient:
  - The dentist is positioned as follows:
    - 8:00–9:00 o'clock for the right side.
    - 11:00–12:00 o'clock for the left side.
  - The patient lies down with his/her head backward, the neck extended (hyperextension), and the mouth open as wide as possible so that the dentist can see the palate directly. The patient's head can turn toward the right for block of the right side and slightly to the left for block of the left side.
- Location of the insertion point. With this technique, it is not necessary to accurately locate the greater palatine foramen, since we are going to block the nerve in front of it.
  - The nerve is found at the junction of the horizontal hard palate with the vertical alveolar process (Westmoreland and Blanton 1982; Malamed and Trieger 1983); *in approximately 85% of cases it lies around the third molar* (Annex 42) (Figure 14.15, Chapter 14). The third molar zone is the area ranging from a point slightly forward of the third molar (between it and the second molar) to a point slightly backward of the third molar and including the third molar zone (Annex 42). Thus, the injection point is in front of the second molar and at the midpoint between the palatal gingival festoon of the second molar and the palatine raphe, in other words, some 15 mm toward the palatine raphe.
  - If the molars are missing, the reference is take as a point 10–15 mm in front of the limit between the hard palate (pale gray mucosa) and the soft palate (dark red mucosa) (Mercuri 1979; Wong and Sved 1991). It is also possible to inject in the area where the fibromucousa of the palate is thicker and the connective tissue laxer.
  - Clinical studies have shown that anesthesia of the soft tissues of the hard palate lasts longer when the anesthetic is administered in front of the greater palatine foramen (Meechan et al. 2000).
- The needle is directed from the opposite side; if it is to be inserted into the right side of the palate, it is directed from the left side and vice versa. If necessary, the lower premolars on the contralateral side can be used for support (Figure 15.7).
- The needle is inserted and injected using the *minimum intervention technique*, as explained above (minimum volume/minimum injection time) to reduce the pain of the injection into the palate.

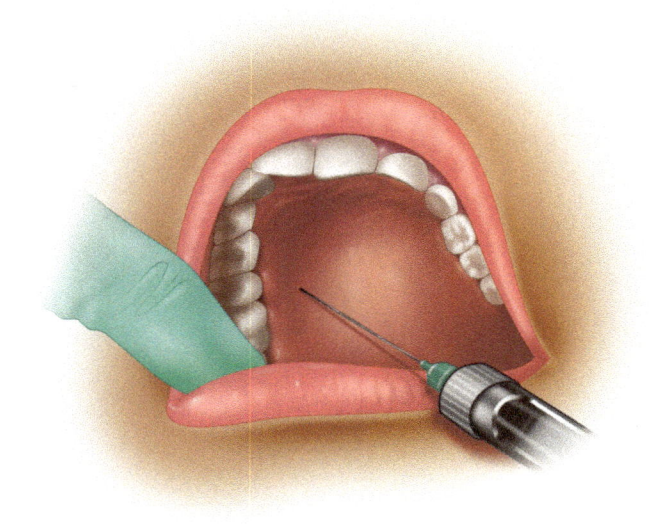

**Figure 15.7** Greater palatine nerve block. The needle is inserted from the opposite side.

  - Warn the patient that he/she will feel some "discomfort" when the anesthetic is injected into the palate, but emphasize that this will be "very quick." Prepare the patient psychologically, given that unexpected painful events are perceived as being more painful; in addition, during the nonpainful periods of administration, allow the patient to relax, reassured by explanations (Jackson 1974; Wepman 1978).
  - Press firmly on the area to be injected with the head of a cotton swab or bar of ice or the end of the shaft of the mirror (see section on methods for making palatal anesthesia less painful).
  - Inject perpendicularly into the palatal fibromucosa where pressure is being applied. Insert the needle a few millimeters (2–5 mm, it is not necessary to reach the bone) (Figure 15.8), inject only a few drops of anesthetic in 1–2 seconds, and wait 60 seconds after withdrawing the needle. This ensures that the soft tissues at the injection site are anesthetized.
  - Repeat the maneuver and then inject one or two drops at the same site (the blood spot created by the first injection is usually visible) in 1–2 seconds and this time wait only 30 seconds.
  - Finally, at the same site, inject a larger amount of anesthetic (±1/8 of a cartridge, ±0.25 ml) slowly in 7–10 seconds after aspiration and wait a further 30 seconds. Note that a large amount is not injected, but

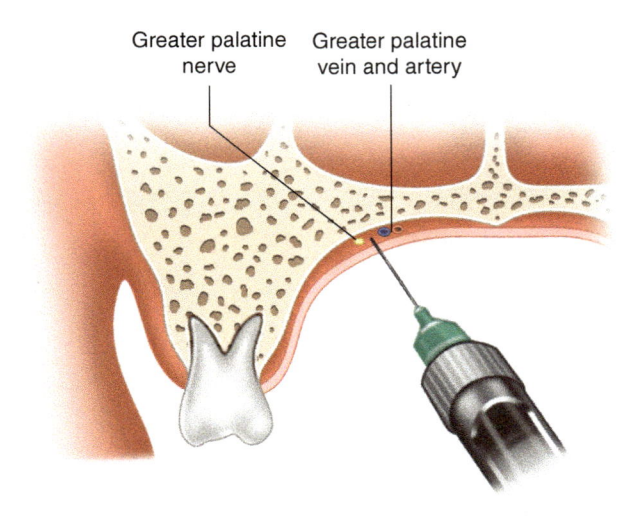

**Figure 15.8** The needle is inserted perpendicularly into the palate. It is not necessary to reach the bone.

rather a small amount to reinforce the previous injections and thus begin anesthesia of the palate.
- The aspiration is positive in approximately 1% of cases (Annex 22).
- The subjective symptoms of anesthesia, i.e. the soft tissue anesthesia that patients define as dullness, numbness, or tingling (Table 13.1, Chapter 13), appear in 1 minute in the hard palate on the same side, from the midline to the area of the molars and premolars. It is important to remember that the tissues of the palate behind the injection site are not anesthetized.
- Anesthesia is completed in 2–3 minutes and lasts around 2 hours (130 minutes). The patient should be told about this.

### Specific Complications of This Technique

While this technique has few complications, the following should be noted.

1) Inflammation and reddening (erythema) at the injection site, which becomes apparent after the procedure. Hematoma resulting from puncture of a vessel is more unusual. Even more uncommon is the appearance of a sterile abscess resulting from necrosis of the mucosa. This is usually caused by injecting too much anesthetic or injecting too quickly, since the capacity of the palatal fibromucosa to distend is limited. The lesions resolve spontaneously in a few days.
2) Injecting too far back and anesthetizing the lesser palatine nerves (previously known as the posterior palatine nerves). In this case, anesthesia affects the velum of the palate, the uvula, the tonsillar pillars (oropharyngeal isthmus), and the soft palate, thus potentially leading the patient to retch, feel nauseous, and experience the subjective sensation of not being able to swallow. In such cases, reassure the patient and inform him/her that it is possible to swallow because the muscular (motor) structures have not been anesthetized or have only been so partially and that only the sensitive part has been anesthetized. In addition, when the anesthetic wears off, the discomfort disappears (Allen 1979; Jastak et al. 1995).

### Partial Variant of the Palate

As we have seen, the area of the palate covering the lateral incisor and first premolar is an area where the fibers of the nasopalatine and greater palatine nerve cross (Phillips and Maxmen 1941; Langford 1989), therefore direct injection here makes it possible to anesthetize the area (Nordenram 1971; Allen 1979).

The technique is practically the same as that used for greater palatine nerve block, although it is performed more anteriorly (Figure 15.9) (Roberts and Sowray 1987).

## Transpapillary Technique in Children

In children, palatal techniques can be very painful, leading to uncontrolled reactions and loss of trust in the dentist (Roberts and Sowray 1987; Jastak et al. 1995). Techniques for making palatal anesthesia less painful

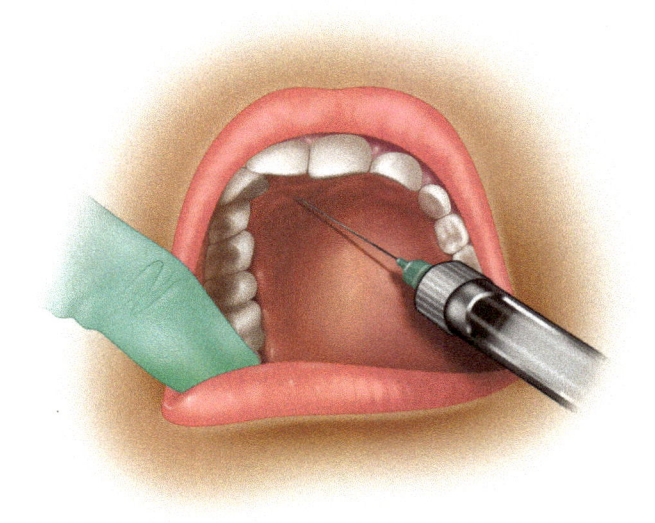

**Figure 15.9** More anterior block in the area where the greater palatine nerve and nasopalatine nerve cross.

may prove ineffective in children (Harbert 1989), therefore an indirect approach from the buccal area across the interdental papilla (intrapapillary technique) is used.

### Technique

- Infiltrate buccally, close to the teeth where the palate is to be treated, using the minimum intervention technique (minimum volume/minimum injection time) (see Chapter 14). Wait 1–2 minutes until the mucosa has been anesthetized.
- Insert the needle into the attached gingiva, close to the area anesthetized using buccal infiltration and infiltrate a few drops while applying pressure. Blanching of the gingiva can be observed. Wait 30 seconds for the anesthetic to take effect.
- Insert the needle at the limit of the blanched attached gingiva and direct it toward the interdental papilla. Slowly infiltrate a few drops of anesthesia while applying pressure and observe the resulting blanching. Wait a further 30 seconds.
- Insert the needle perpendicularly into the papilla from the buccal area toward the palate, immediately above the approximate area of the alveolar ridge (if contact is made with the ridge and the needle cannot advance, repeat the maneuver a little higher up to pass over the bone), but without the needle crossing the palate (Figure 15.10). Inject a few drops under pressure and observe the resulting blanching in the palatal gingiva near the papilla. Wait 30 seconds for the anesthetic to take effect.

An old trick used by some pediatric dentists during this maneuver is to place a thick cotton roll between the teeth and ask the child to bite down on it while the buccal mucosa is being separated. Thus, the child's attention is distracted and the dentist has more buccal space in which to work.

- Repeat the above maneuver, although this time inserting the needle a little further along on the palatal gingiva (Figure 15.11) and slowly injecting a few drops of anesthetic with a certain degree of pressure. It is very important not to perforate the palatal mucous membrane with the needle since this would lead to injection outside and leave a hole in the palatal gingiva that prevents pressure from being applied during the injection (and thus infiltrating the attached tissue appropriately). In addition, perforation favors leakage of the anesthetic solution to the outside.
- As applicable, the area of the palate anesthetized can be widen using the same system by inserting the needle into the peripheral anesthetized area (blanched area) and slowly infiltrating a few drops under pressure and observing how the area of blanching and therefore the anesthetized area extend.

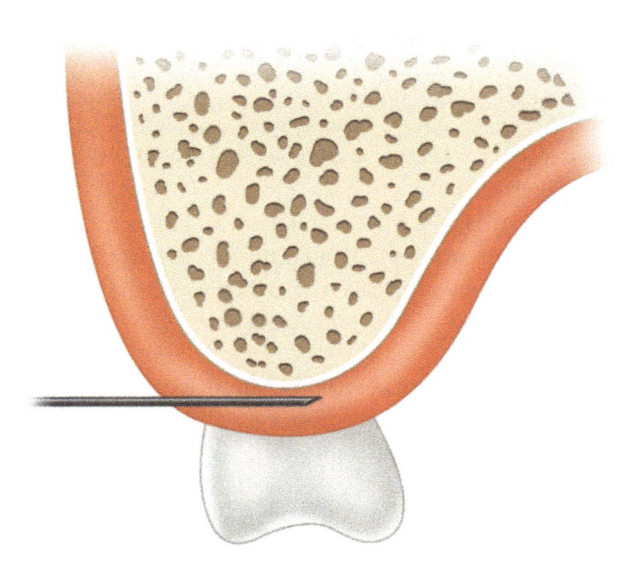

**Figure 15.10** Transpapillary technique. Insert the needle perpendicularly into the papilla but without allowing it to reach the palate.

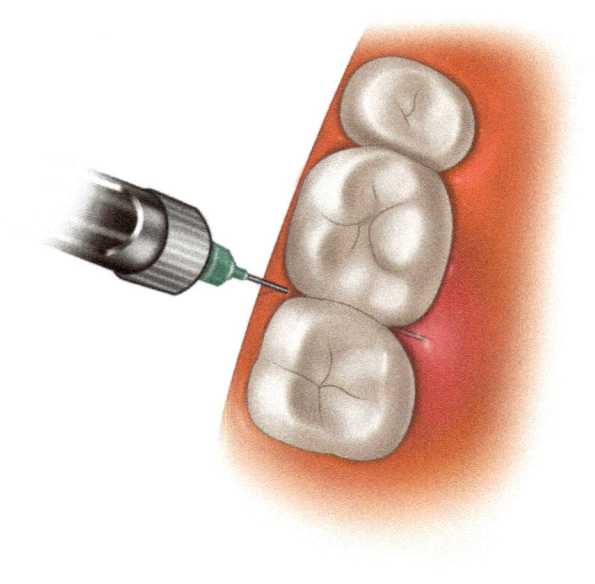

**Figure 15.11** Insert the needle perpendicularly into the palate so that it passes toward the palatal gingiva without perforating the palatine mucosa.

## References

Aggarwal, V., Singla, M., Miglani, S. et al. (2011). A prospective, randomized, single-blind comparative evaluation of anesthetic efficacy of posterior superior alveolar nerve blocks, buccal infiltration, and buccal plus palatal infiltrations in patients with irreversible pulpitis. *J. Endod.* 37 (11): 1491–1494.

Allen, G.D. (1979). *Dental Anesthesia and Analgesia (Local and General)*, 2e. Baltimore: Williams and Wilkins. 108, 140.

Al-Mahalawy, H., Abuohashish, H., Chathoth, S. et al. (2018). Articaine versus lidocaine concentration in the palatal tissues after supraperiosteal buccal infiltration anesthesia. *J. Oral Maxillofac. Surg.* 76 (2): 315.e1–315.e7.

Annex 19. Topical anesthesia I. Results of clinical trials.

Annex 22. Positive aspirations.

Annex 23. Pain resulting from injection techniques.

Annex 41. Nasopalatine canal and foramen.

Annex 42. Greater palatine canal and foramen.

Askari, E.M., Parirokh, M., Nakhaee, N. et al. (2016). The effect of maxillary first molar root length on the success rate of buccal infiltration anesthesia. *J. Endod.* 42 (10): 1462–1466.

Aslin, W.R. (2001). Reduced discomfort during palatal injection. *J. Am. Dent. Assoc.* 132 (9): 1277.

Badcock, M.E., Gordon, I., and McCullough, M.J. (2007). A blinded randomized controlled trial comparing lignocaine and placebo administration to the palate for removal of maxillary third molars. *Int. J. Oral Maxillofac. Surg.* 36 (12): 1177–1182.

Bataineh, A.B. and Al-Sabri, G.A. (2017). Extraction of maxillary teeth using articaine without a palatal injection: a comparison between the anterior and posterior regions of the maxilla. *J. Oral Maxillofac. Surg.* 75 (1): 87–91.

Bataineh, A.B., Nusair, Y.N., and Al-Rahahleh, R. (2019). Comparative study of articaine and lidocaine without palatal injection for maxillary teeth extraction. *Clin. Oral Invest.* 23 (8): 3239–3248.

Bennett, C.R. (1984). *Monheim's local anesthesia and pain control in dental practice*, 7e. St Louis (Mi): The CV Mosby Company. 86, 87.

Bhalla, J., Meechan, J.G., Lawrence, H.P. et al. (2009). Effect of time on clinical efficacy of topical anesthesia. *Anesth. Prog.* 56 (2): 36–41.

Birn, H. and Winther, J.E. (1977). *Atlas de cirugía oral*. Barcelona: Salvat Editores. 92.

Darawade, D.A., Kumar, S., Budhiraja, S. et al. (2014). A clinical study of efficacy of 4% articaine hydrochloride versus 2% lignocaine hydrochloride in dentistry. *J. Int. Oral Health* 6 (5): 81–83.

Dubner, R. (1978). Neurophysiology of pain. *Dent. Clin. N. Am.* 22 (1): 11–30.

Duncan, J.D., Reeves, G.W., and Fitchie, J.G. (1992). Technique to diminish discomfort from the palatal injection. *J. Prosth. Dent.* 67 (6): 901–902.

Evers, H. and Haegerstam, G. (1981). *Handbook of Dental Local Anesthesia.* Copenhagen: Schultz Medical Information. 83.

Fan, S., Chen, W.-L., Yang, Z.-H., and Huang, Z.-Q. (2009). Comparison of the efficiencies of permanent maxillary tooth removal performed with single buccal infiltration versus routine buccal and palatal injection. *Oral Surg. Oral Med. Oral Pathol.* 107 (3): 359–363.

Gill, C.J. and Orr, D.L. II (1979). A double-blind crossover comparison of topical anesthetics. *J. Am. Dent. Assoc.* 98 (2): 213–214.

Guglielmo, A., Drum, M., Reader, A., and Nusstein, J. (2011). Anesthetic efficacy a combination palatal and buccal infiltration of the maxillary first molar. *J. Endod.* 37 (4): 460–462.

Haglund, J. and Evers, H. (1985). *Local Anaesthesia in Dentistry*, 6e. Södertäleje (Sweden): Astra Läkemedel AB. 32.

Harbert, H. (1989). Topical ice: a precursor to palatal injections. *J. Endod.* 15 (1): 27–28.

Hartenian, K.M. and Stenger, T.C. (1976). Postanesthetic palatal ulceration. *Oral Surg. Oral Med. Oral Pathol.* 42 (4): 447–450.

Hicks, K., Reader, A., and Nist, R. (1995). Nasopalatine and labial infiltration in maxillary anterior anesthesia. *J. Dent. Res.* 74 (AADR abstracts); 27 (abstract no. 125).

Jackson, E. (1974). Managing dental fears: a tentative code of practice. *J. Oral Med.* 29 (4): 96–101.

Jastak, J.T., Yagiela, J.A., and Donaldson, D. (1995). *Local Anesthesia of the Oral Cavity.* Philadelphia: WB Saunders Co. 200, 221, 224.

Kandasamy, S., Elangovan, R., John, R.R., and Kumar, N. (2015). Removal of maxillary teeth with buccal 4% articaine without using palatal anesthesia – a comparative double blind study. *J. Oral Maxillofac. Surg. Med. Pathol.* 27 (2): 154–158.

Keller, B.J. (1985). Comparison of the effectiveness of two topical anesthetics and a placebo in reducing injection pain. *Hawaii Dent. J.* 16 (12): 10–11.

Kosaraju, A. and Vandewalle, K.S. (2009). A comparison of a refrigerant and topical anesthetic gel as preinjection anesthetics. A clinical evaluation. *J. Am. Dent. Assoc.* 140 (6): 68–72.

Kramp, L.F., Eleazer, P.D., and Sheetz, J.P. (1999). Evaluation of prilocaine for the reduction of pain associated with trans mucosal anesthetic administration. *Anesth. Prog.* 46 (2): 52–55.

Kravitz, J. (2006). The palatal press and roll anesthesia technique. *Pract. Proc. Aesth. Dent.* 18 (4): 242–245.

Kreider, K.A., Stratmann, R.G., Milano, M. et al. (2001). Reducing children's injection pain: lidocaine patches versus topical benzocaine gel. *Pediatr. Dent.* 23 (1): 19–23.

Kumaresan, R., Srinivasan, B., and Pendayala, S. (2015). Comparison of the effectiveness of lidocaine in permanent maxillary teeth removal performed with single buccal infiltration versus routine and palatal injection. *J. Maxillofac. Oral Surg.* 14 (2): 252–257.

Kuscu, O.O., Scandalli, N., Calgar, E., and Meechan, J.G. (2014). Use of pre-injection diffusion of local anesthesia as a means of reducing needle penetration discomfort. *Acta Stomatol. Croat.* 48 (3): 193–198.

Langford, R.J. (1989). The contribution of the nasopalatine nerve to sensation of the hard palate. *Br. J. Oral Maxillofac. Surg.* 27 (5): 379–386.

Lassemi, E., Motamedi, M.H.K., Jafari, S.M. et al. (2008). Anaesthetic efficacy of a labial infiltration method on the nasopalatine nerve. *Br. Dent. J.* 205 (10): E21.

Lesch, C.A., Squier, C.A., Cruchley, A. et al. (1989). The impermeability of human oral mucosa and skin to water. *J. Dent. Res.* 68 (9): 1345–1349.

Lima-Junior, J.-L., Dias-Ribeiro, E., de Araujo, T.N. et al. (2009). Evaluation of buccal vestibule-palatal diffusion of 4% articaine hydrochloride in impacted maxillary third molar extractions. *Med. Oral Patol. Oral Cir. Bucal* 14 (3): E129–E132.

Lima-Junior, J.-L., Dias-Ribeiro, E., Rocha, J.F. et al. (2013). Comparison of buccal infiltration of 4% articaine with 1:100,000 and 1:200,000 epineophrine for extraction of maxillary third molars with pericoronitis: a pilot study. *Anesth. Prog.* 60 (2): 42–45.

Majid, O.W. and Ahmed, A.M. (2018). The anesthetic efficacy of articaine and lidocaine in equivalent doses as buccal and non-palatal infiltration for maxillary molar extraction: a randomized, double-blinded, placebo-controlled clinical trial. *J. Oral Maxillofac. Surg.* 76 (4): 737–743.

Malamed, S.F. (1986). *Handbook of Local Anesthesia*, 2e. St. Louis (Missouri): The CV Mosby Co. 172–173.

Malamed, S.F. (2004). *Handbook of Local Anesthesia*, 5e. St. Louis (Missouri): Elsevier-Mosby. 202–207.

Malamed, S.F. and Trieger, N. (1983). Intraoral maxillary nerve block: an anatomical and clinical study. *Anesth. Prog.* 30 (2): 44–48.

Martin, M.D., Ramsay, D.S., Whitney, C. et al. (1994). Topical anesthesia: differentiating the pharmacological and psychological contribution to efficacy. *Anesth. Prog.* 41 (2): 40–47.

McArdle, B.F. (1997). Painless palatal anesthesia. *J. Am. Dent. Assoc.* 128 (5): 647.

Meechan, J.G., Day, P.F., and McMillan, A.S. (2000). Local anesthesia in the palate: a comparison of techniques and solutions. *Anesth. Prog.* 47 (4): 139–142.

Meechan, J.G., Howlett, P.C., and Smith, B.D. (2005). Factors influencing the discomfort of intraoral needle penetration. *Anesth. Prog.* 52 (3): 91–94.

Melzack, R. and Wall, P.D. (1965). Pain mechanism: a new theory. *Science* 150 (3699): 971–979.

Mercuri, L.G. (1979). Intraoral second division nerve block. *Oral Surg. Oral Med. Oral Pathol.* 47 (2): 109–113.

Nordenram, A. (1971). *Manuel d'anesthesie locale enpractiquedentaire*. Mölndal (Sweden): Lindgren and Söner. Bofors Nobel-Pharma. 35.

Özec, I., Tasdemir, U., Gümüs, C., and Solak, O. (2010). Is it possible to anesthetize palatal tissues with buccal 4% articaine injection? *J. Oral Maxilllofac. Surg.* 68 (5): 1032–1037.

Paschos, E., Huth, K.C., Benz, C. et al. (2006). Efficacy of intraoral anesthetics in children. *J. Dent.* 34 (6): 398–404.

Phillips, W.H. and Maxmen, H.A. (1941). The nasopalatine block injection as an aid in operative procedures for maxillary incisors. *Am. J. Orthod. Oral Surg.* 27 (8): 426–434.

Primosch, R.E. and Brooks, R. (2002). Influence of anesthetic flow rate delivered by the wand local anesthetic system as pain response to palatal injections. *Am. J. Dent.* 15 (1): 15–20.

Roberts, D.H. and Sowray, J.H. (1987). *Local Analgesia in Dentistry*, 3e. Bristol (UK): Wright. 88, 100, 101.

Salagaray, F. and Salagaray, V.M. (1982). *La anestesia odontoestomatológica*. Barcelona: Hoechst Iberica SA. 82–83.

Sharma, K., Sharma, A., Batta, A. et al. (2014). Maxillary posterior teeth removal without palatal injection – truth or myth: a dilemma for oral surgeons. *J. Clin. Diagn. Res.* 8 (11): ZCO1–ZCO4.

Somuri, A.V., Rai, A.B., and Pillai, M. (2013). Extraction of permanent maxillary teeth by only buccal infiltration of articaine. *J. Maxillofac. Oral Surg.* 12 (2): 130–132.

Uckan, S., Dayangac, E., and Aranz, K. (2006). Is permanent maxillary tooth removal without palatal injection possible? *Oral Surg. Oral Med. Oral Pathol.* 102 (6): 733–735.

Ulusoy, Ö.I.A. and Alacam, T. (2014). Efficacy of single buccal infiltrations for maxillary first molars in patients with irreversible pulpitis: a randomized controlled trial. *Int. Endod. J.* 47 (3): 222–227.

Wahl, M., Overton, D., Howell, J. et al. (2001). Pain on injection of prilocaine plain vs lidocaine with epinephrine.

A prospective double-blind study. *J. Am. Dent. Assoc.* 132 (10): 1396–1401.

Wepman, B.J. (1978). Psychological components of pain perception. *Dent. Clin. N. Am.* 22 (1): 101–113.

Westmoreland, E.E. and Blanton, P.L. (1982). An analysis of the variations in position of the greater palatine foramen in the adult human skull. *Anat. Rec.* 204: 383–388.

Wiswall, A.T., Bowles, W.R., Lunos, S. et al. (2014). Palatal anesthesia: comparison of four techniques for decreasing injection discomfort. *Northwest Dent.* 93 (4): 25–29.

Wong, J.D. and Sved, A.M. (1991). Maxillary nerve block anaesthesia via the greater palatine canal: a modified technique and case reports. *Aust. Dent. J.* 36 (1): 15–21.

# 16

## Mandibular Anesthesia I: Pulpal Anesthesia

Mandibular block is the technique of choice for pulpal anesthesia of the mandibular molars and premolars. Infiltration is much less effective when applied to the mandible, owing to the higher density of the cortical bone in the mandible as compared to the maxilla (Table 3.2, Chapter 3), especially along the external oblique ridge. Mandibular block accounts for nearly 30% of all anesthetic injections performed in dentistry (Annex 1). Although it also known as inferior alveolar nerve block, the term mandibular block is more semantically precise because the block often involves not only the inferior alveolar but also the lingual and buccal nerves, and the nerve to the mylohyoid muscle.

Mental nerve block has been excluded from this chapter because of its two disadvantages:

1) The mental foramen is difficult to locate. In clinical practice, it takes a full minute or longer to find when sought with a needle between the apexes of the two premolars in over 40% of cases (Joyce and Donnelly 1993).
2) The risk of introducing the needle to the mental foramen and injuring the vascular nervous package is high. Clinical studies have shown that there is a 23% risk of hitting (Lustig and Zusman 1999) and a 12% risk of damaging the mental nerve (Joyce and Donnelly 1993). Buccal infiltration with potent a local anesthetic such as 4% articaine with 1:100000 epinephrine (A-100) is a technique more readily mastered that yields good results and entails lower risk.

Indirect mandibular block or the 1-2-3 technique, developed by Heinrich Braun (Lindsay 1929a) and furthered by Guido Fischer since 1910 (Fischer 1910), has likewise been excluded. Known by that name because it consists of a three-phase attempt to reach the groove of the mandibular neck (*sulcus colli*) indirectly by varying the direction of the needle in the soft tissue (Figure 16.1), the technique calls for very thick, stiff caliber 20G needles (no longer in use) that neither break nor bend. It is characterized by major disadvantages, including needle breakage, increased technique sensitivity, and higher probability of injuring the periosteum or the medial (internal) pterygoid muscle (Lindsay 1929b). Although there are more modern variations (Clarke and Holmes 1959; Sittitavornwong et al. 2017), the 1-2-3 technique is of primarily historic interest and is seldom used today.

All the techniques listed below and described in this chapter are intraoral because extraoral approaches are mostly confined to hospital scenarios.

- Mandibular block for pulpal anesthesia of molars and premolars via the:
  - conventional or direct approach
  - Gow-Gates approach
  - Laguardia–Akinosi approach
- Double infiltration for pulpal anesthesia of the anterior mandibular teeth.

## Mandibular Block: General Remarks

The first known mandibular block was performed by William Stewart Halsted on a medical student in 1884, who was administered 0.4 ml of a 4% solution of cocaine (Hall 1884). There is no record of whether the technique was intra- or extraoral, although the three techniques most commonly used today are intraoral.

The primary but not the sole aim of all these techniques is to introduce enough solution to anesthetize the inferior alveolar nerve before it enters the mandibular foramen (Berns and Sadove 1962; Galbreath and Eklund 1970). Given that the inferior alveolar nerve fibers are myelinated, at least three nodes of Ranvier (Blair and Erlanger 1939) or a total of 6 mm must be anesthetized since the nodes in this nerve are spaced at 0.5–1.8 mm (Rood 1978a,b).

---

*Local Anesthesia in Dentistry: A Locoregional Approach*, First Edition. Jesús Calatayud and Mana Saraghi.
© 2024 John Wiley & Sons Ltd. Published 2024 by John Wiley & Sons Ltd.
Companion website: www.wiley.com/go/Calatayud/local

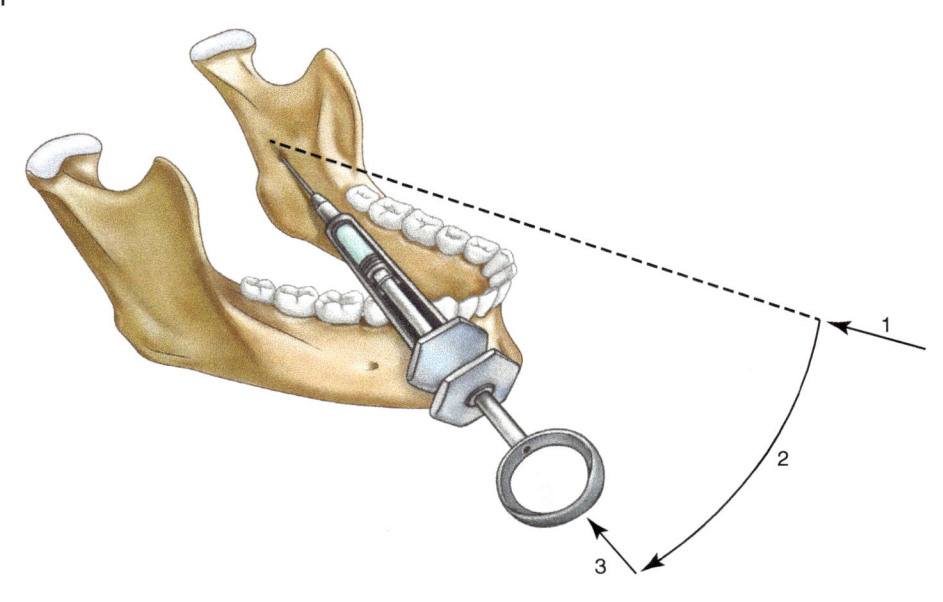

Figure 16.1 Mandibular block, 1-2-3 technique. *Source:* Redrawn from Andlaw and Rock (1994).

## Zone Anesthetized

The various mandibular block techniques anesthetize the following nerve trunks, although to varying degrees.

- The following areas are anesthetized by the inferior alveolar nerve (all in same side, ipsilateral):
  - Teeth, pulp, and periodontal ligament in the entire hemiarch on the respective side; molars and second premolar (via the inferior alveolar nerve itself) and first premolar, canine, and incisors via the incisive nerve, a branch of the inferior alveolar nerve.
  - Interdental papillae, including fibromucosa, bone, and periosteum to the midline.
  - Vestibule, via the mental nerve; fibromucosa (alveolar mucosa and attached gingiva), bone, and periosteum in the area between the premolars and the central incisor, including the molar zone in the 10% of cases where the buccal nerve is scantly developed (Hendy and Robinson 1994); the skin over the ipsilateral half of the chin and in particular *half of the lower lip*, from the corner of the mouth to the midline, denoting successful anesthetization of the alveolar nerve.
- The lingual nerve affects the lingual side fibromucosa (alveolar mucosa and gum), bone, and periosteum of the teeth, along with half of the floor of the mouth and the front two-thirds of the tongue on the side involved.
- The buccal nerve inneravates the following structures (all ipsilaterally): the buccal fibromucosa (alveolar mucosa and attached gingiva), bone, and periosteum of the retromolar triangle; side of the lower molars (reaching the second premolar in 5%) (Hendy and Robinson 1994).
- Other nerves proximal to the inferior alveolar nerve may also be anesthetized:
  - The auriculotemporal nerve, innervating the skin in the temporal region, in some cases as far as the border of the parietal, masseteric, frontal, and supraorbital regions. This nerve is only anesthetized in 20% of cases due to migration of the anesthetic, the odds of which are increased if the patient is in a reclined position (Kim et al. 2003).
  - The mylohyoid nerve, primarily a motor nerve and branch of the mandibular division of the trigeminal nerve, is located on the floor of the mouth. It also innervates the anterior belly of the digastric muscle; when anesthetized, the patient may feel discomfort during swallowing. The nerve to mylohyoid may provide supplemental innervation to the pulp of the posterior and anterior teeth on the side in question and even the contralateral incisors (Chapter 3), as well as sensory innervation to the skin on the chin (Roberts and Harris 1973).This nerve trunk is frequently anesthetized in mandibular blocks.

## Factors to Consider for the Mandibular Block

The factors that affect the scope and limitation of the mandibular block are discussed in this section.

### Efficacy is Correlated to the Location of Tooth in the Mandible

Mandibular block delivers acceptable results in molars and premolars (Table 16.1). Pulpal anesthesia is successful in 60–70% of cases involving the posterior teeth within

Table 16.1 Degree (%) of pulpal anesthesia in lower teeth 10 and 15 minutes after injecting one (1.8 ml) or two (3.6 ml) cartridges of a standard L-100 solution for conventional mandibular block, as well as maximum success rate (%) and time of peak effect electric pulp tester data (see Annex 25).

|  | 1.8 ml | | | 3.6 ml | | |
|---|---|---|---|---|---|---|
|  | Time after injection | | | Time after injection | | |
| Tooth | 10 min | 15 min | Maximum success | 10 min | 15 min | Maximum success |
| Posterior (M and PM) | 60% | 65% | 80%/40 min | 65% | 70% | 80%/40 min |
| Lateral incisor | 30% | 35% | 55%/40 min | 30% | 40% | 55%/40 min |
| Central incisor | 10% | 15% | 25%/30 min | 15% | 25% | 35%/40 min |

M, molar; PM, premolar.

10–15 minutes after injection of 1.8 or 3.6 ml of standard solution (2% lidocaine with 1:100 000 epinephrine, L-100). In contrast, as the results are poor in the anterior teeth (Table 16.1), *mandibular block can be said to be effective in posterior mandibular teeth only*.

### High Failure Rate

As mandibular block is characterized by a high failure rate even in posterior teeth, *it must be reinforced*, as discussed later.

### Unreliability of Lower Lip Anesthesia

An anesthetized lower lip is indicative of anesthesia of the mental nerve which innervates it but not of mandibular dental pulp (Annex 25). A numb lower lip is specific but not sensitive: its absence definitely indicates that the pulps are not anesthetized, but its presence is not a reliable indicator that the pulps are anesthetized (Chavarria-Bolaños et al. 2017). In other words, a numbed lower lip is a necessary but not a sufficient indication of pulpal anesthesia.

### Sequential Nature

The lower lip and teeth are anesthetized sequentially. The lower lip is anesthetized first, followed by pulpal anesthesia of the molars, premolars, and anterior teeth in that order (Table 16.2). The conclusion is that anesthetic onset is longer than previously thought. *Clinicians should wait at least 10–15 minutes after administering the anesthetic*, which is when pulpal anesthetic onset is most rapid. After that time, anesthetic onset continues but much more slowly (Annex 25).

### The Longer the Time, the More Intense the Anesthesia

*In 80% of cases, maximum pulpal anesthesia in posterior teeth is attained after 40 minutes* (Table 16.1), although waiting 40 minutes is not normally practical today. The same applies to the soft tissue anesthesia peaking in the lower lip after 40 minutes (Hersh et al. 1995).

### Minor Effect of the Type of Anesthetic

In mandibular block, *the different local anesthetics available have little impact on success* and all are effective (Annex 24). A mandibular block is effective if the anesthetic is injected close to the inferior alveolar nerve, spanning the lingula and a few aponeurotic membranes, to position the solution in a place from which it can spread passively toward the nerve essentially unobstructed. That is not the case in buccal infiltrations, in which the potency of the anesthetic is instrumental to efficacy because the solution must cross barriers (periosteum, cortical, and spongy bone) to reach the dental apex and anesthetize the pulp. In mandibular blocks, other factors such as accessory pulpal innervation (mylohyoid nerve, buccal nerve), anatomical variations (high lingula, double alveolar ducts), and the greater complexity of the technique affect the outcome, inducing failed pulp anesthesia even when the inferior alveolar nerve is successfully blocked (deeply numbed lower lip).

The anesthetic of choice for mandibular blocks is *2% lidocaine solution with 1:100 000 or 1:80 000 (L-100 or L-80)* for the following reasons:

- It is just as effective as even the most potent solutions (with high anesthetic or vasoconstrictor concentrations) such as 4% articaine with 1:100 000 epinephrine (A-100) or 2% lidocaine with 1:50 000 epinephrine (L-50) (Annex 24).
- Lidocaine is less concentrated, which means that more volume can be administered before reaching the maximum recommended dose (MRD). In more concentrated local anesthetics, such as 3% mepivacaine or 4% articaine, the MRD is achieved at a lower volume. For patients

Table 16.2 Reported and mean electric pulp tester-measured times (minutes) of lower lip and pulpal anesthesia in first molar (first M), first premolar (first PM) and lateral incisor (LI).

| Reference | Sample size | Lower lip | | First M | First PM | LI |
| --- | --- | --- | --- | --- | --- | --- |
| | | Subjective | Objective | | | |
| Vreeland et al. (1989) | 30 | 8.8 | 6.2 | 8.4 | — | 13.2 |
| Chaney et al. (1991) | 30 | 4.7 | 7.7 | 8.2 | 10.2 | 13.0 |
| Hinkley et al. (1991) | 30 | 6.1 | 10.6 | 8.8 | 10.6 | 12.3 |
| McLean et al. (1993) | 30 | 5.0 | 10.7 | 10.8 | 11.8 | 17.8 |
| Kanaa et al. (2006) | 38 | — | — | 5.4 | 8.9 | 13.3 |
| Steinkruger et al. (2006) | 51 | — | — | 8.8 | 10.8 | 13.0 |
| Steinkruger et al. (2006) | 51 | — | — | 9.2 | 10.8 | 13.0 |
| Goldberg et al. (2008) | 40 | — | — | 8.0 | 7.0 | 12.0 |
| Kanaa et al. (2009) | 36 | — | — | 6.8 | 8.9 | 10.9 |
| Mean | | 6.2 | 8.8 | 8.3 | 9.9 | 13.6 |

weighing at least 70 kg, up to 8.5 cartridges (1.8 ml) of 2% lidocaine can be administered as the maximum dose (Annex 10), whereas with other solutions only 5.5 to seven cartridges can be injected. This is especially important when treating small children, as local anesthetic overdose and toxicity is more of a concern.

- It has been listed by the US FDA as pregnancy risk B (safe).
- There is less risk for neurotoxic injury to the inferior alveolar nerves when applied as a block. This is not a property that is inherent to lidocaine, but rather due to the lower lidocaine concentration (2%), as compared to 4% solutions of articaine and/or prilocaine, which has been implicated in such side effects (see Chapter 22).

### Impact of the Volume Injected

As Table 16.1 shows, injecting two cartridges of the standard solution (3.6 ml of L-100) improves pulpal anesthesia after 10–15 minutes in 5% of posterior teeth (Annex 25).

### Minor Effect of the Specific Mandibular Block Technique

The Gow-Gates technique was initially believed to deliver better results than the conventional or direct technique, but as discussed throughout this chapter that has not been proven. Overall, the conventional or direct technique affords the best clinical results of the three mandibular block approaches (Table 16.3) and is the easiest to master.

### Bilateral Mandibular Blocks

Bilateral mandibular blocks (on the right and left sides simultaneously) can be utilized when bilateral mandibular anesthesia is necessary. This procedure was initially believed to entail the risk of serious consequences, such as soft tissue (tongue and lip) injury due to inadvertent biting or discomfort for patients (i.e. dysgeusia, dysphagia as the tongue is anesthetized.) Nonetheless, the only problem reported to date is minor discomfort when swallowing or drinking (Adatia and Gehring 1972). Even in children, bilateral mandibular block has been found (anti-intuitively) to lead to less self-injury than its unilateral counterpart for two reasons: (i) as bilateral blocks entail more extensive, lengthier treatment, the child's soft tissues are anesthetized for less time after leaving the dentist's office and (ii) as the soft tissue anesthesia is felt symmetrically, children are less inclined to explore and bite the tongue and cheeks, as they do not feel a contrast in sensation between the two sides (College et al. 2000).

### Long, Caliber 25G Needles

Mandibular block should be performed using caliber 25G needles (a slightly less optimal alternative is caliber 27G, in as much as 25G needles are not readily available today) for the following reasons (see Chapter 11):

- They deviate less across the linear insertion.
- They ensure good aspiration.
- They do not cause more pain (pain myth, Chapters 11 and 13).
- They are less likely to break.

The 25G needle must be of sufficient length to traverse 20–30 mm of soft tissue before reaching the target and should never be inserted into the soft tissue up to the hub because they are more liable to break.

Table 16.3 Comparison of conventional, Gow-Gates, and Laguardia–Akinosi mandibular block techniques: clinical variables.

| Variable | Mandibular block technique | | | Reference |
|---|---|---|---|---|
| | Conventional | Gow-Gates | Laguardia–Akinosi | |
| % Positive aspirations | 10% | 5–10% | 5% | Annex 22 |
| % Lower lip failure | | | | |
|    After 5 min | 10% | 30% | 30% | Annex 28 |
|    After 10 min | 5% | 5% | 20% | |
| % Lingual nerve anesthesia | 95% | 80% | 85% | Annex 29 |
| % Buccal nerve anesthesia | 60% | 70% | 70% | Annex 29 |
| Grade A anesthetic efficacy | 85% | 80% | 80% | Annex 30 |

### Slow Injection

As noted in Chapter 13, the injection speed presently recommended is 40–60 seconds for a 1.8-ml cartridge to:

- Reduce pain because tissues are not distended abruptly.
- Reduce toxicity in the event of intravascular injection. For some authors this is the single most important measure for preventing adverse reactions, more even than aspiration (Malamed 2004).
- Enhance clinical efficacy. Higher pulpal anesthesia success rates according to clinical trials (Kanaa et al. 2006).

## Mandibular Block: Conventional or Direct Technique

The conventional or direct technique, also denominated the classic or standard (or inferior alveolar nerve block), is much more commonly used than others worldwide because of its greater efficacy and relative simplicity. It consists of inserting the needle, directed from the lower premolars on the opposite side, into the pterygotemporal depression and subsequently into the pterygomandibular space (Figure 3.14, Chapter 3) and from there to the *sulcus colli* in the ramus of the mandible above the lingula (Figure 16.2), where the anesthetic solution is deposited and where the inferior alveolar nerve lies in a wide open mouth. It is called "direct" because the needle is inserted directly to the target, with no need for prior maneuvering.

This technique was initially introduced by Parisian clinician Pageix in 1906, although he directed the needle from a point on the midline too high (15–20 mm) over the occlusal plane (Lindsay 1929a). Boris Levitt (New York) developed the technique as it is known today (Levitt 1924), while Ashley Lindsay (Toronto) was instrumental in its popularization (Lindsay 1929a,b). Nonetheless, a host of minor variations on the technique are in place and each dentist could almost be said to have their own.

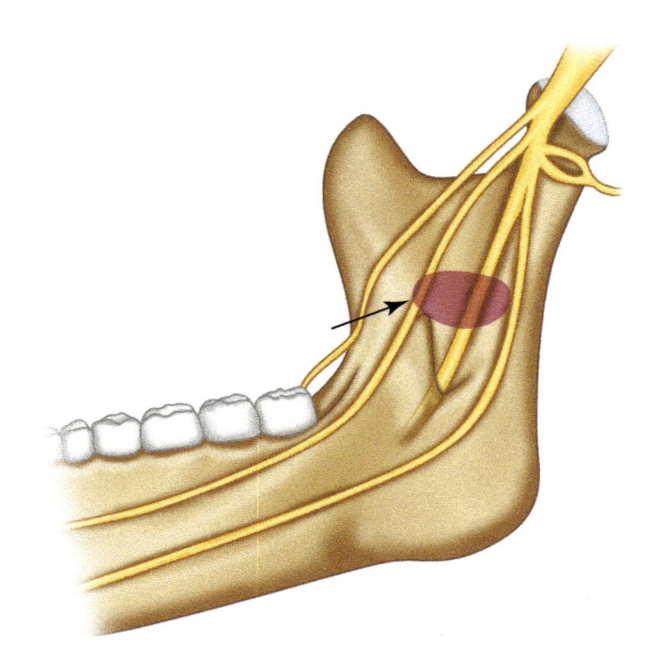

**Figure 16.2** *Sulcus colli* above and behind the lingula, where the anesthetic solution is deposited in conventional mandibular block.

### Distribution of the Anesthetic Solution

The anesthetic solution normally spreads rapidly across the pterygomandibular space and it remains there for several minutes (Petersen 1971). It is confined between the anterior and posterior edges of the ramus of the mandible, although the course taken cannot be predicted because the path of least resistance is determined by the fascial planes and the structures inside the pterygomandibular space (Berns and Sadove 1962; Galbreath and Eklund 1970). That said, it tends to travel upward and backward (sigmoid distribution) (Berns and Sadove 1962; Galbreath and Eklund 1970; Petersen 1971), therefore the success rate is lower if the anesthetic is positioned too high and too far back of the inferior alveolar nerve (Galbreath and Eklund 1970; Petersen 1971). In such situations, while the solution tends to spread to the parapharyngeal space, it does so more slowly (Petersen 1971).

The greatest factor in achieving a successful direct mandibular block is the position of the needle, which must be as close as possible to the beginning of the mandibular foramen and behind and close to the lingula (<5 mm), but this does not guarantee a perfect success rate (Berns and Sadove 1962; Galbreath and Eklund 1970). In contrast, placing the tip of the needle more than 5 mm away from and behind the mandibular foramen is associated with a large number of failures (Berns and Sadove 1962; Galbreath and Eklund 1970; Petersen 1971).

### Zone Anesthetized

The zone anesthetized is as described in the general remarks, although the degree to which each element is numbed varies from one technique to another. All techniques must anesthetize the inferior alveolar nerve, often indicated by soft tissue (the lower lip ipsilateral to the injection site). *In 95% of cases, the lingual nerve is also anesthetized with this technique and the buccal nerve in 60%* (Table 16.3 and Annex 29).

### Technique

- Use a long (35–42 mm) needle, given the depth of the insertion. Caliber 25G is ideal because it affords good aspiration and as it is thick and stiff, it deviates very little. If caliber 25G is not available, 27G can be used, although this is less effective because deflection is somewhat greater.
- Solution. In most cases standard 2% lidocaine with 1:100 000 (L-100) or 1:80 000 (L-80) epinephrine is the option of choice (Annex 24).
- Patient positioning
  - Supine or semisupine in dentist's chair.
  - *Mouth opened maximally* throughout the injection to facilitate direct visualization of intraoral landmarks and ensure that the inferior alveolar nerve lies against the *sulcus colli* on the inner side of the ramus of the mandible (target area).
  - Head turned slightly to the same side as the side being injected (i.e. right in right-side blocks and to the left in left-side blocks).
  - Tongue at rest and low in the posterior part of the mouth (Keetley and Moles 2001).
- Dentist's position and position of the non-dominant hand (i.e. left hand in right-handed clinicians), depending on the side to be anesthetized
  - Right side:
    - Dentist at 8:00 o'clock.
    - *Index finger in the patient's mouth* (Figure 16.3).
    - All other fingers stretching across the patient's face to block their vision and control the position of the mouth.

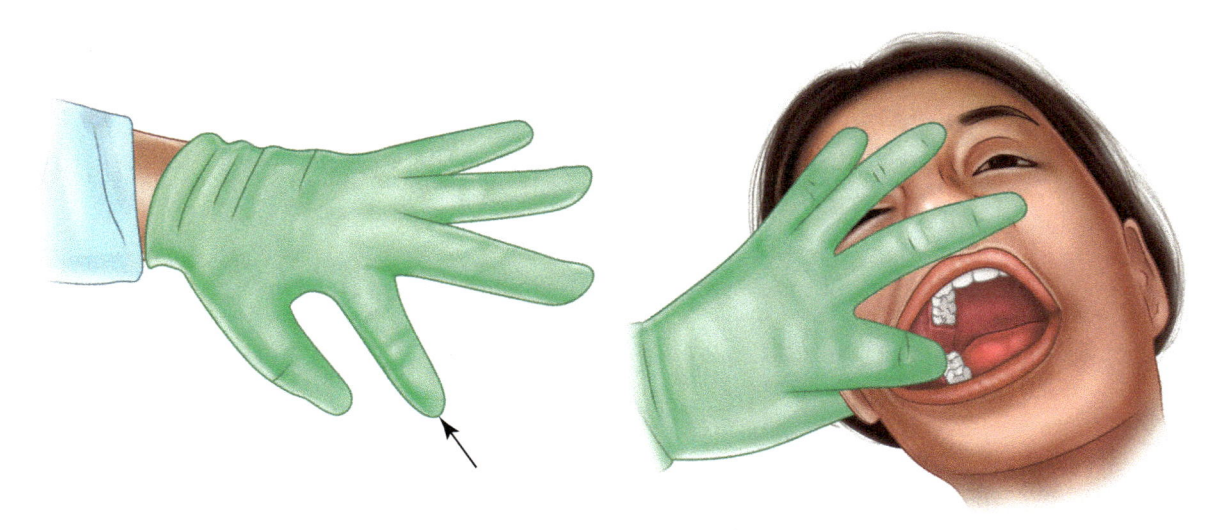

**Figure 16.3** Index figure of non-injection hand inside patient's mouth for approach from right side, with other fingers stretched across patient's face.

- Left side:
  - Dentist at 9:00–10:00 o'clock.
  - *Thumb of the non-dominant hand in the patient's mouth*, requiring the right-handed dentist to pass their left arm over the patient's forehead (Figure 16.4).
  - Dentist's non-injection palm and wrist blocking patient's vision.
- Intraoral finger or thumb. *The finger in the patient's mouth should rest on the anterior edge of the ramus of the mandible*, in the concavity known as the coronoid notch (Figure 16.5). It should also be parallel to the occlusal plane of the mandibular molars to:
  - Bring the pterygotemporal depression into view.
  - Help visualize the zone and locate the needle insertion site.
  - Tighten and stretch the soft tissue to make needle insertion less traumatic.
    In 10% of cases the coronoid notch cannot be readily reached because it is underdeveloped or the adjacent soft tissue is very thick (anterior edge of the temporal muscle or adipose tissue and mucosa) (Angelman 1945). In such cases, clinicians should gently exert greater pressure to palpate the area and identify the anatomic landmarks.
- Insertion zone. The insertion zone lies in the pterygotemporal depression, which consists of a fold or cleft in the oral mucosa that is elliptical and elongated in shape and runs parallel and outside to the pterygomandibular raphe or ligament (medial limit) (Figure 16.6) (Khoury et al. 2011). Its lateral limit is the deep tendon

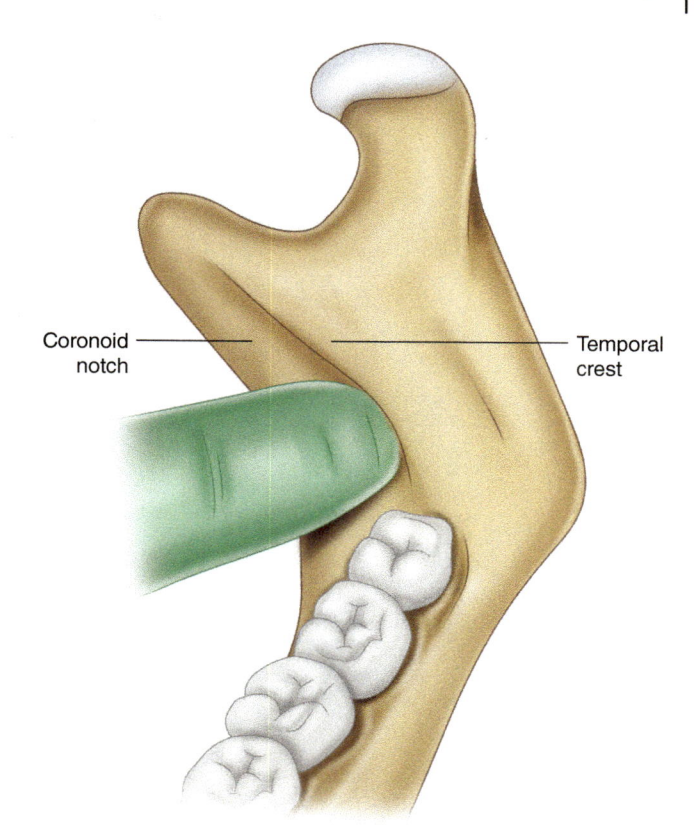

**Figure 16.5** Intraoral index finger or thumb resting on the anterior edge of the mandible in the hollow of the coronoid notch. *Source:* Redrawn from Evers and Haegerstam (1981).

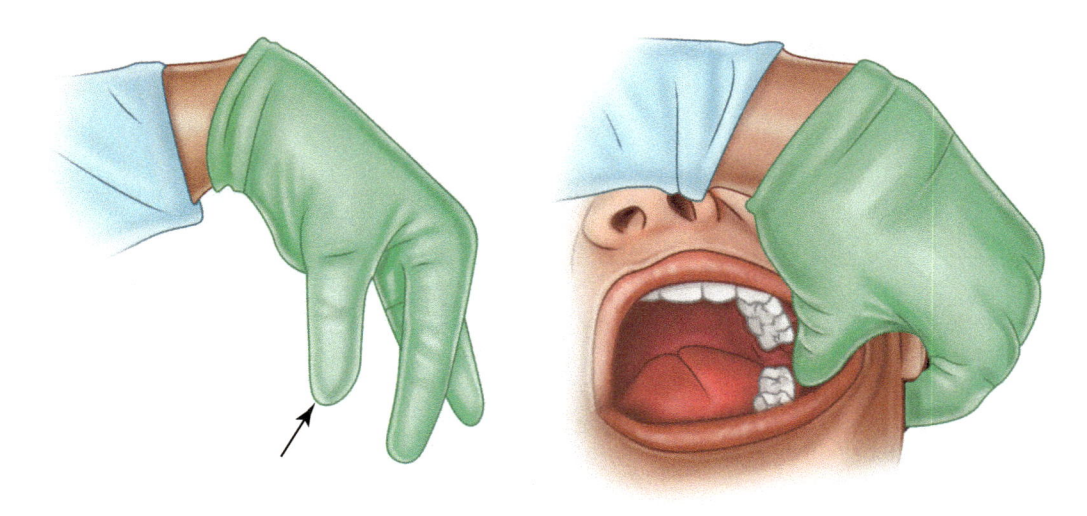

**Figure 16.4** Thumb of non-injection hand inside patient's mouth for approach from left side, with dentist's palm and wrist blocking patient's vision.

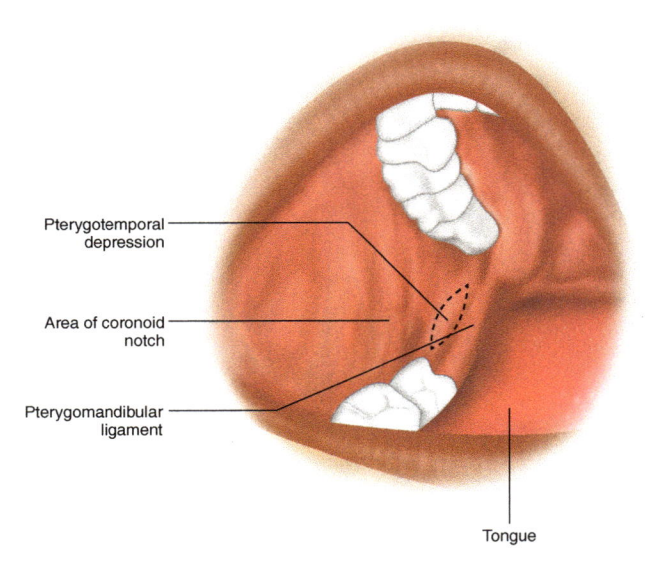

**Figure 16.6** Pterygotemporal depression outward of the pterygomandibular ligament or raphe.

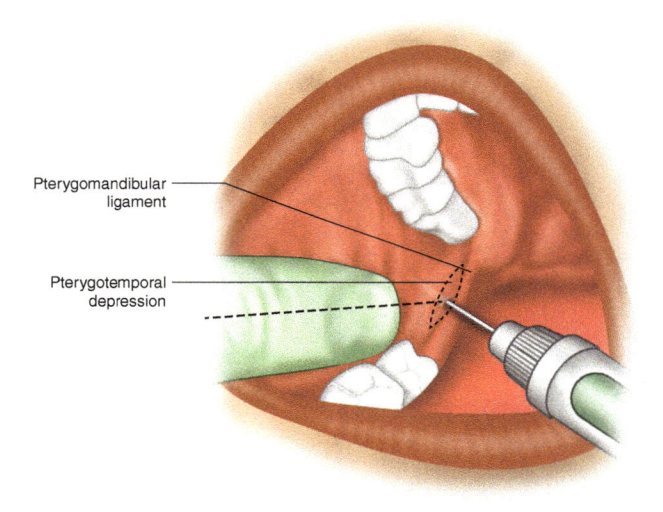

**Figure 16.7** Needle insertion site in conventional technique outside the pterygomandibular ligament, in the pterygotemporal depression, around 10 mm over the occlusal plane of the mandibular molars, with imaginary line projected distally from mid-finger to help find the insertion site.

that attaches the temporal muscle to the temporal crest, exactly where the finger is rested on the coronoid notch (Figure 3.14, Chapter 3) and thus highlights the *pterygotemporal depression*.

Some clinicians draw an imaginary line along the middle of the intraoral finger, parallel to the occlusal plane, and project it distally to pinpoint the insertion site (Figure 16.7).

In children under the age of 7 years (Via 1953) and in 35% of adults (Angelman 1945) this depression and its vertex lie under a mucosal pad and are difficult to distinguish (Lindsay 1929b). In such cases, the tip of the intraoral finger should stretch the proximal buccal mucosa and insert the needle outside the pterygomandibular ligament (always present), in the area where the vertex of the pterygotemporal depression is assumed to lie (Lindsay 1929b).

- Injection height.
  - A site around *10 mm above the occlusal plane of the mandibular molars* is recommended because in 95–100% of cases this ensures by-passing the lingula (Table 3.7, Chapter 3), leaving the path to the *sulcus colli* clear.
  - The exception is the occlusal plane of the third molar (wisdom tooth), unless it is aligned with the other two molars (Bremer 1952). The occlusal plane of the premolars can also be used as a reference if the molars are missing.
  - One aid to finding the insertion height is, as noted earlier, to draw an imaginary line backwards down the middle of the finger on the non-injection hand (that rests on the coronoid notch) toward the pterygotemporal depression (Figure 16.7) (Angelman 1945).
- Modification of the injection height.
  - It should be higher (>10 mm) in:
    - Toothless patients, for as the alveolar ridge is reabsorbed, the lingula is higher.
    - Patients with a wide gonial angle and wide ramus of the mandible, typical of class III Angle's malocclusion with mandibular hyperplasia (Hetson et al. 1988).
  - It should be lower (<10 mm) in:
    - Children under 10 years and especially children under 6 years (Benham 1976) (Table 3.8, Chapter 3) (Figure 16.8).
    - Patients with a narrow gonial angle and ramus of the mandible, typical of class II Angle's malocclusion with mandibular hypoplasia (Hetson et al. 1988).
  - Some clarifications are in order regarding modification in height.
    - In patients with a wide gonial angle and narrow ramus of the mandible or *vice versa*, the needle insertion height should be 10 mm.
    - Between its posterior and anterior the ramus of the mandible is 30 mm wide on average, ranging from 20 to 40 mm (Table 3.6, Chapter 3).
    - The gonial angle is 120° on average, but may range from 93° to 143°.
- Syringe direction.
  - In around 90% of cases the syringe is positioned over the mandibular premolar zone on the opposite side, with the needle traveling toward the pterygotemporal depression and touching bone at the *sulcus colli*.
  - The divergent angle between the ramus of the mandible and the sagittal or medial plane is 0–27°

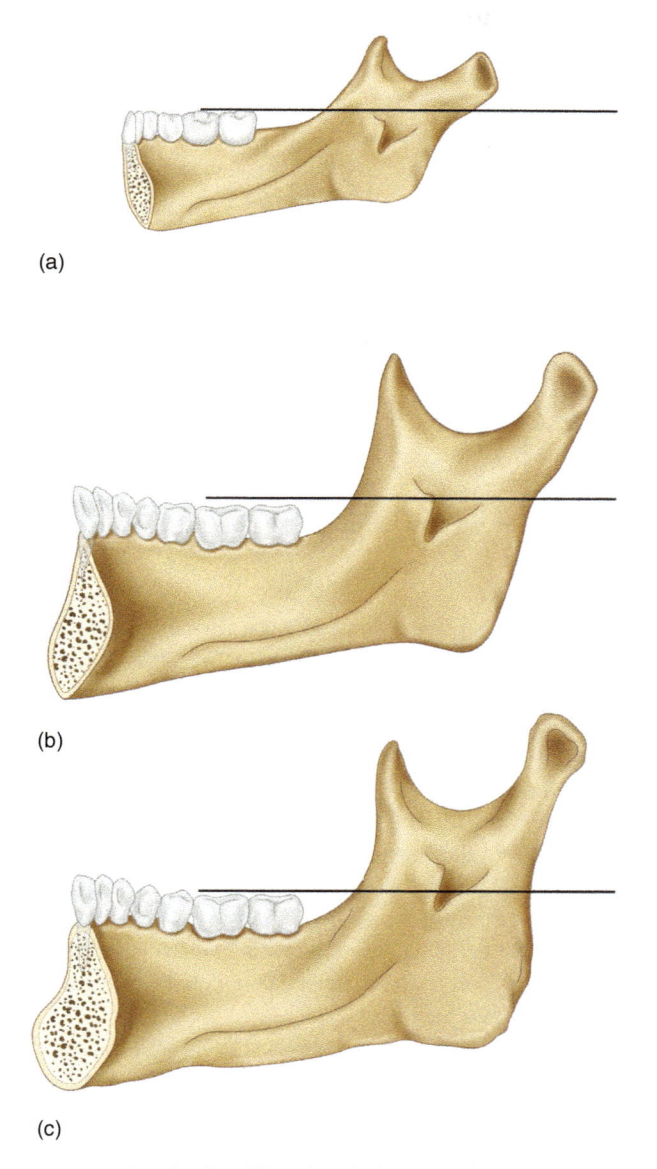

**Figure 16.8** Height of lingula relative to occlusal plane in (a) 4-year-old child, (b) 8-year-old child, and (c) adult.

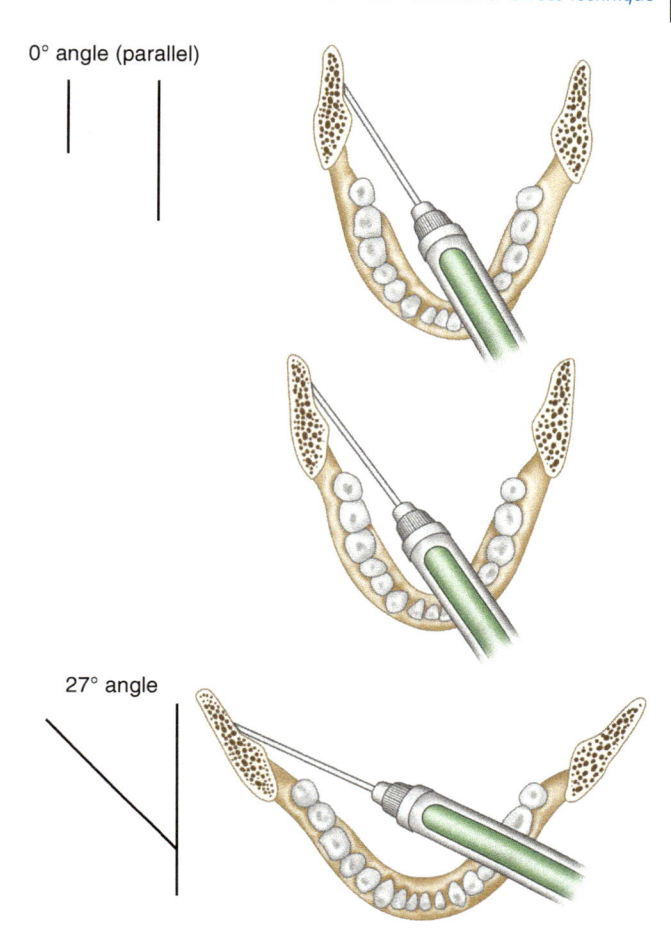

**Figure 16.9** Syringe positioned at contralateral mandibular molars (rather than premolars) when the divergent angle of the ramus of the mandible is >18° (conventional approach). *Source:* Redrawn from Roberts and Sowray (1987).

(Figure 3.11, Chapter 3). In the nearly 10% of cases where it is greater than 18° (Simon and Kömives 1938), the syringe must be positioned further back to reach the *sulcus colli, alongside the mandibular molars*, for with such a wide angle, if it lies above the premolars the needle would run behind the ramus of the mandible without touching bone (Figure 16.9).

- Needle insertion. The following is recommended to minimize discomfort associated with injection:
  - *The intraoral finger should stretch and tighten the mucosa overlying the pterygotemporal depression.*
  - *A light but firm tap followed by quick insertion* is regarded as the optimal technique. The site is lightly but firmly tapped with the non-dominant hand while at the same time quickly inserting the needle to hit bone. This maneuver is crucial because if the pain threshold's peak traumatic stimulus (the needle advancing through the soft tissues) lasts too long it will exceed the initial threshold, giving rise to pain (Fuller et al. 1979). Slower insertion triggers the initial threshold and if a few drops of anesthetic are injected as the needle advances the pain rises (Nusstein et al. 2006; McCartney et al. 2007; Chapter 13 Appendix); moreover, the anesthetic does not take immediate effect. The factor that causes most pain in truncal blocks is needle movement (Annex 23).
- Insertion depth.
  - The insertion depth is the distance between the anterior edge (pterygotemporal depression) and the *sulcus colli*, where the inferior alveolar nerve lies in a wide-open mouth. That distance is *around 20–25 mm*, ranging from 15 to 30 mm (Table 16.4), and in children under 6–8 years old it is 15–20 mm.
  - Inserting the needle into the hub is a technical error for two reasons: this is the weakest area and may result

Table 16.4 Needle insertion depth in soft tissue in conventional mandibular block.

| Reference | Sample size | Factor assessed | Mean (mm) | Range (mm) |
| --- | --- | --- | --- | --- |
| Angelman (1945) | 300 | Patient | — | 18–33 |
| Bremer (1952) | 100 | Dry mandible | 24 ± 3.1 | 16–32 |
| Waikakul and Punwutikorn (1991) | 68 | Patient | 20–25 | — |
| Kronman et al. (1994) | 39 | Corpse | 22 ± 1.8 | 15–28 |
| Delgado-Molina et al. (1999) | 246 | Patient | 21 | 10–34 |
| Hannan et al. (1999) | 40 | Patient | 19 | 18–20 |
| Tofoli et al. (2003) | 20 | Patient | 20–25 | — |
| Simon et al. (2010) | 38 | Patient | 19 ± 3.2 | — |
| | | Mean | 21.7 | 15.4–29.4 |
| | | Rounded mean | **20–25** | **15–30** |

in needle breakage as well as the fact that the depth is excessive to hit the landmarks for anesthesia of the inferior alveolar nerve.
- The insertion depth may vary (Angelman 1945) depending on:
  - The divergent angle between the ramus of the mandible and the sagittal or medial plane; the greater the divergent angle, the deeper the insertion.
  - The width of the ramus of the mandible; the wider, the deeper.
  - The thickness of the mucosa and adipose tissue that comprise the wall of the pterygotemporal depression; the thicker, the deeper.
- Interestingly, the dimensions in a given individual may vary by 1–4 mm between sides (Angelman 1945).
- *If the needle is not successfully inserted* because it fails to touch bone after 30 mm or because it touches bone too soon, in less than 15 mm, the recommendation is to aspirate and slowly remove the needle, *injecting 0.25 to 0.5 of a cartridge (0.5–0.9 ml)* to anesthetize the pterygomandibular space and facilitate a second, less painful maneuver in a second attempt after a 1-minute wait.

- Pre-injection aspiration.
  - *Once bone has been reached with the tip of the needle the clinician should avoid exerting undue pressure* to prevent injury to the periosteum (causing post-injection pain) and barb formation on the tip of the needle. If a barb forms outwardly, when the needle is withdrawn from the pterygomandibular space, the following structures may become injured: nerves (leaving persistent paresthesia in the lingual or inferior alveolar nerves), muscles (trismus due to injury to the medial pterygoid or temporal muscles), and the inferior alveolar artery and vein (hematoma) (Stacy and Hajjar 1994).
  - After touching bone the needle is *drawn back 1–2 mm* to aspirate. Aspiration is *positive in 10% of cases* (Annex 22), one of the highest rates in dental local anesthesia.

- Injection of the anesthetic solution and lingual nerve anesthesia.
  - *A 1.8-ml cartridge should be slowly injected, in 40–60 seconds*. To anesthetize the lingual nerve the needle is slowly withdrawn along the same path as it was inserted through; *at mid-distance and prior to removing the needle*, a second aspiration is performed and the last ±0.3 ml in the cartridge is injected to anesthetize the lingual nerve.
  - In the absence of this maneuver, the lingual nerve is often anesthetized by diffusion across the pterygomandibular space. However, this maneuver ensures anesthesia of the lingual nerve.
  - Many clinicians aspirate every 0.25–0.50 ml, seeking to further guarantee the safety of the injection with a series of negative aspirations (McClure 1968; Lloyd 1992); this also helps retard the injection by curbing the natural tendency to move faster.

- Amount to be injected
  - In adults, teenagers, and older children, a 1.8-ml cartridge is used (1.5 ml during deposition and ±0.3 ml while removing the needle to anesthetize the lingual nerve).
  - *In children <6–8 years old, only ½ of a cartridge is needed.*

- Subjective symptoms of anesthesia.
  - Soft tissue anesthesia appears in the lower lip on the anesthetized side. Soft tissue anesthesia may be described as tingling, numbing, itching, dullness, feeling "pins and needles," and feeling a "fat lip" sensation (Table 13.1, Chapter 13). The onset of soft tissue

Table 16.5 Electric pulp tester readings of anesthesia in first mandibular molar after conventional mandibular block with a supplemental buccal injection using A-100 anesthetic solution.

| Reference | Mandibular block ml/LAS | Supplementary buccal infiltration ml/LAS | Success rate (%) (absolute values) |
|---|---|---|---|
| Haase et al. (2008) | 1.8/A-100 | 1.8/A-100 | 96% (70/73) |
| Kanaa et al. (2009) | 2.0/L-80 | 2.0/A-100 | 92% (33/36) |
| Gazal (2015) | 1.8/M-100 | 1.8/A-100 | 100% (23/23) |
|  |  | Mean | 96% ≈ **95%** |

LAS, local anesthetic solution; A-100, 4% articaine with 1:100 000 (10 μg/ml) epinephrine; L-80, 2 lidocaine with 1:80 000 (12.5 μg/ml) epinephrine; M-100, 2% mepivacaine with 1:100 000 (10 μg/ml) epinephrine.

anesthesia is approximately 2 minutes after injection (Annex 27) and *in nearly 90% of cases in less than 5 minutes* (Annex 28).
- In approximately 10% of cases the lower lip is not anesthetized in the first 5 minutes (Annex 28). Such cases are regarded as failures in practice and a second mandibular block is recommended (Cohen et al. 1993; Reisman et al. 1997; Nusstein et al. 1998; Fan et al. 2009).
- Soft tissue anesthesia is denoted by the following.
  - In the lower lip ipsilateral to the injection site it is a sign of anesthesia of the inferior alveolar nerve, the primary aim of the procedure.
  - In the tongue ipsilateral to the injection site it is an indication of anesthesia of the lingual nerve. In 50% of cases, this precedes lip numbness (Angelman 1945; Ay et al. 2011).
  - In the auricular and temporal region ipsilateral to the injection site it is a sign of anesthesia of the auriculotemporal nerve. With this technique it occurs in only 20% of cases (Kim et al. 2003).
- Supplemental buccal infiltration.
  - After the first 5 minutes soft tissue anesthesia appears in the lower lip (an initial sign of mandibular block onset), verifying anesthesia of the inferior alveolar nerve, and supplementary buccal infiltration is recommended in posterior mandibular teeth requiring good pulpal anesthesia. *This procedure raises the pulpal anesthesia rate from 60–70% (Table 16.1) to 95% (Table 16.5).*
  - The infiltration is performed after 5 minutes to avoid the risk of masking or concealing mandibular block failure due to the overlapping of the effects of mandibular block and infiltration in the soft tissue.
  - The infiltration anesthetics recommended are:
    - In adults a potent solution such as a whole cartridge (1.8 ml) of *4% articaine with 1:100 000 epinephrine (A-100)* on the buccal aspect of the posterior teeth to be treated.
    - In teenagers and older children, a cartridge (1.8 ml) of the standard lidocaine solution (L-100).
    - In children under 6–8 years, half a standard L-100 cartridge (0.9 ml).
    - It takes an additional 5–10 minutes (10–15 minutes in all after starting mandibular block) for pulpal anesthesia to be fully effective.
- Duration of soft tissue anesthesia. This usually lasts 3–4 hours (200 minutes), a fact of which the patient should be notified after treatment.

### Efficacy of this Technique

The efficacy of this technique, measured with an electric pulp tester in posterior teeth after injection of one or two cartridges of standard 2% lidocaine with 1:100 000 epinephrine (L-100), is 60–70% after 10–15 minutes (Table 16.1) and 95% when reinforced by buccal infiltration with 1.8 ml of a potent solution such as 4% articaine with 1:100 000 epinephrine (A-100) (Table 16.5).

When measured with less rigorous methods such as the system to determine grade A anesthesia used for routine procedures (normally extractions), the success rate for non-reinforced mandibular block is 85% (Annex 30).

### Complications Specific to this Technique

- Technical error. Inappropriate maneuvering leads to failed mandibular block and other complications, depending on the injection position (Figures 3.13 and 3.14, Chapter 3).
  - Positioning the needle too deep/too far back (>30 mm) is one of the most common technical errors. In such cases, the anesthetic is injected into the parotid gland and remains in its capsule (Cook 1919; Sicher 1946;

Petersen 1971; Barker and Davies 1972). Occasionally, this results in anesthetizing the portion of the facial nerve (VII cranial nerve) that runs through the parotid gland. The result is temporary facial paralysis of the side involved until the anesthesia is reabsorbed (1–2 hours) (Petersen 1971; Shaw and Fierst 1988). The retromandibular vein may also be punctured (Shaw and Fierst 1988).

- Another common technical error is to insert the needle too deeply and medially, affecting the inner/medial (rather than the outer/lateral) aspect of the pterygomandibular ligament and the medial (internal) pterygoid muscle, with the risk of trismus (lockjaw). When the needle is inserted so deeply, the anesthetic solution injected into the parapharyngeal space (Petersen 1971) and spreads upward and backward behind the ramus of the mandible. In very deep injections that entails the risk of puncturing the internal or external carotid artery and the jugular vein, the vagus nerve (X cranial nerve), the sympathetic plexus or the superior laryngeal nerve (Dobbs 1956; Shaw and Fierst 1988).
- A needle inserted into the pterygomandibular raphe or ligament, that is, overly internally or medially, affects the medial (internal) pterygoid muscle, inducing trismus (Petersen 1971; Barker and Davis 1972; Shaw and Fierst 1988).
- When the needle is positioned too low the anesthetic is injected into and irritates the medial (internal) pterygoid muscle, causing trismus and failure to anesthetize the inferior alveolar nerve because the anesthetic is entrapped in the muscular fascia (Barker and Davies 1972; Shaw and Fierst 1988). Failure may also occur if the needle does not span the lingula because this structure obstructs the path of the anesthetic to the inferior alveolar nerve (Angelman 1945).
- An overly high/cranial needle position also has adverse implications, including:
  - Anesthesia of the auriculotemporal nerve, with soft tissue anesthesia of the skin of the ear, temporal region, and parietal wall, as well as the masseteric and at times the supraorbital zone (Sicher 1946; Shaw and Fierst 1988).
  - Hitting the lateral (outer) pterygoid muscle at the top of the pterygomandibular space, which may cause trismus (Barker and Davies 1972; Coleman and Smith 1982; Shaw and Fierst 1988).
  - Damaging the maxillary artery with hematoma or ischemic facial pallor on the side affected due to irritation of the sympathetic plexus around the artery (Shaw and Fierst 1988).

- Most common complications.
  - Anesthesia is unsuccessful in 10% of cases, with failure of the respective side of the lower lip to numb in the first 5 minutes (Annex 28).
  - In 7% of interventions, the soft tissues (particularly the periosteum) are traumatized. As a consequence, the patient experiences localized pain for 2–4 days that usually disappears spontaneously (Chapter 22).
  - An "electric shock" sensation may occur in 3% of cases, normally around the lingual or inferior alveolar nerves (lower lip on the side affected), if the needle contacts these nerve trunks (Chapter 22).
  - Trismus (lockjaw) may also appear in 3% of cases as a result (usually) of medial (internal) pterygoid muscle spasm (Table 22.11, Chapter 22).
  - Ischemia (manifested as pallor or blanching) appears on the side of the face in 1% of cases (Chapter 22).
  - Facial paralysis, which occurs in less than 0.5% of cases, is the result of facial nerve (VII cranial nerve) anesthesia (Chapter 22).
- Soft tissue anesthesia of the external auditory meatus (the ear). This rare but very irritating complication, which has been reported to date only in connection with mandibular block, generally lasts about 1 hour and disappears spontaneously (Ngeow and Chai 2009).

## Mandibular Block: Gow-Gates Technique

The Gow-Gates technique consists of placing the anesthetic in the (anterior-lateral) neck of the mandible (Figure 16.10), using extraoral reference points to anesthetize the inferior alveolar, lingual, and buccal nerves and their accessory branches in a single maneuver.

The technique was developed in 1947 by Australian dentist George Albert Edward Gow-Gates (1910–2001) (Kafalias and Gow-Gates 1987; Gow-Gates and Watson 1989), who first published a description of his method in 1973 (Gow-Gates 1973).

The Gow-Gates technique is particularly useful when the traditional block poses special difficulties that call for a second injection, such as accessory innervations (Coleman and Smith 1982). Several variations of the technique have been described (Waikakul and Punwutikorn 1991).

### Mechanism

In the Gow-Gates technique the anesthetic is injected into the neck of the mandible, in the upper part of the pterygomandibular space (Sisk 1985), just under the lateral (outer) pterygoid muscle insertion (Watson and Gow-Gates 1976; Levy 1981; Malamed 1981; Kafalias and

**Figure 16.10** Anterior-lateral surface of the neck of the mandible, where the anesthetic solution is deposited in Gow-Gates mandibular blocks.

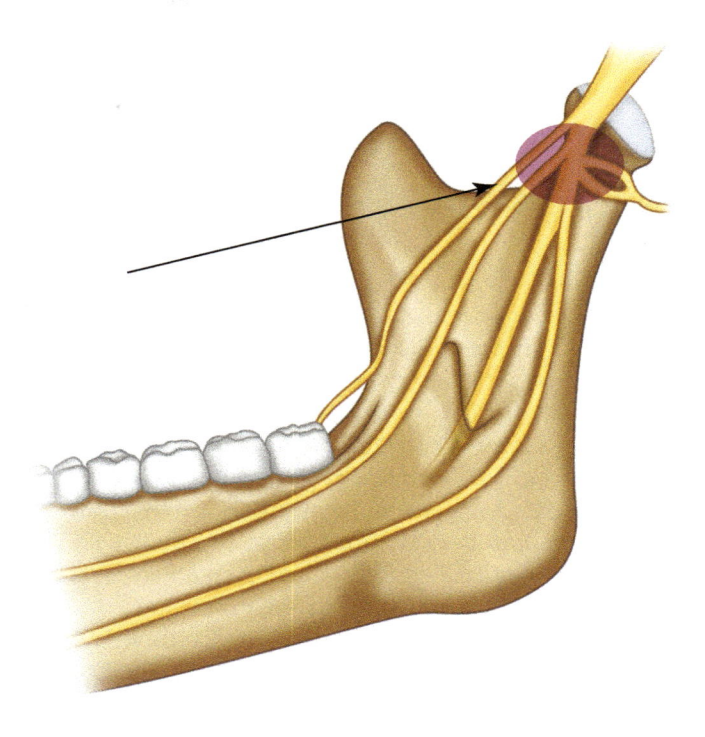

Gow-Gates 1987). It was initially believed to anesthetize the 3–5 mm of the common trunk of the mandibular nerve ($V_2$) after exiting the skull through the oval foramen and prior to branching (Watson 1973). As the oval foramen is located around 20 mm from the neck of the mandible (Gow-Gates and Watson 1977; Agren and Danielsson 1981), the common trunk, which lies higher/more superiorly, medially (internally), and anteriorly (Coleman and Smith 1982), cannot be readily reached by the anesthetic. The solution is obstructed in its pathway toward the common trunk:

- Posteriorly, by the neck of the mandible (Coleman and Smith 1982; Kafalias and Gow-Gates 1987).
- Superiorly, by the lower end of the head of the lateral (external) pterygoid muscle, which is inserted in the highest part of the neck of the mandible (Coleman and Smith 1982; Kafalias and Gow-Gates 1987).
- Medially (internally) by the lateral (external) pterygoid muscle, the temporomandibular joint (TMJ) and interpterygoid fascia (Agren and Danielsson 1981; Kafalias and Gow-Gates 1987).
- Laterally (externally) by the inner side of the ramus of the mandible (Kafalias and Gow-Gates 1987).

The anesthetic solution can only spread forward and downward, bathing the entire pterygomandibular space and its lax connective tissue (Agren and Danielsson 1981; Coleman and Smith 1982; Kafalias and Gow-Gates 1987; Shaw and Fierst 1988) from the top downward, driven by gravity and biophysical forces such as maxillary artery pulsations or muscular movements in the mandible (Kafalias and Gow-Gates 1987). The nerves anesthetized include:

- The inferior alveolar and lingual nerves, lying at around 10 mm from the neck of the mandible (Watson and Gow-Gates 1976; Agren and Danielsson 1981; Malamed 1981; Sisk 1985), which separate from one another in the depths of the lateral (external) pterygoid muscle (Agren and Danielsson 1981).
- The buccal nerve, located around 23 mm from the neck of the mandible (Kafalias and Gow-Gates 1987), separated from the target area by the lateral (external) pterygoid muscle and the lateral and pterygoid fascia (Levy 1981; Coleman and Smith 1982; Shaw and Fierst 1988).
- The accessory innervation encountered (Agren and Danielsson 1981; Levy 1981; Kafalias and Gow-Gates 1987), such as:
  - Accessory branches of the inferior alveolar nerve that pass through the highest and most independent foramina (e.g. the branch that innervates the third molar).
  - The mylohyoid nerve on the side affected if it is separated from and higher than the inferior alveolar nerve and has accessory innervations.
  - Accessory branches of the auriculotemporal nerve that innervate the molars and may pass through the accessory foramina of the neck of the mandible.

Lastly, as demonstrated by contrast radiology studies, the anesthetic descends forward, spreading throughout the pterygomandibular space to the buccinator muscle (Gow-Gates and Watson 1989).

## Advantages, Disadvantages, and Non-advantages

### Advantages
1) The mandibular block Gow-Gates technique anesthetizes the buccal nerve in 70% of cases, compared to 60% with the conventional technique (Annex 29).
2) Theoretically it lowers the risk of trismus (Gow-Gates and Watson 1977; Coleman and Smith 1982; Azagra and Cordoba 1983; Sisk 1985; Shaw and Fierst 1988) because the needle advances along the high lateral area of the pterygomandibular space, between the deep tendon of the temporal muscle and the medial (internal) pterygoid muscle. The most common cause of trismus is related to traumatizing the medial pterygoid muscle, which is avoided in this technique (Gow-Gates and Watson 1977; Coleman and Smith 1982; Kafalias and Gow-Gates 1987; Shaw and Fierst 1988). If the needle is inserted too high, however, the risk of perforating the lateral (external) pterygoid muscle is greater (Coleman and Smith 1982; Shaw and Fierst 1988).
3) The risk of needle-induced nerve injury is minimized as the anesthetic is deposited at a distance from nerve trunks (Azagra and Cordoba 1983; Zandi and Sabounchi 2008).
4) The mandibular block Gow-Gates technique is indicated in patients whose tongue persistently obstructs the view of soft-tissue landmarks used in the conventional mandibular block (Haas 2011).

### Disadvantages
1) Gow-Gates is more difficult to master than the conventional technique (Levy 1981; Malamed 1981; Hung et al. 2006).
2) The patient must open their mouth very wide. Limited ability to do so hinders the technique or rules it out entirely (Haas 2011). As it calls for extraoral markings, extraoral inflammation changes or potentially obscures the points of reference.
3) Onset (time to lower lip anesthesia) is 6 minutes (Table 16.6) compared to 2 minutes with the conventional technique (Annex 27), lengthening the time to anesthesia not only of the soft tissues but also of the

Table 16.6 Onset of lower lip anesthesia with Gow-Gates mandibular block.

| Reference | Sample size | Anesthetic ml/LAS | Onset (min) |
|---|---|---|---|
| Agren and Danielsson (1981) | 12 | 1.8/L-80 | 2.1 |
| Malamed (1981) | 4275 | –/– | 6 (5–7) |
| Yamada and Jasstak (1981) | 11 | 1.8/L-100 | 2 ± 1.2 |
| Sisk (1985) | 40 | 1.8/L-100 | 7.7 ± 1.9 |
| Todorovic et al. (1986) | 30 | 2.0/L-80 | 7 |
| Boué et al. (1987) | 23 | 1.8/M-3 | 7.1 |
| Jofré and Münzenmayer (1998) | 40 | 1.8/L-100 | 8 (7–9) |
| Jofré and Münzenmayer (1998) | 40 | 1.8/L-100 | 16 (8–25) |
| Pratts and Ferres (1999) | 20 | 1.8/L-100 | 4.9 |
| Proaño and Guillen (2005) | 30 | 1.8/L-100 | 2.2 |
| Haghighat et al. (2015) | 63 | 1.8/L-80 | 3.5 |
| Lenka et al. (2014) | 40 | 2.0/L-80 | 3.8 ± 1.2 |
| Dubey et al. (2017) | 50 | 1.8/L-80 | 11.8 ± 2.7 |
| Madan et al. (2017) | 100 | 2.0/L-80 | 6.4 ± 0.9 |
| Kiran et al. (2018) | 70 | 2.8/L-80 | 5.7 ± 2.5 |
| | | Mean | 6.3 |
| | | Rounded mean | 6 |

LAS, local anesthetic solution; L-100, 2% lidocaine with 1:100 000 (10 µg/ml) epinephrine; L-80, 2% lidocaine with 1:80 000 (12.5 µg/ml) epinephrine; M-3, 3% plain mepivacaine.

pulp (Goldberg et al. 2008). As this is believed to be due to the higher position and greater thickness of the nerve trunk, the anesthetic must travel across a longer path (Hung et al. 2006).
4) The lingual nerve is anesthetized in 80% compared to 95% of cases with the conventional technique (Annex 29).

**Non-advantages**

Non-advantages refer to presumed advantages that have not been supported by the literature.

1) Alleged higher efficacy
   - Gow-Gates was initially believed to enhance the anesthetic efficacy of mandibular block relative to the conventional or direct technique (Gow-Gates and Watson 1977; Sisk 1985) for the following reasons.
     - As extraoral landmarks are more stable and reliable than intraoral reference points, the anesthetic is deposited more precisely (Malamed 1981).
     - No interpterygoid or vascular fascias hinder the spread of the anesthetic (Watson 1973).
     - Much of the accessory innervation is blocked because as anesthetic is deposited higher and proceeds downward and forward, it tends to anesthetize all the nerve branches in its path (Agren and Danielsson 1981; Levy 1981; Kafalias and Gow-Gates 1987).
   - Clinical studies conducted in the interim have not confirmed such assumed improvements, however.
     - Grade A clinical efficacy awards Gow-Gates an 80% success rate, compared to 85% for the conventional technique (Table 16.3). Nonetheless, given the fair number of shortcomings and uncontrolled factors associated with this assessment method, its values must be regarded as indicative only (Annex 30).
     - Pulpal anesthesia measurements taken with an electric pulp tester are much more precise and more reliable. Unfortunately, very few clinical studies have been conducted with the Gow-Gates technique. According to the few published studies, its efficacy is similar to or slightly lower than that of the conventional technique (Table 16.7).

2) Alleged fewer positive aspirations
   Gow-Gates was initially thought to be associated with fewer positive aspirations than the conventional technique (Gow-Gates and Watson 1977; Malamed 1981; Azagra and Cordoba 1983; Sisk 1985) as the mandibular neck has fewer vessels and is primarily filled with fatty areolar tissue (Gow-Gates and Watson 1977; Kafalias and Gow-Gates 1987). Due to their inner (medial) position, large vessels (maxillary artery, masseteric artery, and inferior alveolar artery) or vessels running directly to the skull (middle meningeal artery and accessory meningeal arteries) are less likely to be injected. In the event that an aspiration does occur, as anatomical variations are possible, the implications are more severe (Levy 1981; Coleman and Smith 1982; Shaw and Fierst 1988).
   Later clinical studies have reported an incidence of 5–10% for positive aspirations, which is similar than the 10% found for the conventional or direct technique (Annex 22).

Table 16.7 Electric pulp tester-measured percentage of teeth anesthetized with Gow-Gates and conventional mandibular block.

| | | | | Success rate (%) | |
| --- | --- | --- | --- | --- | --- |
| Reference | ml/LAS | Variable analyzed | Tooth | Gow-Gates | Conventional |
| Agren and Danielsson (1981) $n = 12$ | 1.8/L-80 | % anesthesia before 60 min | M | 75% | 92% |
| Montagnese et al. (1984) $n = 40$ | 1.8/L-100 | % anesthesia at 10 min | LI | 35% | 38% |
| Goldberg et al. (2008) $n = 32$ | 3.6/L-100 | % anesthesia lasting 15–60 min | 1PM | 44% | 62% |
| Goldberg et al. (2008) $n = 32$ | 3.6/L-100 | % anesthesia lasting 15–60 min | 1M | 38% | 53% |
| Haghighat et al. (2015) $n = 63/73$ | 2.0/L-80 | % anesthesia at 10 min | PM | 75% | 60% |
| Haghighat et al. (2015) $n = 63/73$ | 2.0/L-80 | % anesthesia at 10 min | C | 41% | 49% |

LAS, local anesthetic solution; L-100, 2% lidocaine with 1:100 000 (10 µg/ml) epinephrine; L-80, 2% lidocaine with 1:80 000 (12.5 µg/ml) epinephrine; M, molar; PM, premolar; LI, lateral incisor; C, canine.

It should also be noted that the early reports that alleged better results with the Gow-Gates technique were conducted by Dr Gow-Gates himself or individuals highly trained and proficient in the technique, using 2.0 or 2.2 ml of local anesthetic instead of the standard 1.8-ml cartridges and plain (vasoconstrictor-free) solutions. These factors may account for the higher clinical efficacy (Annex 30) and lower positive aspiration rate (Annex 22) obtained.

### Zone Anesthetized

The zone anesthetized is as described in the general remarks, although the degree to which each element is numbed varies from one technique to another. All techniques must anesthetize the inferior alveolar nerve, a sure sign of which is soft tissue anesthesia in the lower lip ipsilateral to the side being anesthetized. *In 80% of cases, the lingual nerve is also anesthetized with this technique and the buccal nerve in 70%* (Table 16.3 and Annex 29).

### Technique

- Long (35–42 mm) needle, given the depth of the insertion. Caliber 25G is ideal because aspiration is possible and as it is thick and stiff, it deviates very little. If caliber 25G is not available, 27G can be used, although this is less effective because the degree of deviation is somewhat greater.
- Patient's position.
  - Supine or semisupine in dentist's chair.
  - *Maximum mouth opening* throughout the injection time to facilitate intraoral vision and position the neck of the mandible as far forward as possible (Robertson 1979; Kafalias and Gow-Gates 1987).
  - Head turned slightly to the same side as the side being injected (i.e. right in right-side blocks and left in left-side blocks) and always toward the dentist, who must correlate the intraoral and extraoral reference points with the least possible movement (Robertson 1979).
  - Tongue at rest and in the lower back part of the mouth.
- Dentist's position and position of their non-dominant hand (i.e. the left hand in right-handed clinicians) depending on the side to be anesthetized.
  - Right side:
  - Dentist at 8:00 o'clock.
  - *Left index finger in the patient's mouth.*
  - All other fingers stretching across the patient's face to block their vision and control the position of the mouth (Figure 16.3).
  - Left side:
  - Dentist at 9:00–10:00 o'clock.
  - *Thumb of the nondominant hand in the patient's mouth*, requiring the right-handed dentist to pass their (left) arm over the patient's forehead (Figure 16.4).
  - Dentist's non-dominant palm and wrist blocking patient's vision.
- Intraoral finger or thumb. *The finger in the patient's mouth should rest on the anterior edge of the ramus of the mandible*, in the concavity known as the coronoid notch, although the tip of the finger should rest somewhat more internally/medially on the temporal crest where the deep tendon of the temporal muscle lies (Figure 16.5), ensuring that the cheek is sufficiently withdrawn to:
  - Visualize the area and locate the injection site.
  - Tighten and stretch the soft tissue to make the needle insertion less traumatic.
- Extraoral reference points.
  - All are essential: tragus, intertragal notch of the ear between tragus and antitragus, and labial commissure are all essential (Figure 16.11).
  - These reference points serve a dual purpose:
    - To visualize the line joining the labial commissure to the intertragal notch, the pathway to be followed by the needle. The intraoral target (anterolateral side of the neck of the mandible) lies underneath the tragus (Figure 16.12).
    - To indicate the orientation of the syringe based on the separation of the tragus when the ramus of the mandible is more open or closed.
- Intraoral reference points. Note that intraoral reference points are secondary to the extraoral reference points and if the intraoral reference points seem to contradict the extraoral reference points on a particular patient, then the extraoral reference points supersede the intraoral points of reference. These intraoral points are supplemental and include:
  - Temporal crest, where the deep tendon connects to the temporal muscle.
  - Palatine cusp of the second or third upper molar.
  - Contralateral mandibular canines and premolars.
- Syringe direction and tragus of the ear (Gow-Gates 1973; Gow-Gates and Watson 1977; Levy 1981; Azagra and Cordoba 1983; Kafalias and Gow-Gates 1987) (Figure 16.13 and Figure 3.11, Chapter 3):
  - A tragus (lower part of the ear) flush against the face (flat tragus), the most common configuration, is indicative of a narrow divergent angle of the ramus of the mandible (scant divergence from the mid-sagittal plane). The syringe should be placed over the lower canine on the opposite side (maximum inferior incisive edge).
  - If the tragus projects notably outward from the face (diverget tragus), a configuration found in 10% of

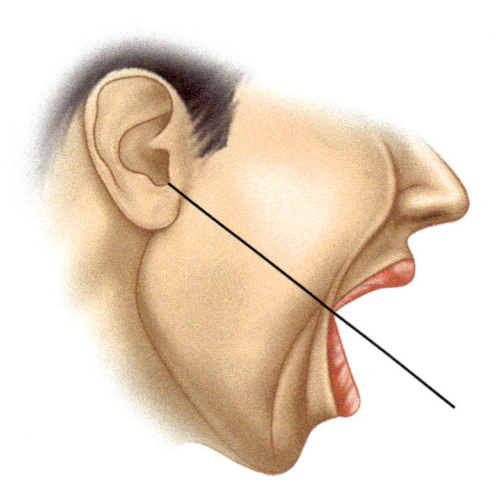

**Figure 16.11** Extraoral references for the Gow-Gates technique.

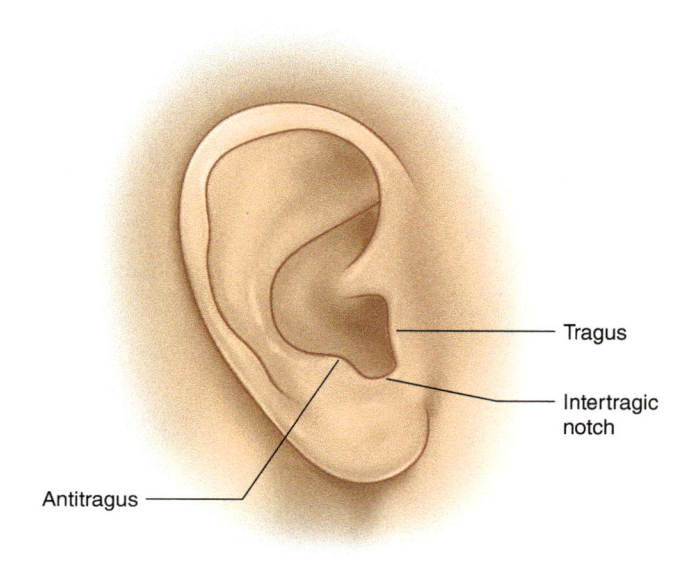

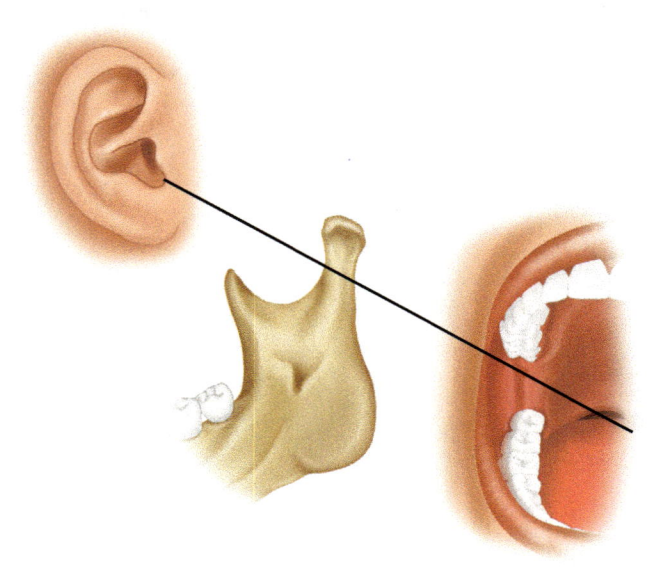

**Figure 16.12** Needle pathway and intra- and extraoral references in the Gow-Gates technique. *Source:* Redrawn from Gow-Gates and Watson (1977).

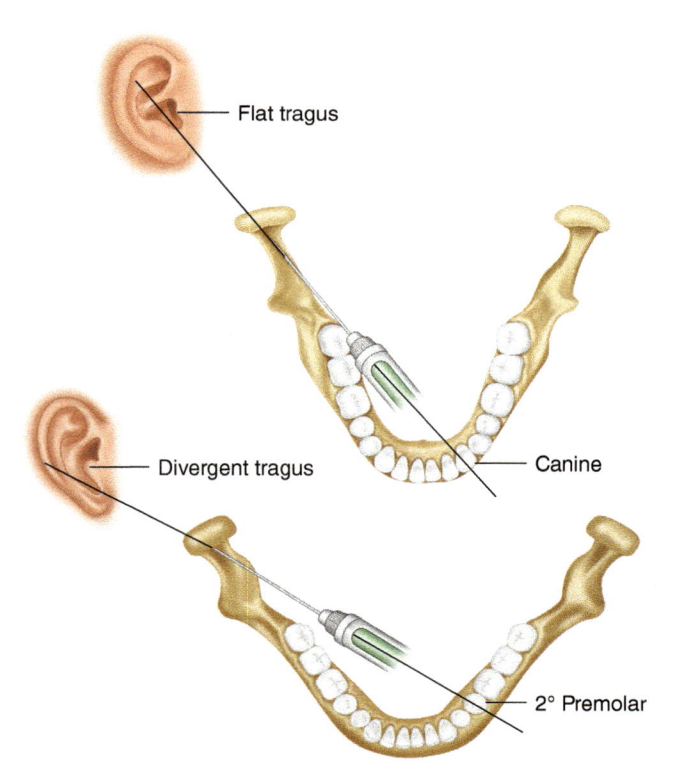

**Figure 16.13** Syringe orientation depending on the tragus position relative to the ear (flat or divergent).

cases (Simon and Kömives 1938), the divergent angle of the ramus of the mandible relative to the midsagittal plane is wide. The syringe should be positioned over the lower premolars on the opposite side (maximum edge of first molar).

- Needle insertion point (intraoral references) is at a much higher level than the conventional technique (Figure 16.14):
  - Horizontally, *the point is lateral to (outward of) the pterygotemporal depression but medial to and near the deep tendon of the temporal muscle* (not to be perforated), which can be felt with the tip of the intraoral finger.
  - Vertically, it is inserted on the distal side of the second molar (or the third if in normal occlusion and aligned with the rest of the arch), or at the height of its palatine cusp in children (Yamada and Jasstak 1981).

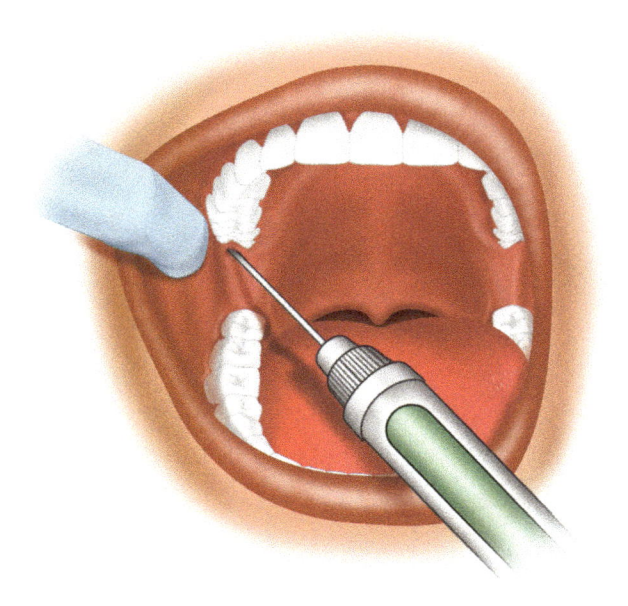

**Figure 16.14** Intraoral needle insertion point in the Gow-Gates technique (higher, more lateral/outward than in the conventional technique, without affecting the deep tendon of the temporal muscle).

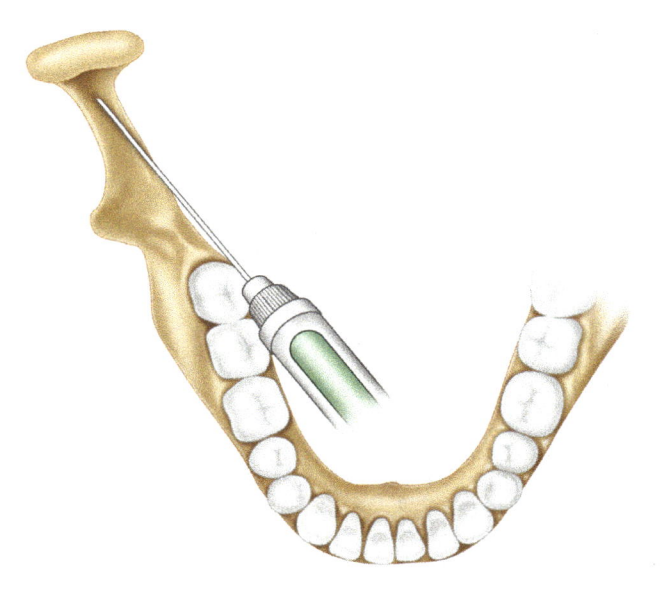

**Figure 16.15** Needle travel, around 25 mm, to the anterior-lateral side of the head of mandible.

- Nonetheless, the exact insertion site ultimately depends on the extraoral reference points. Note that it is higher and slightly more lateral (outward) than in the conventional technique.
- Path taken by the needle.
  - *The needle advances toward the tragus* along the reference plane defined by the line joining the labial commissure to the intertragal notch (Figure 16.15). *The insertion depth is 25 mm* (never over 28 mm) (Gow-Gates and Watson 1977, 1989) and in children 4–16 years old from 18 to 22 mm (Yamada and Jasstak 1981). When approaching the target *the needle must firmly impact the bone* to ensure it is on the anterior-lateral side of the neck of the mandible (Gow-Gates and Watson 1977, 1989; Gow-Gates 1981).
  - During this procedure the dentist must check intraorally and extraorally (the latter by turning the patient's head) to ensure that the needle is correctly directed toward the tragus (Levy 1981). Some authors recommend placing the needle cap on the external auditory meatus or asking the patient to place a finger in their ear to better visualize the orientation of the needle (Malamed 1981; Azagra and Cordoba 1983).
  - If no bone is impacted at 27–28 mm, the needle must be removed and reoriented, resting the hand more toward the premolars or the first mandibular molar on the opposite side (Gow-Gates and Watson 1977).

According to some reports, mandibular block was successful in 20% of first insertions when the anesthetic was injected even without feeling the bone (Goldberg et al. 2008).
  - Needle insertion and advance is fairly painless or slightly uncomfortable because very few nerve endings lie in its path (Gow-Gates 1973; Yamada and Jasstak 1981). Inserting the needle to the hub is a technical error for two reasons: (i) the depth of the needle is in excess of what is needed to provide anesthesia and (ii) the needle is weakest at its hub and may fracture at this point.
- Pre-injection aspiration.
  - *Once bone has been reached with the tip of the needle the clinician should avoid exerting undue pressure* to prevent injury to the periosteum (causing post-intervention pain) and barb formation on the tip of the needle. If a barb forms outwardly, the needle may traumatize muscles, neurovascular bundles, and anything else in its path.
  - *After touching bone the needle is withdrawn 1–2 mm for aspiration, which is positive in 5–10% of cases* (Annex 22).
- Injection of the anesthetic solution.
  - *A 1.8-ml cartridge should be slowly injected, in 40–60 seconds.* Gow-Gates initially used the 2.2-ml cartridges available in Australia (Watson and Gow-Gates 1976), which is why some authors recommend injecting *two cartridges or 3.6 ml* (Levy 1981; Coleman and Smith 1982; Kohler et al. 2008).
  - Many clinicians aspirate every 0.25–0.50 ml, seeking to further guarantee the safety of the injection with a

series of negative aspirations; this also helps slow the speed of administration by curbing the natural tendency to move faster.
    - After injection patients are asked to keep their mouth open for 20–60 seconds for the anesthetic solution to spread more effectively toward the nerve trunks (Gow-Gates 1973; Levy 1981; Montagnese et al. 1984).
    - Only one 1.8-ml cartridge is injected in children under 10 years old (Yamada and Jasstak 1981).
- Buccal nerve anesthesia (optional).
    - As the buccal nerve is anesthetized directly only 70% of the time (Annex 29), anesthesia can be enhanced if the solution is infiltrated directly during needle withdrawal.
    - Just before the needle is removed completely, a few drops of anesthetic are injected. This is effective because in a wide-open mouth, the buccal nerve is located very superficially, along the occlusal plane of the upper molars, where it crosses over the anterior edge of the ramus of the mandible (Coleman and Smith 1982; Montagnese et al. 1984).
- After injection is administered, ask the patients to keep their mouths open for at least 20 seconds if this is possible (Haas 2011).
- Subjective symptoms of anesthesia.
    - Soft tissue anesthesia appears in the lower lip on the anesthetized side around 6 minutes (Table 16.6) after injection and in *nearly 70% of cases in less than 5 minutes* (Annex 28). Soft tissue anesthesia may be described as tingling, numbing, itching, dullness, feeling "pins and needles," and feeling a "fat lip" sensation (Table 13.1, Chapter 13).
    - In around 5% of cases the lower lip is not anesthetized in the first 10 minutes (Annex 28). Such cases are regarded as failures and a second Gow-Gates mandibular block is recommended.
    - Soft tissue anesthesia is denoted by the following.
        - In the lower lip, from the corner of the mouth to the midline on the ipsilateral side to the injection site, it is a sign that the primary aim of the procedure (anesthesia of the inferior alveolar nerve) has been achieved.
        - In the tongue on the ipsilateral side, it is an indication of anesthesia of the lingual nerve, attained in 80% of cases (Table 16.3 and Annex 29).
        - In the area around the ipsilateral periauricular and temporal region, it is a sign of anesthesia of the auriculotemporal nerve, although this is less common.
- Supplemental buccal infiltration. Although no clinical studies have been published in this regard, this measure is recommended here just as it is for the conventional technique.
    - After the first 10 minutes when soft tissue anesthesia appears in the lower lip (sign of effective mandibular block), verifying anesthesia of the inferior alveolar nerve, supplemental buccal infiltration is recommended in posterior mandibular teeth requiring good pulpal anesthesia.
    - The infiltration is performed after 10 minutes to avoid the risk of masking or concealing mandibular block failure due to the overlapping of the effects of mandibular block and infiltration in the soft tissue.
    - Note that this measure anesthetizes the buccal nerve, as observed above.
    - In adults a potent solution such as a whole cartridge (1.8 ml) of *4% articaine with 1:100 000 epinephrine (A-100)* is injected buccal to the posterior teeth to be treated. This procedure aims to increase the number of teeth with pulpal anesthesia.
    - It takes an *additional 5–10 minutes* (15–20 minutes in total after starting mandibular block) for pulpal anesthesia to be fully effective.
- Duration of soft tissue anesthesia. This usually lasts 3–4 hours (200 minutes) (Agren and Danielsson 1981; Madan et al. 2017), and the patient should be notified of this as part of the informed consent process.

### Efficacy of this Technique

As previously noted, the Gow-Gates success rate, measured as Grade A anesthesia, is 80% compared to 85% for the conventional technique (Table 16.3). Nonetheless, given the fair number of shortcomings and uncontrolled factors associated with this assessment method, its values must be regarded as indicative only (Annex 30). The few studies of the degree of pulpal anesthesia conducted with the much more reliable electric pulp tester method appear to indicate that efficacy is similar to or somewhat lower than in the conventional technique (Table 16.7).

### Complications Specific to this Technique

- Technical errors in the Gow-Gates technique. Inappropriate maneuvering, the most common complication, leads to failed mandibular block and other complications, depending on the needle position on injection (Figures 3.13 and 3.14, Chapter 3).
    - Positioning the needle too laterally and too high is the most common technical error (Gow-Gates 1973). This is the result of directing the needle from the mandibular premolar zone on the opposite side (instead of the reference lower canine) and inserting it too high, usually above the palatine cusp of the second upper molar.

- Such maneuvering entails the risk of penetrating the sigmoid notch and injuring the masseteric artery (Shaw and Fierst 1988). The remedy is to remove the needle and re-introduce it, correctly oriented.
  - Starting from the mandibular lateral incisor on the opposite side (instead of the lower canine) positions the needle too far inward/mesially (the opposite of the above). As in the preceding case, it must be removed and re-oriented.
  - A needle positioned too high, above the palatine cusp of the second upper molar, runs the risk of perforating the lateral (external) pterygoid muscle and inducing trismus (Coleman and Smith 1982; Shaw and Fierst 1988).
- Side effects specific to the Gow-Gates technique. *Headaches (cephaleas) attributable to changes in the middle ear* are a rare side effect fairly specific to this technique (Levy 1981; Brodsky and Dower 2001; Madan et al. 2017). They usually appear immediately after injection and may last for up to 10–15 days, after which they disappear spontaneously. They are characterized by a sensation of pressure in the middle ear, an altered sense of balance, (sometimes acute) hearing disorders, or pulsing earache, accompanied by headache. Although the cause is poorly understood, the belief is that while the zone is weakly vascularized, anatomical variations or puncturing the internal maxillary artery or branches of the middle meningeal artery with a needle oriented too inwardly induces hematoma or inflammation in the tissues around the Eustachian tube and middle ear (Levy 1981; Brodsky and Dower 2001).
- Other occasional side effects may appear, the most common being trismus, followed by ischemic pallor (blanching) and more rarely ocular alterations (Norris 1982; Fish et al. 1989; Dryden 1993) (Chapter 22).

### Remark on the Gow-Gates Technique

Based on the authors' own experience and after reviewing the available literature, the Gow-Gates technique is not recommended in routine practice, but only as an alternative to direct or conventional mandibular block for the following reasons:

1) The Gow-Gates technique is difficult to master, irrespective of the special aids that have come to market in recent years to make it easier (Jofré and Münzenmayer 1998; Zandi and Sabounchi 2008).
2) It has a longer onset (Table 16.6) than the conventional method, making it less practical for routine clinical work.
3) It has not been proven to anesthetize posterior mandibular tooth pulp more effectively than the conventional technique (Table 16.7).
4) Lingual nerve anesthesia is less successful than with conventional block (80% vs. 95%) (Table 16.3).
5) Although the buccal nerve is anesthetized at a higher rate with Gow-Gates than with the conventional approach (70% versus 60%) (Table 16.3), that advantage is offset when the latter is supplemented with buccal infiltration to improve pulpal anesthesia.

For these and other reasons the Gow-Gates technique is used by a minority of dentists, even though it is taught and demonstrated in many educational institutions (Johnson et al. 2007).

## Mandibular Block: Laguardia–Akinosi Technique

The Laguardia–Akinosi technique, also known as closed-mouth mandibular block (Akinosi 1977; Gustainis and Peterson 1981), consists of inserting the needle in the mucosa between the ramus of the mandible and the maxillary tuberosity alongside and parallel to the occlusal plane of the second upper molar to reach the pterygomandibular space with the patient's mouth closed (Figure 16.16).

The precedent for this technique was introduced in the early twentieth century by Türkheim (Cieszynski 1914; Carrea 1921) using a 30-mm long, caliber 22G needle with a 45° elbow to reach the *sulcus colli* with the mouth closed (Cieszynski 1914). In 1921, Juan Ubaldo Carrea of Buenos Aires improved the technique by inserting a straight needle at a very high position alongside the lower edge of the malar process (Carrea 1921). The technique as it is known today was developed by Laguardia at Montevideo in 1940 (Laguardia 1940). It was rediscovered in 1960 by Sunder Vazirani in Bombay (Vazirani 1960) and by Akinosi of Lagos in 1977 (Akinosi 1977). In the English-speaking world it is called the Akinosi or the Vazirani–Akinosi technique.

### Advantages and Disadvantages

- Advantages. It is the only technique where the inferior alveolar nerve can be anesthetized with the patient's mouth closed, which is useful in situations where the patient has significant trismus. Another advantage is its simplicity, in particular when compared to the conventional and Gow-Gates techniques.

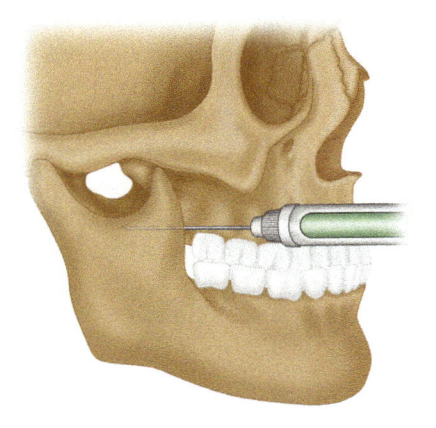

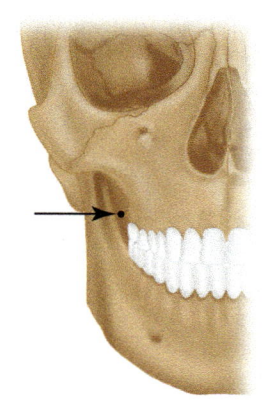

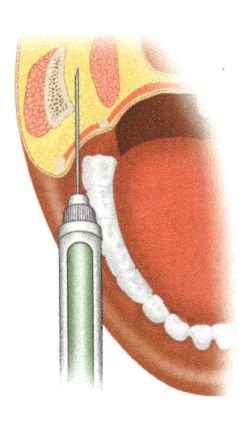

Figure 16.16  Three perspectives of the needle insertion zone in the Laguardia–Akinosi mandibular block. *Source:* Redrawn from Gustainis and Peterson (1981).

- Disadvantages
  - It fails more frequently than the conventional technique. Its Grade A anesthesia success rate is 80–85%, compared to 85% for the conventional technique (Table 16.3).
  - Onset is longer than with the conventional technique, with a 30% incidence of failed blocks within 5 minutes of administration, as compared to a 10% incidence of failed blocks in the conventional technique (Annex 28).
  - Appropriate needle depth is difficult to determine because no contact is made with bone.
  - This method is not reliable in pediatric patients due to the difficulty experienced in estimating the depth to which the needle should penetrate in the growing child (Akinosi 1977; Jendi and Thomas 2019).

## Use

The Laguardia–Akinosi closed-mouth technique is not designed for routine use, but as an alternative with patients:

1) *Unable to open their mouth wholly or partially (trismus)* (Laguardia 1940; Vazirani 1960; Akinosi 1977).
2) In whom having the dentist's fingers in their mouth induces nausea (Small and Waters 1983) or in patients whose tongue persistently obstructs the view of soft-tissue landmarks used in the conventional mandibular block (Haas 2011).

Extraoral techniques may also be used in many of these cases (Roberts and Sowray 1987), although this intraoral technique is currently preferred over the extraoral approaches to mandibular blocks.

## Distribution of the Anesthetic Solution

Diffusion-weighted imaging with contrast studies have shown that the anesthetic spreads well upward, backward, and outward in the pterygomandibular space. Anesthesia fails if the needle is too medial (inward), as this position hinders entry of the solution into the pterygomandibular space, where it spreads upward and inward or downward and outward (Gustainis and Peterson 1981).

## Zone Anesthetized

The zone anesthetized is as described in the general remarks, although the degree to which each element is numbed varies from one technique to another. All techniques must anesthetize the inferior alveolar nerve, a sure sign of which is soft tissue anesthesia of the lower lip on the side in question. *In 85% of cases, the lingual nerve is also anesthetized with this technique and the buccal nerve in 70%* (Table 16.3 and Annex 29).

## Technique

- Use a long (35–42 mm) needle, given the depth of the insertion. A 25G needle is ideal because it affords good aspiration and as it is thick and stiff, it deviates very little. If 25G is not available, 27G can be used, although less effectively (larger degree of deviation).
- Patient's position:
  - Reclining or semireclining in dentist's chair, with head turned slightly toward the dentist.
  - Lips open but teeth occluded or at rest (separation of a few millimeters between upper and lower arches) and chewing muscles relaxed to favor separation of the buccal mucosa and lips.
  - In edentulous patients, upper and lower arches separated to the estimated height of their former teeth (Vazirani 1960; Gustainis and Peterson 1981).

- Dentist's position and position of their non-dominant hand (i.e. the left in right-handed clinicians), depending on the side to be anesthetized.
  - Right side:
    - Dentist at 8:00 o'clock.
    - *Left index finger in the patient's mouth.*
    - All other fingers stretching across the patient's face to block their vision and control the position of the mouth (Figure 16.3)
  - Left side:
    - Dentist at 9:00.10:00 o'clock.
    - *Non-dominant thumb in the patient's mouth*, requiring the right-handed dentist to pass their left arm over the patient's forehead (Figure 16.4).
    - Dentist's non-injection palm and wrist blocking patient's vision.
- Intraoral finger or thumb. *The finger in the patient's mouth should rest on the anterior edge of the ramus of the mandible*, in the concavity known as the coronoid notch (Figure 16.5) to:
  - Retract the upper lip and cheek upward and outward to have a good view of the vestibule.
  - Tighten and stretch the soft tissue to make the needle insertion less traumatic.
- Intraoral syringe position. The syringe should be placed on the buccal side of the maxillary molars to (Figure 16.17):
  - Hold it parallel to the occlusal plane of the maxillary molars.
  - Hold it at either (Table 16.8):
    - A lower height along the cervical or gingival margin of the upper molars.
    - A greater height along the muco-gingival line that separates the inserted or attached gingiva from the alveolar mucosa.
- The needle is inserted into the mucosa between the ramus of the mandible and the maxillary tuberosity beside the second or third upper molar to reach a middle position inside the pterygomandibular space (Figure 16.16).
- *The recommended insertion depth is 25 mm*, but may range from 20 to 30 mm (Table 16.8). Inserting the needle to the hub is a technical error for two reasons: (i) it is the weakest part of the needle (therefore it may break) and (ii) this depth is excessive.
- Pre-injection aspiration. There is a 5% incidence of positive aspiration (Annex 22).
- Injection of the anesthetic.
  - *A 1.8-ml cartridge should be slowly injected in 40–60 seconds* (Table 16.8), although one author (Shaw and Fierst 1988) recommends 3.6 ml or two cartridges.
  - Many clinicians aspirate every 0.25–0.50 ml to further guarantee the safety of the injection with a series of negative aspirations; this also helps retard the injection by curbing the natural tendency to inject rapidly.
- Subjective symptoms of anesthesia.
  - Soft tissue anesthesia appears in the lower lip on the anesthetized side around 5 minutes after injection and in about *80% of cases in less than 10 minutes* (Annex 28), with a mean of 3 minutes (Table 16.9). Soft tissue anesthesia may be described as tingling, numbing, itching, dullness, feeling "pins and needles," and feeling a "fat lip" sensation (Table 13.1, Chapter 13).
  - In around 20% of cases the lower lip is not anesthetized in the first 10 minutes (Annex 28). Such cases are regarded as failures and a second Laguardia–Akinosi mandibular block is recommended.
  - Soft tissue anesthesia is denoted by the following:
    - In the lower lip, from the corner of the mouth to the midline on the ipsilateral side to the injection site it is

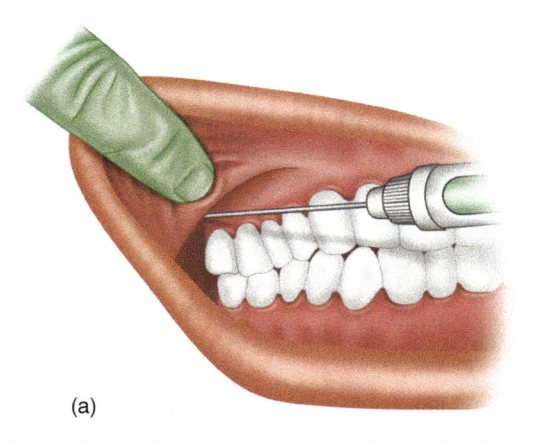

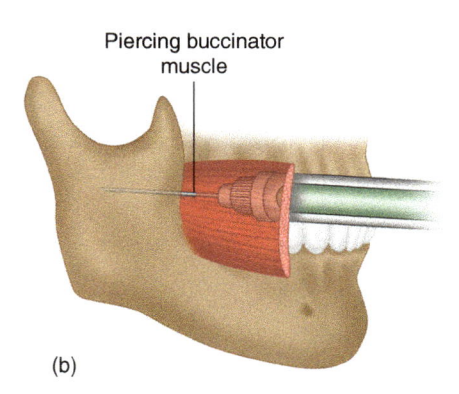

**Figure 16.17** Needle insertion site in the closed mouth technique: (a) at mucogingival margin and (b) crossing the buccinator muscle. *Source:* Redrawn from Roberts and Sowray (1987).

Table 16.8 Insertion depth, site, and volume in Laguardia–Akinosi mandibular block.

| Reference | Insertion depth (mm) | Insertion site | Volume injected (ml) |
| --- | --- | --- | --- |
| Vazirani (1960) | 15 | Cervical margin | — |
| Akinosi (1977) | 25–30 | Cervical margin | 1.5–2.0 |
| Gustainis and Peterson (1981) | 38 | Mucogingival junction | 1.5–1.8 |
| Jasmin et al. (1983) | 20–23 | Mucogingival junction | — |
| Small and Waters (1983) | 25–30 | Mucogingival junction | 1.8 |
| Dewitt (1984) | 25 | Mucogingival junction | 1.8 |
| Vailland (1985) | 25 | Mucogingival junction | — |
| Todorovic et al. (1986) | 25 | Cervical margin | 2.0 |
| Mean | **25 mm** | | **1.8 ml** |

Table 16.9 Onset (minutes) in lower lip with Laguardia–Akinosi mandibular block.

| Reference | Sample size | Latency (min) |
| --- | --- | --- |
| Todorovic et al. (1986) | 30 | 3 |
| Martínez-González et al. (2003) | 28 | 3.8 |
| Lenka et al. (2014) | 40 | 2.8 ± 0.6 |
| Kiran et al. (2018) | 70 | 3.2 ± 1.0 |
| Jendi and Thomas (2019) | 70 | 1.5 ± 0.4 |
| Nakkeeran et al. (2019) | 100 | 3.6 ± 1.6 |
| Mean | | 2.98 |
| Rounded mean | | 3 |

a sign that the primary aim of the procedure (anesthesia of the inferior alveolar nerve) has been achieved.
- In the tongue ipsilateral to the injection site it is an indication of anesthesia of the lingual nerve; this is attained in 85% of cases (Table 16.3 and Annex 29).
- In the area around the ipsilateral periauricular and temporal region it is a sign of anesthesia of the auriculotemporal nerve, although this is less common.

- Supplemental buccal infiltration. Although no clinical studies have been published in this regard, this measure is recommended here just as it is for the conventional technique.
  - It is recommended to wait for both the onset of soft tissue anesthesia in the lower lip (sign of effective mandibular block) and at least 10 minutes following the injection. One should wait to ensure that there is anesthesia of the inferior alveolar nerve and that the block has not been missed. A supplemental buccal infiltration is recommended to enhance anesthesia in posterior mandibular teeth requiring profound pulpal anesthesia.
  - The infiltration is performed after 10 minutes to avoid the risk of masking or concealing mandibular block failure due to the overlapping of the effects of mandibular block and infiltration in the soft tissue.
  - In adults a potent solution such as a whole cartridge (1.8 ml) of *4% articaine with 1:100 000 epinephrine (A-100)* is inserted on the buccal aspect of the posterior teeth to be treated. This procedure aims to increase the number of teeth with pulpal anesthesia.
  - It takes an additional *5–10 minutes* (15–20 minutes after starting mandibular block) for pulpal anesthesia to be fully effective.
- Duration of soft tissue anesthesia. This usually lasts 3–4 hours (200 minutes). The patient should be advised about this in the process of obtaining informed consent prior to treatment.

### Efficacy of this Technique

As noted previously, the Laguardia–Akinosi technique exhibits the same 80% success rates the conventional technique in terms of Grade A anesthesia (Table 16.3). Nonetheless, given the fair number of shortcomings and uncontrolled factors associated with this assessment method, its values must be regarded as indicative only (Annex 30). Unfortunately, no clinical studies on the evaluation of pulpal anesthesia with an electric pulp tester have been published to date for this technique.

### Complications Specific to this Technique

- Technical errors in the Laguardia–Akinosi technique. Inappropriate maneuvering, the most common complication, leads to failed mandibular block and other complications, depending on the injection position (Figures 3.13 and 3.14, Chapter 3).

- o A needle inserted too mesially/internally reaches the pterygomandibular ligament or raphe, which is tantamount to insertion from outside to inside the pterygomandibular space (Gustainis and Peterson 1981; Shaw and Fierst 1988). This is more common when right-handed dentists anesthetize the left side (Gustainis and Peterson 1981).
- o The needle may be too high, injecting the solution over the muco-gingival line, when inserted too slowly (Gustainis and Peterson 1981).
- Non-applicability of the technique in the presence of a large hyperplasia on the lateral maxillary edge that prevents correct needle positioning (Gustainis and Peterson 1981).
- Most common complications:
  1) The upper arch may be anesthetized if the anesthetic solution or part of it is deposited outside the pterygomandibular space. According to some reports symptoms of soft tissue anesthesia of the upper lip appear in nearly 8% of cases and of the infraorbital zone in 2% (Donkor et al. 1990).
  2) The side of the face affected may also pale (blanching) (Donkor et al. 1990).

## Double Infiltration in Anterior Teeth

This technique is also known as double infiltration because the anesthetic is injected twice, first buccally and then lingually. Given that, as noted earlier, mandibular block yields very poor results in the lower anterior incisors and canines (Table 16.1), double injection is deployed to attain pulpal anesthesia (Adatia and Gehring 1972). Infiltration is successful in these teeth for a number of reasons.

- The mandibular cortical bone in the anterior teeth, while thicker than the maxilla, is thinner than at the back of the mandible (Arens et al. 1984; Denio et al. 1992; Gowgiel 1992) (Table 3.2, Chapter 3).
- The mandibular zone has many foramina that favor the spread of the anesthetic (Starkie and Stewart 1931; Sutton 1974; Naitoh et al. 2009).
- In this part of the mandible, the mandibular incisive nerve or its plexus runs adjacent to the buccal aspect of the cortical bone (Annex 4).

Curiously, in the lower premolars the aforementioned is partly attributable to the presence of the mental foramen, with a 2–4 mm diameter, and in 5% of patients to the presence of accessory foramina (Annex 5), which favors the spread of the anesthesia.

### Keys to Success

The following maneuvers can raise the success rate of double injection in the anterior mandibular teeth:

- Infiltrating not only buccally but also lingually with 0.5–0.9 ml (double infiltration) (Meechan and Ledvinka 2002; Jaber et al. 2010; Nuzum et al. 2010) may block the accessory innervation penetrating the many foramina located along the mylohyoid line from the premolars to the mental symphysis (Shiller and Wiswell 1954; Sutton 1974; Chapnick 1980).
- Potent solutions such as 4% articaine with 1:100 000 epinephrine (10 µg/ml) (A-100) can be used instead of the standard lidocaine (L-100) solutions (Annex 31), given cortical thickness.
- Greater volume of anesthetic could be infiltrated, preferably a full cartridge (1.8 ml) instead of 0.9–1.5 ml and distributed between the buccal and lingual zone, either half (0.9 ml) on each side or more buccally and less lingually
- The anesthetic should be allowed more time, from 5 to 10 minutes, to take effect in the dental pulp (Annex 31), given that the cortical bone is thicker and therefore penetrated more slowly.

### Zone Anesthetized

- Tooth (periodontal pulp and ligament) injected, often extending to the mesial and distal adjacent teeth.
- Buccal and lingual zone, including fibromucosa (alveolar mucosa, gum and interdental papillae), bone, and periosteum.
- Lower lip and chin in the injection zone.

### Technique

- A 25G or 27G short (20–25 mm) needle is used, except where the technique is supplemental to mandibular block, in which case a long needle is acceptable.
- The solution of choice for adults is 4% articaine with 1:100 000 (10 µg/ml) epinephrine (A-100) and in children the standard 2% lidocaine with 1:100 000 epinephrine (L-100) (Annex 31).
- Patient's position:
  o Supine or semisupine with head raised slightly and chin tilted downward toward the sternum.
  o Mouth half open with muscles partially relaxed to favor lower lip and buccal mucosa relaxation.
- Dentist's position:
  o For anterior mandibular teeth on the left and even the right side, behind the patient, at 11:00–12:00 o'clock.
  o For anterior mandibular teeth on the right side, if preferred, at 8:00 o'clock.

- Buccal approach:
  - With the non-dominant index finger and thumb (i.e. left hand in right-handed dentists), the lower lip is retracted to view the floor of the vestibule and the mucogingival junction (line separating the darker attached gingiva from the lighter tone oral mucosa) to:
    - Improve visibility.
    - Stretch the oral mucosa to facilitate needle penetration and reduce pain on injection.
  - The needle is inserted (Figure 16.18) into the tensed oral mucosa *about 2–3 mm under the mucogingival junction* (Figure 16.19) (Roberts and Sowray 1987), because:
    - The roots of the mandibular teeth are very short.
    - The technique ensures deposit of the anesthetic in the submucosal connective tissue rather than in the chin muscles, where spread to the bone (and thus pulpal anesthesia) would be less likely and the intravascular absorption of the local anesthetic would be more likely.
- Lingual approach (Figure 16.20):
  - The patient is asked to raise their tongue and where they are unable to do so a mirror is used for retraction of the tongue and visualization of the floor of the mouth.
  - If necessary, the needle stem/shaft of the needle is bent slightly to facilitate insertion, but never at the hub, the weakest part of needles, where they tend to break.
  - The needle is inserted into the lingual vestibule, approximating the apex of the tooth to be treated to a depth of just 2–3 mm to position the anesthetic close to the bone and not in the mylohyoid muscle on the floor of the mouth.
- *Minimal intervention* (minimum volume/minimum injection time). This procedure, which significantly reduces the pain of injection, is implemented in four steps:
  - One or two drops of anesthetic are injected first buccally for 1–2 seconds and then lingually, likewise for 1–2 seconds and then needle is removed to anesthetize the soft tissue around the injection zone.
  - After a 60-second pause to anesthetize the soft tissue, another one or two drops are injected for 1–2 seconds first buccally and then lingually in the same vestibular and lingual sites (normally identifiable by tiny blood droplets caused by the first injection) and the needle is removed.
  - After a 30-second pause and after aspirating, a small amount (1/8 of a cartridge or 0.25 ml) of solution is injected into the same buccal and lingual sites for 7–10 seconds to reinforce the first two steps and begin pulpal anesthesia, waiting a further 30 seconds.
  - Thirty seconds later and again after aspirating, more of the anesthetic remaining in the *1.8-ml cartridge* is injected buccally and the rest lingually. Alternatively, the same amount may be injected on each side.

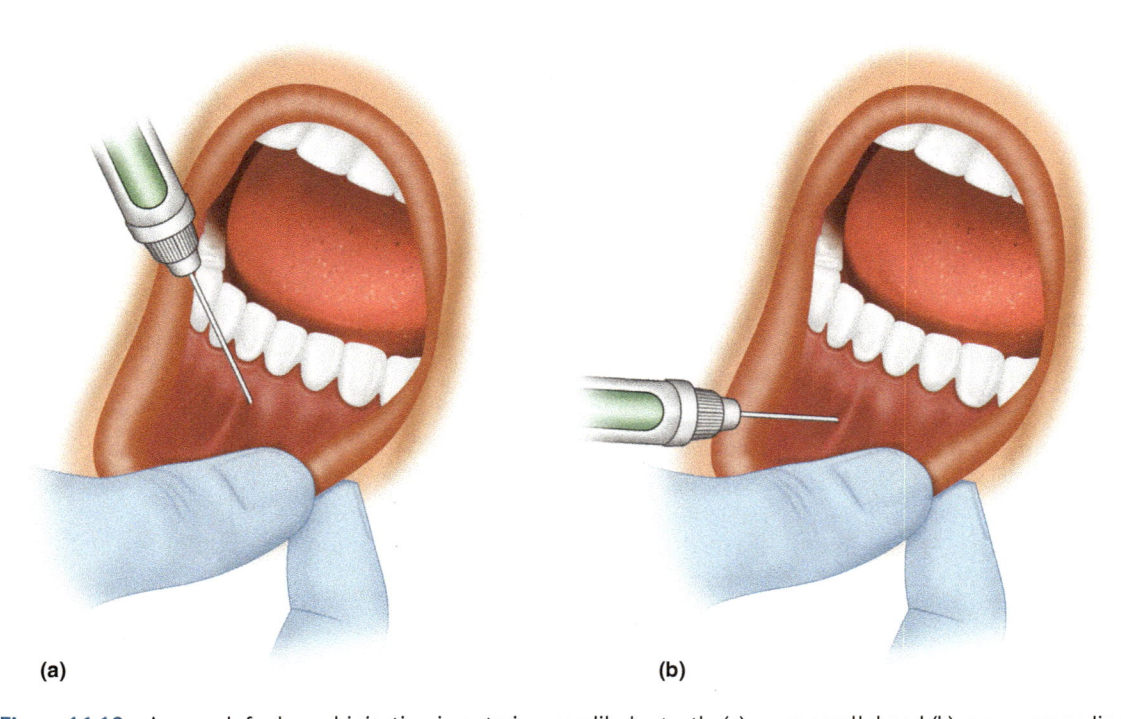

(a)     (b)

**Figure 16.18** Approach for buccal injection in anterior mandibular teeth: (a) more parallel and (b) more perpendicular to tooth.

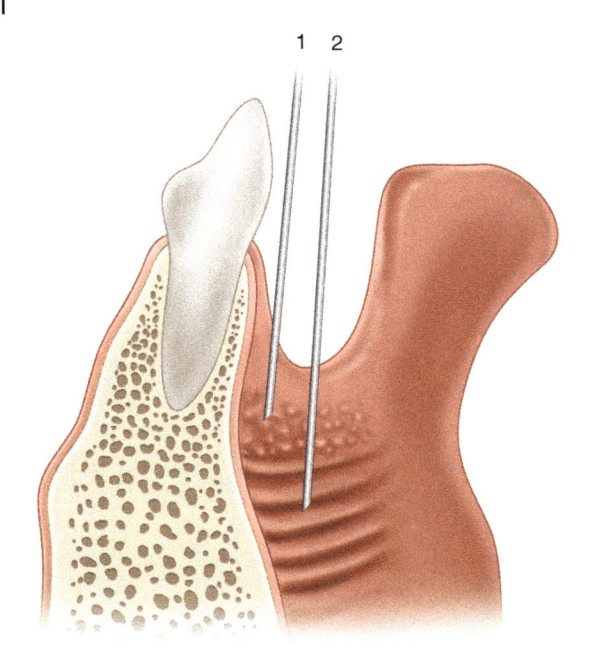

**Figure 16.19** Needle insertion immediately below the mucogingval junction, with millimetric penetration (1) due to shallowness of mandibular incisors and (2) to prevent injection in chin muscles. *Source:* Redrawn from Roberts and Sowray (1987).

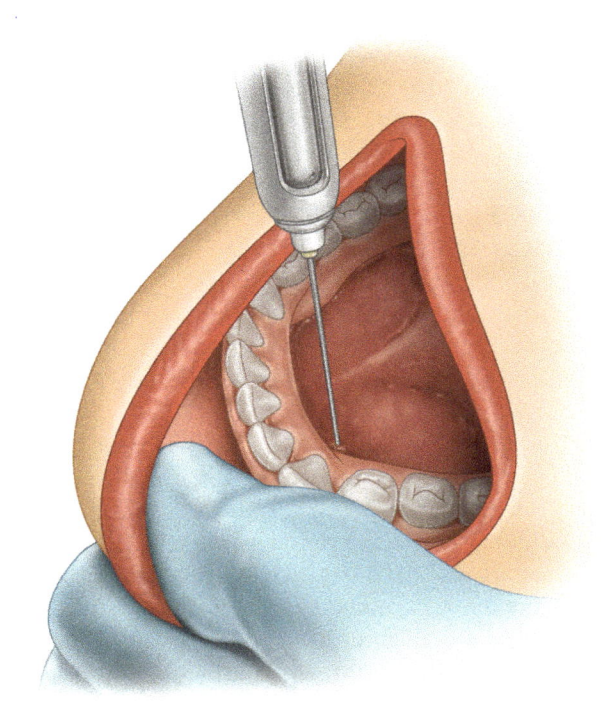

**Figure 16.20** Lingual injection in anterior mandibular teeth.

- Pre-injection aspiration. Positive aspirations appear (Annex 22):
   - In <1% of anterior mandibular teeth.
   - In 5% in the premolar buccal zone due to the proximity of the mental foramen neurovascular bundle.
- *Submucosa lump or blister. This protrusion must not be touched* to enable the anesthetic to spread across the periosteum, cortical, and spongy bone to reach the apex and from there the nerve fibers in the teeth. Massaging the blister forces the anesthetic to spread along the pathway of least resistance, the lax soft tissues, carrying it away from the injection site and lowering the concentration at the target zone and hence the capacity to reach the dental apex.
- Subjective symptoms of anesthesia, for example soft tissue anesthesia, appear in the lower lip after 2–3 minutes. Soft tissue anesthesia may be described as tingling, numbing, itching, dullness, feeling "pins and needles," and feeling a "fat lip" sensation (Table 13.1, Chapter 13). The total waiting period prior to intervening is *5–10 minutes* to ensure pulpal anesthesia since the cortical bone is fairly thick and its penetration slow (Annex 31).
- Duration of soft tissue anesthesia. This usually lasts 3–4 hours (200 minutes). The patient should be advised about this prior to treatment as part of the informed consent process.

## Efficacy of this Technique

Clinical studies conducted with an electric pulp tester and a potent anesthetic solution such as A-100 found the efficacy of this technique to be on the order of 98% in adult mandibular incisors (Table 16.10). The 80% efficacy in premolars can be raised to 93% if two cartridges (3.6 ml) are administered (Dressman et al. 2013).

**Table 16.10** Electric pulp tester-measured degree (%) of pulpal anesthesia after double infiltration in incisors and single infiltration in mandibular premolars and first molars (see Annex 31).

| 1.8 ml of anesthetic solution | Incisors | Premolars | First molar |
|---|---|---|---|
| 4% articaine + 1:100 000 epinephrine (A-100) | 98% | 80% | 65% |
| 2% lidocaine + 1:100 000 epinephrine (L-100) | 91% | 80% | 40% |

## Complications Specific to this Technique

Fortunately, this technique seldom poses complications. The most frequent is a *subcutaneous hematoma*, particularly where the minimum volume/minimum time technique is used, due to the repeated injections in the mucosa. Hematomas, which may arise around the insertion sites due to small vessel damage, are usually asymptomatic and often disappear spontaneously in a few days.

# References

Adatia, A.K. and Gehring, E.N. (1972). Bilateral inferior alveolar and lingual nerve block. *Br. Dent. J.* 133 (9): 377–383.

Agren, E. and Danielsson, K. (1981). Conduction block analgesia in the mandible. *Swed. Dent. J.* 5 (3): 81–89.

Akinosi, J.O. (1977). A new approach to the mandibular nerve block. *Br. J. Oral Surg.* 15 (1): 83–87.

Andlaw, R.J. and Rock, W.P. (1994). *Manual de odontopediatría*, 3e. Mexico: Interamericana. McGraw-Hill. 82 (Translated from the English original: A manual of paedodontics. London: Longman Group. 1993).

Angelman, J. (1945). The inferior dental injection. *Br. Dent. J.* 79 (2): 31–37.

Annex 1. Frequency of use of local anesthesia in dentistry.

Annex 4. Mandibular incisive canal and anterior loop.

Annex 5. Mental foramen.

Annex 10. Maximum doses of dental local anesthetics solutions.

Annex 22. Positive aspirations.

Annex 23. Pain resulting from injection techniques.

Annex 24. Mandibular block I. Efficacy of the standard solution L-100 or L-80.

Annex 25. Mandibular block II. Pulpal anesthesia with the standard solution (L-100).

Annex 26. Mandibular block III. Late, discontinuous and short-term pulpal anesthesia.

Annex 27. Mandibular block IV. Anesthesia of the lower lip and time to first pain.

Annex 28. Mandibular block V. Failure of lower lip anesthesia.

Annex 29. Mandibular block VI. Lingual and buccal nerve anesthesia.

Annex 30. Mandibular block VII. Grade A clinical efficacy.

Annex 31. Mandibular pulpal anesthesia. Infiltrative.

Arens, D.E., Adams, W.R., and De Castro, R.A. (1984). *Cirugía en endodoncia*. Barcelona: Ed Doyma. 38–50.

Ay, S., Kücük, D., Gümüs, C., and Kara, M.I. (2011). Distribution and absorption of local anesthetics in inferior nerve block: evaluation by magnetic resonance imaging. *J. Oral Maxillofac. Surg.* 69 (11): 2722–2730.

Azagra, E. and Cordoba, J.F. (1983). Bloqueo mandibular por la técnica de Gow-Gates. Revisión. *Bol. Inf. Dent. (Madrid)* 43 (331): 35–40.

Barker, B.C.W. and Davies, P.L. (1972). The applied anatomy of the pterigomandibular space. *Br. J. Oral Surg.* 10 (1): 43–55.

Benham, N.R. (1976). The cephalometric position of the mandibular foramen with age. *J. Dent. Child.* 43 (4): 233–237.

Berns, J.M. and Sadove, M.S. (1962). Mandibular block injection: a method of study using an injected radiopaque material. *J. Am. Dent. Assoc.* 65 (6): 735–745.

Blair, E.A. and Erlanger, J. (1939). Propagation, and extension of excitatory effects of the nerve action potential across nonresponding internodes. *Am. J. Phys.* 126 (1): 97–108.

Boué, D., Boué, C., and Charriere, C. (1987). Evaluación clínica de las técnicas de anestesia mandibular en el joven. *Arch. Odontoestomatol. (Barcelona)* 3 (6): 299–304.

Bremer, G. (1952). Measurements of special significance in connection with anesthesia of the inferior alveolar nerve. *Oral Surg. Oral Med. Oral Pathol.* 5 (9): 966–988.

Brodsky, C.D. and Dower, J.S. (2001). Case report. Middle ear problems after Gow-Gates injection. *J. Am. Dent. Assoc.* 132 (10): 1420–1424.

Carrea, J.U. (1921). Procedimientos de anestesias tronculares de los nervios maxilares. *La Odontología (Madrid)* 30 (9): 393–405.

Chaney, M.A., Kerby, R., Reader, A. et al. (1991). An evaluation of lidocaine hydrocarbonate compared with lidocaine hydrochloride for inferior alveolar nerve block. *Anesth. Prog.* 38 (6): 212–216.

Chapnick, L. (1980). A foramen on the lingual of the mandible. *J. Can. Dent. Assoc.* 46 (7): 444–445.

Chavarria-Bolaños, D., Rodríguez-Wong, I., Noguera-Gonález, D. et al. (2017). Sensitivity, specificity, predictive values, and accuracy of three diagnostic tests to predict inferior alveolar nerve blockade failure in symptomatic irreversible pulpitis. *Pain Res. Manag.* 2017: 3108940.

Cieszynski, A. (1914). Technique of intra- and extraoral injection of the mandibular nerves in local anaesthesia. In: *Translations of the Sixth International Dental Congress*. (ed. HRF Brooks). London: Committee of the Sixth International Dental Congress. 729–733.

Clarke, J. and Holmes, G. (1959). Local anaesthesia of the mandibular molar teeth—a new technique. *Dent. Pract.* 10 (2): 36–38.

Cohen, H.P., Cha, B.Y., and Spangberg, L.S.W. (1993). Endodontic anesthesia in mandibular molars: a clinical study. *J. Endod.* 19 (7): 370–373.

Coleman, R.D. and Smith, R.A. (1982). The anatomy of mandibular anesthesia: review and analysis. *Oral Surg. Oral Med. Oral Pathol.* 54 (2): 148–153.

College, C., Feigal, R., Wandera, A., and Strange, M. (2000). Bilateral versus unilateral mandibular block anesthesia in a pediatric population. *Pediatr. Dent.* 22 (6): 453–457.

Cook, W.A. (1919). Anatomical measurement relative to conductive anesthesia with procaine and alcoholic injection for tic douloureux. *J. Nat. Dent. Assoc.* 6 (11): 1030–1038.

Delgado-Molina, E., Bueno-Lafuente, S., Berini-Aytes, L., and Gay-Escoda, C. (1999). Comparative study of different syringes in positive aspiration during inferior alveolar nerve block. *Oral Surg. Oral Med. Oral Pathol.* 88 (5): 557–560.

Denio, D., Torabinejad, M., and Bakland, L.K. (1992). Anatomical relationship of the mandibular canal to its surrounding structures in mature mandibles. *J. Endod.* 18 (4): 161–165.

DeWitt, K. (1984). What...another injection technique? *J. Wis. Dent. Assoc.* 60 (1): 22–23.

Dobbs, A.E. (1956). Alarming sequele of an inferior alveolar nerve block simulates Horner's syndrome. *J. Dent. Assoc. S. Afr.* 11: 358–386.

Donkor, P., Wong, J., and Punnia-Moorthy, A. (1990). An evaluation of the closed mouth mandibular block technique. *Int. J. Oral Maxillofac. Surg.* 19 (4): 216–219.

Dressman, A.S., Nusstein, J., Drum, M., and Reader, A. (2013). Anesthetic efficacy of a primary articaine infiltration and repeated articaine infiltration in the incisive/mental nerve region of mandibular premolars: a prospective, randomized, single-blind study. *J. Endod.* 39 (3): 313–318.

Dryden, J.A. (1993). An unusual complication resulting from a Gow-Gates mandibular block. *Compend. Contin. Educ. Dent.* 14 (1): 94–100.

Dubey, M., Ali, I., Passi, D. et al. (2017). Comparative evaluation of classical inferior dental nerve block and Gow-Gates mandibular nerve block for posterior dentoalveolar surgery: a prospective study and literature review. *Ann. Med. Health Sci. Res.* 7 (1): 92–96.

Evers, H. and Haegerstam, G. (1981). *Handbook of Dental Local Anesthesia.* Copenhagen: Schultz Medical Information. 154.

Fan, S., Chen, W.-L., Pan, C.-B. et al. (2009). Anesthetic efficacy of inferior alveolar nerve block plus buccal infiltration or periodontal ligament injections with articaine in patients with irreversible pulpitis in the mandibular first molar. *Oral Surg. Oral Med. Oral Pathol.* 108 (5): e89–e93.

Fischer, G. (1910). *Di locale Anästhesie in der Zahnheilkunde. Mit spezieller Berück sichtingung der Schleimhaut und Leitungsanästhesie. Kurz gefaβtes lehrbuch für zahnärte, Ärzte und Studierende.* Berlin: Hermann Meusser.

Fish, L.R., McIntire, D.N., and Johnson, L. (1989). Temporary paralysis of cranial nerves III, IV, and VI after a Gow-Gates injection. *J. Am. Dent. Assoc.* 119 (1): 127–130.

Fuller, N.P., Menke, R.A., and Meyers, W.S. (1979). Perception of pain to three different intraoral penetrations of needles. *J. Am. Dent. Assoc.* 99 (5): 822–824.

Galbreath, J.C. and Eklund, M.K. (1970). Tracing the course of the mandibular block injection. *Oral Surg. Oral Med. Oral Pathol.* 30 (4): 571–582.

Gazal, G. (2015). Comparison of speed of action and injection discomfort of 4% articaine and 2% mepivacaine for pulpal anesthesia in mandibular teeth: a randomized, double-blind cross-over trial. *Eur. J. Dent.* 9 (2): 201–206.

Goldberg, S., Reader, A., Drum, M. et al. (2008). Comparison of the anesthetic efficacy of the conventional inferior alveolar, Gow-Gates, and Vazirani–Akinosi techniques. *J. Endod.* 34 (11): 1306–1311.

Gow-Gates, G.A.E. (1973). Mandibular conduction anesthesia: a new technique using extraoral landmarks. *Oral Surg. Oral Med. Oral Pathol.* 36 (3): 321–328.

Gow-Gates, G.A.E. (1981). Gow-Gates mandibular block (letter). *J. Am. Dent. Assoc.* 103 (5): 692.

Gow-Gates, G.A.E. and Watson, J.E. (1977). Gow-Gates mandibular block: further understanding. *Anesth. Prog.* 24 (6): 183–189.

Gow-Gates, G. and Watson, J.E. (1989). Gow-Gates mandibular block—applied anatomy and histology. *Anesth. Prog.* 36 (4–5): 193–195.

Gowgiel, J.M. (1992). The position and course of the mandibular canal. *J. Oral Implamtol.* 18 (4): 383–385.

Gustainis, J.F. and Peterson, L.J. (1981). An alternative method of mandibular nerve block. *J. Am. Dent. Assoc.* 103 (1): 33–36.

Haas, D.A. (2011). Alternative mandibular nerve block techniques. A review of the Gow-Gates and Akinosi–Vazirani closed-mouth mandibular nerve block techniques. *J. Am. Dent. Assoc.* 142 (9 Suppl): 8s–12s.

Haase, A., Reader, A., Nusstein, J. et al. (2008). Comparing anesthetic efficacy of articaine versus lidocaine as a supplemental buccal infiltration on the mandibular first molar after an inferior alveolar nerve. *J. Am. Dent. Assoc.* 139 (9): 1228–1235.

Haghighat, A., Jafari, Z., Hasheminia, D. et al. (2015). Comparison of success rate and onset time of two different anesthesia techniques. *Med. Oral Patol. Oral Cir. Bucal.* 20 (4): e459–e463.

Hall, R.J. (1884). Hydrochlorate of cocaine. *N. Y. Med. J.* 40: 643–644.

Hannan, L., Reader, A., Nist, R. et al. (1999). The use of ultrasound for guiding needle placement for inferior alveolar nerve blocks. *Oral Surg. Oral Med. Oral Pathol.* 87 (6): 658–665.

Hendy, C.W. and Robinson, P.P. (1994). The sensory distribution of the buccal nerve. *Br. J. Oral Maxillofac. Surg.* 32 (6): 384–386.

Hersh, E.V., Hermann, D.G., Lamp, C.J. et al. (1995). Assessing the duration of mandibular soft tissue anesthesia. *J. Am. Dent. Assoc.* 126 (11): 1531–1536.

Hetson, G., Share, J., Frommer, J., and Kronman, J.H. (1988). Statistical evaluation of the position of the mandibular foramen. *Oral Surg. Oral Med. Oral Pathol.* 65 (1): 32–34.

Hinkley, S.A., Reader, A., Beck, M., and Meyers, W.J. (1991). An evaluation of 4% prilocaine with 1:200,000 epinephrine and 2% mepivacaine with 1:20,000 levonordefrin compared with 2% lidocaine with 1: 100,000 epinephrine for inferior alveolar nerve block. *Anesth. Prog.* 38 (3): 84–89.

Hung, P.-C., Chang, H.-H., Yang, P.-J. et al. (2006). Comparison of the Gow-Gates mandibular block and inferior alveolar nerve block using a standardized protocol. *J. Formos. Med. Assoc.* 105 (2): 139–146.

Jaber, A., Whiteworth, J.M., Corbett, I.P. et al. (2010). The efficacy of infiltration anaesthesia for adult mandibular incisors: a randomized double-blind cross-over trial comparing articaine and lidocaine buccal and buccal plus lingual infiltrations. *Br. Dent. J.* 209 (9): E16. (1–6).

Jasmin, J.R., Vailland, J.-P., and Ionesco-Benaiche, N. (1983). L'anesthésie mandibulaire en pédodontie la méthode d'Akinosi. *Chir. Dent. Fr.* 53 (229–230): 61–64.

Jendi, S.K. and Thomas, B.G. (2019). Vazirani–Akinosi block technique: an asset of oral and maxillofacial surgeon. *J. Maxillofac. Oral Surg.* 18 (4): 628–633.

Jofré, J. and Münzenmayer, C. (1998). Design and preliminary of an extraoral Gow-Gates guiding device. *Oral Surg. Oral Med. Oral Pathol.* 85 (6): 661–664.

Johnson, T.M., Badovinac, R., and Shaefer, J. (2007). Teaching alternatives to the standard inferior alveolar nerve block in dental education: outcomes in clinical practice. *J. Dent. Educ.* 71 (9): 1145–1152.

Joyce, A.P. and Donnelly, J.C. (1993). Evaluation of the effectiveness and comfort of incisive nerve anesthesia given inside or outside the mental foramen. *J. Endod.* 19 (8): 409–411.

Kafalias, M.C. and Gow-Gates, G.A.E. (1987). The Gow-Gates technique for mandibular block anesthesia. A discussion and mathematical analysis. *Anesth. Prog.* 34 (4): 142–149.

Kanaa, M.D., Meechan, J.G., Corbett, I.P., and Whitworth, J.M. (2006). Speed of injection influences efficacy of inferior alveolar nerve blocks: a double-blind randomized controlled trial in volunteers. *J. Endod.* 32 (10): 919–923.

Kanaa, M.D., Whitworth, J.M., Corbett, I.P., and Meechan, J.G. (2009). Articaine buccal infiltration enhances the effectiveness of lidocaine inferior alveolar nerve block. *Int. Endod. J.* 42 (3): 238–246.

Keetley, A. and Moles, D.R. (2001). A clinical audit into success rate of inferior alveolar nerve block analgesia in general dental practice. *Prim. Dent. Care* 8 (4): 139–142.

Khoury, J.N., Mihailidis, S., Ghabriel, M., and Townsed, G. (2011). Applied anatomy of the pterygomandibular space: improving the success of inferior alveolar nerve blocks. *Aust. Dent. J.* 56 (2): 112–121.

Kim, H.-K., Lee, Y.-S., Kho, H.-S. et al. (2003). Facial and glossal distribution of anaesthesia after alveolar nerve block. *J. Oral Rehabil.* 30 (2): 189–193.

Kiran, B.S.R., Kashyap, V.M., Uppada, U.K. et al. (2018). Comparison of efficacy of Halstead, Vazirani Akinosi and Gow Gates techniques for mandibular anesthesia. *J. Maxillofac. Oral Surg.* 17 (4): 570–575.

Kohler, B.R., Castellón, L., and Laissle, G. (2008). Gow-Gates technique: a pilot study for extraction procedures with clinical evaluation and review. *Anesth. Prog.* 55 (1): 2–8.

Kronman, J.H., El-Bermani, A.-W., Wongwatana, S., and Kumar, A. (1994). Preferred needle lengths for inferior alveolar anesthesia. *Gen. Dent.* 42 (1): 74–76.

Laguardia, H.J. (1940). Uber die Leitungsanaesthesie und eine neue Methode der Mandibularanaesthesie. *Korrespondenzblatt für Zahnärzte (Berlin)* 64 (9): 283–291.

Lenka, S., Jain, N., Mohanty, R. et al. (2014). A clinical comparison of three techniques of mandibular local anesthesia. *Adv. Hum. Biol.* 4 (1): 13–19.

Levitt, B. (1924). A few departures from the standard technique in conduction anesthesia. *Dent. Cosmos* 66 (11): 1168–1176.

Levy, T.P. (1981). An assessment of the Gow-Gates mandibular block for third molar surgery. *J. Am. Dent. Assoc.* 103 (1): 37–41.

Lindsay, A.W. (1929a). The direct approach technic in mandibular block anesthesia. *J. Am. Dent. Assoc.* 16 (12): 2284–2286.

Lindsay, A.W. (1929b). The direct approach technique in mandibular block anesthesia. Thesis, Faculty of Dentistry, The University of Toronto.

Lloyd, J.M. (1992). Aspiration in dental local anaesthesia (letter). *Br. Dent. J.* 172 (4): 136.

Lustig, J.P. and Zusman, S.P. (1999). Immediate complications of local anesthetic administrated to 1,007 consecutive patients. *J. Am. Dent. Assoc.* 130 (4): 496–499.

Madan, N., Kamath, K.S., Gopinath, A.L. et al. (2017). A randomized controlled study comparing efficacy of classical and Gow-Gates technique for providing anesthesia during surgical removal of impacted mandibular third molar: a split mouth design. *J. Maxillofac. Oral Surg.* 16 (2): 186–191.

Malamed, S.F. (1981). The Gow-Gates mandibular block. *Oral Surg. Oral Med. Oral Pathol.* 51 (5): 463–467.

Malamed, S.F. (2004). *Handbook of Local Anesthesia*, 5e. St. Louis (Missouri): Elsevier-Mosby. 310–311.

Martínez-González, J.M., Benito-Peña, B., Fernández-Cáliz, F. et al. (2003). A comparative study of direct mandibular nerve block and the Akinosi technique. *Med. Oral* 8 (2): 143–149.

McCartney, M., Reader, A., and Beck, M. (2007). Injection pain of the inferior alveolar nerve block in patients with irreversible pulpitis. *Oral Surg. Oral Med. Oral Pathol.* 104 (4): 571–575.

McClure, D.B. (1968). Local anesthesia for the preschool child. *J. Dent. Child.* 35 (6): 441–448.

McLean, C., Reader, A., Beck, M., and Meyers, W.J. (1993). An evaluation of 4% prilocaine and 3% mepivacaine compared with 2% lidocaine (1:100,000 epinephrine) for inferior alveolar nerve block. *J. Endod.* 19 (3): 146–150.

Meechan, J.G. and Ledvinka, I.M. (2002). Pulpal anaesthesia for mandibular central incisor teeth: a comparison of infiltration and intraligamentary injections. *Int. Endod. J.* 35 (7): 629–634.

Montagnese, T.A., Reader, A., and Melfi, R. (1984). A comparative study of the Gow-Gates technique and a standard technique for mandibular anesthesia. *J. Endod.* 10 (4): 158–163.

Naitoh, M., Nakahara, K., Hiraiwa, Y. et al. (2009). Observation of buccal foramen in mandibular body using cone-beam computed tomography. *Okajimas Folia Anat. Jpn.* 86 (1): 25–29.

Nakkeeran, K.P., Ravi, P., Doss, G.T., and Raja, K.K. (2019). Is the Vazirani–Akinosi nerve block a better technique than the conventional inferior alveolar nerve block for beginners? *J. Oral Maxillofac. Surg.* 77 (3): 489–492.

Ngeow, W.C. and Chai, W.L. (2009). Numbness of the ear following inferior alveolar nerve block: the forgotten complication. *Br. Dent. J.* 207 (1): 19–21.

Norris, L. (1982). Eye complications following Gow-Gates block technique. *Dent. Anesth. Sedat.* 11 (2): 59–60.

Nusstein, J., Reader, A., Nist, R. et al. (1998). Anesthetic efficacy of the supplemental intraosseous injection of 2% lidocaine with 1:100,000 epinephrine in irreversible pulpitis. *J. Endod.* 24 (7): 487–491.

Nusstein, J., Steinkruger, G., Reader, A. et al. (2006). The effects of a 2-stage injection technique on inferior alveolar nerve block injection pain. *Anesth. Prog.* 53 (4): 126–130.

Nuzum, F.M., Drum, M., Nusstein, J. et al. (2010). Anesthetic efficacy of articaine for combination labial plus lingual infiltrations versus labial infiltration in the mandibular lateral incisor. *J. Endod.* 36 (6): 952–956.

Petersen, J.K. (1971). The mandibular foramen block. A radiographic study of the spread of the local analgesic solution. *Br. J. Oral Surg.* 9 (21): 126–138.

Pratts, J. and Ferres, E. (1999). Estudio comparativo entre las técnicas del bloqueo anestésico de la tercera rama del trigémino (convencional, de Gow-Gates y de Akinosi) en 120 exodoncias quirúrgicas de terceros molares inferiores. *Quintesence (Edición española)* 12 (3): 167–174.

Proaño, D. and Guillen, M.F. (2005). Comparación de las técnicas anestésicas de bloqueo mandibular troncular convencional directa y Gow-Gates en exodoncia de molares mandibulares. *Rev. Estomatol. Herediana* 15 (1): 30–35.

Reisman, D., Reader, A., Nist, R. et al. (1997). Anesthetic efficacy of the supplemental intraosseous injection of 3% mepivacaine in irreversible pulpitis. *Oral Surg. Oral Med. Oral Pathol.* 84 (6): 672–682.

Roberts, G.D. and Harris, M. (1973). Neuropraxia of the mylohyoid nerve and submental analgesia. *Br. J. Oral Surg.* 11 (2): 110–113.

Roberts, D.H. and Sowray, J.H. (1987). *Local Analgesia in Dentistry*, 3e. Bristol (UK): Wright. 95, 116, 121–123, 127, 128.

Robertson, W.D. (1979). Clinical evaluation of mandibular conduction anesthesia. *Gen. Dent.* 27 (5): 49–51.

Rood, J.P. (1978a). Some anatomical and physiological causes of failure to achiev mandibular analgesia. *Br. J. Oral Surg.* 15 (1): 75–82.

Rood, J.P. (1978b). The diameters on intermodal lengths of the myelinated fibers in human inferior alveolar nerve. *J. Dent.* 6 (4): 311–315.

Shaw, M.D. and Fierst, P. (1988). Clinical prosection for dental gross anatomy: a medial approach to the pterygomandibular space. *Anat. Rec.* 222 (3): 305–308.

Shiller, W.R. and Wiswell, O.B. (1954). Lingual foramina of the mandible. *Anat. Rec.* 119 (3): 387–390.

Sicher, H. (1946). The anatomy of the mandibular anesthesia. *J. Am. Dent. Assoc.* 33 (23): 1541–1557.

Simon, B. and Kömives, O. (1938). Dimensional and positional variations of the ramus of the mandible. *J. Dent. Res.* 17 (2): 125–149.

Simon, F., Reader, A., Drum, M. et al. (2010). A prospective, randomized single-blind study of the anesthetic efficacy of the inferior alveolar nerve block administered with a peripheral nerve stimulator. *J. Endod.* 36 (3): 429–433.

Sisk, A.L. (1985). Evaluation of the Gow-Gates mandibular block for oral surgery. *Anesth. Prog.* 32 (4): 143–146.

Sittitavornwong, S., Babston, M., Denson, D. et al. (2017). Lingual nerve measurements in cadaveric dissections: clinical applications. *J. Oral Maxillofac. Surg.* 75 (6): 1104–1112.

Small, S.C. and Waters, B.G. (1983). An alternative approach to mandibular block anaesthesia. *Oral Health* 73 (2): 21–23.

Stacy, G.C. and Hajjar, G. (1994). Barbed needle and inexplicable paresthesias and trismus after dental regional anesthesia. *Oral Surg. Oral Med. Oral Pathol.* 77 (6): 585–588.

Starkie, C. and Stewart, D. (1931). The intra-mandibular course of the inferior dental nerve. *J. Anat.* 65 (Pt 3): 319–323.

Steinkruger, G., Nusstein, J., Reader, A. et al. (2006). The significance of needle bevel orientation in achieving a successful inferior nerve block. *J. Am. Dent. Assoc.* 137 (12): 1685–1691.

Sutton, R.N. (1974). The practical significance of mandibular accessory foramina. *Aust. Dent. J.* 19 (3): 167–173.

Todorovic, L., Stajcic, Z., and Petrovic, V. (1986). Mandibular versus inferior dental anaesthesia: clinical assessment of 3 different techniques. *Int. J. Oral Maxillofac. Surg.* 15 (6): 733–738.

Tofoli, G.R., Ramacciato, J.C., de Oliveira, P.C. et al. (2003). Comparison of 4% articaine associated with 1:100,000 or 1:200,000 epinephrine in inferior alveolar nerve block. *Anesth. Prog.* 50 (4): 164–168.

Vailland, J.-P. (1985). Use technique originale d'anesthésie mandibulaire la méthode d'Akinosi. *Inform. Dent.* 67 (18): 1851–1852.

Vazirani, S.J. (1960). Closed mouth mandibular nerve block: a new technique. *Dent. Digest.* 66 (1): 10–13.

Via, W.F. (1953). The pterigomandibular space relation to effective mandibular block anesthesia for children. *J. Dent. Child.* 20: 105–110.

Vreeland, D.L., Reader, A., Beck, M. et al. (1989). An evaluation of volumes and concentrations of lidocaine in human inferior alveolar nerve block. *J. Endod.* 15 (1): 6–12.

Waikakul, A. and Punwutikorn, J. (1991). A comparative study of the extra-intraoral landmark technique and the direct technique for inferior alveolar nerve block. *J. Oral Maxillofac. Surg.* 49 (8): 804–808.

Watson, J.E. (1973). Appendix: some anatomic aspects of the Gow-Gates technique for mandibular anesthesia. *Oral Surg. Oral Med. Oral Pathol.* 36 (3): 328–330.

Watson, J.E. and Gow-Gates, G.A.E. (1976). A clinical evaluation of the Gow-Gates mandibular block technique. *N. Z. Dent. J.* 72 (330): 220–223.

Yamada, A. and Jasstak, J.T. (1981). Clinical evaluation of the Gow-Gates block in children. *Anesth. Prog.* 28 (4): 106–109.

Zandi, M. and Sabounchi, S.S. (2008). Design and development a device for facilitation of Gow-Gates mandibular block and evaluation of its efficacy. *Oral Maxillofac. Surg.* 12 (3): 149–153.

## 17

# Mandibular Anesthesia II: Complementary Anesthesia

## Introduction

Mandibular block does not always lead to anesthesia of the lingual nerve, and, therefore, of the tissue in the area of the tongue. Similarly, it does not anesthetize the buccal nerve or the tissues of the buccal area of the molars (Annex 29). Consequently, when working on the soft and hard tissue in this area, it is appropriate to anesthetize these nerve trunks.

The potency of anesthetic solutions – in terms of the anesthetic itself and the concentration of anesthetic and vasoconstrictor – is not important for surgery will be successful, since the buccal and lingual nerves are very superficial and not covered by periosteum, cortex, or aponeurosis. They therefore become anesthetized with a small volume of anesthetic solution. In this chapter, we review the following techniques:

- lingual nerve block
- buccal nerve block.

## Indications

These techniques do not aim to achieve pulpal anesthesia but rather complementary anesthesia for mandibular block in the following cases:

1) Oral surgery and extractions.
2) Scaling and root planning.
3) Subgingival preparations in the following cases:
   o Subgingival restorations.
   o Restorations by cervical caries.
   o Placement of a retraction cord.
   o Retraction of the gingiva at the level of the papilla.
4) Insertion of subgingival matrix bands.
5) Placement of clamps for a rubber dam that penetrate or pinch the gum in the buccal or lingual area.

## Lingual Nerve Block

The lingual nerve is generally anesthetized using mandibular block techniques (Annex 29). However, when this approach is unsuccessful or it is necessary to anesthetize the lingual nerve only, the technique is simple and almost 100% successful because the nerve is both superficial and accessible.

### Anesthetized Area

The anesthetized area corresponds to the whole area supplied by the lingual nerve (see Chapter 3). This includes the following:

- Fibromucosa (alveolar mucosa and attached gum), bone, and periosteum in the lingual area of the whole ipsilateral hemimandible up to the midline.
- Fibromucosa of the floor of the mouth on the ipsilateral side up to the midline.
- Anterior two-thirds of the tongue, on the ipsilateral side up to the midline. The nerve also provides proprioceptive sensation to the musculature of the tongue (Barker and Davies 1972).

### Technique

- Use a long needle (35 mm) owing to the very posterior position to be reached (here, the depth of the insertion is not important). The caliber used is 25G or 27G: as the technique is often complementary to mandibular block, we generally use the same needle.
- Position of the dentist and patient.
  o Dentist at 8:00–9:00 o'clock.
  o Patient semireclined with the head slightly turned toward the dentist. The patient's mouth is held wide open so that the dentist can reach the floor of the mouth.

*Local Anesthesia in Dentistry: A Locoregional Approach*, First Edition. Jesús Calatayud and Mana Saraghi.
© 2024 John Wiley & Sons Ltd. Published 2024 by John Wiley & Sons Ltd.
Companion website: www.wiley.com/go/Calatayud/local

- Separation of the tongue. Using a mirror in the support hand (left hand in right-handed persons), the dentist gently separates the tongue from the lingual surface of the second and third mandibular molars, thus revealing the floor of the mouth at this level (Figure 17.1).
- The point of insertion of the needle is located on the *floor of the mouth alongside the second and third molars* (Sicher 1946) because at this level the lingual nerve enters the floor of the mouth relatively close to the lingual bone plate. The nerve then courses forward within the floor of the mouth, pulling away from the lingual bony plates, and advances toward the center/interior to reach the base of the tongue (Figure 17.2).
- The needle is inserted 2–4 mm into the floor of the mouth. The insertion is short since the nerve runs below the mucous membrane but above the mylohyoid muscle (Figure 3.4, Chapter 3), which forms the base of the floor of the mouth.
- The injection is performed following the *minimum intervention technique* (minimum volume/minimum injection time), which considerably reduces the pain caused by the injection. The procedure is as follows:
  1) Initially inject only one or two drops of anesthetic solution in 1–2 seconds and wait 60 seconds after withdrawing the needle. Thus, the soft tissue is anesthetized at the injection site.
  2) Perform a second injection at the same site (the blood spot formed by the first injection may be visible). Again, inject one or two drops over 1–2 seconds. This time wait only 30 seconds after removing the needle.
  3) After aspiration, perform a third injection at the same site. However, this time the amount of anesthetic is

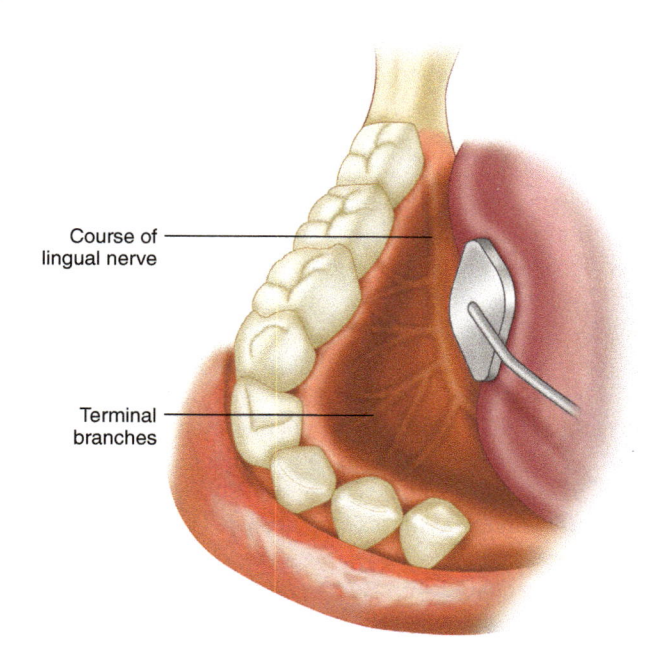

Figure 17.2 Course of the lingual nerve along the floor of the mouth and its terminal branches.

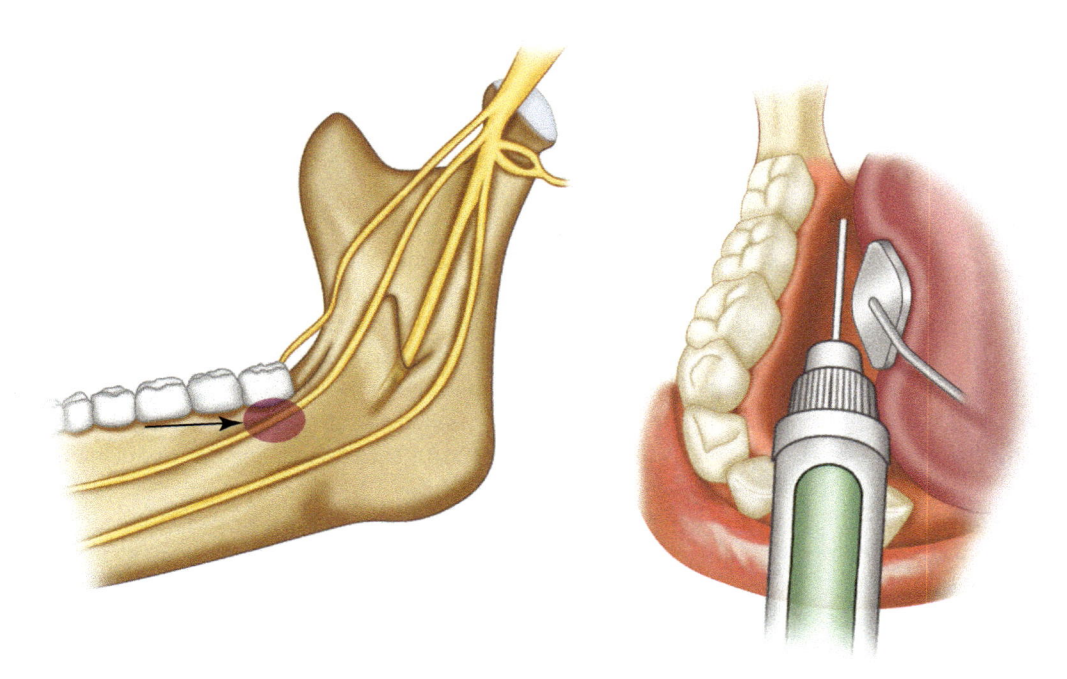

Figure 17.1 Anesthesia of the lingual nerve. Injection site.

larger (±1/8 of a cartridge, 0.2–0.25 ml) and is injected slowly over 7–10 seconds. Wait 30 seconds.
- Aspiration is positive in 1% of cases (Annex 22).
- Subjective symptoms of soft tissue anesthesia, defined by patients as dullness, numbing, tingling, and swollen tongue sensation (Table 13.1, Chapter 13) in the anterior and lateral areas of the tongue, appears after a few minutes and lasts 1–2 hours.

### Complications of this Technique

1) Local hematoma at the injection site owing to extravasation of blood from a vessel injured by the tip of the needle. The lesion is asymptomatic and resolves in a few days.
2) Rarely, the patient may experience an intense burning or electric shock sensation that appears suddenly on half of the tongue or at the tip on the same side as the injection. This is caused by contact between the needle and the lingual nerve. There are no sequelae.
3) Very rarely the parapharyngeal area is reached. This occurs when the needle is placed deep in the mouth, the insertion is behind the second mandibular molar on the floor, and the injection is made under a certain degree of pressure, with the mouth wide open. In this situation, the tip of the needle passes behind the posterior border of the mylohyoid muscle, and the anesthetic spreads throughout the area of the carotid triangle, thus anesthetizing the hypoglossal nerve (XII cranial nerve), the thyroid nerve, and the internal and external pharyngeal nerves far as the carotid body. This leads to a sensation of anesthesia and swelling in the neck on the relevant side, thus making it difficult to swallow and creating a sensation of chest tightness. The heart rate may also increase (palpitations), as may arterial blood pressure (Dormer and Barker 1976).

### Partial Variant as Complementary Anesthesia

The lingual nerve can be partially anesthetized by anesthetizing the floor of the mouth as far as the distal part of the tooth or the area to be treated (Allen 1979; Haglund and Evers 1985; Roberts and Sowray 1987). To do so, it is useful to deflect the needle a little along the shaft to reach the relevant areas easily, especially in the area of the mandibular incisors, and to insert the needle into the floor of the mouth alongside the lingual surface of the alveolar process of the tooth to be reinforced.

This complementary measure is frequently used in the area of the anterior teeth (Nordenram 1971) (Figure 17.3) owing to the presence of cross-innervation and supplementary innervation (see Chapter 19). The injection can also be performed

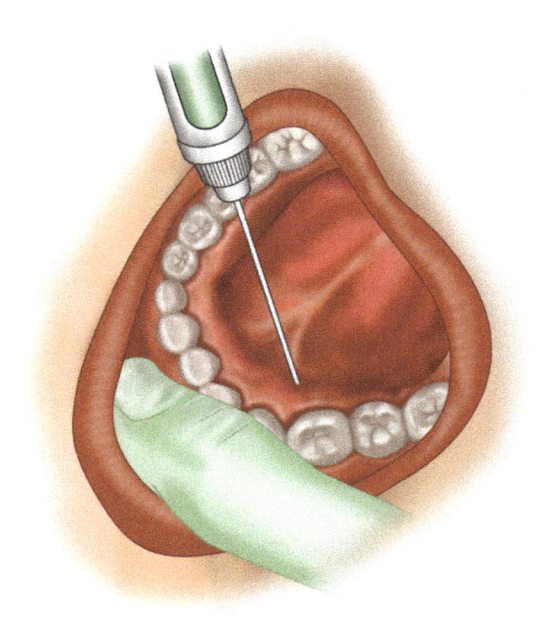

**Figure 17.3** Anesthesia of the lingual nerve, more anterior partial variant.

at the level of the premolars (Sutton 1974) or second molar (Murnane 1971) to block – in addition to the lingual nerve – the mylohyoid nerve, which courses in contact with the bone along a canal in the internal surface of the mandibular body and immediately under the mylohyoid muscle, which is the floor of the mouth (Figure 3.4, Chapter 3).

In any case, complementary lingual anesthetic is precisely that, a complement, since it is fairly unsuccessful as a technique for achieving pulpal anesthesia (Table 17.1).

## Buccal Nerve Block

In some older books, this technique is also known as long buccal nerve block (Sloman 1939; Roberts and Sowray 1987) and buccinator nerve block (Sloman 1939), both of which names are incorrect. The buccal nerve is frequently anesthetized using mandibular block techniques (Annex 29), although when anesthesia is not achieved or only this nerve must be anesthetized, the technique is simple and almost 100% successful because the nerve is both superficial and accessible.

This technique is usually applied as a complement to mandibular block, therefore it is administered *after confirming soft tissue anesthesia in the lower lip* (sign that the inferior alveolar nerve has been anesthetized and that mandibular block is successful). Previously blocking the buccal nerve carries a risk of overlap with anesthesia of the lower lip and may mask a possible failure of mandibular block.

Table 17.1 Percentage of pulpal anesthesia achieved by complementary lingual anesthesia at the level of the mandibular molars, when used as the only anesthetizing technique.

| Tooth | Reference | Sample size | ml/LAS | Pulpal anesthesia (%) |
|---|---|---|---|---|
| Second molar | Clark et al. (1991) | 30 | 1.8/L-100 | 7% |
|  | Clark et al. (1991) | 30 | 1.8/L-100 | 17% |
| First molar | Sillanpää et al. (1988) | 29 | 1.8/P-03 | 21% |
|  | Clark et al. (1999) | 30 | 1.8/L-100 | 7% |
| Second premolar | Clark et al. (1999) | 30 | 1.8/L-100 | 10% |

LAS, local anesthetic solution; L-100, lidocaine 2% with epinephrine 1:100 000 (10 µg/ml); P-03, prilocaine 3% with felypressin 0.03 IU/ml (0.54 µg/ml).

## Anesthetized Area

The anesthetized area corresponds to the area supplied by the buccal nerve (see Chapter 3), as follows:

- Fibromucosa (alveolar mucosa and gum), bone, and periosteum in the buccal area of the lower molars, although this can vary. Thus, in 10% of cases the nerve only supplied the buccal area of the retromolar trigone (Hendy and Robinson 1994); in contrast, in less than 1% of cases it can reach the buccal area of the lower canine (Stewart and Wilson 1928; Stewart 1932; Sicher 1950; Singh 1981) (Figure 3.3, Chapter 3).
- The buccal mucosa of the posterior part of the mouth and the upper part of this area in many cases.
- In 80–90% of cases, this nerve is mainly sensitive, providing a motor supply to the lateral pterygoid muscle (external) (Kim et al. 2003).
- It can occasionally give off branches to supply the pulp of the mandibular molars (Schejtman et al. 1967; Sutton 1974; Ossenberg 1986).

## Technique

- The technique requires a long needle (35 mm) owing to the need to reach back into the oral cavity (depth of insertion is not important). The caliber can be 25G or 27G. Since the technique very often complements mandibular block, the same needle is generally used.
- Position of the dentist and patient.
  - Dentist at 8:00–9:00 o'clock.
  - Patient semireclined with the head turned slightly toward the dentist. The mouth is moderately open in order to separate the cheek tissue.
- The dentist uses the fingers of his/her support hand (left hand in right-handed dentists) to separate the buccal mucosa in order to better view the area.
  - On the patient's right side, the dentist puts the index finger inside the mouth.
  - On the left side of the patient, the dentist puts his thumb inside the mouth and tends to embrace the patient's head with his arm.
- The syringe is placed parallel to the occlusal plane of the molars.
- Insertion point. Various approaches are possible (Sloman 1939), although we have selected the most common (Figure 17.4):
  - High insertion point. The needle is inserted into the anterior border of the ramus of the mandible, close to and within the oblique line (external) and at the level of the occlusal plane of the inferior molars or somewhat higher. In this area, the buccal nerve crosses the anterior border of the ascending branch and is superficial, at some 2 mm below the mucous membrane (Sloman 1939; Phillips 1943).
  - Low insertion point. The needle is inserted into the bottom of the buccal area alongside the inferior molars, generally in the alveolar mucosa below the mucogingival line of the last molar, although it can be inserted below any of the molars. This block usually anesthetizes terminal branches.
- Insert the needle 2–4 mm. If it touches the bone, it should be withdrawn 1–2 mm.
- Inject the solution following the *minimum intervention technique* (minimum volume/minimum injection time), which considerably reduces the pain caused by the injection. The procedure is as follows:
  1) Initially inject only one or two drops of anesthetic solution in 1–2 seconds and wait 60 seconds after withdrawing the needle. Thus, the soft tissue is anesthetized at the injection site.
  2) Perform a second injection at the same site (the blood spot formed by the first injection is sometimes visible). Again, inject one or two drops over 1–2 seconds. This time wait only 30 seconds after removing the needle.
  3) Then perform a third injection at the same site. However, this time the amount of anesthetic is larger (±1/8 of a cartridge, 0.2–0.25 ml) and is injected slowly over 7–10 seconds after aspiration. Wait 30 seconds.
- Aspiration is positive in 1% of cases (Annex 22).

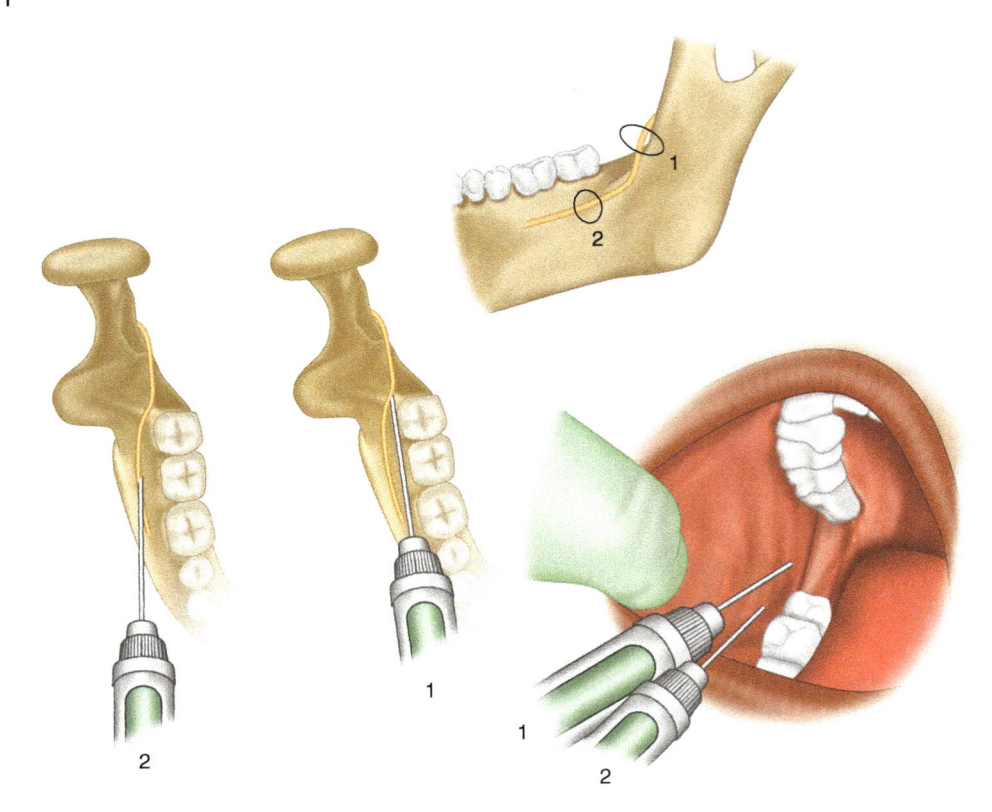

**Figure 17.4** Anesthesia of the buccal nerve. (1) High insertion in the anterior border of the ramus; (2) low insertion in the buccal area of the inferior molars.

- Subjective symptoms of soft tissue anesthesia, defined by patients as dullness, numbing, tingling, and swollen lip sensation (Table 13.1, Chapter 13), are rarely felt by the patient or are only felt weakly in the lower lip, therefore it is advisable to wait 2–3 minutes for the anesthetic to take full effect. The duration of anesthesia is 1–2 hours

### Specific Complications of this Technique

The most common complication is hematoma at the injection site resulting from extravasation from a vessel injured by the tip of the needle. The lesion is asymptomatic and resolves spontaneously in a few days.

## References

Allen, G.D. (1979). *Dental Anesthesia and Analgesia (Local and General)*, 2e. Baltimore: Williams and Wilkins. 114.

Annex 22. Positive aspirations.

Annex 29. Mandibular block VI. Lingual and buccal nerve anesthesia.

Barker, B.C.W. and Davies, P.L. (1972). The applied anatomy of the pterygomandibular space. *Br. J. Oral Surg.* 10 (1): 43–55.

Clark, S., Reader, A., Beck, M., and Meyers, W. (1991). Evaluation of mylohyoid and myloyoid/IAM blocks in human mandibular anesthesia. *J. Endod.* 17 (4): 194. (abstract no. 28).

Clark, S., Reader, A., Beck, M., and Meyers, W.J. (1999). Anesthetic efficacy of the mylohyoid nerve block and combination inferior alveolar nerve block/mylohyoid nerve block. *Oral Surg. Oral Med. Oral Pathol.* 87 (5): 557–563.

Dormer, B.J. and Barker, B.C.W. (1976). A rare local anesthetic misadventure. Case report and anatomic considerations. *Oral Surg. Oral Med. Oral Pathol.* 41 (3): 300–307.

Haglund, J. and Evers, H. (1985). *Local Anaesthesia in Dentistry*, 6e. Södertäleje (Sweden): Astra Läkemedel AB. 46, 49.

Hendy, C.W. and Robinson, P.P. (1994). The sensory distribution of the buccal nerve. *Br. J. Oral Maxillofac. Surg.* 32 (6): 384–386.

Kim, H.J., Kwak, H.H., Hu, K.S. et al. (2003). Topographic anatomy of the mandibular nerve branches distributed on the two heads of the lateral pterygoid. *Int. J. Oral Maxillofac. Surg.* 32 (4): 408–413.

Murnane, T.W. (1971. Cited by: Frommer J, Mele FA, and Monroe CW (1972).). The possible role of the mylohyoid nerve in mandibular posterior teeth sensation. *J. Am. Dent. Assoc.* 85 (1): 113–117.

Nordenram, A. (1971). *Manuel d'anesthesie locale enpractiquedentaire*. Mölndal (Sweden): Lindgren and Söner. Bofors Nobel-Pharma. 29.

Ossenberg, N.S. (1986). Temporal crest canal: case report and statistics on a rare mandibular variant. *Oral Surg. Oral Med. Oral Pathol.* 62 (1): 10–12.

Phillips, W.H. (1943). Anatomic considerations in local anesthesia in dental surgery. *Anesth. Analg.* 22 (1): 5–14.

Roberts, D.H. and Sowray, J.H. (1987). *Local Analgesia in Dentistry*, 3e. Bristol (UK): Wright. 124.

Schejtman, R., Devoto, F.C.H., and Arias, N.H. (1967). The origin and distribution of the elements of the human mandibular retromolar canal. *Archs. Oral Biol.* 12 (11): 1261–1267.

Sicher, H. (1946). The anatomy of mandibular anesthesia. *J. Am. Dent. Assoc.* 33 (23): 1541–1557.

Sicher, H. (1950). Aspects in the applied anatomy of local anesthesia. *Int. Dent. J.* 1 (1): 70–82.

Sillanpää, M., Vuori, V., and Lehtinen, R. (1988). The mylohyoid nerve and mandibular anesthesia. *Int. J. Oral Maxillofac. Surg.* 17 (3): 206–207.

Singh, S. (1981). Aberrant buccal nerve encountered at the third molar surgery. *Oral Surg. Oral Med. Oral Pathol.* 52 (2): 142.

Sloman, E.G. (1939). Anatomy and anesthesia of the buccinator (long buccal) nerve. *J. Am. Dent. Assoc.* 26 (3): 428–434.

Stewart, D. (1932). The innervations of the dental tissues and its importance in regional anaesthesia. *Br. Dent. J.* 53 (6): 277–284.

Stewart, D. and Wilson, S.L. (1928). Regional anaesthesia and innervations of the teeth. *Lancet* 212 (5486): 809–811.

Sutton, R.N. (1974). The practical significance of mandibular accessory foramina. *Aust. Dent. J.* 19 (3): 167–173.

# 18

# Supplementary Techniques in Cases of Failure

## Introduction

Supplementary techniques are applied only in the case of failure of conventional local anesthetic techniques, such as those mentioned above, therefore they are not first-choice, primary techniques. All of these techniques have special characteristics:

1) They are sufficiently powerful to achieve pulpal anesthesia.
2) They are self-limiting in their extension and their effect is very localized (they cover very few adjacent tissues), therefore they are not efficacious as primary techniques in the case of wider procedures that involve both soft and hard tissue.
3) Their action is independent of anatomical variations, such as accessory innervations or cortical thickness, which usually affect the efficacy of conventional techniques.
4) Anesthetic solutions enter the bloodstream easily and quickly, therefore it is important to take into account the following:
   - The total dose administered is limited. Their advantage is that the dose required is very low.
   - Aspiration is unnecessary since this is very often positive (almost intravascular).
5) Anesthetics with a long-lasting effect in the soft tissues, such as bupivacaine, etidocaine, and ropivacaine, are contraindicated because they do not improve the efficacy of pulpal anesthetic (Johnson et al. 1985; McLean et al. 1992; Hull and Rothwell 1998; Meechan 2002). In addition, since they enter the systemic bloodstream easily, they increase toxicity.
6) They are usually painful when used as primary techniques.

In this chapter, we shall address four techniques. However, the intraseptal technique can be considered a hybrid of the periodontal ligament technique (PDL) and intraosseous techniques. The techniques are as follows:

- Intrapulpal.
- PDL.
- Intraseptal.
- Intraosseous.

## Intrapulpal Anesthesia

This supplementary technique is applied when traditional methods fail, therefore the adjacent tissues are usually anesthetized, even if the dental pulp remains sensitive. The method consists of the injection of anesthetic solution directly into the dental pulp when the chamber is open. This approach is indicated in two situations:

1) In endodontic treatments, where the pulp chamber is open and remains sensitive to contact with instruments (the most common situation).
2) In surgical extractions in which the tooth is cut and remains sensitive (Berini and Gay 1997).

Below, we analyze two intrapulpal techniques, as follows:

- The traditional technique (the most frequent).
- The topical anesthesia technique.

### Traditional Technique

#### Keys to a Successful Approach

1) *The pressure* of the injection of anesthetic solution on the pulp (Birchfield and Rosenberg 1975; Van Gheluwe and Walton 1997). Experiments have shown that 100% of injections are unsuccessful if there is no pressure (Van Gheluwe and Walton 1997) and that injection of saline solution under pressure can be effective in a high percentage of patients (Birchfield and Rosenberg 1975; Van Gheluwe and Walton 1997).
2) An anesthetic solution with vasoconstrictor such as the *standard solution* of lidocaine 2% with epinephrine 1:100000 (10μg/ml) (L-100). Experiments have shown that a 90% success rate is achieved with saline solution,

*Local Anesthesia in Dentistry: A Locoregional Approach*, First Edition. Jesús Calatayud and Mana Saraghi.
© 2024 John Wiley & Sons Ltd. Published 2024 by John Wiley & Sons Ltd.
Companion website: www.wiley.com/go/Calatayud/local

but that a 100% success rate is achieved with L-100 (Van Gheluwe and Walton 1997). Higher concentrations of anesthetic and/or vasoconstrictor are not recommended because the anesthetic solution passes easily into the systemic bloodstream (Lamian and Simard-Savoie 1979; Smith and Smith 1983a), although this step is limited by apical constriction and residual pulp (Smith and Smith 1983a).

These recommendations enable 100% pulpal anesthesia, even in patients with irreversible, anesthetic-resistant acute pulpitis (Dreven et al. 1987; Cohen et al. 1993; Nusstein et al. 1998: Parente et al. 1998).

### Intrapulpal Technique

- 27G or 30G short needle (20–25 mm). If the needle is to be inserted into the radicular pulp canal, then the finer the better. It is usually necessary to bend the needle along its stem to facilitate insertion. The needle should not be bent at the hub, which is the weakest part and where it most commonly breaks.
- A little hole should be made in the pulp chamber to insert the needle. If the hole is too big, the anesthetic cannot be inserted under pressure and the solution will leak from the chamber. This can be avoided by *placing a cotton wool ball* in tweezers and pressing it against the needle inserted into the chamber to prevent reflux and maintain pressure (Walton 1990) (Figure 18.1).
- The patient should be warned that he/she will feel "intense discomfort" at the beginning of the injection, although this will be very brief (Miles 1983).
- *The needle should be placed firmly* with the fingers in the orifice and *a few drops should be injected under pressure* into the pulp chamber. In the case of multirooted teeth, if discomfort is felt in a canal as result of the instruments, the tip of the needle is inserted into the entrance of the canal, the needle is held firmly, and the solution is injected under pressure in such a way that it reaches the apex (Smith and Smith 1983a). If it is not possible to maintain pressure, place a cotton ball (see above) to maintain pressure and prevent reflux.
- After the injection, wait 30 seconds before starting to work. The anesthetic is working if the instruments can be introduced into the canals without pain. If the patient continues to experience discomfort, repeat the maneuver with emphasis on maintaining pressure (Van Gheluwe and Walton 1997).

### Topical Anesthetic Technique

This approach involves placing topical anesthetic gel (generally benzocaine 20%) into the root canals with endodontic files (DeNunzio 1998). Although this technique can be used as an alternative to the traditional technique, it is mainly used in cases of sensitive, twisted, and narrow canals where the needle cannot be appropriately positioned to maintain injection pressure.

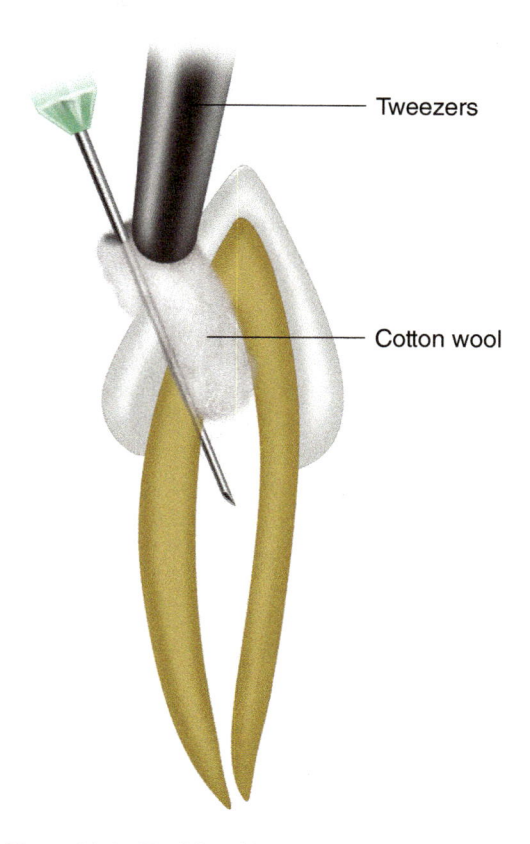

**Figure 18.1** Traditional intrapulpal technique in which a cotton wool ball has been placed in the pulp chamber to prevent reflux and maintain pressure during the injection.

### Technique

- Cover the tip of a no. 10 or 15 file with benzocaine 20% gel. It is very important for the gel to be viscous so that it adheres to the metal, therefore it should be kept at a low temperature. If the gel is very thin, having a liquid-like consistency due to high ambient temperatures, it can be placed in the refrigerator.
- Insert the file into the canal and file for a few seconds. One or two applications is usually sufficient, except in extremely sensitive patients, who may require more time and more applications.
- Any benzocaine gel remaining in the chamber can act as a reservoir for anesthesia of other canals in multirooted teeth.
- Once anesthesia is achieved, abundant irrigation can be applied to remove any remaining anesthetic from the canal. If irrigation is with hypochlorite, the benzocaine can turn a *dark reddish-orange color*. This also occurs if benzocaine mixes with blood. The color has no clinical relevance.

## Periodontal Ligament Technique (PDL)

This technique is also known as the intra-alveolar, intra-periodontal, intrasulcular, intraperiosteal, transligamentary, intraligamentary, or peridental technique (Nevin and Puterbaugh 1949; Mulkey 1976). The method involves trying to inject the anesthetic solution under pressure across the periodontal ligament and cancellous bone to reach the apex.

According to Nevin and Puterbaugh, this technique was first used in 1895 (Nevin and Puterbaugh 1949). The oldest reference we were able to find was by Emilie Sauvez from Paris in 1905 (Sauvez 1905), although it is not referenced as the original. Cassamani wrote a doctoral thesis on this technique in 1924 (Cassamani 1924), but this remained outside the scientific literature until the 1970s, when it was discussed in the studies of Robert Lafargue and Chenaux (Lafargue 1973; Chenaux et al. 1976). In 1981, a study by Richard Walton and Bernard Abbott made this technique known in English (Walton and Abbott 1981). Since then the number of his published scientific studies has increased.

### Indications and Contraindications

#### Indications

1) When the habitual anesthetic techniques fail (Council on Dental Materials, Instruments, and Equipment 1983; Johnson et al. 1985; Cowan 1986; Walton 1990; Meechan 1992). This is the basic indication since the duration of pulpal anesthesia is short and post-injection discomfort is common, as is the risk of periodontal lesions (see below).
2) In patients with severe hemophilia-associated coagulation disorders (Sachs et al. 1978; Pin 1987; Spuller 1988) or patients with high international normalized ratio (INR) taking anticoagulants (see Chapter 8), truncal block techniques (such as mandibular block, high-tuberosity technique, or transpalatal technique) can be replaced by the PDL technique.

#### Contraindications

1) In primary teeth (Brännström et al. 1984). Even though experimental studies in animals have demonstrated that solution injected using this procedure is distributed between the bony crypt and the enamel organ without penetrating the organ and with minimal apparent risk (Tagger et al. 1994a), experiments in monkeys revealed increased enamel abnormalities in the permanent teeth below the primary teeth that are injected using the PDL technique (Brännström et al. 1984), although these abnormalities are minimal. The exceptions to this contraindication are as follows:
   - Children with severe coagulation abnormalities (Spuller 1988) (see above).
   - Computer-controlled PDL injections (The Wand) because pressure is controlled (Table 18.2) and there are no enamel abnormalities (Ashkenazi et al. 2010).
2) Teeth with advanced periodontal disease (Rakusin et al. 1986), given that this can compromise periodontal support. Logically, teeth with periodontal disease that are to be extracted are an exception.
3) Infection at an injection site with cellulitis or abscess, given that this can be very painful and it may not be possible to achieve deep anesthesia (Reader et al. 2011; Council on Clinical Affairs 2015).

### Diffusion of the Solution

With the needle inserted in the gingival sulcus and firmly placed between the alveolar crest and the neck of the root of the tooth, the strong pressure exerted on the anesthetic solutions leads the solution to diffuse through two sites (Figure 18.2):

1) The periodontal ligament (Dreyer et al. 1983; Fuhs et al. 1983). Small quantities pass through to the periodontal ligament. Larger quantities cannot pass in humans, the width of the ligament is 0.13–0.21 mm (Coolidge 1937), the interval ranges from 0.06 to 0.35 mm (Kronfeld 1931), and the finest 30G needle has a caliber of 0.3 mm, thus restricting direct passage to the ligament. However, part of the solution penetrates via

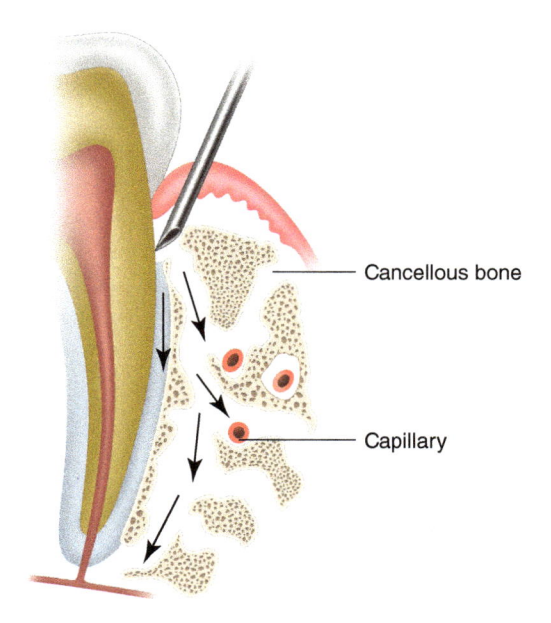

**Figure 18.2** Diffusion of the anesthetic solution along the periodontal ligament and along the fenestrations of the alveolar bone wall and of the subperiosteal orifices.

the alveolar wall fenestrations to reach the medullary cavities of the alveolar bone (Garfunkel et al. 1983).
2) Along the outer surface of the alveolar bone, below the periosteum and crossing through the cortical cavities to the medullary cavities of the alveolar cancellous bone (Tagger et al. 1994a; Tagger et al. 1994b).

In both cases, the anesthetic penetrates the medullary cavities of the alveolar cancellous bone (Fuhs et al. 1983; Dreyer et al. 1983; Garfunkel et al. 1983; Smith and Walton 1983b; Tagger et al. 1994a, 1994b), thus infiltrating wide areas of the bone under pressure and moving toward the apex at some distance from the injection site (Garfunkel et al. 1983; Smith and Walton 1983b). Furthermore, as it reaches the vessels and capillaries of the medullary cavities, it is considered to be equivalent with an intravascular injection (Smith et al. 1983c; Rawson and Orr II 1985; Pashley 1986), although experiments in humans have found that, compared with intravascular injection, blood levels are 25–40% without a vasoconstrictor, 10–15% with epinephrine, and 10–50% with felypressin (Cannell et al. 1993). In summary, the PDL technique functions in much the same way as the intraosseous technique (Garfunkel et al. 1983; Smith and Walton 1983b; Smith et al. 1983c; Pashley 1986), but with lower levels of anesthetic.

## Factors that Determine Efficacy

### Major Factors

1) *The pressure exerted is essential for successful anesthesia.* Resistance during injection is highly indicative of successful anesthesia (Walton and Abbott 1981; Smith and Smith 1983a) because the pressure is necessary for the anesthetic solution to be distributed along the periodontal ligament and bone marrow to reach the apex (Edwards and Head 1989).

2) Use of *pressure syringes (pistol-type)*. This type of syringe is more successful than traditional cartridge-type syringes (Table 18.1), thus reinforcing point 1 above. This point reinforces the first point, since pressure syringes are designed to exert more pressure during the injection (Pashley 1986; D'Souza et al. 1987; Walmsley et al. 1989), to the extent that it is almost double (Table 18.2).

3) Use of *local anesthetic solutions with epinephrine*. The best results are observed with standard solutions of lidocaine 2% with epinephrine 1:100 000 (Malamed 1982; Johnson et al. 1985; Kim 1986; Schleder et al. 1988) and 1:80 000 (Gray and Rood 1987; Meechan 2002), and articaine 4% with epinephrine 1:100 000 (Berlin et al. 2005).

Lidocaine 2% with epinephrine 1:50 000 (high concentration of epinephrine) also yields favorable results, which are even better and last longer than pulpal anesthesia, although they also increase the risk of adverse effects (such as tachycardi, palpitations, or tremors) (Kaufman et al. 1984). This better result is due not only to the fact that the vasoconstrictor retains the anesthetic by preventing its absorption, but also to the fact that epinephrine partially reduces blood flow in the dental pulp, thus leading to a partial reduction in A delta nerve fiber impulses (Edwards and Head 1989).

Poorer results are observed with anesthetic solutions that do not contain epinephrine (Malamed 1982; Kaufman et al. 1984; Kim 1986; Gray and Rood 1987; Meechan 2002), have low doses of epinephrine (1:200 000), or contain weaker vasoconstrictors (norepinephrine, levonordefrin, felypressin) (Malamed 1982; Kaufman et al. 1984, 1994; Johnson et al. 1985).

### Minor Factors

1) Treatments where efficacy is evaluated.
   - The best results are observed with extractions, obturations, and periodontal procedures (Malamed 1982;

Table 18.1 Percentage of success with intraligamentary (periodontal ligament technique) anesthesia achieved with high-pressure syringes (pistol-grip) or traditional cartridge syringes.

| | Success (proportion) | | |
| --- | --- | --- | --- |
| Reference | High-pressure syringe | Standard syringe | Treatment |
| Malamed (1982) | 89% (54/61) | 82% (32/39) | Ob, En, Ex, C |
| Smith and Walton (1983b) | 65% (39/60) | 62% (55/88) | En |
| D'Souza et al. (1987) | 72% (13/18) | 50% (12/24) | Cold |
| Proportion | 75% | 65% | |

Ob, obturation; En, endodontics; Ex, extraction; C, cutting.
Cold, dry ice stimulation.
$\chi^2 = 3.9537$ ($P < 0.05$).

Table 18.2 Maximum pressures achieved with standard high-pressure syringes (pistol-type) in the PDL and infiltrative techniques.

| Factors evaluated | | Pressure | | |
| --- | --- | --- | --- | --- |
| | | PSI | kg/cm$^2$ | Reference |
| Maximum pressure achieved | | | | |
| Anesthetic technique | Type of syringe | | | |
| PDL | Traditional | 340 | 23.9 | Pashley et al. (1981) |
| | Traditional | 325 | 22.8 | Walmsley et al. (1989) |
| | The Wand | 232 | 16.0 | Nusstein et al. (2005a) |
| | The Wand STA[a] | 294 | 20.3 | Hochman et al. (2006) |
| | High-pressure | 616 | 43.3 | Walmsley et al. (1989) |
| Infiltrative | Traditional | 153 | 10.8 | Maita and Horiuchi (1984) |
| | The Wand STA[a] | 11.5 | 0.8 | Hochman et al. (2006) |
| Palatal injection | The Wand STA[a] | 68 | 4.7 | Hochman et al. (2006) |
| Mandibular block | The Wand STA[a] | 5 | 0.35 | Hochman et al. (2006) |
| Cartridges: resistance to breakage | | | | |
| | Glass | 1474 | 101.2 | Meechan et al. (1990) |
| | Plastic | 655 | 45.2 | " |

kg/cm$^2$, kilograms per square centimeter; PDL, periodontal ligament; PSI, pounds per square inch.
1 kg/cm$^2$ = 14.5 PSI; 1 PSI = 0.069 kg/cm$^2$.
[a] The Wand STA injection 0.005 ml/second, mean pressure values.

Faulkner 1983; Kaufman et al. 1983; Miller 1983; Grundy 1984; Gray and Rood 1987), undoubtedly because these procedures require less deep pulpal anesthesia (Handler and Albers 1987; Walton 1990).

- The poorest results are observed with endodontic procedures (Malamed 1982; Faulkner 1983; Kaufman et al. 1983; Miller 1983; Grundy 1984) and tooth cutting (Malamed 1982; Kaufman et al. 1983; Miller 1983) because these approaches require deep pulpal anesthesia.

2) Teeth in which a PDL injection is made. Thus, the worst results are noted for the anterior teeth (incisors and canines) and the best results in the posterior teeth (molars and premolars) (Kaufman et al. 1983; White et al. 1988; Meechan 2002). These data are also shown in Table 18.3.
3) The clinician's experience with this technique also improves on the results of clinical trials (Grundy 1984).

## Instrument Set

The PDL technique can be performed with the traditional instrument set or with a more specific set, which is worthy of analysis in terms of both syringes and needles.

**Syringes**

1) Traditional syringe. This is the classic cartridge-type metal syringe, although it has certain disadvantages with respect to the PDL technique: (i) it exerts half the pressure of a high-pressure syringe (pistol-type) (Table 18.2), therefore its anesthetic effect is reduced (Table 18.1) given that pressure is a key factor for the success of this technique; (ii) women tend to exert 30% less pressure than men with the traditional syringe (Walmsley et al. 1989); and (iii) if the cartridge breaks because of excess pressure, the syringe does not have the security foil that high-pressure syringes have to prevent glass fragments from falling into the patient's mouth (Malamed 1982; Miller 1983).
2) Pen-type high-pressure syringe (Citoject®) (Figure 18.3). This type of high-pressure syringe is easier to hide in the hand, with the result that it is less "threatening" for the patient (Primosch 1986), although it is less stable and requires considerable pressure with the fingers (Cowan 1986). Each trigger pull injects 0.06 ml. In terms of clinical efficacy, this syringe is 65% successful as a primary technique (Cowan 1986).

Table 18.3 Percentage of pulpal anesthesia, evaluated using an electrical pulp tester, after administration of the standard solution (L-100) with the PDL technique and a high-pressure pistol-type syringe in the maxillary teeth (max) and mandibular teeth (mand).

| Tooth | Reference | Sample size | Pulpal anesthesia | Duration (min) | Adjacent teeth Mesial | Adjacent teeth Distal |
|---|---|---|---|---|---|---|
| **Molars and premolars (M and PM)** | | | | | | |
| First M max | White et al. (1988) | 20 | 75% | 7 | 45% | 60% |
| First M mand | White et al. (1988) | 38 | 79% | 6 | 33% | 62% |
|  | Cohen et al. (1993)[a] | 10 | 80% | — | — | — |
| First PM max | White et al. (1988) | 24 | 58% | 4 | 17% | 42% |
| First PM mand | Handler and Albers (1987) | 7 | 57% | 22 | — | — |
|  | Moore et al. (1987) | 19 | 79% | 10 | 16% | 63% |
|  | Schleder et al. (1988) | 75 | 87% | 20 | 45% | 78% |
|  | White et al. (1988) | 39 | 63% | 8 | 21% | 45% |
|  | McLean et al. (1992) | 24 | 38% | 12 | — | — |
|  | Meechan (2002) | 16 | 79% | 16 | — | — |
| Second PM | D'Souza et al. (1987)[b] | 42 | 60% | — | — | — |
|  |  | Average | 68.6% | 11.7 | 30% | 58% |
|  |  | Rounded average | **70%** | **10** | | |
| **Incisors and canines (LI, C)** | | | | | | |
| C max | Johnson et al. (1985) | 20 | 35% | 10 | — | — |
| LI max | White et al. (1988) | 23 | 39% | 16 | 30% | 26% |
|  | Kaufman et al. (1994) | 40 | 50% | 5 | — | — |
|  | Meechan (2002) | 16 | 75% | 16 | — | — |
| LI mand | White et al. (1988) | 22 | 18% | 7 | 9% | 9% |
| C max | Johnson et al. (1985) | 20 | 55% | 17 | — | — |
|  |  | Average | 45.3% | 11.8 | 20% | 18% |
|  |  | Rounded average | **45%** | **10** | | |

The table also shows the extension to adjacent teeth both mesially and distally.
L-100 is the standard solution of lidocaine 2% with epinephrine 1:100 000 (10 μg/ml).
[a] Cold stimulus with dichlorodifluoromethane in irreversible pulpitis, instead of an electric pulp tester.
[b] Cold stimulus with carbon dioxide, instead of an electric pulp tester.

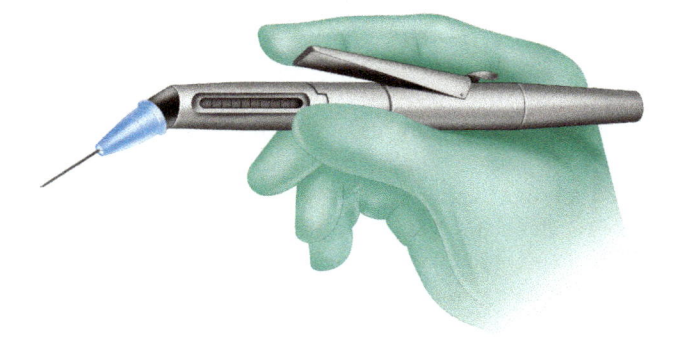

Figure 18.3 High-pressure pen-type syringe (Citojet®).

3) *Pistol-type high-pressure syringe* (Ligmaject® and Peripress® or similar syringes) (Figure 18.4).

This type of syringe first appeared in the 1970s. It has a pistol grip and a barrel with a lateral window that enables the clinician to see how much solution remains in the cartridge and any possible breakage in the cartridge (Primosch 1986). The syringe has a Mylar sheath that encases the cartridge in the barrel to prevent pieces of glass from entering the patient's mouth in the case of breakage (Khedari 1982; Malamed 1982; Miller 1983; Saadoun and Malamed 1985; Primosch 1986). It is important to remember that with this technique the cartridge can break in 1.5%

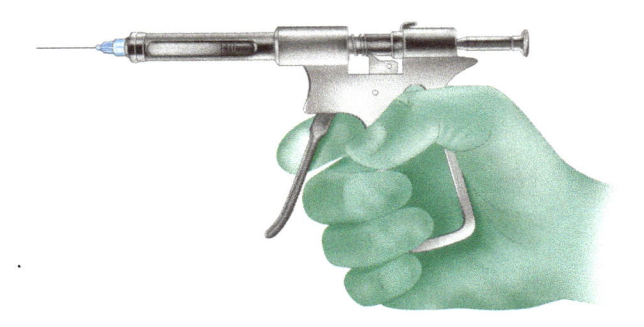

**Figure 18.4** High-pressure pistol-type syringe (Ligmaject® or Peripress®).

of cases (Primosch 1986). Each trigger pull injects 0.2 ml of the anesthetic solution (Council on Dental Materials, Instruments, and Equipment 1983).

The pistol grip provides better control and stability, thus enabling the following: (i) application of considerable pressure (Chenaux et al. 1976; Khedari 1982; Pashley 1986; D'Souza et al. 1987), almost twice that of a traditional syringe (Table 18.2), and (ii) a measurable difference in applied pressures between male and female providers has not been detected (Walmsley et al. 1989). Therefore, as a primary technique, this type of syringe has a success rate of 75% (Table 18.1).

### Needles

Traditional cartridge-type syringes require 27G or 25G short needles (20–25 mm). Since 25G needles are more rigid, they are easier to manage (Walton and Abbott 1981; Malamed 1982; Walton 1990).

High-pressure syringes require 30G or 27G extrashort needles (8–12 mm), and although the 30G needle is the most widely used, it is also the caliber that most frequently bends under the pressure applied during injection (Malamed 1982; Smith and Smith 1983a). Therefore, the extrashort 27G needle (8 mm) is preferable, since it bends less and is sufficiently fine to fit between the tooth and the alveolar crest.

### Cartridges

Glass cartridges are preferred because they can bear twice as much pressure as plastic cartridges before breaking (Table 18.2). Plastic cartridges do not break, although they deform at half the pressure of a glass cartridge, thus enabling the anesthetic solution to leak out (Meechan et al. 1990).

### Anesthetized Area

The area anesthetized with the PDL technique is well-defined, as in all supplementary techniques.

- Tooth (pulp and periodontal ligament) on which the technique is performed, extending mesially – and more often distally – to the adjacent teeth.
- Vestibule and tongue area, both the fibromucosa (alveolar mucosa, gum, and interdental papillae) and the bone and periosteum of the anesthetized tooth. It is important to remember that this technique is applied in a very well-defined area.

### Technique

- If a dental dam is in place, then it *must not* be removed (Nusstein et al. 2003). This is an advantage.
- As a primary technique, this approach is considered painful (Annex 23), but it is not painful in practice because it is used as a supplementary technique when all other approaches have failed and therefore all the adjacent tissues, but not the dental pulp, are anesthetized.
- Given our previous comments, the most advisable approach would be to use a pistol-type high-pressure syringe with an extrashort 27G needle (8 mm) and a local anesthetic solution with epinephrine (if there are no contraindications), similar to the one being used in the area (remember not to mix two different anesthetic solutions at the same site). For example, if articaine 4% with epinephrine 1:100 000 (A-100) is used in a buccal maxillary infiltration, then the same solution should be injected; if a mandibular block is performed with standard lidocaine 2% with epinephrine 1:100 000 (L-100) and then reinforced with a buccal infiltration a of A-100, then the procedure should be continued with A-100 in the intraligamentary technique.
- Clean the gingival area of food particles, debris, plaque, or tartar beforehand (Chenaux et al. 1976; Brännström et al. 1982; Kaufman et al. 1983; Council on Dental Materials, Instruments, and Equipment 1983; Faulkner 1983) to prevent them from entering the tissues.
- Insert the needle into the gingival sulcus. This is the most important step, and often the most difficult (Council on Dental Materials, Instruments, and Equipment 1983).
  - Insert the needle mesially into the mesial-buccal and mesial-lingual angles, distally into the distal-vestibular and distal-lingual angles (Figure 18.5).
  - With an angle of approximately 30° with respect to the axis of the tooth to respect the convexity of the enamel of the neck of the tooth (Figure 18.6).
  - The bevel should be facing outwards.
  - *The needle should be forced firmly between the alveolar crest and the cervical surface of the root of the tooth*, pressing toward the apex.
  - It is occasionally necessary to bend the stem of the needle to reach the most posterior teeth (Chenaux et al. 1976; Khedari 1982; Primosch 1986).

Orr II 1985). Some clinical trials report positive aspirations in 94% of cases (Medvedev et al. 2012).
- Inject under pressure.
  - *Pressure is very important for the success of the technique* and is a sign that the needle has been inserted correctly (Walton and Abbott 1981; Smith and Smith 1983a). If the injection is made at several points in a tooth, then there should be resistance to the injection in at least one point. If there is no resistance, then the anesthetic solution has been distributed through the soft tissue but has not reached the apex.
  - *If there is no resistance, remove the needle and reposition it* by reinserting it and forcing it toward the apex (Khedari 1982).
  - *Pressure should be maintained at each point for 10–20 seconds while injecting slowly* (Meechan 1992) in order to:
    - Prevent excess pressure from breaking the cartridge.
    - Ensure that the anesthesia penetrates the tissue, preventing reflux of the anesthetic into the mouth. Despite these measures, some of the anesthetic often flows back into the patient's mouth, and in 70% of cases he/she notices the bitter taste of the solution (Grundy 1984).
  - The gum adjacent to the injection point turns white and pale owing to the ischemic effect of the pressure and the vasoconstrictor.
- Amount to be injected.
  - Each trigger pull injects 0.2 ml (Chenaux et al. 1976; Council on Dental Materials, Instruments, and Equipment 1983). Thus:
    - In monoradicular teeth, the solution is injected into one or two of the abovementioned sites mesially and/or distally (total 0.2–0.4 ml).
    - In the case of multirooted teeth, the solution is injected at two or four sites mesially and distally (total 0.4–0.8 ml).
  - These amounts are indeterminate since an unknown quantity of solution flows back into the patient's mouth.
- *Onset of pulpal anesthesia is very fast (10–30 seconds)* (Walton and Abbott 1981; Kaufman et al. 1983; Gray and Rood 1987; White et al. 1988; Childers et al. 1996). In 93% of cases where anesthesia is successful, the pulp is already anesthetized at 15 seconds (Walton and Abbott 1981). *The anesthetic effect has a short duration, on average 10 minutes* (Table 18.3) and generally less than 20 minutes (Childers et al. 1996).
  - As the effect is very localized and there are scarcely any subjective symptoms (soft tissue anesthesia), the only guarantee of success is treatment. If the technique is used as a supplementary approach (the most common situation), the soft tissue anesthesia is from the techniques that have failed.

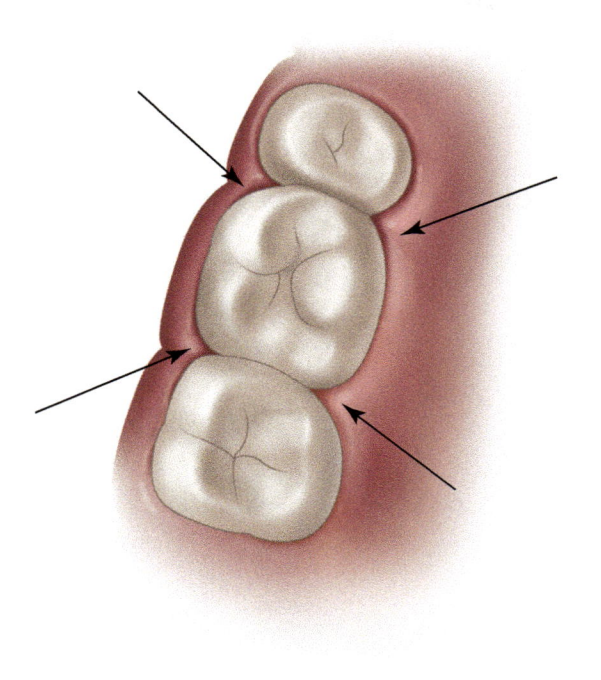

Figure 18.5 Mesio-vestibular, mesio-lingual, disto-vestibular, and disto-lingual angles where the needle is inserted.

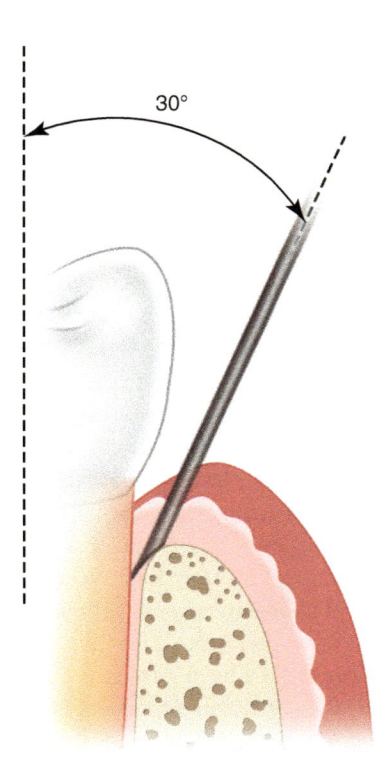

Figure 18.6 30° angle with respect to the axis of the tooth for insertion of the needle. Note that the bevel is turned outwards.

- Aspiration is not necessary since the anesthetic solution, once injected, is thought to reach the systemic bloodstream quickly (Smith and Walton 1983b; Rawson and

○ As primary anesthesia (very uncommon), anesthesia of the soft tissues lasts 25–40 minutes (Johnson et al. 1985).
- If the approach fails, a new attempt can be made after 30–60 seconds (Cohen et al. 1993), thus improving the results (Table 18.4). There is generally no risk of toxicity, even though the technique is considered to inevitably result in intravascular administration, since the dose administered is small and the technique is only used in specific teeth when standard techniques have failed. Moreover, part of the injected solution flows back into the mouth.

### Efficacy of This Technique

The efficacy of the technique is evaluated using an electric pulp tester, which tells us that the success rate is 70% in posterior teeth and 45% in anterior teeth, with a duration of around 10 minutes (Table 18.3). These data are for pistol-type high-pressure syringes and a single injection of standard solution (L-100). Furthermore, we can observe that the neighboring teeth are also anesthetized, especially the distal teeth (Table 18.3). Evaluation of clinical success (more subjective and less rigorous method) reveals a success rate of 90%, although this can be with one or two injections (two if the first fails) (Tables 18.4 and 18.5).

### Specific Complications of the Technique

#### Complications Due to Performance of the Technique

1) 30G needles usually bend because they are not very rigid and it is necessary to apply a certain degree of pressure (Malamed 1982; Kaufman et al. 1983; Smith and Smith 1983a), therefore it is more appropriate to use extrashort 27G needles in high-pressure syringes because these are more rigid and resistant. If the needle bends, it should be replaced.
2) Reflux of the anesthetic solution into the patient's mouth is common. The patient experiences the bitter taste in the case of solutions that contain vasoconstrictor (Malamed 1982; Kaufman et al. 1983). This occurs in 70% of cases in some series (Primosch 1986).
3) Breakage of a glass cartridge due to excess pressure (Malamed 1982; Kaufman et al. 1983). This has been reported in 1.5% of cases (Primosch 1986). Thus, with traditional cartridge-type syringes, pieces of glass may fall into the patient's mouth (especially if the cartridges do not have a transparent adhesive plastic protective sleeve [security foil] that limits splintering; Rawson and Orr II 1985). The problem of glass entering the patient's mouth does not affect the high-pressure syringes used in the PDL technique because they have a transparent plastic sleeve that encases the cartridge in the barrel of the syringe (Khedari 1982; Malamed 1982; Miller 1983).

#### Periodontal Abnormalities

The periodontium can be damaged for three reasons (Brännström et al. 1982; Peterson et al. 1983): (i) mechanical damage caused by the needle, (ii) pressure of the injected solution, and (iii) toxic effect of the solution.

Table 18.4 Percentage of successful clinical outcome after the first injection and after the first and second injections, both with pistol-type syringes.

| Reference | Treatment | Success First injection | First and second injection |
|---|---|---|---|
| Smith and Walton (1983b) | En | 65% | 85% |
| Gray and Rood (1987) | Ob, Ex, En | 71% | 92% |
| Cohen et al. (1993) | En | 80% | 90% |
| Cohen et al. (1993) | En | 70% | 100% |
| Average | | 72% | 92% |
| Rounded average | | **70%** | **90%** |

Ob, obturation; En, endodontics; Ex, extraction.

Table 18.5 Percentage of clinical success with the periodontal ligament injection using a pistol-type syringe and the standard injection solution (L-100).

| Reference | Sample size | Treatment | Success |
|---|---|---|---|
| Malamed (1982) | 100 | Ob, Ex, En, C | 86% |
| Faulkner (1983)[a] | 200 | Ob, Ex, En | 86% |
| Kaufman et al. (1983) | 258 | Ob, Ex, En | 84% |
| Miller (1983) | 361 | Ob, Ex, En, C | 96% |
| Smith and Smith (1983a) | 60 | En | 85% |
| Matthews and Stables (1985) | 100 | — | 86% |
| Rakusin et al. (1986) | 30 | Ob | 97% |
| Gray and Rood (1987) | 48 | Ob, Ex, En | 92% |
| Edwards and Head (1989) | 14 | Ex | 80% |
| Average | | | 88% |
| Rounded average | | | **90%** |

L-100, lidocaine 2% with epinephrine 1 : 100 000; Ob, obturation; En, endodontics; Ex, extraction; C, cutting.
Success after one or two injections.
[a] Local anesthetic solution unknown.

Studies with animals (mainly dogs and monkeys) and gum dissection have shown lesser damage, mainly in the bony crest and cementum and in the more coronal areas, with reabsorption of the root (Roahen and Marshal 1984, 1990; Nakane and Kamayama 1987). This type of damage reverses in a few weeks (Brännström et al. 1982; Walton and Garnick 1982; Dreyer et al. 1983; Fuhs et al. 1983; Peterson et al. 1983; Galili et al. 1984; Albers and Ellinger 1988).

Clinical studies in humans have shown that there are no periodontal sequelae after a few weeks (Malamed 1982; Moore et al. 1987; Schleder et al. 1988). However, complications and exceptional cases may arise, as follows:

1) Pain after a PDL injection is very common (Kaufman et al. 1984; D'Souza et al. 1987) and occurs in around 80% of cases (Schleder et al. 1988; White et al. 1988; Nusstein et al. 2004). It is very intense in 5% of cases (Table 18.6), although it usually resolves spontaneously in 2–3 days.
2) Twenty percent of patients report feeling that the tooth is high during occlusion (Table 18.6), although this resolves spontaneously in a few days. If the feeling does not improve, occlusion can be adjusted (Malamed 1982). There have been reports of two extreme cases of teeth that were ejected after the PDL injection: a first mandibular premolar (Nelson 1981) and a mandibular molar (Council on Dental Materials, Instruments, and Equipment 1983), both of which were healthy.
3) A certain degree of gingival inflammation appears in 5% of cases (Table 18.6). This resolves spontaneously in a few days, and, if it lasts longer, chlorhexidine mouth rinses and antibiotics can be administered. Three extreme cases have been reported: an upper molar with recession of the root that required endodontic treatment (White et al. 1988), a molar with marginal papillitis and necrosis (Kaufman et al. 1983), and a molar with inflammation of the gum, loss of 50% of bone, and pockets measuring 6–8 mm treated with scaling and root planning and antibiotics for 8 months (Childers et al. 1996).

**Pulpal Abnormalities**

Dissections of teeth in experimental animals revealed no histological changes or damage in dental pulp (Roahen and Marshall 1984, 1990; Peurach 1985; Albers and Ellinger 1988; Walton 1990; Plamondon et al. 1990). The same observation was reported for humans (Torabinejad et al. 1993). Some experimental studies revealed reduced pulpal blood flow due to the action of epinephrine in the injection (Kim 1986).

Clinical studies in humans have not reported pulpal abnormalities (Malamed 1982; Moore et al. 1987; Schleder et al. 1988), except for the case of pulpal abnormality in a cut tooth (Kim 1986). We do not know whether the PDL or the cutting caused the problem.

Table 18.6 Percentage of periodontal complications with the periodontal ligament injection.

| Reference | Sample size | Severe postinjection pain | High tooth feeling | Gum inflammation |
| --- | --- | --- | --- | --- |
| Malamed (1982) | 100 | 3% | 2% | — |
| Kaufman et al. (1983) | 258 | 2% | — | 0.4% |
| Faulkner (1983) | 200 | — | — | 2.5% |
| Grundy (1984) | 361 | 9% | — | — |
| Matthews and Stables (1985) | 100 | 11% | — | — |
| Johnson et al. (1985) | 20 | — | — | 5% |
| Rakusin et al. (1986) | 32 | 10% | — | — |
| Davidson and Craig (1987) | 100 | 8% | — | — |
| List (1988) | 22 | — | 27% | — |
| Schleder et al. (1988) | 75 | 5% | 49% | 5% |
| Spuller (1988) | 28 | — | 3.5% | — |
| White et al. (1988) | 147 | 2% | — | — |
| McLean et al. (1992) | 48 | 2% | 13% | — |
| Nusstein et al. (2004) | 51 | 3% | 27% | 8% |
| Average | | 5.5% | 20.2% | 4.2% |
| Rounded average | | **5%** | **20%** | **5%** |

### Cardiovascular Abnormalities

The PDL technique is considered almost intravenous since the anesthetic solution passes very quickly to the bloodstream. Experiments with dogs revealed a 20% fall in arterial pressure and a 20% increase in heart rate (Smith and Pashley 1983d; Pashley 1986).

Clinical trials with anesthetic solutions containing epinephrine 1:100000 (10 μg/ml) (Kaufman et al. 1994; Nusstein et al. 2004) and 1:80000 (12.5 μg/ml) (Gray and Rood 1987) did not reveal appreciable modifications in arterial pressure or heart rate. However, the use of higher concentrations of epinephrine (1:50000, 20 μg/ml) leads to an increase in heart rate (tachycardia), which patients describe as palpitations, in 20% of cases (Kaufman et al. 1984).

## Intraseptal Technique

The intraseptal technique, also known as the crestal technique (Giffin 1994) or papillary technique (Marthaler 1970), involves inserting the needle into the interdental papilla to reach the septum (where the cortical plate is very narrow or has disappeared [Marthaler 1970] and which is the exit for a large number of miniperforations that finish in the medullary cavity [Saadoun and Malamed 1985]) and penetrating a few millimeters with the tip of the needle to inject the anesthetic solution under pressure into the cancellous bone so that it spreads quickly to the apex of the tooth. In practical terms, *this approach is a variant of the PDL injection*; in addition, during the PDL injection, the needle very often becomes stuck in the alveolar crest instead of in the gingival sulcus, and the solution is injected into the interdental septum under pressure.

The intraseptal technique was already well known in the 1940s (Nevin and Puterbaugh 1949). It was recovered by Marthaler in the 1970s (Marthaler 1970).

### Factors Underlying a Successful Technique

1) The use of pistol-type high-pressure syringes, such as those used in the PDL (Ligmaject® or Peripress®), because they enable high-pressure continuous and uniform injection (Saadoun and Malamed 1985).
2) 27G extrashort needles (8–12 mm), which are somewhat thicker than the 30G needles, since these are sufficiently rigid so as not to bend during injection under pressure and sufficiently fine to penetrate the intraseptal bone (Saadoun and Malamed 1985; Giffin 1994).
3) The use of local anesthesia solutions with vasoconstrictor, such as lidocaine 2% with epinephrine 1:100000 (Giffin 1994) or 1:50000 (Saadoun and Malamed 1985).

### Contraindications

The contraindications are the same as those of the PDL technique, as follows:

1) In primary teeth, there is a risk of permanently damaging the tooth (Alantar 1993).
2) In the case of teeth with advanced periodontal disease, the periodontal structures may be affected. This point is under debate because some authors consider it a contraindication (Alantar 1993), whereas others do not (Saadoun and Malamed 1985). As is the case with the PDL injection, teeth affected by periodontal disease that are to be extracted constitute an exception.
3) Infection at the injection site.

### Anesthetized Area

- Tooth (pulp and periodontal ligament) on which the technique is applied, although the area anesthetized frequently extends to the adjacent teeth mesially and distally. The results are not known with any degree of accuracy, although they are considered to be similar to those of the PDL technique (Giffin 1994), with a lower percentage of success in the anterior teeth (Giffin 1994) and a shorter duration of pulpal anesthesia.
- Vestibule and lingual area, both in the fibromucosa (alveolar mucosa, gum, and interdental papillae) and in the bone and periosteum along a limited band measuring approximately 20–25 mm in length (Saadoun and Malamed 1985). Anesthesia lasts less than an hour.

### Technique

- Select the insertion site *in the center of the interdental papilla* close to the tooth to be anesthetized. The insertion site is at the midpoint of the papilla between the teeth and *exactly 2 mm under the cusp of the papilla*.
- Place the needle vertically at an angle of approximately 45° with respect to the axis of the tooth and horizontally perpendicular to the papilla (Figure 18.7).

In posterior mandibular teeth, it may be necessary to bend the needle some 45° along the stem to ensure correct positioning.

- Insertion of the needle:
  o Inject a few drops into the fibromucosa of the papilla after inserting the needle.
  o Advance the needle until it makes contact with the alveolar bone crest and continue to apply pressure so that the needle crosses the weak point of the cortical plate at this level and reaches the cancellous bone. In

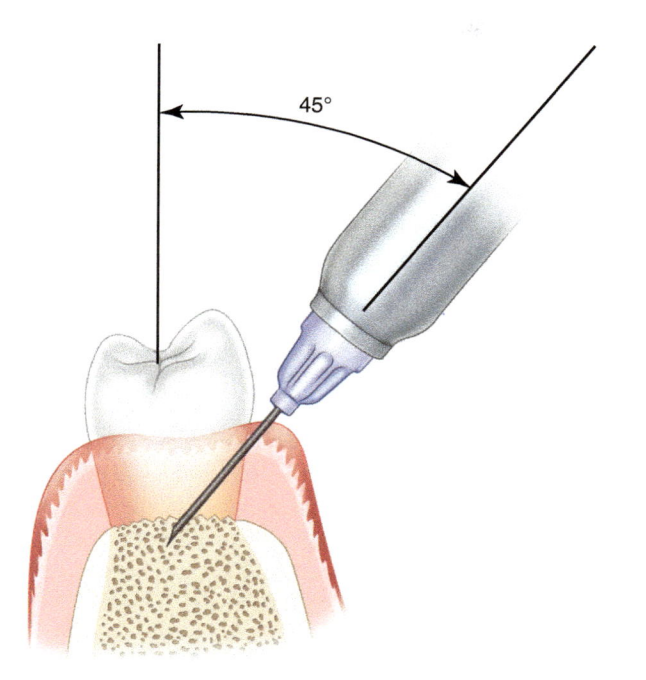

**Figure 18.7** Insertion of the needle into the interdental septum at an approximate angle of 45°, with penetration of the cancellous bone.

total, the needle can penetrate 2–3 mm into the bone tissue (Figure 18.7).
- Withdrawing the needle 1 mm and rotating the syringe helps the needle to penetrate the bone (Saadoun and Malamed 1985).
- Inject 0.2–0.4 ml of anesthetic solution (Saadoun and Malamed 1985; Alantar 1993; Giffin 1994).
  - The solution is *injected under pressure* so that the anesthetic penetrates the medullary spaces. In addition, *it is injected slowly* (0.2 ml in 20–30 seconds) to prevent excess pressure from breaking the cartridge.
  - The ischemia caused by the pressure of the injection and the vasoconstrictor in the solution leads to blanching.
  - If the injection is very fluid and there is no pressure, then the needle is not penetrating the bone and the distribution of the solution is limited to the soft tissue or may even flow back into the mouth (in this case the patient notices the bitter taste of the solution [Saadoun and Malamed 1985]). The needle should then be withdrawn and repositioned in the papilla before starting the procedure again.
  - If the injection seems difficult and the needle does not advance despite pressure, then it has reached an area of thick cortex or is poorly angled, thus preventing it from entering the cancellous bone. In this case, the needle should be withdrawn and repositioned in the papilla before starting the procedure again.

- Aspiration is not performed, since this technique, as with the PDL injection, is considered almost intravascular.
- Anesthesia is almost immediate, less than 15 seconds (Saadoun and Malamed 1985). It is restricted to the tooth and the surrounding area, and the patient has no subjective sensation of paresthesia in the soft tissues. If anesthesia has not been achieved after 30 seconds, then the technique has failed and must be restarted (Saadoun and Malamed 1985).

### Specific Complications of the Technique

1) Pain during the injection in more than 25% of cases, when it is used as the primary technique (Saadoun and Malamed 1985), although in practice it is used as a supplementary technique in cases of failure, when the tissues are already anesthetized.
2) Patients often complain of palpitations (tachycardia) owing to the use of anesthetic solutions containing epinephrine (Saadoun and Malamed 1985; Giffin 1994).
3) Postinjection pain at the injection site in 20% of cases, although this disappears spontaneously in 1 or 2 days (Giffin 1994).

## Intraosseous Technique

This technique is also known as the intradiploic or transcortical technique. It involves crossing the cortex with a drill and using a needle to inject the anesthesia into the cancellous bone close to the tooth to be anesthetized in such a way that it spreads rapidly toward the apex.

The technique was first applied by Otte in 1896 (Smith 1920) or by R. Nogué in 1907 (Nogué 1907) (we were unable to verify which of the two was first) and then by Masselink in 1910 (Masselink 1910). In these early techniques, the bone was perforated with round burrs (thus making it difficult to maintain the perforation straight) and the solution was injected with a thick cannula to prevent reflux (Masselink 1910; Parrot 1914). During the 1930s, the method became popular and dentists started to drill at the level of the attached gingiva with straight burrs (Schmitt 1936; Nevin and Puterbaugh 1949). In the 1940s, Beutelrock perforators became popular; however, as these were relatively long, they broke easily, and it was difficult to extract them (Nevin and Puterbaugh 1949). Consequently, the Van den Berg system was developed (Leonard 1995; Dunbar et al. 1996; Peñarrocha et al. 1997); this involved 5-mm perforators with a stop to prevent overpenetration and extrashort needles of the same caliber. Unfortunately, the perforator was too short (5 mm) and, very often, it was not possible to completely perforate the cortical plate (Roberts and Sowray 1987). During the 1960s and 1970s, few studies based on this technique were published (Magnes 1968; Bourke 1974; Lilienthal 1976).

The modern era began in 1991, when Frank Dillon developed the *Stabident® system*, which incorporated new designs and disposable materials, with a 9-mm drill and a needle of the same caliber and length (Leonard 1995; Dunbar et al. 1996; Peñarrocha et al. 1997). Later, in 1999, Arthur Weather developed the *X-Tip® system*, with characteristics that are very similar to those of Stabident® but which incorporates a guide sleeve so as not to lose the perforation when inserting the needle (Hawkins and Moore 2002). Some time later, Stabident® also incorporated an optional guide sleeve. Other less popular variants began to appear, such as a hand-held device designed for this technique, IntraFlow® (Kleber 2003; Remmers et al. 2008) or Anesto (Graetz et al. 2013), and the hybrid system known as QuickSleeper (Villette 2003) (see Chapter 20).

In this section, we provide a careful analysis of the Stabident® and X-Tip® systems because these are the most important and most widely used.

## Indications, Contraindications, and Disadvantages

We have already mentioned the indications. The intraosseous technique is a supplementary technique that is only used when standard techniques fail. In addition, it has two disadvantages: (i) it requires a perforator and an extrashort needle, and (ii) rubber dams must be removed to apply the technique (one advantage of the PDL injection is that this is not necessary). The contraindications of the technique are as follows:

1) Primary teeth, since the permanent tooth buds may be damaged, although some authors have used the approach in children (Magnes 1968; Bourke 1974).
2) Teeth with advanced periodontal disease since the tooth may fall out accidentally during the procedure (Parente et al. 1998). Teeth to be extracted are an exception.
3) Infection with cellulitis or an abscess in the area to be perforated since this would be very painful and deep anesthesia may not be achieved (Reader et al. 2011; Council on Clinical Affairs 2015).
4) Areas with little cancellous bone, such as those between the upper and lower central incisors (Lilienthal 1975a) and areas with very crowded teeth. As it is difficult to drill in these areas, it is recommended to use the nearest distal space. An alternative is to use the PDL injection and not the intraosseous technique.

## Instrument Set

In this section, we analyze the instruments used in the two main systems, Stabident® and X-Tip®.

### Stabident®

This system is based on two elements, as follows (Stabident instruction manual 2001) (Figure 18.8):

1) The perforator, or drill, which comprises a plastic shank and has the following parts:
    - Plastic shank that is inserted into the contra-angle hand piece.
    - Plastic stop that marks the depth of perforation and is, at the same time, an adapter for the plastic protective cap that covers the metal needle of the perforator.
    - Solid 27G metal needle (0.43 × 9 mm) that comes out of the plastic stop and is the active part of the perforator used to penetrate the cortical layer.
    - Plastic protective cap that covers the solid metal needle (or active end) and adapts to the plastic stop.
2) Extrashort 27G needle (0.4 × 8 mm) with dimensions that are identical to those of the perforator and covered by its corresponding sleeve.

The instrument is sufficiently long to cross the gum and cortical bone, and thus reach the cancellous bone in most cases. Table 18.7 shows the thicknesses to be crossed by the perforator. Since the distance would be greater than 8 mm in only 2.5% of cases, the system has a longer reach than the 5 mm of the old Van den Berg system.

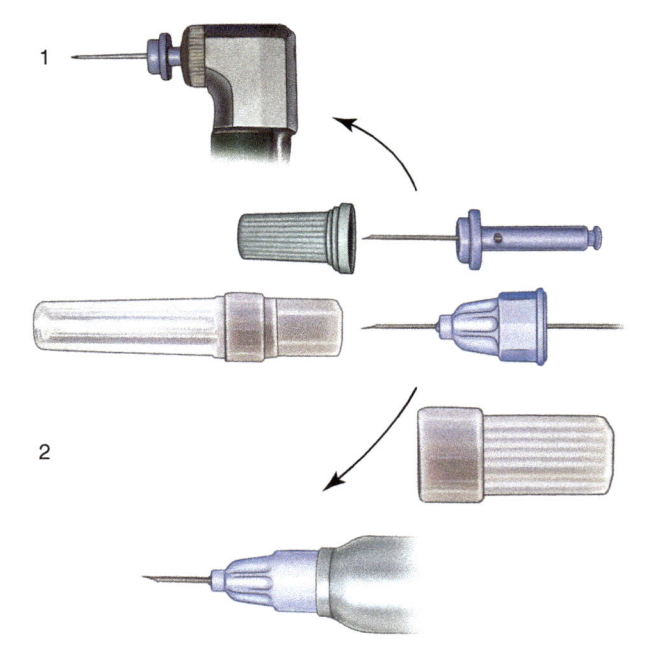

**Figure 18.8** Stabident® system with the perforator (1) and needle (2).

Table 18.7 Thickness (mm) of the gum and cortical plate in the mandibular vestibule.

| Anatomic part | | $\bar{x} \pm SD$ | 95% CI |
|---|---|---|---|
| Attached gingiva (Goaslind et al. 1977) | | 1.22 ± 0.4 | 0.5–2 |
| Cortical bone (Denio et al. 1992) | First PM | 1.8 ± 0.3 | 1–2 |
| | Second PM | 2.0 ± 3.1 | 0–5 |
| | First M | 2.7 ± 0.5 | 2–4 |
| | Second M | 3.2 ± 0.7 | 2–5 |

CI, confidence interval; PM, premolar; M, molar; SD, standard deviation.

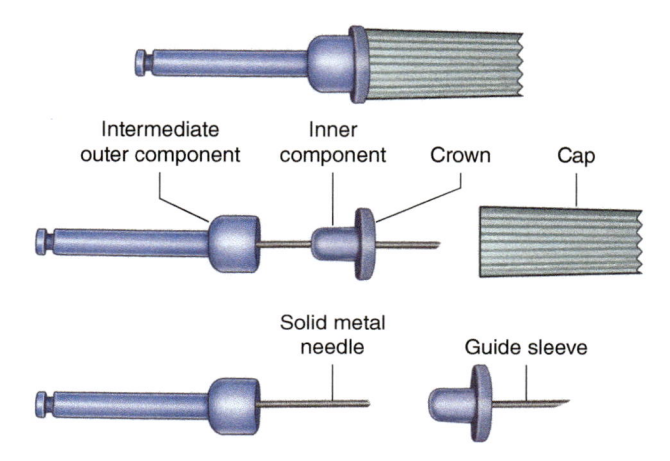

Figure 18.9 X-Tip® with the perforator and guide sleeve. Note how the perforator and guide sleeve are presented as a unit with the protective cap (upper image).

### X-Tip®

This system comprises four elements (X-Tip 2010) (Figure 18.9):

1) Perforator, which is formed by a plastic shank with various parts:
   - Plastic shank that is introduced into the contra-angled hand piece.
   - Intermediate outer component to hold the guide sleeve (cup).
   - Solid metal 27G needle (0.4×9 mm) that comes out of the center of the female component and is the active part that perforates the cortical plate.
2) Guide sleeve, which is composed of the following parts:
   - Plastic inner component, which fits into the outer component of the perforator and has a mark at the top where the needle is introduced.
   - Crown, a plastic outer component surrounding the inner component and marking the depth stop for perforation.
   - Hollow metal guide measuring 0.63×7 mm (the active part), which contains the perforator and which, once placed in the mouth, serves as a guide for the needle (Gallatin et al. 2003b).
3) Protective cap (generally in a bright color, red) that covers the active part of the complex or perforator-catheter-guide sleeve block. This set is presented together in a plastic ampoule inside a blister pack.
4) Extrashort 27G needle (0.4×9 mm), with measurements identical to those of the perforator to be able to penetrate the guide sleeve.

### Anesthetic Solutions

Clinical trials show that local anesthetic solutions with epinephrine yield better results than those that do not contain vasoconstrictor (Lilienthal and Reynolds 1975b; Replogle et al. 1997) or those that contain felypressin (Lilienthal 1976). In addition, no statistically significant differences have been found between the use of solutions containing articaine 4% and lidocaine 2%, both of which contain epinephrine 1:100 000 (Bigby et al. 2006).

Despite containing epinephrine, the anesthetic enters the bloodstream very quickly with this technique (Cannell and Cannon 1976), although the vasoconstrictor attenuates the increase in plasma concentrations (Wood et al. 2005). This technique is therefore considered to be equivalent to an intravascular administration, with positive aspirations in 60–85% of cases (Peñarrocha et al. 1996, 2012).

Finally, when epinephrine is contraindicated, we can use vasoconstrictor-free solutions, such as mepivacaine 3% (Reisman et al. 1997; Replogle et al. 1999) and prilocaine 3% with felypressin 0.03 IU/ml (Lilienthal 1976), although the results for these agents are somewhat poorer.

### Anesthetized Area

The area anesthetized with the intraosseous technique is very well defined, as is the case in all supplementary techniques.

- Tooth (pulp and periodontal ligament) on which the technique is performed distally and frequently extended to the adjacent tooth mesially.
- Vestibule and lingual area, both the fibromucosa (alveolar mucosa, gum, and interdental papillae) and the bone and periosteum of the anesthetized tooth. It is important to remember that this technique is used in a very well-defined area.
- In the mandibula, the lower lip is also anesthetized in 65% of cases (Table 18.8), as is the tongue on many occasions.

Table 18.8 Variables to be considered in the intraosseous technique with Stabident® and X-Tip®.

| Study data | | | Study variables | | |
|---|---|---|---|---|---|
| Reference | System | Sample size | Tachycardia | No attached gingiva | Anesthesia lower lip |
| Lilienthal (1976) | — | 9 | — | — | 55% |
| Leonard (1995) | Stabident® | 89 | — | — | 0% |
| Coggins et al. (1996) | Stabident® | 40 | 78% | 8% | 58% |
| Dunbar et al. (1996) | Stabident® | 20–40 | 80% | 5% | — |
| Replogle et al. (1997) | Stabident® | 42 | — | 7% | 76% |
| Reitz et al. (1998) | Stabident® | 38 | 68% | 2.5% | — |
| Guglielmo et al. (1999) | Stabident® | 40 | 78% | 7.5% | — |
| Replogle et al. (1999) | Stabident® | 42 | 67% | — | — |
| Gallatin et al. (2003a) | Stabident® | 41 | 85% | 5% | 100% |
| Gallatin et al. (2003a) | X-Tip® | 41 | 93% | — | 94% |
| Nusstein et al. (2003) | X-Tip® | 33 | 73% | — | — |
| Bigby et al. (2006) | Stabident® | 37 | 81% | — | — |
| | | Average | 78.1% | 5.8% | 64% |
| | | Rounded average | **80%** | **5%** | **65%** |

Values are shown as percentages. The percentage of anesthesia in the lower lip only applies to use of the technique in the mandible.

## Intraosseous Technique

- Rubber dams must be removed (Nusstein et al. 2003).
- This technique is not very painful as a primary technique (Annex 23), although in practice it is not painful because it is used as a supplementary technique when all other approaches have failed and the adjacent tissues – but not the dental pulp – are therefore anesthetized. If this approach is used as the primary technique, then we advise the following:
  o The Stabident® or X-Tip® extrashort needle can be used.
  o Injecting 0.2–0.6 ml in the area to be drilled (Lilienthal 1975a; Pearce 1976; Leonard 1995; Dunbar et al. 1996; Coggins et al. 1996; Replogle et al. 1997; Gallatin et al. 2003a, 2003b).
  o Waiting 1 minute for the gum, periosteum, and cortical plate to become anesthetized before perforating (Leonard 1995; Peñarrocha et al. 1996).
- The best advice is to use a local anesthetic solution containing epinephrine (if there are no contraindications), similar to the one we are already using in the area (remember the principle of not mixing two anesthetics at the one site). For example, if articaine 4% with epinephrine 1:100 000 (A-100) is used in the maxilla in a buccal infiltration, then this same solution can be used; if mandibular block is performed with the standard solution of lidocaine 2% with epinephrine 1:100 000 (L-100) and then reinforced with A-100 in buccal area, then the intraosseous technique should be continued with A-100.
- Advise the patient that he/she may experience palpitations:
  o When solutions with epinephrine are used, *80% of patients have an increased heart rate* that is felt as palpitations (Table 18.8), which last 2–4 minutes (Lilienthal and Reynolds 1975b); in 20% of cases, they may last 4–6 minutes (Replogle et al. 1999; Guglielmo et al. 1999).
  o No palpitations are observed with epinephrine-free anesthetic solutions (Replogle et al. 1999; Guglielmo et al. 1999). Similarly, palpitations do not appear if the injection rate is very slow (around 5 minutes) (Susi et al. 2008). This is difficult to ensure manually, although it is easy with computer-controlled delivery systems.
- Selection of the perforation site.
  o *Perforate distally to the tooth to be treated* (Leonard 1995); however, perforation may be mesial in certain cases:
    ▪ Second permanent molar because it is located toward the back of the mouth.
    ▪ Very crowded teeth because there is little cortical bone between them.
  o Perforate buccally, with an equal distance between the two teeth (Figure 18.10).

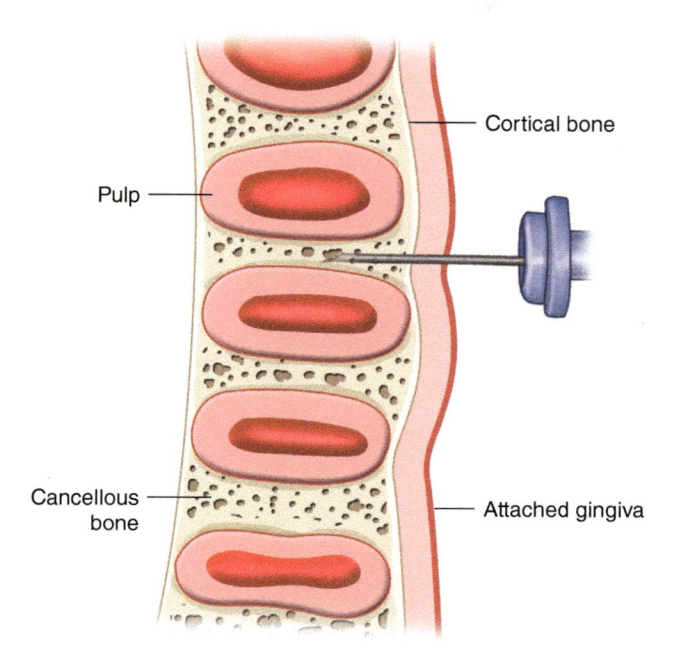

**Figure 18.10** Perforation via the buccal area at an equal distance between the teeth. Source: Redrawn from Leonard (1995) and Reader et al. (2011).

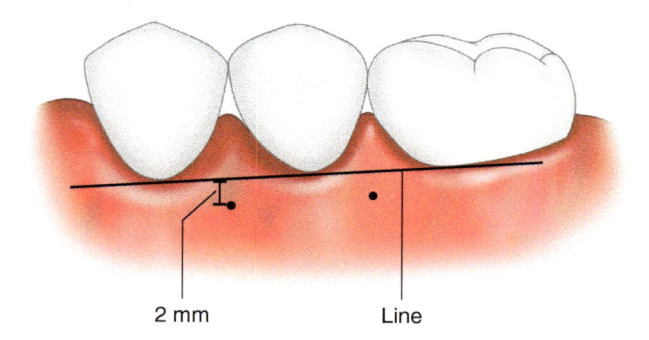

**Figure 18.11** In the Stabident® system, the dentist perforates 2 mm apically from the imaginary horizontal line that passes through the gingival margin into the attached gingiva. Notice how the horizontal line traverses the gingival margins of the adjacent teeth and the vertical line bisects the interdental papilla.

| Stabident® | X-Tip® |
|---|---|
| • At 2 mm toward the apical part of the imaginary horizontal line that passes through the gingival margin (Figure 18.11). | • Identical to Stabident®, although we can even go a further 3–7 mm toward the apex. |
| • Always on the attached gingiva. If this is missing (5%, Table 18.8), then at 1 mm above the mucogingiv aljunction.[a] | • On attached gingiva or even on the alveolar mucosa (Gallatin et al. 2003a; Nusstein et al. 2003) since this approach has a guide sleeve. |

[a] Always on attached gingiva, since if the technique is performed on the alveolar mucosa, which is mobile, there is movement above the perforation in the cortical plate and the placement of the insertion point is then very difficult (Bourke 1974). Remember that the teeth where the attached gingiva is usually less narrow in the area of the canines and maxillary and mandibular first premolar (Bowers 1963).

- In edentulous areas, the perforation is made vertically, on the alveolar crest, where the cortical layer is thinner (Figure 18.12).
- Observations on the perforation point:
  - If the perforation is made in areas close to the papilla (Stabident®), distant from the apex, the bone may be fragile and the intraosseous technique may fail.
  - If the perforation is made in very apical areas (X-Tip®), where the cortical layer is very thick, structures may be damaged (mental nerve, mandibular canal, etc.) or the intraosseous technique may fail because the needle does not penetrate the cancellous bone (maxillary sinus).

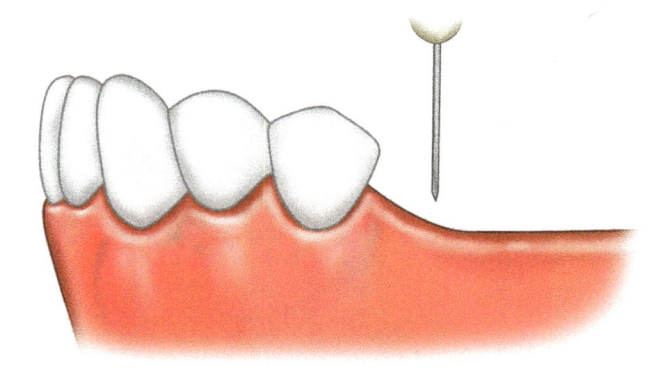

**Figure 18.12** Perforation is vertical in edentulous areas.

- Place the perforator in the contra-angle and proceed as follows:

| Stabident® | X-Tip® |
|---|---|
| Remove the protective cap from the active part | When the protective cap is removed from the active part, *hold the crown of the guide sleeve with one finger* so that the guide sleeve does not come out of the perforator. |

- Perforate the cortical layer with the perforator placed at a contra-angle, as follows:
  - Place the drill perpendicular to the area to be perforated without activating the handpiece.
  - Insert the drill by pushing it until the tip touches the bone after crossing the gum or mucosa (Figure 18.13).

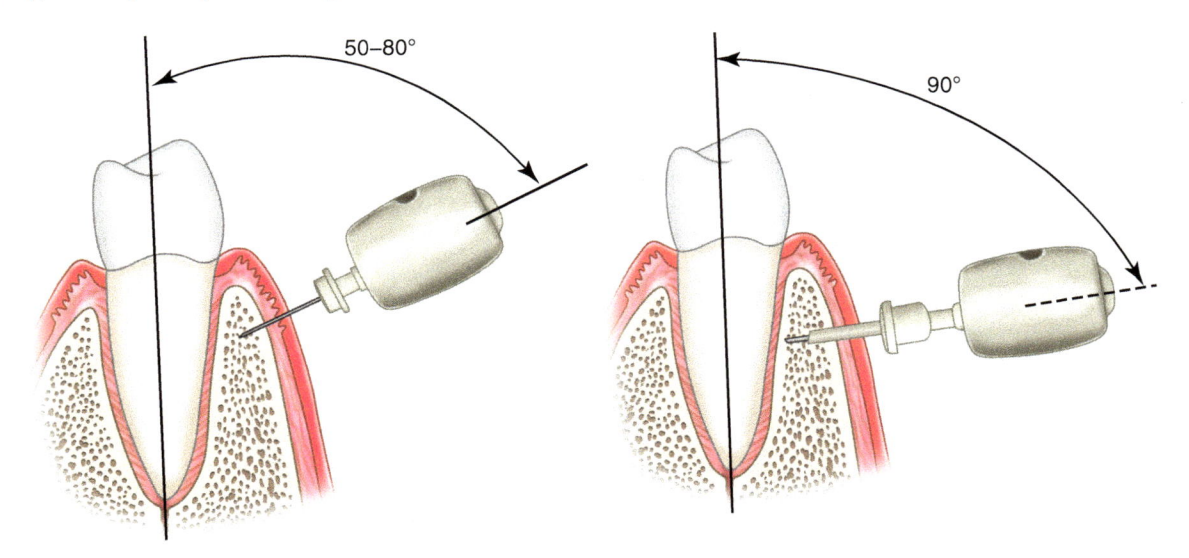

**Figure 18.13** Approximate angle at which the perforator is inserted with Stabident® (note that it is in the attached gingiva) and X-Tip® (note that, in this case, it is in the alveolar mucosa).

| Stabident® | X-Tip® |
|---|---|
| The angle over the vertical axis of the tooth varies:<br>• Upper teeth 60–80°<br>• Lower teeth 50–60° | • The angle over the vertical axis of the tooth will be ≤90°.<br>• *If the alveolar mucosa is involved, it should be pulled taut with a finger of the other hand* to minimize the possibility that the perforator will become stuck in the mobile mucosa on activation and detach it. |

- ○ The handpiece is activated at low speed (15 000–20 000 rpm):
  - ▪ With irrigation to prevent overheating of the bone and thus reduce postoperative pain.
  - ▪ With short, intermittent impulses, by applying a slight pressure. When the perforator reaches the cancellous bone, we feel it "give" as the resistance of the cortical bone cedes (Schmitt 1936; Bourke 1974; Pearce 1976). Sometimes, the patient feels a vibration such as that felt during tartar removal (Peñarrocha et al. 1997).
  - ▪ *The maneuver lasts 2–5 seconds* (Bourke 1974; Dunbar et al. 1996; Coggins et al. 1996; Replogle et al. 1997). If it takes more than 5 seconds, the procedure should be stopped and the area selected checked. The greater the hardness or thickness of the cortical layer, the longer it will take, for example in the posterior parts of the mandibula or when a dental root is perforated (serious problem).

- Insert the extrashort needle.
  - ○ Hold the syringe with the needle in place with a pen grip, with the fingers near the hub to help with insertion (Lilienthal 1975a) (Figure 18.14).

| Stabident® | X-Tip® |
|---|---|
| • Remove perforator.<br>• *Identify the orifice of the perforation.* This is done by drying and blotting the area with gauze to clean up any blood and reveal the *little blood spot* on the inserted gingiva (Schmitt 1936).<br>• Insert the needle across the perforation, in exactly the same direction as the perforation in order not to touch the walls of the orifice. *This maneuver may prove difficult and have to be tried a few times* (Figure 18.16). | • After perforation, and with the handpiece stopped, *use tweezers to hold the crown surrounding the inner component of the sleeve guide* against the gum so that when the perforator is removed from the bone, it does not drag the guide sleeve and pull it out of the bone (Figure 18.15).<br>• Insert the needle across the orifice in the cusp of the inner component of the guide sleeve (Figure 18.16). |

- ○ The needle should be bent in posterior teeth:
  - ▪ Approximately 45° to facilitate insertion (Dunbar et al. 1996; Coggins et al. 1996; Replogle et al. 1997; Parente et al. 1998) and even 60–80° (Gallatin et al. 2003a; Nusstein et al. 2003).
  - ▪ Squeeze a few drops of anesthetic out of the tip of the needle to ensure that bending the needle has not obstructed the lumen.

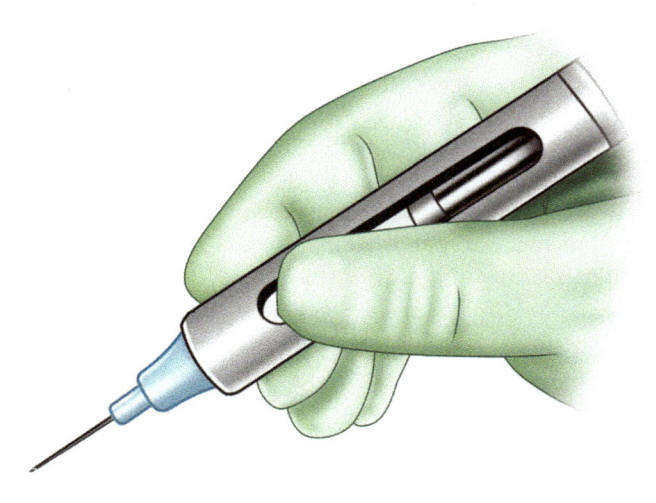

**Figure 18.14** Holding the syringe with a pen grip.

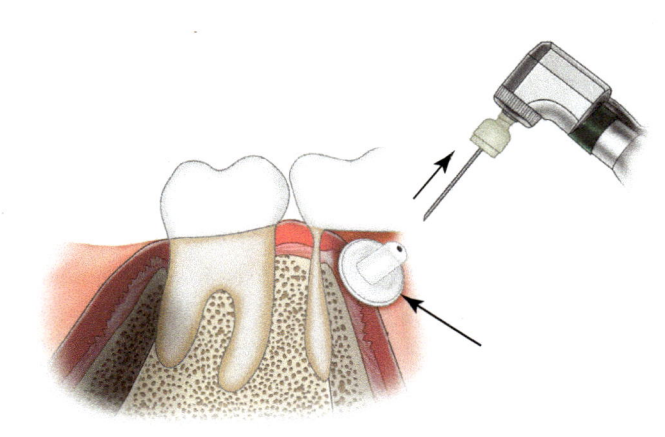

**Figure 18.15** In the X-Tip® system, when the perforator is withdrawn after perforation, the crown (marked with an arrow) should be held so that the guide sleeve remains inserted in the gingiva and bone.

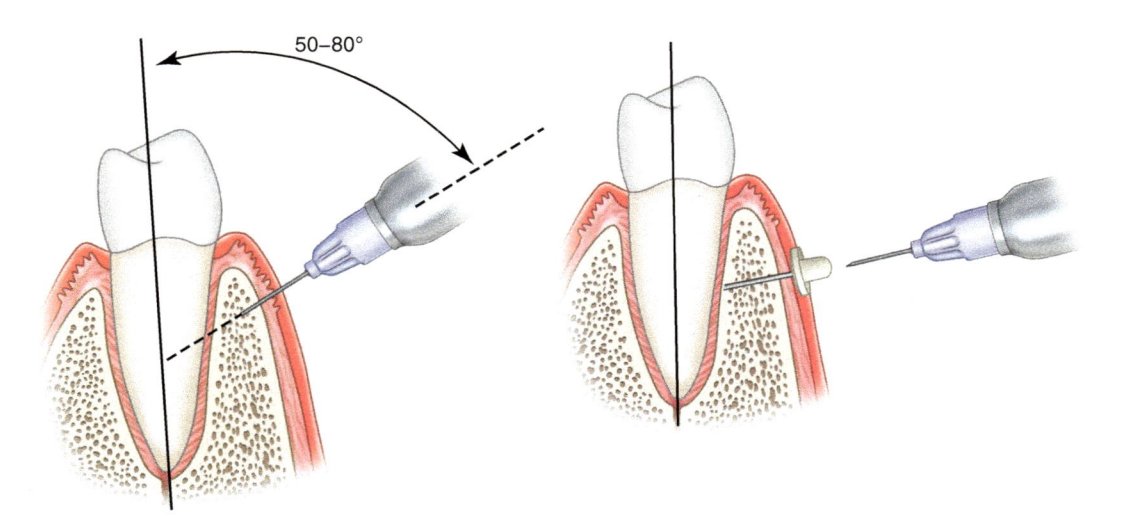

**Figure 18.16** Insert the needle for injection.

- Remember that inserting the needle at the level of the second molar can prove difficult owing to the lack of accuracy and of angulation (Leonard 1995).
- *Slow injection* of half a cartridge (0.9 ml) in 30 seconds (Lilienthal and Reynolds 1975b) or even more slowly up to 2 minutes (Pereira et al. 2013), and a whole cartridge (1.8 ml) in 1–2 minutes. The most common approach is to inject the whole cartridge (Coggins et al. 1996; Reisman et al. 1997; Replogle et al. 1997, 1999; Guglielmo et al. 1999; Gallatin et al. 2003a).
  - Inject slowly since the solution enters the bloodstream very quickly (Cannell and Cannon 1976; Wood et al. 2005).
  - *Little resistance is noted on injecting* since the solution is entering the cancellous bone.
  - When the injection finishes, the needle should be pressed for a few seconds to prevent reflux and enable the anesthetic to spread and reach the apexes (Pearce 1976).
  - The needle is not aspirated: we know that aspiration is positive in 60–85% of cases because it is inevitably intravascular (Peñarrocha et al. 1996, 2012).
- Withdraw the needle.

| Stabident® | X-Tip® |
|---|---|
| Withdrawal of the needle leaves a blood spot on the gum. | • Withdraw the needle from the guide sleeve.<br>• Then, withdraw the guide sleeve from the bone with a hemostat or pliers. |

- Note (X-Tip®): Before withdrawing the guide sleeve, ensure that the tooth is anesthetized in order to be able to reinject if necessary, without having to start over.

- Pulpal anesthesia takes effect quickly (Leonard 1995; Parente et al. 1998; Peñarrocha et al. 1996), generally *in about 2 minutes* (Gallatin et al. 2003a; Nusstein et al. 2005b; Pereira et al. 2013), and *lasts about 25 minutes* (Nusstein et al. 2005b).
  - If the tooth remains sensitive after 2 minutes, we can reinject (Magnes 1968; Reisman et al. 1997; Parente et al. 1998).
  - Anesthesia is restricted to the tooth and adjacent teeth, therefore the patient generally experiences few symptoms in the soft tissues. If this approach is used only as the primary technique, the soft tissue anesthesia can last 25–30 minutes (Lilienthal 1976).
  - When an intraosseous injection has been performed in the mandibula, the lower lip is affected by soft tissue anesthesia in 65% of cases (Table 18.8).

## Efficacy

The efficacy of this technique evaluated using electrical pulp testing shows that *it is successful in 95% of cases in maxillary teeth and in 85% of cases in mandibular teeth* (anterior and posterior) (Table 18.9); the effect of pulpal anesthesia lasts for around 25 minutes (Nusstein et al. 2005b). Evaluation of clinical success (more subjective and less rigorous) reveals a success rate of around 95%, although this may be with one or two injections (two if the first one fails) (Magnes 1968; Pearce 1976).

### Specific Complications

**Complications Due to Mechanical Aspects**

1) Pain during perforation of the cortical plate in approximately 10% of cases (Annex 23). This may be due to the following:
   - Inappropriate anesthesia of the gum, alveolar mucosa, and periosteum. This can be improved by increasing infiltrative anesthesia.
   - Teeth with irreversible acute pulpitis. In such cases, the tissues are very sensitive despite the infiltrative anesthesia and anesthesia of the soft tissues. In some series, moderate-to-intense pain is recorded in around 50% of cases (Nusstein et al. 2003).
   - Perforation of the periodontal ligament or lamina dura of any of the adjacent teeth. In these cases, we must remove the drill and modify the angle of perforation or search for an alternative interdental space mesially or distally.

2) Not perforating the cortical plate in less than 5 seconds and not feeling that the perforator has reached the cancellous bone. This may be caused by the following:
   - Lack of cancellous bone because the teeth are close together. The solution is to move the perforation point mesially or distally.
   - The root of an adjacent tooth is being perforated (Coggins et al. 1996; Dunbar et al. 1996; Replogle et al. 1997). In terms of touch, a difference can be felt

Table 18.9 Percentage of pulpal anesthesia, evaluated using an electric pulp tester after the intraosseous technique with standard lidocaine 2% with epinephrine 1:100 000 solution (L-100) and in mesial and distal tooth.

| Tooth | Reference | Sample size | Pulpal anesthesia | Anesthesia Mesial | Anesthesia Distal |
| --- | --- | --- | --- | --- | --- |
| **Maxillary arch** | | | | | |
| First M | Coggins et al. (1996) | 40 | 93% | 68% | 93% |
| LI | Coggins et al. (1996) | 40 | 90% | 73% | 88% |
|  | Nusstein et al. (2005b) | 40 | 98% | — | — |
|  |  | Average | 93.6% | 70% | 90% |
|  |  | Rounded average | **95%** | | |
| **Mandibular arch** | | | | | |
| First M | Coggins et al. (1996) | 40 | 75% | 52% | 90% |
|  | Replogle et al. (1997) | 42 | 74% | 57% | 76% |
|  | Gallatin et al. (2003a) | 41 | 93% | 81% | 95% |
|  | " | " | 93% | 83% | 95% |
| LI | Coggins et al. (1996) | 40 | 78% | 52% | 58% |
|  |  | Average | 82.6% | 65% | 83% |
|  |  | Rounded average | **85%** | | |

First M, first molar; LI, lateral incisor.

between the bone and the root, and it takes considerable strength to perforate the root (Coggins et al. 1996). The solution in these cases is to reorient the perforation or change the perforation site.
- Cortical layer excessively thick (>8 mm). This situation arises in 2.5% of cases (Table 18.7), although it has arisen in 8% of cases in some series (Peñarrocha et al. 1996). In these situations, the direction of the perforation can be changed or, if this does not work, an alternative technique, such as the PDL injection, can be applied. Remember that with Stabident®, the angle of perforation may be excessively open or closed, with the result that the cortical layer becomes thicker.

3) Excessive pressure is needed to inject the anesthetic solution. This situation may arise in 10% of cases (Table 18.10) because of the lack of cancellous bone, obstruction of a bent needle, or insufficient perforation of the cortical layer (Lilienthal 1975a). The measures to be taken are as follows (Gallatin et al. 2003a):
- Rotate the needle a quarter turn to inject via a different part of the bevel, where there may be cancellous bone or the cortical plate has been perforated.
- If this does not work, remove the needle and verify that it is not obstructed. This situation is more common with bent needles.
- If the all of the above fail, start again.

4) Specific complications of the Stabident® system:
- Breakage of the perforator with separation of the metal needle from the plastic shank (2% of cases) (Table 18.10). In this case, the needle can be removed easily with pliers or a hemostat (Coggins et al. 1996; Replogle et al. 1997; Parente et al. 1998). This situation is now uncommon because of improvements in the materials used.
- Inability to locate the perforation site to insert the needle in 8% of patients (Table 18.10). This may arise for two reasons:
  1) The alveolar mucosa has been perforated instead of the attached gingiva, with the result that the soft tissues move above the perforation in the cortical plate, thus making the insertion site difficult to locate. If the site is not located after several attempts, the only solution is to make a second perforation, only this time in the attached gingiva.
  2) The needle is not inserted into the perforation at the same angle, therefore it makes contact with the lateral walls and does not cross the cancellous bone. This situation is common in mandibular molars (Replogle et al. 1997). The solution is one of trial and error, in which the dentist attempts to redirect the needle. In the case of posterior teeth, it could prove useful to bend the needle to reach the opening more easily. If these approaches fail, we can start again with a fresh perforation.

5) Specific complications of the X-Tip® system:
- There are two reports of breakage of the guide sleeve, which separated from the metal cannula of the plastic inner component (Gallatin et al. 2003a; Pereira et al. 2013). The solution is to withdraw the metal part with a hemostat or pliers, given that it projects by 3 mm. The procedure should be restarted or the opening should be used as if we were working with the Stabident® system.
- As the openings are larger, reflux of anesthetic solution via the guide sleeve is observed in approximately 10% of cases (Gallatin et al. 2003a; Nusstein et al. 2003). This can be avoided by pressing the needle in the top part of the inner component of the guide sleeve for a few seconds after the injection to enable the solution to spread through the cancellous bone without reflux.

Note: When the perforation is repeated close to the initial site as a result of a problem, there is some reflux of the anesthetic solution through the first opening (Peñarrocha et al. 1996).

**Postoperative Complications**

Postoperative complications are caused by injury to tissue resulting from drilling and the maneuvers applied in this technique. However, they are not associated with the anesthetic solutions used (Replogle et al. 1997).

1) Moderate to severe pain at the perforation site in 10% of cases (Table 18.10). This usually disappears spontaneously in 1–3 days (Peñarrocha et al. 1996; Gallatin et al. 2003b).
2) The tooth feels high during occlusion in around 10% of cases (Table 18.10) owing to damage to the periodontal ligament and inflammation of the bone. This disappears spontaneously in 1–3 days (Replogle et al. 1997; Gallatin et al. 2003b). Occlusion can always be adjusted.
3) Injection site lesions in 5% of cases (Table 18.10) with inflammation, reddening, pain, and even purulent exudate, which may require treatment with antibiotics, disinfectant solution, and analgesics (Coggins et al. 1996; Peñarrocha et al. 1996; Replogle et al. 1997). This may last up to 14 days (Coggins et al. 1996; Replogle et al. 1997). In addition, these lesions are thought to be caused by overheating of the bone and pressure during drilling. Hematomas have also been reported (Dunbar et al. 1996), as have aphthous ulcers (Replogle et al. 1997), which resolve spontaneously in a few days.
4) Osteonecrosis. There is one report of osteonecrosis that resulted in extraction of the two mandibular molars in an HIV-infected patient who was taking antiretroviral

Table 18.10 Percentage of complications of the intraosseous technique during the procedure and afterwards.

| Reference | System | Sample size | Excessive pressure | Perforator breakage | Failure to locate perforation | Severe pain | High teeth | Local lesions |
|---|---|---|---|---|---|---|---|---|
| Leonard (1995) | Stabident® | 89 | 11% | — | 4% | — | — | — |
| Coggins et al. (1996) | Stabident® | 40–160 | 9% | 0.6% | — | 2–15% | 4% | 3% |
| Dunbar et al. (1996) | Stabident® | 40 | 15% | — | — | 2% | 10% | 3% |
| Peñarrocha et al. (1996) | Stabident® | 50 | — | — | 10% | 24% | — | 2% |
| Replogle et al. (1997) | Stabident® | 44–84 | 19% | 4% | 10% | 2–10% | 13% | 5% |
| Parente et al. (1998) | Stabident® | 37 | — | 3% | — | — | — | — |
| Reitz et al. (1998) | Stabident® | 38 | — | — | — | 11% | 0% | 0% |
| Guglielmo et al. (1999) | Stabident® | 80 | — | — | — | 10–13% | 9% | 3% |
| Gallatin et al. (2003a) and Gallatin et al. (2003b) | Stabident® | 41 | 12% | 0% | — | 7% | 5% | 5% |
| Gallatin et al. (2003b) | X-Tip® | 41 | 2.5% | 2.5% | — | 25% | 15% | 22% |
| Nusstein et al. (2003) | X-Tip® | 33 | 18% | 0% | — | — | — | — |
| Peñarrocha-Oltra et al. (2012) | Stabident® | 100 | — | 6% | 6% | 11% | — | — |
| Pereira et al. (2013) | X-Tip® | 60 | — | 1.5% | — | — | — | 1.5% |
| | | Average | 12.4% | 2.2% | 7.5% | 11% | 8% | 4.9% |
| | | Rounded average | **10%** | **2%** | **8%** | **10%** | **10%** | **5%** |

drugs. In this case, the X-Tip® system was used by a young, inexperienced dentist who may have applied the technique without irrigation. These factors may have contributed to the accident (Woodmansey et al. 2009).

Final note: The intraosseous technique has fewer adverse effects than the PDL injection.

**Pulpal Abnormalities**

Pulpal abnormalities have not been detected in humans in clinical studies to date (Dunbar et al. 1996; Replogle et al. 1997; Reitz et al. 1998; Guglielmo et al. 1999; Gallatin et al. 2003b).

# Final Remarks

When performed with pressure, the intrapulpal technique is 100% effective (see above). However, in endodontic treatments, it is often necessary to reach the pulp (this may be impossible because of the pain in acute pulpitis) and the technique is of no use in nonpulpal treatments (e.g. cutting or a very deep cavity). In these cases, we can use the PDL injection and intraosseous technique, both of which require special equipment and have advantages and disadvantages, as follows:

- Advantages of the intraosseous technique over the PDL injection:
  - Greater pulpal anesthesia in the first injection (85% vs. 65% in acute pulpitis [Annex 35]).
  - Greater duration of pulpal anesthesia (25 minutes vs. 10 minutes).
  - Fewer postoperative adverse events.
- Disadvantages of the intraosseous technique with respect to PDL injection:
  - Later onset of pulpal anesthesia (2 minutes vs. 30 seconds), although this is of little clinical relevance.
  - The rubber dam has to be removed during endodontic treatments.
  - In central incisors (upper and lower) with little cancellous bone, it is not possible to use the intraosseous technique, therefore the PDL injection must be used.

# References

Alantar, A. (1993). L'anesthésie intraseptale. A propos de sept cas cliniques. *Rev. Odonto Stomatol. (Paris)* 22 (2): 105–112.

Albers, D.D. and Ellinger, R.F. (1988). Histologic effects of high pressure intraligamental injections on the periodontal ligament. *Quintessence Int.* 19 (5): 361–363.

Annex 23. Pain resulting from injection techniques.

Annex 35. Irreversible acute pulpitis (hot tooth). Efficacy of dental local anesthesia.

Ashkenazi, M., Blumer, S., and Eli, I. (2010). Effect of computerized delivery intraligamental injection in primary molars on their corresponding permanent tooth buds. *Int. J. Paediatr. Dent.* 20 (4): 270–275.

Berini, L. and Gay, C. (1997). *Anestesia odontológica*. Madrid: Ediciones Avances Médico-Dentales SL. 201.

Berlin, J., Nusstein, J., Reader, A. et al. (2005). Efficacy of articaine and lidocaine in a primary intraligamentary injection administered with a computer-controlled local anesthetic delivery system. *Oral Surg. Oral Med. Oral Pathol.* 99 (3): 361–366.

Bigby, J., Reader, A., Nusstein, J. et al. (2006). Articaine for supplemental intraosseous anesthesia in patients with irreversible pulpitis. *J. Endod.* 32 (11): 1044–1047.

Birchfield, J. and Rosenberg, P.A. (1975). Role of the anesthetic solution in intrapulpal anesthesia. *J. Endod.* 1 (1): 26–27.

Bourke, K. (1974). Intra-osseous anaesthesia. *Dent. Anaesth. Sedat.* 3 (2): 13–19.

Bowers, G.M. (1963). A study of the width of attached gingiva. *J. Perodontol.* 34 (3): 201–209.

Brännström, M., Nordenvall, K.-J., and Hedström, K.G. (1982). Periodontal tissue changes after intraligamentary anesthesia. *J. Dent. Child.* 49 (6): 417–423.

Brännström, M., Lindskog, S., and Nordenvall, K.-J. (1984). Enamel hypoplasia in permanent teeth induced by periodontal ligament anesthesia of primary teeth. *J. Am. Dent. Assoc.* 109 (5): 735–736.

Cannell, H. and Cannon, P.D. (1976). Intraosseous injections of lignocaine local anaesthetics. *Br. Dent. J.* 141 (2): 48–50.

Cannell, H., Kerawala, C., Webster, K., and Whelpton, R. (1993). Are intraligamentary injections intravascular? *Br. Dent. J.* 175 (8): 281–284.

Cassamani C. Une nouvelle technique d'anesthesia intraligamentaire. Theses de Doctorat. Paris. 1924.

Chenaux, G., Castagnola, L., and Colombo, A. (1976). L'anesthésie intraligamentaire avec la seringue "Péripress". *Scheweiz Monatsschr. Zahnheilkd.* 86 (11): 1165–1173.

Childers, M., Reader, A., Nist, R. et al. (1996). Anesthetic efficacy of the periodontal ligament injection after an inferior alveolar nerve block. *J. Endod.* 22 (6): 317–320.

Coggins, R., Reader, A., Nist, R. et al. (1996). Anesthetic efficacy of the intraosseous injection in maxillary and mandibular teeth. *Oral Surg. Oral Med. Oral Pathol.* 81 (6): 634–641.

Cohen, H.P., Cha, B.Y., and Spangberg, L.S.W. (1993). Endodontic anesthesia in mandibular molars: a clinical study. *J. Endod.* 19 (7): 370–373.

Coolidge, E.D. (1937). The thickness of the human periodontal membrane. *J. Am. Dent. Assoc. Dent. Cosmos* 24 (8): 1260–1270.

Council on Clinical Affairs (2015). Guideline on use of local anesthesia for pediatric dental patients. *Pediatr. Dent.* 37 (Special issue): 199–205.

Council on Dental Materials, Instruments, and Equipment (1983). Status report: the periodontal ligament injection. *J. Am. Dent. Assoc.* 106 (2): 222–224.

Cowan, A. (1986). A clinical assessment of the intraligamentary injection. *Br. Dent. J.* 161 (8): 296–298.

D'Souza, J.E., Walton, R.E., and Peterson, L.C. (1987). Periodontal ligament injection: an evaluation of the extent of anesthesia and postinjection discomfort. *J. Am. Dent. Assoc.* 114 (3): 341–344.

Davidson, L. and Craig, S. (1987). The use of the periodontal ligament injection in children. *J. Dent.* 15 (5): 2004–2008.

Denio, D., Torabinejad, M., and Bakland, L.K. (1992). Anatomical relationship of the mandibular canal to its surrounding structures in mature mandibles. *J. Endod.* 18 (4): 161–165.

DeNunzio, M. (1998). Topical anesthetic as an adjunct to local anesthesia during pulpectomies. *J. Endod.* 24 (3): 202–203.

Dreven, L.J., Reader, A., Beck, M. et al. (1987). An evaluation of an electric pulp tester as a measure of analgesia in human vital teeth. *J. Endod.* 13 (5): 233–238.

Dreyer, W.P., Heerden, J.D., and Joubert JJ de V. (1983). The route of periodontal ligament injection of local anesthetic solution. *J. Endod.* 9 (11): 471–474.

Dunbar, D., Reader, A., Nist, R. et al. (1996). Anesthetic efficacy of the intraosseous injection after an inferior alveolar nerve block. *J. Endod.* 22 (9): 481–486.

Edwards, R.W. and Head, T.W. (1989). A clinical trial of intraligamentary anesthesia. *J. Dent. Res.* 68 (7): 1210–1214.

Faulkner, R.K. (1983). The high-pressure periodontal ligament injection. *Br. Dent. J.* 154 (4): 103–105.

Fuhs, Q.M., Walker, W.A. III, Gough, R.W. et al. (1983). The periodontal ligament injection: histological effects on the periodontium in dogs. *J. Endod.* 9 (10): 411–415.

Galili, D., Kaufman, E., Garfunkel, A.A., and Michael, Y. (1984). Intraligamentary anesthesia – a histological study. *Int. J. Oral Surg.* 13 (6): 511–516.

Gallatin, J., Reader, A., Nusstein, J. et al. (2003a). A comparison of two intraosseous anesthetic techniques in mandibular posterior teeth. *J. Am. Dent. Assoc.* 134 (11): 1476–1484.

Gallatin, J., Nusstein, J., Reader, A. et al. (2003b). Comparison of injection pain and postoperative pain of two intraosseosus anesthetic techniques. *Anesth. Prog.* 50 (3): 111–120.

Garfunkel, A.A., Kaufman, E., Marmary, Y., and Galili, D. (1983). Intraligamentary – intraosseous anesthesia. A radiographic demonstration. *Int. J. Oral Surg.* 12 (5): 334–339.

Giffin, K.M. (1994). Providing intraosseous anesthesia with minimal invasion. *J. Am. Dent. Assoc.* 125 (8): 1119–1121.

Goaslind, G.D., Robertson, P.B., Mahan, C.J. et al. (1977). Thickness of facial gingiva. *J. Periodontol.* 48 (12): 768–771.

Graetz, C., Fawzy-El-Sayed, K.-M., Graetz, N., and Dörfer, C.-E. (2013). Root damage induced by intraosseous anesthesia – an in vitro investigation. *Med. Oral Patol. Oral Cir. Bucal* 18 (1): e130–e134.

Gray, R.J.M. and Rood, J.P. (1987). Periodontal ligament injection: with or without a vasoconstrictor. *Br. Dent. J.* 162 (7): 263–265.

Grundy, J.R. (1984). Intraligamentary anaesthesia. A survey of use by general practitioners and by staff and students in a dental school. *Restorative Dent.* 1 (2): 36–42.

Guglielmo, A., Reader, A., Nist, R. et al. (1999). Anesthetic efficacy and heart rate effects of the supplemental intraosseous injections of 2% mepivacaine with 1:20,000 levonordefrin. *Oral Surg. Oral Med. Oral Pathol.* 87 (3): 284–293.

Handler, L.E. and Albers, D.D. (1987). The effects of the vasoconstrictor epinephrine on the duration of pulpal anesthesia using the intraligamentary injection. *J. Am. Dent. Assoc.* 114 (6): 807–809.

Hawkins, J.M. and Moore, P.A. (2002). Local anesthesia: advances in agents and techniques. *Dent. Clin. N. Am.* 46 (4): 719–732.

Hochman, M.N., Friedman, M.J., Williams, W., and Hochman, C.B. (2006). Interstitial tissue pressure associated with dental injections: a clinical study. *Quintessence Int.* 37 (6): 469–476.

Hull, T.E. and Rothwell, B.R. (1998). Intraosseous anesthesia comparing lidocaine and etidocaine. *J. Dent. Res.* 77 (Special issue A): 197. (abstract no. 733).

Johnson, G.K., Hlava, G.L., and Kalkwarf, K.L. (1985). A comparison of periodontal intraligamental anesthesia using etidocaine HCL and lidocaine HCL. *Anesth. Prog.* 32 (5): 202–205.

Kaufman, E., Valli, D., and Garfunkel, A.A. (1983). Intraligamentary anesthesia: a clinical study. *J. Prost. Dent.* 49 (3): 337–339.

Kaufman, E., Dworkin, S.F., LeResche, L. et al. (1984). Intraligamentary anesthesia: a double-blind comparative study. *J. Am. Dent. Assoc.* 108 (2): 175–178.

Kaufman, E., Solomon, V., Rozen, L., and Peltz, R. (1994). Pulpal anesthesia efficacy of four lidocaine solutions injected with an intraligamentary syringe. *Oral Surg. Oral Med. Oral Pathol.* 78 (1): 17–21.

Khedari, A.J. (1982). Alternative to mandibular block injections through intraligamental anesthesia. *Quintessence Int.* 13 (2): 231–237.

Kim, S. (1986). Ligament injection: a physiological explanation of its efficacy. *J. Endod.* 12 (10): 486–491.

Kleber, C.H. (2003). Intraosseous anesthesia. Implications, instrumentation and techniques. *J. Am. Dent. Assoc.* 134 (4): 487–491.

Kronfeld, R. (1931). Histologic study of the influence of function on the human periodontal membrane. *J. Am. Dent. Assoc.* 18: 1242–1274.

Lafargue, R. (1973). Anesthésie intraligamentaire possibilitésd´une nouvelle technique. *Actual Odontostomatol. (Paris)* 27 (103): 551–573.

Lamian, L. and Simard-Savoie, S. (1979). The effect of intrapulpal injections on the systemic blood pressure. *J. Dent. Res.* 58 (A): 209. (abstract no. 465).

Leonard, M.S. (1995). The efficacy of an intraosseous injection system of delivering local anesthetic. *J. Am. Dent. Assoc.* 126 (1): 81–86.

Lilienthal, B. (1975a). A clinical appraisal of intraosseous dental anesthesia. *Oral Surg. Oral Med. Oral Pathol.* 39 (5): 692–697.

Lilienthal, B. (1976). Cardiovascular responses to intraosseous injections of prilocaine containing vasoconstrictors. *Oral Surg. Oral Med. Oral Pathol.* 42 (5): 552–556.

Lilienthal, B. and Reynolds, A.K. (1975b). Cardiovascular responses to intraosseous injections containing catecholamines. *Oral Surg. Oral Med. Oral Pathol.* 40 (5): 574–583.

List, G., Meister, F.J., Nery, E.B., and Prey, J.H. (1988). Gingival crevicular fluid response to various solutions using the intraligamentary injection. *Quintessence Int.* 19 (8): 559–563.

Magnes, G.D. (1968). Intraosseous anesthesia. *Anesth. Prog.* 15 (9): 264–267.

Maita, E. and Horiuchi, H. (1984). Measurements of pressures developed in the syringe during dental infiltration anaesthesia. *Br. Dent. J.* 156 (11): 399–400.

Malamed, S.F. (1982). The periodontal ligament (PDL) injection: an alternative to inferior alveolar nerve block. *Oral Surg. Oral Med. Oral Pathol.* 53 (2): 117–121.

Marthaler (1970). Pulp anaesthesia of lower teeth through intraseptal injection. *Quintessence Int.* 1 (2): 21–23. (Note. No initial provided).

Masselink, B.H. (1910). The advent of painless dentistry. *Dent. Cosmos* 52 (8): 868–872.

Matthews, R.W. and Stables, D.K. (1985). Intraligamentary dental analgesia by dental therapists. *Br. Dent. J.* 159 (10): 329–330.

McLean, M.E., Wayman, B.E., and Mayhew, R.B. (1992). Duration of anesthesia using the periodontal ligament injection: a comparison of bupivacaine to lidocaine. *Anesth. Pain Control Dent.* 1 (4): 207–213.

Medvedev, D., Petrikas, A., and Dyubaylo, M. (2012). Aspiration in intra-ligamental anaesthesia of lower first molar teeth: a pilot study. *Oral Health Dent. Manag.* 11 (3): 95–99.

Meechan, J.G. (1992). Intraligamentary anesthesia. *J. Dent.* 20 (6): 325–332.

Meechan, J.G. (2002). A comparison of ropivacaine and lidocaine with epinephrine for intraligamentary anesthesia. *Oral Surg. Oral Med. Oral Pathol.* 93 (4): 469–473.

Meechan, J.G., McCabe, J.F., and Carrick, T.E. (1990). Plastic dental local anaesthetic cartridges: a laboratory investigation. *Br. Dent. J.* 169 (2): 54–56.

Miles, T.S. (1983). Dental pain: self-observations by a neurophysiologist. *J. Endod.* 19 (12): 613–615.

Miller, A.G. (1983). A clinical evaluation of the Ligmaject periodontal ligament injection syringe. *Dent. Update* 10 (10): 639–643.

Moore, K.D., Reader, A., Meyers, W.J. et al. (1987). A comparison of the periodontal ligament injection using 2% lidocaine with 1:100,000 epinephrine and saline in human mandibular premolars. *Anesth. Prog.* 34 (5): 181–186.

Mulkey, T.F. (1976). Outpatient treatment of hemophiliacs for dental extractions. *J. Oral Surg.* 34 (5): 428–434.

Nakane, S. and Kamayama, Y. (1987). Root resorption caused by mechanical injury of the periodontal soft tissues in rats. *J. Periodont. Res.* 22 (5): 390–395.

Nelson, P.W. (1981). Injection system (letter). *J. Am. Dent. Assoc.* 103 (5): 692.

Nevin, M. and Puterbaugh, P.G. (1949). *Conduction, Infiltration and General Anesthesia in Dentistry*, 5e. New York: Dental Items of Interest Publishing Co Inc. 235–243.

Nogué, R. (1907). L'anesthésie diploique – exposé de la méthode – technique –résultats. *Rev. Stomatol. (Paris)* 13: 191–196.

Nusstein, J., Reader, A., Nist, R. et al. (1998). Anesthetic efficacy of the supplemental intraosseous injection of 2% lidocaine with 1:100,000 epinephrine in irreversible pulpitis. *J. Endod.* 24 (7): 487–491.

Nusstein, J., Kennedy, S., Reader, A. et al. (2003). Anesthetic efficacy of the supplemental X-Tip intraosseous injection in patients with irreversible pulpitis. *J. Endod.* 29 (11): 724–728.

Nusstein, J., Berlin, J., Reader, A. et al. (2004). Comparison of injection pain, heart rate increase, and postinjection pain of articaine and lidocaine in a primary intraligamentary injection administered with a computer-controlled local anesthetic delivery system. *Anesth. Prog.* 51 (4): 126–133.

Nusstein, J., Claffey, E., Reader, A. et al. (2005a). Anesthetic effectiveness of the supplemental intraligamentary injection, administered with a computer controlled local anesthetic delivery system, in patients with irreversible pulpitis. *J. Endod.* 31 (5): 354–358.

Nusstein, J., Wood, M., Reader, A. et al. (2005b). Comparison of the degree of pulpal anesthesia achieved with the intraosseous injection and infiltration injection using 2% lidocaine with 1:100,000 epinephrine. *Gen. Dent.* 53 (1): 50–53.

Parente, S.A., Anderson, R.W., Herman, W.W. et al. (1998). Anesthetic efficacy of the supplemental intraosseous injection for teeth with irreversible pulpitis. *J. Endod.* 24 (12): 826–828.

Parrot, A.H. (1914). *Injection (intra-alveolar) anaesthesia in conservative work. Translations of the six International Dental Congress*. London: Published by the Committee of Organization. 561–567.

Pashley, D.H. (1986). Systemic effects of intraligamental injections. *J. Endod.* 12 (10): 501–504.

Pashley, E.L., Nelson, R., and Pashley, D.H. (1981). Pressures created by dental injections. *J. Dent. Res.* 60 (10): 1742–1748.

Pearce, J.H. (1976). Intraosseous injection for profound anesthesia of the lower molar. *J. Colo Dent. Assoc.* 54 (2): 25–26.

Peñarrocha, M., Oltra, M.J., Estarelles, B. et al. (1996). Estudio comparativo entre la anestesia intraósea y las técnicas de anestesia oral convencionales. *Av. Odontoestomatol. (Madrid)* 12 (9): 597–609.

Peñarrocha, M., Oltra, M.J., Gay, C., and Berini, L. (1997). Anestesia intraósea oral. *Av. Odontoestomatol. (Madrid)* 13 (1): 19–30.

Peñarrocha-Oltra, D., Ata-Ali, J., Oltra-Moscardó, M.J. et al. (2012). Side effects and complications of intraosseous anesthesia and conventional oral anesthesia. *Med. Oral Patol. Oral Cir. Bucal* 17 (3): e430–e434.

Pereira, L.A.P., Groppo, F.C., Bergamaschi, C.C. et al. (2013). Articaine (4%) with epinephrine (1:100,000 or 1:200,000) in intraosseous injections in symptomatic irreversible pulpitis of mandibular molars: anesthetic efficacy and cardiovascular effects. *Oral Surg. Oral Med. Oral Pathol.* 116 (2): e85–e91.

Peterson, J.E., Matsson, L., and Nation, W. (1983). Cementum and epithelial attachment response to the sulcular and periodontal ligament injection techniques. *Pediatr. Dent.* 5 w(4): 257–260.

Peurach, J.C. (1985). Pulpal response to intraligamentary injection in the cynomologus monkey. *Anesth. Prog.* 32 (2): 73–75.

Pin, P.J.A. (1987). The use of intraligamental injections in haemophiliacs. *Br. Dent. J.* 162 (4): 151–152.

Plamondon, T.J., Walton, R., Graham, G.S. et al. (1990). Pulp response to the combined effects of cavity preparation and periodontal ligament injection. *Oper. Dent.* 15 (3): 86–93.

Primosch, R.E. (1986). The role of pressure syringes in the administration of intraligamentary anesthesia. *Comp. Cont. Edu. Dent.* 7 (5): 340–348.

Rakusin, H., Lemmer, J., and Gutmann, J.L. (1986). Periodontal ligament injection: clinical effects on tooth and periodontium of young adults. *Int. Endod. J.* 19 (5): 230–236.

Rawson, R.D. and Orr, D.L. II (1985). Vascular penetration following intraligamental injection. *J. Oral Maxillofac. Surg.* 43 (8): 600–604.

Reader, A., Nusstein, J., and Drum, M. (2011). *Successful Local Anesthesia. For Restorative Dentistry and Endodontics*. Chicago: Quintessence Publishing Co, Inc. 99, 114.

Reisman, D., Reader, A., Nist, R. et al. (1997). Anesthetic efficacy of the supplemental intraosseous injection of 3% mepivacaine in irreversible pulpitis. *Oral Surg. Oral Med. Oral Pathol.* 84 (6): 676–682.

Reitz, J., Reader, A., Nist, R. et al. (1998). Anesthetic efficacy of the intraosseous injection of 0.9 mL of 2% lidocaine (1:100,000 epinephrine) to augment an inferior alveolar nerve block. *Oral Surg. Oral Med. Oral Pathol.* 86 (5): 516–523.

Remmers, T., Glickman, G., Spears, R., and He, J. (2008). The efficacy of IntraFlow intraosseous injection as a primary anesthesia technique. *J. Endod.* 34 (3): 280–283.

Replogle, K., Reader, A., Nist, R. et al. (1997). Anesthetic efficacy of the intraosseous injection of 2% lidocaine (1:100,000 epinephrine) and 3% mepivacaine in mandibular first molars. *Oral Surg. Oral Med. Oral Pathol.* 83 (1): 30–37.

Replogle, K., Reader, A., Nist, R. et al. (1999). Cardiovascular effects of intraosseous injections of 2 percent lidocaine with 1:100,000 epinephrine and 3 percent mepivacaine. *J. Am. Dent. Assoc.* 130 (5): 649–657.

Roahen, J. and Marshall, F.J. (1984). Pulpal and periodontal tissue effects of the periodontal ligament injection. *J. Endod.* 10 (3): 122. (abstract no. 18).

Roahen, J.O. and Marshall, F.J. (1990). The effects of periodontal ligament injection on pulpal and periodontal tissues. *J. Endod.* 16 (1): 28–33.

Roberts, D.H. and Sowray, J.H. (1987). *Local Analgesia in Dentistry*, 3e. Bristol (UK): Wright. 90–93.

Saadoun, A.P. and Malamed, S. (1985). Intraseptal anesthesia in periodontal surgery. *J. Am. Dent. Assoc.* 111 (2): 249–256.

Sachs, S.A., Lipton, R., and Frank, R. (1978). Management of ambulatory oral surgical patients with hemophilia. *J. Oral Surg.* 36 (1): 25–29.

Sauvez, E. (1905). *L'anesthésie locale pour l'extraction des dents*. Paris: Vigot Fréres Editeurs. 1–34, 178. (Note. The author's name is Emil. Not provided in the bibliography).

Schleder, J.R., Reader, A., Beck, M., and Meyers, W.J. (1988). The periodontal ligament injection: a comparison of 2% lidocaine, 3% mepivacaine, and 1:100,000 epinephrine to 2% lidocaine with 1:100,000 epinephrine in human mandibular premolars. *J. Endod.* 14 (8): 397–404.

Schmitt, E. (1936). Intraseptal anesthesia. *Dent. Cosmos* 78: 1190–1192.

Smith, A.E. (1920). *Block Anesthesia and Allied Subjects. With Special Chapters on the Maxillary Sinus, the Tonsils, and Neuralgias of the Nervous Trigeminus for Oral Surgeons, Dentists, Laryngologists, Rhinologists, Otologists, and Students*. St Louis (Mo): CV Mosby Co. 439.

Smith, G.N. and Pashley, D.H. (1983d). Periodontal ligament injection: evaluation of systemic effects. *Oral Surg. Oral Med. Oral Pathol.* 56 (6): 571–574.

Smith, N. and Smith, S.A. (1983a). Intrapulpal injection: distribution of an injected solution. *J. Endod.* 9 (5): 167–170.

Smith, G.N. and Walton, R.E. (1983b). Periodontal ligament injection: distribution of injected solutions. *Oral Surg. Oral Med. Oral Pathol.* 55 (3): 232–238.

Smith, G.N., Walton, R.E., and Abbott, B.J. (1983c). Clinical evaluation of periodontal ligament anesthesia using a pressure syringe. *J. Am. Dent. Assoc.* 107 (6): 953–956.

Spuller, R.L. (1988). Use of the periodontal ligament injection in dental care of the patient with haemophilia – a clinical evaluation. *Spec. Care Dent.* 81 (1): 28–29.

Stabident instruction manual. Miami; Fairfax Dental Inc. 2001.

Susi, L., Reader, A., Nusstein, J. et al. (2008). Heart rate effects of intraosseous injections using slow and fast rates of anesthetic solution deposition. *Anesth. Prog.* 55 (1): 9–15.

Tagger, E., Tagger, M., Sarnat, H., and Mass, E. (1994a). Periodontal ligament injection in the dog primary dentition: spread of local anaesthetic solution. *Int. J. Paediatr. Dent.* 4 (3): 159–166.

Tagger, M., Tagger, E., and Sarnat, H. (1994b). Periodontal ligament injection: spread of the solution in the dog. *J. Endod.* 20 (4): 283–287.

Torabinejad, M., Peters, D.L., Peckham, N. et al. (1993). Electron microscopic changes in human pulp after intraligamental injection. *Oral Surg. Oral Med. Oral Pathol.* 76 (2): 219–224.

Van Gheluwe, J. and Walton, R. (1997). Intrapulpal injection. *Oral Surg. Oral Med. OralPathol.* 83 (1): 38–40.

Villette, A. (2003). Untersuchungs-bilanzaus 500 in erster Intention durchgeführten Trans-kortikalelis-Anästhesien. *Schweitz Monatsschr. Zahnmed.* 113 (11): 1211–1214.

Walmsley, A.D., Lloyd, J.M., and Harrington, E. (1989). Pressures produced in vitro during intraligamentary anaesthesia. *Br. Dent. J.* 167 (10): 341–344.

Walton, R.E. (1990). The periodontal ligament injection as a primary technique. *J. Endod.* 16 (2): 62–66.

Walton, R.E. and Abbott, B.J. (1981). Periodontal ligament injection: a clinical evaluation. *J. Am. Dent. Assoc.* 103 (4): 571–575.

Walton, R.E. and Garnick, J.J. (1982). The periodontal ligament injection: histological effects on the periodontium in monkeys. *J. Endod.* 8 (1): 22–26.

White, J.J., Reader, A., Beck, M., and Meyers, W.J. (1988). The periodontal ligament injection: a comparison of the efficacy in human maxillary and mandibular teeth. *J. Endod.* 14 (10): 508–514.

Wood, M., Reader, A., Nusstein, J. et al. (2005). Comparison of intraosseous and infiltration injections for venous lidocaine blood concentrations and heart rate changes after injection of 2% lidocaine with 1:100,000 epinephrine. *J. Endod.* 31 (6): 435–438.

Woodmansey, K.F., White, R.K., and He, J. (2009). Osteonecrosis relates it intraosseous anesthesia: report of a case. *J. Endod.* 35 (2): 288–291.

X-Tip (2010). *X-Tip Intraosseous Anesthesia Delivery System.* Ballaigues (Switzerland): Dentsply Mailleffer.

# 19

## Failure of Dental Local Anesthesia

Despite scientific advances, there is, unfortunately, no infallible technique for ensuring local anesthesia in dentistry, and failures generally reflect specific situations such as anatomical variations, pathological abnormalities (e.g. local inflammation), considerable patient anxiety, and failures associated with the dentist. In this chapter, we address the area of failure of dental anesthesia and its causes and examine the means at our disposal to overcome it.

## Frequency

It is difficult to quantify how often dental local anesthesia fails because pulpal anesthesia, the most difficult type of anesthesia to achieve, is hampered by various factors.

1) Type of stimulus. The pain stimulus differs depending on whether the procedure is obturation (especially if it is not very deep), extraction, incision of soft tissue, or an endodontic procedure in a vital tooth. It is much easier to anesthetize the soft tissues or alveolar process than the dental pulp (Phillips 1943). We believe that the electric pulp meter is the most reliable experimental stimulus for evaluating the efficacy of local pulpal anesthesia since it reaches deep levels and its findings are reproducible. Therefore, in this book, we have selected studies whose results are based on the application of this approach.
2) Type of local anesthetic solution. Different outcomes are achieved by varying the concentration of anesthetic and/or vasoconstrictor, as well as by using different local anesthetics or vasoconstrictors. This is particularly important in infiltrative techniques (Annex 21), although generally of little relevance in mandibular block (Annex 24). Therefore, we have selected the two most widely used solutions today: the one we have referred to throughout the book as the standard solution, i.e. lidocaine 2% with epinephrine 1:100000 (10 μg/ml) (L-100) or 1:80000 (12.5 μg/ml) (L-80), and a potent solution, i.e. articaine 4% with epinephrine 1:100000 (10 μg/ml) (A-100).
3) The amount of solution administered (in milliliters [ml]). We selected the standard quantities on which current clinical evaluations are based (generally slightly higher than recommended in textbooks) and which are those used in daily clinical practice.
4) Area of the mouth. The results are very different for the maxillary and the mandibular arches and are very different for the anterior teeth (canines and incisors) and posterior teeth (molars and premolars). Therefore, we have drawn a distinction between these four areas and have taken the lateral incisor and first molar as a reference.

Table 19.1 summarizes the percentage of failures in healthy teeth that respond to an electric stimulus despite being anesthetized. A study from 2002 in patients receiving dental treatment over 5 years found that treatment was painful in more than 40%. In addition, the pain was moderate or intense in more than half (20% of the total) (Maggirias and Locker 2002). Consequently, dental local anesthesia could be improved.

## Consequences of Failure

Failure of dental locoregional anesthesia is important for various reasons:

1) Dental treatment cannot be administered.
2) Patients lose trust not only in their dentist, but also in modern dental techniques for controlling pain (Kaufman et al. 1984).
3) Failure is especially important in children because traumatic experiences (e.g. pain during dental procedures resulting from insufficient anesthesia) generate psychological effects, i.e. patients become very fearful of dental treatment and may develop phobias during adulthood (Molin and Seeman 1970; Kleinknecht et al. 1973; Cohen et al. 1993; Berggren and Meynert 1984).

---

*Local Anesthesia in Dentistry: A Locoregional Approach*, First Edition. Jesús Calatayud and Mana Saraghi.
© 2024 John Wiley & Sons Ltd. Published 2024 by John Wiley & Sons Ltd.
Companion website: www.wiley.com/go/Calatayud/local

Table 19.1 Summary of failures.

| Tooth | Anesthetic technique | ml/LAS/time (min) | Failure | Reference |
|---|---|---|---|---|
| **Maxillary teeth** | | | | |
| Incisors | Buccal infiltration | 1.0/L-100/5′ | 5% | Annex 21 |
| | Buccal infiltration | 1.0/A-100/5′ | **2%** | Annex 21 |
| First molar | Buccal infiltration | 1.8/L-100/5′ | 13% | Annex 21 |
| | | 1.8/A-100/5′ | **5%** | Annex 21 (estimated) |
| **Mandibular teeth** | | | | |
| Incisors | Buccal infiltration | 1.8/L-100/5–10′ | 45% | Annex 31 |
| | Buccal infiltration | 1.8/A-100/5–10′ | 20% | Annex 31 |
| | Double infiltration | 1.8/L-100/5–10′ | 10% | Annex 31 |
| | Double infiltration | 1.8/A-100/5–10′ | **2%** | Annex 31 |
| | Mandibular block | 1.8/L-100/10–15′ | 65–70% | Annex 25 |
| | Mandibular block | 3.6/L-100/10–15′ | 60–70% | Annex 25 |
| First molar | Mandibular block | 1.8/L-100/10–15′ | 35–40% | Annex 25 |
| | Mandibular block | 3.6/L-100/10–15′ | 30–35% | Annex 25 |
| | Mandibular block + complementary buccal infiltration | 1.8/L-100/10–15′<br>1.8/A-100/5–10′ | **5%** | Table 16.5<br>Chapter 16 |

Percentage of failures with the most frequently used techniques in healthy teeth. The lowest percentages of failure are shown in bold. Evaluation is with electrical stimulation.
ml/LAS/time, milliliters/local anesthetic solution/time in minutes; L-100, lidocaine 2% with epinephrine 1:100 000 (10 µg/ml); A-100, articaine 4% with epinephrine 1:100 000 (10 µg/ml).

## Failures: General Causes

Many failures are associated with patient-specific situations.

### Highly Anxious Patients

As we saw in Chapter 8, around 10% of patients are highly anxious and fear dental treatment. Anxiety reduces the pain threshold and increases the possibility that nonpainful stimuli are interpreted as being painful (Pinkham and Schroeder 1975; Wepman 1978; Woolgrove 1983; Sokol et al. 1985; Van Wijk and Makkes 2008). It is therefore important to bear in mind that local anesthetics are very effective for anesthetizing painful stimuli but are much less effective with sensations of temperature and pressure. In addition, they are poorly effective with the nerve fibers that transmit proprioceptive stimuli (de Jong 1977; Wildsmith 1986). In such patients, it is necessary to follow various steps:

1) Inform the patient that he/she should distinguish between "painful" stimuli, which can be easily anesthetized, and sensations of touch, pressure, and temperature, which are more difficult to anesthetize. Thus, we can help the patient to interpret these sensations in two ways:
- Extraorally:
  - The dentist can take the patient's hand by the wrist in his/her own hand, move it from side to side, and ask the patient if he/she notices this and if it hurts. The patient will reply that he/she does notice it but that it does not hurt.
  - The dentist presses the patient's hand with his/her own and asks if the patient notices pressure and if this is painful. The patient will reply that he/she does notice the pressure but that it is not painful.
  - The dentist asks the patient if his/her hand is cold or warm. The patient replies that it is warm.
  - Finally, the dentist points out to the patient that he/she felt the movement of the hand, the pressure, and the temperature, but no pain. The same will be true of the mouth, that is, the patient will notice sensations (movement, pressure, temperature) but not pain.
- Intraorally. The word "pain" is now taboo, and the euphemism "discomfort" is used instead.
  - The dentist shows the patient his/her right hand with the fist closed and the index finger extended and says, "Look at my finger."

- The dentist then inserts the finger into the patient's mouth and presses on the injection site and says "Here is where I'll place the anesthesia. Can you feel where I'm touching you? The patient will reply that he/she does notice it. Observe that the dentist says "place" the anesthesia and not "inject," which is taboo.
- The dentist says that when the anesthetic is placed in this area, the patient will notice it or perhaps will feel some "discomfort" (euphemism for pain, now a taboo word).

2) The dentist must exercise great care when administering local anesthetic to minimize the pain of the injection (see sections "Insertion of the Needle" and "Injection", Chapter 13). In addition, it is advisable to administer a larger quantity of anesthetic.
3) If necessary, the patient should receive an anxiolytic or sedative drug, although therapy of this type is beyond the scope of this book.
4) If the patient continues to feel pain for any reason during treatment, supplementary techniques can be applied to address failure (see Chapter 18).

However, if the level of anxiety is very high or the patient is phobic (irrational and uncontrolled fear), then he/she must be treated by a psychologist or psychiatrist. Such patients may require psychiatric drugs or general anesthesia, both of which approaches are beyond the scope of this book.

### Patients with Drug Addiction and Alcoholism

Patients who are addicted to alcohol or other drugs such as heroin, cocaine, or tranquilizers have a very low tolerance of stress (nervousness) and pain because of psychological and physiological abnormalities affecting the central nervous system (Scheutz 1982; Chemical 1987; Stewart and Finn 1995; Fiset et al. 1997; Lindroth et al. 2003). These patients require greater amounts of anesthesia, and anesthesia fails twice as often as in patients who do not have addictions (Scheutz 1982; Chemical 1987; Stewart and Finn 1995). In addition, they are often difficult to manage and require both medical and psychological treatment.

This group of patients should be treated in the same way as highly anxious patients (see above).

### Teeth Affected by Irreversible Acute Pulpitis

The pulp of teeth affected by acute pulpitis (symptomatic irreversible pulpitis) is both inflamed and hypersensitive (called a "hot tooth"). The frequency of failure of local anesthetic is higher, i.e. double or triple that of patients without pulpitis (Table 19.2), given that the tooth is more difficult to anesthetize. In Table 19.2, failure in healthy molars is evaluated based on an electric pulp meter; however, in molars affected by irreversible acute pulpitis, failure is evaluated in endodontic procedures when the pulp chamber is opened and during cleaning because negative electrical stimulation is no guarantee of a painless endodontic procedure in these cases (Dreven et al. 1987; Reisman et al. 1997; Nusstein et al. 1998; Tortamano et al. 2009). It is also important to highlight that the more severe the symptoms are in teeth with pulpitis (more pain), the greater the percentage of failures will be (Aggarwal et al. 2015).

**Table 19.2** Percentage of failures after local anesthesia in molars with irreversible acute pulpitis compared with healthy molars.

| Anesthetic technique | ml/LAS/time (min) | Failure healthy molars | Failure molars with pulpitis |
|---|---|---|---|
| **Maxillary teeth** | | | |
| Buccal infiltration | 1.8/L-100/5–10′ | 13% | 35% |
| " | 1.8/**A-100**/5–10′ | 5% | 25% |
| **Mandibular teeth** | | | |
| Mandibular block | 1.8/L-100/10–15′ | 35–40% | 70% |
| Mandibular block | **3.6**/L-100/10–15′ | 30–35% | 55% |
| | Reference | Table 19.1 | Annex 35 |

ml/LAS/time, milliliters/local anesthetic solution/time in minutes; L-100, lidocaine 2% with epinephrine 1:100 000 (10 μg/ml); A-100, articaine 4% with epinephrine 1:100 000 (10 μg/ml).

**Reasons for Failure of Anesthesia in Acute Pulpitis**
1) Structural abnormalities affecting peripheral nerves. These nerves are affected by inflammation (Kimberly and Byers 1988; Byers et al. 1990; Taylor and Byers 1990; Sorensen et al. 2004), and their thresholds of excitability and of electrolyte exchange in the membrane are altered, thus rendering the membrane hyperexcitable (Brown 1981; Rood and Pateromichelakis 1981). These *neurodegenerative changes* affect not only the axonal membrane exposed to inflammation, but also the *whole nerve pathway*, therefore truncal block at some distance from the inflammation also fails (Najjar 1977; Wallace et al. 1985; Luo et al. 2008).
2) Local factors:
   - Tissue pH in inflamed or purulent areas is lower and may reach 5–6.6 (Schade et al. 1921; de Jong and Cullen 1963) instead of the 7.4 observed in healthy

tissue, therefore the acid environment leaves very little free base for the anesthetic to penetrate the cell membrane (Bieter 1936; de Jong 1977; Walton and Torabinejad 1992; Wong and Jacobsen 1992).
- Increase of inflammatory mediators (such as prostaglandins, calcitonin gene-related peptide, substance P, neurokinin A, neuropeptide Y, vasoactive intestinal polypeptide) that sensitize the sodium channels of the free nerve endings by facilitating depolarization with less intense stimuli (hyperalgesia), therefore local anesthetics are less efficacious for blocking them (Bowles et al. 2003; Lai et al. 2004; Caviedes-Bucheli et al. 2006).
- Modifications in the sodium channels of the dental pulp lead to a threefold multiplication of the subtype or isoform $Na_v$ 1.9 (Wells et al. 2007), which requires 2.5–5 times more anesthetic for the block to be effective (Scholz et al. 1998); six to eightfold of the subtype $Na_v$ 1.8 (Renton et al. 2005; Warren et al. 2008) and also the subtype $Na_v$ 1.7 (Luo et al. 2008).
- Regional vasodilation favors rapid removal of the anesthetic solution at the affected site as a result of it entering the systemic circulation (Kramer and Mitton 1973; Meechan 1999).

**Approach**

1) Administer a nonsteroidal anti-inflammatory drug (NSAID) 45–60 minutes before local anesthesia. The most widely used NSAID is ibuprofen at 400–800 mg, although any NSAID can be used (Annex 35; Modaresi et al. 2006). When NSAIDs cannot be used (e.g. in patients with gastrointestinal ulcer, pregnant women, patients taking oral anticoagulants, aspirin-sensitive asthmatics), acetaminophen can be administered at 1000 mg, although the outcome is somewhat more modest (Annex 35; Modaresi et al. 2006). In addition, two meta-analyses have shown that NSAIDs taken 1 hour before the procedure improve anesthesia in mandibular block. This finding was statistically significant (Li et al. 2012; Shirvani et al. 2017).

2) Administration of local anesthesia (Annex 35).
   - Use potent solutions such as articaine 4% with epinephrine 1:100 000 (10 µg/ml) (A-100) instead of the standard solution of lidocaine (Annex 35). Three meta-analyses have demonstrated the superiority of A-100 over the standard lidocaine solution (L-100 or L-80) in patients with irreversible acute pulpitis (Kung et al. 2015; Su et al. 2016; de Geus et al. 2020).
   - In maxillary teeth:
     - Anterior teeth. Buccal infiltration with 1.8 ml of A-100 complemented by a small amount administered via the area of the palate. Wait a little longer, 5–10 minutes.
     - Posterior teeth. Buccal infiltration with more than 1.8 ml of A-100 (75% success rate [Annex 35]) and complement with 0.3–0.4 ml via the palate to enhance anesthesia of the palatal roots (Ulusoy and Alacam 2014; Askari et al. 2016).
   - In mandibular teeth:
     - Anterior teeth. Double infiltration (buccal and lingual) of 1.8–3.6 ml of A-100. Wait 5–10 minutes for the anesthetic to take effect.
     - Posterior teeth. Mandibular block with 1.8 ml of A-100. Wait 5 minutes to ensure that the lower lip is anesthetized. At this point, inject a further 1.8 ml of A-100 as mandibular block (two cartridges, 3.6 ml, have now been injected) and use complementary anesthesia in the buccal region with a further 1.8 ml of A-100 (three cartridges have now been injected). Wait 5–10 minutes longer (10–15 minutes in total). It is important to take two aspects into account:
       - If the second mandibular block is performed using the Gow-Gates technique instead of the conventional technique used for the first block, it increases efficacy and the number of teeth anesthetized (Saatchi et al. 2018).
       - It is interesting to observe that mandibular block is more painful in these cases (McCartney et al. 2007; Fan et al. 2009; Kreimer et al. 2012; Annex 23), therefore the technique should be performed meticulously.

3) Anesthesia with supplementary techniques. If the above approach is insufficient and the anesthetic fails to take effect.

Failure of mandibular block affects the dentine in 30% of cases (pain is felt when the burr reaches the dentine), therefore it is too early to apply the intrapulpal technique and it is necessary to turn to other supplementary techniques (Annex 35).

We can turn to the periodontal ligament technique (PDL) and the intraosseous technique (IO), again using A-100, which we have used so far (it is important to remember not to mix two local anesthetics at the same point of action, Chapter 5). The initial success with the first injection is greater with the IO technique than with the PDL (85% vs. 65%), although the cumulative effect after the second injection (if the first fails) is very similar (almost 100%) (Annex 35). However, the supplementary technique may sometimes have to be repeated as many as three times (Nusstein et al. 1998). The PDL has the advantage that if a rubber dam is in place, it is not necessary to remove it for administration (Walton and

Abbott 1981; Khedari 1982); the advantage of the IO technique is that is has fewer adverse effects (Chapter 18).

In patients with irreversible acute pulpitis, supplementary techniques can be painful because of the high sensitivity of the teeth, even if all the tissue is anesthetized (Nusstein et al. 2003).

It is also noteworthy that other methods are currently being sought, such as inhalation of nitrous oxide, for which data seem promising (Fullmer et al. 2014; Chompu-inwai et al. 2018).

Finally, remember that endodontic procedures are considered to be successful when the anesthetized teeth do not hurt or only do so minimally, so that the procedure can be performed with the drill able to penetrate the enamel and dentine and reach the pulp chamber (Annex 35). These teeth may subsequently require intrapulpal anesthesia.

### Resistance to Local Anesthetics

Cases of resistance to the action of various local anesthetics have been reported. In both medical practice (Miller et al. 1981; Kavlock and Ting 2004) and in dental practice (Beckett and Gilmour 1990), resistance takes the form of short duration of effect or insufficient effect. In dental practice (Beckett and Gilmour 1990) this cannot be attributed to the traditional causes of failure addressed in this chapter, but rather to genetic abnormalities that lead to structural abnormalities in some of the isoforms of the sodium channels (Panigel and Cook 2011; Clendenen et al. 2016). The frequency of resistance is unknown, although it must be low, and in some cases it has been overcome using local anesthetics in which the concentration of the anesthetic component is high (Beckett and Gilmour 1990).

### Other Causes of Failure

Other proposed causes of failure include hematoma in mandibular block that could dilute the anesthetic solution in the pterygomandibular space (Traeger 1979), although this seems highly unlikely.

## Specific Failures After Maxillary Infiltration

Failure of local anesthesia is less frequent after infiltration in maxillary teeth than after mandibular block. Below, we present the causes and the means to overcome them.

### Causes of Maxillary Failure

1) Excessive thickening of the maxillary bone cortex. This mainly affects the superior central incisors via the anterior nasal spine (Figure 19.1) if this is very wide and covers the apices. However, such a situation is highly unlikely (Jastak et al. 1995). This situation may also arise in the first molars owing to thickening of the zygomatic crest (Evers and Haegerstam 1981; Roberts and Sowray 1987; Jastak et al. 1995) or thickening of the outer bone plate, which is typical of patients with bruxism.

2) Excessive separation of the palatal roots of the molars, premolars, and lateral incisor as they course toward the palate. In the posterior teeth, the distance separating the palatal roots and the buccal roots may be very great. In fact, the maxillary sinus may even lie between the palatal and the buccal roots (Figure 19.2), thus hampering diffusion of the anesthetic solution toward the palatal root (Evers and Haegerstam 1981; Haglund and Evers 1985). Very rarely, the root of the lateral incisor may be inclined toward the palate.

3) Accessory innervation via the nasopalatine nerve to the pulp of the incisors and, occasionally, the canines. This branch of the nasopalatine root was proposed initially by Otto Hofer from Vienna (Hofer 1922) and supported, albeit without demonstration, by various authors (Phillips and Maxmen 1941; Cook 1949). In 1943, the Department of Anatomy of the University of Wayne reported having found this branch in dissections (Phillips 1943), although other studies based on dissection did not (Olsen et al. 1955), therefore these contradictory results created an atmosphere of distrust (FitzGerald and Scott 1958; Westwater 1960; Sicher 1950). More recently, it was suggested that fibers

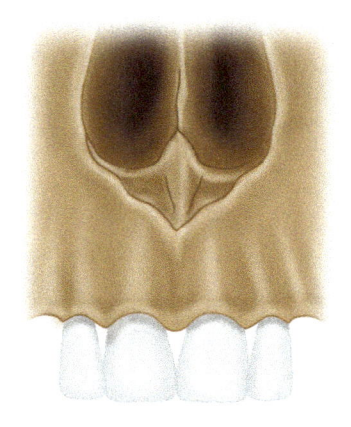

**Figure 19.1** Thickening of the anterior nasal spine covering the apices of the maxillary central incisors.

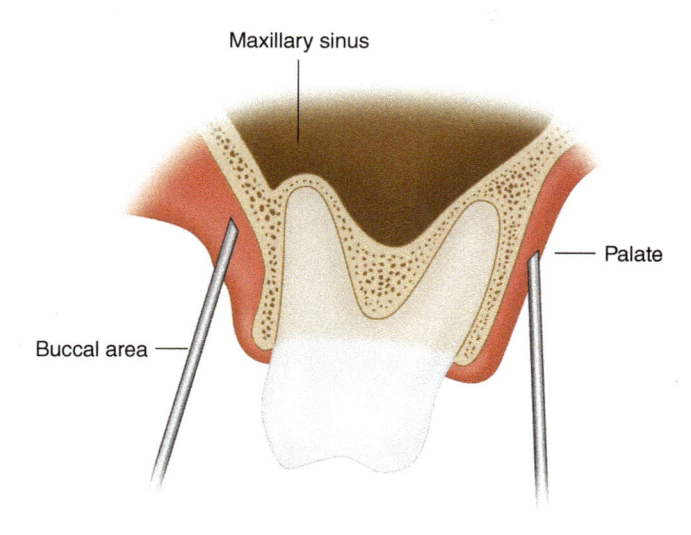

**Figure 19.2** Maxillary sinus entering the space between the palatal and buccal roots.

of the superior dental plexus can join the nasopalatine nerve right at the nasal floor and reach the apices of the central incisors (Roda and Blanton 1994).
4) Accessory innervations of the pulp via branches of the greater palatine nerve of the palatal roots of the molars and premolars (Ulusoy and Alacam 2014).

### Approach

If pulpal anesthesia has not been achieved 5 minutes after injection, the available options are as follows:

1) Complementary anesthesia:
   - Adults. If articaine 4% with epinephrine 1:100 000 (A-100) was used, i.e. the first choice in adults, repeat the injection with a greater quantity at the same sites.
   - Children. If the standard solution of lidocaine 2% with epinephrine 1:100 000 (10 μg/ml) (L-100) was used, i.e. the solution indicated for children, repeat the injection with a greater quantity at the same sites, but use *lidocaine 2% with epinephrine 1:50 000 (20 μg/ml) (L-50)*, which contains double the amount of epinephrine, thus rendering its effect more potent. Note that the anesthetic is the same, since two different anesthetics should not be mixed at the same site.
2) Complementary palatal anesthesia.
   - Adults. Complementary anesthesia administered via the palate in small amounts (±0.2–0.3 ml) of A-100 increases both the efficacy and the duration of pulpal anesthesia, especially in posterior teeth with palatal roots (Aggarwal et al. 2011a, 2011b; Guglielmo et al. 2011; Ulusoy and Alacam 2014).
   - Children. Complementary anesthesia can also be administered via the palate, but using L-50 and trans-papillary injection, which is typical in children (Chapter 15).
3) Supplementary techniques. If the two methods proposed above fail after a further 5 minutes (complementary anesthesia and complementary anesthesia administered via the palate), then the PDL and/or the IO technique is used.

In children, supplementary techniques such as the PDL or the IO technique can be used, although only in permanent teeth (not in temporary teeth, so as not to affect the buds of the underlying permanent teeth).

## Specific Failures After Mandibular Block

As we have seen, mandibular block is only used to achieve pulpal anesthesia in molars and premolars (posterior teeth), where the results are acceptable (Annex 25). Below, we present the reasons for failure and the means to address it.

### Reasons for Failure After Mandibular Block

#### Failure Owing to Inappropriate Technique

This failure arises when soft tissue anesthesia of half of the ipsilateral lower lip is not achieved 5 minutes after injection (Cohen et al. 1993; Hersh et al. 1995; Nusstein et al. 1998). This is the most frequent cause and may arise in up to 10% of cases (Annex 28).

Logically, this failure is particularly common among dentistry students (Rood and Sowray 1980) since the technique is not easy to apply and requires the acquisition of appropriate skills. Failure may also arise among experienced professionals, although it has been demonstrated that the frequency of this type of failure decreases with experience and the number of years the dentist has been working (Keetley and Moles 2001). Nonetheless, cases of failure are reported.

#### Failure for Anatomical Reasons

*Accessory Mandibular Foramina* Most accessory mandibular foramina are found in the region of the condyle and the mandibular foramen (Barker 1972a; Haveman and Tebo 1976). In some cases, accessory branches, which are smaller than the inferior alveolar nerve, may enter some foramina at higher levels and supply the inferior molars. These branches may not be affected by conventional mandibular block.

***Very High Lingula*** A very high lingula means that the inferior alveolar nerve does not come into contact with the solution because the anesthetic cannot be appropriately placed in the pterygomandibular space, as in conventional mandibular block (Coleman and Smith 1982). The finding of a lingula greater than 11 mm occurs in 0.1% of cases (Kay 1974) and in up to 5% of cases (Bremer 1952). To avoid this, it is recommended that the level of needle contact with bone should be slightly superior to the lingula.

***Double (Bifid) Mandibular Canal and/or Foramen*** Bifid mandibular canal and/or foramen was initially described in isolated cases (Kiersch and Jordan 1973; Patterson and Funke 1973). Trifid canal/foramen is even rarer (Mizbah et al. 2012). It is important to remember that this situation arises because the mandibular canal originates from the junction of three separate canals during embryonic development (Chavez-Lomeli et al. 1996). Such anatomical anomalies are thought to hamper the efficacy of conventional mandibular block (Kiersch and Jordan 1973; Grover and Lorton 1983; Neves et al. 2013), especially in cases of bifid foramina (Nortjé et al. 1977; Langlais et al. 1985; Bogdan et al. 2006; Correr et al. 2013). Modern tomography-based techniques have made it possible to identify these anomalies (mean length of 10–15 mm) in 30% of mandibular canals (Annex 34).

Bifid mandibular canals are important because they can sometimes escape mandibular block (Grover and Lorton 1983; Neves et al. 2013).

***Sphenomandibular Ligament*** Sometimes, deposition of local anesthetic where it is separated from the inferior alveolar nerve by the sphenomandibular ligament (Figure 3.14, Chapter 3) or other fibrous tissue in the pterygomandibular space may impede diffusion (Barker and Davies 1972b; Garg and Townsend 2001; Shiozaki et al. 2007; Khoury et al. 2010, 2011; Simonds et al. 2017). To avoid this, it is recommended that the level of needle contact with bone should be slightly superior to the lingula (Khoury et al. 2010, 2011).

**Failure Arising from Accessory Innervation**

***Mylohyoid Nerve*** The mylohyoid nerve is mainly a motor nerve that supplies the mylohyoid muscle and the anterior belly of the digastric muscle, therefore anesthesia of this nerve causes some discomfort when swallowing (Barker and Davies 1972b). The nerve emerges from the inferior alveolar nerve before entering the mandibular foramen. It was initially thought to emerge at a very low level, some 5 mm before entering the mandibular foramen (Jeffries 1944; Barker and Davies 1972b), therefore it was systematically anesthetized during mandibular block.

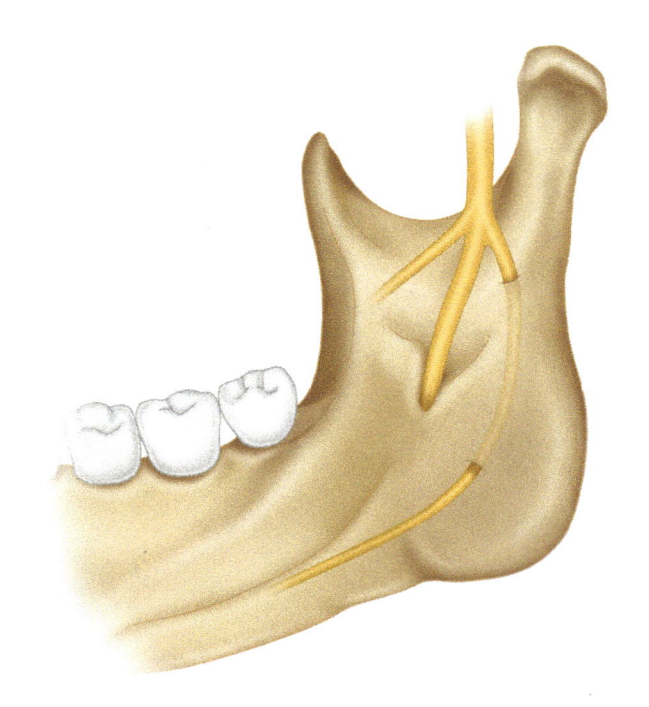

**Figure 19.3** Variant of the mylohyoid nerve emerging at a high level and penetrating a specific canal.

Thanks to meticulous dissection studies, we now know that it emerges much higher, at around 15 mm (5–23 mm) (Wilson et al. 1984; Bennett and Townsend 2001). Consequently, it is often not anesthetized (Figure 19.3); furthermore, it may be protected from the anesthetic solution by the interpterygoid fascia (i.e. it penetrates the fascia) or by the sphenomandibular ligament (Stein et al. 2007).

In 1904, in Vienna, Schumacher proposed that the mylohyoid nerve could give off branches to the mandibular symphysis to supply the inferior incisors (Schumacher 1904). Dissection studies have shown that up to 20% of its fibers are sensitive to pain and temperature, and supply the skin of the chin (Sicher 1946; Frommer et al. 1972; Roberts and Harris 1973). In 15–50% of cases, it may also supply the pulp of the mandibular teeth (Novitzky 1938; Sicher 1946; Carter and Keen 1971; Madeira et al. 1978; Wilson et al. 1984). The pulpal branches penetrate the bone via the foramina along the mylohyoid groove of the internal aspect of the mandible, along which the nerve courses. Thus, we have the following (Figure 19.4):

- Branches for *molars* (Frommer et al. 1972), which penetrate via the posterior foramina and are found in more than 80% of mandibles (Haveman and Tebo 1976).
- Branches for *premolars* (Carter and Keen 1971; Chapnick 1980; Bennett and Townsend 2001), which penetrate via the foramina in the area of the bicuspids of

## Specific Failures After Mandibular Block

**Buccal Nerve** The buccal nerve is involved in the innervation of the mandibular molars because it gives off a series of variants:

- Foramen at the level of the retromolar fossa. The buccal nerve or any of its branches penetrates via this foramen and reaches the apices of the molars via an accessory canal (Figure 19.5). This variant was suggested by Stewart in 1932 (Stewart 1932) and supported by clinical experience (Jeffries 1944). The dissection-based explanation of the anatomy was put forward by Sutton in 1974 (Sutton 1974). The variant may occasionally escape mandibular block.
- Retromolar canal. The buccal nerve or any of its branches can emerge at a very low level and become separated from the inferior alveolar nerve in the mandibular canal itself and emerge in the retromolar fossa (Figure 19.6) via a foramen measuring 0.2–1.7 mm in diameter (Turner 1864; Schejtman et al. 1967; Singh 1981). Before emerging behind the molars, it may give off a branch that reaches the apices of the inferior molars via an accessory canal (Schejtman et al. 1967). The frequency of this variant in the general population is unknown, although it is found in 63% of Amazonian Indians (Schejtman et al. 1967) and in 12% of Nordic Europeans (Löfgren 1957). It is usually anesthetized with mandibular block.

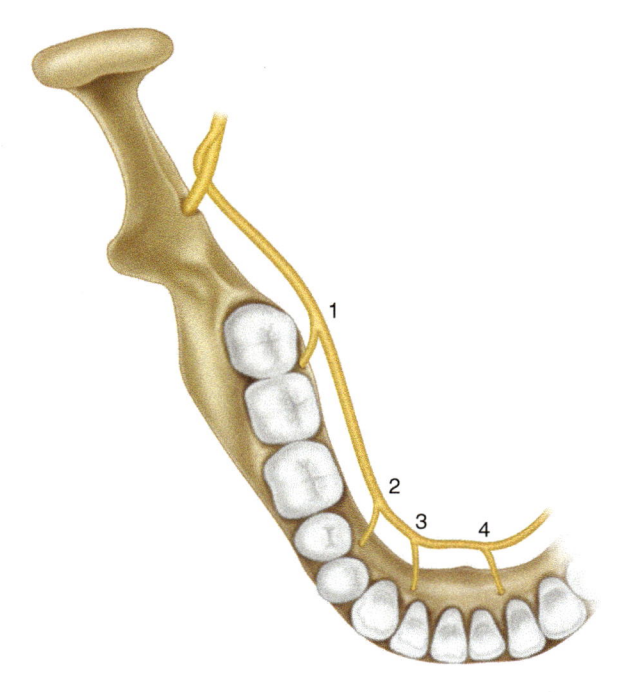

**Figure 19.4** Branches of the mylohyoid nerve that supply the molars (1), premolars (2), incisors and canines (3), and even contralateral anterior teeth (4).

the mylohyoid groove and are found in 60–70% of mandibles (Shiller and Wiswell 1954; Chapnick 1980).

- Branches for the *ipsilateral mandibular incisors* (Novitzky 1938; Sicher 1946; Carter and Keen 1971; Sutton 1974; Madeira et al. 1978; Wilson et al. 1984) and *contralateral incisors* (Madeira et al. 1978). These penetrate via the foramina of the mandibular symphysis and appear in 90% of mandibles (Shiller and Wiswell 1954; Sutton 1974; Madeira et al. 1978). They have been observed in 30% of dissections (Table 19.3).

Finally, the mylohyoid nerve is one of the best documented accessory innervations and is widely accepted by most authors (Barker and Davies 1972b; Rood 1976; Chapnick 1980; Coleman and Smith 1982).

**Table 19.3** Percentage of cases of mylohyoid nerve in mandibular symphysis.

| Reference | Percentage |
| --- | --- |
| Sicher (1946) | 10% |
| Carter and Keen (1971) | 12.5% |
| Madeira et al. (1978) | 50% |
| Wilson et al. (1984) | 43% |
|  | 30% |

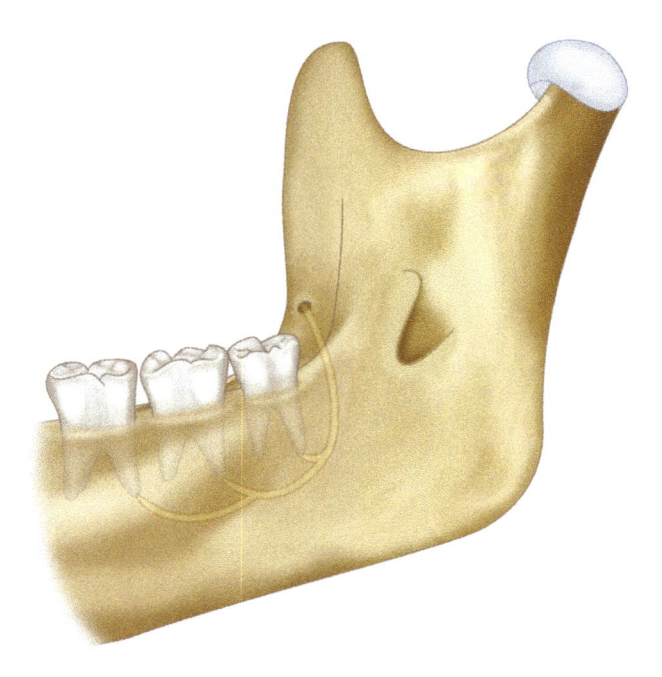

**Figure 19.5** Branches of the buccal nerve penetrating via a foramen of the retromolar fossa and an accessory channel can reach the apex of the molars. *Source:* Redrawn from Ossenberg (1986).

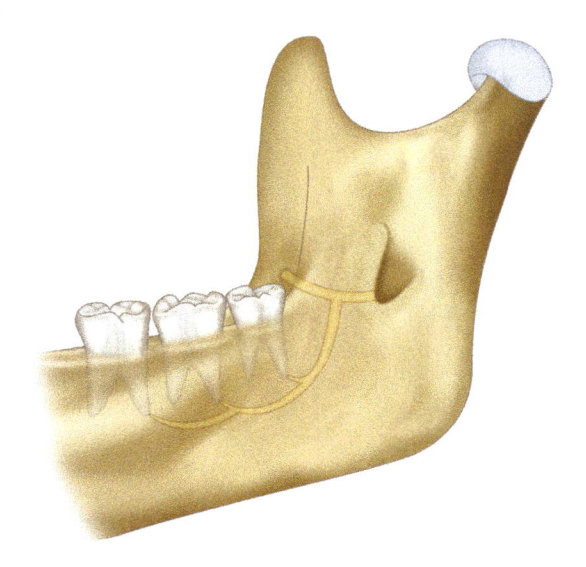

**Figure 19.6** Branches of the buccal nerve emerge at a low level, within the mandibular channel itself, and emerge in the retromolar fossa by giving off a branch to the apices of the molars. *Source:* Redrawn from Ossenberg (1986).

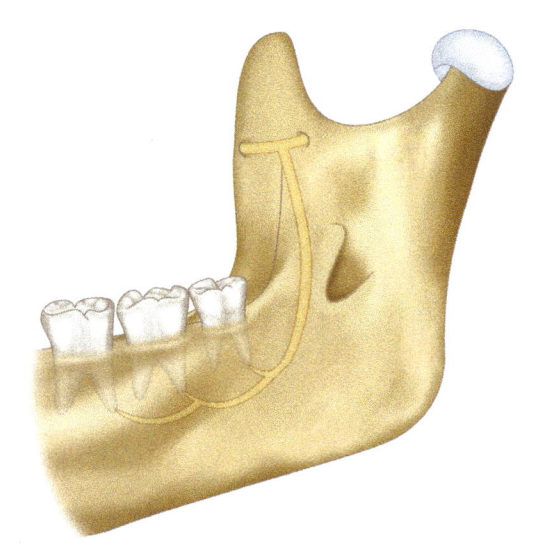

**Figure 19.7** The buccal nerve can course through a high foramen in the temporal crest, with some branches diverting through an accessory channel that reaches the apex of the molars. *Source:* Redrawn from Ossenberg (1986).

- Temporal crest canal. The buccal nerve or any of its branches can penetrate via a high foramen of the ascending branch behind the temporal crest (formerly the internal oblique line) and continue along a canal measuring 0.5–3mm in diameter that opens just as it passes the temporal crest at the anterior border of the mandibular ascending ramus (Figure 19.7). In many cases, an accessory canal emerges and reaches the apices of the mandibular molars. The frequency of this variant in the general population is 1.7% (Ossenberg 1986). The variant is not usually affected by mandibular block.

***Accessory Branch for the Wisdom Teeth*** In 40% of cases, the inferior alveolar nerve gives off a specific branch for the third molar immediately before or after it enters the mandibular foramen (Sicher 1946; Barker and Davies 1972b). There is a possibility that this branch will emerge at a high level, penetrating via its own foramen into the area of the condyle (Figure 19.8), where most foramina are concentrated (Carter and Keen 1971; Barker 1972a; Haveman and Tebo 1976), and thus remaining unaffected by mandibular block.

***Auriculotemporal Nerve*** The auriculotemporal nerve emerges from the common trunk of the third branch of the trigeminal (mandibular nerve, $V_3$) and crosses behind and outside in the highest part of the pterygomandibular space. This sensory nerve supplies the skin in the temporal region (which can reach the limits of the parietal, masseter, frontal, and supraorbital region), pinna with the tragus, external auditory canal, and posterior part of the temporomandibular joint capsule. Branches of this nerve have occasionally been found to penetrate via the foramina in the region of the condylar neck and the retromolar fossa and reach the apices of the mandibular molars (Carter and Keen 1971; Sutton 1974). It is worth remembering the high number of foramina present in the retromolar region (Carter and Keen 1971; Haveman and Tebo 1976) and the fact that nerve fibers have been found in 40% of these (Carter and Keen 1971).

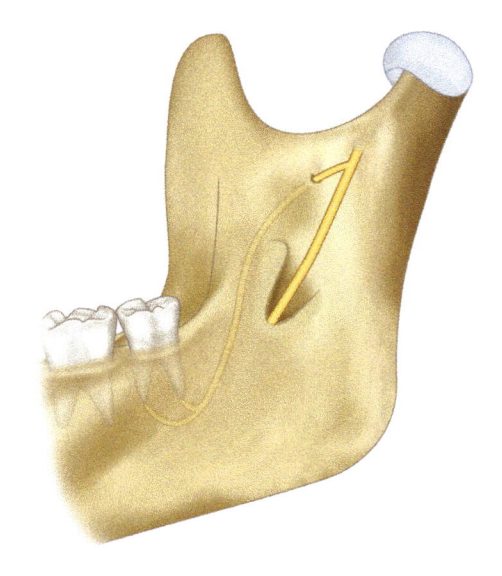

**Figure 19.8** Branch for the wisdom tooth that emerges at a very high level and penetrates via its own foramen.

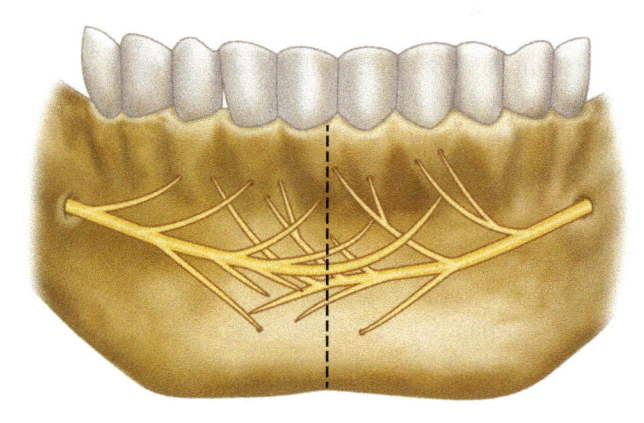

**Figure 19.9** Labial plexus with branches that cross the midline and may enter via the buccal foramina to supply the anterior teeth. *Source:* Redrawn from Rood (1977).

***Crossed Innervation in the Region of the Incisors (Labial Plexus)*** For embryological reasons (mandibular symphyseal cartilage) and anatomical reasons, the incisive nerve does not pass the midline of the mandible, therefore there is no contralateral crossed innervation (Olivier 1927; Sicher 1946) (Note: In only one case, in 535 patients, was the mandibular incisive canal found to pass the symphysis area in one series; Zhang et al. 2019.). However, the mental nerve gives off branches that form the labial plexus in the area of the mucosa and the anterior soft tissues, and these branches do cross the midline (Figure 19.9). Some of these branches can penetrate via the buccal mandibular foramina and innervate the contralateral canines and incisors (Starkie and Stewart 1931; Rood 1977; Pogrel et al. 1997).

***Other Uncertain Innervations*** Other nerve branches have been involved in the accessory innervation, although these have not been verified.

- The transverse nerve of the neck, or transverse cervical nerve (previously known as the cutaneous colli nerve), is a branch of the cervical plexus that innervates the skin between the sternocleidomastoid and the mandible. At the beginning of the twentieth century, Marshall proposed that it was a source of accessory innervation (Stewart 1932), and the theory became very popular with various authors (Phillips 1943; Jeffries 1944; Cook 1951; Bremer 1952; Sutton 1974; Rood 1976) who claimed that branches of this nerve penetrated via the inferior border of the mandible and thus innervated the teeth. Evidence for this accessory innervation is only clinical, since complementary buccal and lingual infiltration often complete the pulpal anesthesia of mandibular block in the anterior teeth.

Meticulous dissection studies have shown that branches of the transverse nerve of the neck approach the inferior border of the mandible. However, these have never demonstrated contact with the periosteum or penetration via foramina in which only feeder vessels have been found (Novitzky 1938; Sicher 1946, 1950; Cook 1951; Rizzolo et al. 1988). Furthermore, embryologic data demonstrates that the third branchial arch is the territory of the trigeminal nerve and that the passage of the transverse cervical nerve to the area of the trigeminal nerve contradicts the basic principles of embryology (Barker and Davies 1972b; Rizzolo et al. 1988), therefore this accessory innervation is thought to be unlikely (Chapnick 1980; Coleman and Smith 1982) and is probably confused with other nerve trunks, particularly with the accessory innervation of the mylohyoid nerve or the labial plexus.

Note: The transverse cervical nerve innervated the posterior inferior border of the mandible in one of two cadavers in one study (Lin et al. 2013).

- The lingual nerve may occasionally innervate the inferior incisors (Stewart and Wilson 1928; Jeffries 1944; Rood 1976; Chapnick 1980), although there is little anatomical evidence to support this hypothesis (Coleman and Smith 1982). In 1932, Stewart reported how Wilfred Ellison, in his anatomical dissections, found that branches of the lingual nerve penetrated via the alveolar vessels of the neck of the molars and premolars, supposedly with the aim of Innervating them (Stewart 1932). This data has not been confirmed.

Finally, Table 19.4 provides a summary of the accessory innervations of each tooth, with emphasis on cross-innervation in the area of the incisors and, to a lesser extent, of the canines, possibly owing to the course of the mylohyoid nerve (Madeira et al. 1978) and the labial plexus (Starkie and Stewart 1931; Rood 1977; Pogrel et al. 1997).

**Table 19.4** Summary of accessory innervation in mandibular teeth.

| Teeth | Possible accessory innervation |
|---|---|
| Molars | Mylohyoid nerve |
| | Variant branches of the inferior alveolar nerve |
| | Accessory branches for wisdom teeth |
| | Buccal nerve |
| | Auriculotemporal nerve |
| Premolars | Mylohyoid nerve |
| Incisors and canines | Mylohyoid nerve ⎫ |
| | ⎬ **Even contralateral** |
| | Labial plexus ⎭ |

This anatomical finding has been clinically verified by increasing pulpal anesthesia of these teeth with bilateral mandibular block (Yonchak et al. 2001).

## Approach

Unfortunately, since the cause of failure is unknown in most cases, the course of action in the posterior mandibular teeth will be as follows:

1) Absence of anesthesia of the lower lip. If injection of mandibular block is not followed by anesthesia of half of the lower lip within 5 minutes, the technique is considered to have failed (Cohen et al. 1993; Hersh et al. 1995; Nusstein et al. 1998) and should therefore not be repeated.
2) Complementary buccal anesthesia. If soft tissue anesthesia of the lower lip can be verified after 5 minutes (sign that the mandibular block is taking effect), complementary buccal infiltration should be applied in posterior mandibular teeth that require full pulpal anesthesia. *This maneuver considerably improves pulpal anesthesia.* The recommended approach is infiltration with a potent solution such as *articaine 4% with epinephrine 1:100 000 (A-100)*. A whole cartridge should be used for the buccal area in the posterior teeth to be treated (1.8 ml) (Haase et al. 2008; Kanaa et al. 2009; Gazal 2015).

After this infiltration, *wait a further 5–10 minutes* (total 10–15 minutes from initiation of mandibular block) to ensure that pulpal anesthesia has taken full effect.

3) Complement this approach with a second injection in the pterygomandibular space. If pain continues to be present after mandibular block with the standard solution (L-100) and the lower lip is fully anesthetized (indicating that the inferior alveolar nerve has been anesthetized), and after administering complementary buccal anesthesia with A-100 and waiting 10–15 minutes, then a second injection of L-100 into the pterygomandibular space is recommended (now 3.6 ml instead of 1.8 ml) and then wait an additional 5 minutes. This measure increases the efficacy of pulpal anesthesia by 5% (Annex 25).

If the second injection, after a conventional approach, is Gow-Gates technique (Haas 2011; Saatchi et al. 2018) or Laguardia–Akinosi (Haas 2011), the outcome improves as this different approach can overcome some anatomical variability and/or accessory innervations (Haas 2011).

4) Supplementary techniques. If the above approach is not sufficient and anesthesia fails after waiting a further 5 minutes, use supplementary techniques, namely, the PDL and the intraosseous technique (IO). If complementary buccal anesthesia has been administered with a potent solution such as A-100, then the same solution should be used in the periodontal ligament or IO technique so as not to mix two different anesthetics at the same site.

## References

Aggarwal, V., Singla, M., Miglani, S. et al. (2011a). A prospective, randomized, single-blind comparative evaluation of anesthetic efficacy of posterior superior alveolar nerve blocks, buccal infiltration, and buccal plus palatal infiltrations in patients with irreversible pulpitis. *J. Endod.* 37 (11): 1491–1494.

Aggarwal, V., Singla, M., Rizvi, A., and Miglani, S. (2011b). Comparative evaluation of local infiltration of articaine, articaine plus ketorolac, and dexamethasone on anesthetic efficacy of inferior alveolar nerve block with lidocaine in patients with irreversible pulpitis. *J. Endod.* 37 (4): 445–449.

Aggarwal, V., Singla, M., Subbiya, A. et al. (2015). Effect of preoperative pain on inferior alveolar nerve block. *Anesth. Prog.* 62 (4): 135–139.

Annex 21. Maxillary pulpal anesthesia: buccal infiltration.

Annex 23. Pain resulting for injection techniques.

Annex 24. Mandibular block I. Efficay of standard solution L-100 o L-80.

Annex 25. Mandibular block II. Pulpal anesthesia with the standard solution (L-100).

Annex 28. Mandibular block V. Failure of lower lip anesthesia.

Annex 31. Mandibular pulpal anesthesia: infiltrative.

Annex 34. Bifid (double) mandibular canals.

Annex 35. Irreversible acute pulpitis (hot tooth). Efficacy of dental local anesthesia.

Askari, E.M., Parirokh, M., Nakhaee, N. et al. (2016). The effect of maxillary first molar root length on the success rate of buccal infiltration anesthesia. *J. Endod.* 42 (10): 1462–1466.

Barker, B.C.W. (1972a). Multiple canals in the rami of a mandible. *Oral Surg. Oral Med. Oral Pathol.* 34 (3): 384–389.

Barker, B.C.W. and Davies, P.L. (1972b). The applied anatomy of the pterygomandibular space. *Br. J. Oral Surg.* 10 (1): 43–55.

Beckett, H.A. and Gilmour, A.G. (1990). Resistance to local analgesia – report of a case treated using 5% lignocaine solution. *Br. Dent. J.* 169 (10): 327–328.

Bennett, S. and Townsend, G. (2001). Distribution of the mylohyoid nerve: anatomical variability and clinical implications. *Aust. Endod. J.* 27 (3): 109–111.

Berggren, U. and Meynert, G. (1984). Dental fear and avoidance: causes, symptoms, and consequences. *J. Am. Dent. Assoc.* 109 (2): 247–251.

Bieter, R.N. (1936). Applied pharmacological of local anesthetics. *Am. J. Surg.* 34 (3): 500–510.

Bogdan, S., Pataky, L., Barabas, J. et al. (2006). Atypical course of the mandibular canal: comparative examination of dry mandibles and X-rays. *J. Craniofac. Surg.* 17 (3): 487–491.

Bowles, W.R., Withrow, J.C., Lepinski, A.M., and Hargreaves, K.M. (2003). Tissues levels of immunoreactive substance P are increased in patients with irreversible pulpitis. *J. Endod.* 29 (4): 265–267.

Bremer, G. (1952). Measurements of special significance in connection with anesthesia of the inferior alveolar nerve. *Oral Surg. Oral Med. Oral Pathol.* 5 (9): 966–988.

Brown, R.D. (1981). The failure of local anaesthesia in acute inflammation. Some recent concepts. *Br. Dent. J.* 151 (2): 47–51.

Byers, M.R., Taylor, P.E., Khayat, B.G., and Kimberly, C.L. (1990). Effects of injury and inflammation on pulpal and periapical nerves. *J. Endod.* 16 (2): 78–84.

Carter, R.B. and Keen, E.N. (1971). The intramandibular course of the inferior alveolar nerve. *J. Anat.* 108 (3): 433–440.

Caviedes-Bucheli, J., Lombana, N., Azuero-Holguin, M.M., and Munoz, H.R. (2006). Quantification of neuropeptides (calcitonin gene-related peptide, substance P, neurokinin A, neuropeptide Y and vasoactive intestinal polypeptide) expressed in healthy and inflamed human pulp. *Int. Endod. J.* 39 (5): 394–400.

Chapnick, L. (1980). A foramen on the lingual of the mandible. *J. Can. Dent. Assoc.* 46 (7): 444–445.

Chavez-Lomeli, M.E., Lory, J.M., Pompa, J.A., and Kjaer, I. (1996). The human mandibular canal arises from three separate canals innervating different tooth groups. *J. Dent. Res.* 75 (8): 1540–1544.

Chemical Dependency and Dental Practice (1987). Council on Dental Practice. *J. Am. Dent. Assoc.* 114 (4): 509–515.

Chompu-inwai, P., Simprasert, S., Chuveera, P. et al. (2018). Effect of nitrous oxide on pulpal anesthesia: a preliminary study. *Anesth. Prog.* 65 (3): 156–161.

Clendenen, N., Cannon, A.D., Porter, S. et al. (2016). Whole-exome sequencing of a family with local anesthetic resistance. *Minerva Anesthesiol.* 82 (10): 1089–1097.

Cohen, H.P., Cha, B.Y., and Spangberg, L.S.W. (1993). Endodontic anesthesia in mandibular molars: a clinical study. *J. Endod.* 19 (7): 370–373.

Coleman, R.D. and Smith, R.A. (1982). The anatomy of mandibular anesthesia: review and analysis. *Oral Surg. Oral Med. Oral Pathol.* 54 (2): 148–153.

Cook, W.A. (1949). The nerve supply to the maxillary incisors. *J. Oral Surg. (Chicago)* 7 (2): 149–154.

Cook, W.A. (1951). The cervical plexus and its probable role in the oral operator's field. *Dent. Items Interest* 73 (4): 356–361.

Correr, G.M., Iwanko, D., Leonardi, D.P. et al. (2013). Classification of bifid mandibular canals using cone beam computed tomography. *Braz. Oral Res.* 27 (6): 510–516.

De Geus, J.L., da Costa, J.K.N., Wambier, L.M. et al. (2020). Different anesthetics on the efficacy of inferior alveolar nerve block in patients with irreversible pulpitis. A network systemic review and meta-analysis. *J. Am. Dent. Assoc.* 151 (2): 87–97.

De Jong, R.H. (1977). *Local Anesthetics*, 2e. Springfield (Il): Charles C Thomas Publisher. 43–44, 57–59.

De Jong, R.H. and Cullen, S.C. (1963). Buffer-demand and pH of local anesthetic solutions containing epinephrine. *Anesthesiology* 24 (6): 801807.

Dreven, L.J., Reader, A., Beck, M. et al. (1987). An evaluation of an electric pulp tester as a measure of analgesia in human vital teeth. *J. Endod.* 13 (5): 233–238.

Evers, H. and Haegerstam, G. (1981). *Handbook of Dental Local Anesthesia*. Copenhagen: Schultz Medical International. 104.

Fan, S., Chen, W.-L., Pan, C.-B. et al. (2009). Anesthetic efficacy of inferior alveolar nerve block plus buccal infiltration or periodontal ligament injections with articaine in patients with irreversible pulpitis in the mandibular first molar. *Oral Surg. Oral Med. Oral Pathol.* 108 (5): e89–e93.

Fiset, L., Leroux, B., Rothen, M. et al. (1997). Pain control in recovering alcoholics: effects of local anesthesia. *J. Stud. Alcohol* 58 (3): 291–296.

FitzGerald, M.J.T. and Scott, J.H. (1958). Observations on the anatomy of the superior dental nerves. *Br. Dent. J.* 104 (6): 205–208.

Frommer, J., Mele, F.A., and Monroe, C.W. (1972). The possible role of the mylohyoid nerve in mandibular posterior tooth sensation. *J. Am. Dent. Assoc.* 85 (1): 113–117.

Fullmer, S., Drum, M., Reader, A. et al. (2014). Effect of preoperative acetaminophen/hydrocodone on the efficacy of the inferior alveolar nerve block in patients with symptomatic irreversible pulpitis: a prospective, randomized, double-blind, placebo-controlled study. *J. Endod.* 40 (1): 1–5.

Garg, A. and Townsend, G. (2001). Anatomical variation of the sphenomandibular ligament. *Aust. Endod. J.* 27 (1): 22–24.

Gazal, G. (2015). Comparison of speed of action and injection discomfort of 4% articaine and 2% mepivacaine for pulpal anesthesia in mandibular teeth: a randomized, double-blind cross-over trial. *Eur. J. Dent.* 9 (2): 201–206.

Grover, P.J. and Lorton, L. (1983). Bifid mandibular nerve as a possible cause of inadequate anesthesia in the mandible. *J. Oral Maxillofac. Surg.* 41 (3): 177–179.

Guglielmo, A., Drum, M., Reader, A., and Nusstein, J. (2011). Anesthetic efficacy of a combination palatal and buccal infiltration of the maxillary first molar. *J. Endod.* 37 (4): 460–462.

Haas, D.A. (2011). Alternative mandibular nerve block techniques. A review of the Gow-Gates and Akinosi-Vazirani closed-mouth mandibular nerve block techniques. *J. Am. Dent. Assoc.* 142 (9 Suppl): 8s–12s.

Haase, A., Reader, A., Nusstein, J. et al. (2008). Comparing anesthetic efficacy of articaine versus lidocaine as a supplemental buccal infiltration on the mandibular first molar after an inferior alveolar nerve. *J. Am. Dent. Assoc.* 139 (9): 1228–1235.

Haglund, J. and Evers, H. (1985). *Local Anaesthesia in Dentistry*, 6e. Södertäleje (Sweden): Astra Läkemedel AB. 37.

Haveman, C.W. and Tebo, H.G. (1976). Posterior accessory foramina of the human mandible. *J. Prosth. Dent.* 35 (4): 462–468.

Hersh, E.V., Hermann, D.G., Lamp, C.J. et al. (1995). Assessing the duration of mandibular soft tissue anesthesia. *J. Am. Dent. Assoc.* 126 (11): 1531–1536.

Hofer, O. (1922). Die Leitungsanästhesie des nervus nasopalatinus Scarpae bei stomatologischen eingriffen. *Z. Stomatol.* 20: 411–416.

Jastak, J.T., Yagiela, J.A., and Donaldson, D. (1995). *Local Anesthesia of the Oral Cavity*. Philadelphia: WB Saunders Co. 203, 284.

Jeffries, C.N. (1944). The inferior alveolar injection for fillings. *Br. Dent. J.* 77: 153–159.

Kanaa, M.D., Whitworth, J.M., Corbett, I.P., and Meechan, J.G. (2009). Articaine buccal infiltration enhances the effectiveness of lidocaine inferior alveolar nerve block. *Int. Endod. J.* 42 (3): 238–246.

Kaufman, E., Weinstein, P., and Milgrom, P. (1984). Difficulties in achieving local anesthesia. *J. Am. Dent. Assoc.* 108 (2): 205–208.

Kavlock, R. and Ting, P.H. (2004). Local anesthetic in a pregnant patient with lumbosacral plexopathy. *BMC Anesthesiol.* 4: 1.

Kay, L.W. (1974). Some anthropologic investigations of interest to oral surgeons. *Int. J. Oral Surg.* 3 (6): 363–379.

Keetley, A. and Moles, D.R. (2001). A clinical audit into the success rate of inferior alveolar nerve block analgesia in general dental practice. *Prim. Dent. Care* 8 (4): 139–142.

Khedari, A.J. (1982). Alternative to mandibular block injections through intraligamental anesthesia. *Quintessence Int.* 13 (2): 231–237.

Khoury, J.N., Mihailidis, S., Ghabriel, M., and Townsed, G. (2010). Anatomical relationship within the human pterygomandibular space: relevance to local anesthesia. *Clin. Anat.* 23 (8): 936–944.

Khoury, J.N., Mihailidis, S., Ghabriel, M., and Townsed, G. (2011). Applied anatomy of the pterygomandibular space: improving the success of inferior alveolar nerve blocks. *Aust. Dent. J.* 56 (2): 112–121.

Kiersch, T.A. and Jordan, J.E. (1973). Duplication of the mandibular canal. *Oral Surg. Oral Med. Oral Pathol.* 35 (1): 133–134.

Kimberly, C.L. and Byers, M.R. (1988). Inflammation of rat molar pulp and periodontium causes increased calcitonin gene-related peptide and axonal sprouting. *Anat. Rec.* 222 (3): 289–300.

Kleinknecht, R.A., Keplac, R.K., and Alexander, L.D. (1973). Origins and characteristics of fear of dentistry. *J. Am. Dent. Assoc.* 86 (4): 842–848.

Kramer, H.S. and Mitton, V.A. (1973). Complications of local anesthesia. *Dent. Clin. N. Am.* 17 (3): 443–460.

Kreimer, T., Kiser, R., Reader, A. et al. (2012). Anesthetic efficacy of combinations of 0.5 mol/L mannitol and lidocaine with epinephrine for inferior alveolar nerve blocks in patients with symptomatic irreversible pulpitis. *J. Endod.* 38 (5): 598–603.

Kung, J., McDonagh, M., and Sedgley, C.M. (2015). Does articaine provide an advantage over lidocaine in patients with symptomatic irreversible pulpitis? A systematic review and meta-analysis. *J. Endod.* 41 (11): 1784–1794.

Lai, J., Porreca, F., Hunter, J.C., and Gold, M.S. (2004). Voltage-gated sodium channels and hyperalgesia. *Annu. Rev. Pharmacol. Toxicol.* 44: 371–397.

Langlais, R.P., Broadus, R., and Glass, B.J. (1985). Bifid mandibular canals in panoramic radiographs. *J. Am. Dent. Assoc.* 110 (6): 923–926.

Li, C., Yang, X., Ma, X. et al. (2012). Preoperative oral nonsteroidal anti-inflammatory drugs for the success of the inferior alveolar nerve block in irreversible pulpitis treatment: a systematic review and meta-analysis based on randomized controlled trials. *Quintessence Int.* 43 (3): 209–219.

Lin, K., Feldman, D.U., and Barbe, M.F. (2013). Transverse cervical nerve: implications for dental anesthesia. *Clin. Anat.* 26 (6): 688–692.

Lindroth, J.E., Herren, M.C., and Falace, D.A. (2003). The management of acute dental pain in the recovering alcoholic. *Oral Surg. Oral Med. Oral Pathol.* 95 (4): 432–436.

Löfgren, A. (1957). Foramina retromolaria mandibulae. A study on human skulls of nutrient foramina situated in the mandibular retromolar fossa. *Odontol. Tidskr.* 65: 552–573.

Luo, S., Perry, G.M., Levinson, S.R., and Henry, M.A. (2008). $Na_v$ 1.7 expression is increased in painful human pulp. *Mol. Pain* 4: 16–29.

Madeira, M.C., Percinoto, C., and Silva, M.C. (1978). Clinical significance of supplementary innervations of the lower incisor teeth: a dissection study of the mylohyoid nerve. *Oral Surg. Oral Med. Oral Pathol.* 46 (5): 608–614.

Maggirias, J. and Locker, D. (2002). Psychological factors and perception of pain associated with dental treatment. *Commun. Dent. Oral Epidemiol.* 30 (2): 151–159.

McCartney, M., Reader, A., and Beck, M. (2007). Injection pain of the inferior alveolar nerve block in patients with irreversible pulpitis. *Oral Surg. Oral Med. Oral Pathol.* 104 (4): 571–575.

Meechan, J.G. (1999). How to overcome failed local anaesthesia. *Br. Dent. J.* 186 (1): 15–20.

Miller, G.L., Scurlock, J.E., Covino, B.G. et al. (1981). Letters to the editor. *Reg. Anesth.* 6 (3): 122–125.

Mizbah, K., Gerlach, N., Maal, T.J. et al. (2012). The clinical relevance of bifid and trifid mandibular canals. *Oral Maxillofac. Surg.* 16 (1): 147–151.

Modaresi, J., Dianat, O., and Mozayeni, M.A. (2006). The efficacy comparison of ibuprofen, acetaminophen-codeine, and placebo premedication therapy on the depth of anesthesia during treatment of inflamed teeth. *Oral Surg. Oral Med. Oral Pathol.* 102 (3): 399–403.

Molin, C. and Seeman, K. (1970). Disproportionate dental anxiety. Clinical and nosological considerations. *Acta Odontol. Scand.* 28 (2): 197–212.

Najjar, T.A. (1977). Why can't you achieve adequate regional anesthesia in the presence of infection? *Oral Surg. Oral Med. Oral Pathol.* 44 (1): 7–13.

Neves, F.S., Nascimiento, M.C.C., Oliveira, M.L. et al. (2013). Comparative analysis of mandibular anatomical variations between panoramic radiograph and cone beam computed tomography. *Oral Maxillofac. Surg.* 18 (4): 419–424.

Nortjé, C.J., Farman, A.G., and de V Joubert, J.J. (1977). The radiographic appearance of the inferior dental canal: an additional variation. *Br. J. Oral Surg.* 15 (2): 171–172.

Novitzky, J. (1938). Sensory nerves and anesthesia of the teeth and jaws. *Mod. Dent.* 5 (1): 5–10.

Nusstein, J., Reader, A., Nist, R. et al. (1998). Anesthetic efficacy of the supplemental intraosseous injection of 2% lidocaine with 1:100 000 epinephrine in irreversible pulpitis. *J. Endod.* 24 (7): 487–491.

Nusstein, J., Kennedy, S., Reader, A. et al. (2003). Anesthetic efficacy of the supplemental X-Tip intraosseous injection in patients with irreversible pulpitis. *J. Endod.* 29 (11): 724–728.

Olivier, E.L. (1927). Canal dentaire inferiéur et son nerf chez l'adulte. *Ann. Anat. Path. Anat. Norm. Med-Chir. (Paris)* 4 (9): 975–987.

Olsen, N.H., Teuscher, G.W., and Vehe, K.L. (1955). A study of the nerve supply to the upper anterior teeth. *J. Dent. Res.* 34 (3): 413–420.

Ossenberg, N.S. (1986). Temporal crest canal: case report and statistics on a rare mandibular variant. *Oral Surg. Oral Med. Oral Pathol.* 62 (1): 10–12.

Panigel, J. and Cook, S.P. (2011). A point mutation at F1737 of the human $Na_v$ 1.7 sodium channel decreases inhibition by local anesthetics. *J. Neurogenet.* 25 (4): 134–139.

Patterson, J.E. and Funke, F.W. (1973). Bifid inferior alveolar canal. *Oral Surg. Oral Med. Oral Pathol.* 36 (2): 287–288.

Phillips, W.H. (1943). Anatomic considerations in local anesthesia in dental surgery. *Anesth. Analg.* 22 (1): 5–14.

Phillips, W.H. and Maxmen, H.A. (1941). The nasopalatine block injection as an aid in operative procedures for maxillary incisors. *Am. J. Orthod. Oral Surg.* 27 (8): 426–434.

Pinkham, J.R. and Schroeder, C.S. (1975). Dentist and psychologist: practical consideration for team approach to the intensely anxious dental patient. *J. Am. Dent. Assoc.* 90 (5): 1022–1026.

Pogrel, M.A., Smith, R., and Ahani, R. (1997). Innervation of the madibular incisors by the mental nerve. *J. Oral Maxillofac. Surg.* 55 (9): 961–963.

Reisman, D., Reader, A., Nist, R. et al. (1997). Anesthetic efficacy of supplemental intraosseous injection of 3% mepivacaine in irreversible pulpitis. *Oral Surg. Oral Med. Oral Pathol.* 84 (6): 676–682.

Renton, T., Yiangour, Y., Plumpton, C. et al. (2005). Sodium channel $Na_v$ 1.8 immunoreactivity in painful human dental pulp. *BMC Oral Heath* 5: 5.

Rizzolo, R.J.C., Madeira, M.C., Bernaba, J.M., and de Freitas, V. (1988). Clinical significance of the supplementary innervation of the mandibular teeth: a dissection study of the transverse cervical (cutaneous colli) nerve. *Quintessence Int.* 19 (2): 167–169.

Roberts, G.D. and Harris, M. (1973). Neuropraxia of the mylohyoid nerve and submental analgesia. *Br. J. Oral Surg.* 11 (2): 110–113.

Roberts, D.H. and Sowray, J.H. (1987). *Local Analgesia in Dentistry*, 3e. Bristol (UK): Wright. 84–85.

Roda, R.S. and Blanton, P.L. (1994). The anatomy of local anesthesia. *Quintessence Int.* 25 (1): 27–38.

Rood, J.P. (1976). The analgesia and innervation of the mandibular teeth. *Br. Dent. J.* 140 (7): 237–238.

Rood, J.P. (1977). Some anatomical and physiological causes of failure to achieve mandibular analgesia. *Br. J. Oral Surg.* 15 (1): 75–82.

Rood, J.P. and Pateromichelakis, S. (1981). Inflammation and peripheral nerve sensitization. *Br. J. Oral Surg.* 19 (1): 67–72.

Rood, J.P. and Sowray, J.H. (1980). Clinical experience with 5 per cent lignocaine solution. *J. Dent.* 8 (2): 128–131.

Saatchi, M., Shafiee, M., Khademi, A., and Memarzadeh, B. (2018). Anesthetic efficacy of Gow-Gates nerve block, inferior alveolar nerve block, and their combination in mandibular molars with symptomatic irreversible pulpitis: a prospective, randomized clinical trial. *J. Endod.* 44 (3): 384–388.

Schade, H., Neukrich, P., and Halpert, A. (1921). Ueber lokale Acidose des Gewebes und die Methodik ihner intravitalen Messung, zugleich ein Beitrag zur Lehre der Entzündung. *Z. Gesamte Exp. Med. (Berlin)* 24: 11–56.

Schejtman, R., Devoto, F.C.H., and Arias, N.H. (1967). The origin and distribution of the elements of the human mandibular retromolar canal. *Arch. Oral Biol.* 12 (11): 1261–1267.

Scheutz, F. (1982). Drug addicts and local anesthesia – effectivity and general side effects. *Scand. J. Dent. Res.* 90 (4): 299–305.

Scholz, A., Kuboyama, N., Hempelmann, G., and Vogel, W. (1998). Complex blockade of TTX-resistant $Na^+$ currents by lidocaine and bupivacaine reduce firing frequency in DRG neurons. *J. Neurophysiol.* 79 (4): 1746–1754.

Schumacher, S. (1904). Der Nervus mylohyoideus des Menschen und der Säugetiere. *Kais Akad. Wiss. Wien.* 113: 241–275.

Shiller, W.R. and Wiswell, O.B. (1954). Lingual foramina of the mandible. *Anat. Rec.* 119 (3): 387–390.

Shiozaki, H., Abe, S., Tsumori, N. et al. (2007). Macroscopic anatomy of the sphenomandibular ligament related to the inferior alveolar nerve block. *Cranio* 25 (3): 160–165.

Shirvani, A., Shamszadeh, S., Eghbal, M.J. et al. (2017). Effect of preoperative oral analgesics on pulpal anesthesia in patients with irreversible pulpitis – a systematic review and metaanalysis. *Clin. Oral Invest.* 21 (1): 43–52.

Sicher, H. (1946). The anatomy of the mandibular anesthesia. *J. Am. Dent. Assoc.* 33 (23): 1541–1557.

Sicher, H. (1950). Aspects in the applied anatomy of local anesthesia. *Int. Dent. J.* 1 (1): 70–82.

Simonds, E., Iwanaga, J., Oskouian, R.J., and Tubbs. R.S. (2017). Dupilcation of the sphenomandibular ligament. *Cureus* 9 (10): e1783.

Singh, S. (1981). Aberrant buccal nerve encountered at third molar surgery. *Oral Surg. Oral Med. Oral Pathol.* 52 (2): 142.

Sokol, D.J., Sokol, S., and Sokol, C.K. (1985). A review of nonintrusive therapies used to deal with anxiety and pain in the dental office. *J. Am. Dent. Assoc.* 110 (2): 217–222.

Sorensen, H.J., Skidmore, L.J., Rzasa, R.S. et al. (2004). Comparison of pulp sodium channel density in normal teeth to diseased teeth with severe spontaneous pain. *J. Endod.* 30 (4): 287. (abstract no. PR 55).

Starkie, C. and Stewart, D. (1931). The intra-mandibular course of the inferior dental nerve. *J. Anat.* 65 (Pt 3): 319–323.

Stein, P., Brueckner, J., and Milliner, M. (2007). Sensory innervations of mandibular teeth by the nerve to the mylohyoid: implications in local anesthesia. *Clin. Anat.* 20 (6): 591–595.

Stewart, D. (1932). The innervations of the dental tissues and its importance in regional anaesthesia. *Br. Dent. J.* 53 (6): 277–284.

Stewart, S.H. and Finn, P.R. (1995). A dose-response study of the effects of alcohol on the perceptions of pain and discomfort due to electric shock in men at high familial-genetic risk of alcoholism. *Psychopharmacology (Berlin)* 119 (3): 261–267.

Stewart, D. and Wilson, S.L. (1928). Regional anaesthesia and innervations of the teeth. *Lancet* 212 (5486): 809–811.

Su, N., Li, C., Wang, H. et al. (2016). Efficacy and safety of articaine versus lidocaine for irreversible pulpitis treatment: a systematic review and meta-analysis of randomized controlled trials. *Aust. Dent. J.* 42 (1): 4–15.

Sutton, R.N. (1974). The practical significance of mandibular accessory foramina. *Aust. Dent. J.* 19 (3): 167–173.

Taylor, P.E. and Byers, M.R. (1990). An immunocytochemical study of the morphological reaction of nerves containing calcitonin gene-related peptide to microabscess formation and healing in rat molars. *Arch. Oral Biol.* 35 (8): 629–638.

Tortamano, I.P., Siviero, M., Costa, C.G. et al. (2009). A comparison of the anesthetic efficacy of articaine and lidocaine in patients with irreversible pulpitis. *J. Endod.* 35 (2): 165–168.

Traeger, K.A. (1979). Hematoma following inferior alveolar injection: a possible cause for anesthetic failure. *Anesth. Prog.* 26 (5): 122–123.

Turner, M.B. (1864). LXXIII. On some variations in the arrangement of the nerves of the human body. *Nat. Hist. Rev.* 4: 612–617.

Ulusoy, Ö.I.A. and Alacam, T. (2014). Efficacy of single buccal infiltrations for maxillary first molars in patients with irreversible pulpitis: a randomized controlled trial. *Int. Endod. J.* 47 (3): 222–227.

Van Wijk, A.J. and Makkes, P.C. (2008). Highly anxious dental patients report more pain during dental injections. *Br. Dent. J.* 205 (3): 142–143.

Wallace, J.A., Michanowicz, A.E., Mundell, R.D., and Wilson, E.G. (1985). Pilot study of the clinical problem of regionally anesthetizing the pulp of an acutely inflamed mandibular molar. *Oral Surg. Oral Med. Oral Pathol.* 59 (5): 517–521.

Walton, R.E. and Abbott, B.J. (1981). Periodontal ligament injection: a clinical evaluation. *J. Am. Dent. Assoc.* 103 (4): 571–575.

Walton, R.E. and Torabinejad, M. (1992). Managing local anesthesia problems in the endodontic patient. *J. Am. Dent. Assoc.* 123 (5): 97–102.

Warren, C.A., Mok, L., Gordon, S. et al. (2008). Quantification of neural protein in extirpated tooth pulp. *J. Endod.* 34 (1): 7–10.

Wells, J.E., Bingham, V., Rowland, K.C., and Hatton, J. (2007). Expression of Nav1.9 channels in human dental pulp and trigeminal ganglion. *J. Endod.* 33 (10): 1172–1176.

Wepman, B.J. (1978). Psychological components of pain perception. *Dent. Clin. N. Am.* 22 (1): 101–113.

Westwater, L.A. (1960). The innervation of the pulps of the teeth. *Br. Dent. J.* 109 (10): 407–410.

Wildsmith, J.A.W. (1986). Peripheral nerve and local anesthetic drugs. *Br. J. Anaesth.* 58 (7): 692–700.

Wilson, S., Johns, P., and Fuller, P.M. (1984). The inferior alveolar and mylohyoid nerves: an anatomical study and relationship to local anesthesia of the anterior mandibular teeth. *J. Am. Dent. Assoc.* 108 (3): 350–352.

Wong, M. and Jacobsen, P.L. (1992). Reasons for local anesthesia failure. *J. Am. Dent. Assoc.* 123 (1): 69–73.

Woolgrove, J. (1983). Pain perception and patient management. *Br. Dent. J.* 154 (8): 243–246.

Yonchak, T., Reader, A., Beck, M., and Meyers, W.J. (2001). Anesthetic efficacy of unilateral and bilateral inferior alveolar nerve blocks to determine cross innervations in anterior teeth. *Oral Surg. Oral Med. Oral Pathol.* 92 (2): 132–135.

Zhang, Y.Q., Yan, X.B., Zhang, L.Q. et al. (2019). Prevalence and morphology of mandibular incisive canal: comparison among healthy, periodontitis and edentulous mandibles in a population of the Beijing area using cone beam computed tomography. *Chin. J. Dent. Res.* 22 (4): 241–249.

# 20

# Alternatives to Conventional Techniques

In this chapter, we review four types of technique that can be used instead of the traditional methods discussed so far, although, as we will see, some of these methods yield poorer results. Nevertheless, they do have a series of advantages. The methods we review are the following:

- Jet injection.
- Electronic dental anesthesia.
- Computer-controlled injection systems.
- Intranasal maxillary local anesthesia (Kovanaze®).

## Jet Injection

This alternative injection technique is based on injecting the local anesthetic solution *without a needle*. The solution is propelled at speed in a fine, high-pressure jet in such a way that it crosses the oral mucosa to reach the subcutaneous tissue *painlessly*; this is why it is also known as high-pressure jet injection.

This technique arose from a workplace accident. Fuel oil under pressure accidentally penetrated the fingers of a diesel mechanic. The oil passed deep under the skin, leading to the loss of fingers owing to its toxic effect. However, the liquid did not hurt when it penetrated the skin (Figge and Scherer 1947; Stephens and Kramer 1964).

Marshall Lockhart is said to have patented the first high-speed jet injection machine in 1936 (Warren et al. 1955; Bennett et al. 1971). However, it was first used in cadavers by Figge and Scherer (1947). In the same year, it was applied in clinical practice for the injection of procaine with epinephrine into the skin (Hingson and Hughes 1947). In 1958, Margetis used it for the first time to administer local dental anesthetic (Margetis et al. 1958). The device in all these cases was the Hypospray (Stephens and Kramer 1964; Schmidt 1966), which was first introduced in 1947 (Kutscher and Zegarelli 1965). Hypospray was followed by many other commercial devices (Annex 33), of which the most widely used today are Syrijet® and Injex®.

### Distribution of the Solution

Distribution of the solution has been studied in cadavers (Figge and Scherer 1947; Kramer 1962; Whitehead and Young 1968), rats (Bennett et al. 1971; Ikehara et al. 1972; ElGeneidy et al. 1974), and dogs (Bell et al. 1971). Once discharged, the local anesthetic solution crosses the mucosa and tends to spread through the connective tissue laterally in parallel to the mucosa (Kramer 1962; Stephens and Kramer 1964; Bennett et al. 1971) and manages to cover 10–40 mm in 90% of cases (Whitehead and Young 1968). The amplitude also depends on the area of discharge (Garellek 1967), in such a way that it can reach 15 mm in the buccal, 10 mm in the palate, and only 5 mm in the mandibular sulcus.

The entry wound is round or slightly irregular, with a diameter similar to that of the needle as it enters tissue (Stephens and Kramer 1964). The solution enters the area of least resistance and therefore penetrates better in looser connective tissue (Bell et al. 1971; Bennett et al. 1971; ElGeneidy et al. 1974). However, it does not penetrate or does so slightly in barrier structures such as bone, periosteum, nerve stem, vessels, salivary glands, and muscle (Stephens and Kramer 1964; Kutscher and Zegarelli 1965; Bennett et al. 1971; Epstein 1971; ElGeneidy et al. 1974). When it penetrates the muscles, it does so across fascial planes but not within the muscle structure (Bennett et al. 1971).

Deep penetration depends on the following: (i) the discharge area – penetration is 5 mm in the buccal and 10–15 in the mandibular sulcus (Garellek 1967; Bennett et al. 1971 oral); and (ii) the quantity injected – penetration is 5 mm with 0.05 ml and 15 mm with 0.2 ml (Bennett et al. 1971).

Microlesions may remain after discharge (Stephens and Kramer 1964) with subcutaneous edema, separation of collagen fibers (Ikehara et al. 1972), and inflammatory reaction (ElGeneidy et al. 1974), which differ little from the microlesions caused by a needle. Furthermore, while the

*Local Anesthesia in Dentistry: A Locoregional Approach*, First Edition. Jesús Calatayud and Mana Saraghi.
© 2024 John Wiley & Sons Ltd. Published 2024 by John Wiley & Sons Ltd.
Companion website: www.wiley.com/go/Calatayud/local

most concentrated anesthetic solutions (5% vs 2%) increase the frequency of tissue lesions (Bennett et al. 1971), they also enhance clinical outcomes (Lambrianidis et al. 1979–1980).

When we compare high-pressure jet injection with conventional injection, we see that a needle makes it possible to place the anesthetic solution at the required depth and to administer the required quantity of solution at this level in such a way that it leaves a deposit (Stephens and Kramer 1964). However, with jet injection, we can see how it loses strength from the moment it crosses the mucosa and cannot reach very deep areas. In addition, the solution penetrates deeper, therefore a smaller quantity of anesthetic is administered (Stephens and Kramer 1964; Epstein 1971). Since it is injected suddenly, it mixes more with tissues without leaving a deposit from which it can then spread out (Bell et al. 1971). The microlesions produced by both systems are similar (Stephens and Kramer 1964; Ikehara et al. 1972; ElGeneidy et al. 1974).

### Indications

As we have seen, this technique does not ensure deep anesthesia because the solution does not penetrate deeply into the tissue or, if it does, it delivers a small quantity of anesthetic. It can therefore prove useful in the following situations:

1) As topical anesthetic it is very useful (Kutscher and Zegarelli 1965; Garellek 1967; Bennett and Monheim 1971; Epstein 1971; Boj 1992), especially in the palate (Stephens and Kramer 1964) since it can be injected using the conventional technique after a minute (Kutscher et al. 1964).
2) For supra- and sub-gingival anesthesia during scaling and root planning procedures, respectively. (Kutscher and Zegarelli 1965; Epstein 1971).
3) Placement of rubber dam clamps, especially if subgingival clamp placement is necessary for appropriate isolation of the teeth (Garellek 1967; Epstein 1971; Boj 1992; Arapostathis et al. 2010).
4) Simple surgical techniques such as extraction of mobile primary teeth (Saravia and Bush 1991; Boj 1992), lancing fluctuant abscesses (Garellek 1967; Epstein 1971), gingivectomy limited to one tooth (Epstein 1971), excision of small lesions such as papillomas and fibromas (Greenfield and Karpinski 1972), removal of bone spurs, etc.
5) Placement and removal of fixed orthodontic devices that can irritate the gingival (Epstein 1971; Greenfield and Karpinski 1972), such as fixed space maintainers, bands, orthodontic arches and ligature ties, subgingival matrix bands, etc.

### Disadvantages

The technique has various disadvantages owing to the characteristics of distribution of local anesthetic solution (see above):

1) *Insufficient depth of anesthesia* to ensure pulpal anesthesia (Dabarakis et al. 2007): Björn used an electric pulp tester to show that pulpal anesthesia is achieved in 13% of cases (Lethinen 1979). Anesthesia of deeper tissues is also poorer, therefore it yields poorer results in surgical techniques, extractions (Kutscher and Zegarelli 1965; Saravia and Bush 1991; Boj 1992; Arapostathis et al. 2010), endodontics, pulpotomy (Epstein 1971; Boj 1992), crown cutting and bridges in vital teeth (Kutscher and Zegarelli 1965), obturations in permanent teeth (Epstein 1971; Saravia and Bush 1991; Boj 1992) and primary teeth – although there may be some success in the latter (Saravia and Bush 1991; Boj 1992; Grau et al. 1997; Miegimolle et al. 2005; Arapostathis et al. 2010) – and mandibular block (Stephens and Kramer 1964; Bennett and Monheim 1971; Boj 1992).
2) Cost, since many of the devices used are very expensive.

### Advantages

The advantages to this technique can be summarized as follows:

1) The absence of a needle means could be a very positive attribute for those patients who fear needles, therefore it could prove very useful in children and fearful adults (Stephens 1962; Stephens and Kramer 1964; Greenfield and Karpinski 1972, Miegimolle et al. 2005).
2) When this technique can be used, patients prefer it to conventional techniques in 75% of cases (Table 20.1).
3) Injection is not painful in 85% of cases (Table 20.1).
4) The risk of transmission of blood-borne pathogens to the provider or dental assistant is reduced because there are no sharps or infectious waste.

### Equipment

Annex 33 discusses the main devices used in dentistry. The main ones are Syrijet® (designed exclusively for dentistry) and Injex®, which is the smallest. We comment on both devices below.

#### Syrijet®

This device was introduced in 1971 (Annex 33) and is still in use (Figure 20.1). It can be purchased online. As it is specially designed for dentistry, it has no anesthetic solution deposit, but uses 1.8-ml dental cartridges. The nozzle

Table 20.1 Percentage of patients who do not feel pain, prefer the *pressure jet injection technique*, and have hematoma at the injection site in various clinical trials.

| Study data | | | Variables analyzed | | |
|---|---|---|---|---|---|
| Reference | Device | Patients | No pain | Preference | Hematoma |
| Hingson and Hughes (1947) | Hypospray | Children/adults | 94% | — | — |
| Margetis et al. (1958) | Hypospray | Children/adults | 100% | — | 72% |
| Kutscher et al. (1964) | Hypospray | Children/adults | 100% | — | — |
| Kutscher and Zegarelli (1965) | Hypospray | Children/adults | — | — | 42% |
| Schmidt (1966) | Hypospray | Children | 95% | 81% | 10% |
| Whitehead and Young (1968) | Panjet | Children/adults | 84% | 78% | 81% |
| Bennett and Monheim (1971) | Syrijet® | Children/adults | — | 90% | 1.5% |
| Lambrianidis et al. (1979–1980) | Panjet | Children/adults | 98% | 98% | 10% |
| Saravia and Bush (1991) | Syrijet® | Children/adults | — | 73% | — |
| Grau et al. (1997) | Syrijet® | Children | 76% | — | 33% |
| Grau et al. (1997) | Syrijet® | Adults | 96% | — | 24% |
| Dabarakis et al. (2007) | Injex® | Adults | — | 18% | 15% |
| Arapostathis et al. (2010) | Injex® | Children | 30% | — | 61% |
| | | Average | 86% | 73% | 35% |
| | | Rounded average | **85%** | **75%** | **35%** |

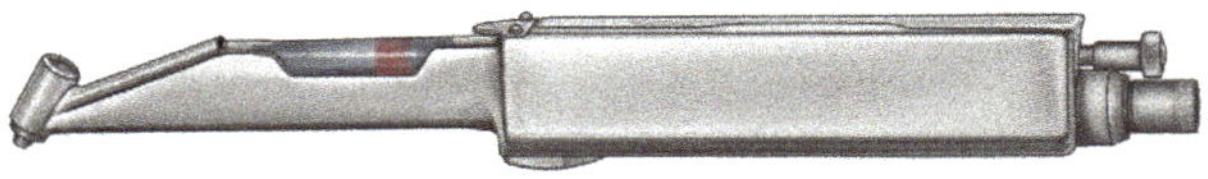

Figure 20.1 Syrijet®: high-speed jet injection system.

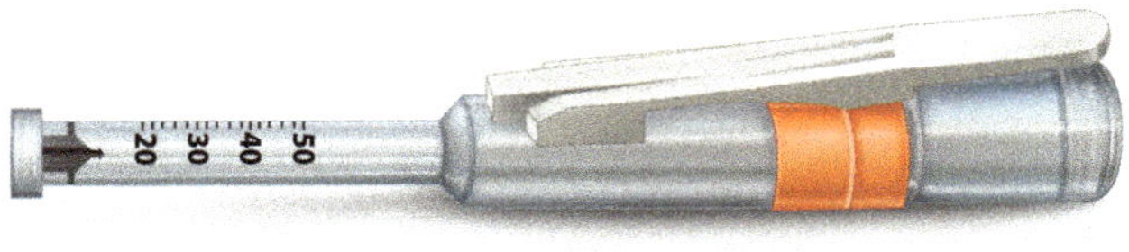

Figure 20.2 Injex®: high-speed jet injection system.

pressure is 2000 pounds per square inch (psi), which is lower than that of other devices designed to cross the skin (Stephens and Kramer 1964). In this case, it is applied to the oral mucosa with little or no damage. The solution can be administered gradually in doses of 0.05 ml, from a minimum of 0.05 ml to a maximum of 0.2 ml (Annex 33).

The head of the device is contra-angled to facilitate access to the different areas of the oral cavity. The nozzle of the jet has a rubber ring that can be adapted to the mucosa so that when the device is discharged, the rubber ring reduces the sensation of pressure (Epstein 1971). The ring is replaceable and can be sterilized. The problem with this device is its size (245 mm long) and weight (550 g) (Annex 33).

### Injex®

Injex® first appeared in 1999 and has the advantage that it is small (only 75 g) (Annex 33) (Figure 20.2). It comes with a fixed ampoule reservoir (0.3 ml), but also has a transporter and adapter that makes it possible to load the reservoir with anesthetic solution in 1.8-ml dental cartridges. The discharge is set at 0.15 ml, and the solution cannot be dosed. It is used only for anterior teeth (maxillary and mandibular) in the buccal area (Arapostathis et al. 2010) since it cannot be adapted to the posterior part of the mouth. Given that the device is used for injection of insulin into the skin, it has a nozzle pressure of 3000 psi (Annex 33).

### Technique

- Preparation of the device for high-pressure jet injection.
  - Syrijet®. A 1.8-ml dental cartridge is loaded. The dose is selected and the spring is activated to discharge.
  - Injex®. The ampoule is loaded with the transporter and the spring is activated to inject with the "reset-box."
- Anesthetic solution. Any dental anesthetic solution can be used; the most common is the standard lidocaine with epinephrine. Epinephrine-free solutions yield poorer results (Dabarakis et al. 2007); those with a higher

concentration of anesthetic achieve better results, although they also lead to greater irritation of tissue (Lambrianidis et al. 1979–1980).

- Preparation of the patient.
  - Show the device to the patient (Lambrianidis et al. 1979–1980; Saravia and Bush 1991; Munshi et al. 2000a).
  - Inform the patient that during the discharge, he/she will hear a sound. We can avoid language with a high emotional content by not using the term "discharge," but rather "jet." Similarly, try to avoid the term "sound," but rather euphemisms, such as "pop" or "click."
  - Advise the patient that he/she should not move during this stage.
- Dry and clean the area where the jet is to be applied (Bennett and Monheim 1971; Greenfield and Karpinsky 1973; Lambrianidis et al. 1979–1980; Saravia and Bush 1991).
- Apply the device to the mucosa.
  - Hold the device so that it does not move during the discharge. Remember that the Syrijet® is fairly heavy (Bennett and Monheim 1971; Greenfield and Karpinsky 1973; Boj 1992).
  - Place the mouth of the device *against the attached mucosa* and rest it on the bone to avoid tearing during the discharge (Greenfield and Karpinsky 1973; Boj 1992) and *at a right angle, perpendicular to the point of discharge* (Margetis et al. 1958; Kutscher and Zegarelli 1965; Bennett and Monheim 1971; Lambrianidis et al. 1979–1980) (Figure 20.3). Remember that it may be difficult to position the Syrijet® device correctly in the areas of the tongue and molars (Arapostathis et al. 2010).
- Discharge.
  - Advise the patient to remain still and inform him/her that the process will only take a second (Stephens and Kramer 1964; Kutscher and Zegarelli 1965; Garellek 1967).
  - The noise of the discharge causes the patient to react with a slight involuntary movement (Kutscher et al. 1964; Whitehead and Young 1968; Epstein 1971). He/she may also feel a slight jolt against the gingiva (Grau et al. 1997; Miegimolle et al. 2005).
  - This maneuver is painless in 85% of cases (Table 20.1).
  - The dose to be injected varies with the site:
    - Palate, 0.1–0.15 ml (Stephens and Kramer 1964; Epstein 1971).
    - Buccal infiltration, 0.15–0.3 ml (Schmidt 1966; Greenfield and Karpinsky 1973; Boj 1992).
- After the discharge:
  - A small mucosal lesion with mild hematoma appears at the site of the discharge. There may sometimes be slight bleeding and mild blanching around the hematoma. Occasionally, we observe slight elevation of the area.
  - Wait 1–3 minutes (Kutscher et al. 1964; Stephens and Kramer 1964; Garellek 1967), sometimes 5 minutes (Lambrianidis et al. 1979–1980) to the onset of anesthesia.
  - It is important to remember that the patient barely notices the soft tissue anesthesia (tingling, dullness, fat lip, etc.) (Stephens and Kramer 1964), although the area of anesthetized soft tissue can vary depending on the site:
    - Palate, 10 mm (Garellek 1967).
    - Buccal area, 10–40 mm (Garellek 1967; Whitehead and Young 1968).
- If anesthesia is insufficient, we have two options:
  1) Discharge more anesthetic, although more discharges and a larger quantity of anesthetic do not generally improve the results (Greenfield and Karpinsky 1973; Boj 1992).
  2) Inject more anesthetic using the conventional technique, with the advantage that the superficial-topical anesthesia prevents the discomfort normally associated with the conventional injection.

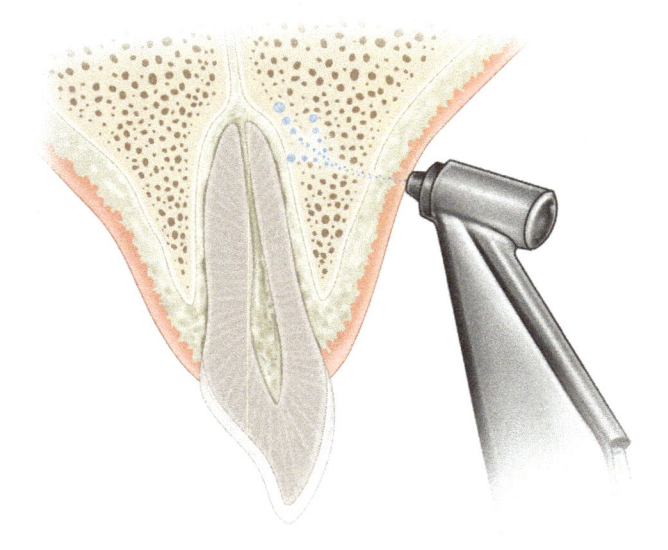

**Figure 20.3** Discharge of Syrijet® with the nozzle of the jet supported against the inserted gingiva. *Source:* Redrawn from Andlaw and Rock (1994).

## Complications of this Technique

1) Bleeding and sometimes hematoma at the injection site in 35% of cases (Table 20.1), especially when several discharges are made at the same site (Greenfield and Karpinski 1972, 1973).

2) Blanching in 90% of cases (Whitehead and Young 1968; Grau et al. 1997). This may be tender on palpation and inflamed (Margetis et al. 1958; Whitehead and Young 1968; Grau et al. 1997), especially when various discharges have been made at the same site (Greenfield and Karpinsky 1973).
3) Laceration (cut in the mucosa) at the discharge site, especially when the patient moves his/her head as the discharge is made (Margetis et al. 1958; Kramer 1962; Stephens and Kramer 1964; Kutscher and Zegarelli 1965; Schmidt 1966; Garellek 1967).
4) Bitter taste is reported if some of the anesthetic solution flows into the patient's mouth. In some series, this occurs in more than 50% of cases (Arapostathis et al. 2010). To reduce the possibility of this complication, it is best to adapt the nozzle of the device to the tissues where the discharge is to be made.
5) The patient may become startled owing to the surprise at the noise of the discharge, especially with Injex®. This occurs in around one-third of cases (Dabarakis et al. 2007).
6) Postoperative pain at the injection site in a small percentage of patients (Dabarakis et al. 2007). This usually resolves spontaneously in a few days.

## Electronic Anesthesia: Electronic Dental Anesthesia

Electronic dental anesthesia (EDA) is a totally different system. We have previously discussed types of local anesthetic injection by various methods; however, EDA is based on electrical stimulation to generate anesthesia.

Transcutaneous electrical nerve stimulation (TENS) is used in general medicine. In dentistry, TENS is used to control chronic pain such as trigeminal neuralgia or atypical facial pain (Yap and Ong 1996; Cho et al. 1998). EDA is a variant of TENS that is used in dentistry to achieve anesthesia. It is based on a lower current and higher frequency (Cho et al. 1998).

The first references to the use of electrodes to relieve dental pain were by James Ferguson in 1770 (Ferguson 1770), although in 1858, the College of Dentists of London advised against the technique because electricity did not have an anesthetic effect and increased pain, and the few favorable outcomes achieved were the result of "distraction" (Kane and Taub 1975). However, operative systems began to be developed after the publication of the gate control theory in 1965 (see Chapter 11) (Melzack and Wall 1965), with the appearance of the first clinical trials in dentistry (Shane and Kessier 1967; Brooks et al. 1970; Laster and Pressman 1975). The first practical system marketed for dental use was UltraCalm, which appeared in 1989. The system was very expensive and required placement of an intraoral electrode in the area of the vestibule to be treated (Clark et al. 1987; Malamed et al. 1989). It was therefore necessary to dry the mucosa well to ensure successful placement (Cho et al. 1998). In addition, the electrode blocked the dentist's vision and hampered the procedure (Cho et al. 1998; Baghdadi 1999). The other electrode was placed in the patient's hand.

In 1993, the company 3M marketed a smaller device for use in dentistry known as the Dental Electronic Anesthesia System 8670 (Burke 1997; Baghdadi 1999). This was much more affordable and had the huge advantage that it involved placement of electrodes extraorally on the patient's face. The system was introduced in the United Kingdom in 1997 (Burke 1997).

### Mechanism of Action

The mechanism of action of EDA is unknown, although several factors have been shown to be associated with it (Munshi et al. 2000b):

1) The gate control theory blocks the transmission of painful messages to the highest levels of the central nervous system (CNS) (Katch 1986; Clark et al. 1987; Hochman 1988; Silverstone 1989) (see Chapter 11, instrumental, vibrators).
2) Release of serotonin, a neurotransmitter that is derived from tryptophan (Clark et al. 1987; Hochman 1988; Silverstone 1989; Cho et al. 1998). Adding 2–3 g of tryptophan to the diet, per day, 3 days before TENS is applied can approve the results (Hochman 1988).
3) Release of β-endorphins by the periaqueductal gray substance of the CNS (Clark et al. 1987; Hochman 1988; Silverstone 1989; Yap and Ong 1996; Cho et al. 1998). Endorphins are endogenous opioids and can produce analgesia.
4) Placebo effect, because the patient controls the intensity of the current applied with his/her hand, thus keeping him/her distracted (Hochman 1988; Silverstone 1989; Mellor 1993; Modaresi et al. 1996).

### Indications

- Conventional indications:
  1) Topical anesthesia, since this is very useful for reducing the pain resulting from the needle prick and injection of conventional anesthesia (Croll and Simonsen 1994; Quarnstrom and Libed 1994; Meechan and Winter 1996; Vongsavan and Vongsavan 1996; Meechan et al. 1998).

2) Calculus removal in sensitive teeth and scaling and root planing (Bishop 1986; Clark et al. 1987; Hochman 1988; Pirkner et al. 1995; Yap and Ong 1996; Burke 1997).
3) Placement of rubber dams, especially if the prongs of the clamp are placed subgingivally (te-Duits et al. 1993; Baghdadi 1999).
4) Cavities of small or moderate, barely invasive obturations (Malamed et al. 1989; Yap and Ho 1996; Cho et al. 1998). According to Table 20.2, the efficacy is 80%, although it is important to take into account that successful cases include those in which patients experienced with mild discomfort or pain but were able to complete treatment without the addition of conventional local anesthetic by injection. Some authors report that outcomes are better for primary teeth than for permanent teeth (Cho et al. 1998).
5) Cementing of fixed prosthesis in vital teeth (Yap and Ong 1996; Burke 1997).

- Special indications for this technique:
  - Allergy to local anesthetics or their components because this technique does not involve drugs (Jedrychowski and Duperon 1993; Yap and Ong 1996; Burke 1997; Munshi et al. 2000b).
  - Hemophiliac patients because there is no need for an injection and, above all, there is no need for truncal block, with the result that there is no risk of asphyxiating hematomas (Savage 1982).

Note: It is noteworthy that EDA is more successful in children aged 5–12 years; in contrast, the results are not so good in anxious and/or skeptical patients (Quarnstrom and Quinn 1995).

Table 20.2 Percentage of patients in whom cavity cutting is successful (mildly aggressive) and who prefer EDA to conventional systems (results from clinical trials).

| | Study data | | Variables analyzed | |
|---|---|---|---|---|
| Reference | Device | Patients | Successful cavities | Preference |
| Bradley et al. (1974) | Special air turbine[a] | Adults | 75% | — |
| Savage (1982) | HM-100 PSU | Adults | 92% | — |
| Clark et al. (1987) | HFNM | Adults | 93% | — |
| Donaldson et al. (1989) | TENS | Adults | 33% | — |
| Malamed et al. (1989) | EDA | Adults | 86% | — |
| Esposito et al. (1993) | UltraCalm | Adults | 80% | 70% |
| Jedrychowski and Duperon (1993) | UltraCalm | Children | 83% | — |
| Mellor (1993) | UltraCalm | Adults | 100% | 60% |
| te-Duits et al. (1993) | Spectrum Max-SD | Children | 78% | 78% |
| Pirkner et al. (1995) | DEAS 3M (8670) | Adults | — | 56% |
| Sasa and Donly (1995) | DEAS 3M (8670) | Children | — | 40% |
| Segura et al. (1995) | DEAS 3M (8670) | Children | — | 93% |
| Jones and Blinkhorn (1996) | Cedeta | Children | 73% | 61% |
| Yap and Ho (1996) | DEAS 3M (8670) | Adults | 93% | — |
| Burke (1997) | DEAS 3M (8670) | Adults | — | 41% |
| Öztas et al. (1997) | U-TENS plus | Children | 68% | 56% |
| Cho et al. (1998) | DEAS 3M (8670) | Children | 81% | 63% |
| Baghdadi (1999) | DEAS 3M (8670) | Children | 75% | 53% |
| Munshi et al. (2000b) | MES | Children | 94% | — |
| | | Average | 80% | 61% |
| | | Rounded average | **80%** | **60%** |

HFNM, high-frequency neural modulator; MES, Madras Engineering Services; TENS, transcutaneous electrical nerve stimulation; EDA, electronic dental anesthesia; DEAS, Dental Electronic Anesthesia System.
[a] Miniature electrical generator within turbine head.

## Disadvantages

This technique has several disadvantages, the most important of which are as follows:

1) *Inadequate depth of anesthesia* (Harvey and Elliott 1995; Sasa and Donly 1995; Modaresi et al. 1996; Yap and Ong 1996; Burke 1997). Consequently, outcomes in oral surgery and extractions are poor (Bishop 1986; Katch 1986; Clark et al. 1987), as are those of endodontic procedures (Bishop 1986; Clark et al. 1987), cutting of crowns and bridges in vital teeth (Hochman 1988; Burke 1997), and deep scaling and root planing (Pirkner et al. 1995). Furthermore, the technique is not recommended in procedures where moderate or severe postoperative pain is expected (surgery, endodontics) (Malamed et al. 1989).
2) The cost of the system and devices. While this has decreased over time, it continues to be high compared to traditional local anesthetic. In addition, single-use adhesive electrodes are necessary for each new patient.
3) The time taken to explain the technique to the patient and to try it, given that the patient's cooperation is necessary (Modaresi et al. 1996; Yap and Ong 1996; Burke 1997).

## Advantages

The advantages of the technique can be summarized as follows:

1) No needle or injection, with the result that:
   - There are no injections to fear (Jedrychowski and Duperon 1993; Yap and Ong 1996; Burke 1997). Some authors recommend this technique in patients with needle phobia (Hochman 1988; Malamed et al. 1989; Burke 1997; Munshi et al. 2000b), however, efficacy was not as well established in anxious or skeptical patients (Quarnstrom and Quinn 1995).
   - It can be used in patients with bleeding dyscrasias because there are no injections. Moreover there is no need for truncal block and no risk of hematoma (Savage 1982), as seen previously.
2) Patients prefer this technique to conventional techniques in 60% of cases, when it can be used (Table 20.2).
3) Since no drugs are involved (local anesthetics, vasoconstrictors), there are no associated risks (Jedrychowski and Duperon 1993; Yap and Ong 1996; Burke 1997; Munshi et al. 2000b) such as the following:
   - Toxicity induced by accidental intravascular injection or overdose.
   - Allergy to any of the components in the anesthetic solution. This is one of the indications for this technique.
4) No long-term postoperative paresthesia (Hochman 1988; Malamed et al. 1989; Silverstone 1989; Jedrychowski and Duperon 1993; Yap and Ong 1996; Burke 1997; Munshi et al. 2000b) since the effect disappears once the device is switched off and there is no electric current:
   - There is no risk of self-injury resulting from biting the lips, tongue, or jugal mucosa or of burning oneself with hot food.
   - The patient can eat and drink after treatment.
   - Bite adjustment is easier because the patient's perception is not altered by the anesthesia of the soft tissues.

## Contraindications

While some contraindications are well established, others are empirical. However, in case of doubt, we include all possibilities:

1) Abnormalities of the heart:
   - Pacemaker, to prevent electromagnetic interference (Katch 1986; Hochman 1988; Donaldson et al. 1989; Malamed et al. 1989; Croll and Simonsen 1994; Quarnstrom and Libed 1994; Yap and Ho 1996; Yap and Ong 1996; Burke 1997; Meechan et al. 1998).
   - Arrhythmias, to prevent alterations to heart rate caused by electrical depolarization (Donaldson et al. 1989).
2) Abnormalities of the CNS and head:
   - Cerebrovascular abnormalities such as stroke, transient ischemic attacks, and aneurysms since EDA can increase the risks of these occurring (Katch 1986; Hochman 1988; Donaldson et al. 1989; Malamed et al. 1989; Croll and Simonsen 1994; Quarnstrom and Libed 1994; Yap and Ho 1996; Yap and Ong 1996).
   - Epileptic seizures or convulsions, owing to the risk of triggering them (Katch 1986; Hochman 1988; Quarnstrom and Libed 1994; Yap and Ho 1996; Yap and Ong 1996; Burke 1997; Meechan et al. 1998).
   - Brain tumors, owing to the risk of worsening them (Croll and Simonsen 1994; Yap and Ho 1996).
   - Neuralgia of the head and neck such as trigeminal neuralgia, postherpetic neuralgia, multiple sclerosis, Bell's palsy, owing to the risk of worsening them (Croll and Simonsen 1994; Yap and Ho 1996; Yap and Ong 1996; Burke 1997; Meechan et al. 1998).
   - Cochlear implants (Croll and Simonsen 1994; Yap and Ho 1996).
3) Pregnancy, mainly because the effects on the fetus are unknown (Katch 1986; Hochman 1988; Donaldson et al. 1989; Malamed et al. 1989; Croll and Simonsen 1994; Quarnstrom and Libed 1994; Yap and Ho 1996; Yap and Ong 1996; Burke 1997; Meechan et al. 1998).

4) Placement of electrodes is totally contraindicated at the following sites:
   - Skin on the face affected by abnormalities (Croll and Simonsen 1994; Yap and Ho 1996; Yap and Ong 1996; Burke 1997).
   - Eyes (Katch 1986; Burke 1997).
   - Neck, because of stimulation of the carotid baroreceptors may induce bradycardia and subsequent reductions of cardiac output may not be tolerated in some patients (Yap and Ong 1996).
5) Other possible contraindications:
   - Fear of electrocution in patients who previously had a serious electrical accident (Quarnstrom and Libed 1994).
   - Patients with communication barriers since they must understand the instructions to be able to cooperate (Donaldson et al. 1989; Yap and Ong 1996; Burke 1997).
   - Arterial hypotension or bradycardia because EDA can worsen it (Hochman 1988).

## Equipment

Annex 33 shows the main devices used in dentistry. Below, however, we refer to the Dental Electronic Anesthesia System 8670, manufactured by 3M Dental (Figure 20.4), since this was specially designed for dental anesthesia. Its technical features are shown in Table 20.3.

The device has a modern and attractive design, uses a 9 V battery, and is easy to handle, with manual controls:

- Switch, with three positions: M transmits smooth intermittent impulses, R transmits impulses in bursts, and C transmits continuous impulses and is the most commonly used option.
- Two buttons: R to set the frequency at 140 Hz and W to set the pulse width at 250 µs.
- Current intensity controller. Controlled by the patient, with a current that ranges from 0 to 60 milliamperes (mA).
- "On" button. When the device is turned on, a LED light advises us that the device is operational.

At both sides of the main box, we can find an input for the cables of the two electrodes. These electrodes are extraoral (this is an advantage because they do not interfere with interventions in the mouth) and are attached by means of spongy adhesive patches: green, main electrode, which is placed on the skin above the treatment area; brown, complementary electrode. The cables of the electrodes are reusable, therefore they should be cleaned after use. Each one goes with its respective color (green or brown).

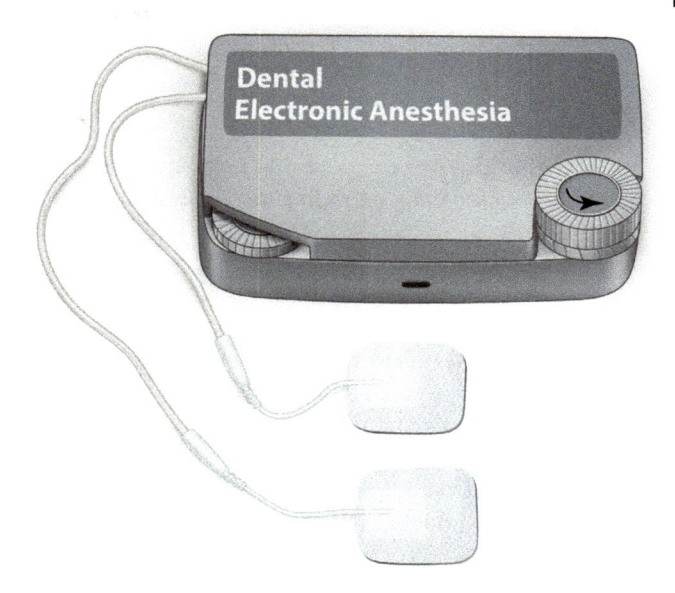

**Figure 20.4** Dental Electronic Anesthesia System 8670 device from 3M dental, with adhesive extrabuccal electrodes.

**Table 20.3** Technical characteristics of the Dental Electronic Anesthesia System 8670 from 3M Dental.

| Variable | Measurement | Value |
| --- | --- | --- |
| Cycle frequency | Hertz (Hz) | 140 |
| Current/amplitude | Milliamperes (mA) | 0–60 |
| Volts | Volts (V) | 9 |
| Bandwidth/pulse | Microseconds | 250 |

*Source:* Data obtained from: Croll and Simonsen (1994), Yap and Ong (1996), Burke (1997), Domínguez et al. (1998), and Cho et al. (1998).

## Technique

As stated above, here we address the Dental Electronic Anesthesia System 8670, manufactured by 3M Dental.

- Pre-operative phase. Explain to the patient how the device works and show him/her the equipment and the single-use adhesive electrodes.
- Children. While the child is in the dental chair, apply the "tell-show-do" technique and show pictures of children with the electrodes. Let the child touch the device and tell him/her that it "gives you tickles on your face" (Domínguez et al. 1998), which is a nice way of describing paresthesia.
- Place the extraoral adhesive electrodes (with the device off):
   o Clean the skin of the face with alcohol to remove grease and sweat that might interfere with the transmission of the electrical current.
   o Instruct the patient to open his/her mouth as wide as possible. This maneuver stretches the skin and brings

the apex of the teeth closer. Thus, we can locate the area where the electrodes will be placed; the goal is to approximate the electrodes to the apices of the teeth being anesthetized.
- ○ Place the adhesive electrodes on the skin. Each electrode symmetrically on each side of the skin, at least 1 mm apart.
  - In the maxilla:
    – Anterior teeth, more forward.
    – Posterior teeth, more backward.
  - Mandible, on the skin in the area of the chin:
    – Anterior teeth, more forward.
    – Posterior teeth, more backward.
  - Try to ensure that the electrode is at the level of the apex of the tooth to be treated.
- Connect the electrodes to the cables on the box.
  - ○ Green connector. For the green electrode in the area of the apice of the teeth to be treated.
  - ○ Brown connector. For the electrode on the opposite side.
- Explain to the patient how to use the manual control (only the on–off button and intensity control button).

Note: In children aged under 8 years, the dentist and/or the assistant manages the device since children can increase intensity suddenly. While this does not damage tissue, it can be uncomfortable and surprise children, thus causing them to alter their behavior (Jedrychowski and Duperon 1993; Croll and Simonsen 1994).

- The patient should increase the intensity (mA) little by little until he/she feels a slight tingling sensation (Clark et al. 1987; Croll and Simonsen 1994). Small muscle contractions (fasciculations) also appear on the face and muscles near the electrodes (sign that the minimum therapeutic level has been reached).
  - ○ The fasciculations usually appear at levels 5–10 (Croll and Simonsen 1994: Yap and Ho 1996; Domínguez et al. 1998), which is between 15 seconds and 2–4 minutes (Yap and Ho 1996; Domínguez et al. 1998).
  - ○ With children, it is a good idea to use a mirror so that they can see the fasciculations.
- The patient can increase the intensity during the treatment. Most do so to levels 10–20 in 3–5 minutes. Smooth increases every 20 seconds are recommended.
- If the effect of the anesthesia is not sufficient during treatment, then we can use the following:
  - ○ Nitrous oxide ($N_2O/O_2$), which provides sedation and enhances analgesia (Donaldson et al. 1989; Croll and Simonsen 1994).
  - ○ Let the children listen to their favorite music through headphones, thus providing a distraction and increasing the pain threshold (Croll and Simonsen 1994).
  - ○ Administer injections of conventional local anesthetic, which do not hurt now because the patient is already feeling the anesthetic effect of EDA (Croll and Simonsen 1994; Quarnstrom and Libed 1994; Meechan and Winter 1996).
- When treatment has finished:
  - ○ Switch off the device. Warn the patient that he/she may feel fasciculations for another few minutes.
  - ○ Remove the electrodes from the skin of the face. The skin may be red. Explain to the patient that this will disappear in a few minutes (10–20 minutes).

### Complications of this Technique

- During treatment:
  - ○ Increased salivation. This can be resolved easily by using a rubber dam, isolating with cotton wool (Croll and Simonsen 1994), or increasing suction.
  - ○ Muscle twitching may appear in the eyes and eyelids (Yap and Ong 1996; Yap and Ho 1996). This has no clinical relevance.
- After treatment:
  - ○ Reddening of the skin the electrodes were adhered to (Burke 1997) caused by increased blood flow to the area. This situation may occur in around 15% of cases (Yap and Ho 1996) and usually disappears in 15–20 minutes (Domínguez et al. 1998). Burns on the skin have been reported rarely, although these were with older EDA devices (Katch 1986).
  - ○ The sensation of soft tissue anesthesia on the face, where the electrodes were placed, lasts a few minutes longer in over 35% of patients (Yap and Ho 1996).

### Computer-Controlled Injection Systems (The Wand®)

The first computer-controlled injection system was The Wand, whose prototype appeared and was first examined in a clinical trial in 1997 (Hochman et al. 1997), the same year that the clinical model for professionals also appeared (Friedman and Hochman 1997), before being acceptance by the American Dental Association (ADA) in 1998 (Anonymous 2002).

The main objective of this system (and of the variants discussed below) is that *the injection is painless or involves minimal discomfort* (Lee et al. 2004), as corroborated in clinical trials with The Wand (Annex 32). The system manages to separate the rate of injection from the pressure (impossible with a manual syringe), thus enabling an extremely low injection rate.

The Wand is a genuine novelty and an alternative to conventional injection techniques. Below, we describe the device in detail, the specific anesthetic techniques developed (palatal approach to the anterior and middle superior alveolar nerves [P-AMSA] and palatal approach to the anterior superior alveolar nerve [P-ASA]), as well as some variations with conventional techniques when they are applied using The Wand.

## Description of the Device

Although the device is basically the same as when it first appeared, a series of modifications have been introduced (Clark and Yagiela 2010):

- 1997. The Wand. The first device.
- 2000. The Wand plus. With some modifications in the foot control.
- 2005. CompuDent Wand. With a high-speed injection function.
- 2007. The Wand STA (Single Tooth Anesthesia). With a modification for optimizing periodontal ligament injection (STA 2015).
- The features of The Wand are continuously updated with regular minor modifications.

### Central Processing Unit

The central processing unit (CPU) is as large as a thick book, with an attractive, brightly colored design (Figure 20.5). It contains a microprocessor with an electric motor to control the injection of local anesthetic solution, thus removing the need for manual pressure from the operator to administer the injection. This ensures the following:

1) *A constant flow*, regardless of tissue resistance because *the microprocessor automatically adjusts the pressure* on the plunger in such a way that if the resistance increases, the force on the plunger increases, although the same injection rate is maintained at all times, therefore there is less tissue distension and less pain. As the maximum pressure of the device is 450 psi (31.6 kg/cm$^2$) (STA 2015), it does not break glass cartridges (Froum et al. 2000) (Table 18.2, Chapter 18). It is important to note that with the hand, it is impossible to maintain a constant flow with increased resistance (Hochman et al. 1997).
2) *Very slow injection rate* of approximately one drop per second (Friedman and Hochman 2001; Nusstein et al. 2004a,b) to ensure that the anesthetic is injected below the pain threshold. Such a rate is almost impossible to achieve with the conventional manual technique owing to factors such as muscle fatigue.

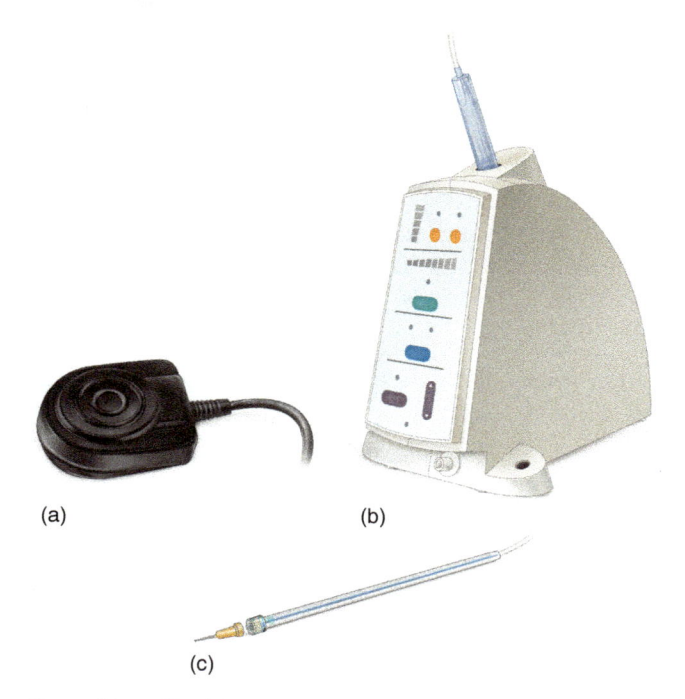

**Figure 20.5** The Wand STA: (a) foot control pedal; (b) central processing unit, and (c) handpiece (The Wand).

**Table 20.4** Injection rate in milliliters (ml) injected per unit of time (seconds, s or minutes, min) and seconds per milliliter with The Wand.

| Rate | Milliliters (ml) per second | Seconds per milliliter (ml) | Injection time 1.4 ml | Injection time 1.8 ml |
|---|---|---|---|---|
| Very fast TurboFlo | 0.06 | 17 | 23 s | 30 s |
| Fast RapidFlo | 0.031 | 35 | 45 s | 1 min |
| Slow ControlFlo | 0.005 | 207 | 4 min, 45 | 6 min |

Approximate date (±15%).
*Source:* Data from Friedman and Hochman (2001), Nusstein et al. (2004b), and STA (2015).

The system initially had three rates (Table 20.4), although the slow rate is truly novel: the plunger advances at 1/200 in. per second (0.005 in. per second = 0.1235 mm) (Hochman et al. 1997).

Studies have shown that control of the injection, a slow injection rate, and control of pressure are impossible with manual systems based on conventional metal syringes (Tzafalia and Sixou 2011).

### Foot Control

The foot control serves to control the injection rate and enable aspiration:

1) Injection flow rate, from very fast to slow.
2) Aspiration, after activation of this function by pressing a button on the CPU (aspiration button). In the original devices, aspiration lasted 14 seconds (Goodell et al. 2000). In more modern devices, however, this time has been reduced to 5 seconds (Saloum et al. 2000; Nicholson et al. 2001).

The injection flow rate also warns us using acoustic and visual signals:

1) Acoustic. A soft "beep" sounds every time a drop is injected.
2) Visual. The original devices had lights on the front part of the CPU. Today's devices have a screen that tells us the exact volume of solution administered and the pressure of the injection.

The huge advantage of the foot control is that it leaves the hands free throughout the injection and aspiration procedure so that the dentist can concentrate on guiding and controlling the needle. Furthermore, during aspiration, traction on the plunger with the thumb on the ring in the conventional technique meant that, for a second, the needle moved uncontrollably and almost imperceptibly. An *in vitro* study performed in 2016 showed how this movement of the tip of the needle was 2.5 mm with conventional cartridge syringes, but less than 1 mm with The Wand, precisely because of the control provided by the foot control (Kämmerer et al. 2016).

### Handpiece

The handpiece is made of single-use plastic in the form of an ultralight pencil. It looks like a wand, with a long, fine shaft that is held in a pen grasp and with a type of head at the most anterior part, where a needle with a Luer lock fitting is screwed into its nozzle (Figure 20.6).

This shape makes for a highly precise, maneuverable, and flexible device that increases tactile sensitivity (Hochman et al. 1997) and ensures that the needle is in contact with the fingers, almost an extension of them. Therefore, it is easier to use than conventional syringes, in which the fingers are far from the needle in order to support the body of the syringe and retract the plunger (Krochak and Friedman 1998).

A 60-in. (5 ft or 1.5 m) sterile microtubing enters the posterior part of the head and connects the cartridge, which is located on the upper part of the CPU, with the nozzle of the head of the wand, into which the needle is screwed. To prevent cross-contamination, the microtubing, the handpiece, and the cartridge are single use (Nusstein et al. 2004a).

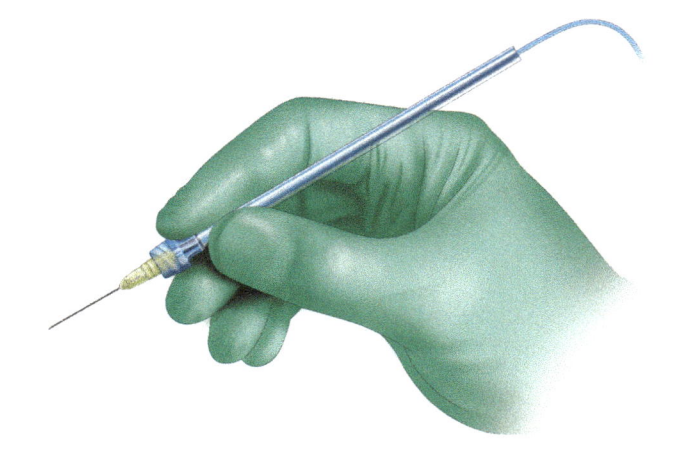

**Figure 20.6** Method of holding the handpiece in a pen grip. Fingers close to the head of the handpiece.

The long posterior shaft of the handpiece can be broken down to only the head with the needle and its connection to the microtubing in such a way that it is even more manageable, as if the needle was being held with the fingers.

### Needles

The handpiece accepts needles that are compatible with a Luer lock. These are screwed into the nozzle on the head. While various brands are available, the most widely used are those from Becton-Dickinson Co. Table 20.5 shows the different calibers and lengths of needle.

### Set-up

The system uses conventional 1.8-ml cartridges, which are loaded into the plastic cartridge support and adjusted to an opening in the upper part of the CPU. This houses the piston, which is controlled by the microprocessor so that the

**Table 20.5** Caliber and lengths of needles from brands used with The Wand.

| Needle | Caliber | Length | | Brand |
| --- | --- | --- | --- | --- |
| | | Millimeters | Inches | |
| Extrashort | 30G | 12 | ½ | Becton Dickson Co |
| | 32G | 12 | ½ | Misana-Dental |
| | 27G | 12 | ½ | Monojet (Tyco Healthcare) |
| Short | 30G | 25 | 1 | Becton Dickson Co |
| | 30G | 25 | 1 | J. Morita |
| | 30G | 25 | 1 | Sherwood Medical |
| Long | 27G | 30 | $1^{1/4}$ | Becton Dickson Co |

head of the piston fits into the plunger of the cartridge (Krochak and Friedman 1998).

The single-use microtubing that crosses the diaphragm of the nozzle of the cartridge holder socket is inserted into the far end of the plastic support. The microtubing reaches the head of the handpiece (wand) to deliver the anesthetic solution.

Once the system is set up, it is started by pressing on the foot control. The system primes the microtubing with local anesthetic, purging the system from any air. The priming volume (of the microtubing) is 0.4 ml, leaving only 1.4 ml in the first cartridge for administration to the patient.

As with conventional systems, the cartridge, needle, and microtubing are disposed of, since they are contaminated with blood, plasma, or tissue fluids in each aspiration, even when the aspiration is negative (Trapp and Davies 1980).

### Advantages and Disadvantages
- Disadvantages:
  1) The device is expensive, and new microtubing and handpiece must be used for each patient.
  2) Lost volume of 0.4 ml of local anesthetic solution from the first cartridge when priming the microtubing.
  3) The injection process takes several minutes.
  4) The operator must undergo a learning curve – albeit short – before mastering the hand-foot technique.
- Advantages:
  1) The injection method is almost painless in most cases, or at least less so than with conventional methods (Annex 32).
  2) The needle moves very little during aspiration (<1 mm) (Kämmerer et al. 2016).
  3) As we will see below, new anesthetic techniques can be used, namely, P-AMSA and P-ASA. The outcomes of these techniques are more favorable with The Wand than with conventional manual syringes (Lee et al. 2004).

## P-AMSA

P-AMSA stands for palatal approach to the anterior and middle superior alveolar nerves. The technique was devised by Ronald P. Spinello in 1996 during the development of the prototypes of The Wand, specifically for this device (Friedman Friedman and Hochman 1997, 1998). The technique can also be applied using conventional techniques, although it is not as successful (Lee et al. 2004) and is more painful (Nusstein et al. 2004b).

The P-AMSA technique aims to anesthetize the anterior and middle superior alveolar nerves from the palate, with a slow and pressurized injection that enables the anesthetic solution to penetrate through the many small accessory foramina of the palate (Friedman and Hochman 1999). The objective is to achieve pulpal anesthesia of the incisors, canines, and premolars, as well as of the palatal fibromucosa on the same side.

### Anesthetized Area
- Teeth, pulp, and periodontal ligament of the central and lateral incisor, canine, and maxillary premolars on one side (Friedman and Hochman 1998, 2001; Fukayama et al. 2003; Lee et al. 2004).
- Palate, including fibromucosa, periosteum, and bone of the whole palatine hemiarch, up to the midline, from the central incisor to the area of the molars (Lee et al. 2004).
- Vestibule. Fibromucosa of the gingiva and interdental papillae and periosteum of the teeth where pulpal anesthesia is achieved.

*Note*: We do not anesthetize the alveolar mucosa, lips, nose, or the muscles of facial expression. If the solution is administered bilaterally, anesthesia is, in theory, from the second maxillary premolar to the contralateral second maxillary premolar.

### Technique
- Use extrashort 30G needles (12 mm) compatible with a Luer lock (Friedman and Hochman 1997, 1998, 2001) or short 27G needles (25 mm) (Lee et al. 2004; Nusstein et al. 2004b).
- Position of dentist and patient:
  o The dentist places him/herself at 7:00–8:00 o'clock for block on the right side and at 11:00 o'clock for block on the left side.
  o The patient lies back horizontally, with his/her head back, the neck well extended (hyperextension), and the mouth open as far as possible so that the dentist can see the palate clearly. The patient's head can be turned right or left depending on the approach.
- Warn the patient about the following (Lee et al. 2004; Nusstein et al. 2004b):
  o Administration of the anesthetic may take 4–5 minutes.
  o He/she will hear sounds during administration; these are only warnings from the computer.
  o There may be some discomfort in the palate. This affects only one area, is over quickly (1–2 seconds), and is followed by a sensation of pressure.
- The handpiece (wand) is held in a pen grasp (Figure 20.6), with the right hand (for right-handed operators), and the palate is approached from the area of the contralateral maxillary premolars (Friedman and Hochman 2001).
- The needle is inserted at the midpoint between the palatal gingival margin between the first and second premolars and the midline of the palate (Figure 20.7).

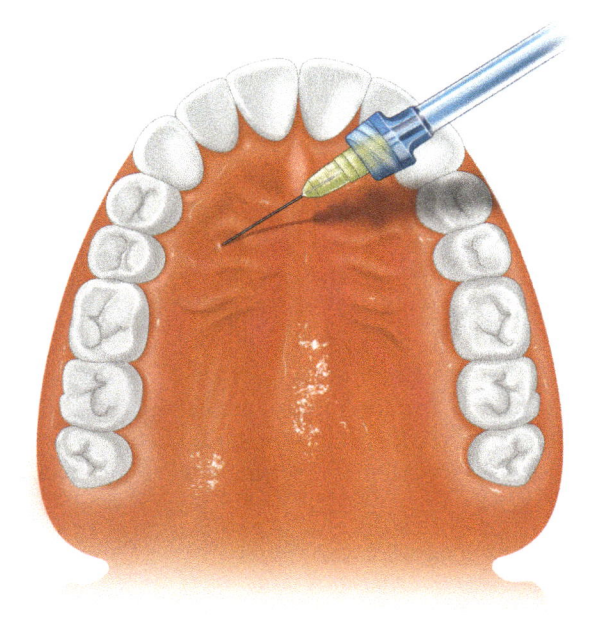

**Figure 20.7** Needle injection site in P-AMSA.

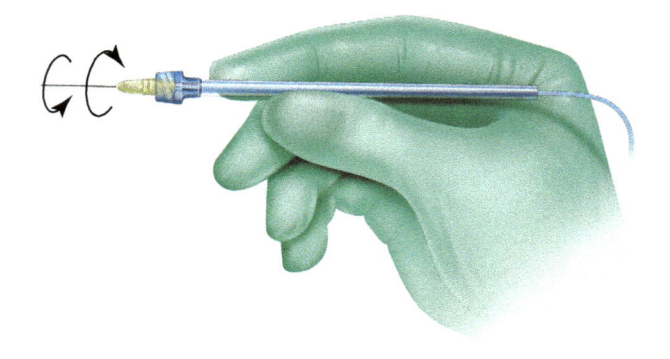

**Figure 20.8** Biaxial and bidirectional rotation of the needle with the fingers approximately 45° clockwise and 45° anticlockwise while advancing the needle.

- In the palate, the needle is directed toward the teeth (premolars) with the bevel parallel to the palate and an approximately 45° angle between the needle and the palate.
- Insertion of the needle using two similar approaches:
  1) After the first contact with the mucosa, the solution is injected slowly, drop by drop, to ensure that the anesthetic penetrates from the start.
  2) Alternatively, a cotton swab can be used to press firmly down on the palatal mucosa during insertion to reduce discomfort and absorb the excess anesthetic that oozes out during the first drops of the injection.
- Advancing the needle. Once the needle is inside the palatal fibromucosa and while the solution is being injected drop by drop, we can advance it in two ways. However, the needle should be rotated biaxially with the fingers (45° clockwise, 45° anticlockwise) (Figure 20.8):
  1) Advancing with pauses (Lee et al. 2004; Nusstein et al. 2004b), together with pressure from a cotton swab:
     - Advance 1–2 mm.
     - Short pause and injection of three or four drops in more or less 4 seconds (four beeps).
     - Advance a further 2–4 mm until the needle is just touching the bone, then smoothly withdraw the needle by 1 mm.
     - Short pause and injection of a further four drops in more or less 4 seconds (four beeps).
     - Withdraw the swab. Palatal blanching can be observed.
  2) Continuous advance (Friedman and Hochman 1997, 1998):
     - Advance smoothly and slowly while injecting drop by drop until the bone is reached. Then withdraw the needle slowly by 1 mm (Friedman and Hochman 2001).
     - Palatal blanching will be observed as the anesthetic solution enters the palate.
- The aspiration cycle is activated with the foot control.
- Slow injection, drop by drop:
  o The amount to be injected can be:
     - Up to 1 ml in children.
     - 0.6–0.9 ml in adults (Friedman and Hochman 1997, 1998) or up to 1.4 ml (Friedman and Hochman 1997; Lee et al. 2004; Nusstein et al. 2004b). Remember that the maximum amount in the first cartridge is 1.4 ml.
  o If anesthetic solution leaks out, then the needle should be repositioned.
  o Monitor excess blanching by periodically pausing the injection so that the solution can spread and there is no risk of palatal ulcer due to excessive pressure.
- After the injection, which takes 3–5 minutes, wait 5–10 seconds before withdrawing the needle, since:
  o This reduces reflux of the anesthetic to the exterior. If the needle is withdrawn quickly, residual pressure in the tissues tends to expel part of the solution through the opening left by the needle (Nusstein et al. 2004b).
  o Observe how blanching of the palate extends first forward toward the incisive papilla and then backwards toward the soft palate but without passing the midline (Lee et al. 2004).
- Pulpal anesthesia takes a further 10–20 minutes to achieve (Corbett et al. 2010).

- Final remarks:
  - This technique must sometimes be reinforced with an extra 0.9 ml of solution.
  - Talk to the patient throughout the process to distract him/her and verify how he/she is feeling.

### Efficacy of the P-AMSA Technique

The clinical outcomes are similar to those of conventional techniques (Annex 32). Studies on pulpal anesthesia evaluated using an electrical pulp tester yield more modest results (Table 20.6), with approximately 40% in the central incisor and *around 70% in the lateral incisor, canine, and first and second premolars.*

Another important factor to take into account is that *onset of pulpal anesthesia is slow, i.e. 15–20 minutes* (Fukayama et al. 2003; Lee et al. 2004; Corbett et al. 2010), possibly because the anesthetic solution has to cover some distance from the palatine process to the apexes of the tooth.

### Specific Complications of this Technique

1) The technique causes moderate or severe pain in 20% of patients during the procedure (Table 20.7).
2) Inflammation of the palate at the injection site in less than 10% of cases, and postoperative pain in less than 10%, which lasts 1–2 days before resolving spontaneously (Nusstein et al. 2004b). Palatal ulceration is rare but may occur.

Table 20.6 Percentage of pulpal anesthesia, evaluated using an electric pulp tester, after injection of standard solution (L-100) with the *P-AMSA technique* and The Wand.

| Tooth | Fukayama et al. (2003) 1.4 ml | Lee et al. (2004) 1.4 ml | Corbett et al. (2010) 1 ml |
| --- | --- | --- | --- |
| Central incisor | 45% | 35% | 43% |
| Lateral incisor | 65% | 58% | 75% |
| Canine | 85% | 52% | 77% |
| First premolar | 65% | 42% | 68% |
| Second premolar | 75% | 55% | 86% |

L-100 is lidocaine 2% with epinephrine 1:100 000 (10 µg/ml).

Table 20.7 Percentage of pain caused by P-AMSA with The Wand.

| Reference | Pain |
| --- | --- |
| Friedman and Hochman (1997) | 4% |
| Fukayama et al. (2003) | 15% |
| Nusstein et al. (2004b) | 38% |
| Average | 20% |

### Advantages of the P-AMSA Technique

1) Only 20% of patients complain that the P-AMSA technique using The Wand was painful or uncomfortable (Table 20.7), even though it was in the palate, the most painful area for injection in the mouth (Annex 23).
2) There is no soft tissue anesthesia affecting the lips, face, or muscles of facial expression, therefore it is very useful in aesthetic evaluations of the teeth and lips along the smile line (Friedman and Hochman 1998; Fukayama et al. 2003; Lee et al. 2004). It has been reported that only 15% of patients experienced soft tissue anesthesia lasting under 2 hours in the upper lip (Corbett et al. 2010).
3) It achieves pulpal anesthesia of five maxillary teeth (central incisor, lateral incisor, canine, first and second premolars) with a single injection and a low dose of anesthetic solution (Friedman and Hochman 1998; Gibson et al. 2000).

## P-ASA

P-ASA is the acronym for palatal approach to the anterior superior alveolar nerve. The technique was developed by Mark J. Friedman in 1999 specifically for The Wand (Friedman and Hochman 1999) and is a variation of nasopalatine nerve block that is applied to try to anesthetize the dental pulp of six anterior teeth, from canine to canine. The P-ASA technique is used to anesthetize the nasopalatine nerve and anterior superior alveolar nerves by means of a slow injection at a constant pressure that enables the anesthetic to reach the dental pulp painlessly. Therefore, this technique is different from conventional injection of the nasopalatine nerve, in that the needle penetrates more deeply, and a higher quantity of anesthetic is injected to anesthetize the dental pulp (Nusstein et al. 2004a).

### Anesthetized Area

- Teeth, pulp, and periodontal ligament of the central incisor, lateral incisor, maxillary canine on both sides, that is, the six anterior teeth (Friedman and Hochman 1999, 2001).
- Palate, including the fibromucosa, periosteum, and bone of the whole anterior third of the palate supplied by nasopalatine nerve.
- Buccal. Fibromucosa of the gingiva and interdental papillae, bone, and periosteum of the six anterior and maxillary teeth.

Note that there is no anesthesia of the alveolar mucosa, upper lip, nose, or muscles of facial expression (Ram and Kaissirer 2006).

**Technique**

- Use Luer Lock–compatible 30G extrashort needles (12 mm) (Friedman and Hochman 1999, 2001; Ram and Kaissirer 2006) or 25-mm needles (Burns et al. 2004; Nusstein et al. 2004a).
- Position of the dentist and patient:
  - Right-handed dentist at 10:00–12:00 o'clock.
  - Patient reclining horizontally with the head backwards, the neck extended (hyperextension), and the mouth open as wide as possible so that the dentist has a clear, direct view of the palate (Friedman and Hochman 1999).
- Warn the patient of the following (Nusstein et al. 2004a):
  - Administration of the anesthetic solution takes some time, 4–5 minutes.
  - The patient will hear sounds during administration. These are warnings from the computer.
  - The palate will be anesthetized but not the upper lip or face.
  - The patient may initially notice some small and short discomfort in the palate (1–2 seconds) and then a certain feeling of pressure.
- The dentist takes the handpiece (The Wand) in a pen grasp, using the right hand (for right-handed dentists), and approaches the incisive papilla between the two central incisors in the on the right side (Figure 20.9).
- Insertion of the needle:
  - Press the papilla firmly with a cotton swab from the left side with the supporting hand (that is, the left hand in right-handed dentists).
  - Insert the needle into the lateral groove of the incisive papilla on the right-hand side, with the bevel parallel to the palate just below the point where the cotton swab is being pressed.
  - Start a slow flow with the foot pedal (drop by drop) while maintaining pressure with the cotton swab for 6–8 seconds (six to eight beeps).

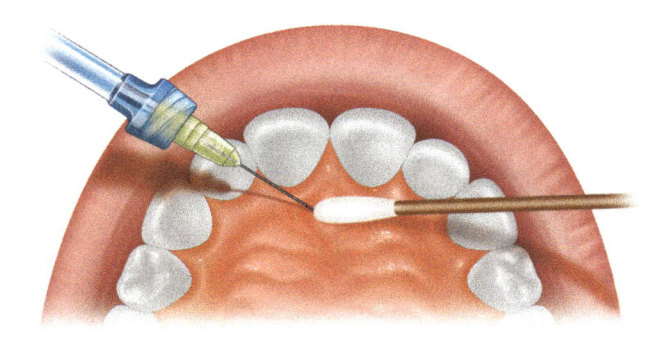

**Figure 20.9** Injection site with P-ASA.

Note: The cotton swab helps to do the following:
1) Reduce the discomfort from needle insertion and the injection.
2) Absorb the anesthetic that flows back into the mouth during the injection.

- Advancing the needle:
  - Rotate the needle biaxially with the fingers (45° clockwise, 45° anticlockwise) (Friedman and Hochman 1999; Burns et al. 2004). This is also known as bidirectional rotation and helps the needle to penetrate the tissues (Figure 20.8) with minimal resistance and discomfort as it advances slowly:
    - With advance-pause cycles. Thus, advancing 1–2 mm, followed by a pause of 4–5 seconds (four or five beeps), advancing a further 1–2 mm followed by a pause of 4–5 seconds.
    - Throughout this period, the solution is injected steadily and slowly (drop by drop).
  - After this maneuver, withdraw the cotton swab. Blanching of the papilla is observed.
- Reorientation of the needle to enter the incisive canal.
  - Slightly withdraw the needle and redirect it parallel to the axes of the maxillary central incisors. Solution is not injected during this maneuver.
  - Advance in the new direction:
    - By rotating the needle biaxially (see above).
    - By advancing in advance-pause cycles, i.e. advancing 1–2 seconds followed by a pause of 2–6 seconds.
    - The solution is injected steadily and slowly throughout this period.
  - If the needle makes contact with the bone (25% of cases) (Burns et al. 2004; Nusstein et al. 2004a), stop injecting and redirect the needle to ensure that it is in the canal.
  - During the maneuver, it is useful for the assistant to have the suction cannula near the needle to aspirate the drops of anesthetic that flow back, thus stopping them from entering the patient's mouth.
- Final injection and position:
  - The needle is advanced with advance-pause cycles some 6–10 mm in adults (Friedman and Hochman 2001; Nusstein et al. 2004a) or 3–5 mm in small children (Ram and Kaissirer 2006).

Note: It is not recommended to penetrate further, since this may perforate the floor of the nose (Friedman and Hochman 1999).

  - Activate the 5-second aspiration cycle with the foot control before injecting the final amount. Aspiration is rarely positive with this technique (Friedman and Hochman 1999; Burns et al. 2004; Nusstein et al. 2004a).

- Slowly inject 0.9–1.4 ml (Friedman and Hochman 1999, 2001; Burns et al. 2004; Nusstein et al. 2004a; Ram and Kaissirer 2006). Remember, with the first injection, the maximum amount of anesthetic is 1.4 ml.
- Blanching of the whole anterior palate is observed.
- After the injection, wait 5–10 seconds before withdrawing the needle so that the pressure of the injected solution can reach all the tissues and does not flow back into the mouth (Burns et al. 2004; Ram and Kaissirer 2006).
- Throughout the process, distract the patient by talking and checking on how he/she feels.
- Dental pulp becomes anesthetized in around 5 minutes (3–7 minutes) (Friedman and Hochman 1999, 2001).

Final remark: Slow injection (drop-by-drop) prevents the transmission of excessive pressure to the tissue and gives time for the solution to be absorbed.

### Efficacy of P-ASA

While the clinical outcomes are similar to those of conventional techniques (Annex 32), studies on pulpal anesthesia evaluated using an electric pulp tester yield more modest results (Table 20.8), with approximately *55% in the four incisors and a third in the canines*. Furthermore, pulpal anesthesia is achieved fairly quickly, *in about 5 minutes* (Friedman and Hochman 1999, 2001; Burns et al. 2004), in contrast with P-AMSA.

### Specific Complications with this Technique

1) The technique is painful despite being slow and careful since it produces moderate to severe pain in 55% of patients during the procedure (Nusstein et al. 2004a).
2) It leaves the incisive papilla inflamed in 25% of cases and postoperative pain at the same site in 15% of patients. This usually resolves spontaneously in 1–3 days (Nusstein et al. 2004a). Rarely (approx. 2%), the incisive papilla becomes ulcerated at 2–4 days and resolves spontaneously in 7–10 days (Friedman and Hochman 1999; Nusstein et al. 2004a).
3) Excessive penetration by the needle can accidentally perforate the floor of the nose (Friedman and Hochman 1999).
4) Pulpal anesthesia of the canines is often unsuccessful (Table 20.8), therefore it may be necessary to inject a further 0.4 ml with P-ASA or inject buccally using the conventional technique.

### Advantages of P-ASA

1) The technique causes "relatively little discomfort" when used with The Wand, especially considering that it is used in the anterior palate, the most painful site for injection in the mouth (Annex 23).
2) There is no soft tissue anesthesia of the lips, face, or muscles of facial expression, therefore the technique is very useful in cosmetic evaluations of the lips and teeth on the smile line (Friedman and Hochman 1999; Ram and Kaissirer 2006).
3) With P-ASA, we can anesthetize six maxillary teeth (incisors and canines) using a single injection and a reduced dose of anesthetic (Friedman and Hochman 1999).

## The Wand and Conventional Techniques

The system makes it possible to perform all the conventional techniques with the same results, given that we inject the same drugs at the same sites; the only variation is that The Wand enables greater control of the injection rate, especially for a slow, drop-by-drop injection, which cannot be achieved with conventional syringes (Tzafalia and Sixou 2011). However, the periodontal ligament technique and mandibular block present some variations.

### Periodontal Ligament Technique
*Technique*

- Use extrashort 27G needles (12 mm) (Nusstein et al. 2004c) or 30G (Ram and Peretz 2003; Ashkenazi et al. 2005).
- The needle is inserted into the gingival groove at a mesio-vestibular or distal-vestibular angle with the bevel toward the tooth.
- Approximately 0.6 ml is injected slowly (drop by drop) into each angle of the monoradicular teeth (Ram and Peretz 2003) and 0.7–0.9 ml into each angle of the multirooted teeth (Nusstein et al. 2004c; Ashkenazi et al. 2005) at 0.7 ml every 2 minutes (Nusstein et al. 2004c).
- Once the injection is complete, it is advisable to maintain the needle in place for a further 10 seconds so that the injected solution can disperse and be distributed through the tissues and not reflux to the exterior. Nevertheless, it is thought that around 0.05 ml flows back (Nusstein et al. 2004c).

Table 20.8 Percentage of pulpal anesthesia, evaluated using an electric pulp meter after injection of standard solution (L-100) using the *P-ASA technique* with The Wand.

| Tooth | Right side | Left side |
| --- | --- | --- |
| Canine | 35% | 32% |
| Lateral incisor | 48% | 58% |
| Central incisor | 58% | 58% |

L-100 is lidocaine 2% with epinephrine 1:100 000 (10 μg/ml).
*Source:* Data from Burns et al. (2004).

***Results*** In children, The Wand has been shown to be less painful in the periodontal ligament technique (PDL) than the conventional approach and as effective as maxillary buccal infiltrations (Ram and Peretz 2003). However, when compared with mandibular block, the discomfort caused by the injection is worse, and clinical efficacy is poorer with the PDL using The Wand (Öztas et al. 2005).

***Specific Complications of this Technique*** Experimental studies in animals have shown The Wand to produce limited inflammation of the periodontium that lasts 24 hours and disappears after around 7 days (Froum et al. 2000).

*In children, application in primary teeth has not been proven to increase hypoplasia in permanent teeth*, possibly because slow injection reduces pressure on the tooth buds of the permanent teeth (Ashkenazi et al. 2010).

### Mandibular Block

Mandibular block is applied as in the conventional technique, although The Wand makes it possible to *insert the needle using bidirectional or biaxial rotation* (Hochman and Friedman 2000). The method requires the head of the handpiece to be held in a pen grasp and, as the needle is inserted into the tissue of the pterygomandibular space, it is turned with the fingers 45° clockwise and 45° anticlockwise, in the same way as endodontic files are turned during instrumentation of root canals (Figure 20.8) in such a way that:

- The needle enters the tissue with minimum resistance (40–50% less) and therefore with minimum discomfort.
- We avoid deviation of the tip of the needle from the objective, as is the case with linear insertion (as is usual with conventional syringes). This maneuver is very effective for preventing deviation independently of the caliber of the needle or the characteristics of its manufacture.

The maneuver is very difficult to perform with conventional syringes that are held in a thumb-palm grasp, which are designed for linear insertion.

## Other Computer-controlled Injection Systems

The launch of The Wand onto the market was followed by other systems like the Calaject controlled-flow system (Romero-Galvez et al. 2016). In the coming years, we expect to see variations, with improvements, the disappearance of some systems, and the appearance of new approaches. The two most important at the moment are the Comfort Control Syringe system from Midwest and QuickSleeper.

### Comfort Control Syringe from Midwest

This system, designed by Mark Smith from Ontario (Canada), first appeared in 2001 (Hawkins and Moore 2002). It does not have a foot control and consists of two components (Hawkins and Moore 2002; Clark and Yagiela 2010):

- The base unit, which is modern in design and makes it possible to select five injection speeds depending on the technique: blocks, infiltrations, periodontal ligament injection, intraosseous injection, and palatal injection (Figure 20.10).
- The hand piece. The cartridge is inserted into the hand piece in a special sheath and the needle is adjusted. This component is operated using the hand that holds it by pressing the button for injection and aspiration (Figure 20.11).

On activation, the system begins to inject the solution at an extremely low rate, 0.007 ml per second (Friedman and Hochman 2001), which increases after 10 seconds depending on the program preselected in the base unit (Hawkins

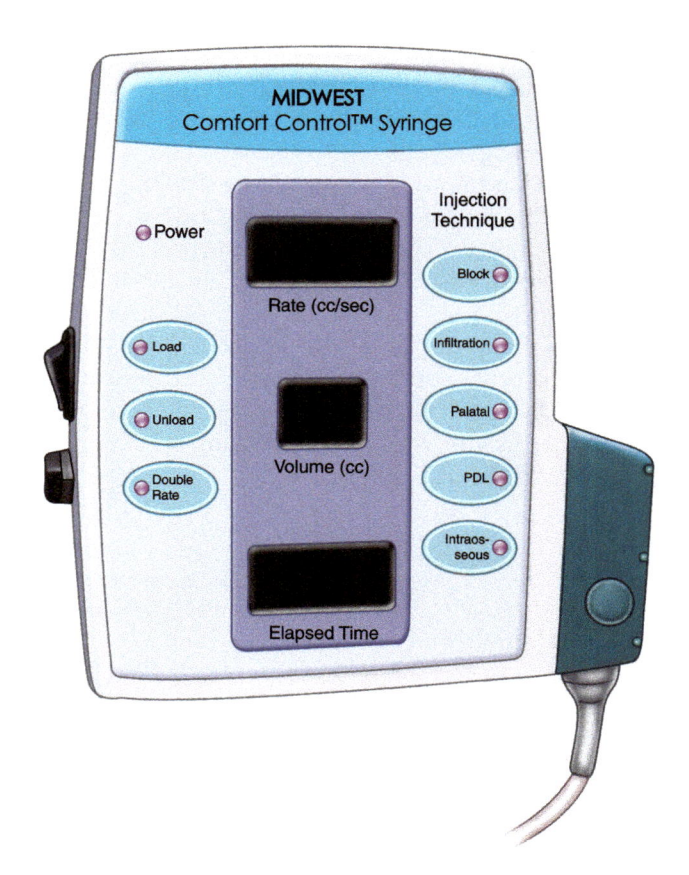

**Figure 20.10** Base unit of the Midwest Comfort Control Syringe system.

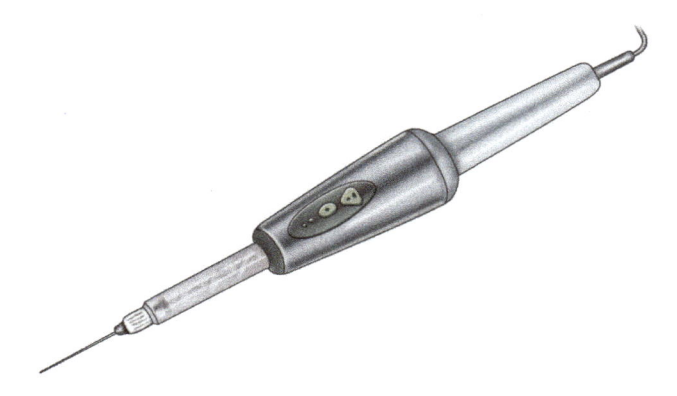

**Figure 20.11** Handpiece of the Midwest Comfort Control Syringe system.

and Moore 2002; Clark and Yagiela 2010). This device presents a series of advantages:

1) The learning curve is smoother, since it is managed in much the same way as conventional techniques (Clark and Yagiela 2010).
2) As there is no microtubing, there is no need to prime it for each patient and it is not contaminated by aspiration.

However, it also has some disadvantages:

1) It is expensive, and a new cartridge sheath must be used for each patient (Clark and Yagiela 2010).
2) The handpiece is bulky, and the injection is activated with the buttons of the hand that holds it, thus rendering it less manageable than The Wand.

Finally, initial clinical studies have provided promising results (Grace et al. 2000, 2003; Langthasa et al. 2012; Rogers et al. 2014), although more randomized clinical trials are necessary to demonstrate its advantages over conventional systems. Other less popular variants have begun to appear, like Smartject (Ghaderi and Ahmadbeigi 2018).

## Quicksleeper

This system, known as transcortical anesthesia, was first developed by Alain Villette in France in 1984 (Villette 1984). The first study with the modern device was published in 2003 (Villette 2003). QuickSleeper is a special device for administering computer-controlled intraosseous and infiltrative injections. Version 2, which was available in 2006, was improved on by Version 5 in 2016.

With QuickSleeper, one instrument makes it possible to administer infiltrative anesthesia, perforate the bone (by rotating a special needle), and perform a controlled slow injection that gradually speeds up with a force that can reach 25 kg. The whole process is regulated using a foot control. The idea is to achieve painless intraosseous anesthesia very quickly by anesthetizing the dental pulp in under 3 minutes. As the technique is intraosseous, it is contraindicated in primary teeth so as not to affect the tooth buds of the permanent teeth (Sixou et al. 2009).

### Equipment

The equipment and device comprise the following elements (Figure 20.12):

- Hand piece (QuickSleeper5), where the cartridge is loaded. The hand piece contains the plunger and nozzle, into which a special needle is screwed. The needle rotates in the hand piece to perforate the cortical plate. Currently there is a new hand piece call SleeperOne5, also bulky but very light (71 g).
- Foot control, with three functions:
  1) Rotation of the special needle for perforation, although the rotation is discontinuous: 1 second with rotation, 1 second without so as not to overheat the bone and thus ensure painless anesthesia.
  2) Slow, progressive anesthesia: 61 seconds for half a cartridge and 93 seconds for the remainder of the cartridge. Thus, anesthesia is painless.
  3) Rapid injection: 32 seconds for half a cartridge and 64 seconds for the remainder.

Note: These actions emit beeps during functioning, and lights go on in the base unit.

- Special Transcort-S needles, with asymmetric bevels that enable not only the injection, but also perforation of the cortical plate. These are of two types (Sixou et al. 2009):
  o 27G extrashort (12 mm).
  o 30G extrashort (9 mm).

### Anesthetized Area

- In the maxilla: three teeth mesially and two distally from the injection site.
- In the mandible: two teeth mesially and one distally from the injection site.

### Transcortical Technique

- If local anesthetic solutions containing epinephrine are injected, the patient should be warned that he/she may experience palpitations (tachycardia) but that these will disappear spontaneously in 2–4 minutes.
- Injection site. Between the teeth, mesially or distally from the tooth selected, into the attached gingiva 2–10 mm from the neck of the tooth. The injection is always into the attached gingiva since if it is into the alveolar mucosa, which is mobile, then this becomes caught in the drill and can tear.

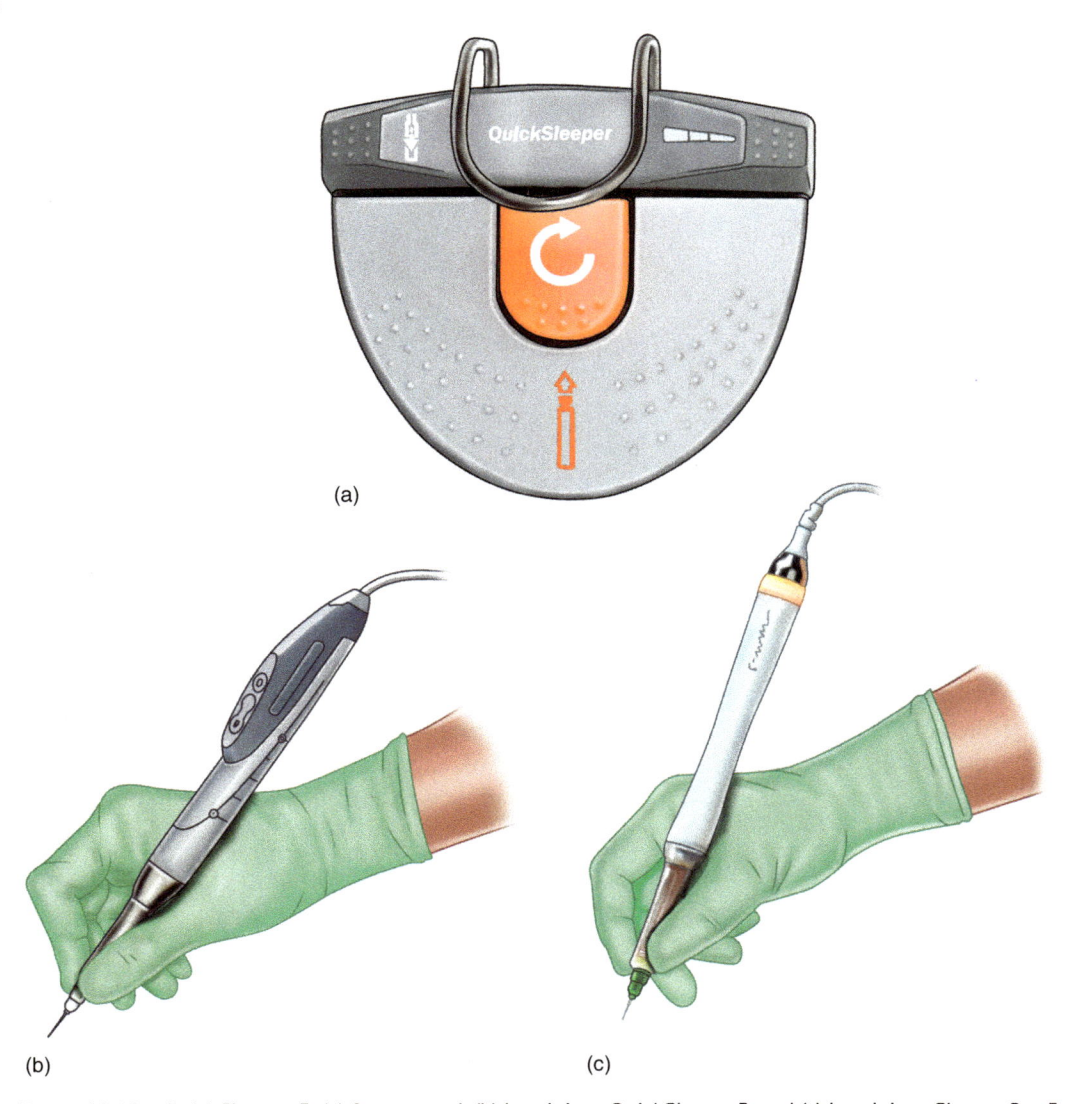

**Figure 20.12** QuickSleeper 5: (a) foot control, (b) handpiece QuickSleeper5, and (c) handpiece SleeperOne5.

- Anesthetize the attached gingiva:
  - Insert the needle over the gingiva with the bevel flat or parallel to it, that is, with an angle of 15–20° over the axis of the needle.
  - Advance the needle approximately 1–3 mm.
  - Using the foot control, activate the slow injection to place some drops of anesthesia in the gingiva.
  - Observe the gradual blanching of the gingiva and mucosa and wait 30 seconds until the anesthesia takes effect.
- Perforate the cortical plane:
  - Turn the needle so that it is perpendicular to the bone plate with a 90° angle.
  - Activate the foot control so that the needle rotates and perforates the cortical plate. A "click" is felt as the needle penetrates the trabecular bone. At this point the needle has crossed the cortical plate.
  - It generally takes from 1 to a maximum of 6 seconds to perforate the cortical plate (Villette 2003). In children it takes around 1 second (Sixou and Barbosa-Rogier 2008; Sixou et al. 2009) and in adults usually 2–3 seconds (Villette 2003).
- Injection of the anesthetic:
  - Withdraw the needle a few millimeters (although remaining within the trabecular bone) to leave space so that the anesthetic can spread.
  - Start a slow progressive injection with the foot control. In general, half a cartridge is injected.

Note: The whole process usually takes 3 minutes.

### Efficacy of QuickSleeper

Although clinical trials have been performed in adults (Villette 2003; Benito-Brotons et al. 2012) and in children

(Sixou and Barbosa-Rogier 2008; Sixou et al. 2009), randomized controlled trials are still required to fully evaluate the efficacy of this system. Nevertheless, current results do seem promising. Trials have shown satisfactory results in 75–85% of extractions and 90–95% of endodontic procedures in primary and permanent teeth (Sixou and Barbosa-Rogier 2008), although there is less efficacy in permanent teeth and mandibular teeth.

Trials comparing QuickSleeper with conventional techniques have shown how anesthesia is very quick (less than a minute), although its duration is short (a few minutes) and the injection is usually more painful than with conventional techniques; however, 70% of patients prefer QuickSleeper (Benito-Brotons et al. 2012).

### Disadvantages
1) The device is expensive.
2) The hand piece is large and bulky, thus making it less manageable than The Wand.
3) More clinical trials are necessary, since the duration of anesthesia is short, although the initial results seem promising.

## Intranasal Maxillary Local Anesthesia (Kovanaze®)

Kovanaze® (intranasal 3% tetracaine and 0.05% oxymetazoline spray) is a needle-free means of achieving dental local anesthesia. The first clinical studies began in 2012 (Giannakopoulos et al. 2012; Ciancio et al. 2013), when the drug was known as K305 (Ciancio et al. 2016; Hersh et al. 2016b). Kovanaze® was approved by the United States Food and Drug Administration (US FDA) in June 2016 for anesthesia of the anterior teeth superior and maxillary premolars. Kovanaze® is a formulation of two well-known medications, tetracaine and oxymetazoline (Saraghi and Hersh 2017). Local anesthetic and vasoconstrictor for intranasal administration were combined based on the fact that these medications have been used for many years to provide local anesthesia for surgical and diagnostic procedures in the nasal cavity (Hersh et al. 2017).

### Composition of the Solution
1) Tetracaine (hydrochloride) is an ester local anesthetic (Chapter 12). It has been used for many years by ear, nose, and throat (ENT) surgeons to provide local anesthesia of the nasal mucosa for diagnostic and surgical procedures (Hersh et al. 2016a, 2017). The main characteristics of tetracaine are summarized in Table 12.7 (Chapter 12).
2) Oxymetazoline (hydrochloride) is a sympathomimetic drug that was developed in Germany in 1961 (Vardanyan and Hruby 2006). It is a selective adrenergic receptor $\alpha_1$ agonist and an $\alpha_2$ adrenergic receptor partial agonist that induces vasoconstriction (Ciancio et al. 2016) to compensate for the marked vasodilatory effect of tetracaine (Chapter 5). Oxymetazoline is a commonly used nasal decongestant and the active ingredient in Afrin® nasal spray. It has traditionally been used with tetracaine for ENT procedures to enhance hemostasis and lower the risk of bleeding (Ciancio et al. 2013: Hersh et al. 2016a, 2017).
3) Benzyl alcohol is the vehicle by which the drug is formulated (Hersh et al. 2016b; Saraghi and Hersh 2017).

### Zone Anesthetized

On entering the maxillary sinus (Hersh et al. 2016a: Saraghi and Hersh 2017), intranasal maxillary local anesthesia targets the afferent sensory nerves, namely, the anterior superior and the middle superior alveolar nerve (it is important to remember that the middle superior alveolar nerve is only found in 55% of cases (Table 2.2, Chapter 2). Kovanace® can be used to anesthetize the following:

- Teeth. All maxillary primary (baby) teeth in children (who weigh at least 40 kg) and permanent maxillary teeth from the second premolar to the second premolar (canines and incisors, from one side to the other) in teenagers and adults, i.e. the smile zone.
- Soft tissues. A unique feature of this delivery system is that the cheeks, lips (15–20 minutes), and nose retain their sensation. The anterior palatal mucosa is anesthetized for about 30 minutes (Ciancio et al. 2013). Soft tissue anesthesia was sufficient for restoration of interproximal caries and for the patient to tolerate the placement of matrix bands and wedges (Hersh et al. 2016a,b; Saraghi and Hersh 2017).

### Indications and Contraindications

#### Indications
Intranasal tetracaine (Kovanaze®) is indicated for regional anesthesia when performing a *restorative procedure* (drilling and filling) on *maxillary teeth* from the second premolar to the second premolar (from one side to the other) in adults and children for all maxillary primary (baby) teeth who weigh 40 kg or more.

Intranasal local anesthetic obviates the need for injection and is therefore highly desirable in *patients who have needle phobia and experience fear and anxiety associated with intraoral injections* (Hersh et al. 2016a; Saraghi and Hersh 2017).

**Contraindications (Hersh et al. 2016b; US Food and Drug Asministration 2019)**
- General contraindications:
  - Allergy to any of the components of the solution – ester local anesthetics, (tetracaine, benzocaine, procaine and para-aminobenzoic acid), oxymetazoline, and benzyl alcohol – is an absolute contraindication.
  - Children who weigh less than 40 kg (generally children aged under 12 years).
  - Epistaxis. Intranasal maxillary local anesthesia is not advised in patients with five or more nose bleeds per month.
- Contraindications for oxymetazoline. It is important to remember that the drug has a long half-life (2 hours) (Giannakopoulos et al. 2012):
  - Uncontrolled hypertension. There is potential for a hypertensive event due to the vasoconstrictive effects of oxymetazoline. Nevertheless, the provider is advised to monitor blood pressure.
  - Uncontrolled or active thyroid disease (Ciancio et al. 2013).
  - Interactions with the following medications may lead to a hypertensive reaction (Chapter 10):
    - Nonselective beta-adrenergic blocking agents (Table 10.4, Chapter 10).
    - Tricyclic antidepressants (Table 10.5, Chapter 10).
    - Monoamine oxidase inhibitor antidepressants (Table 10.5, Chapter 10).
  - Administration of other intranasal medications and/or products containing oxymetazoline in the previous 24 hours.
- Contraindications for tetracaine:
  - History of congenital or idiopathic methemoglobinemia because although the literature suggests a lower association with tetracaine, the risk still exists (Levergne et al. 2006; Guay 2009).

**Equipment**

Kovanaze® comes in a prepackaged spray device (similar to a syringe without the needle), known as a *prefilled sprayer* or nasal spray (Figure 20.13). The device consists of 3% tetracaine hydrochloride (30 mg/ml) and 0.05% oxymetazoline chloride (0.5 mg/ml) delivered as a single 0.2-ml dose. In other words, each intranasal spray contains 6 mg of tetracaine hydrochloride and 0.1 mg of oxymetazoline hydrochloride. Each sprayer is intended for a single use and is not to be refilled (Hersh et al. 2016a,b; Saraghi and Hersh 2017).

The sprayers should be stored in the *refrigerator at 36–46 °F (2–8 °C)* and in a dark place if possible. Devices that have been at room temperature for 5 days should not be used. The device should not be autoclaved, wiped with disinfectant, or used if dropped on the ground. It should not be placed in a cartridge warmer (Highlights 2016).

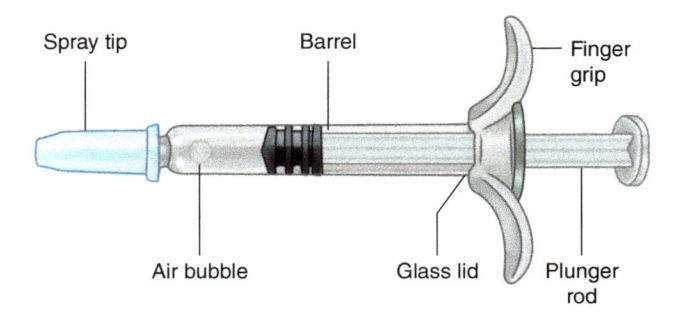

**Figure 20.13** Parts of the prefilled sprayer. *Source:* Redrawn, with modifications, from Kovanaze® instructions for use.

**Preparation**
- Remove two or three prefilled sprayers from the packet using the finger grip. We remove two or three because this is the quantity to be used during the session (see below).
- Check the expiration date (on both the carton and the sprayer label). Check that the solution is clear and colorless. *Note: The presence of a bubble is normal* and does not interfere with the product or dosing. Do not expel the air bubble prior to dosing patient (Figure 20.13).
- Install the finger grip. Snap the finger grip onto the top of the sprayer barrel next to the glass lip (Figure 20.14a,b).
- Remove the gray cap from the prefilled sprayer (Figure 20.14c). The device is now ready for use.

**Technique**

The technique for using Kovanaze® follows a well-established protocol for administration, which we describe below (Ciancio et al. 2013, 2016; Hersh et al. 2016b; Highlights 2016):

- Patient position:
  - The patient must be sitting upright for administration of Kovanaze®.
  - The patient's nose should be perfectly clear and free of mucus.
- *Application of the first prefilled sprayer.* The objective of this stage is for the solution to reach the inferior meatus.
  - Positioning the prefilled sprayer. Place the white tip inside the nostril on the same side as the planned dental procedure (ipsilateral):
    - As parallel as possible to the nasal floor, along the horizontal plane (ala-tragus) at an angle of approximately 90° with respect to the line that joins the nasion and the subnasale (vertical plane) (Figure 20.15a).
    - Parallel toward the septum (midline) of the nasal cavity (Figure 20.15b).

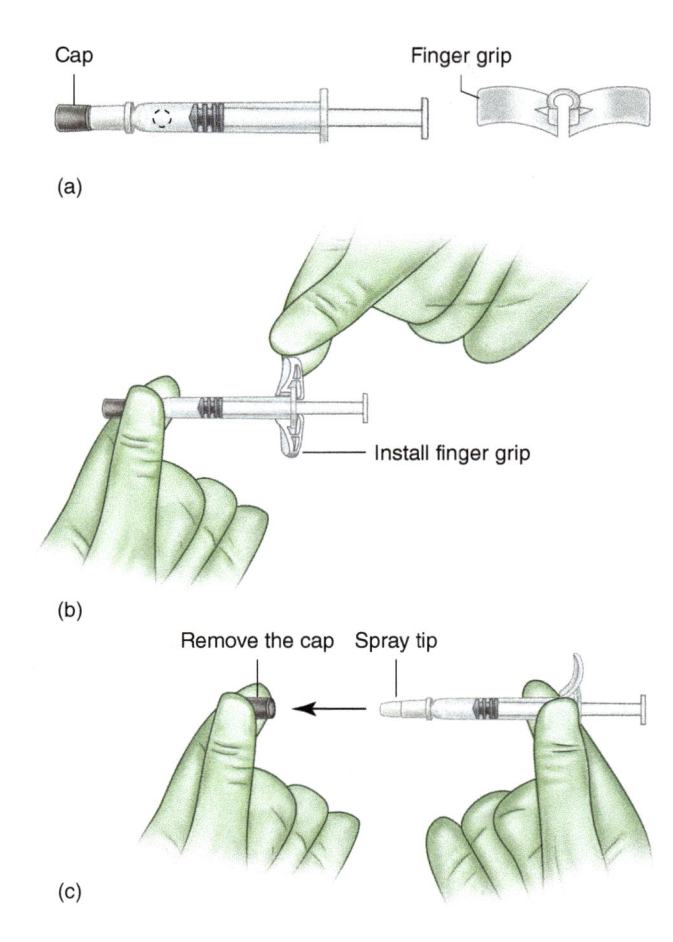

**Figure 20.14** The finger grips and the prefilled sprayer are separate (a). Snap the finger grip onto the top of the sprayer barrel next to the glass lip (b) and remove the gray cap from the prefilled sprayer (c). *Source:* Redrawn, with modifications, from Kovanaze® instructions for use.

- Kovanaze® must be *sprayed rapidly, therefore push hard and fast* on the plunger rod (expel the spray in 0.5 second or less) to create a mist or a plume that can reach and anesthetize the nerves, and wait 4–5 minutes.

Note: Pushing slowly will create a stream (liquid) and not a mist.

- *Application of the second prefilled spray.* The objective here is for the solution to reach the middle meatus. After waiting the necessary time, repeat the maneuver with the other nasal spray, although this time at 45° to the line that joins the nasion with the subnasale (vertical plane) (Figure 20.16a,b) and wait an additional 4–5 minutes.
- After waiting 8–10 minutes in total, we apply the test drill into the dentin to ascertain whether the patient responds. If the patient does not respond (no pain), then continue with the procedure.

- If patient reports discomfort, administer a *third nasal spray*, at the same angle as the second spray (45°) (total 18 mg of tetracaine and 0.3 mg of oxymetazoline), and wait an additional 10 minutes (total 18–20 minutes).

Note: The third spray is contraindicated in children and adolescents (12–18 years) (total of only 12 mg of tetracaine and 0.2 mg of oxymetazoline). At present, Kovanaze® is contraindicated in children weighing less than 40 kg (generally children aged under 12 years).

- If the third nasal spray has failed (or the second in children and adolescents), we can then use a rescue strategy based on standard local anesthesia administered via buccal infiltration.

## Efficacy of the Technique

Clinical success has been evaluated in dental restorative procedures (drilling and filling), where the drill is operated at high speed to penetrate dentin. Table 20.9 shows the success rate to be 85%, although this tends to be greater in incisors and canines (95–100%) than in premolars (60–75%) (Ciancio et al. 2016; Hersh et al. 2016b). However, rigorous assessment with an electric pulp tester shows that *pulpal anesthesia is achieved in 30%*. This is also higher in the incisors and premolars (Capetillo et al. 2019). The success of the technique is low in comparison with buccal infiltration with the standard solution of lidocaine 2% with epinephrine 1:100 000, which has success rates of 90–95% (Capetillo et al. 2019; Annex 21). Consequently, the use of this technique is limited in more invasive procedures such as extractions and endodontic dentistry.

Capetillo reported that these poor results could be explained, at least in part, by the fact that the buccal cortical plate of the first premolar apices is only 0.7–1.8 mm thick (Capetillo et al. 2019). Therefore, during an infiltration, the local anesthetic is delivered very close to the apices of the teeth; in contrast, the apices are 8–9 mm from the sinus floor (Jang et al. 2017).

## Complications Specific to this Technique

Around 70% of patients experience an adverse effect, although, fortunately, these are mild and usually resolve in a few hours (Table 20.10). This section is intended to guide dentists with respect to the most important and frequent signs and symptoms (data shown as rounded percentages), as follows:

- Local complications:
  - Increased secretion of the nasal mucosa (rhinorrhea) in 50%. Nasal dryness is rare (5% of cases).

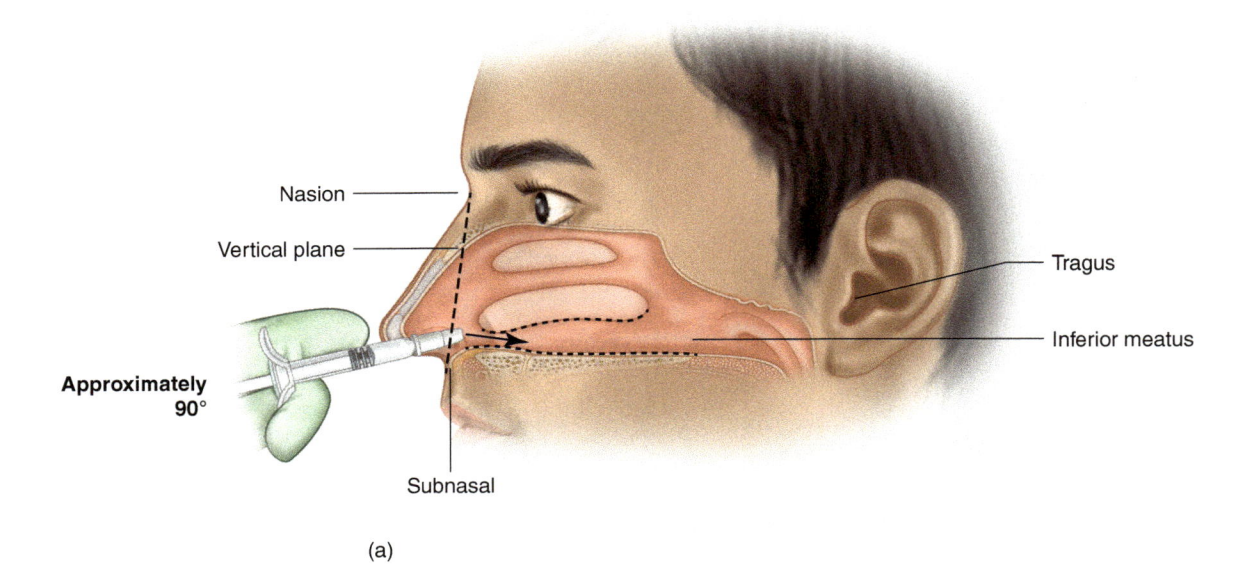

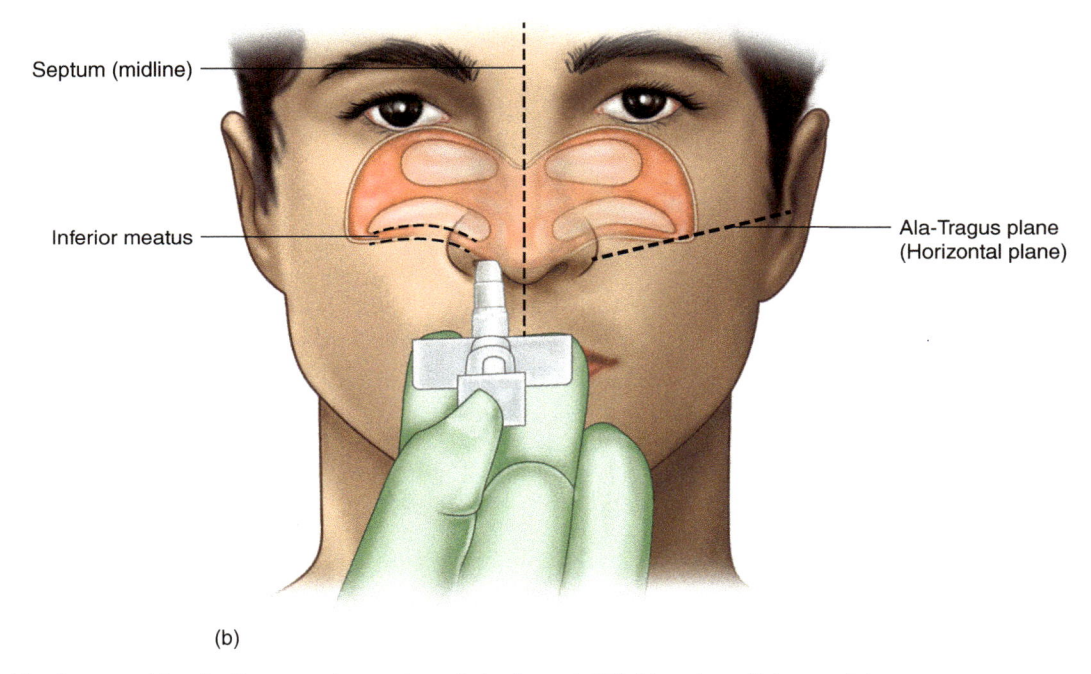

**Figure 20.15** Spray position for first spray (approximately horizontal, 90°) (a) and parallel toward the septum (middle) of the nasal cavity (b). Source: Redrawn, with modifications, from Kovanaze® instructions for use.

- Nasal congestion in 40% of cases with nasal discomfort, stuffy nose, sensation of pressure, and even – albeit more rarely – rhinalgia and nose bleed (epistaxis), both in 5% of cases.
- Throat irritation in 10% of cases, with itching, numbness, burning sensation, and, more rarely, oropharyngeal pain.
- Increased tearing in 10% of cases.
- Sneezing in 3%.

Note: Although most of these complications resolve in minutes or hours, some series have shown epistaxis to persist for 24–48 hours and rhinorrhea and nasal congestion to last a week (Capetillo et al. 2019).

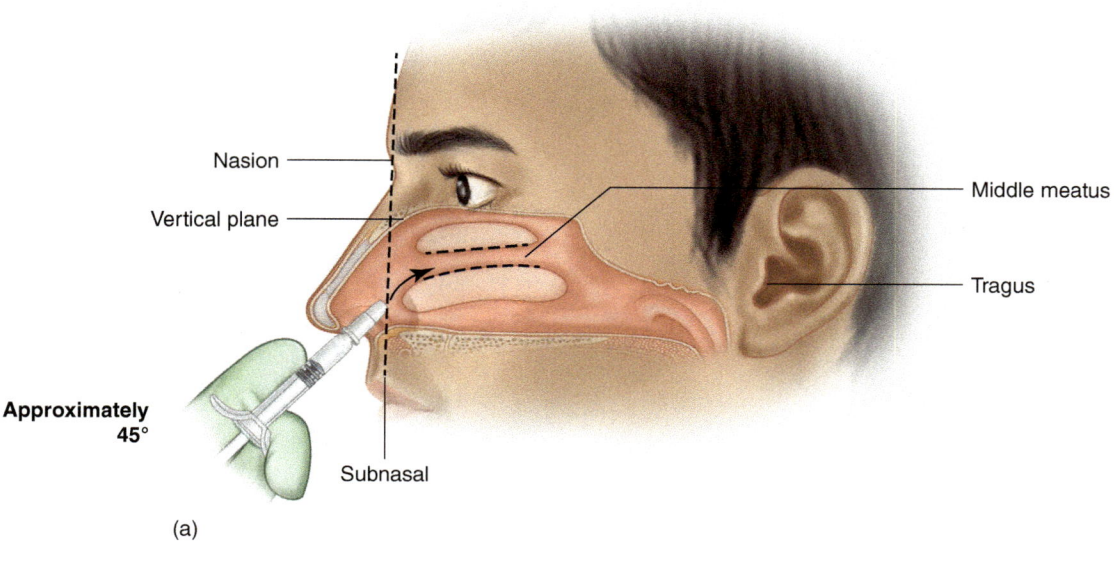

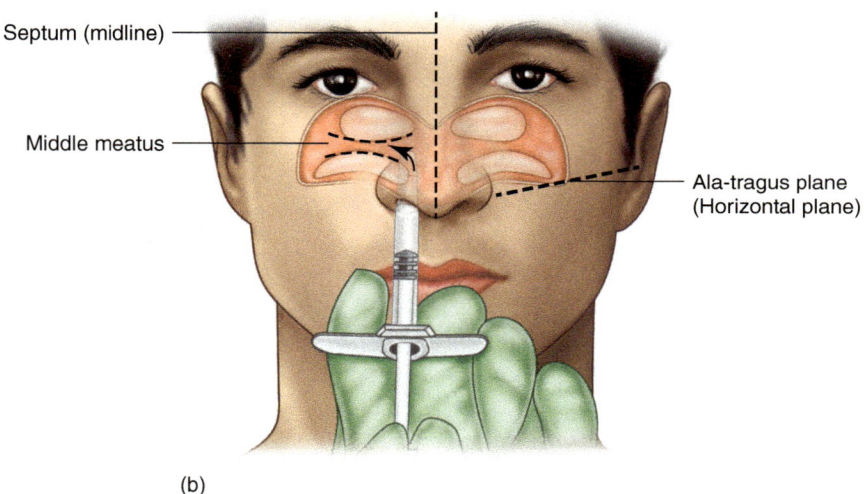

**Figure 20.16** Spray position for second spray (approximately 45°) (a) and parallel toward the septum (midline) of the nasal cavity (b). *Source:* Redrawn, with modifications, from Kovanaze® instructions for use.

**Table 20.9** Percentage of clinical success with Kovanaze® in restorative procedures in the anterior maxillary teeth.

| Reference | Sample size | Success |
|---|---|---|
| Ciancio et al. (2013) | 30 | 83% |
| Ciancio et al. (2016) | 44 | 84% |
| Hersh et al. (2016b) | 100 | 88% |
|  | Rounded | 85% |

- General complications:
  - Headache (cephalea) in 15% of cases.
  - Cardiovascular abnormalities with increased systolic and diastolic arterial pressure, as well as tachycardia and bradycardia in 5–10% of cases.

It is interesting to note that, owing to its vasoconstrictive effect, oxymetazoline enhances the anesthetic efficacy of tetracaine but also increases local and general adverse effects (Ciancio et al. 2016), probably because of its long half-life (2 hours) (Giannakopoulos et al. 2012).

### Advantages and Disadvantages

**Advantages**
1) This system can be used in patients who feel *fear or anxiety associated with intraoral injections and in needle-phobic patients*.
2) Elimination of adverse effects associated with injections. These include hematoma, needle breakage, paresthesia, and trismus.

Table 20.10 Complications specific to this technique (Kovanaze®) as recorded from five clinical trials (percentage of patients affected).

| | Giannakopoulos et al. (2012) N = 12 | Ciancio et al. (2013) N = 30 | Hersh et al. (2016b) N = 100 | Ciancio et al. (2016) N = 44 | Capetillo et al. (2019) N = 50 |
|---|---|---|---|---|---|
| Patients affected | 50% | 37% | 88% | — | 86% |
| Rhinorrhea | 50% | 13% | 57% | 39% | 86% |
| Nasal dryness | 8% | — | 4% | — | — |
| Nasal congestion | 33% | 20% | 24% | 34% | 80% |
| Rhinalgia | — | — | 5% | 7% | — |
| Epistaxis | 17% | — | 3% | — | 6% |
| Throat irritation | 8% | — | 15% | 14% | — |
| Sneezing | — | 3% | 4% | — | — |
| Lacrimation | — | — | 8% | 16% | — |
| Headache | 25% | — | 9% | 14% | — |
| Arterial hypertension | 8% | 3% | 8% | 9% | — |
| Tachycardia/bradycardia | 8% | — | — | 16% | — |

The terms used by the authors to define specific signs and symptoms often differ, with the result that there may be a certain degree of overlap and differences in interpretation, for example nasal discomfort, nasal congestion, and sinus congestion (Ciancio et al. 2016; Hersh et al. 2016b). Similarly, we cannot know whether the same patient presents more than one sign or symptom.

In addition, some signs and symptoms that presented very low frequencies have been eliminated and appear in a single series. Such is the case, for example, of ringing ear (tinnitus) (Giannakopoulos et al. 2012).

3) The absence of an injection means that there is no risk of transmitting infections via the blood (e.g. hepatitis B, hepatitis C, and human immunodeficiency virus).
4) This system reduces the risk of accidental needlestick injuries in clinicians.

**Disadvantages**

The technique has various disadvantages owing to the characteristics of this new method, as previously seen:

1) The *absence of deep pulpal anesthesia*. Evaluation with an electric pulp tester reveals pulpal anesthesia of 30%, which is poor compared with buccal infiltration with the standard solution (Capetillo et al. 2019). Consequently, the technique cannot be used in more invasive procedures such as oral surgery, extractions, endodontic procedures, and preparation of crowns and bridges in vital teeth.
2) The time needed to apply the technique, 10–20 minutes, plus the time necessary for explanations is longer than the 5 minutes (or little more) necessary for a simple buccal infiltration to take effect (Capetillo et al. 2019).
3) The technique is subject to a high frequency of adverse effects. Fortunately, these are of little relevance and resolve in a few minutes or hours.
4) Cost. As with most new medications and technologies, it is more costly than a standard local anesthetic injection. In addition, it can be 30–60 times more expensive than a standard local anesthetic cartridge and needle (Capetillo et al. 2019).
5) Kovanaze® is contraindicated in children weighing less than 40 kg (generally children aged under 12 years).

# References

Andlaw, R.J. and Rock, W.P. (1994). *Manual de odontopediatría*, 3e. Mexico: Interamericana. McGraw-Hill. 85 (Translation: A manual of paedodontics. London: Longman Group. 1993).
Annex 21. Maxillary pulpal anesthesia: buccal infiltration.
Annex 23. Pain resulting from injection techniques.
Annex 32. Computer-controlled injection systems (The Wand).
Annex 33. Jet-injection devices and electronic dental anesthesia.
Anonymous (2002). Local anesthetic delivery system. *J. Am. Dent. Assoc.* 133 (1): 106–107.

Arapostathis, K.N., Dabarakis, N.N., Coolidge, T. et al. (2010). Comparison of acceptance, preference, and efficacy between jet injection Injex and local infiltration anesthesia in 6 to 11 year old dental patients. *Anesth. Prog.* 57 (1): 3–12.

Ashkenazi, M., Blumer, S., and Eli, I. (2005). Effectiveness of computerized delivery of intrasulcular anesthetic in primary molars. *J. Am. Dent. Assoc.* 136 (10): 1418–1425.

Ashkenazi, M., Blumer, S., and Eli, I. (2010). Effect of computerized delivery intraligamental injection in primary molars on their corresponding permanent tooth buds. *Int. Paediatr. Dent.* 20 (4): 270–274.

Baghdadi, Z.D. (1999). Evaluation of electronic dental anesthesia in children. *Oral Surg. Oral Med. Oral Pathol.* 88 (4): 418–423.

Bell, W.A., Traeger, K.A., and Hansen, L.S. (1971). Histologic evaluation of a jet injection of 2 percent lidocaine solution on the oral mucosa of a mixed-breed dog. *Oral Surg. Oral Med. Oral Pathol.* 31 (1): 79–86.

Benito-Brotons, R., Peñarrocha-Oltra, D., Ata-Ali, J., and Peñarrocha, M. (2012). Intraosseous anesthesia with solution injection controlled by a computerized system versus conventional oral anesthesia: a preliminary study. *Med. Oral Patol. Oral Cir. Bucal.* 17 (3): e426–e429.

Bennett, C.R. and Monheim, L.M. (1971). Production of local anesthesia by jet injection. A clinical study. *Oral Surg. Oral Med. Oral Pathol.* 32 (4): 526–530.

Bennett, C.R., Mudell, R.D., and Monheim, L.M. (1971). Studies on tissue penetration characteristics produced by jet injection. *J. Am. Dent. Assoc.* 83 (3): 625–629.

Bishop, T.S. (1986). High frequency neural modulation in dentistry. *J. Am. Dent. Assoc.* 112 (2): 176–177.

Boj, J.R. (1992). La jeringa sin aguja syrijet y su utilidad en pacientes infantiles. *Odontol. Pediatr. (Madrid)* 1 (2): 85–88.

Bradley, J.F., Brooks, B., and Umans, R. (1974). Electroanalgesia in restorative dentistry. *J. Prosthet. Dent.* 32 (2): 171–177.

Brooks, B., Reiss, R., and Umans, R. (1970). Local electroanesthesia in dentistry. *J. Dent. Res.* 49 (2): 298–300.

Burke, F.J.T. (1997). Dentist and patient evaluation of an electronic dental analgesia system. *Quintessence Int.* 28 (9): 609–613.

Burns, Y., Reader, A., Nusstein, J. et al. (2004). Anesthetic efficacy of the palatal-anterior superior alveolar injection. *J. Am. Dent. Assoc.* 135 (9): 1269–1276.

Capetillo, J., Drum, M., Reader, A. et al. (2019). Anesthetic efficacy of intranasal 3% tetracaine plus 0.05% oxymetazoline (Kovanaze) in maxillary teeth. *J. Endod.* 45 (3): 257–262.

Cho, S., Drummond, B.K., Anderson, M.H., and Williams, S. (1998). Effectiveness of electronic dental anesthesia for restorative care in children. *Pediatr. Dent.* 20 (2): 105–111.

Ciancio, S.G., Hutcheson, M.C., Ayoub, F. et al. (2013). Safety and efficacy of a novel nasal sparay for maxillary dental anesthesia. *J. Dent. Res.* 92 (Suppl 1): 43S–48S.

Ciancio, S.G., Marberger, A.D., Ayoub, F. et al. (2016). Comparison of 3 intranasal mists for anesthetizing maxillary teeth in adults: a randomized, double-masked, multicenter phase 3 clinical trial. *J. Am. Dent. Assoc.* 147 (5): 339–347.

Clark, T.M. and Yagiela, J.A. (2010). Advanced techniques and armamentarium for dental local anesthesia. *Dent. Clin. N. Am.* 54 (4): 757–768.

Clark, M.S., Silverstone, L.M., Lindenmuth, J. et al. (1987). An evaluation of the clinical analgesia/anesthesia efficacy on acute pain using the high frequency neural modulator in various dental settings. *Oral Surg. Oral Med. Oral Pathol.* 63 (4): 501–505.

Corbett, I.P., Jaber, A.A., Whitworth, J.M., and Meechan, J.G. (2010). A comparison of the anterior middle superior alveolar nerve block and infraorbital nerve block for anesthesia of maxillary anterior teeth. *J. Am. Dent. Assoc.* 141 (12): 1442–1448.

Croll, T.P. and Simonsen, R.J. (1994). Dental electronic anesthesia for children: technique and report of 45 cases. *J. Dent. Child.* 61 (2): 97–104.

Dabarakis, N.N., Alexander, V., Tsirlis, A.T. et al. (2007). Needle-less local anesthesia: clinical evaluation of the effectiveness of the jet anesthesia Injex in local anesthesia in dentistry. *Quintessence Int.* 38 (10): E572–E576.

Domínguez, A., Aznar, T., and Galán, A. (1998). Anestesia dental electrónica en pacientes preescolares. *Odontol. Pediátr. (Madrid)* 6 (1): 7–11.

Donaldson, D., Quarnstrom, F., and Jastak, J.T. (1989). The combined effect of nitrous oxide and oxygen and electrical stimulation during restorative dental treatment. *J. Am. Dent. Assoc.* 118 (6): 733–736.

te-Duits, E., Goepferd, S., Donly, K. et al. (1993). The effectiveness of electronic dental anesthesia in children. *Pediatr. Dent.* 15 (3): 191–196.

ElGeneidy, A.K., Bloom, A.A., Skerman, J.H., and Stallard, R.E. (1974). Tissue reaction to jet injection. *Oral Surg. Oral Med. Oral Pathol.* 38 (4): 501–511.

Epstein, S. (1971). Pressure injection of local anesthetics: clinical evaluation of an instrument. *J. Am. Dent. Assoc.* 82 (2): 374–377.

Esposito, C.J., Shay, J.S., and Morgan, B. (1993). Electronic dental anesthesia: a pilot study. *Quintessence Int.* 24 (3): 167–170.

Ferguson, J. (1770). *An Introduction to Electricity. In Six Sections*. London: Printed for W. Straham and T. Cadell. 73.

Figge, F.H.J. and Scherer, R.P. (1947). Anatomical studies on jet penetration of human skin for subcutaneous medication without the use of needles. *Anat. Rec.* 97 (3): 335. (abstract no. 17).

Friedman, M.J. and Hochman, M.N. (1997). A 21st century computerized injection system for local pain control. *Compendium* 18 (10): 995–1003.

Friedman, M.J. and Hochman, M.N. (1998). The AMSA injection: a new concept for local anesthesia of maxillary teeth using a computer-controlled injection system. *Quintessence Int.* 29 (5): 297–303.

Friedman, M.J. and Hochman, M.N. (1999). P-ASA block injection: a new palatal technique to anesthetize maxillary anterior teeth. *J. Esthet. Dent.* 11 (2): 63–71.

Friedman, M.J. and Hochman, M.N. (2001). Using AMSA and P-ASA nerve blocks for esthetic restorative dentistry. *Gen. Dent.* 49 (5): 506–511.

Froum, S.J., Tarnow, D., Caiazzo, A., and Hochman, M.N. (2000). Histologic response to intraligament injections using a computerized local anesthetic delivery system. A pilot study in mini-swine. *J. Periodontol.* 71 (9): 1453–1459.

Fukayama, H., Yoshikawa, F., Kohase, H. et al. (2003). Efficacy of anterior middle superior alveolar (AMSA) anesthesia using a new injection system: the wand. *Quintessence Int.* 34 (7): 537–541.

Garellek, A.L. (1967). Clinical evaluation of a jet injector for local anaesthesia. *J. Can. Dent. Assoc.* 33 (6): 329–332.

Ghaderi, F. and Ahmadbeigi, M. (2018). Pain perception due to dental injection by Smartject: split mouth design study. *J. Dent. (Shiraz)* 19 (1): 57–62.

Giannakopoulos, H., Levin, L.M., Chou, J.C. et al. (2012). The cardiovascular effects and pharmacokinetics of intranasal tetracaine plus oxymetazoline. Preliminary findings. *J. Am. Dent. Assoc.* 143 (8): 872–880.

Gibson, R.S., Allen, K., Hutfless, S., and Beiraghi, S. (2000). The Wand vs. traditional injection: a comparison of pain related behaviors. *Pediatr. Dent.* 22 (6): 458–462.

Goodell, G.G., Gallagher, F.J., and Nicoll, B.K. (2000). Comparison of a controlled injection pressure system with a conventional technique. *Oral Surg. Oral Med. Oral Pathol.* 90 (1): 89–94.

Grace, E.G., Barnes, D.M., Macek, M.D., and Tatum, N. (2000). Patient and dentist satisfaction with computerized local anesthetic injection system. *Compendium* 21 (9): 746–752.

Grace, E.G., Barnes, D.M., Reid, B.C. et al. (2003). Computerized local dental anesthetic systems: patient and dentist satisfaction. *J. Dent.* 31 (1): 9–12.

Grau, T., Ernst, C.-P., and Willerhausen, B. (1997). Eine nadellose, intraorale Injektionstechnik. *Schweiz. Monatsschr. Zahnmed.* 107 (11): 993–998.

Greenfield, W. and Karpinski, J.F. (1972). Needleless jet injection in comprehensive pain control and applications to oral surgery. *Anesth. Prog.* 19 (4): 94–97.

Greenfield, W. and Karpinsky, J.F. (1973). Clinical application of jet injection to comprehensive pain control. *Anesth. Prog.* 20 (4): 110–112.

Guay, J. (2009). Methemoglobinemia related to local anesthetics: a summary of 242 episodes. *Anesth. Analg.* 108 (3): 837–845.

Harvey, M. and Elliott, M. (1995). Transcutaneous electrical nerve stimulation (TENS) for pain management during cavity preparations in pediatric patients. *J. Dent. Child.* 62 (1): 49–51.

Hawkins, J.M. and Moore, P.A. (2002). Local anesthesia: advances in agents and techniques. *Dent. Clin. N. Am.* 46 (4): 719–732.

Hersh, E.V., Saraghi, M., and Moore, P.A. (2016a). Intranasal tetracaine and oxymetazoline: a newly approved drug formulation that provides maxillary dental anesthesia without needles. *Curr. Med. Res. Opin.* 32 (11): 1919–1925.

Hersh, E.V., Pinto, A., Saraghi, M. et al. (2016b). Double-masked, randomized, placebo-controlled study to evaluate the efficacy and tolerability of intranasal K305 (3% tetracaine plus 0.05% oxymetazoline) in anesthetizing maxillary teeth. *J. Am. Dent. Assoc.* 147 (4): 278–287.

Hersh, E.V., Saraghi, M., and Moore, P.A. (2017). Two recent advances in local anesthesia: intranasal tetracaine/oxymetazoline and liposomal bupivacaine. *Curr. Oral Health Rep.* 4: 189–196.

Highlights of Prescribing Information (2016). *Kovanaze (Tetracaine HCL and Oxymetazoline HCL) Nasal Spray*. Fort Colins (Colorado): St. Renatus.

Hingson, R.A. and Hughes, J.G. (1947). Clinical studies with jet injection. A new method of drug administration. *Anesth. Analg.* 26 (6): 221–230.

Hochman, R. (1988). Neurotransmitter modulator (TENS) for control of dental operative pain. *J. Am. Dent. Assoc.* 116 (2): 208–212.

Hochman, M.N. and Friedman, M.J. (2000). In vitro study of needle deflection: a linear insertion technique versus a bidirectional rotation insertion technique. *Quintessene Int.* 31 (1): 33–39.

Hochman, M., Chiarello, D., Hochman, C.B. et al. (1997). Computerized local anesthesia delivery vs traditional syringe technique. Subjective pain response. *N. Y. Stat. Dent. J.* 63 (7): 24–29.

Ikehara, N.K., McKibben, D.H., Pechersky, J.L., and Rapp, R. (1972). Comparison of jet injection and needle-syringe injection techniques in production of edema. *J. Dent. Res.* 51 (2): 573–576.

Jang, J.K., Kwak, S.W., Ha, J.H., and Kim, H.C. (2017). Anatomical relationship of maxillary posterior teeth with the sinus floor and buccal cortex. *J. Oral Rehabil.* 44 (8): 617–625.

Jedrychowski, J.R. and Duperon, D.F. (1993). Effectiveness and acceptance of electronic dental anesthesia by pediatric patients. *J. Dent. Child.* 60 (3): 186–192.

Jones, C.M. and Blinkhorn, A.S. (1996). Dental electro-anaesthesia in children: a pilot study. *Int. J. Paediatr. Dent.* 6 (2): 107–110.

Kämmerer, P.W., Schneider, D., Pacyna, A.A., and Daunbländer, M. (2016). Movement control during aspiration with different injection systems via video monitoring – an in vitro model. *Clin. Oral Investig.* 21 (1): 105–110.

Kane, K. and Taub, A. (1975). A history of local electrical analgesia. *Pain* 1 (2): 125–138.

Katch, E.M. (1986). Applications of transcutaneous electrical nerve stimulation in dentistry. *Anesth. Prog.* 33 (3): 156–160.

Kramer, I.R.H. (1962). Distribution in the tissues of fluid injected by high-pressure jet. *J. Dent. Res.* 41 (6): 1255. (abstract no. 17).

Krochak, M. and Friedman, N. (1998). Using a precision-metered injection system to minimize dental injection anxiety. *Compendium* 19 (2): 137–148.

Kutscher, A.H. and Zegarelli, E.V. (1965). An intraoral jet injection technique: clinical impressions. *N. Y. J. Dent.* 35 (6): 219–222, 224.

Kutscher, A.H., Zegarelli, E.V., Cain, E.A. et al. (1964). Jet injection as a means of obtaining oral mucosal anesthesia: a preliminary report. *J. Oral Surg. Anesth. Hosp. Dent. Serv.* 22: 310.

Lambrianidis, T., Rood, J.P., and Sowray, J.H. (1979–1980). Dental analgesia by jet injection. *Br. J. Oral Surg.* 17: 227–231.

Langthasa, M., Yeluri, R., Jain, A.A., and Munshi, A.K. (2012). Comparison of the pain perception in children using comfort control syringe and a conventional injection technique during pediatric dental procedures. *J. Indian Pedod. Prev. Dent.* 30 (4): 323–328.

Laster, A.M. and Pressman, R.S. (1975). An evaluation of an electroanesthetic device. *J. Am. Dent. Assoc.* 90 (4): 816–821.

Lee, S., Reader, A., Nusstein, J. et al. (2004). Anesthetic efficacy of the anterior middle superior alveolar (AMSA) injection. *Anesth. Prog.* 51 (3): 80–89.

Lethinen, R. (1979). Efficiency of jet injection technique in production of local anesthesia. *Proc. Finn. Dent. Soc.* 75 (1): 13–14.

Levergne, S., Darmon, M., Levy, V., and Azoulay, E. (2006). Methemoglobinemia and acute hemolysis after tetracaine lozenge use. *J. Crit. Care* 21 (1): 112–114.

Malamed, S.F., Quinn, C.L., Torgersen, R.T., and Thompson, W. (1989). Electronic dental anesthesia for restorative dentistry. *Anesth. Prog.* 36 (4–5): 195–198.

Margetis, P.M., Quarantillo, E.P., and Lindberg, R.B. (1958). Jet injection local anesthesia in dentistry. *U.S. Armed Forces Med. J.* 9 (5): 625–634.

Meechan, J.G. and Winter, R.A. (1996). A comparison of topical anaesthesia and electronic nerve stimulation for reducing the pain of intra-oral injections. *Br. Dent. J.* 181 (9): 333–335.

Meechan, J.G., Gowans, A.J., and Welbury, R.R. (1998). The use of patient-controlled transcutaneous electronic nerve stimulation (TENS) to decrease the discomfort of regional anaesthesia in dentistry: a randomized controlled clinical trial. *J. Dent.* 26 (5–6): 417–420.

Mellor, A.C. (1993). A comparison of injectable local anesthesia and electronic dental anesthesia in restorative dentistry. *Anesth. Pain Control Dent.* 2 (3): 177–179.

Melzack, R. and Wall, P.D. (1965). Pain mechanisms: a new theory. *Science* 150 (3699): 971–979.

Miegimolle, M., Martínez, E.V., Gallegos, L., and Planells, P. (2005). Evaluación del sistema de anestesia Injex® en el paciente odontopediátrico. Estudio piloto. *Odontol. Pediatr. (Madrid)* 13 (2): 45–53.

Modaresi, A., Lindsay, S.J.E., Gould, A., and Smith, P. (1996). A partial double-blind, placebo-controlled study of electronic dental anaesthesia in children. *Int. J. Paediatr. Dent.* 6 (4): 245–251.

Munshi, A.K., Hegde, A.M., and Girdhar, D. (2000a). Clinical evaluation of electronic dental anesthesia for various procedures in pediatric dentistry. *J. Clin. Pediatr. Dent.* 24 (3): 199–204.

Munshi, A.K., Hegde, A., and Bashir, N. (2000b). Clinical evaluation of the efficacy of anesthesia and patient preference using the needle-less jet syringe in pediatric dental practice. *J. Clin. Pediatr. Dent.* 25 (2): 131–136.

Nicholson, J.W., Berry, T.G., Summitt, J.B. et al. (2001). Pain perception and utility: a comparison of the syringe and computerized local injection techniques. *Gen. Dent.* 49 (2): 167–173.

Nusstein, J., Burns, Y., Reader, A. et al. (2004a). Injection pain and postinjection pain of the palatal-anterior superior alveolar injection, administered with the wand plus® systemcomparing 2% lidocaine with 1:100,000 epinephrine to 3% mepivacaine. *Oral Surg. Oral Med. Oral Pathol.* 97 (2): 164–172.

Nusstein, J., Lee, S., Reader, A. et al. (2004b). Injection pain and postinjection pain of the anterior middle superior alveolar injection administered with the Wand® or conventional syringe. *Oral Surg. Oral Med. Oral Pathol.* 98 (1): 124–131.

Nusstein, J., Berlin, J., Reader, A. et al. (2004c). Comparison of injection pain, heart rate increase, and postinjection pain of articaine and lidocaine in primary intraligamentary injection administered with a computer-controlled local anesthetic delivery system. *Anesth. Prog.* 51 (4): 126–133.

Öztas, N., Ölmez, A., and Yel, B. (1997). Clinical evaluation of transcutaneous electronic nerve stimulation for pain control during tooth preparation. *Quintessence Int.* 28 (9): 603–608.

Öztas, N., Ulsun, T., Bodur, H., and Dogan, C. (2005). The Wand in pulp therapy: an alternative to inferior alveolar nerve block. *Quintessence Int.* 36 (7–8): 559–564.

Pirkner, A., Pimlott, J.F.L., and Tritscher, H. (1995). Electronic anesthesia: it's suitable and application to dental hygiene practice. *J. Dent. Res.* 74 (AADR abstracts): 193. (abstract no. 1452).

Quarnstrom, F. and Libed, E.N. (1994). Electronic anesthesia versus topical anesthesia for the control of injection pain. *Quintessence Int.* 25 (10): 713–716.

Quarnstrom, F.C. and Quinn, C.L. (1995). Electronic dental analgesia (Chapter 14). In: *Local Anesthesia of Oral Cavity* (ed. J.T. Jastak, J.A. Yagiela, and D. Donaldson). Philadelphia: WB Saunders Co. 313–327.

Ram, D. and Kaissirer, J. (2006). Assessment of a palatal approach—anterior superior alveolar (P-ASA) nerve block with the Wand® in paediatric dental patients. *Int. J. Paediatr. Dent.* 16 (5): 348–351.

Ram, D. and Peretz, B. (2003). Assessing the pain reaction of children receiving periodontal ligament anesthesia using a computerized device (Wand). *J. Clin. Pediatr. Dent.* 27 (3): 247–250. (NB. In the study, the first author's name appears as "Ran" when it is actually "Ram").

Rogers, B.S., Botero, T.M., McDonald, N.J. et al. (2014). Efficacy of articaine versus lidocaine as a supplemental buccal infiltration in mandibular molars with irreversible pulpitis: a prospective, randomized, double-blind study. *J. Endod.* 40 (6): 753–758.

Romero-Galvez, J., Berini-Aytes, L., Figueiredo, R., and Amabat-Dominguez, J. (2016). A randomized Split-mouth clinical trial comparing pain experienced during palatal injections with traditional syringe versus controlled-flow delivery Calaject technique. *Quintessence Int.* 47 (9): 797–802.

Saloum, F.S., Braumgartner, J.C., Marshall, G., and Tinkle, J. (2000). A clinical comparison of pain perception to the Wand and a traditional syringe. *Oral Surg. Oral Med. Oral Pathol.* 89 (6): 691–695.

Saraghi, M. and Hersh, E.V. (2017). Intranasal tetracaine and oxymetazoline spray for maxillary local anesthesia without injections. *Gen. Dent.* 65 (2): 16–19.

Saravia, M.E. and Bush, J.P. (1991). The needleless syringe: efficacy of anesthesia and patient preference in child dental patients. *J. Clin. Pediatr. Dent.* 15 (2): 109–112.

Sasa, I. and Donly, K.J. (1995). Extraoral electronic dental anesthesia for invasive restorative procedures in children. *J. Dent. Res.* 74 (AADR abstracts): 27. (abstract no. 124).

Savage, M. (1982). Clinical use of dental electro-analgesia. *Br. Dent. J.* 152 (7): 242–244.

Schmidt, D.A. (1966). Anesthesia by jet-injection in the practice of pedodontics. *J. Dent. Child.* 33 (6): 340–352.

Segura, A., Kenellis, M., and Donly, K.J. (1995). Extraoral electronic dental anesthesia for moderate procedures in pediatric patients. *J. Dent. Res.* 74 (AADR abstracts): 27. (abstract no. 123).

Shane, S.M. and Kessier, S. (1967). Electricity for sedation in dentistry. *J. Am. Dent. Assoc.* 75 (6): 1369–1375.

Silverstone, L.M. (1989). Electronic dental anaesthesia. *Dent. Pract.* 27 (11): 1–2.

Sixou, J.-L. and Barbosa-Rogier, M.E. (2008). Efficacy of intraosseous injections of anesthetic in children and adolescents. *Oral Surg. Oral Med. Oral Pathol.* 106 (2): 173–178.

Sixou, J.-L., Marie-Cousin, A., Huet, A. et al. (2009). Pain assessment by children and adolescents during intraosseous anaesthesia using a computerized system (QuickSleeper™). *Int. J. Paediatr. Dent.* 19 (5): 360–366.

STA (Single Tooth Anesthesia) system (2015). *Featuring the Wand STA Handpiece*. Livingston (NJ): Milestone Scientific Inc.

Stephens, R.R. (1962). Jet injection of local anesthetic solutions for dental procedures. *J. Dent. Res.* 41 (6): 1255. (abstract no. 16).

Stephens, R.R. and Kramer, I.R.H. (1964). Intra-oral injections by high pressure jet. *Br. Dent. J.* 117 (11): 465–481.

Trapp, L.D. and Davies, R.O. (1980). Aspiration as a function of hypodermic needle internal diameter in the in vivo human upper limb. *Anesth. Prog.* 49 (2): 49–51.

Tzafalia, M. and Sixou, J.-L. (2011). Administration of anesthetics using metal syringes. An ex vivo study. *Anesth. Prog.* 58 (2): 61–65.

US Food and Drug Asministration. Drugs@FDA: FDA approved Drug Products. Kovanaze. http://www.accessdata.fda.gov/scripts/ceder/daf/index.cfm?event=overview. Process & Appl No =208032 (accessed March 1 2019).

Vardanyan, R.S. and Hruby, V.J. (2006). Adrenergic (sympathomimetic) drugs. Chapter 11. In: *Synthesis of Essential Drugs* (ed. R.S. Vardanyan and V.J. Hruby). Amsterdan: Elsevier BV. 142–159.

Villette, A. (1984). L'anesthésie intradiploïque (transcorticale), ses moyens, ses possibilities. *Chir. Dent. Fr.* 54 (239): 45–51.

Villette, A. (2003). Untersuchungs-bilanzaus 500 in erster Intention durchgeführten Trans-Kortikalis-Anásthesien. *Schweiz Monatsschr Zahnmed* 113 (11): 1211–1214.

Vongsavan, K. and Vongsavan, N. (1996). Comparison of topical anesthesia gel and TENS in reducing pain. *J. Dent. Res.* 75 (Special Issue): 248. (abstract no. 1841).

Warren, J., Ziherl, F.A., Kish, A.W., and Ziherl, L.A. (1955). Large-scale administration of vaccines by means of an automatic jet injection syringe. *JAMA* 157 (8): 633–637.

Whitehead, F.I.H. and Young, I. (1968). An intra-oral jet injection instrument. A histological, bacteriological and clinical assessment. *Br. Dent. J.* 125 (10): 437–440.

Yap, A.U.J. and Ho, H.C.W. (1996). Electronic and local anesthesia: a clinical comparison for operative procedures. *Quintessence Int.* 27 (8): 549–553.

Yap, A.U.J. and Ong, G. (1996). An introduction to dental electronic anesthesia. *Quintessence Int.* 27 (5): 325–331.

# 21

## Local Anesthesia in Children

This short chapter examines the special case of children undergoing dental local anesthesia treatment. For all of the techniques addressed in this book, we have provided data on the methodological and anatomical variations and specific details that must be taken into account when treating children. Here, we bring together the most important aspects of this patient group, even though most have been addressed elsewhere in the book.

## The Problem with Children and Adolescents

Control of pain during dental treatment in children and adolescents is essential, not only to be able to carry out the procedure, but also because trauma at this age *determines the patient's attitude to dental treatment in the future*. It is in this age group that patients *develop high levels of anxiety and phobias* that lead them to avoid treatment in the future (McClure 1968; Molin and Seeman 1970; Lautch 1971; Cohen et al. 1982; Berggren and Meynert 1984; Rankin and Harris 1984).

Table 21.1 shows that pain is poorly controlled in 15% of children. The problem is even more serious because dentists tend to think that pain is poorly controlled in fewer cases than actually occurs (Nakai et al. 2000). Various circumstances favor failure of dental local anesthesia in children and adolescents, as follows:

1) Preschool age (<5–6 years) (Wright et al. 1991; Sharaf 1997; Tyrer 1999; Lind-Strömberg 2001). Children in this age group are unable to understand the need to cooperate with the dentist (Pinkham and Schroeder 1975), even though their bones are more porous and thus facilitate diffusion of the anesthetic solution.
2) High levels of anxiety. Treatment fails in 55% of patients who experience excess anxiety (Nakai et al. 2000). Remember that seeing the syringe and needle and feeling the needle prick are the most anxiety-inducing aspects of treatment (Lautch 1971; Gale 1972; Meldman 1972; Berggren and Meynert 1984; Scott et al. 1984; LeClaire et al. 1988).
3) Probability of failure of local anesthesia. This can reach 20% in patients who have previously experienced symptoms of pain (Nakai et al. 2000).

## Local Anesthetic Solutions

The most commonly used anesthetic solutions in children and adolescents are as follows:

- Standard lidocaine 2% with epinephrine 1:100 000 (10 µg/ml) or 1:80 000 (12.5 µg/ml) (L-100 or L-80) is the solution most commonly used to achieve pulpal anesthesia in children, both for mandibular block and for maxillary and mandibular buccal infiltration. There are various reasons for this choice:
  - As children's bones are smaller and more porous, the standard solution is very well diffused and successful pulpal anesthesia is achieved.
  - The standard solution makes it possible to administer a greater volume of the solution in milliliters depending on the child's weight, since the maximum limits are greater than with most anesthetic solutions used in dentistry (Annex 10). This makes the approach much safer.
- Lidocaine 2% with epinephrine 1:50 000 (20 µg/ml) (L-50), which contains twice the amount of epinephrine as the standard solution, is used to *complement buccal infiltration* of lidocaine 2% with epinephrine 1:100 000 (10 µg/ml) when pulpal anesthesia is not achieved (Gruber 1950). It is important to remember the criterion of not mixing two anesthetics at the same site (see Chapter 5). In this case, the anesthetic is the same; only the concentration of epinephrine varies. As this is double and thus more potent, pulpal anesthesia is more efficacious (Annex 21).

---

*Local Anesthesia in Dentistry: A Locoregional Approach*, First Edition. Jesús Calatayud and Mana Saraghi.
© 2024 John Wiley & Sons Ltd. Published 2024 by John Wiley & Sons Ltd.
Companion website: www.wiley.com/go/Calatayud/local

Table 21.1 Failure of local anesthetic in children.

| Reference | Sample size | Failure |
|---|---|---|
| Kuster and Rakes (1987) | 4134 | 12.8% |
| Kaufman et al. (1991) | 151 | 27% |
| Jones et al. (1995) | 308 | 20.5% |
| Nakai et al. (2000) | 361 | 11.6% |
| Naidu et al. (2004) | 101 | 9% |
|  |  | 16.2% |
|  | Rounded average | 15% |

- Articaine 4% with epinephrine 1:100 000 (10 μg/ml) (A-100) is recommended *only for buccal infiltration* in anterior and posterior teeth in the maxilla and mandible in special cases:
  o To achieve successful pulpal anesthesia in children, which is difficult with the standard solution (e.g. anterior mandibular teeth with irreversible acute pulpitis).
  o To achieve anesthesia of primary mandibular molars with periapical infiltration when mandibular block is contraindicated (e.g. patients with hemophilia) (Dudkiewicz et al. 1987; Donohue et al. 1993).
  o To reinforce mandibular block (with the standard solution) in mandibular molars that are particularly difficult to anesthetize (e.g. irreversible acute pulpitis).
- This solution of articaine has some disadvantages:
  o *It is contraindicated in children aged under 4 years* because, although its safety has been demonstrated in clinical trials (Wright et al. 1989), it must be verified with more data and clinical studies (Malamed et al. 2000, 2001; Katyal 2010).
  o There may be more cases of self-injury of the lips, tongue, and buccal mucosa because of the longer duration of soft tissue anesthesia (Adewuni et al. 2008; Chopra et al. 2016; Annex 21).

Other anesthetic solutions can also be administered (mepivacaine, prilocaine), although they are much less effective (Annex 21). Solutions with long-lasting anesthesia, such as bupivacaine, are contraindicated in children aged under 12 years owing to the risk of self-injury (Laskin et al. 1977; Jensen et al. 1981; Moore 1984).

## Anesthetic Technique in Children

Here, we would like to draw attention to the most relevant aspects of the techniques applied with children:

1) Topical anesthetics in aerosolized form are not recommended for children (especially children under 6-year age) because they may lead to sudden uncooperative behavior owing to the noise they make and a bad taste as the anesthetic spreads through the mouth (Frasier 1967; Evers and Haegerstam 1981), and thus yield poor results (Chapter 12 and Annex 19). The preferred form is gel, ointment, cream, or paste (Annex 19).

2) In each technique, the quantity of solution administered to children younger than 6–8 years is *usually half that administered to adults* to avoid overdosage. For example, if we were injecting the standard solution of lidocaine 2% with epinephrine 1:100 000 (10 μg/ml) in the conventional mandibular block technique (inferior alveolar nerve block), then our approach would be as follows:

   In an adult weighing 52 kg and in another weighing 86 kg, we would inject 1 cartridge (i.e. 1.8 ml) to achieve mandibular block. If we had to administer additional injections in these adults, for example maxillary and mandibular buccal infiltrations, the absolute maximum dose would be 6.2 cartridges for the patient weighing 52 kg and 8.5 cartridges for the patient weighing 86 kg (Annex 10).

   In a 5-year-old child weighing 20 kg, we would inject half a cartridge (i.e. 0.9 ml) to achieve mandibular block (*half the adult dose*). If we had to administer additional injections, for example maxillary and mandibular buccal infiltrations, the absolute maximum dose would be 2.5 cartridges (Annex 10).

3) The injection should not take long. When an injection takes too long, the child becomes nervous and subjectively associates the injection with pain (Jones et al. 1995). This problem is partly resolved in little children because they receive half the dose and therefore the injection takes half the time.

4) Vasovagal syncope is uncommon. The frequency of vasovagal syncope in children aged under 14 years is very low (1 per 2000 = 0.05%) because children react to emotional tension differently from adults; they do not repress the fight-or-flight response, but rather scream, cry, throw a tantrum, or resist the injection, therefore a vasovagal reaction does not occur (Kuster and Udin 1985). In young adults, on the other hand, one-third are thought to be susceptible to this type of reaction (Yjipaavalniemi and Sane 1981).

5) Self-injury may be more frequent. Self-injury is a problem with children since after dental treatment the soft tissue remains anesthetized and, in some cases, the patient may bite and injure his/her lip, buccal mucosa, and tongue. Thus, the main associated factors are as follows:
   - Age. Owing to the child's immaturity, the frequency of self-injury increases with younger age (College et al. 2000; Adewuni et al. 2008).

- The duration of anesthesia in the soft tissues. Since the frequency of self-injury increases with the duration of anesthesia (Adewuni et al. 2008), it is not recommended to use articaine 4% solution with epinephrine 1:100 000 (10 µg/ml), even though it is not contraindicated. As seen above, bupivacaine 0.5% with epinephrine 1:200 000 is contraindicated.

Interestingly, bilateral mandibular block leads to self-injury less frequently than unilateral mandibular block (counterintuitive). This may be due to the following two factors (College et al. 2000):
- Bilateral mandibular block is performed in longer, more extensive treatments, therefore the child's soft tissues are anesthetized for shorter periods after leaving the dentist's office.
- The sensation of symmetrical soft tissue anesthesia on both sides leaves the child less likely to explore the mouth and bite him/herself.

The measures dentists can take to prevent these lesions or at least reduce their frequency in children are as follows:
- Explain to the parents that the child should not chew or take very hot drinks while the lips remain anesthetized (tingling, numbness, dullness, tickling, or fat lip). This point should be emphasized to both parents and children.
- Place a cotton roll between the lips and the cheek. Pediatric dentists use this trick with children for the duration of soft tissue anesthesia. The child should be reminded not to chew.
- Injection of phentolamine (OraVerse®) may prove useful in the areas where the anesthetic solution was injected to reduce the duration of anesthesia in the soft tissues after treatment (Tavares et al. 2008; Zurfluh et al. 2015; Hersh et al. 2017, 2019) (see Chapter 6).

6) Supplementary techniques. If the conventional techniques is not sufficient and anesthesia fails, we can turn to supplementary techniques (mainly periodontal ligament [PDL] technique), but in children, we can use supplementary techniques *only in permanent teeth*, not in primary teeth, so as not to affect the buds of the underlying permanent teeth (Brännström et al. 1984), although these abnormalities are minimal (Chapter 18). The exceptions to this contraindication are as follows:

   o Children with severe coagulation abnormalities (Spuller 1988). The PDL technique is an alternative to mandibular block.
   o Computer-controlled PDL injections (The Wand), since pressure is controlled and there are no enamel abnormalities (Ashkenazi et al. 2010).

## Anesthesia of the Primary Mandibular Molars

The primary mandibular molars can be anesthetized in several ways:

1) Standard mandibular block. Children aged 6–8 years receive half a cartridge (0.9 ml) with the standard solution of lidocaine L-100 or L-80. After waiting 5 minutes, onset of soft tissue anesthesia in the lower lip (a sign that the mandibular block is taking effect) should be verified, thus indicating that the inferior alveolar nerve has been anesthetized. Complementary buccal infiltration with a further half a cartridge of standard lidocaine solution is recommended in the posterior mandibular molars, which require good pulpal anesthesia.

   It is important to note that complementary anesthesia is applied after 5 minutes to avoid the risk of overlapping anesthesia of the lower lip via mandibular block with that of the infiltration and thus masking failure of the block.

2) Buccal infiltration of the primary molars with the more potent articaine solution (A-100) in half a cartridge to a full cartridge (0.9–1.8 ml) to avoid using mandibular block. This method has some advantages:
   - As it is easier to administer, it could prove useful in children who are more difficult to manage, such as small children (McClure 1968).
   - As there is no anesthesia of the tongue, the risk of self-injury is reduced (Dudkiewicz et al. 1987).
   - It is a good option for hemophiliac patients, as we have seen, since mandibular block is usually contraindicated in this population (Dudkiewicz et al. 1987; Donohue et al. 1993).

   The disadvantage of this approach is that it may be less effective than mandibular block, especially in the second primary molar, possibly because the cortical layer is thicker at this level and we use standard lidocaine solution as complementary buccal anesthesia (Wright et al. 1991; Sharaf 1997), therefore articaine solution with epinephrine 1:100 000 is preferred because it is effective even in irreversible acute pulpitis (Veena and Mytri 2015; Chopra et al. 2016).

3) Traditional mandibular block with the standard solution of lidocaine (L-100 or L-80). After verifying that the lower lip has been anesthetized, we wait 5 minutes before injecting complementary buccal anesthesia with a potent solution such as articaine (A-100) or lidocaine (L-50).

It is important to note that in this case, when we apply complementary buccal anesthesia with articaine, we follow the criterion of not mixing two local anesthetics at the same site (see Chapter 5). Thus, we use standard lidocaine solution in the pterygomandibular space and articaine in the buccal region. When complementary anesthesia is with L-50, we are using the same anesthetic, albeit at greater potency, since it contains double the amount of epinephrine (Annex 21).

This option is used in cases where it is difficult to anesthetize the patient, such as in acute pulpitis, to guarantee successful anesthesia, although we do not recommend it as routine practice.

### Needles and Mandibular Block

A survey in the United States indicated that 40% of pediatric dentists use 30G needles for mandibular block and that almost 80% used short needles (Kohli et al. 2001). If we review cases of needle breakage in mandibular block, we can observe the following:

1) *In more than 70% of cases, the needles used were inappropriate for the technique* as they were 30G or short or both (Annex 37).
   - 30G needles (0.3 mm in diameter) are the finest, and many dentists still think that these needles make injection and anesthesia less painful than thicker calibers (27G, 0.4 mm and 25G, 0.5 mm) (Smith 1968; Cooley and Robinson 1979; Fuller et al. 1979); however, clinical trials have not shown that 30G needles are less painful than the other two, which are thicker but more resistant to breakage (Table 11.3, Chapter 11).
   - In mandibular block, short needles (≤25 mm) are easily inserted into the soft tissues as far as the hub, which is the weakest part and the point at which the needle breaks (Pietruszka et al. 1986; Bhatia and Bounds 1998; Zelster et al. 2002; Ethunandan et al. 2007; Pogrel 2009; Shah et al. 2009).
2) *In 30% of cases of needle breakage, the patients are children* (Annex 37): of note, children aged under 18 years account for 16% of the population in Spain (INE 2015) and for 23% of the population in the United States (Census 2015). This observation is closely associated with the possible lack of cooperation among children (around 20% of cases involved patients aged <8 years [Annex 37]) and the habitual use of short 30G needles for mandibular block by pediatric dentists (Kohli et al. 2001).

Chapter 22 provides a more careful analysis of needle breakage. *In conclusion, long 27G or 25G needles should be used for mandibular block in children.*

### Remarks on Buccal Infiltration

- Many authors report that mandibular block is more painful than buccal infiltration (Jones et al. 1995; Oulis et al. 1996; Sharaf 1997; Chopra et al. 2016), although other clinical trials have not found this to be the case (Brownbill et al. 1987). We believe that there is no difference if we follow the indications for mandibular block shown in Chapter 16.

- Many clinical studies have shown more soft tissue anesthesia with mandibular block than with buccal infiltration and therefore a greater risk of self-injury (Wright et al. 1991; Donohue et al. 1993; Oulis et al. 1996). However, it is also important to note that if A-100 solution is used as complementary buccal anesthesia, then the effect of the anesthetic takes longer to wear off in soft tissues than with the standard solution (Annex 21).

## References

Adewuni, A., Hall, M., Guelmann, M., and Riley, J. (2008). The incidence of adverse reactions following 4% septocaine (articaine) in children. *Pediatr. Dent.* 30 (5): 424–428.

Annex 10. Maximum doses of dental local anesthetic solutions.

Annex 19. Topical anesthesia I. Results from clinical trials.

Annex 21. Maxillary pulpal anesthesia: buccal infiltration.

Annex 37. Needle breakage.

Ashkenazi, M., Blumer, S., and Eli, I. (2010). Effect of computerized delivery intraligamental injection in primary molars on their corresponding permanent tooth buds. *Int. J. Paediatr. Dent.* 20 (4): 270–275.

Berggren, U. and Meynert, G. (1984). Dental fear and avoidance: causes, symptoms, and consequences. *J. Am. Dent. Assoc.* 109 (2): 247–251.

Bhatia, S. and Bounds, G. (1998). A broken needle in the pterygomandibular space: report of a case and review of the literature. *Dent. Update* 25 (1): 35–37.

Brännström, M., Lindskog, S., and Nordenvall, K.-J. (1984). Enamel hypoplasia in permanent teeth induced by periodontal ligament anesthesia of primary teeth. *J. Am. Dent. Assoc.* 109 (5): 735–736.

Brownbill, J.W., Walker, P.O., Bourcy, B.D., and Keenan, K.M. (1987). Comparison of inferior dental nerve block injections in child patients using 30-gauge and 25-gauge short needles. *Anesth. Prog.* 34 (6): 215–219.

Census (2015). www.census.gov (accessed July 10 2017).

Chopra, R., Marwaha, M., Bansal, K., and Mittal, M. (2016). Evaluation of buccal infiltration with articaine and inferior alveolar nerve block with lignocaine for pulp therapy in mandibular primary molars. *J. Clin. Pediatr. Dent.* 40 (4): 301–305.

Cohen, L.A., Snyder, T.L., and LaBelle, A.D. (1982). Correlates of dental anxiety in a university population. *J. Public Health Dent.* 42 (3): 228–235.

College, C., Feigal, R., Wandera, A., and Strange, M. (2000). Bilateral versus unilateral mandibular block anesthesia in a pediatric population. *Pediatr. Dent.* 22 (6): 453–457.

Cooley, R.L. and Robinson, S.F. (1979). Comparative evaluation of the 30-gauge dental needle. *Oral Surg. Oral Med. Oral Pathol.* 48 (5): 400–404.

Donohue, D., García-Godoy, F., King, D.L., and Barnwell, G.M. (1993). Evaluation of mandibular infiltration versus block anesthesia in pediatric patients. *J. Dent. Child.* 60 (2): 104–106.

Dudkiewicz, A., Schwartz, S., and Laliberté, R. (1987). Effectiveness of mandibular infiltration in children using the local anesthetic Ultracaine® (articaine hydrochloride). *J. Can. Dent. Assoc.* 53 (1): 29–31.

Ethunandan, M., Tran, A.L., Anand, R. et al. (2007). Needle breakage following inferior alveolar nerve block: implications and management. *Br. Dent. J.* 2002 (7): 395–397.

Evers, H. and Haegerstam, G. (1981). *Handbook of Dental Local Anesthesia*. Copenhagen: Schultz Medical International. 65, 171.

Frasier, I.M. (1967). Local anesthetics. In: *Premedication, Local and General Anesthesia in Dentistry* (ed. A.B. Jorgensen and J. Hayden). Philadelphia: Lea and Febiger. 89–96.

Fuller, N.P., Menke, R.A., and Meyers, W.J. (1979). Perception of pain of three different intraoral penetrations of needles. *J. Am. Dent. Assoc.* 99 (5): 822–824.

Gale, E.M. (1972). Fears of the dental situation. *J. Dent. Res.* 51 (4): 964–966.

Gruber, L.W. (1950). Preliminary report in the use of xylocaine as a local anesthetic in dentistry. *J. Dent. Res.* 29 (2): 137–142.

Hersh, E.V., Lindemeyer, R., Berg, J.H. et al. (2017). Phase four, randomized, double-blinded, controlled trial of phentolamine mesylate in two- to five-year-old patients. *Pediatr. Dent.* 39 (1): 39–45.

Hersh, E.V., Moore, P.A., and Saraghi, M. (2019). Phentolamine mesylate: pharmacology, efficacy, and safety. *Gen. Dent.* 67 (3): 12–17.

INE (2015). www.ine.es (accessed July 10 2017).

Jensen, O.T., Upton, L.G., Hayward, J.R., and Sweet, R.B. (1981). Advantages of long-acting local anesthetic using etidocaine hydrochloride. *J. Oral Surg.* 39 (5): 350–353.

Jones, C.M., Heimann, J., and Gerrish, A.C. (1995). Children's ratings of dental injection and treatment pain, and the influence of the time taken to administer the injection. *Int. J. Pediatr. Dent.* 4 (2): 81–85.

Katyal, V. (2010). The efficacy and safety of articaine versus lidocaine in dental treatments: a meta-analysis. *J. Dent.* 38 (4): 307–317.

Kaufman, E., Holan, G., Goodman-Topper, E., and Eidelmen, E. (1991). Evaluation of students' performance in obtaining local anaesthesia in children. *Int. J. Paediatr. Dent.* 1 (3): 147–150.

Kohli, K., Ngan, P., Crout, R., and Linscott, C.C. (2001). A survey of local and topical anesthesia use by pediatric dentists in the United States. *Pediatr. Dent.* 23 (39): 256–269.

Kuster, C.G. and Rakes, G. (1987). Frequency of inadequate local anaesthesia in child patients. *J. Paedtr. Dent.* 3 (1): 7–9.

Kuster, C. and Udin, R.D. (1985). Vasopressor syncope in children: incidence and treatment. *J. Pedod.* 9 (3): 210–217.

Laskin, J.L., Wallace, W.R., and De Leo, B. (1977). Use of bupivacaine hydrochloride in oral surgery – a clinical study. *J. Oral Surg.* 35 (1): 25–29.

Lautch, E. (1971). Dental phobia. *Br. J. Psychiatry* 119 (549): 151–158.

LeClaire, A.J., Skidmore, A.E., Griffin, J.A. Jr., and Balaban, F.S. (1988). Endodontic fear survey. *J. Endod.* 14 (11): 560–564.

Lind-Strömberg, U. (2001). Rectal administration of midazolam for conscious sedation of uncooperative children in need of dental treatment. *Swed. Dent. J.* 25 (3): 105–111.

Malamed, S.F., Gagnon, S., and Leblanc, D. (2000). A comparison between articaine HCl and lidocaine HCl in pediatric dental patients. *Pediatr. Dent.* 22 (4): 307–311.

Malamed, S.F., Cagnon, S., and Leblanc, D. (2001). Articaine hydrochloride: a study of the safety of a new amide local anesthetic. *J. Am. Dent. Assoc.* 132 (2): 177–185.

McClure, P.B. (1968). Local anesthesia for the preschool child. *J. Dent. Child.* 35 (6): 441–448.

Meldman, M.J. (1972). The dental-phobia test. *Psychosomatics* 13 (6): 371–372.

Molin, C. and Seeman, K. (1970). Disproportionate dental anxiety. Clinical and nosological considerations. *Acta Odontol. Scand.* 28 (2): 197–212.

Moore, P.A. (1984). Bupivacaine: a long-acting local anesthetic for dentistry. *Oral Sug. Oral Med. Oral Pathol.* 58 (4): 369–374.

Naidu, S., Loughlin, P., Coldwell, S.E. et al. (2004). A randomized controlled trial comparing mandibular local anesthesia techniques in children receiving nitrous oxide-oxygen sedation. *Anesth. Prog.* 51 (1): 19–23.

Nakai, Y., Milgrom, P., Mancl, L. et al. (2000). Effectiveness of local anesthesia in pediatric dental practice. *J. Am. Dent. Assoc.* 131 (12): 1699–1705.

Oulis, C.J., Vadiakas, G.P., and Vasilopoulou, A. (1996). The effectiveness of mandibular infiltration compared to mandibular block anesthesia in treating primary molars in children. *Pediatr. Dent.* 18 (4): 301–305.

Pietruszka, J.F., Hoffman, D., and McGivern, B.E. Jr. (1986). A broken dental needle and its surgical removal: a case report. *N. Y. State Dent. J.* 52 (7): 28–31.

Pinkham, J.R. and Schroeder, C.S. (1975). Dentist and psychologist: practical consideration for team approach to the intensely anxious dental patient. *J. Am. Dent. Assoc.* 90 (5): 1022–1026.

Pogrel, M.A. (2009). Broken local anesthetic needles. A case series of 16 patients, with recommendations. *J. Am. Dent. Assoc.* 140 (12): 1517–1522.

Rankin, J.A. and Harris, M.B. (1984). Dental anxiety: the patient's point of view. *J. Am. Dent. Assoc.* 109 (1): 43–47.

Scott, D.S., Hirschman, R., and Schroeder, K. (1984). Historical antecedents of dental anxiety. *J. Am. Dent. Assoc.* 108 (1): 42–45.

Shah, A., Mehta, N., and Von Arx, D.P. (2009). Fracture of a dental needle during administration of an interior alveolar nerve block. *Dent. Update* 36 (1): 20–25.

Sharaf, A.A.T. (1997). Evaluation of mandibular infiltration versus block anesthesia in pediatric dentistry. *J. Dent. Child.* 64 (4): 276–281.

Smith, N.A. (1968). An investigation of the influence of gauge on some physical properties of hypodermic needles. Part I. The relation between gauge and flexibility of the needle. *Aust. Dent. J.* 13: 158–161.

Spuller, R.L. (1988). Use of the periodontal ligament injection in dental care of the patient with haemophilia – a clinical evaluation. *Spec. Care Dent.* 81 (1): 28–29.

Tavares, M., Goodson, J.M., Student-Pavlovich, D. et al. (2008). Reversal of soft-tissue local anesthesia with phentolamine mesylate in pediatric patients. *J. Am. Dent. Assoc.* 139 (8): 1095–1104.

Tyrer, G.L. (1999). Referrals for dental general anaesthetics – how many really need GA? *Br. Dent. J.* 187 (8): 440–443.

Veena, A. and Mytri, P. (2015). Anaesthetic efficacy of 4% articaine mandibular buccal infiltration compared to 2% lignocaine inferior alveolar nerve block in children with irreversible pulpitis. *J. Clin. Diagn. Res.* 9 (4): 65–67.

Wright, G.Z., Weinberger, S.J., Friedman, C.S., and Plotzke, O.B. (1989). Use of articaine local anesthesia in children under 4 years of age – a retrospective report. *Anesth. Prog.* 36 (6): 268–271.

Wright, G.Z., Weinberg, S.J., Martin, R., and Plotzke, O. (1991). The effectiveness of infiltration anesthesia in mandibular primary molar region. *Pediatr. Dent.* 13 (5): 278–283.

Yjipaavalniemi, P. and Sane, J. (1981). Changes in heart rate during injection of local anesthetics. *Proc. Finn. Dent. Soc.* 77 (6): 346–349.

Zelster, R., Cohen, C., and Casap, N. (2002). The complications of a broken needle in the pterygomandibular space: clinical guidelines for prevention and retrieval. *Pediatr. Dent.* 24 (2): 153–156.

Zurfluh, M.A., Daubländer, M., and Van Waes, H.J.M. (2015). Comparison of two epinephrine concentrations in an articaine solution for local anesthesia in children. *Swiss Dent. J.* 125 (6): 698–703.

**Complications**

# 22

## Local Complications of Dental Local Anesthesia

Local complications caused by or associated with dental local anesthesia can be classified according to onset (Laskin 1984; Vega 1998): (i) as immediate or accidental complications, when they appear during treatment in the office, or (ii) as late complications, or simply complications, when they appear after the patient has left the office.

Local complications are more frequent than general complications, although, fortunately, the vast majority resolve spontaneously without severe problems for the patient and without leaving sequelae (Laskin 1984). Table 22.1 shows these complications, their association with onset (immediate or late), and their severity.

In 1997 (Vega 1998) and during 2000–2010 (Perea-Perez et al. 2014), 4% of adverse effects (local or general) recorded in Spain were associated with dental local anesthesia.

## Persistent Post-injection Pain

Disappearance of local anesthesia effect is sometimes followed by slight discomfort at the injection site, which is usually of little clinical relevance (Jorkjend and Skoglund 1999); however, persistent moderate-to-severe pain may be present and may last several days.

Persistent post-injection pain is unusual in maxillary buccal infiltration and affects approximately 1% of cases of persistent pain (Table 22.2). This is natural, given the low degree of trauma involved in this technique at this level (Kennedy et al. 2001; Evans et al. 2008), and the pain disappears spontaneously within 3 days (Evans et al. 2008). Post-injection pain is much more frequent in mandibular block and is thought to affect 5% of cases (Table 22.2), possibly because it is a much more traumatic technique. This complication usually resolves spontaneously within 3–4 days (Dunbar et al. 1996; Ridenour et al. 2001; Mikesell et al. 2005).

## Self-inflicted Injury

Anesthesia of the soft tissue persists after the dental treatment session, and some patients (mainly young children and developmentally disabled patients) may bite and injure their lips, jugal mucosa, and tongue.

The frequency of these lesions was unknown until recently, not because they were uncommon, but because of the few problems they generally cause. Pediatric dentists estimate their *frequency to be 5%* or slightly greater (College et al. 2000; Ram and Amir 2006), and studies based on case series agree, reporting the frequency to be around 7% (Table 22.3). However, this percentage only refers to the most severe cases, given that clinical studies focusing on self-inflicted injury report a frequency of 13% (College et al. 2000; Adewuni et al. 2008), possibly because they include small lesions such as redness or swelling that are noticed by the dentist but not by parents (College et al. 2000). The lesions affect the lips (13%), buccal mucosa (10%) (cheeks), and tongue (6%) (Adewuni et al. 2008).

Once soft tissue anesthesia resolves, red and inflamed lesions appear on the affected tissues and, in the more severe cases, may become ulcerated and painful. The lesions heal spontaneously in less than 2 weeks. We have already seen that the cause is accidental biting of the anesthetized tissues. Occasional cases of burning by cigarette smoke have been recorded in adults. The associated factors are as follows:

1) Age. Smaller children are more likely to experience self-inflicted injury because of their age (College et al. 2000; Adewuni et al. 2008). The same applies to patients with intellectual disability.
2) The duration of anesthesia in soft tissues. The longer the duration, the greater the frequency of self-inflicted injuries (Adewuni et al. 2008).

---

*Local Anesthesia in Dentistry: A Locoregional Approach*, First Edition. Jesús Calatayud and Mana Saraghi.
© 2024 John Wiley & Sons Ltd. Published 2024 by John Wiley & Sons Ltd.
Companion website: www.wiley.com/go/Calatayud/local

**Table 22.1** Local complications of dental local anesthesia: severity and onset.

|  | Severity | | Onset | |
| --- | --- | --- | --- | --- |
| Complication | Mild | Severe | Immediate | Late |
| 1) Persistent pain | + | | | + |
| 2) Self-inflicted injury | + | | | + |
| 3) Facial blanching | + | | + | |
| 4) Delay cutaneous lesion | + | | | + |
| 5) Facial hematoma | + | | + | + |
| 6) Nerve lesions | + | + | + | + |
| 7) Trismus | + | + | + | + |
| 8) Facial palsy | + | + | + | + |
| 9) Ocular complications | + | + | + | + |
| 10) Infections | | + | | + |
| 11) Mucosal ulceration | + | + | | + |
| 12) Breakage of needles | | + | + | |
| 13) Breakage of cartridges | + | + | + | |
| 14) Aural complications | + | + | + | |

**Table 22.2** Moderate to severe pain after maxillary buccal infiltration and mandibular block.

| Reference | Sample size | Persistent pain |
| --- | --- | --- |
| **Maxillary infiltration** | | |
| Kennedy et al. (2001) | 120 | 0% |
| Evans et al. (2008) | 80 | 0% |
| Hersh et al. (2008) | 122 | 2.5% |
| | | 0.83% ≈ **1%** |
| **Mandibular block** | | |
| Krafft and Hickel (1994) | 12 104 | 0.32% |
| Dunbar et al. (1996) | 40 | 5% |
| Reitz et al. (1998) | 38 | 0% |
| Ridenour et al. (2001) | 30 | 14% |
| Mikesell et al. (2005) | 57 | 5% |
| Mikesell et al. (2005) | 57 | 21% |
| Goodman et al. (2006) | 46 | 7% |
| Hersh et al. (2008) | 122 | 5% |
| Willett et al. (2008) | 25 | 8% |
| | | 7% ≈ **5%** |

3) Bilateral mandibular block. Surprisingly, bilateral block has a lower incidence of self-inflicted lesions than unilateral block, possibly for two reasons (College et al. 2000):
   - Bilateral mandibular block is used in more extensive and longer treatments, therefore duration of soft

**Table 22.3** Percentage of lesions resulting from biting after dental local anesthesia.

| Reference | Age (years) | Lesions |
| --- | --- | --- |
| College et al. (2000) | 2–18 | 13% |
| Malamed et al. (2001) | <13 | 0.07% |
| Ram and Amir (2006) | 5–13 | 5% |
| Adewuni et al. (2008) | 2–14 | 13% |
| Peñarrocha-Oltra et al. (2012) | 11–55 | 4% |
| Hersh et al. (2017) | 2–5 | 2% |
| | | 6.2% ≈ **5%** |

tissue anesthesia is shorter when the child leaves the dentist's office.
   - The sensation of symmetrical paresthesia on both sides means that the patient is less likely to explore and bite the tissue.

The measures that dentists can take to prevent, or at least reduce, the probability of these lesions in children are as follows:

1) Explain to patients (especially children and their caregivers) that they cannot chew or have very hot drinks while the lips continue to feel numb (tingling sensation, numbness, dullness, swollen or fat lip).
   - Adults should be advised not to smoke.
   - Some patients claim that they can chew with the other (nonanesthetized) side, although it must be stressed that both sides tend to be used unconsciously when chewing and that chewing may be more difficult than the patients perceive it to be.
   - This must be emphasized to both children and parents.
2) Place a cotton roll between the lips and cheek. This is a commonly utilized practice in pediatric dentistry; the cotton roll is left in place for as long as the soft tissue anesthesia persists, reminding the patient not to chew their lips or cheeks.
3) Phentolamine (OraVerse®) could prove very useful in the areas where the anesthetic solution has been injected to reduce numbness in the soft tissue after treatment (Tavares et al. 2008; Zurfluh et al. 2015; Hersh et al. 2017) (Chapter 6).

## Facial Blanching

Although the real frequency of this condition is unknown, it is thought to be frequent and has been reported to account for 1% of all cases of numbness caused by dental local anesthetic (Lustig and Zusman 1999).

Blanching (ischemic paling) is characterized by blood loss during the injection or immediately after. It affects the skin of the face (cheek) on the maxilla and disappears spontaneously after 10–30 minutes without sequelae (Kronman and Giunta 1987; Heasman and Reid 1995; Aravena et al. 2016).

## Anesthetic Techniques Involved

- Mandibular block with the conventional or direct technique (Kronman and Giunta 1987; Heasman and Reid 1995; Webber et al. 2001; Uckan et al. 2006; Paul et al. 2009; Aravena et al. 2016), the Gow-Gates technique (Dryden 1993) or the Laguardia–Akinosi technique (Donkor et al. 1990).
- In the maxillary arch, the techniques involved are buccal infiltration, posterior superior alveolar nerve block, the high tuberosity technique (Kronman and Giunta 1987; Lustig and Zusman 1999), and the transpalatal (greater palatine canal) approach (Mercuri 1979).

## Clinical Manifestations

Blanching appears on the same side of the face as the injection, with the following:

1) Facial blanching, which is characterized by the following:
   - Onset on the skin of the face below the lower eyelid (infraorbital), malar or zygomatic region, side of the nose, and above the nasolabial fold (cheek). It manifests as a continuous white patch (Figure 22.1) or occasionally two patches (Kronman and Giunta 1987). Blanching is easily observed in persons whose skin is not black (Mercuri 1979) and disappears spontaneously after 10–30 minutes (Kronman and Giunta 1987; Heasman and Reid 1995; Paul et al. 2009; Aravena et al. 2016; Kumaresan et al. 2018).
   - The patch can sometimes extend intraorally to the maxillary gingiva (Heasman and Reid 1995; Aravena et al. 2016), hard palate (Dryden 1993; Heasman and Reid 1995; Aravena et al. 2016; Kumaresan et al. 2018), or even to the lower lip (Webber et al. 2001).
   - An asymptomatic sign (only observed by the dentist), although the patient may initially feel numbness, itching, a burning sensation, or even shooting pain, in the affected area (Mercuri 1979; Webber et al. 2001; Uckan et al. 2006; Paul et al. 2009; Aravena et al. 2016; Kumaresan et al. 2018).
2) While rare, ocular complications (see section "Ocular Complications") of the have been described (Dryden 1993; Webber et al. 2001; Chiappelli and Cajulis 2002; Uckan et al. 2006) and include the following:
   - Double vision (diplopia).
   - Sensation of numbness, burning, or even pain in the eye and periorbital area.
   - Drooping of the upper eyelid (ptosis).
   - Ischemic paling may extend to the eyelids and forehead (Webber et al. 2001; Uckan et al. 2006).

   In these cases, ocular manifestations are the main event, with blanching no more than an accompanying sign.

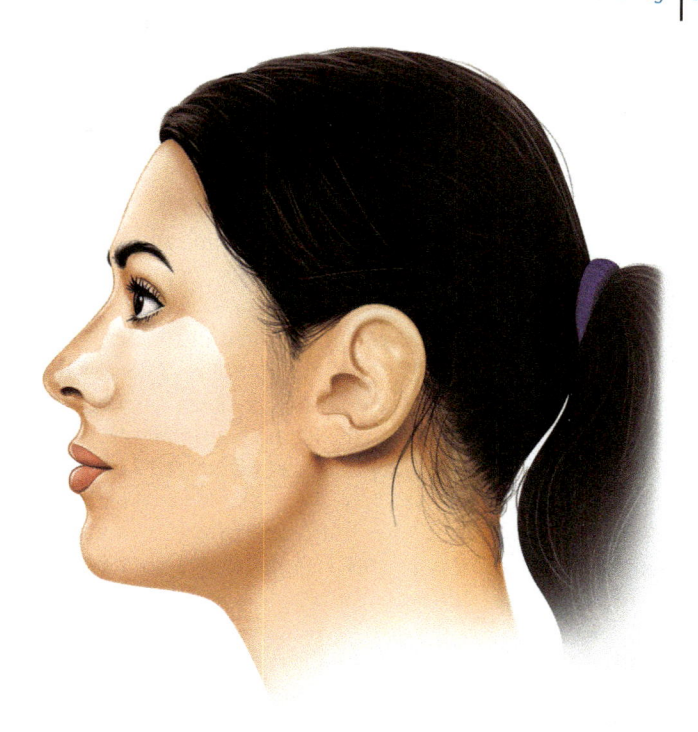

**Figure 22.1** Area affected by facial blanching.

## Causes and Pathophysiology

### Proposed Causes

1) Irritation of sympathetic fibers surrounded the arteries (perivascular sympathetic plexus) by the tip of the needle at the injection site can cause reflex vasoconstriction along the terminal branches, in this case at the level of the skin (this may occur internally, although we do not see it). Since aspiration is negative in most cases, this seems to be the most common explanation (Laskin 1984; Kronman and Giunta 1987; Lustig and Zusman 1999).
2) Epinephrine from the local intravascular anesthetic injected is transported to the terminal peripheral branches of the skin of the face (Kumaresan et al. 2018).

### Pathophysiology

Vasoconstriction follows the path of the superior alveolar arteries (in injections into the superior arch) or of the lower alveolar arteries (in mandibular block) to the maxillary artery, from where it will reach the infraorbital artery, whose branches perfuse the skin (zygoma, infraorbital border, wing of the nose). One variant is from the maxillary artery to the greater palatine artery (palate).

Injecting directly into the maxillary artery (not from the alveolar arteries) is also possible (Kronman and Giunta 1987; Heasman and Reid 1995). It is important to remember the anatomical variations of the maxillary artery, which runs superficially and laterally to the lateral (external) pterygoid muscle at this level (Pretterklieber et al. 1991). The maxillary artery varies widely in diameter (2–6 mm) (Biermann 1943) and often descends to the mandibular foramen (Lacouture et al. 1983) (Figure 3.13, Chapter 13).

Another possibility is the retrograde flow of the anesthesia, and especially the vasoconstrictor, from the alveolar arteries to the maxillary artery. This option is less probable (Heasman and Reid 1995).

## Localized Late-onset Skin Lesion

The frequency of this type of lesion, which affects the skin of the lips, is unknown, although it is thought to be exceptional, given that very few cases have been reported. It is noteworthy that most occur after mandibular block in children aged 7–10 years (Table 22.4).

### Clinical Manifestations

The affected skin depends on the region where the anesthesia is injected. Thus, in cases of mandibular block, the skin of the lower lip is affected above the chin or adjacent to the commissure; the skin of the upper lip is affected in maxillary infiltrations.

Clinical manifestations appear during the first hours (30 minutes to 3 hours) after administration of the anesthetic (rarely before 3 days) (Table 22.4) and are characterized by the appearance of a reddish patch (*erythematous macule*), which is usually accompanied by itching (*pruritus*) or a burning sensation. Occasionally, it first manifests as a pale patch that progresses to an erythematous macule within a few hours (Torrente-Castells et al. 2008).

During the following days or weeks, the lesion progresses to necrosis of the skin with formation of a crust that leaves a *pigmented or hypopigmented* area or simply a scar on healing. Sensory alterations on the chin are a potential sequela (Krüger and Nehse 1991).

### Causes and Pathophysiology

The causes are not well known, although two possible mechanisms have been posited (Curley and Baxter 1987):

#### Ischemic Necrosis Due to Vasospasm

Vasoconstriction results from needle-induced irritation of the sympathetic fibers surrounding the arterial wall, thus leading to vasoconstriction along the terminal branches, in

Table 22.4 Characteristics of cases of localized delayed skin lesion

| Reference | Age/sex | Technique | Skin affected | Anesthetic ml/LAS | Time to onset |
|---|---|---|---|---|---|
| Lederman et al. (1980) | 7/♀ | MB left | Lower lip Chin | 1.8/L-100 | 30 min |
|  | 8/♀ | MB left | Lower lip Chin | <1.8/L-100 | 1 h |
|  | 7/♀ | MB left | Lower lip near commissure | 1.8/L-100 | 45 min |
|  | 9/♀ | MB left | Lower lip near commissure | –/L-100 | 2 h |
| Curley and Baxter (1987) | 7/♀ | InfP left | Upper lip | 2.2/L-50-50 | Hours |
| Krüger and Nehse (1991) | 33/♀ | MB left + inf mental | Lower lip Chin | 5.4/A-100 | 3 days |
| Torrente-Castells et al. (2008) | 10/♀ | MB left + inf mental | Lower lip Chin | 1.8/A-100 | 3 h |

MB, mandibular block; inf mental, infiltration in mental nerve; InfP, buccal infiltration in posterior upper arch (molars); ml, injected milliliters; LAS, local anesthetic solution: L-100, lidocaine 2% with epinephrine 1:100 000; A-100, articaine 4% with epinephrine 1:100 000; L-50-50, lidocaine with epinephrine 1:50 000 and with norepinephrine 1:50 000.

this case at the level of the skin. It may also be caused by exogenous epinephrine injected intravascularly that is transported toward the terminal peripheral branches of the skin of the face.

In mandibular block, the path covered by the vasoconstrictor effect runs from the inferior alveolar artery (branch of the maxillary artery) to its mental branch and from here by anastomosis (Kawai et al. 2006) with the submandibular and inferior labial arteries (both branches of the facial artery), leading to vasoconstriction of the vessels of the skin of the chin (Torrente-Castells et al. 2008). Direct injection into the area of the mental nerve is an aggravating factor, leading to vasospasm of the arteries that supply the skin of the chin and the intraoral mucosa in the region of the lower canine and first mandibular premolar (Krüger and Nehse 1991; Torrente-Castells et al. 2008).

### Type III Allergic Reaction

A type III allergic reaction, or immune complex–mediated reaction (e.g. Arthus reaction or serum sickness), is an antigen–antibody reaction in the walls of the blood vessels that leads to acute vasculitis with tissue necrosis. This reaction manifests *locally within a few hours*. It very rarely occurs with local anesthetics (Lederman et al. 1980).

In cases of type III allergic reaction, skin allergy tests usually yield negative results (Lederman et al. 1980; Curley and Baxter 1987), although when the same drug is applied at the same site, the late skin eruption re-occurs. However, when another solution is used, the reaction does not appear (Lederman et al. 1980).

## Facial Hematomas

A hematoma is caused by extravasation of blood from a vessel to the surrounding tissue as a result of needle injury (Kuster and Udin 1984). If the vessel is an artery, blood accumulates quickly; if it is a vein, blood accumulates slowly (Laskin 1984). In all cases, bleeding is self-limiting because of pressure from the surrounding tissue.

Many techniques can lead to hematoma, for example mandibular block, although given that the vessels are very deep, the hematoma is not clinically visible (Kuster and Udin 1984). Even so, small hematomas are common on the oral mucosa as a result of techniques involving maxillary infiltration into the lateral incisors and first molars: hematoma has been estimated to appear in 1% of cases (Evans et al. 2008), although with the minimum volume/minimum injection time technique, this frequency is multiplied since several injections are made at the same site.

In this section, we will examine hematomas that appear on the skin of the face, but not the smaller yet common hematomas that appear on the mucosa.

### Technical Factors Contributing to Hematomas

The techniques that most frequently lead to hematomas on the face are as follows:

1) Injections into the area of the upper molars in buccal infiltration, posterior superior alveolar nerve block, and high tuberosity approaches (Bennett 1984; Laskin 1984; Roberts and Sowray 1987; Jastak et al. 1995; Malamed 2004). At this level, 0.5% of injections can lead to facial hematoma (Kuster and Udin 1984), especially when the needle is inserted higher and deeper, since it is easier to inject into a branch of the pterygoid venous plexus or the posterior superior alveolar artery (Harn et al. 2002).
2) Block applied at the level of the foramina (infraorbital and mental) (Laskin 1984; Roberts and Sowray 1987; Joyce and Donnelly 1993; Jastak et al. 1995; Malamed 2004; Karkut et al. 2010). With some exceptions and specific cases such as those already discussed, these techniques are not recommended in current practice (Evers and Haegerstam 1981; Kleier et al. 1983; Haglund and Evers 1985; Joyce and Donnelly 1993).

### Clinical Manifestations

- *Swelling*, which appears in the area of the upper molars (Kuster and Udin 1984) and can appear on the skin of the *malar region or masseter*. This swelling is very large and cosmetically undesirable because a large quantity of blood can accumulate in the infratemporal space, thus highlighting the resulting facial asymmetry (Malamed 2004). Swelling appears rapidly if the lesion affects an artery, such as a branch of the facial artery or a buccogingival branch of the posterior superior alveolar artery, which follows an irregular path along the maxillary tuberosity (Jastak et al. 1995; Harn et al. 2002; Malamed 2004), or slowly if the lesion affects a vein of the pterygoid venous plexus (Jastak et al. 1995; Malamed 2004).
- *Skin discoloration*, also known as ecchymosis (Bennett 1984; Kuster and Udin 1984; Roberts and Sowray 1987; Malamed 2004), progresses downwards and forwards along the muscle planes of the cheek until it reabsorbs spontaneously after 10–15 days (Malamed 2004).
- Other occasional manifestations include the following:
  - Sensation of tightness, but not pain, in the area affected (Jastak et al. 1995).
  - Difficulty opening the mouth (trismus) if the tip of the needle has irritated the lateral (external) pterygoid muscle (Malamed 2004).

### Management by the Dentist

- The patient should be advised that the hematoma reabsorbs within 10–15 days (Bennett 1984; Malamed 2004). *Often no interventions are recommended* and invasive measures such as drainage are contraindicated (Bennett 1984; Roberts and Sowray 1987; Jastak et al. 1995; Malamed 2004).
- If the swelling is detected early, the dentist may attempt to control it by pressing on the affected area for 15 minutes (Kuster and Udin 1984; Laskin 1984) and/or applying ice to the skin for its vasoconstrictive effect (Kuster and Udin 1984; Jastak et al. 1995; Malamed 2004). In the case of a hematoma affecting the region of the upper molars, it is difficult to apply direct pressure, therefore a finger should be inserted directly into the mouth and pressure applied at the bottom of the vestibular surface of the upper molars, whereas on the outside pressure can be applied to the skin of the malar region (Malamed 2004).
- As an option, some authors recommend that the patient apply heat to the affected area 24 hours after the procedure to aid reabsorption of the hematoma (Laskin 1984; Jastak et al. 1995; Malamed 2004). Heat causes vasodilation, favors withdrawal of the extravasated blood, and has an analgesic effect.
- Some authors suggest reassessing the lesion at 48 hours to determine whether an infection has developed (very unusual) and prescribe antibiotics (Laskin 1984).

## Nerve Lesions

This section includes nerve lesions caused by injection of dental local anesthesia. Thus, we can mention the following:

1) Electric shock sensation on insertion of the needle.
2) Long-term paresthesia caused by persistent neuropathy.
3) Alterations of the sense of taste caused by injury to the chorda tympani.
4) Hoarseness by block of recurrent laryngeal nerve.

### Anatomical Lesions

In 1943, Seddon described three basic types of lesion of the peripheral nerves (Seddon 1943):

- Neurapraxia. When there is no axonal degeneration, although the axons are intact, they do not conduct electrochemical impulses. There is no loss of axonal continuity. In these cases, recovery is spontaneous (10 days to 3 weeks).
- Axonotmesis. When there is axonal degeneration. There is no anatomical damage to the nerve, and although the axon is split, the nerve stem remains intact thanks to the supporting connective tissue. Recovery is spontaneous (6–8 weeks or 2–6 months).
- Neurotmesis. When there is axonal degeneration and anatomical damage to the nerve and therefore complete rupture of the nerve stem. The resulting lesion is permanent and a scar neuroma may form as a result of interference in neuronal regeneration.

### General Causes

1) Needle injury (physical effect). The tip of the needle, especially if barbed outwards (typical in mandibular block after pressing the needle against the bone) (Stacy et al. 1994), can directly injure the nerve stem and lead to intraneural hemorrhage (Haas and Lennon 1995; Pogrel and Thamby 2000) (Figure 22.2), which in turn could increase pressure on the nerve fibers, thus altering metabolism and nerve function (Haas and Lennon 1995). The situation is aggravated by the subsequent intra- and extraneural fibrosis (Pogrel and Thamby 2000).

   Repeating the number of injections, especially in mandibular block, increases the risk of this type of

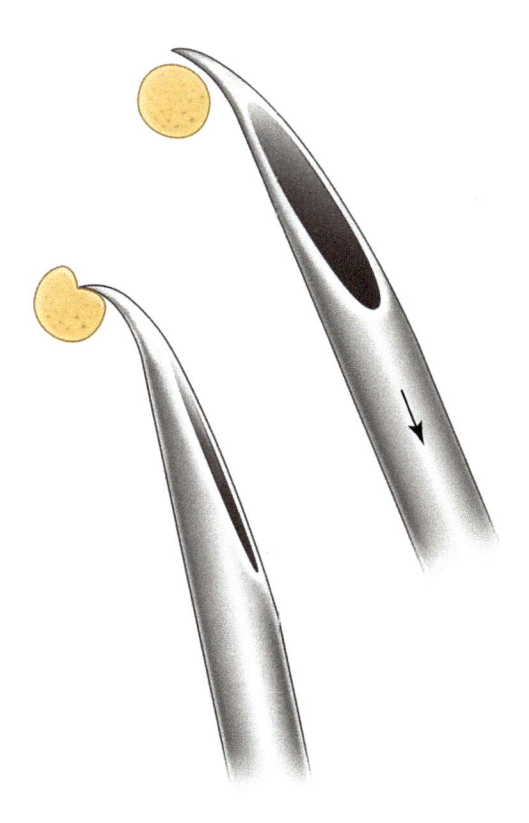

**Figure 22.2** Nerve injury caused by a needle barbed outward. *Source:* Redrawn from Stacy et al. (1994).

lesion (Pogrel et al. 1995; Pogrel and Thamby 2000; Hillerup and Jensen 2006). In some series, 35% of patients report having received more than two injections at the same site (Hillerup and Jensen 2006).

Note: It is interesting that, in five cases involving exploratory surgery, no evidence of needle-induced microtrauma was observed, although the area was slightly pale and there were adhesions around the nerve (Pogrel and Thamby 2000).

2) Neurotoxicity caused by contamination of anesthetic solution (chemical effect). For some time, professionals had a bad habit of submerging the local anesthesia cartridges in surface disinfectants, often alcohol, with the result that the disinfectant entered the cartridge through the diaphragm or the rubber plunger (made from semipermeable membranes), thus making the injection more painful and irritating the tissues and, more importantly, the nerve (Shannon and Feller 1972; Shannon and Wescott 1974).

3) Neurotoxicity caused by the individual components of the local anesthesia solution (chemical effect). Experiments with animals (Lundy et al. 1933; Tui et al. 1944; Skou 1954; Fink and Kish 1976; Myers et al. 1986; Kalichman et al. 1993) have demonstrated the neurotoxic effect of local anesthetics, especially when these are used at high concentrations. Clinical studies have also demonstrated this adverse effect in medical practice (Rigler et al. 1991) and in dental practice (Nickel 1990; Haas and Lennon 1995; Miller and Haas 2000; Van Eeden and Patel 2002; Hillerup and Jensen 2006; Garisto et al. 2010), especially when high concentrations are administered, as is the case with lidocaine 5% (Rigler et al. 1991), articaine 4% (Haas and Lennon 1995; Miller and Haas 2000; Van Eeden and Patel 2002; Hillerup and Jensen 2006; Hillerup et al. 2011; Garisto et al. 2010), and prilocaine 4% (Haas and Lennon 1995; Miller and Haas 2000; Garisto et al. 2010).

## Immediate Electric Shock Sensation

Immediate electric shock sensation (cramp) is mainly felt in mandibular block. When the needle is inserted, the patient experiences a sudden and short electric shock sensation, which is like an intense burning sensation along the nerve that has been touched by the tip of the needle (lingual nerve or inferior alveolar nerve). The sensation lasts a second but is very unpleasant for the patient, although it has the advantage of producing deep and quick anesthesia with a small amount of anesthetic solution.

The frequency of electric shock sensation in mandibular block is around 3% (Table 22.5), and this is more common in the lingual nerve than in the inferior alveolar nerve

Table 22.5 Percentage of cases of electrical shock sensation after mandibular block and recovery.

| Reference | Sample size (cases/total) | Nerves affected | Electric shock | Total recovery |
|---|---|---|---|---|
| Harn and Durham (1990) | 347/9587 | Lingual | 3.6% | 85% |
| Krafft and Hickel (1994) | 856/12104 | Lingual | 7% | 98% |
| Lustig and Zusman (1999) | 40/731 | Lingual and inferior alveolar | 5.5% | 100% |
| Pogrel and Thamby (2000) | 1/80 | Lingual | 1.3% | — |
| Pogrel and Thamby (2000) | 1/320 | Inferior alveolar | 0.3% | — |
| Nooh and Abdullah (2010) | 2/5000 | Lingual | 0.04% | 100% |
| Morris et al. (2010)[a] | 2/44 | Lingual | 4.5%[a] | — |
| | Average | | 3.2% | 95.7% |
| | Rounded average | | 3% | 95% |

[a] Cadaver, contact the needle with the nerve.

(ratio 4:1). In the case of the lingual nerve, the area affected by the sensation is the tongue on the side the anesthetic is injected; in the case of the inferior alveolar nerve, the area affected is the half of the lower lip on the side which the anesthetic is injected.

When faced with these situations in the office, we advise the following:

- Show the patient that you are aware how unpleasant the sensation is and state that this happens because the anesthetic was injected immediately above the nerve, when the normal approach is to inject it to the side.
- Tell the patient that the discomfort has the advantage that the anesthetic effect is quicker and stronger.
- In cases where this accident is repeated in the same patient, we advise against using mandibular block because it indicates a possible anatomical abnormality and repeated injury could carry a risk of long-term paresthesia. As alternatives, we propose the use of another mandibular block technique such as Gow-Gates (Chapter 16) or infiltrative techniques accompanied by intraligamentary or intraosseous approaches (Chapter 18).

### Electric Shock Sensation After the Transpalatal Approach

An interesting variation of this problem is in the transpalatal (greater palatine canal) approach, which in 1% of cases can lead to an intense sensation of electric discharge or burning in the palate on the side of the injection (Sved et al. 1992). This occurs because the needle is inserted into the greater palatine canal, which leads to the pterygopalatine fossa, where the maxillary division of the trigeminal nerve (CN $V_2$) is located.

No permanent or long-term lesions have been reported at this level, probably because the technique is rarely used.

## Long-Term Paresthesia

The frequency of long-term paresthesia or nonsurgical neuropathy caused by dental local anesthesia is unknown (Pogrel and Thamby 2000; Hillerup and Jensen 2006); however, some authors provide estimates, although these vary widely, ranging from 1:5000 injections to 1:14 million injections (Table 22.6). Clinical experience tells us that cases of long-term paresthesia are not often seen in clinical practice, therefore a frequency ranging from 1:5000 to 1:10 000 seems excessive. Furthermore, the study by Garisto et al. (2010), which reported a frequency of 1:14 million, recognizes that this is improbable and that the frequency may be even greater. We believe that the true value lies somewhere between the figures reported (Table 22.6), that is, a median of 1:100 000 injections.

Table 22.6 Frequency of long-term paresthesia after mandibular block, as estimated by various authors

| Reference | Nerves affected | Estimated number | Round number |
|---|---|---|---|
| Harn and Durham (1990) | Lingual | 1:4743 | 1:5000 |
| Krafft and Hickel (1994) | Lingual | 1:12 104 | 1:10 000 |
| Pogrel and Thamby (2000)[a] | Lingual and inferior alveolar | 1:26 762 | 1:25 000 |
| Sambrook and Goss (2011)[b] | Lingual and inferior alveolar | 1:48 956 | 1:50 000 |
| Pogrel and Thamby (2000)[a] | Lingual and inferior alveolar | 1:160 571 | 1:160 000 |
| Ehrenfeld et al. (1992) | Lingual and inferior alveolar | 1:200 000 | 1:200 000 |
| Haas and Lennon (1995) | Lingual and inferior alveolar | 1:785 000 | 1:800 000 |
| Garisto et al. (2010) | Lingual and inferior alveolar | 1:13 800 970 | 1:14 000 000 |

Data ordered by estimated frequency.
[a] Data from Pogrel and Thamby (2000) (two series of patients).
[b] Estimated 30% of mandibular block (data from Annex 1).

By far the most frequently involved technique is mandibular block (99%) (Table 22.7) and the most frequently involved nerves are the lingual nerve (70%, tongue involvement), the inferior alveolar nerve (20%, involvement of half of the lower lip), and both nerves (10%) (Table 22.7). The reason for more frequent involvement of the lingual nerve seems to be that in 33% of cases it is composed of a single bunch of nerve fibers (possibly one to eight), whereas the inferior alveolar nerve is composed of three to 14 bundles, therefore injury is offset by the remaining healthy bundles (Pogrel et al. 2003; Khoury et al. 2010). Also, the inferior alveolar nerve may be partially protected from oncoming the needles by a crest of thickened bone, which bulges anteriorly in the sulcus colli, and the protection of the lingula (Khoury Mihailidis et al. 2011). In contrast, the lingual nerve is quite bare, with no bony protection, exposing it to an increased risk of direct contact during needle insertion due to its anteromedial position (Khoury Mihailidis et al. 2011) (Figure 3.14, Chapter 3).

### Causes of Long-term Lesions

1) Needle-tip injury, given that in 40% of cases there is a history of electric shock sensation, although this data varies widely between authors (Table 22.7).
2) Neurotoxicity of local anesthetic solutions, especially those administered at high concentrations. Thus, articaine 4% has a 9-fold higher risk than average and a 22-fold greater risk than solutions with lidocaine 2%, which is the standard local anesthetic (Table 22.8). The same is true of prilocaine 4%, which carries a 4-fold greater risk than average and a 35-fold greater risk than lidocaine 2% (Table 22.8). Therefore, some authors do not recommend these two solutions for mandibular block (Hillerup and Jensen 2006; Hillerup et al. 2011), especially since the standard solution of lidocaine 2% with epinephrine yields similar efficacy for inferior alveolar nerve (Annex 24), under the usual conditions of dental work.

### Clinical Manifestations

1) *Paresthesia and dysesthesia*. These are the main manifestations; they occur in the area innervated by the affected nerve (half of the tongue for the lingual nerve or half of the lower lip and the chin for the inferior alveolar nerve). The sensation is abnormal and generally unpleasant, and may involve heat, loss of feeling, tingling, numbness, burning sensation, prickling, and even pain. The most characteristic sensation of paresthesia is tingling or numbness (Girard 1979) and dysesthesia (abnormal sense of touch).

There are variations with respect to pain, such as more increased sensitivity to a stimulus (hyperalgesia),

Table 22.7 Long-term paresthesia: most frequently involved techniques, most affected nerves, and history of electric shock sensation.

| | Basic study data | | | | Technique used | | | Nerves affected | | | | | | | History of electric shock | |
|---|---|---|---|---|---|---|---|---|---|---|---|---|---|---|---|---|
| | | | | | | | | Lingual | | Inferior alveolar | | Both | | | | |
| Reference | Origin | Cases | Sample size | Years of study | Mandibular block | Other | | N | % | N | % | N | % | | Proportion | Percentage |
| Gerlach et al. (1989) | Germany | 12 | — | 1985–1988 | 100 | 0 | | 7 | 58 | 5 | 42 | 0 | 0 | | — | — |
| Harn and Durham (1990) | United States | 51 | 41 | 1985–1990 | 100 | 0 | | 51 | 100 | 0 | 0 | 0 | 0 | | 52/52 | 100 |
| Ehrenfeld et al. (1992) | Germany | 9 | 8 | 1987–1991 | 100 | 0 | | 8 | 89 | 1 | 11 | 0 | 0 | | 4/9 | 44 |
| Krafft and Hickel (1994) | Germany | 18 | 18 | 1987–1990 | 100 | 0 | | 18 | 100 | 0 | 0 | 0 | 0 | | 0/18 | 0 |
| Haas and Lennon (1995) | Canada | 143 | — | 1973–1993 | 100 | 0 | | 92 | 65 | 42 | 30 | 9 | 6 | | 31/143 | 22 |
| Pogrel and Thamby (2000) | United States | 93 | 83 | 1983–2000 | 100 | 0 | | 57 | 69 | 18 | 22 | 9 | 11 | | 47/83 | 57 |
| Hillerup and Jensen (2006) | Denmark | 54 | 52 | 1997–2004 | 100 | 0 | | 40 | 77 | 10 | 19 | 2 | 4 | | 20/36 | 55 |
| Alcaina et al. (2010) | Spain | 2 | 2 | — | 100 | 0 | | 1 | 50 | 0 | 0 | 1 | 50 | | 1/2 | 50 |
| Garisto et al. (2010) | United States | 226 | — | 1997–2008 | 95[a] | 5 | | 170 | 89 | 14 | 7 | 7 | 4 | | 18/191 | 10 |
| Hillerup et al. (2011) | Denmark | 115 | — | 2001–2007 | 94 | 6 | | — | — | — | — | — | — | | — | — |
| Sambrook and Goss (2011) | Australia | 8 | 8 | 2009 | 100 | 0 | | 2 | 25 | 4 | 50 | 2 | 25 | | — | — |
| | | | Average | | 99% | 1% | | | 72% | | 18% | | 10% | | | 42% |
| | | | Rounded average | | | | | | 70% | | 20% | | 10% | | | 40% |

[a] Garisto et al. (2010) also report 4% high tuberosity block and 1% mental block (in total 5% other techniques).

Table 22.8 Greater risk of long-term paresthesia after mandibular block with articaine 4% and prilocaine 4% with respect to the general average risk and lidocaine 2%, which is the standard anesthetic.

| Anesthetic | Greater risk than | Times greater | Reference |
|---|---|---|---|
| Articaine 4% | General risk | 3.6 | Garisto et al. (2010) |
| | | 5 | Hillerup et al. (2011) |
| | | 5 | Miller and Haas (2000) |
| | | 11 | Legarth (2005) |
| | | 20 | Hillerup and Jensen (2006) |
| | Mean | 9 | |
| | Lidocaine 2% | 6.3 | Hillerup et al. (2011) |
| | | 15[a] | Haas and Lennon (1995) |
| | | 45 | Garisto et al. (2010) |
| | Mean | 22 | |
| Prilocaine 4% | General risk | 0 | Legarth (2005) |
| | | 5 | Miller and Haas (2000) |
| | | 7.5 | Garisto et al. (2010) |
| | Mean | 4 | |
| | Lidocaine 2% | 0 | Legarth (2005) |
| | | 11[a] | Haas and Lennon (1995) |
| | | 90 | Garisto et al. (2010) |
| | Mean | 35 | |

[a] Estimated based on data from 1993 with consumption of lidocaine forecast from 1973 and of articaine from 1983 and averaging the total number of years.

pain with normally painless stimuli (allodynia), or absence of pain with stimuli that are normally painful (analgesia).

There are also variations with respect to stimuli in general, for example loss of sensitivity to stimuli (anesthesia), reduced sensitivity to stimuli (hypoesthesia), or increased sensitivity to stimuli (hyperesthesia).

2) *Altered sense of taste in 50% of cases* in which the lingual nerve is involved, owing to its association with the

Table 22.9 Occurrence altered taste in patients with injuries to the lingual nerve.

| Reference | Sample size (cases/total) | Percentage |
|---|---|---|
| Ehrenfeld et al. (1992) | 5/8 | 63% |
| Haas and Lennon (1995) | 22/101 | 22% |
| Hillerup and Jensen (2006) | 33/42 | 79% |
| Garisto et al. (2010) | 44/170 | 26% |
| Average | | 48% ≈ **50%** |

chorda tympani nerve (Table 22.9). The alterations the patient perceives are as follows:
- Reduced perception of taste (hypogeusia) and, more rarely, absence of taste (ageusia) (Haas and Lennon 1995; Hillerup and Jensen 2006).
- Altered perception of taste with a burning sensation on the tongue, bitter taste, or bad taste (dysgeusia) (Haas and Lennon 1995; Hillerup and Jensen 2006).

Of clinical interest, there are no differences in involvement between the right and left sides (Harn and Durham 1990; Haas and Lennon 1995; Pogrel and Thamby 2000).

3) These symptoms may very occasionally be accompanied by painful ulceration on the dorsum of the tongue, which usually resolves after a few weeks when the paresthesia disappears (Martis 1969), or late-onset trismus (Smyth and Marley 2010).

**Management by the Dentist**

The recommendations are as follows:

1) Reassure the patient, given that 60% of cases resolve without sequelae within 6 months (Table 22.10).
2) Prescribe vitamin $B_{12}$ for a few weeks since this helps the nerve to recover (Tamaddonfard et al. 2014; Horasanli et al. 2017; Hasegawa et al. 2018).
3) If the patient does not recover within 2–3 weeks, *refer to a neurologist* with a full report.

Around 60% of cases resolve within 6 months (Table 22.10). This period is generally accepted, although some authors recommend waiting 2 years (Girard 1979).

In some countries, such as Denmark, these complications are not considered malpractice, but rather accidents or adverse effects of local anesthesia (Hillerup and Jensen 2006). Finally, in cases that do not resolve and cases of pain and severe dysesthesia, the patient should be referred to a pain clinic since surgery does not lead to improvement and may worsen the patient's condition (Ehrenfeld et al. 1992; Pogrel and Thamby 2000).

Table 22.10 Occurrence of long-term paresthesia that resolved within 6 months.

| Reference | Sample size | Nerves affected | Resolved |
|---|---|---|---|
| Harn and Durham (1990) | 51 | Lingual | 96% |
| Ehrenfeld et al. (1992) | 9 | Lingual Alveolar inferior | 23% |
| Krafft and Hickel (1994) | 18 | Lingual | 95% |
| Pogrel et al. (1995); Pogrel and Thamby (2000) | 12 | Lingual Alveolar inferior | 33% |
| Hillerup and Jensen (2006) | 22 | Alveolar inferior | 23% |
| Alcaina et al. (2010) | 2 | Alveolar inferior | 100% |
| Garisto et al. (2010) | 108 | Alveolar inferior | 32% |
| Sambrook and Goss (2011) | 8 | Alveolar inferior | 75% |
| | | | 60% |

## Alterations of the Sense of Taste

Ten percent of the fibers of the facial nerve (CN VII) leave the nerve 15 mm after exiting the stylomastoid foramen. After a varied course, they join the upper border of the lingual nerve to form the chorda tympani, which also carries special visceral afferent (taste) fibers from the anterior two-thirds of the tongue as well as general visceral efferent parasympathetic fibers that synapse at the submandibular ganglion and go on to provide innervation of the sublingual and submandibular glands.

Injury to these fibers leads to reduced sense of taste (hypogeusia) on the affected side of the tongue or even total disappearance of the sense of taste (ageusia) for sugar-sweet, salty, bitter, and acid-lemon flavors, as assessed using gustometry (Paxton et al. 1994; Hillerup and Jensen 2006). Atrophy of the fungiform papillae on the affected side of the tongue may also be observed (Cowan 1990).

Of note, there have been three cases of involvement of the sense of taste only, with no other nervous abnormality. None of the three recovered within a year (Paxton et al. 1994; Pogrel and Thamby 2000).

## Hoarseness

There have been few reports of hoarseness immediately after injection in mandibular block. Hoarseness was accompanied by dysphagia and breathing difficulty, which lasted 2–3 hours before resolving without sequelae. The cause is thought to be recurrent laryngeal nerve block (branch of the vagus nerve, CN X) because of an anatomical variation (Cilasun et al. 2012).

## Trismus

Trismus is a limitation of mouth opening. The frequency of trismus *caused by local anesthesia is around 1–3%* (Table 22.11) and, as we will see, the disorder is associated mainly with mandibular block (Table 22.12), therefore by weighting the average, with respect to all the other dental local anesthesia techniques – mandibular block accounts for 30% of the techniques used (Annex 1) – the frequency of trismus is around 1%.

### Local Anesthetic Techniques Implicated in the Development of Trismus

1) Mandibular block, which irritates the medial (internal) pterygoid muscle (Stone and Kaban 1979; Stacy et al. 1994). The technique leads to trismus in 3% of cases (Table 22.11) and accounts for 95% of all cases of trismus (Table 22.12).
2) In the upper arch, posterior superior alveolar nerve block or the high tuberosity approach. When applied in the area of the maxillary molars, these techniques can irritate the lateral (external) pterygoid muscle (Stone and Kaban 1979; Shaner et al. 2007) and account for 5% of all cases (Table 22.12) as compared to trismus following mandibular block.

Table 22.11 Occurrence of trismus after mandibular block.

| Reference | Sample size (cases/total) | Percentage |
|---|---|---|
| Krafft and Hickel (1994) | 49/12 104 | 0.4% |
| Kaufman et al. (2000) | 3/179 | 1.6% |
| Ridenour et al. (2001) | 1/30 | 3% |
| Mikesell et al. (2005) | 10/114 | 9% |
| Moore et al. (2006) | 2/187 | 1.1% |
| Lenka et al. (2014) | 1/40 | 2.5% |
| Mohajerani et al. (2014) | 2/80 | 2.5% |
| Dubey et al. (2017) | 3/50 | 6% |
| Kiran et al. (2018) | 0/70 | 0% |
| Average | | 3% |

Table 22.12 Cases of trismus caused by mandibular block and techniques involving the upper molars

| Reference | Mandibular block | Maxillary techniques involving upper molars |
|---|---|---|
| Campbell (1954) | 1 | 0 |
| Brown (1976a) | 19 | 1 |
| Brooke (1979) | 16 | 0 |
| Stone and Kaban (1979) | 3 | 1 |
| Adam et al. (1995) | 1 | 0 |
| Shaner et al. (2007) | 0 | 1 |
|  | 40 | 3 |
| Rounded percentage | **95%** | **5%** |

Table 22.13 Day of onset of late chronic trismus due to the presence of a fibrous band

| Day | Brown (1976a) $n = 20$ | Brooke (1979) $n = 16$ |   |
|---|---|---|---|
| 1 | 4 | 5 |  |
| 2 | 7 | 3 | 70% |
| 3 | 2 | 4 |  |
| 4 | 2 | 0 |  |
| 5 | 1 | 1 |  |
| 6 | 1 | 3 |  |
| 7 | 1 | 0 |  |
| 9 | 1 | 0 |  |
| 14 | 1 | 0 |  |

## Causes of Trismus

1) Mechanical injury or irritation of the pterygoid muscles (medial and lateral) by the *tip of the needle*, especially if it is barbed outwards (Stacy et al. 1994).
2) Mechanical irritation of the muscles mentioned above by residue of silicone or aluminum, which can enter the lumen of the needle when this is inserted through the membrane of the cartridge. It is important to remember that such residue has been found in around 10% of needles (Kelly and Cohen 1984) (see Chapter 13).
3) The toxic-chemical effect of local anesthetics and vasoconstrictors on the muscles. *In vivo* experimental studies in animals demonstrate this effect (Brun 1959; Libelius et al. 1970; Benoit and Belt 1972; Dolwick et al. 1977; Benoit 1978; Fort et al. 1979; Foster and Carlson 1980; Tal 1982). The effect is one of muscular alteration and degeneration that, fortunately, is reversible within 15–30 days (Libelius et al. 1970; Dolwick et al. 1977; Fort et al. 1979; Foster and Carlson 1980; Tal 1982). Increased concentrations worsen the situation (Bennett et al. 1971).

## Clinical Types of Trismus

### Acute Early-onset Trismus

Acute early-onset trismus appears immediately or almost immediately after the effect of the anesthetic wears off. Acute-onset trismus is the most frequent type by far and is characterized by pain when trying to force the mouth open, and pain or painful sensitivity during palpation and exploration of the pterygoid muscles with the fingers at the injection site.

### Chronic Late-onset Trismus Due to Fibrous Band Formation

Chronic late-onset trismus is much less common and is caused by an injury to a small artery that causes a hematoma that fibroses to form a fibrous band within or adjacent to the pterygoid muscles (Campbell 1954; Killey and Kay 1967; Brown 1976a; Brooke 1979; Stone and Kaban 1979; Adam et al. 1995).

Its symptoms are characterized (Killey and Kay 1967; Brown 1976a; Brooke 1979) by late onset (during the first 3 days in 70% of cases, although it can take up to 14 days) (Table 22.13) and absence of pain when forcing or palpating the injection site (only a mechanical limitation to the range of motion in mouth opening). Very rarely, it may be accompanied by long-term paresthesia (Smyth and Marley 2010) (see section "Long-Term Paresthesia").

### Chronic Late-onset Trismus Due to Infection

This type of trismus is due to infection caused by microorganisms injected via the needle (e.g. contamination by saliva, food remains, contact between the needle and skin) into the tissue adjacent to the pterygoid muscles. Both the pterygomandibular space and the lateral pharynx are infected (Brown 1976a; Brooke 1979; Cohen and Quinn 1988; Kitay et al. 1991).

Clinically, onset is late, 2–3 days after administration of the anesthetic (Cohen and Quinn 1988; Kitay et al. 1991), with pain while trying to close the mouth, pain on palpation of the injection site, and, in more advanced cases, complications in the form of sublingual inflammation, inflammation of the soft palate, inflammation of cervical lymph nodes (adenopathy), or fever (Cohen and Quinn 1988; Kitay et al. 1991). Acute trismus can occasionally become chronic (Adam et al. 1995).

## Treatment of Trismus

### Conservative Treatment (Mechanical Therapy)

This is the treatment of choice owing to its success both in acute trismus and in chronic trismus (Campbell 1954;

Brown 1976b; Berry 1976; Nicholls 1976). The key component of treatment involves exercises to open and close the mouth (physical therapy) that prevent a clot from forming and subsequent fibrosis and ankylosis (Stone and Kaban 1979). The main recommendations are as follows:

- *Vigorous exercises to open and close the mouth* accompanied by lateral movements (Campbell 1954; Nicholls 1976; Brooke 1979) for 5–10 minutes two or three times per day. The patient can help by using his/her fingers to force the mouth to open or by using devices such as clothes pegs. The devices designed by Kaban may prove useful in uncooperative children (Kaban et al. 1977). The condition improves in 5–7 days.
- Exercise may initially be quite painful, and adjunctive measures include analgesics and/or anti-inflammatory drugs (Stone and Kaban 1979), muscle relaxants such as diazepam (Valium®) (Stone and Kaban 1979), and heat, because of its relaxing effect on muscles, which makes exercise easier. The heat may be dry or wet and should be applied to the face and the angle of the mandible several times per day or accompanied by shortwave or ultrasound therapy in 10-minute sessions three times weekly (Campbell 1954; Stone and Kaban 1979; Brooke 1979). Sugar-free chewing gum may also be used.
- Antibiotics may be administered in cases of suspected infection, provided that no major improvement is observed after 2–3 days of exercise (Stone and Kaban 1979).

Treatment should be maintained until the patient recovers and may take several days. It generally takes less than a week (Nicholls 1976).

### Forced Opening Under General Anesthesia

Forced opening under general anesthesia is indicated when conservative measures such as physical therapy fail (Brown 1976b; Berry 1976; Brooke 1979; Adam et al. 1995), as occurs in 20% of cases in some series (Brooke 1979), although the consensus is that it only affects a minority of patients (Brown 1976b). Treatment can be considered to have failed *when no improvement has been observed after 3 weeks* or the improvement is negligible (Brooke 1979). These findings are important because if trismus is prolonged over time, it can lead to ankylosis of the bones of the temporomandibular joint (Stone and Kaban 1979). The available options are as follows:

- Surgery (by an oral and maxillofacial surgeon). An instrument is placed over the occlusal surface of the molars on both sides in order to slowly force the mouth open (Brown 1976a; Stone and Kaban 1979) while trying to avoid damaging the dentition or displacement of the second premolar to the maxillary sinus (Killey and Kay 1967; Brown 1976a). A sensation of mechanical limitation and resistance to opening is observed (Killey and Kay 1967), followed by a sudden opening in the mouth as if a fibrous band was breaking and overcoming the resistance (Killey and Kay 1967; Brown 1976a).
- The mouth is opened 3.5–6 cm (the opening is measured from the incisal edge of the upper and lower central incisors) (Stone and Kaban 1979), the mandible is moved so that it opens and closes and is moved in to lateral excursive movements for 10–15 minutes (Stone and Kaban 1979). Finally, a dental jaw-opening device is placed on one side to maintain the gained opening until the patient emerges from anesthesia (Stone and Kaban 1979). It is ideal if the opener is in place during the first post-operative night.
- Complications (Brown 1976a): (i) Pain is relatively frequent in the affected temporomandibular joint owing to traumatic arthritis of the condyle and glenoid fossa (treated with analgesics). (ii) The intervention is followed by some loss of the gained opening because the forced opening is inherently traumatic and induces a degree of muscle spasm. (iii) Trismus recurs in 10% of cases, with the result that the procedure has to be repeated.
- Post-operative measures. During the following days, conservative, physical therapy exercises should be continued, with opening and closing exercises and analgesics (Stone and Kaban 1979).
- Findings of interest. There is no association between the duration of trismus and the efficacy of the intervention with forced opening under general anesthesia (Brown 1976a). Prognosis is more favorable for patients with good lateral mobility immediately after surgery (Stone and Kaban 1979).

### Surgical Drainage

In patients with severe antibiotic-resistant infection with pus, surgery should be performed to drain the pus (Brown 1976a; Cohen and Quinn 1988; Kitay et al. 1991), therefore the patient *must be referred to an oral and maxillofacial surgeon*. In these cases, the abscess should be identified using magnetic resonance imaging and computed tomography, high doses of antibiotics should be administered, and physical therapy should be continued after surgery (opening/closing exercises, analgesics).

## Facial Palsy

Facial palsy is caused by involvement of the facial nerve (CN VII) and is known as Bell's palsy after the Scottish surgeon Charles Bell, who first described it in 1830 (Van Gijn 2011).

## Clinical Manifestations

The paralysis affects the side of the face where the anesthetic was injected (ipsilateral), with the following manifestations:

- Eye: owing to involvement of the temporal branch of the facial nerve.
  - A strange sensation such as numbness may initially be noted in the eye (Cooley and Coon 1978).
  - *Difficulty closing the eye*. The most important sign (Figure 22.3).
  - Occasional tearing or, on the contrary, hyposecretion (Genthon et al. 1987).
  - Bell's sign, when the patient closes eye, the eye globe turns upwards and there is slight movement of upper eyelid (García-Fernández 1969; Bernsen 1993).
  - Rapid, uncontrolled, and repetitive horizontal (side to side) or vertical (up and down) movements may rarely be observed in both eyes (nystagmus). Nystagmus is caused by a central nervous system effect (Parsons-Smith and Roberts 1970).
- Face: owing to involvement of the zygomatic branch of the facial nerve.
  - A strange sensation such as numbness may initially be noted on the face (Cooley and Coon 1978).
  - *Disappearance of the nasolabial fold* and flattening of the face with disappearance of the physiognomic traits (García-Fernández 1969) (Figure 22.3).
  - *Deviation of the commissure* to the healthy side of the face owing to the predominance of the muscles on this side (García-Fernández 1969) (Figure 22.3).
  - The sign is even more noticeable when the patient tries to force a gesture such as laughing, speaking, or blowing (the paralyzed cheek is inflated). (Bernsen 1993); when the patient wrinkles his/her brow, no lines are seen on the affected side.
- Other less common manifestations include the following:
  - Altered sense of taste (Droter 1959; García-Fernández 1969; Genthon et al. 1987; Bernsen 1993).
  - Altered hearing (Tiwari and Keane 1970; Genthon et al. 1987), noises and ringing (tinnitus) (Droter 1959), and even ear pain (Stoy and Gregg 1951; García-Fernández 1969; Genthon et al. 1987; Bernsen 1993).
  - The auriculotemporal nerve may occasionally be anesthetized, with the result that the skin around the ear and temporal region is also anesthetized (Stoy and Gregg 1951; García-Fernández 1969).
  - Although very rare, vertigo and dizziness resulting from central nervous system involvement have been reported (Droter 1959; Parsons-Smith and Roberts 1970).

## Facial Palsy Associated with Mandibular Block

Facial palsy is generally associated with mandibular block, and, although uncommon, it is thought to occur in *1 in 200 mandibular block procedures* (Table 22.14). There are two forms of presentation.

### Immediate Onset and Short Duration

This is the most common situation by far in clinical practice. The paralysis is observed immediately or within 5 minutes following the injection and lasts from minutes to a few hours (generally 30 minutes to 2 hours, rarely 7 hours) (Table 22.15). The clinical manifestations are partial and slight, since the facial nerve is for motor supply and local anesthetics affect motor nerves to a lesser extent than sensory nerves. For the same reason, facial palsy disappears

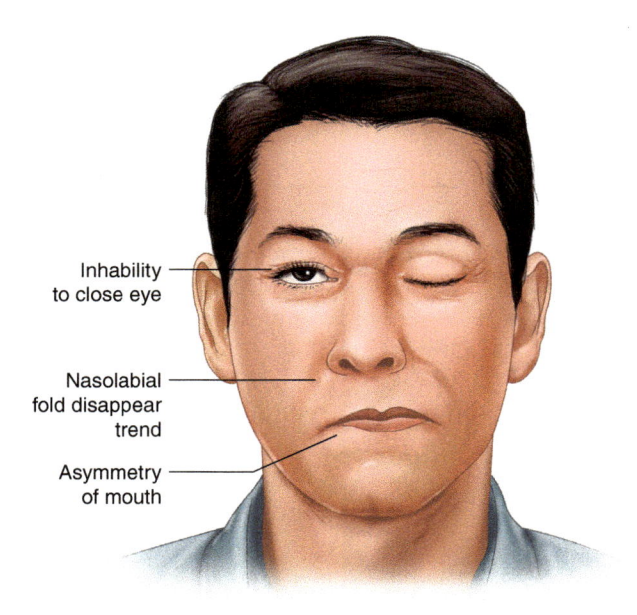

**Figure 22.3** Inability to close eye and Bell's sign. Trend to disappearance of the nasolabial fold, and deviation of the commissure with asymmetry of mouth.

**Table 22.14** Occurrence of facial paralysis after mandibular block.

| Reference | Percentage | Sample size (cases/total) |
|---|---|---|
| Kaufman et al. (2000) | 1.1% | 1/179 |
| Keetley and Moles (2001) | 0.3% | 2/580 |
| Nooh and Abdullah (2010) | 0.02% | 1/5000 |
|  | 0.45% → **1/200** |  |

Table 22.15 Clinical cases with facial paralysis after mandibular block.

| Reference | Patient | | | Time | |
|---|---|---|---|---|---|
| | Age | Sex | Side of block | Onset | Duration |
| **1. Immediate paralysis of short duration** | | | | | |
| Droter (1959) | 24 | ♀ | Left | 2 min | 3.5 h |
| Haugen (1966) | 38 | ♀ | Left | <5 min | 50 min |
| Haugen (1966) | 28 | ♀ | Left | <5 min | 40 min |
| Gray (1978) | 44 | ♀ | Left | 3 min | 2 h |
| Gray (1978) | 29 | ♀ | Left | 3 min | 7 h |
| Gray (1978) | 16 | ♀ | Left | 2 min | 1.5 h |
| Cooley and Coon (1978) | 18 | ♀ | Right | 5 min | 25 min |
| Cooley and Coon (1978) | 22 | ♀ | Left | 5 min | 1.5 h |
| Cooley and Coon (1978) | 30 | ♂ | Right | <5 min | 1 h |
| **2. Late-onset paralysis of long duration** | | | | | |
| Stoy and Gregg (1951) | 45 | ♀ | Left | >Minutes | 6 weeks |
| Parsons-Smith and Roberts (1970) | 25 | ♂ | Left | 1 h | 3 weeks |
| Tiwari and Keane (1970) | ? | ♂ | Left | Hours | 5.5 weeks |
| Ling (1985) | 22 | ♂ | Left | 13 days | 4 weeks |
| Shuaib and Lee (1990)[a] | 26 | ♂ | Left | 24 h | 2 weeks |
| Shuaib and Lee (1990)[a] | 26 | ♂ | Right | 24 h | 2 weeks |
| Tzermpos et al. (2012) | 20 | ♀ | Left | 24 h | 8 weeks |

[a] The same patient on two different occasions.

before the effect of the anesthesia on the lower lip (Cooley and Coon 1978).

The paralysis is caused by anesthesia of the facial nerve or any of its main branches because the needle is inserted too deep or posterior, potentially leading to injection of the anesthetic into the parotid gland, with the needle trapped in the capsule, thus numbing the facial nerve on its path (Figure 3.14, Chapter 3) (Sicher 1950; García-Fernández 1969; Petersen 1971; Cooley and Coon 1978). Occasionally, the facial nerve follows an anomalous course and remains in the retromandibular space, thus leaving it more exposed to the anesthetic solution (Sicher 1950; García-Fernández 1969; Gray 1978).

The dentist can manage this situation as follows: (i) informing the patient, to reassure him/her, that the effect only lasts as long as the anesthetic; (ii) protecting the eye from desiccation of the ocular surface (risk of erosion and ulceration) by closing it with the fingers and placing a damp gauze for the duration of the paralysis.

**Late Onset and Long Duration**

This situation is extremely uncommon in clinical practice. The paralysis appears late (hours or days) after injection and generally lasts 2–8 weeks (Table 22.15). The causes are not well known, although the following have been proposed:

1) Abnormality of the facial nerve resulting from delayed reflex vasospasm caused by the epinephrine in the local anesthetic solution or mechanical irritation by the tip of the needle in the external carotid plexus (Figure 3.14, Chapter 3), which communicates with the stylomastoid artery to produce vasoconstriction in the vasa nervorum of the facial nerve, leading to ischemic neuritis (Stoy and Gregg 1951; Tiwari and Keane 1970; Gray 1978; Ling 1985). The duration of the paralysis depends on the degree of ischemia and nerve damage (Tiwari and Keane 1970).
2) Paralysis resulting from a latent viral infection (Shuaib and Lee 1990) or a previous neurological disorder triggered and revealed by the mandibular block (Parsons-Smith and Roberts 1970).

The dentist can manage these situations as follows: (i) reassuring the patient because most cases resolve spontaneously, although it may take weeks; (ii) protecting the eye from desiccation (risk of erosion and ulceration) by closing it with the fingers and placing a damp gauze over it at night and wearing dark glasses during the day, and referring the patient to a *opthalmologist*; (iii) *referring the patient to a neurologist* with a full report so that the patient can receive an exhaustive neurology work-up and treatment (Tzermpos et al. 2012). In these cases, the neurologist often administers corticosteroids (Parsons-Smith and Roberts 1970; Tiwari and Keane 1970; Ling 1985; Shuaib and Lee 1990).

### Facial Palsy Associated with Maxillary Infiltration

The very few case reports of facial palsy associated with maxillary injection are all of late onset (24–72 hours) and long duration (one to several weeks) (Genthon et al. 1987; Bernsen 1993). Although the causes are unknown, two explanations can be postulated:

1) Retrograde injection of the anesthetic solution (with vasoconstrictor), which runs to the posterior superior alveolar artery and thereby to the middle meningeal artery until it reaches the vasa of the facial nerve through the petrous branches and causes ischemic neuritis.
2) Immunoallergy (Bernsen 1993), but with poor quality of evidence.

The dentist can manage these situations in the same way as for cases of late onset and long duration after mandibular block. Both situations are quite unusual in clinical practice.

## Ocular Complications

Ophthalmological complications are rare after dental local anesthesia. Some authors estimate that they affect 1 in 1000 patients who receive injections of anesthetic (Steenen et al. 2012); however, we estimate that this figure is less frequent, and, as indicated in Table 22.16, it could be closer to *one in every 2000 patients*.

Many of these situations may go unnoticed because visual disorders affecting a single eye are not very intense and may even be asymptomatic for the patient since they are compensated by the healthy eye (Blaxter and Britten 1967; Leopard 1971).

We assessed this problem by reviewing 110 cases published in the international literature between 1936 and 2019 (Annex 36). Ages ranged from 4 to 73 years, with a mean of 33 years (Peñarrocha-Diago and Sanchis-Bielsa 2000; Rishiraj et al. 2005). Females accounted for 70% of cases and males 30% (Annex 36), which is consistent with the fact that more women than men attend clinics (Annex 1). In addition, children aged 4–16 years account for over 10% of patients, and in this case the proportion of males and females is similar (50%) (Annex 36). It must be noted that the data obtained from these series may be biased as only the most dramatic cases are published.

**Table 22.16** Frequency of ocular complications after injection of local dental anesthesia.

| Reference | Sample size | Cases | Proportion |
|---|---|---|---|
| Bartlett (1972) | 3727 | 1 | 1:3727 |
| Hidding and Khoury (1991) | 1518 | 2 | 1:759 |
| Peñarrocha-Diago and Sanchis-Bielsa (2000) | 50 000 | 14 | 1:3571 |
| Kaufman et al. (2000) | 179 | 3 | 1:60 |
| Malamed et al. (2001) | 1325 | 1 | 1:1325 |
| Nooh and Abdullah (2010) | 5000 | 2 | 1:2500 |
| | | Average | 1:1990 |
| | | Rounded average | **1:2000** |

### Anesthetic Techniques Involved

Although ocular complications can occur with any dental local anesthetic (Marinho 1995), they have a higher incidence in the following cases (Annex 36):

- Injections into the maxillary arch (this accounts for close to half of all cases), both through buccal infiltration (most through infiltrations in posterior teeth, mainly molars) and through transpalatal techniques, high tuberosity techniques, and techniques involving infraorbital nerve block. Ocular complications are even more frequent with the latter three techniques (Chapter 14).
- Mandibular block accounts more than 50% of cases, and not only with the conventional or direct technique, but also with the Gow-Gates technique (Norris 1982; Fish et al. 1989; Dryden 1993).

### Clinical Manifestations

Most clinical manifestations affect the eye on the side of the injection (ipsilateral), although the contralateral eye may be involved in some cases. This indicates a poor prognosis and will be commented on below. Thus, we can describe the following complications (Annex 36):

- Visual disorders in over 80% of patients:
  - Double vision (diplopia) in approximately 60%.
  - Impairment of vision, with blurred vision or loss of visual acuity in 20%.
  - Blindness (amaurosis) in 20%.

- Pupillary disorders in 30% of cases, with dilation of the pupil (mydriasis) in more than two-thirds (Figure 22.4) and, much less frequently, with contraction of the pupil (miosis).
- Eye disorders:
  - Drooping of the upper eyelid (ptosis) in 30%.
  - Periorbital and/or orbital sensation ranging from numbness to burning sensation or even pain in 15%.
  - Orbital and/or periorbital blanching in 10%.
  - Other much less frequent disorders include the following:
    - Rapid, uncontrolled, and repetitive horizontal (side to side) or vertical (up and down) movements observed in both eyes (nystagmus).
    - Posterior displacement of the eyeball within the orbit (enophthalmos).
- Eye examination:
  - Partial paralysis due to inability to move the eye in a particular direction or complete paralysis (ophthalmoplegia) in around 40%:
    - Inability to move the affected eye outward (away from the nose), that is, loss of abduction, affecting 30% (Figure 22.4).
    - Other movements, without taking into account loss of abduction or complete paralysis in 10%.
  - Deviation in the alignment of the eye in relation to the other eye (strabismus) in 10% (both convergent and divergent).
  - Absence of contraction when the pupil is exposed to light in 10%.
- Extraocular manifestations in 30%:
  - Dizziness or sensation of vertigo in 10%, rarely accompanied by nausea (Cooley and Cottingham 1979).
  - Facial blanching in 10%. This may occasionally affect the hard palate (Dryden 1993; Wilkie 2000). Reddening of the face (flushing) is much rarer.
  - Facial sensation in 10% of cases, ranging from numbness to burning sensation to pain.
  - Other less common extraocular manifestations include the following:
    - Headache (cephalea).
    - Speech disorders (dysarthria), hoarse voice (Campbell et al. 1979), ranging from partial loss (dyslalia) to total loss (aphasia).
    - Other much less common manifestations such as fever, headache, nausea, and vomiting usually appear in infections of the cavernous sinus, generally one to several days after the injection (Okamoto et al. 2012; Simsek et al. 2013).

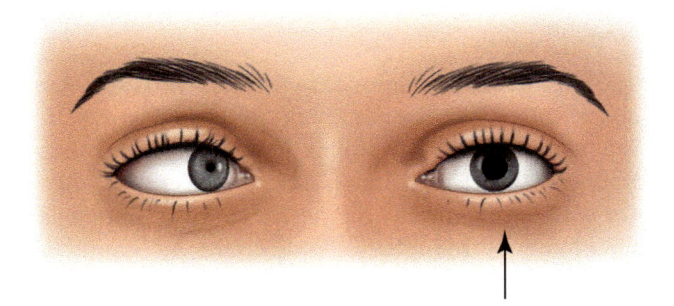

**Figure 22.4** Affected eye (arrow) with a dilated pupil (mydriasis) that does not move outward to accompany the healthy eye (loss of abduction).

## Other Clinical Aspects of Interest

Other clinical manifestations and aspects are not frequent, although they are of particular interest (Annex 36):

- There are five case reports in which clinical manifestations appeared only when the patient went to bed (Kronman and Kabani 1984) or got up (Goldenberg 1990; Magliocca et al. 2006; Yoon and Chussid 2012; Verma et al. 2013). The reasons for this are unknown, although the manifestations were thought to be due to arteriovenous anastomosis or bone disorders.
- There are two case reports where ophthalmological complications occurred in the same patient at different times (Goldberg 1978; Williams et al. 2011) and one case where the complication occurred on three occasions (Petrelli and Steller 1980). The causes involved were bone or anatomical disorders and a history of myositis in the external muscles of the eye.
- In children younger than 16 years, more than 90% of cases are caused by mandibular block, appear after a few minutes (rarely before 2 hours), and last minutes to a few hours. There have been no reports of sequelae, except for one case that lasted 4 days (Hales 1970) and was due to maxillary infiltration in the molars.

## Onset and Duration

The onset and duration of complications can be summarized as follows (Annex 36):

- Onset
  - Around 90% appear between the first few minutes and 1 hour after the injection.
  - A small percentage appear after 24 hours.
- Duration
  - More than 80–90% resolve in a few minutes, although they may take up to 6 hours.
  - A small percentage take several days or weeks to resolve.
  - Long-term sequelae may occur in a small percentage of patients.

### Predictors of Sequelae

Analysis of the cases in Annex 36 revealed a series of indicators that serve to guide us with respect to the outcome of ocular complications.

- Factors indicative of a *favorable outcome*:
  - If the complications appear within an hour of the injection, nearly all patients recovered.
  - If the complications affect children or adolescents younger than 16 years, all patients recovered.
- Factors indicative of a *poor outcome*:
  - If complications appear after 24 hours, then long-term involvement or sequelae are observed in 100% of cases.
  - If ophthalmological complications appear after an hour, then sequelae or long-term complications are observed in 65% of cases.
  - If the contralateral eye is the affected eye then sequelae or long-term complications are observed in 60% of cases. Involvement of the contralateral eye is unusual.
  - If the complication lasts more than 6 hours, irrespective of when it started, then sequelae are observed in 50% of cases.

Blindness (amaurosis) is the most common sequela, affecting 50% of cases with poor outcome. Other sequelae include mild paralysis (ophthalmoplegia) or mild drooping of the upper eyelid (ptosis).

### Management by the Dentist

When faced with such a case, the dentist should act as follows:

1) Stop treatment and reassure the patient that the event is usually temporary and resolves without sequelae after a few minutes or hours in most cases.
2) Examine the affected eye.
3) Cover the affected eye for as long as the disorder persists to protect it and ensure correct vision with the contralateral healthy eye, as this compensates for the visual defect.
4) Advise the patient not to drive or use dangerous machinery. The patient should be accompanied home.
5) Call the patient the same day/night in order to determine his/her status.
6) *Refer the patient to an ophthalmologist* for an evaluation of the eye and supervision of the recovery process. The patient should always be given a full report of the event. This is particularly important in cases indicative of a poor outcome.

### Pathophysiology of Complications

Table 22.17 summarizes the main complications and the structures of the eye involved and mechanisms proposed (Von Arx et al. 2014). It should be noted that the exact mechanisms and causes of these alterations after injection of the anesthetic are not completely clear (Walker et al. 2004; Dogan and Dora 2005; Rishiraj et al. 2005; Huang et al. 2013). A more detailed explanation is found in Annex 36. In any case, we propose the following explanations.

### Retrograde Arterial Flow

The concept of retrograde arterial flow seems counterintuitive owing to arterial pressure; however, it seems valid if we consider that the anesthetic solution is injected under pressure and that arterial pressure falls during the diastolic phase (Williams et al. 2011). This route of intra-arterial injection with retrograde flow was demonstrated in *in vivo* experiments with monkeys (Aldrete et al. 1977, 1978).

Figures 22.5 and 22.6 show the pathway followed by anesthetic from the mouth to the eye. The flow of the anesthetic solution runs backwards under pressure to the maxillary artery, which, via retrograde flow, enables the anesthetic to reach the orbit along two routes:

- The short route, via the *middle meningeal artery*, which enters the cranium through the spinous foramen. From here it joins the *ophthalmic artery* (by anastomosis) (Hayreh and Dass 1962), which enters the orbit to supply various structures through its branches. These include the central retinal artery or the lacrimal artery, which supplies the lateral rectus muscle and the levator muscle, or the ciliary artery, which supplies the ciliary ganglion.
- The long route, via the external carotid artery up to the carotid bifurcation, at which point the anesthetic solution ascends via the internal carotid. From here, it reaches the ophthalmic artery.

Furthermore, the maxillary artery gives off branches to the infraorbital artery, thus accounting for facial blanching, and the descending palatine artery, which, after crossing the greater palatine foramen, becomes the major palatine artery, thus accounting for blanching of the palate (Wilkie 2000).

In addition to retrograde arterial flow of local anesthetic, other variants affecting the arteries have been suggested, as follows:

- The anesthetic solution reaches the orbit via a vascular abnormality of the alveolar arteries or the middle meningeal artery (Blaxter and Britten 1967; Goldenberg 1990; Koumoura and Papageorgiou 2001; Uckan et al. 2006).
- On entering the artery, the needle causes a thrombus that, by retrograde arterial flow, reaches the orbit and retina and leads to permanent blindness (Tomazzoli-Gerosa et al. 1988).

### Retrograde Venous Flow

The case of retrograde venous flow is more obvious, given that there is no arterial pressure and the veins of the head

Table 22.17 Main ocular complications and the structures of the affected eye, as well as pathophysiology and mechanism of production.

| Ophthalmic complications | Anatomical structure involved | Mechanism and pathophysiology |
|---|---|---|
| Diplopia (double vision) | External muscles of the eye (especially the lateral rectus) Oculomotor nerve (CN III) Trochlear nerve (CN IV) Abducens nerve (CN VI) | 1) Block of the motor nerves of the eye (oculomotor, trochlear, abducens) 2) Block or ischemia of the muscles of the eye |
| Amaurosis (blindness) | Optic nerve (CN II) Retina | 1) Block of the optic nerve or the retina 2) Vasospasm of the ophthalmic artery or the central retinal artery |
| Accommodation disorder (blurred vision) | Lens Ciliary muscle Parasympathetic fibers of the ciliary ganglion and of the oculomotor nerve (CN III) | 1) Block of the parasympathetic fibers of the oculomotor nerve and ciliary ganglion 2) Block or ischemia of the ciliary muscle |
| Mydriasis (dilated pupil) | Pupillary sphincter muscle Parasympathetic fibers of the stellate ganglion and oculomotor nerve (CN III) | 1) Block of the parasympathetic fibers of the oculomotor nerve and stellate ganglion 2) Block or ischemia of the papillary sphincter muscle |
| Miosis (constricted pupila) | Pupillary dilator muscle Parasympathetic fibers of the stellate and ciliary ganglion | Block of the parasympathetic fibers (Horner-like syndrome) |
| Ptosis (drooping upper eyelid) | Elevator muscle of the upper eyelid Oculomotor nerve (CN III) Superior tarsal muscle Sympathetic fibers of the ciliar ganglion and stellate ganglion | Oculomotor nerve block Elevator muscle of the eyelid block or ischemia Sympathetic fiber block Superior tarsal muscle block or ischemia |
| Periorbital ischemia (ischemic blanching around the eye) | Infraorbital artery Zygomaticofacial artery Superior labial artery Posterior superior alveolar artery Greater palatine artery Sympathetic fibers | Stimulation of sympathetic fibers |
| Ophthalmoplegia (paralysis of the eye) | All muscles involved in eye movement Oculomotor nerve (CN III) Trochlear nerve (CN IV) Abducens nerve (CN VI) | Oculomotor, trochlear, and abducens nerve block Eye muscle block or ischemia |
| Nystagmus | Vestibulocochlear nerve (VIII cranial nerve) External muscles of the eye | Vestibulocochlear nerve block |
| Enophthalmos (posterior displacement) | Orbital muscle Sympathetic fibers of the stellate and ciliary ganglion | Sympathetic fiber block (Horner-like syndrome) |

*Source:* Table modified from Von Arx et al. (2014).

and neck lack valves, therefore there is no mechanism to prevent the retrograde flow of blood. Furthermore, the veins are more numerous and anatomically more variable than the arteries and their walls are easily penetrated by the needle. Figure 22.7 shows the path followed by the anesthetic solution from the mouth to the eye.

The cavernous sinus warrants a separate comment. This large group of fine-walled veins is located in the middle cranial fossa, on both sides of the sella turcica of the sphenoid. The anesthetic solution that reaches it can affect the eye through various pathways:

- Within the cavernous sinus, along the central part, lie the internal carotid artery and the abducens nerve (CN VI), which at this level are very vulnerable to the action of the anesthetic owing to the fine walls that separate them (Walker et al. 2004; Magliocca et al. 2006). This area is also home to the oculomotor nerve (CN III), the

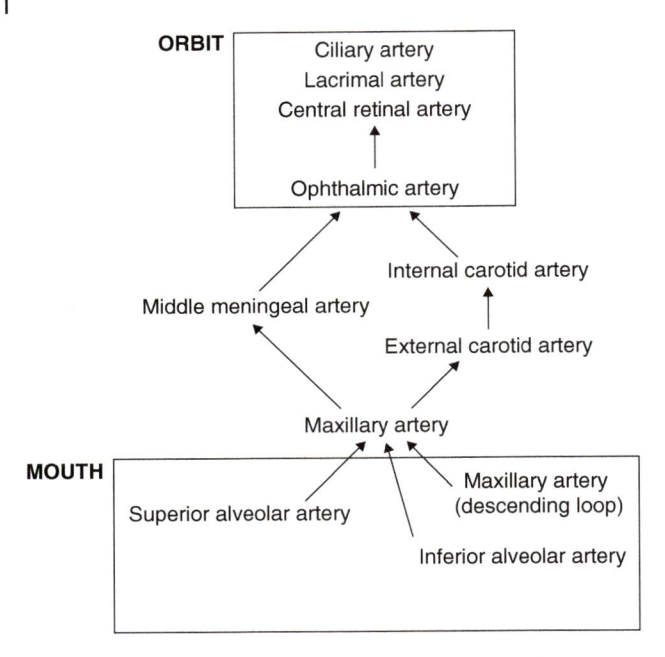

**416** | *Local Complications of Dental Local Anesthesia*

**Figure 22.5** Schematic representation of the arterial retrograde pathway from the mouth to the eye.

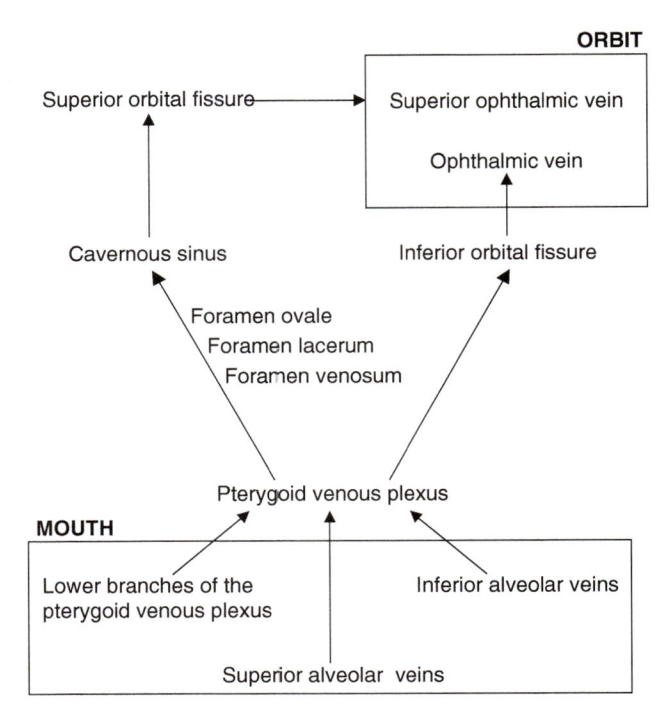

**Figure 22.7** Schematic representation of the venous retrograde pathway from the mouth to the eye.

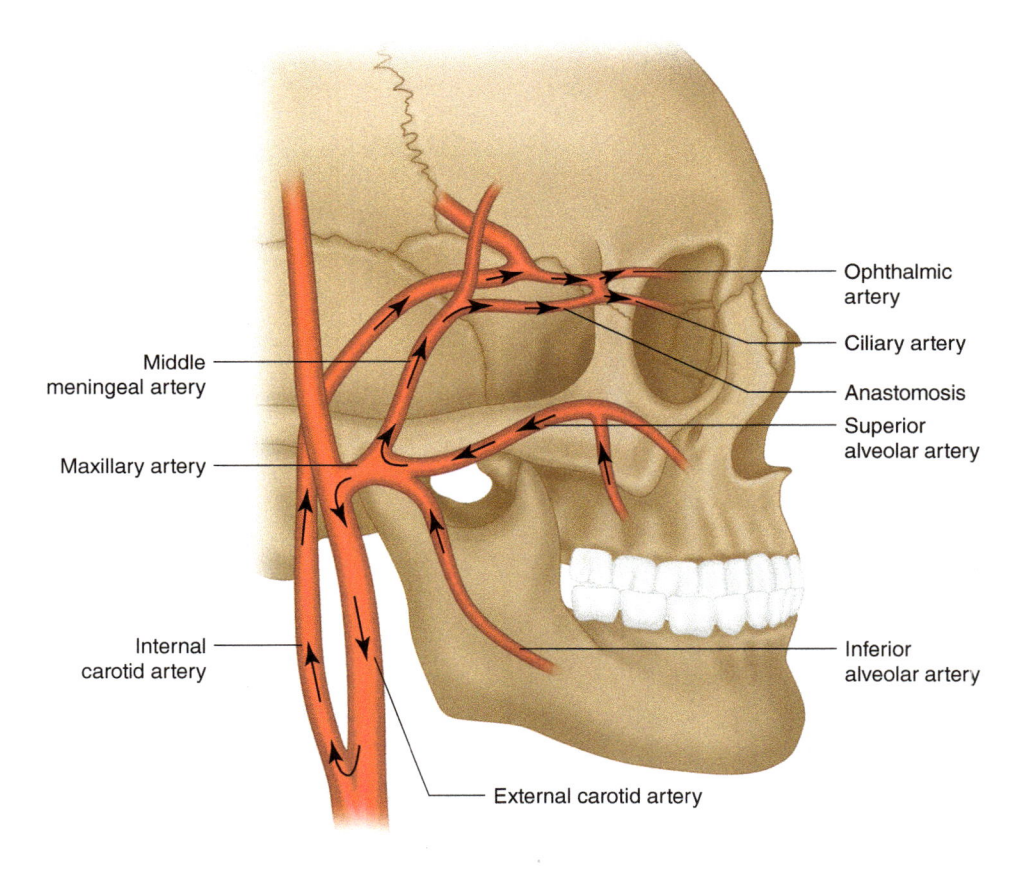

**Figure 22.6** Arterial retrograde pathway of the local anesthetic solution from the mouth to the eye. *Source:* Redrawn from Rood (1972).

trochlear nerve (CN IV), and the ophthalmic and maxillary nerves (CN V$_1$ and CN V$_2$, respectively), although the latter are in contact with the external wall of the cavernous sinus (dura mater), which is thicker and more difficult for the anesthetic solution to cross (Figure 22.8).

- In addition, the superior ophthalmic vein drains into the cavernous sinus via the superior orbital fissure. The anesthetic solution can flow along this pathway by reflux to the orbit.

In addition to filling with anesthetic and vasoconstrictor, the cavernous sinus may also become infected by bacteria from the mouth that enter via a contaminated needle (Okamoto et al. 2012) and then inflamed (thrombophlebitis), thus leading to Tolosa-Hunt syndrome (Simsek et al. 2013), which usually appears after 24 hours or several days and is accompanied by periorbital pain, greater or lesser eye paralysis (ophthalmoplegia), and general involvement with headache, fever, nausea, and vomiting. This complication may take weeks or months to resolve after medical treatment.

**Passive Diffusion to the Orbit**

It is difficult for the anesthetic solution to reach the orbit by diffusion (Steenen et al. 2012); however, maxillary buccal infiltrations in the area of the molars, the technique for blocking the posterior superior alveolar nerve (Holmgreen et al. 1979; Peñarrocha-Diago and Sanchis-Bielsa 2000; Koumoura and Papageorgiou 2001; Horowitz et al. 2005; Magliocca et al. 2006), the high tuberosity technique (Collon 1946; Forloine et al. 2010), and the transpalatal technique (Dickson and Coates 1945; Saborido 1977; Mercuri 1979) may enable diffusion to the orbit via two pathways:

- In the posterior part of the maxilla, in the area of the tuberosity, the solution can spread to the pterygopalatine fossa and, at its highest part, may enter the orbit via the inferior orbital fissure. This is the most frequent pathway.
- Via anatomical abnormalities or defects (Magliocca et al. 2006; Williams et al. 2011) such as an altered wall in the maxillary sinus (Petrelli and Steller 1980) or by vascular or lymphatic defects or defects of the connective tissue (Boynes et al. 2010). This pathway is extremely unusual.

Once the solution enters the orbit, it is distributed via intraorbital fat and various fascia, thus leaving some of the organs at the apex of the orbit more vulnerable, as is the case of the abducens nerve (CN VI) and the lateral rectus muscle (Peñarrocha-Diago and Sanchis-Bielsa 2000; Steenen et al. 2012), and favoring onset of double vision (diplopia) and abduction deficit.

**Irritation of the Sympathetic System**

Irritation of the sympathetic system occurs because the tip of the needle can injure the superior or inferior alveolar artery and irritate the sympathetic plexus that surrounds them. This irritation spreads throughout the vascular wall to the maxillary artery until it reaches the sympathetic plexus of the internal carotid artery, from where it reaches the peripheral branches (Kronman and Kabani 1984). It then reaches the orbit by the ophthalmic artery, causing ischemia by vasospasm in some of the tissues and organs it supplies (Horowitz et al. 2005), which generally leads to

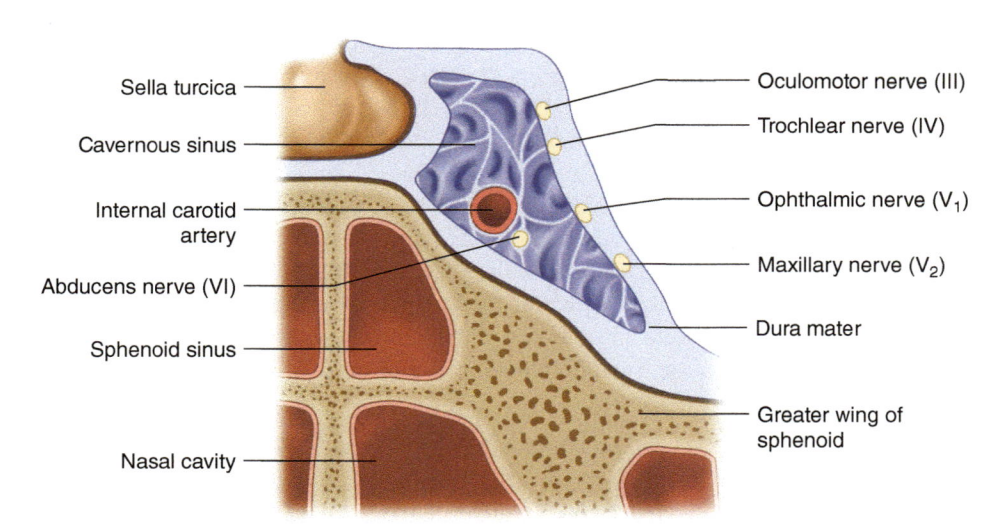

**Figure 22.8** Schematic representation of a cross-section (coronal plane) of the cavernous sinus, in the middle cranial fossa, and its association with the cranial nerves and the internal carotid artery. *Source:* Redrawn with modifications from Koumoura and Papageorgiou (2001) and Pragasm and Managutti (2011).

blanching (Uckan et al. 2006) and other complications (Steenen et al. 2012). In one case of mandibular block, the needle did not touch the bone and led to an electric shock sensation in the lower lip, on touching the nerve stem of the inferior alveolar nerve (Wilkie 2000).

### Sympathetic System Block (Horner-like Syndrome)

Sympathetic system block is the opposite of the previous situation: instead of irritation of the sympathetic system, the anesthetic solution induces selective block of the sympathetic fibers.

The most typical manifestations in these cases are Horner-like syndrome with contraction of the pupil (miosis), vasodilation of the vessels of the face (flushing), and posterior displacement of the eyeball in the orbit (enophthalmos). Other typical manifestations of this syndrome, although not exclusive to sympathetic block and that can be caused by other factors (see above), include drooping of the upper eyelid (ptosis), tearing, and, more rarely, dizziness or alterations of the voice.

The mechanisms proposed to explain this selective block of the sympathetic fibers are as follows:

1) Stellate ganglion block. In mandibular block, the solution descends via the neck to the pterygomandibular space by the lateral wall of the pharynx (parapharyngeal space) before passing the paravertebral space and reaching the stellate ganglion via the alar fascia (Campbell et al. 1979). Some authors consider this possibility highly unlikely because of the distance between the injection site and the stellate ganglion (Peñarrocha-Diago and Sanchis-Bielsa 2000).
2) The anesthetic solution reaches the sympathetic plexus of the internal carotid artery (Dodds 1956). This is at some distance and thus less likely.
3) The sympathetic fibers that accompany the internal carotid artery are blocked selectively when this is inside the cavernous sinus (Walker et al. 2004; Dogan and Dora 2005).
4) The sympathetic fibers are only blocked in the ciliary ganglion within the orbit (Peñarrocha-Diago and Sanchis-Bielsa 2000).
5) Compression and/or traction of the sympathetic fibers due to the prolonged position of the neck and head of the dental chair (Ostergaard and Faix 2001). However, this explanation seems somewhat unlikely.

### Other Proposed Causes

Other causes have been proposed to explain special situations. Although some are very unlikely, others are interesting, for example, hysteria in a 10-year-old girl (Clarke and Clarke 1987), immune response to mepivacaine (Goldberg 1978), vasospasm at the level of the vertebrobasilar vessels leading to contralateral involvement (Machado et al. 1999), or revelation of underlying multiple sclerosis that manifests with alterations in the contralateral eye (Kocer et al. 2009).

## Needle-induced Infection

The needle of the syringe can introduce bacteria into deep tissues and thus cause infection. Infections are now very rare thanks to modern disposable needle systems and sterile cartridges that are ready for use. Infection can arise from several sources (Connor and Edelson 1988):

1) Contamination by the injection equipment itself (needle, cartridge, syringe). This possibility is remote, since the material is sterile before use.
2) Contamination of the tip of the needle through accidental contact with microorganisms on the skin or hair before injection.
3) Contamination through the patient's own flora. This risk is real, since it is impossible to maintain the oral cavity sterile, although it can be reduced by applying topical antiseptic before injecting the needle. Most published studies on post-anesthesia infections confirm infection of the oral cavity by saprophytes (Popowich and Brooke 1979; Connor and Edelson 1988; Kitay et al. 1991).

### Clinical Manifestations

The first manifestations appear after 8–10 hours (Popowich and Brooke 1979; Connor and Edelson 1988) or during the first 2–3 days (Cohen and Quinn 1988; Kitay et al. 1991), with localized pain and inflammation.

Fever appears in more advanced phases and may worsen with general malaise, chills, and vomiting (Popowich and Brooke 1979; Cohen and Quinn 1988; Connor and Edelson 1988), local inflamed lymph nodes (adenopathy) (Popowich and Brooke 1979; Cohen and Quinn 1988), and difficulty swallowing (dysphagia) if the infection reaches the pterygomandibular space after mandibular block. Examination of the area may reveal a fluctuant abscess at the injection site. If the infection is not addressed, advances, or if complications arise, then the following may be observed:

- Trismus, with pain on forced opening (Cohen and Quinn 1988; Kitay et al. 1991).
- Paresthesia of the mental nerve (Barnard 1976).
- Cellulitis of the neighboring skin due to extension to the soft tissue (Popowich and Brooke 1979).
- Osteomyelitis due to extension to bone tissue (Barnard 1976).

### Management by the Dentist

- Initial management includes the following (Popowich and Brooke 1979; Connor and Edelson 1988; Kitay et al. 1991):
  - Antibiotics, which act mainly against anaerobic flora, such as amoxicillin, tetracyclines, clindamycin, or metronidazole.
  - Incision and drainage of the fluctuant abscess.
- Where the clinical course is not clear, the patient should be sent to an oral and maxillofacial surgeon for a more in-depth examination, including blood culture, computed tomography, magnetic resonance, biopsy (cancer screening) (Barnard 1976; Popowich and Brooke 1979; Cohen and Quinn 1988; Connor and Edelson 1988; Kitay et al. 1991), and treatment.

## Post-injection Mucosal Ulceration

Although rare, necrosis of the mucosa may be observed at the injection site. It usually occurs in the palatal mucosa, where there is less tissue elasticity (Hartenian and Stenger 1976) and more rarely in the buccal attached gingiva (Carroll 1980). Curiously, a case of mucosal ulceration was reported in the pterygotemporal depression after mandibular block (Giunta et al. 1975).

### Clinical Manifestations

Symptoms appear at 1–4 days after injection and usually last 1–2 weeks (Allen 1979; Jastak et al. 1995). They are characterized by the following:

- Loss of mass on the mucosal surface, leading to ulceration that may be accompanied by a grayish surface (Giunta et al. 1975; Hartenian and Stenger 1976), which rarely affects the bone and causes a sequestrum that appears on the ulcer some weeks later (Carroll 1980).
- Pain on palpation and frequent reddening of the borders of the ulcer (Hartenian and Stenger 1976; Carroll 1980).

### Proposed Causes

1) Ischemia caused by the vasoconstrictor in the anesthetic solution or by excessive pressure when the injection is too fast and/or the volume injected too great (Giunta et al. 1975; Hartenian and Stenger 1976; Carroll 1980).
2) Trophic alteration of the mucosa caused by needle injury or ischemia caused by the factors mentioned above, leading to lack of irrigation and irreparable necrosis (Hartenian and Stenger 1976; Jastak et al. 1995). In such cases, the ulcer may last for more than a month (Hartenian and Stenger 1976; Carroll 1980).
3) Inadvertent injection of anesthetic solution contaminated with disinfectant (Hartenian and Stenger 1976; Jastak et al. 1995). This is now unlikely since the cartridges come in blister packs and no longer have to be placed in disinfectant solutions.

### Management by the Dentist

- Management is essentially based on monitoring to ensure that a scar forms within 1–2 weeks. In cases of discomfort, symptomatic treatment can be administered. The patient should try to avoid brushing the area by applying rinses with a disinfectant such as chlorhexidine and administering analgesics if the procedure is painful.
- *If the lesion has not healed within a month*, the patient may have a trophic ulcer, in which case a *biopsy* is necessary to screen for cancer and stimulate scarring, as is habitual in trophic ulcers (Giunta et al. 1975; Hartenian and Stenger 1976).

## Breakage of the Needle

At the beginning of the twentieth century, dental needles broke easily. Theodor Blum, from New York, published 120 cases collected between 1914 and 1931 (Blum 1932) showing that 90% of breakages were in what was considered to be at the time a fine-gauge needle (23G and 25G) and that there were no differences between the left and right sides. Fortunately, the frequency of needle breakage has decreased for several reasons:

1) New stainless-steel alloys introduced after the Second World War (Harrison 1948) made needles much more resistant than those that had previously been made of steel, platinum, or platinum-iridium at the start of the twentieth century (Blum 1932; Bump and Roche 1973).
2) The introduction of disposable needles in 1959 (Dobbs 1965) and the early 1960s (Bedrock et al. 1999; Pogrel 2009). These needles removed the need for reuse and resterilization, processes that weaken the metal (Blum 1932; Fraser-Moodie 1958; Bump and Roche 1973).
3) Disuse of the Fischer mandibular block method, or 1-2-3 method, by which the needle changes direction within the tissue, thus increasing the risk of breakage (Blum 1924). Consequently, 80% of breakages occurred during mandibular block (Blum 1932).

The frequency of needle breakage is currently extremely low, and although no exact figures are available, one author considers it to be *one case per 14 million mandibular blocks* (Pogrel 2009).

The data presented below was retrieved from 84 cases published between 1960 and 2020 in patients with a mean age of 29 years (range 3–72 years) (Annex 37). In 1960, more resistant stainless-steel alloy, double-tipped, sterile disposable needles were introduced into clinical practice. As a result, studies prior to 1960 were excluded from this data.

### Anesthetic Techniques Involved

All cases except one (Armbrecht and Schwetz 1962) occurred during techniques applied deep in the mouth, as follows (Annex 37):

1) *Mandibular block. This accounted for 90% of cases.* Involvement of this technique is logical, if we consider that the needle has to be inserted into the soft tissue to an average depth of 20–25 mm (Table 16.4, Chapter 16) and there is a risk of a sudden pain if the lingual nerve or inferior alveolar nerve is touched (electric shock sensation) (Chrcanovic et al. 2009; Kim and Moon 2013). It is important to remember that only around 30% of dental local anesthetic injections are for mandibular block (Annex 1).
2) Maxillary infiltrations accounted for more than 10%, and of these 90% were applied in the region of the molars, including infiltrations, posterior superior alveolar nerve block, and the high tuberosity approach. In the latter two techniques, the needle has to penetrate the soft tissue to an average of 15 mm and to as much as 35 mm in the high tuberosity approach (Chapter 14).

### Causes of Needle Breakage

1) Use of inappropriate needles in truncal block in general and in mandibular block in particular.

    30G needles were used in 60% of cases (Annex 37). These are the thinnest (0.3 mm) and proved more fragile in *in vitro* tests, since they break more easily (Oikarinen and Perkki 1975; Robinson et al. 1984). Fine needles are widely used because many dentists still think that 30G needles make injection and anesthesia less painful than other, thicker calibers (27G, 0.4 mm and 25G, 0.5 mm) (Smith 1968; Cooley and Robinson 1979; Fuller et al. 1979); however, clinical trials have not demonstrated that the 30G needle is less painful than the other two, which are slightly thicker but more resistant (Table 11.3, Chapter 11).

    Furthermore, short needles, measuring 25 mm or less, are used in around 50% of cases (Annex 37), therefore very often the needle is inserted into the soft tissue up to the cone (hub), which is the weakest part of the needle, where it breaks (Wigand 1960; Pietruszka et al. 1986; Bhatia and Bounds 1998; Zelster et al. 2002; Thompson et al. 2003; Ethunandan et al. 2007; Pogrel 2009; Shah et al. 2009). Of note, a survey in the United States showed that 40% of pediatric dentists used 30G needles for mandibular block and that around 80% used short needles (Kohli et al. 2001).

    A review of the cases of needle breakage in mandibular block shows that *in 75% of cases, inappropriate needles were used*, that is, 30G or short or both (Annex 37).
2) Sudden movement by the patient in 60% of cases (Annex 37). This may be caused by a lack of cooperation, especially in children (Bacci et al. 2012) and by a sudden pain when the needle touches the lingual nerve or inferior alveolar nerve (electric shock sensation) in mandibular block (Chrcanovic et al. 2009; Kim and Moon 2013).
3) Incorrect injection technique (Annex 37):
    - Bending the needle before insertion, generally at the hub, which is the weakest part. This can occur in more than 30% of cases.
    - Inserting the needle right up to the hub in soft tissue, which, as seen above, is the weakest part of the needle and the part where breakage occurs. This can occur in 10% of cases and is typical of truncal block.
    - Varying the direction of the needle once it is inserted into the soft tissue. This way of redirecting the needle that causes breakage can occur in 5% of cases.
4) Manufacturing defects in needle production. This possibility is highly unlikely owing to the high quality of the instruments available today, although isolated cases have been reported in Spain (Álvarez 2005) and Italy (Catelani et al. 2013).

### Associated Factors of Interest

Two factors are particularly interesting (Annex 37):

1) Approximately 70% of cases involve males, who generally account for 40% of patients seen at the office (Annex 1).
2) *More than 30% of cases involve children*, when persons aged <18 years account for 16% of the Spanish population (INE 2015) and 23% in the USA (Census 2015). This finding is closely associated with the lack of cooperation by children (around 20% of cases involved children aged under 8 years) and with the use of 30G and short needles for mandibular block by pediatric dentists (Kohli et al. 2001).

## Clinical Manifestations

The vast majority of cases are asymptomatic during the first hours or days, or authors do not record them. Symptoms are worse in adults than in children. Nevertheless, when clinical manifestations do appear, they include the following (Annex 37):

- Pain and/or tenderness at the site of the breakage, accompanied by symptoms in around 70% of cases. The pain may extend to the ear (otalgia) (Rahman et al. 2013; Ribeiro et al. 2014; Casey et al. 2015).
- Difficulty opening the mouth (trismus) in around 50% of cases.

Other manifestations may also be recorded, mainly in adults, for example:

- Reduced auditory acuity or deafness on the affected side (Wigand 1960; Casey et al. 2015).
- Noise or ringing in the ears (tinnitus) (Casey et al. 2015).
- Swollen lower lip (Bump and Roche 1973; Rifkind 2011).
- Pus abscess at the site of the broken needle (Burke 1986).
- Dysphagia (Brooks and Murphy 2016).

Furthermore, in 20% of cases, the patient may be asymptomatic for months or years, with sudden manifestations of pain, trismus, otalgia, and deafness (Annex 37).

## Decision to Retrieve (or Not)

At present, the most widespread solution is to retrieve the needle as quickly as possible, generally within the first days or weeks, although there are exceptions.

- Reasons for retrieving the needle as soon as possible:
  1) Medico-legal (Kennett et al. 1972; Orr 1983; Marks et al. 1984; Bedrock et al. 1999; Akhtar and Ali 2012; Lee and Zaid 2015).
  2) The risk of migration as a result of movement of the muscles and visceral tissue (Okumura et al. 2015; Brooks and Murphy 2016; Giurintano et al. 2017) as well as the cutting nature of the bevel (Brooks and Murphy 2016), which can transport the needle to adjacent anatomical structures. The longer the needle remains in the body, the farther it can move away from the initial site toward more compromised areas that are difficult to access (Dudani 1971). These include the following:
     - Temporal muscle (Crouse 1970).
     - Infratemporal fossa (Armbrecht and Schwetz 1962).
     - Parapharyngeal space (Okumura et al. 2015).
     - Area adjacent to the ascending pharyngeal artery (Augello et al. 2009), descending pharyngeal artery (Faura-Sole et al. 1999) or facial artery (Queiroz et al. 2016).
     - Area adjacent to the external carotid artery (Faura-Sole et al. 1999) or internal carotid artery (Moore et al. 2017; Giurintano et al. 2017).
     - Cochlea (Casey et al. 2015) or medial wall of the external auditory canal (Ribeiro et al. 2014).
     - Base of the cranium (Sen et al. 2006; Prado et al. 2010; Marinheiro et al. 2019).
     - Area adjacent to the skin behind the ear (Rahman et al. 2013; Altay et al. 2014; Karakida et al. 2020). In these cases, the needle is easily retrieved from the skin.
     - Perivertebral space, within the paraspinal muscles (Sahin et al. 2017).
     - Skull base into carotid space (internal carotid artery) (Brooks and Murphy 2016).
  3) Clinical manifestations (e.g. pain, trismus) (Lee and Zaid 2015).
  4) Psychological reasons. The presence of the needle increases anxiety (Armbrecht and Schwetz 1962; Kennett et al. 1972; Orr 1983; Marks et al. 1984; Zelster et al. 2002; Akhtar and Ali 2012; Kim and Moon 2013; Lee and Zaid 2015).
- Reasons for not retrieving the needle have also been proposed, as follows:
  1) When it is a casual finding in an asymptomatic patient who has been carrying the needle for many years. In these cases, the needle is encapsulated by fibrous tissue and attached to the adjacent area and is therefore stabilized (Faura-Sole et al. 1999); even so, the patient should be informed so that he or she can decide.
  2) When the needle has migrated to a critical area, for example the base of the cranium, and retrieving it could leave irreversible sequelae (loss of sensitivity on the tongue, loss of mobility of the lower lip) and the patient is asymptomatic (Prado et al. 2010). Again, the patient should be informed of the risks and benefits of attempting to retrieve the needle from a critical area as compared to leaving the needle in place.

## Management by the Dentist

Two situations are possible: the broken needle is sticking out of the soft tissue or the needle is submerged in the soft tissue. In both cases, it is important to stop the procedure, as this is an emergency situation (Burke 1986).

- *When the end of the needle is visible*, the dentist should act quickly to prevent the needle from becoming

submerged in the soft tissue and disappearing (Burke 1986):
1) Advise the patient not to move.
2) Do not remove the supporting hand (left hand in right-handed people) from the patient's mouth so that the mouth remains open (Malamed 2004) and keep the visible end of the needle in sight (Orr 1983).

    It is important to remember that there is a limited period (5–7 seconds) during which the end of the needle is visible, after which time movements of the head, swallowing, or movement of the fingers can lead the end to become submerged in the soft tissue (Fraser-Moodie 1958; Bhatia and Bounds 1998).
3) We can use clinical tweezers or mosquito forceps (either to hand or provided by the assistant) to withdraw the needle by holding it by the visible end (Fraser-Moodie 1958; Armbrecht and Schwetz 1962; Orr 1983; McDonough 1996). It is important to remember to have these instruments as part of the routine set-up for the procedure (Fraser-Moodie 1958; Pietruszka et al. 1986; Burgess 1988) or to ensure that an assistant is present (Orr 1983).

    *If we have no instruments to hand and the visible end is long, we can retrieve it carefully with the fingers of the dominant hand* (i.e. the right hand in a right-handed persons).
4) After retrieval, the needle should be inspected to determine whether it has manufacturing defects (Orr 1983; Rahman et al. 2013) and photographed (Rahman et al. 2013).

- *When the needle is not visible* because it is submerged in the soft tissue:
1) Do not try to examine the area with the fingers to feel the needle under the tissue. This maneuver rarely enables us to palpate the needle, but rather pushes it further inside, submerging it completely (Zelster et al. 2002; Augello et al. 2009).
2) Reassure the patient (Orr 1983; Zelster et al. 2002), explaining that the needle "can be retrieved later" and that there is "no immediate danger."
3) Advise the patient to avoid moving the jaw (opening-closing, speaking, chewing) to prevent movement and migration of the needle. Swallowing is allowed (Bump and Roche 1973; McDonough 1996; Zelster et al. 2002; Augello et al. 2009; Pogrel 2009).
4) Prescription of antibiotics and analgesics is another option (Pogrel 2009; Altay et al. 2014; Stein 2015).
5) Refer the patient to an oral and maxillofacial surgeon so that the needle can be retrieved under general anesthesia (Fitzpatrick 1967; Burke 1986; McDonough 1996; Bhatia and Bounds 1998; Zelster et al. 2002; Pogrel 2009).

- Consult a surgeon experienced in locating and removing foreign bodies in the maxillofacial area (Leelanuntakit 1974; Orr 1983; Pietruszka et al. 1986).
- Many authors consider this situation an emergency and recommend that the needle be removed as soon as possible (within a few days or weeks) (Annex 37).
6) Once the fragment has been retrieved, it should be kept and note should be taken of the manufacturer and lot number to evaluate possible manufacturing defects (Roberts and Sowray 1987; Álvarez 2005). The fragment should also be photographed (Rahman et al. 2013).
7) Draft a detailed report of the incident (e.g. day, time, technique used, type of needle, lot number, and manufacturer) in preparation for a possible malpractice case (Jastak et al. 1995; Malamed 2004; Rahman et al. 2013). The report should be made as soon as possible so as not to forget any details.

### Preventive Measures

A review of the above information enables us to propose a series of preventive measures distributed in three groups:

- General measures:
  o Evaluate patient cooperation, especially in children. It is important to remember that sudden movements can break the needle (Bacci et al. 2012).
  o Support the patient's head with the free hand (left hand for a right-handed person) during the injection to control sudden and unexpected movements, especially in children (Marks et al. 1984).
  o Remember that repeating injections in the same area increases the risk of breakage (Bedrock et al. 1999; Prado et al. 2010).
- Measures related to the needle:
  o Examine the needle before the injection for defects or damage (Bedrock et al. 1999; Zelster et al. 2002).
  o Avoid bending the needle before the injection (Pietruszka et al. 1986; McDonough 1996; Zelster et al. 2002; Prado et al. 2010). If it is necessary to bend it to gain access to an area of the mouth that is difficult to reach, then it should be bent at the shaft and never at the hub (Burgess 1988; Pogrel 2009), since this is the weakest part, and needles should not be inserted into soft tissues to a depth of greater than 5 mm at the hub (Council on Clinical Affairs 2015).
  o When administering truncal block (mandibular block, high tuberosity technique), never use 30G needles since these are the thinnest and most fragile and break more often than others (27G and 25G are better).

Never use short needles since these often have to be inserted up to the hub, which is where they are prone to break (use long needles).

- Measures related to the anesthetic:
  o Do not insert the needle to the hub, which is the weakest part and where the needle is prone to break (see above).
  o Do not change direction when the needle is inserted in the tissue. The needle is introduced in a straight line and is withdrawn in the same direction. If it is necessary to change direction, the needle is withdrawn almost as far as the mucosal surface, from where, almost fully withdrawn, it is redirected (Prado et al. 2010).
  o Do not force the needle across resistant tissue (e.g. bone and cartilage) unless strictly necessary (Zelster et al. 2002).

## Breakage of the Cartridge in the Mouth

Breakage of the glass cartridge during intraoral injection can be a serious problem because pieces of glass can fall into the mouth and be swallowed. When this occurs, the pieces of glass should be suctioned immediately. If the patient swallows the glass, he/she should be sent to hospital emergency department for immediate evaluation and treatment. The causes of broken cartridge are as follows:

1) In the intraligamentary technique, where the anesthetic is injected under pressure (Malamed 1982; Kaufman et al. 1983; Miller 1983; Rawson and Orr 1985), some series report a 1.5% frequency of breakage (Primosch 1986). With this technique, it is advisable to use specially designed high-pressure syringes, since these have a transparent protective sheath covering the cartridge (Chapter 18).
2) Cartridges with scratched or cracked glass (generally as the result of a knock during transport or careless handling) that have gone unnoticed. While not excessive, the force applied to the plunger can shatter the cartridge at the weak point (American Dental Association 1983).
3) Bending of the harpoon of the plunger. When the plunger is depressed and the harpoon moves forward, it can scratch the glass of the barrel, causing it to shatter (American Dental Association 1983; Malamed 2004).
4) Bent needles, where bending obstructs the lumen. The dentist applies excessive force to the syringe to move the plunger (Malamed 2004).

The glass cartridges used today have a see-through plastic label covering half of the barrel to limit fracturing (Rawson and Orr 1985). Plastic cartridges are better in these cases since they neither break nor fracture (Meechan et al. 1990).

## Aural Complications

Aural complications are very unusual, with only six case reports associated with dental local anesthesia, therefore their frequency is unknown. The causes are unclear. Table 22.18 shows the structures of the ear that are affected and the possible causes that have been put forward.

### Techniques Responsible

1) Mandibular block, both by the direct or conventional technique (Ngeow and Chai 2009) and the Gow-Gates technique (Levy 1981; Brodsky and Dower 2001). Prognosis is good in all of these cases, although in some cases, the clinical manifestations can last up to 10 days (Brodsky and Dower 2001).
2) Maxillary infiltrations in the area of the upper molars, although prognosis is poor in this case and there may be sequelae (Kansu and Yilmaz 2013).

### Clinical Manifestations

The ear is affected on the side the anesthetic was injected into. Symptoms appear quickly as follows (Levy 1981; Brodsky and Dower 2001; Ngeow and Chai 2009; Kansu and Yilmaz 2013):

- *Sensation in the ear ranging from numbness to pressure* and block in the inner ear, or even pain.
- Difficulty hearing, owing to loss of auditory acuity, and even deafness.
- Balance disorders, with a dizziness and vertigo.

Table 22.18 Anatomical structures affected and proposed causes in aural complications by dental local anesthesia.

| Structure affected | Cause proposed |
|---|---|
| External ear (Ngeow and Chai 2009) | Auriculotemporal nerve block (Ngeow and Chai 2009) |
| Middle meningeal artery or its branches (Brodsky and Dower 2001) | Reflex spasm from sympathetic (Kansu and Yilmaz 2013) |
| Internal maxillary artery or its branches (Brodsky and Dower 2001) | Spasm due to epinephrine (Kansu and Yilmaz 2013) |
| | Microembolism (Kansu and Yilmaz 2013) |
| Eustachian tube (Brodsky and Dower 2001) | Hematoma (Brodsky and Dower 2001) |
| Internal ear (Brodsky and Dower 2001) | Inflammation (Brodsky and Dower 2001) |
| | Anatomical variations (Brodsky and Dower 2001) |

- Headache (cephalea). Associated with a good prognosis.
- Noises in the ear (tinnitus). Associated with a poor prognosis.

### Management by the Dentist

Aural complications generally resolve in a few hours or days (<10 days) (Brodsky and Dower 2001). If the patient does not recover after 1–2 days, he/she *should be sent to an ear nose and throat (ENT) specialist* for assessment with an exhaustive detailed report on the event (day, time, technique used, type of needle, cartridge lot number, anesthetic solution used). ENT specialists sometimes administer intratympanic corticosteroids within the first week to prevent sequelae (Kansu and Yilmaz 2013).

## References

Adam, P., Prechenet-Munoz, A.S., Moreau, A. et al. (1995). Limitation d'ouverture buccale par fibrose musculaire après anesthesia locorégionale. *Rev. Stomatol. Chir. Maxillofac. (Paris)* 96 (3): 166–170.

Adewuni, A., Hall, M., Guelmann, M., and Riley, J. (2008). The incidence of adverse reactions following 4% septocaine (articaine) in children. *Pediatr. Dent.* 30 (5): 424–428.

Akhtar, M.U. and Ali, K. (2012). Removal of a broken needle in the pterygomandibular space: a case report. *Arch. Orofac. Sci.* 7 (1): 34–36.

Alcaina, M.A., Cortes, O., German, C., and Castejon, I. (2010). Paresthesia following the use of local anesthetic. A report of two cases. *Odontol. Pediatr. (Madrid)* 18 (3): 205–208.

Aldrete, J.A., Narang, R., Sada, T. et al. (1977). Reverse carotid blood flow – a possible explanation for some reactions to local anesthetics. *J. Am. Dent. Assoc.* 94 (6): 1142–1145.

Aldrete, J.A., Romo-Salas, F., Arora, S. et al. (1978). Reverse arterial blood flow as a pathway for central nervous system toxic responses following injection of local anesthetics. *Anesth. Analg.* 57 (4): 428–433.

Allen, G.D. (1979). *Dental Anesthesia and Analgesia (Local and General)*, 2e. Baltimore: William and Wilkins. 135.

Altay, M.A., Lyu, D.J.-H., Collette, D. et al. (2014). Transcervical migration of a broken dental needle: a case report and literature review. *Oral Surg. Oral Med. Oral Pathol.* 118 (6): e161–e165.

Álvarez, A. (2005). Una demanda civil por rotura de aguja. Juzgado de primera instancia n° 2 de Langreo. Juicio ordinario 472/01. Dentistas (revista de opinión de la Organización Colegial). Organización Colegial. Madrid. no. 6: 42.

American Dental Association (1983). *Dentists' Desk Reference: Materials, Instruments and Equipment*, 2e. Chicago: American Dental Association. 356.

Annex 1. Frequency of use of local dental anesthesia in dentistry.

Annex 24. Mandibular block I. Efficay of standar solution L-100 or L-80.

Annex 36. Ocular complications after dental local anesthesia.

Annex 37. Needle breakage.

Aravena, P.C., Veleria, C., Nuñez, N. et al. (2016). Skin and mucosal ischemia as a complication after inferior alveolar nerve block. *Dent. Res. J. (Isfahan)* 13 (6): 560–563.

Armbrecht, E.C. and Schwetz, W.S. (1962). A case report: recovery of a broken needle. *W. V. Dent. J.* 36: 120–122.

Augello, M., von Jackowski, J., and Dannemann, C. (2009). Nadelbruch als Komplikation bei der intraoralen Leitungsanästhesie im Unterkiefer. *Quintessenz (Berlin)* 60 (11): 1263–1267.

Bacci, C., Mariuzzi, M.L., Ghirotto, C., and Fustti, S. (2012). Local anesthesia needle breakage in 5-year-old child during inferior alveolar nerve block with the Vazirani–Akinosi technique. *Minerva Stomatol.* 62 (7–8): 337–340.

Barnard, J.D.W. (1976). Osteomyelitis of the jaws as a sequel to dental local anaesthetic injections. *Br. J. Oral Surg.* 13 (3): 264–270.

Bartlett, S.Z. (1972). Clinical observations of the effects of injections of local anesthetic preceded by aspiration. *Oral Surg. Oral Med. Oral Pathol.* 33 (4): 520–526.

Bedrock, R.D., Skigen, A., and Dolwick, M.F. (1999). Retrieval of a broken needle in the pterygomandibular space. *J. Am. Dent. Assoc.* 130 (5): 685–687.

Bennett, C.R. (1984). *Monheim's Local Anesthesia and Pain Control in Dental Practice*, 7e. St Louis (MI): The CV Mosby Company. 244.

Bennett, C.R., Mudell, R.D., and Monheim, L.M. (1971). Studies on tissue penetration characteristics produced by jet injection. *J. Am. Dent. Assoc.* 83 (3): 625–629.

Benoit, P.W. (1978). Reversible skeletal muscle damage after administration of local anesthetics with and without epinephrine. *J. Oral Surg.* 36 (3): 198–201.

Benoit, P.W. and Belt, W.B. (1972). Some effects of local anesthetic agents on skeletal muscles. *Exp. Neurol.* 34 (2): 264–278.

Bernsen, P.L.J.A. (1993). Peripheral facial nerve paralysis after local upper dental anaesthesia. *Eur. Neurol.* 33 (1): 90–91.

Berry, D.C. (1976). Persistent limitation of opening following inferior alveolar nerve block injections (letter). *Br. Dent. J.* 141 (9): 264–265.

Bhatia, S. and Bounds, G. (1998). A broken needle in the pterygomandibular space: report of a case and review of the literature. *Dent. Update* 25 (1): 35–37.

Biermann, H. (1943). Die chirurgische Bedentung der Lagevariationen der Arteria maxillaries. *Anat. Anz.* 94 (18–19): 289–309.

Blaxter, P.L. and Britten, M.J.A. (1967). Transient amaurosis after mandibular nerve block. *Br. Med. J.* 1 (5541): 681.

Blum, T. (1924). Further observations with hypodermic needles broken during the administration of oral local anesthesia. *Dent. Cosmos.* 66 (3): 322–328.

Blum, T. (1932). The problem of the hypodermic needles broken in the region of the mandible and maxilla; report of a case. *J. Am. Dent. Assoc.* 19 (7): 1204–1212.

Boynes, S.G., Echevarria, Z., and Abdulwahab, M. (2010). Ocular complications associated with local anesthesia administration in dentistry. *Dent. Clin. N. Am.* 54 (4): 677–686.

Brodsky, C.D. and Dower, J.S. (2001). Case report. Middle ear problems after Gow-Gates injection. *J. Am. Dent. Assoc.* 132 (10): 1420–1424.

Brooke, R.I. (1979). Postinjection trismus due to formation of fibrous band. *Oral Surg. Oral Med. Oral Pathol.* 47 (5): 424–426.

Brooks, J. and Murphy, M.T. (2016). A novel case of a broken dental anesthetic needle transecting the right internal carotid artery. *J. Am. Dent. Assoc.* 147 (9): 739–742.

Brown, A.E. (1976a). Persistent limitation of opening following inferior alveolar nerve block injections. *Br. Dent. J.* 141 (6): 186–190.

Brown, A.E. (1976b). Persistent limitation of opening following inferior alveolar nerve block injections (letter). *Br. Dent. J.* 141 (9): 265.

Brun, A. (1959). Effect of procaine, carbocain and xylocaine on cutaneous muscle in rabbits and mice. *Acta Anaestesiol. Scand.* 3 (2): 59–73.

Bump, R.L. and Roche, W.C. (1973). A broken needle in the pterygomandibular space. Report of case. *Oral Surg. Oral Med. Oral Pathol.* 36 (5): 750–752.

Burgess, J.O. (1988). The broken dental needle-a hazard. *Spec Care Dent.* 8 (2): 71–73.

Burke, R.H. (1986). Management of broken anesthetic injection needle in the maxilla. *J. Am. Dent. Assoc.* 112 (2): 209–210.

Campbell, J. (1954). Trismus following inferior dental block anaesthesia: an analysis of a personal experience. *Dent. Rec.* 74: 180–185.

Campbell, R.L., Mercuri, L.G., and Van Sickels, J. (1979). Cervical sympathetic block following intraoral local anesthesia. *Oral Surg. Oral Med. Oral Pathol.* 47 (3): 223–226.

Carroll, M.J. (1980). Tissue necrosis following a buccal infiltration. *Br. Dent. J.* 149 (7): 209–210.

Casey, J.T., Lupo, E., and Jenkins, H.A. (2015). Retained dental needle migration across the skull base to the cochlea presenting as hearing loss. *Otol. Neurotol.* 36 (2): e42–e45.

Catelani, C., Valente, A., Rossi, A., and Bertolai, R. (2013). Broken anesthetic needle in the pterygomandibular space. Four cases report. *Minerva Stomatol.* 62 (11–12): 455–463.

Census (2015). www.census.gov (accessed 10 July 2017).

Chiappelli, F. and Cajulis, O.S. (2002). Intra-arterial injections (letter). *J. Am. Dent. Assoc.* 133 (9): 1166–1170.

Chrcanovic, B.R., Menezes, D.C. Jr., and Custodio, A.L.N. (2009). Complication of local dental anesthesia – a broken needle in the pterygomandibular space. *Braz. J. Oral Sci.* 8 (3): 159–162.

Cilasun, U., Sinanoglu, E.A., Yilmaz, S. et al. (2012). An unusual laryngeal complication following inferior alveolar nerve block. *Balkan J. Stomatol.* 16 (3): 179–180.

Clarke, J.R. and Clarke, D.J. (1987). Hysterical blindness during dental anaesthesia. *Br. Dent. J.* 162 (7): 267.

Cohen, S.G. and Quinn, P.D. (1988). Facial and myofascial pain associated with infectious and malignant disease. Report of five cases. *Oral Surg. Oral Med. Oral Pathol.* 65 (5): 538–544.

College, C., Feigal, R., Wandera, A., and Strange, M. (2000). Bilateral versus unilateral mandibular block anesthesia in a pediatric population. *Pediatr. Dent.* 22 (6): 453–457.

Collon, D. (1946). Maxillary block anesthesia. *J. Am. Dent. Assoc.* 33 (15): 989–992.

Connor, J.P. and Edelson, J.G. (1988). Needle tract infection. *Oral Surg. Oral Med. Oral Pathol.* 65 (4): 401–403.

Cooley, R.L. and Coon, D.E. (1978). Transient Bell's palsy following mandibular block – a case report. *Quintesence Int.* 9 (10): 9–13.

Cooley, R.L. and Cottingham, A.J. Jr. (1979). Ocular complications from local anesthetic injections. *Gen. Dent.* 27 (4): 40–43.

Cooley, R.L. and Robinson, S.F. (1979). Comparative evaluation of the 30-gauge dental needle. *Oral Surg. Oral Med. Oral Pathol.* 48 (5): 400–404.

Council on Clinical Affairs (2015). Guideline on use of local anesthesia for pediatric dental patients. *Pediatr. Dent.* 37 (Special issue): 199–205.

Cowan, P.W. (1990). Atrophy of fungiform papillae following lingual nerve damage – a suggested mechanism (letter). *Br. Dent. J.* 168 (3): 95.

Crouse, V.L. (1970). Migration of a broken anesthesia needle: report of a case. *S. C. Dent. J.* 28 (9): 16–19.

Curley, R.K. and Baxter, P.W. (1987). An unusual cutaneous reaction to lignocaine. *Br. Dent. J.* 162 (3): 113–114.

Dickson, G.C. and Coates, R.H. (1945). Regional anaesthesia of the maxillary nerve by the palatal method. *Br. Dent. J.* 79: 242–244.

Dobbs, E.C. (1965). A chronological history of local anesthesia in dentistry. *J. Oral Ther. Pharmacol.* 1 (5): 546–549.

Dodds, A.E. (1956). Alarming sequelae of an inferior alveolar nerve block simulates Horner's syndrome. *J. Dent. Assoc. S. Afr.* 11: 385–386.

Dogan, A.E. and Dora, B. (2005). Transient partial ophthalmoplegia and Horner's syndrome after intraoral local anesthesia. *J. Clin. Neurosci.* 12 (6): 696–697.

Dolwick, M.F., Bush, F.M., Seibel, H.R., and Burke, G.W. Jr. (1977). Degenerative changes in masseter muscle following injection of lidocaine: a histochemical study. *J. Dent. Res.* 56 (11): 1395–1402.

Donkor, P., Wong, J., and Punnia-Moorthy, A. (1990). An evaluation of the closed mouth mandibular block technique. *Int. J. Oral Maxillofac. Surg.* 19 (4): 216–219.

Droter, J.A. (1959). Transitory Bell's phenomenon after mandibular injection: report of case. *J. Oral Surg. Anesth. Hosp. Dent. Serv.* 17 (4): 57–58.

Dryden, J.A. (1993). An unusual complication resulting from a Gow-Gates mandibular block. *Compend. Contin. Educ. Dent.* 14 (1): 94–100.

Dubey, M., Ali, I., Passi, D. et al. (2017). Comparative evaluation of classical inferior dental nerve block and Gow-Gates mandibular nerve block for posterior dentoalveolar surgery: a prospective study and literature review. *Ann. Med. Health Sci. Res.* 7 (1): 92–96.

Dudani, I.C. (1971). Broken needles following mandibular injections. *J. Indian Dent. Assoc.* 43 (1): 14–17.

Dunbar, D., Reader, A., Nist, R. et al. (1996). Anesthetic efficacy of the intraosseous injection after an inferior alveolar nerve block. *J. Endod.* 22 (9): 481–486.

Ehrenfeld, M., Cornelius, C.P., Altenmüller, E. et al. (1992). Nervinjektionsschäden nach Leitungsanästhesie im Spatium pterygomandibulare. *Dtsch. Zahnärztl. Z.* 47 (1): 36–39.

Ethunandan, M., Tran, A.L., Anand, R. et al. (2007). Needle breakage following inferior alveolar nerve block: implications and management. *Br. Dent. J.* 2002 (7): 395–397.

Evans, G., Nusstein, J., Drum, M. et al. (2008). A prospective, randomized, double-blind comparison of articaine and lidocaine for maxillary infiltrations. *J. Endod.* 34 (4): 389–393.

Evers, H. and Haegerstam, G. (1981). *Handbook of Dental Local Anesthesia*. Copenhagen: Schultz Medical Information. 74.

Faura-Sole, M., Sánchez-Garcés, M.A., Berini-Aytes, L., and Gay-Escoda, C. (1999). Broken anesthetic injection needles: report of 5 cases. *Quintessence Int.* 30 (7): 461–465.

Fink, B.R. and Kish, S.J. (1976). Reversible inhibition of rapid axonal transport in vivo by lidocaine hydrochloride. *Anesthesiology* 44 (2): 139–146.

Fish, L.R., McIntire, D.N., and Johnson, L. (1989). Temporary paralysis of cranial nerves III, IV, and VI after Gow-Gates injection. *J. Am. Dent. Assoc.* 119 (2): 127–130.

Fitzpatrick, B. (1967). The broken dental needle. *Aust. Dent. J.* 12 (3): 243–245.

Forloine, A., Drum, M., Reader, A. et al. (2010). A prospective, randomized, double-blind comparison of the anesthetic efficacy two percent lidocaine 1:100,000 epinephrine and three percent mepivacaine in the maxillary high tuberosity second division nerve block. *J. Endod.* 36 (11): 1770–1777.

Fort, N.F., Yagiela, J.A., and Benoit, P.W. (1979). Mechanism of epinephrine enhancement of lidocaine-induced skeletal muscle necrosis. *J. Dent. Res.* 58: (A): 208 (abstract n° 461).

Foster, A.H. and Carlson, B.M. (1980). Myotoxicity of local anesthetics and regeneration of the damaged muscle fibers. *Anesth. Analg.* 59 (10): 727–736.

Fraser-Moodie, W. (1958). Recovery of broken needles. *Br. Dent. J.* 105 (3): 79–85.

Fuller, N.P., Menke, R.A., and Meyers, W.J. (1979). Perception of pain of three different intraoral penetrations of needles. *J. Am. Dent. Assoc.* 99 (5): 822–824.

García-Fernández, E. (1969). Parálisis facial y sus causas. *An. Esp. Odontoestomatol. (Madrid)* 28 (5): 419–430.

Garisto, G.A., Gaffen, A.S., Lawrence, H.P. et al. (2010). Occurrence of paresthesia after dental local anesthetic administration in the United States. *J. Am. Dent. Assoc.* 141 (7): 836–844.

Genthon, R., Mas, J.L., Bouche, P., and Derouesne, C. (1987). Paralyse faciale péripherique aprés anesthésie dentaire (letter). *Presse Med.* 16 (21): 1056.

Gerlach, K.L., Hoffmeister, B., and Walz, C. (1989). Dysästhesien und Anästhesien des N. mandibularis nach zahnärztlicher Behandlung. *Dtsch. Zahnärztl. Z.* 44 (12): 970–972.

Girard, K.R. (1979). Considerations in the management of damage to the mandibular nerve. *J. Am. Dent. Assoc.* 98 (1): 65–71.

Giunta, J., Tsamsouris, A., Cataldo, E. et al. (1975). Postanesthetic necrotic defect. *Oral Surg. Oral Med. Oral Pathol.* 40 (5): 590–593.

Giurintano, J.P., Somerville, J., Sebelik, M. et al. (2017). Endovascular extraction of a needle from the internal carotid artery: a novel approach to a controversial dental misadventure. *J. Neurol. Surg. Rep.* 78 (3): e106–e108.

Goldberg, R.T. (1978). Vertical pendular nystagmus in chronic myositis of medial lateral rectus. *Ann. Ophthalmol.* 10 (12): 1697–1702.

Goldenberg, A.S. (1990). Transient diplopia from a posterior alveolar injection. *J. Endod.* 16 (11): 550–551.

Goodman, A., Reader, A., Nusstein, J. et al. (2006). Anesthetic efficacy of lidocaine/meperidine for inferior alveolar nerve blocks. *Anesth. Prog.* 53 (4): 131–139.

Gray, R.L.M. (1978). Peripheral facial nerve paralysis of dental origin. *Br. J. Oral Surg.* 16 (2): 143–150.

Haas, D.A. and Lennon, D. (1995). A 21 year retrospective study of reports of paresthesia following local anesthesia administration. *J. Can. Dent. Assoc.* 61 (4): 319–330.

Haglund, J. and Evers, H. (1985). *Local Anaesthesia in Dentistry*, 6e. Södertälje (Sweden): Astra Läkemedel AB. 31.

Hales, R.H. (1970). Ocular injuries sustained in the dental office. *Am J. Ophthalmol.* 70 (2): 221–223.

Harn, S.D. and Durham, T.M. (1990). Incidence of lingual nerve trauma and postinjection complications in conventional mandibular block anesthesia. *J. Am. Dent. Assoc.* 121 (4): 519–523.

Harn, S.D., Durham, T.M., Callahan, P.P., and Kent, D.K. (2002). The triangle of safety: a modified posterior superior alveolar injection technique based on the anatomy of the PSA artery. *Gen. Dent.* 50 (6): 554–557.

Harrison, S.M. (1948). Regional anesthesia for children. *Dent. Rec.* 68: 146–155.

Hartenian, K.M. and Stenger, T.G. (1976). Postanesthestic palatal ulceration. *Oral Surg. Oral Med. Oral Pathol.* 42 (4): 447–450.

Hasegawa, T., Yamada, S.I., Ueda, N. et al. (2018). Treatment modalities and risk factors associated with refractory neurosensory disturbances of the inferior alveolar nerve following oral surgery: a multicentre retrospective study. *Int. J. Oral Maxillofac. Surg.* 47 (6): 794–801.

Haugen, L.K. (1966). Facialisparalyse ved mandibularisanesthesi. *Nor. Tannlaegeforen. Tid.* 76 (9): 633–637.

Hayreh, S.S. and Dass, R. (1962). The ophthalmic artery. I. Origin and intracranial and intra-canalicular course. *Br. J. Ophthalmol.* 46 (2): 65–98.

Heasman, P.A. and Reid, G. (1995). An unusual sequel to an inferior dental injection. *Br. Dent. J.* 179 (3): 97–98.

Hersh, E.V., Moore, P.A., Papas, A.S. et al. (2008). Reversal of soft-tissue local anesthesia with phentolamine mesylate in adolescents and adults. *J. Am. Dent. Assoc.* 139 (8): 1080–1093.

Hersh, E.V., Lindemeyer, R., Berg, J.H. et al. (2017). Phase four, randomized, double-blinded, controlled trial of phentolamine mesylate in two- to five-year-old patients. *Pediatr. Dent.* 39 (1): 39–45.

Hidding, J. and Khoury, F. (1991). Allgemine Komplikationen bei der zahnärztlichen lokalanästhesie. *Dtsch. Zahnartl. Z.* 46 (12): 834–836.

Hillerup, S. and Jensen, R. (2006). Nerve injury caused by mandibular block analgesia. *Int. J. Oral Maxillofac. Surg.* 35 (5): 437–443.

Hillerup, S., Jensen, R.H., and Ersboll, B.K. (2011). Trigeminal nerve injury associated with injection of local anesthetics. *J. Am. Dent. Assoc.* 142 (5): 531–539.

Holmgreen, W.C., Baddour, H.M., and Tilson, H.B. (1979). Unilateral mydriasis during general anesthesia. *J. Oral Surg.* 37 (10): 740–742.

Horasanli, B., Hasturk, A.E., Atikan, M. et al. (2017). Comparative evaluation of the electrophysiological, functional and ultrastructural effects of alpha lipoic and cyanocobalamin administration in a rat model of scietic nerve injury. *J. Back Musculoskelet. Rehabil.* 30 (5): 967–974.

Horowitz, J., Almong, Y., Wolf, A. et al. (2005). Ophthalmic complications of dental anesthesia: three new cases. *J. Neuroophthalmol.* 25 (2): 95–100.

Huang, R.-Y., Chen, Y.-J., Fang, W.-H. et al. (2013). Concomitant Horner and Harlequin syndromes after inferior alveolar nerve block anesthesia. *J. Endod.* 39 (12): 1654–1657.

INE 2015. Available from www.ine.es (accessed 10 July 2017).

Jastak, J.T., Yagiela, J.A., and Donaldson, D. (1995). *Local Anesthesia of the Oral Cavity*. Philadelphia: WB Saunders Co. 303–307.

Jorkjend, L. and Skoglund, L.A. (1999). Infiltrated lidocaine 2% with epinephrine 1:80,000 causes more postoperative pain than lidocaine 2% after soft tissue surgery. *Anesth. Prog.* 46 (2): 71–76.

Joyce, A.P. and Donnelly, J.C. (1993). Evaluation of the effectiveness and comfort of incisive nerve anesthetic given inside or outside the mental foramen. *J. Endod.* 19 (8): 409–411.

Kaban, L.B., Swanson, L.T., Murray, J.E., and Sheridan, W. (1977). Postoperative physiotherapy device for mandibular hypomobility. *Oral Surg. Oral Med. Oral. Pathol.* 43 (4): 513–516.

Kalichman, M.W., Moorhouse, D.T., Powell, H.C., and Myers, R.R. (1993). Relative neural toxicity of local anesthetics. *J. Neuropathol. Exp. Neurol.* 52 (3): 234–240.

Kansu, L. and Yilmaz, I. (2013). Sudden hearing loss after dental treatment. *J. Oral Maxillofac. Surg.* 71 (8): 1318–1321.

Karakida, K., Takahashi, M., Sakamoto, H. et al. (2020). Subcutaneous migration of a broken dental needle from the mandibular gingival to the neck: a case report. *Tokai J. Exp. Clin. Med.* 45 (3): 108–112.

Karkut, B., Reader, A., Drum, M. et al. (2010). A comparison of the local anesthetic efficacy of the extraoral versus the intraoral infraorbital nerve block. *J. Am. Dent. Assoc.* 141 (2): 185–192.

Kaufman, E., Valli, D., and Garfunkel, A.A. (1983). Intraligamentary anesthesia: a clinical study. *J. Prost. Dent.* 49 (3): 337–339.

Kaufman, E., Goharian, S., and Katz, Y. (2000). Adverse reactions triggered by dental local anesthetics: a clinical survey. *Anesth. Prog.* 47 (4): 134–138.

Kawai, T., Sato, I., Yosue, T. et al. (2006). Anastomosis between the inferior alveolar artery branches and submental artery in human mandible. *Surg. Radiol. Anat.* 28 (3): 308–310.

Keetley, A. and Moles, D.R. (2001). A clinical audit into success rate of inferior alveolar nerve block analgesia in general dental practice. *Prim. Dent. Care* 8 (4): 139–142.

Kelly, J.R. and Cohen, M.E. (1984). Injectable debris associated with dental anesthetic delivery. *J. Am. Dent. Assoc.* 108 (4): 621–624.

Kennedy, M., Reader, A., Beck, M., and Weaver, J. (2001). Anesthetic efficacy of ropivacaine in maxillary anterior infiltration. *Oral Surg. Oral Med. Oral Pathol.* 91 (4): 406–412.

Kennett, S., Curran, J.B., and Jenkins, G.R. (1972). Management of a broken hypodermic needle: report of a case. *J. Can. Dent. Assoc.* 38 (11): 414–416.

Khoury Mihailidis, S., Ghabriel, M., and Townsend, G. (2011). Applied anatomy of the pterygomandibular space: improving the success of inferior alveolar nerve blocks. *Aust. Dent. J.* 56 (2): 112–121.

Khoury, J.N., Mihailidis, S., Ghabriel, M., and Townsed, G. (2010). Anatomical relationship within the human pterygomandibular space: relevance to local anesthesia. *Clin. Anat.* 23 (8): 936–944.

Killey, H.C. and Kay, L.W. (1967). Trismus following inferior dental nerve block (letter). *Br. Med. J.* 3 (5558): 173–174.

Kim, J.-H. and Moon, S.-Y. (2013). Removal of a broken needle using three-dimensional computed tomography: a case report. *J. Korean Assoc. Oral Maxillofac. Surg.* 39 (5): 251–253.

Kiran, B.S.R., Kashyap, V.M., Uppada, U.K. et al. (2018). Comparison of efficacy of Halstead, Vazirani Akinosi and Gow Gates techniques for mandibular anesthesia. *J. Maxillofac. Oral Surg.* 10: https://doi.org/10.1007/s2663-018-1092-5.

Kitay, D., Ferrano, N., and Sonis, S.T. (1991). Lateral pharyngeal space abscess as a consequence of regional anesthesia. *J. Am. Dent. Assoc.* 122 (7): 56–59.

Kleier, D.J., Deeg, D.K., and Averbach, R.E. (1983). The extraoral approach to the infraorbital nerve block. *J. Am. Dent. Assoc.* 107 (5): 758–760.

Kocer, B., Ergan, S., and Nazliel, B. (2009). Isolated abducens nerve palsy following mandibular block articaine anesthesia, a first manifestation of multiple sclerosis: a case report. *Quintessence Int.* 40 (3): 251–256.

Kohli, K., Ngan, P., Crout, R., and Linscott, C.C. (2001). A survey of local and topical anesthesia use by pediatric dentists in the United States. *Pediatr. Dent.* 23 (39): 256–269.

Koumoura, F. and Papageorgiou, G. (2001). Diplopia as a complication of local anesthesia: a case report. *Quintessence Int.* 32 (3): 232–234.

Krafft, T.C. and Hickel, R. (1994). Clinical investigation into the incidence of direct damage to the lingual nerve caused by local anesthetic. *J. Craneomaxillofac. Surg.* 22 (5): 294–296.

Kronman, J.H. and Giunta, J.L. (1987). Reflex vasoconstrictor following dental injections. *Oral Surg. Oral Med. Oral Pathol.* 63 (5): 542–544.

Kronman, J.H. and Kabani, S. (1984). The neuronal basis for diplopia following local anesthetic injections. *Oral Surg. Oral Med. Oral Pathol.* 58 (5): 533–534.

Krüger, U. and Nehse, G. (1991). Nekrosen und Hämatome – zwei lokale Komplikation bei der intraoralen Leitungsanästhesie. *Dtsch. Zahnärztl. Z.* 46 (12): 830–831.

Kumaresan, R., Rajeev, V., Karthikeyan, P., and Arunachalam, R. (2018). An unusual complication after administration an inferior alveolar nerve block – a case report. *J. Oral Maxillofac. Surg. Med. Pathol.* 30 (2): 151–153.

Kuster, C.G. and Udin, R.D. (1984). Frequency of hematoma formation subsequent to injection of dental local anesthetics in children. *Anesth. Prog.* 31 (3): 130–132.

Lacouture, C., Blanton, P.L., and Hairston, L.E. (1983). The anatomy of the maxillary artery in the infratemporal fossa in relationship to oral injections. *Anat. Rec.* 205 (3): 104A.

Laskin, D.M. (1984). Diagnosis and treatment of complications associated with local anesthesia. *Int. Dent. J.* 34 (4): 232–237.

Lederman, D.A., Freedman, P.D., Kerpel, S.M., and Lumerman, H. (1980). An unusual skin reaction following local anesthesia injection. Review of the literature and report of four cases. *Oral Surg. Oral Med. Oral Pathol.* 49 (1): 28–33.

Lee, T.Y.T. and Zaid, W. (2015). Broken dental needle retrieval using a surgical navigation system: a case report and literature review. *Oral Surg. Oral Med. Oral Pathol.* 119 (2): e55–e59.

Leelanuntakit, C. (1974). A broken needle in the pterygomandibular space. *J. Dent. Assoc. Thai.* 24 (4): 205–212.

Legarth, J. (2005). Skader pa nervus lingualis opstaet i forbindelse med mandibularanalgesi. Anmeldt til dansk tandlaegeforenings patientskadeforsikring 2002–2004. *Tandlaegebladet* 109 (10): 786–788.

Lenka, S., Jain, N., Mohanty, R. et al. (2014). A clinical comparison of three techniques of mandibular local anesthesia. *Adv. Hum. Biol.* 4 (1): 13–19.

Leopard, P.J. (1971). Diplopia following injection of local anaesthetic. *Dent. Pract.* 22 (3): 92–94.

Levy, T.P. (1981). An assessment of the Gow-Gates mandibular block for third molar surgery. *J. Am. Dent. Assoc.* 103 (1): 37–41.

Libelius, R., Sonesson, B., Stamenovic, B.A., and Thesleff, S. (1970). Denervation-like changes in skeletal muscle after treatment with local anesthetic (Marcaine®). *J. Anat. (London)* 106 (2): 297–309.

Ling, K.C. (1985). Peripheral facial nerve paralysis after local dental anesthesia. *Oral Surg. Oral Med. Oral Pathol.* 60 (1): 23–24.

Lundy, J.S., Essex, H.E., and Kernohan, J.W. (1933). Experiments with anesthetics. IV. Lesions produced in the spinal cord of dogs by a dose of procaine hydrochloride sufficient to cause permanent and fatal paralysis. *JAMA* 101 (20): 1546–1550.

Lustig, J.P. and Zusman, S.P. (1999). Immediate complications of local anesthetic administered to 1,007 consecutive patients. *J. Am. Dent. Assoc.* 130 (4): 496–499.

Machado, D.M.S., Gomez, R.S., and Gomez, R.S. (1999). Vertebrobasilar ischemia after a dental procedure. *J. Oral Maxillofac. Surg.* 57 (12): 1463–1465.

Magliocca, K.R., Kessel, N.C., and Cortright, G.W. (2006). Transient diplopia following maxillary local anesthetic injection. *Oral Surg. Oral Med. Oral Pathol.* 101 (6): 730–703.

Malamed, S.F. (1982). The periodontal ligament (PDL) injection: an alternative to inferior alveolar nerve block. *Oral Surg. Oral Med. Oral Pathol.* 53 (2): 117–121.

Malamed, S.F. (2004). *Handbook of Local Anesthesia*, 5e. St. Louis (Missouri): Elsevier-Mosby. 116, 287, 294–295.

Malamed, S.F., Cagnon, S., and Leblanc, D. (2001). Articaine hydrochloride: a study of the safety of a new amide local anesthetic. *J. Am. Dent. Assoc.* 132 (2): 177–185.

Marinheiro, B.H., Araujo, R.T.E., Sverzut, T.F.V. et al. (2019). Migration and surgical retrieval of a broken dental needle: a literature review and case report. *Gen. Dent.* 67 (6): 43–37.

Marinho, R.O.M. (1995). Abducent nerve palsy following dental local analgesia. *Br. Dent. J.* 179 (2): 69–70.

Marks, R.B., Carlton, D.M., and McDonald, S. (1984). Management of a broken needle in the pterygomandibular space: report of case. *J. Am. Dent. Assoc.* 109 (2): 263–264.

Martis, C.S. (1969). An unusual case of neurotrophic ulcer of the tongue. *Oral Surg. Oral Med. Oral Pathol.* 28 (2): 172–174.

McDonough, T. (1996). An unusual case of trismus and dysphagia. *Br. Dent. J.* 180 (12): 465–466.

Meechan, J.G., McCabe, J.F., and Carrick, T.E. (1990). Plastic dental local anaesthetic cartridges: a laboratory investigation. *Br. Dent. J.* 169 (2): 54–56.

Mercuri, L.G. (1979). Intraoral second division nerve block. *Oral Surg. Oral Med. Oral Pathol.* 47 (2): 109–113.

Mikesell, P., Nusstein, J., Reader, A. et al. (2005). A comparison of articaine and lidocaine for inferior alveolar nerve blocks. *J. Endod.* 31 (4): 265–270.

Miller, A.G. (1983). A clinical evaluation of the ligmaject periodontal ligament injection syringe. *Dent. Update* 10 (10): 639–643.

Miller, P.A. and Haas, D.A. (2000). Incidence of local anesthetic-induced neuropathies in Ontario from 1994–1998. *J. Dent. Res.* 79: (IADR abstracts): 627 (abstract no. 3869).

Mohajerani, H., Pakravan, A.-H., Bamdadian, T., and Bidart, P. (2014). Anesthetic efficacy of inferior nerve block: conventional versus Akinosi technique. *J. Dent. School* 32 (4): 210–215.

Moore, P.A., Boynes, S.G., Hersh, E.V. et al. (2006). The anesthetic efficacy of 4% articaine 1:200,000 epinephrine. Two controlled clinical trials. *J. Am. Dent. Assoc.* 137 (11): 1572–1581.

Moore, K., Khan, N.R., Michael, L.M., and Arthur, A.S. (2017). Endovascular retrieval of dental needle retained in the internal carotid artery. *BMJ Case Rep.* https://doi.org/10.1136/bcr-2016-012771.

Morris, C.D., Rasmunssen, J., Throckmorton, G.S., and Finn, R. (2010). The anatomic basis of lingual nerve trauma associated with inferior alveolar block injections. *J. Oral Maxillofac. Surg.* 68 (11): 2833–2836.

Myers, R.R., Kalichman, M.W., Reisner, L.S., and Powell, H.C. (1986). Neurotoxicity of local anesthetic altered perineural permeability, edema, and nerve fiber injury. *Anesthesiology* 64 (1): 29–35.

Ngeow, W.C. and Chai, W.L. (2009). Numbness of the ear following inferior alveolar nerve block: the forgotten complication. *Br. Dent. J.* 207 (1): 19–21.

Nicholls, J. (1976). Persistent limitation of opening following inferior alveolar nerve block injections (letter). *Br. Dent. J.* 141 (8): 233.

Nickel, A.A. Jr. (1990). A retrospective study of paresthesia of the dental alveolar nerves. *Anesth. Prog.* 37 (1): 42–45.

Nooh, N. and Abdullah, W.A. (2010). Incidence of complications of inferior alveolar nerve block injection. *J. Med. Biomed. Sci.* 1 (1): 52–56.

Norris, L. (1982). Eye complications following Gow-Gates block technique. *Dent. Anaesth. Sedat.* 11 (2): 59–60.

Oikarinen, V.J. and Perkki, K. (1975). A metallurgic and bacteriological study of disposable injection needles in dental and oral surgery practice. *Proc. Finn. Dent. Soc.* 71 (5): 147–161.

Okamoto, H., Ogata, A., Kosugi, M. et al. (2012). Cavernous sinus thrombophlebitis related to dental infection. Two case reports. *Neurol. Med. Chir. (Tokyo)* 52 (10): 757–760.

Okumura, Y., Hidaka, H., Seiji, K. et al. (2015). Unique migration of a dental needle into the parapharyngeal space: successful removal by an intraoral approach and simulation for tracking visibility in X-ray fluoroscopy. *Ann. Otol. Rhinol. Laryngol.* 124 (2): 162–167.

Orr, D.L. 2nd (1983). The broken needle: report of case. *J. Am. Dent. Assoc.* 107 (4): 603–604.

Ostergaard, C. and Faix, D.J. (2001). Horner syndrome from the dentist's chair. *J. Am. Board Fam. Pract.* 14 (5): 386–388.

Parsons-Smith, G. and Roberts, J.M.N. (1970). Facial paralysis after local dental anesthesia (letter). *Br. Med. J.* 4 (5737): 745–756.

Paul, R., Anand, R., Wray, P. et al. (2009). An unusual complication of an inferior dental nerve block: a case report. *Br. Dent. J.* 206 (1): 9–10.

Paxton, M.C., Hadley, J.N., Hadley, M.N. et al. (1994). Chorda tympani nerve injury following inferior alveolar injection: a review of two cases. *J. Am. Dent. Assoc.* 125 (7): 1003–1006.

Peñarrocha-Diago, M. and Sanchis-Bielsa, J.M. (2000). Ophthalmologic complications after intraoral local anesthesia with articaine. *Oral Surg. Oral Med. Oral Pathol.* 90 (1): 21–24.

Peñarrocha-Oltra, D., Ata-Ali, J., Oltra-Moscardó, M.J. et al. (2012). Side effects and complications of intraosseous anesthesia and conventional oral anesthesia. *Med. Oral Patol. Oral Cir. Bucal.* 17 (3): e430–e434.

Perea-Perez, B., Labajo-Gonzalez, E., Santiago-Saez, A. et al. (2014). Analysis of 415 adverse events in dental practice in Spain from 2000 to 2010. *Med. Oral Patol. Oral Cir. Bucal.* 19 (5): e500–e505.

Petersen, J.K. (1971). The mandibular foramen block. A radiographic study of the spread of the local analgesic solution. *Br. J. Oral Surg.* 9 (21): 126–138.

Petrelli, E.A. and Steller, R.E. (1980). Medial rectus muscle palsy dental anesthesia. *Am J. Ophthalmol.* 90 (3): 422–424.

Pietruszka, J.F., Hoffman, D., and McGivern, B.E. Jr. (1986). A broken dental needle and its surgical removal: a case report. *N. Y. State Dent. J.* 52 (7): 28–31.

Pogrel, M.A. (2009). Broken local anesthetic needles. A case series of 16 patients, with recommendations. *J. Am. Dent. Assoc.* 140 (12): 1517–1522.

Pogrel, M.A. and Thamby, S. (2000). Permanent nerve involvement resulting from inferior alveolar nerve blocks. *J. Am. Dent. Assoc.* 131 (7): 901–907.

Pogrel, M.A., Bryan, J., and Regezi, J. (1995). Nerve damage associated with inferior alveolar nerve blocks. *J. Am. Dent. Assoc.* 126 (8): 1150–1155.

Pogrel, M.A., Schmidt, B.L., Sambajon, V., and Jordan, R.C.K. (2003). Lingual nerve damage due to inferior alveolar nerve blocks. A possible explanation. *J. Am. Dent. Assoc.* 134 (2): 195–199.

Popowich, L.D. and Brooke, R.I. (1979). Postinjection infection – two unusual cases. *J. Oral Surg.* 37 (7): 494–495.

Prado, F.B., Caria, P.H.F., Silva, R.F. et al. (2010). Dental broken needle migration to the skull base. A case of dental broken needle migration to the skull base. Anatomical considerations and prevention. *J. Morphol. Sci.* 27 (2): 98–101.

Pragasm, M. and Managutti, A. (2011). Diplopia with local anesthesia. *Natl. J. Maxillofac. Surg.* 2 (1): 82–85.

Pretterklieber, M.L., Skopakoff, C., and Mayr, R. (1991). The human maxillary artery reinvestigated: I. Topographical relations in the infratemporal fossa. *Acta Anat.* 142 (4): 281–287.

Primosch, R.E. (1986). The role of pressure syringes in the administration of intraligamentary anesthesia. *Comp. Cont. Educ. Dent.* 7 (5): 340–348.

Queiroz, S.B.F., Lima, V.N., Amorin, P.H.G.H. et al. (2016). Retrieval of a broken dental needle close to the facial artery after cervical migration. *J. Craniofac. Surg.* 27 (4): e338–e340.

Rahman, N., Clark, M., and Stassen, L.F. (2013). Case report: management of broken dental needles in practice. *J. Ir. Dent. Assoc.* 59 (5): 241–245.

Ram, D. and Amir, E. (2006). Comparison of articaine 4% and lidocaine 2% in paediatric dental patients. *Int. J. Paediatr. Dent.* 16 (4): 252–256.

Rawson, R.D. and Orr, D.L. II. (1985). Vascular penetration following intraligamental injection. *J. Oral Maxillofac. Surg.* 43 (8): 600–604.

Reitz, J., Reader, A., Nist, R. et al. (1998). Anesthetic efficacy of the intraosseous injection of 0.9 mL of 2% lidocaine (1:100,000 epinephrine) to augment an inferior alveolar nerve block. *Oral Surg. Oral Med. Oral Pathol.* 86 (5): 516–523.

Ribeiro, L., Ramalho, S., Gerós, S. et al. (2014). Needle in the external auditory canal: an unusual complication of inferior alveolar nerve block. *Oral Surg. Oral Med. Oral Pathol.* 117 (6): e436–e437.

Ridenour, S., Reader, A., Beck, M., and Weaver, J. (2001). Anesthetic efficacy of a combination of hyaluronidase and lidocaine with epinephrine in inferior alveolar nerve blocks. *Anesth. Prog.* 48 (1): 9–15.

Rifkind, J.B. (2011). Management of a broken needle in the pterygomandibular space following a Vaziani-Akinosi block: case report. *J. Can. Dent. Assoc.* 77: b64.

Rigler, M.L., Drasner, K., Krejcie, T.C. et al. (1991). Cauda equina syndrome after continuous spinal anesthesia. *Anesth. Analg.* 72 (3): 275–281.

Rishiraj, B., Epstein, J.B., Fine, D. et al. (2005). Permanent vision loss in one eye following administration of local anesthesia for a dental extraction. *Int. J. Oral Maxillofac. Surg.* 34 (2): 220–223.

Roberts, D.H. and Sowray, J.H. (1987). *Local Analgesia in Dentistry*, 3e. Bristol (UK): Wright. 148–151.

Robinson, S.F., Mayhew, R.B., Cowan, R.D., and Hawley, R.J. (1984). Comparative study of deflection characteristics and fragility of 25-, 27-, and 30-gauge short dental needles. *J. Am. Dent. Assoc.* 109 (6): 920–924.

Rood, J.P. (1972). Ocular complication of inferior dental nerve block. A case report. *Br. Dent. J.* 132 (1): 23–24.

Saborido, G. (1977). Anestesia troncular del nervio maxilar superior por vía transpalatina. *Bol. Inf. Dent. (Madrid)* 37 (287): 37–47.

Sahin, B., Yildirimturk, S., Sirin, Y., and Basaran, B. (2017). Displacement of a broken dental injection needle into the perivertebral space. *J. Craniofac. Surg.* 28 (5): e474–e477.

Sambrook, P.J. and Goss, A.N. (2011). Severe adverse reactions to dental local anaesthetics: prolonged mandibular and lingual nerve anaesthesia. *Aust. Dent. J.* 56 (2): 154–159.

Seddon, H.J. (1943). Three types of nerve injury. *Brain* 66 (4): 17–288.

Sen, P., Waith, C., and Clark, S. (2006). (P.016) Fractured dental needle at the base of skull. *J. Cranio-Maxillofac. Surg.* 34 (Suppl 1): 136–137.

Shah, A., Mehta, N., and Von Arx, D.P. (2009). Fracture of a dental needle during administration of an inferior alveolar nerve block. *Dent. Update* 36 (1): 20–25.

Shaner, J.W., Saini, T.S., Kimmes, N.S. et al. (2007). Transitory paresis of the lateral pterygoid muscle during a posterior superior alveolar nerve block – a case report. *Gen. Dent.* 55 (6): 532–536.

Shannon, I.L. and Feller, R.P. (1972). Contamination of local anesthetic carpules by storage in alcohol. *Anesth. Prog.* 19 (1): 6–8.

Shannon, I.L. and Wescott, W.B. (1974). Alcohol contamination of local anesthetic cartridges. *J. Acad. Gen. Dent.* 22 (1): 20–21.

Shuaib, A. and Lee, M.A. (1990). Recurrent peripheral facial nerve palsy after dental procedures. *Oral Surg. Oral Med. Oral Pathol.* 70 (6): 738–740.

Sicher, H. (1950). Aspects in the applied anatomy of local anesthesia. *Int. Dent. J.* 1 (1): 70–82.

Simsek, I.B., Kiziloglu, O.Y., and Ziylan, S. (2013). Painful ophthalmoplegia following dental procedure. Case report. *Neuro-Ophthalmology* 37 (4): 165–168.

Skou, J.C. (1954). Local anesthetics. II. Toxic potencies of some local anesthetics and of butyl alcohol, determined on peripheral nerves. *Acta Pharmacol. Toxicol.* 10 (3): 292–296.

Smith, N.A. (1968). An investigation of the influence of gauge on some physical properties of hypodermic needles. Part I. The relation between gauge and flexibility of the needle. *Aust. Dent. J.* 13: 158–161.

Smyth, J. and Marley, J. (2010). An unusual delayed complication of inferior alveolar nerve block. *Br. J. Oral Maxillofac. Surg.* 48 (1): 51–52.

Stacy, G.C., Orth, D., and Hajjar, G. (1994). Barbed needle and inexplicable paresthesias and trismus after dental regional anesthesia. *Oral Surg. Oral Med. Oral Pathol.* 77 (6): 585–588.

Steenen, S.A., Dubois, L., Saeed, P., and de Lange, J. (2012). Ophthalmologic complications after intraoral local anesthesia: case report and review of literature. *Oral Surg. Oral Med. Oral Pathol.* 113 (6): e1–e5.

Stein, K.M. (2015). Use of intraoperative navigation for minimally invasive retrieval of a broken dental needle. *J. Oral Mexillofac. Surg.* 73 (10): 1911–1916.

Stone, J. and Kaban, L.B. (1979). Trismus after injection of local anesthetic. *Oral Surg. Oral Med. Oral Pathol.* 48 (1): 29–32.

Stoy, P.J. and Gregg, G. (1951). Bell's palsy following local anaesthesia. *Br. Dent. J.* 91 (11): 292–293.

Sved, A.M., Wong, J.D., Donkor, P. et al. (1992). Complications associated with maxillary nerve block anaesthesia via the greater palatine canal. *Aust. Dent. J.* 37 (5): 340–345.

Tal, M. (1982). The effect of long-acting local anaesthetic agent (Marcaine®) on the masticatory muscle in rats. *Int. J. Oral Surg.* 11 (2): 101–105.

Tamaddonfard, E., Farshid, A.A., Samadi, F., and Eghdami, K. (2014). Effect of vitamin B 12 on functional recovery and histopathologic changes on tibial nerve-crushed rats. *Drug. Res. (Stuttg)* 64 (9): 470–475.

Tavares, M., Goodson, J.M., Student-Pavlovich, D. et al. (2008). Reversal of soft-tissue local anesthesia with phentolamine mesylate in pediatric patients. *J. Am. Dent. Assoc.* 139 (8): 1095–1104.

Thompson, M., Wright, S., Cheng, L.H.H., and Starr, D. (2003). Locating broken needles. *Int. J. Oral Maxillofac. Surg.* 32 (6): 642–644.

Tiwari, I.B. and Keane, T. (1970). Hemifacial palsy after inferior dental block for dental treatment (letter). *Br. Med. J.* 1 (5699): 798.

Tomazzoli-Gerosa, L., Marchini, G., and Monaco, A. (1988). Amaurosis and atrophy of the optic nerve: an unusual complication of mandibular-nerve anesthesia. *Ann. Ophthalmol.* 20 (5): 170–171.

Torrente-Castells, E., Gargallo-Albiol, J., Rodriguez-Baeza, A. et al. (2008). Necrosis of the chin. A possible complication of inferior alveolar nerve block injection. *J. Am. Dent. Assoc.* 139 (12): 1625–1630.

Tui, C., Preiss, A.L., Barcham, I., and Nevin, M.I. (1944). Local nervous tissue changes following spinal anesthesia in experimental animals. *J. Pharmacol. Exp. Ther.* 81: 209–217.

Tzermpos, F.H., Cocos, A., Kleftogiannis, M. et al. (2012). Transient delayed facial nerve palsy after inferior alveolar nerve block anesthesia. *Anesth. Prog.* 59 (1): 22–27.

Uckan, S., Cilasun, U., and Erkman, O. (2006). Rare ocular and cutaneous complication of inferior alveolar nerve block. *J. Oral Maxillofac. Surg.* 64 (4): 719–721.

Van Eeden, S.P. and Patel, M.F. (2002). Prolonged paresthesia following inferior alveolar nerve block using articaine (letter). *Br. J. Oral Maxillofac. Surg.* 40 (6): 519–521.

Van Gijn, J. (2011). Charles Bell (1774–1842). *J. Neurol.* 258 (6): 1189–1190.

Vega, J.M. (1998). *Estudio de las quejas presentadas en la Comisión Deontológica del Colegio de la 1° Región (periodo 1982-1997)*. Madrid: Uniteco Profesional. 8, 9, 20.

Verma, D.K., Rajan, R., and Prabhu, S. (2013). Ipsilateral, isolated amaurosis after inferior alveolar nerve block: report of two rare cases. *Oral Maxillofac. Surg.* 17 (1): 73–75.

Von Arx, T., Lozanoff, S., and Zinkernagel, M. (2014). Ophthalmologische Komplikationen und Lokalanästhesie. *Swiss Dent. J.* 124 (11): 1189–1196.

Walker, M., Drangsholt, M., Czartoski, T.J., and Longstreth, W.T. Jr. (2004). Dental diplopia with transient abducens palsy. *Neurology* 63 (12): 1449–1450.

Webber, B., Orlansky, H., Lipton, C., and Stevens, M. (2001). Case report. Complications of an intra-arterial injection from an inferior alveolar nerve block. *J. Am. Dent. Assoc.* 132 (12): 1702–1704.

Wigand, F.T. (1960). Otalgia caused by a broken needle in the pterygomandibular space: report of case. *J. Oral Surg. Anesth. Hosp. Dent. Serv.* 18: 439–440.

Wilkie, G.J. (2000). Temporary unilocular blindness and ophthalmoplegia associated with a mandibular block injection. A case report. *Aust. Dent. J.* 45 (2): 131–133.

Willett, J., Reader, A., Drum, M. et al. (2008). The anesthetic efficacy of diphenhydramine and the combination diphenhydramine/lidocaine for the inferior alveolar nerve block. *J. Endod.* 34 (12): 1446–1450.

Williams, J.V., Williams, L.R., Colbert, S.D., and Revington, P.J. (2011). Amaurosis, ophthalmoplegia, ptosis, mydriasis and periorbital blanching following inferior alveolar nerve anaesthesia. *Oral Maxillofac. Surg.* 15 (1): 67–70.

Yoon, R.K. and Chussid, S. (2012). Ocular complications following an inferior alveolar nerve block on a child patient: a review of the literature and report of a case. *Pediatr. Dent.* 34 (4): 343–346.

Zelster, R., Cohen, C., and Casap, N. (2002). The complications of a broken needle in the pterygomandibular space: clinical guidelines for prevention and retrieval. *Pediatr. Dent.* 24 (2): 153–156.

Zurfluh, M.A., Daubländer, M., and Van Waes, H.J.M. (2015). Comparison of two epinephrine concentrations in an articaine solution for local anesthesia in children. *Swiss Dent. J.* 125 (6): 698–703.

# 23

# General Complications of Dental Local Anesthesia

General or systemic complications are less common during dental treatment than local complications, and it is estimated that *fewer than 1% of patients treated are affected* (see Tables 23.1 and 23.2). General complications or systemic toxicity can result in serious harm or even death, but fortunately most cases are of little consequence. Approximately *75% of cases are caused or associated with dental local anesthesia* (Table 23.3), and it has been observed that there are situations in which the frequency of general complications is increased, as follows:

- After multiple administrations of local anesthetic in the same patient (Persson 1969).
- Failure of local anesthetic (Persson 1969).
- Patients with a history of complications during administration of local anesthetic (Persson 1969).
- Patients at risk (ASA III) when treatment takes more than 30 minutes, especially patients with cardiovascular conditions (Hughes et al. 1966; Daubländer et al. 1997).
- Endodontic treatment and extractions increase the risk (Matsuura 1989; Malamed 1993).

**Table 23.1** Vasovagal syncope as a percentage of general complications that appear during dental treatment.

| Reference | Origin | Complications observed | Years of study | Vasovagal syncope (%) |
|---|---|---|---|---|
| Fast et al. (1986) | United States | 16.773 | 10 | 67 |
| Matsuura 1989 | Japan | — | 5 | 63 |
| Malamed (1993) | United States | 13.835 | 10 | 30 |
| Girdler and Smith (1999) | UK | 814 | 1 | 73 |
| | | | Mean | 58 ≈ **60** |

**Table 23.2** Percentage of patients who experience vasovagal syncope in the office, excluding patients aged <14 years.

| Reference | Sample size | No. of cases of vasovagal syncope | Cases of vasovagal syncope (%) |
|---|---|---|---|
| **First part, pre-1980** | | | |
| Moose (1959) | 1636 | 25 | 1.5 |
| Hannington-Kiff (1969) | 3000 | 60 | 2 |
| McGimpsey (1977) | 9513 | 100 | 1.1 |
| Edmondson et al. (1978) | 6265 | 135 | 2.2 |
| | | Mean | 1.7 ≈ **1.5** |
| **Second part, post-1980** | | | |
| Lemay et al. (1984) | 108 | 1 | 0.9 |
| Meechan and Blair (1989) | 440 | 1 | 0.2 |
| Hidding and Khoury (1991) | 1518 | 12 | 0.8 |
| Salins et al. (1992) | 1500 | 10 | 0.7 |
| D'Eramo (1992) | 199 045 | 278 | 0.4 |
| Daubländer et al. (1997) | 2731 | 12 | 0.4 |
| D'Eramo (1999) | 158 061 | 1114 | 0.7 |
| Lustig and Zusman (1999) | 1007 | 1 | 0.1 |
| Kaufman et al. (2000) | 179 | 1 | 0.6 |
| Moore et al. (2006) | 187 | 1 | 0.5 |
| | | Mean | 0.53 ≈ **0.5** |

Many patients in the first part (pre-1980) were treated while seated in the chair, therefore we took the values in the second part because patients were lying back in the dentist's chair (leading to fewer cases). The second part (post-1980) is the current data.

---

*Local Anesthesia in Dentistry: A Locoregional Approach*, First Edition. Jesús Calatayud and Mana Saraghi.
© 2024 John Wiley & Sons Ltd. Published 2024 by John Wiley & Sons Ltd.
Companion website: www.wiley.com/go/Calatayud/local

Table 23.3 Percentage of general complications during dental treatment caused by or associated with dental local anesthesia.

| Reference | Percentage of complications during Local anesthesia (%) | Dental treatment (%) | Total (%) |
|---|---|---|---|
| Hannington-Kiff (1969) | 36 | 48 | 84 |
| Edmondson et al. (1978) | 45 | 22 | 67 |
| Matsuura 1989 | 55 | 23 | 78 |
| Malamed (1993) | 55 | 22 | 77 |
| | | Mean | 76.5 |
| | | Rounded mean | **75** |

The two main causes or triggers of complications associated with local anesthetic are as follows: (i) psychogenic reaction because of anxiety and needle phobia, and (ii) adverse reactions to the components of the local anesthetic solution.

Death is the most severe complication that can arise in the dentist's office. Dental local anesthesia has proven to be very safe. Table 23.4 shows that when dental local anesthesia is administered with a minimum standard of recommended care, mortality is *one case in 100 million injections*, whereas with general anesthetic or deep sedation it is *one case in 500 000*, that is, a 200-fold greater risk. Furthermore, death during general anesthesia is recorded mainly in healthy patients graded as ASA I or II, whereas cases of death as a result of dental local anesthesia usually involve patients graded as ASA III or IV (Driscoll 1974). Finally, general complications, especially those caused by local anesthesia in the dental clinical setting are as follows:

1) Psychogenic reaction:
   - Vasovagal syncope.
   - Hyperventilation syndrome.
   - Allergic-like reactions.
2) Toxicity induced by sympathomimetic vasoconstrictors (epinephrine and norepinephrine).
3) Systemic toxicity induced by local anesthetics.
4) Toxic methemoglobinemia caused by some local anesthetics.
5) Allergic reactions to components of local anesthetic solutions.

Table 23.4 Frequency of death after dental local anesthesia and general anesthesia and deep sedation in dentistry.

| Reference | Origin | Study period | Deaths/patients | Frequency of death |
|---|---|---|---|---|
| **Local anesthesia** | | | | |
| Selding and Recant (1955) | USA | 1943–1952 | 2/90 million | 1/45 million |
| Cawson et al. (1983) | UK | 1970–1979 | 10/700 million | 1/70 million |
| Matsuura 1989 | Japan | 1984–1985 | 9/300 million[a] | 1/33 million |
| Perea et al. (2014) | Spain | 2000–2010 | 1/385 million[a] | 1/385 million |
| | | | Mean | 1/130 million |
| | | | Rounded mean | **1/100 million**[a] |
| **General anesthesia and deep sedation** | | | | |
| Driscoll (1974) | USA | — | 11/5 285 750 | 1/480 000 |
| Tomlin (1974) | UK | 1963–1968 | 26/7 956 000 | 1/300 000 |
| Coplans and Curson (1982) | UK | 1970–1979 | 99/15 168 000 | 1/150 000 |
| Lytle and Stamper (1989) | USA | 1968–1988 | 7/4 700 000 | 1/670 000 |
| Nkansah et al. (1997) | Canada | 1990–1995 | 4/2 830 000 | 1/700 000 |
| D'Eramo (1992, 1999), D'Eramo et al. (2003) | USA | 1984–1999 | 8/5 377 000 | 1/670 000 |
| | | | Mean | 1/495 000 |
| | | | Rounded mean | **1/500 000** |

[a] The data for Japan are estimated based on double the population of the UK since Japan has twice as many inhabitants. The data for Spain are based on 35 million cartridges per year (Rosso 2015). The figures for Japan may be underestimated and those for Spain may be overestimated, therefore we established the figure of 1/100 million.

## Preventive Measures

The main preventive measures we can take when administering local anesthetic in the office are as follows:

1) A complete *clinical history and health questionnaire* to obtain information about the patient's illnesses (e.g. diabetes, hypertension, history of myocardial infarction), current medications (e.g. beta-blockers, digoxin, insulin, tricyclic antidepressants), or general reactions to previous local anesthetics that the patient has experienced and require anesthetic techniques or solutions to be modified or reactions that simply contraindicate local anesthetic (Chapters 8–10).
2) *Reassure the patient* (Abasi 1987). The methods for administering local anesthetic are discussed in the chapter on basic injection techniques (Chapter 13). It is important to remember the repercussions of anxiety (Annex 17). Other techniques (e.g. pharmacologic therapy, hypnosis) in patients with considerable anxiety or medical problems are beyond the scope of this book.
3) *Prevent pain* (Abasi 1987), both during administration of the local anesthesia and during the dental procedure (in cases where deep anesthesia is necessary). It is important to remember the repercussions of pain (Annex 17).
4) *Aspirate before the injection* to prevent inadvertent intravascular injection of solution entering the bloodstream (Chapter 13). Although some authors have not found an association between positive and negative aspirations and systemic reactions (Forrest 1959; Goldman and Gray 1963; Persson et al. 1974; Blair and Meechan 1985; Lipp et al. 1988), possibly because toxic reactions to anesthetics are often confused with other types of reaction (e.g. vasovagal syncope), there is general consensus that aspirating reduces the risk of intravascular injection (Malamed 2004; Horowitz et al. 2005). Furthermore, aspiration is recommended at each stage to prevent intravascular injection (Lloyd 1992). It is important to remember that intravascular injection can sometimes increase toxicity by up to 200-fold (Meechan and Rood 1992).

    To ensure correct aspiration, it is very important to use 25G or 27G needles (25G is better) since they enable evaluation of the blood that colors the cartridge; this is not possible with 30G needles because the smaller lumen of the needle makes detection of aspiration unreliable and difficult, thus little blood enters the cartridge (see Chapter 11).
5) *The injection should be administered slowly*. The currently recommended rate is 1.8 ml in 40–60 seconds (Chapter 13), which enables us to reduce the toxicity of the anesthetic solution since fast injections can lead to rapid increases in plasma levels, especially in the case of inadvertent intravascular injections (Adriani and Campbell 1956; Adriani et al. 1959; Campbell and Adriani 1958; Scott and Hirschman 1982). Slow injections enable the anesthetic solution to dilute in the bloodstream (Adriani and Campbell 1956; Campbell and Adriani 1958; Forrest 1959), in turn enabling the lungs to retain some of the drug and attenuate the toxic effect (Tucker and Mather 1979; Scott 1986). Some authors consider slow injections to be the most important factor for preventing adverse reactions in dental local anesthesia, even more than aspiration (Malamed 2004).
6) *Do not exceed the maximum dose for dental treatment*. Remember the patient's weight and height, especially in preschool children and children younger than 6–8 years (Annex 10) and in low-weight adults with reduced body mass, who are very often elderly, to minimize the risk of overdose (Goodson and Moore 1983; Hersh et al. 1991; Virts 1999). It is also important to remember that topical anesthesia contributes to the dose administered and should be added to the total dose (Cannell 1996; Meechan 1998). It is very useful to keep the empty cartridges until the procedure has finished to know at all times the dose administered, especially in the case of repeated injections.

## Basic Management of Complications

This book does not address the management of general complications in the office: the reader can consult the several excellent texts available (Bennett and Rosenberg 2002; Malamed 2007; Grimes 2013) and guidelines such as those of the European Resuscitation Council (Monsieurs et al. 2015; European Resuscitation Council 2020) and the American Heart Association (Panchal et al. 2020; Topjian et al. 2020). However, we do wish to provide accepted guidelines on how to manage general complications.

### Initial Measures

The steps to be taken in the case of a general complication associated with local anesthesia are as follows:

1) Suspend the dental treatment being administered to address the complication that has arisen.
2) Patient position.
   - If the patient is conscious and is having difficulty breathing and/or shows signs of chest discomfort or is anxious or nervous, the best approach is to allow

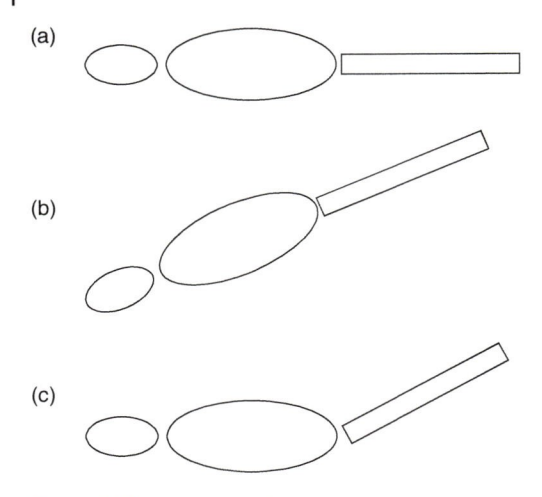

**Figure 23.1** (a) Patient lying in the horizontal position (supine decubitus). (b) Patient in the Trendelenburg position. (c) Correct position, horizontal with the legs raised.

him/her to find a position that is comfortable. This generally involves the patient *sitting up*.
- If the patient becomes dizzy and it seems that he/she is going to lose consciousness, the best position is lying down (supine decubitus), with the head at the same height as the rest of the body and heart, to help blood reach the brain. In addition, the legs should be raised 15–30° to favor venous return of the peripheral blood to the heart (Figure 23.1c).
- Two important observations about posture:
  o Do not place the patient in the Trendelenburg position, with the whole body in a straight line with the head pointing downwards (Figure 23.1b). In this posture, even though the head is lower than the heart, the abdominal organs exert pressure on the diaphragm, which in turn exerts pressure on the lungs, thus restricting respiration.
  o Pregnant women in the third trimester should not be placed horizontally face up, since the gravid uterus exerts pressure on the inferior vena cava, which ascends pressing against the spinal column, leading to aortocaval compression syndrome. In these cases, the best approach is to place the patient in the *left lateral recumbent position* (McGimpsey 1977).
3) Loosen tight clothing such as belts, ties, and shirt collars so as not to interfere with blood flow (Edmonson et al. 1978; Kuster and Udin 1985).

## Unconscious Patient

A loss of consciousness indicates a more dangerous phase, when we should adopt the PABC approach (Malamed 2007; Haas 2010) or the PCAB approach (Field et al. 2010).

**P: Posture**

The approach described is for a patient who reports dizziness, lightheadedness, or feeling faint, among other signs of impending unconsciousness, namely, lying down with the feet raised 15–30°. If the patient does not recover consciousness after a few seconds with this maneuver, then we should suspect a more severe underlying condition (i.e. arrhythmia, myocardial infarction, cerebrovascular accident, hypoglycemia) (Greenwood 2008; Sambrook et al. 2011).

**A: Airway**

1) Remove any apparatus from the mouth, for example gauze, cotton rolls, removable dental prosthesis, removable orthodontics devices, rubber dam, clamps, etc.
2) Clear the airway of obstruction by soft tissue, mainly a closed tongue, which falls backwards. Leave the patient's head in a horizontal position by removing the extra head supports before performing the following maneuvers:
   - Head tilt-chin lift maneuver (standard maneuver) (Figure 23.2).
     o The dentist places him/herself to the side of the patient's head and, with the palm of the hand on the forehead, pulls downward. With the index and middle finger of the other hand placed on the symphysis menti, the dentist pulls upward until the imaginary line that joins the earlobe with the chin is perpendicular to the floor. Thus, the head is turned backward and the neck extended.
     o During this maneuver, we should ensure that the patient's mouth is not fully closed and that the full extension of the neck does not obstruct the airway.
   - Jaw-thrust technique (Figure 23.3). Sometimes, the previous technique may not be sufficient to clear the upper airway. The head tilt-chin lift maneuver may not be applicable if the patient has a limited range of motion, such as one acquired by having a cervical spinal fusion or cervical disc herniation. The jaw-thrust technique allows manipulation of the airway without movement of the head or cervical spine. The technique is as follows:
     - The dentist places him/herself behind the patient's head and places his/her index and middle fingers behind the posterior border of the mandibular ramus, with one hand on each side, and pulls the mandible upward.
     - The lower lip can be pulled back with the thumbs to help the patient exhale through the mouth and nose.
     - This maneuver is uncomfortable. However, any audible complaint from the patient is a positive sign because it shows that the degree of unconsciousness is not so deep.

Basic Management of Complications | **437**

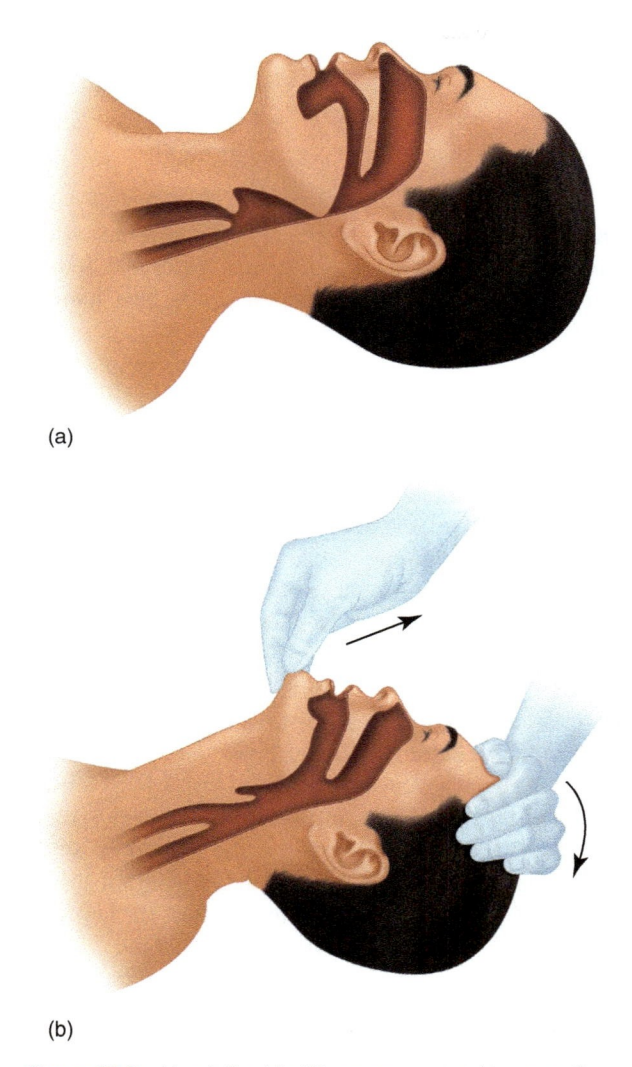

**Figure 23.2** Head tilt-chin lift maneuver, used to open the airways: (a) airway closed and (b) airway open.

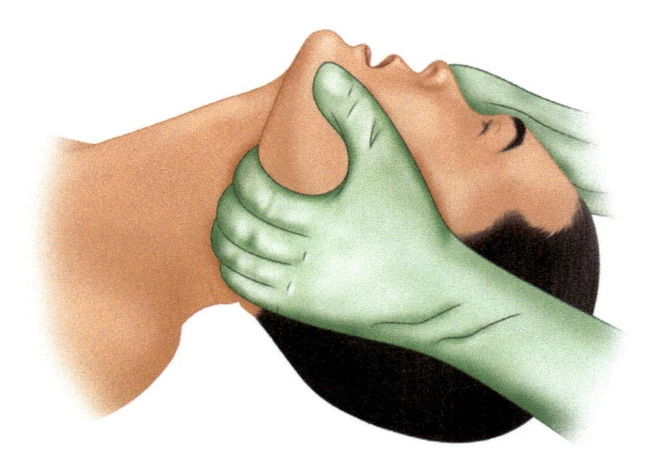

**Figure 23.3** Jaw-thrust technique, used to open the airways.

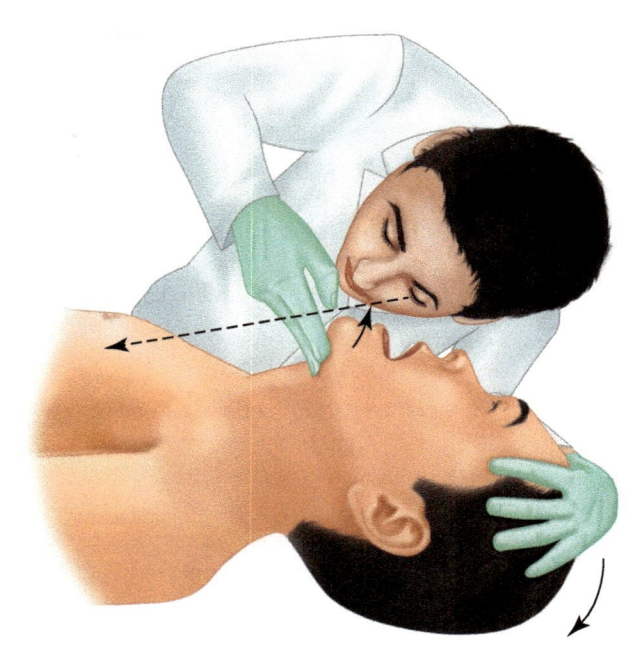

**Figure 23.4** With the patient in the head tilt-chin lift position, the dentist places his/her head with the ear approximately 2 cm from the patient's nose and mouth, with the face looking toward the patient's chest.

**B: Breathing**

1) With the hands on the patient's face to maintain the head tilt-chin lift position, the dentist places his/her head with the ear approximately 2 cm from the patient's nose and mouth and with the face looking toward the patient's chest. This position enables the following (Figure 23.4):
   - The dentist can hear and feel air entering and leaving the patient's nose and mouth (very reliable).
   - The dentist can see the movements of the patient's chest. This is not as reliable since, while it shows that the patient is trying to breathe, it does not guarantee that gas exchange is taking place (as the diaphragm may be working against an obstructed upper airway). Sometimes, the patient's clothing prevents the dentist from observing the movement of the chest.

2) A bubbling/gurgling noise indicates that the airway is partially obstructed by blood, saliva, water, secretions, or vomit and should be cleared. The approach to adopt is as follows:
   - The dentist positions the head downward and places the patient's head turned to one side to facilitate expulsion and prevent the aspiration of liquids and debris.
   - The dentist opens the patient's mouth with the index and middle finger and inserts an aspirator to suck out liquids and debris. The cannula can even be

inserted – carefully – in the posterior part of the mouth and lower pharynx to remove any remaining debris. The cannular should be plastic (not metal) so as not to further damage soft and hard tissue.

3) If the patient is not breathing and there is no debris, the dentist should undertake artificial respiration maneuvers (not covered in this book). Please consult guidelines such as those of the European Resuscitation Council and the American Heart Association.

### C: Circulation

At this point, the most important action is to *palpate the carotid artery*. With the patient in the low head tilt-chin lift position, remove the hand from the chin and, as the patient has his/her neck stretched, palpate the thyroid cartilage (Adam's apple). The carotid pulse is checked by placing the index and middle fingers between the thyroid cartilage and the sternocleidomastoid muscle.

If the pulse is weak but present, maintain the position until the patient recovers or until the emergency services arrive (see below) in the case of a patient whose condition remains unchanged or worsens.

If no pulse is felt for 10 seconds, start cardiopulmonary resuscitation. These maneuvers are beyond the scope of this book, although they are very well explained in other books and guidelines (Bennett and Rosenberg 2002; Malamed 2007; Monsieurs et al. 2015; Panchal et al. 2020; Topjian et al. 2020).

Note: The assistant can place a stethoscope on the patient's chest to evaluate the heart rate and take the patient's blood pressure with a sphygmomanometer. If the situation persists, the patient should be assessed every 5 minutes (heart rate, blood pressure, and breathing rate).

### Routes of Administration of Drugs

Specific maneuvers may be necessary depending on the complication, and it may even be necessary to administer drugs. We can make a series of comments on the routes of administration:

- Intravenous route. While this route is the fastest, it also requires specific training. It is necessary to apply a tourniquet and to find the appropriate vein in the arm, hand, forearm, or antecubital fossa.
- Sublingual route (Mercurio 1967). The drug is injected into the floor of the mouth underneath the tongue if the injection is intraoral (Figure 23.5a); if the injection is extraoral, the submental technique is used (Figure 23.5b). This technique has somewhat slower onset than the intravenous technique, although it is faster than the intramuscular technique (Sklar and Schwartz 1965; Nichols and Cutright 1971). In some cases, it may be a good alternative to the intravenous technique for dentists who find it difficult to insert an intravenous line. One important caveat to this is that injecting into a highly vascular area, such as the floor of the mouth, can result in a hematoma that can worsen an already obstructed airway (Weaver 2011).
- Intramuscular route. This route is slower than the others. The drug can be injected into the deltoid muscle (shoulder), gluteus muscle (upper lateral quadrant so as not to inject the sciatic nerve or the vessels of the leg), or the vastus lateralis muscle of the leg (medial-lateral area of the thigh), which is the preferred route in children. This route is one of the best for dentists.
- Subcutaneous route. This is the slowest route.

Parenteral injection techniques are addressed in various texts (Bennett and Rosenberg 2002; Malamed 2007).

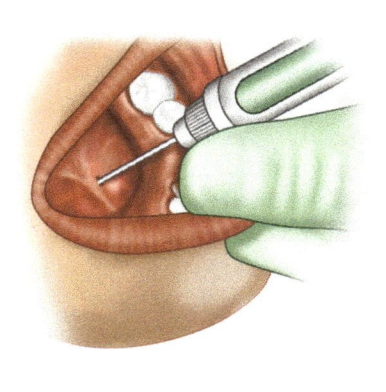

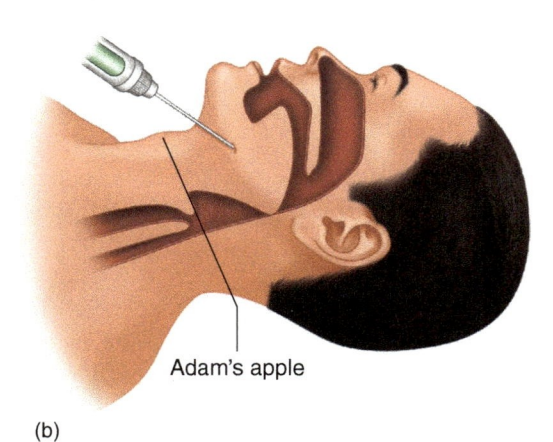

(a) (b)

**Figure 23.5** Sublingual injection techniques. (a) Injection into the floor of the mouth under the tongue if the drug is administered intraorally. (b) Submental approach if the drug is injected extraorally.

### Calling the Emergency Services

If the dentist observes that (i) the patient does not improve and the situation does not resolve, (ii) the patient's condition worsens, or (iii) his/her instinct indicates that the course of the complication is problematic, then the emergency services should be called so that the patient can be treated in situ by specialized staff with specialized equipment or taken to a hospital. *The emergency telephone number is 911 in the United States, 112 in the European Union, and 999 in the UK.*

## Psychogenic Reactions

Psychogenic, or psychosomatic, reactions are the most frequent general complications and can be classified into three types:

1) Vasovagal syncope: the most common.
2) Hyperventilation syndrome.
3) Allergic-like reaction: this is exceptional.

### General Causes

In all of the psychogenic reactions to be discussed, we can identify two key factors:

1) The emotional situation of anxiety, tension, fear, or panic. This is the basic factor.
2) The onset of intense and unexpected pain. This factor is closely associated with the first one because it triggers the emotional situation by creating a profound emotional experience of anxiety (McGimpsey 1977; Edmondson et al. 1978; Salins et al. 1992).

Anxiety is such an important factor that it is worth pointing out some associated characteristics:

- People who are naturally anxious. Approximately 10% of people have high levels of anxiety and fear when receiving dental treatment and a further 5% suffer from a phobia (Table 8.1, Chapter 8).
- Dental local anesthesia is the factor related to dental treatment that causes the highest levels of anxiety. Seeing the syringe and needle and feeling the prick of the needle generate the most anxiety (Chapter 8).
- It is difficult to differentiate between the behavior of anxious and non-anxious adults in the office (McGimpsey 1977; Kleinknecht and Bernstein 1978; Ayer et al. 1983; Scott et al. 1984), therefore the health questionnaire should contain a direct question on fear of dental treatment, which could be classified into five categories (from none to considerable fear) to identify the most anxious patients and to consider the risk of general complications and the need for concomitant treatment to sedate the patient and control anxiety (Kleinknecht and Bernstein 1978; Scott and Hirschman 1982; Ayer et al. 1983).

It is interesting to highlight how nervousness before dental treatment can induce vasovagal syncope, even before the treatment is administered (D'Eramo 1999).

### Vasovagal Syncope

Vasovagal syncope (neurocardiogenic syncope) is defined as a sudden and marked drop in blood pressure (hypotension) and heart rate (bradycardia) caused by anxiety, fear, and pain that is accompanied by weakness, sweating, and pallor. In its most severe form it involves a sudden, transitory loss of consciousness (syncope or faint) due to the drastic reduction in blood flow to the brain.

Vasovagal syncope is the most common complication during administration of dental anesthesia and dental treatment, *accounting for 60% or more of all general complications* (Table 23.1) and affecting *0.5% of patients treated* (one in every 200) (Table 23.2). Other authors report a frequency of one case every 6 months (Girdler and Smith 1999).

It is important to draw attention to the fact that this type of reaction is easily confused with toxic reactions to local anesthetics or vasoconstrictors and with allergic reactions (Verrill 1975; McCarthy 1982; Milgrom and Fiset 1986; Daubländer et al. 1997; Batinac et al. 2013).

#### Pathophysiology

The severe emotional reaction induced by anxiety leads to three types of reaction:

1) Severe hypotension. This is the main type of syncope. The emotional reaction and pain activate the parasympathetic nervous system in the brain (cholinergic), which acts via the vagus nerve (cranial nerve X), leading to the following:
   - Dilation of the vessels of the abdominal viscera (splanchnic circulation) (Bourne 1980).
   - Dilation of the vessels of the skeletal muscles in the absence of physical activity due to the lack of a fight or flight reaction (Harrison 1973; Edmondson et al. 1978; Bourne 1980).
   - Reduction in heart rate (bradycardia).
   
   These factors in turn lead to a severe reduction in blood pressure and therefore a reduction in blood flow to the brain. Curiously, the effect of this reaction can be triggered by stimulation of the autonomic nervous system (Taggart et al. 1976).

2) Hyperventilation syndrome. This syndrome does not always accompany vasovagal syncope, although when it does, the level of carbon dioxide ($CO_2$) falls, leading to a marked reduction in the concentration of this gas in blood (hypocapnia) and respiratory alkalosis caused by the increase in pH resulting from the reduction in carbonic acid. $CO_2$ is a key factor in the self-regulation of cerebral blood flow, which is independent of arterial pressure, therefore the reduction in $CO_2$ causes cerebral vasoconstriction, reducing blood flow to this organ (Harrison 1973; Campbell et al. 1976; Noble 1977; Salins et al. 1992) and peripheral vasodilation (Noble 1977).
3) Hypoglycemia. The parasympathetic reaction leads to increased insulin levels, which in turn reduces the blood glucose level (hypoglycemia). This also deteriorates because the hyperglycemic effect of epinephrine is reduced in situations of respiratory alkalosis due to hyperventilation, as reported elsewhere (Salins et al. 1992). Interestingly, blood sugar levels tend to self-regulate after the vasovagal syncope (Salins et al. 1992).

### Predisposing Factors

As we have seen, anxiety, fear, and pain are the main triggers of vasovagal syncope, although other factors can favor its appearance. Here, we classify them as more important and less important:

- More important, main factors (Table 23.5):
  o Patient age. In general, patients aged under 30–35 years account for 80% of cases. However, in children aged <14 years, the frequency of this type of reaction is very low (one per 2000 = 0.05%) because children react to emotional tension differently than adults. They do not repress the fight or flight response, but rather scream, cry, and kick up a fuss. They resist the injection and therefore do not experience a vasovagal reaction (Kuster and Udin 1985). It is estimated that around one-third of young adults are prone to this type of reaction (Yjipaavalniemi and Sane 1981).
  o Male sex. This is the main factor in 75% of cases. It is important to remember that males account for 40% of visits (Annex 1). The reason is that society teaches males not to show emotions such as fear or pain, therefore they repress the fight or flight reaction, thus leaving themselves open to vasovagal syncope.
  o Previous history. Patients with a history of fainting or syncope in other dental treatments or injections, blood donation, and vaccination. This is the case in almost half of all patients treated.
- Less important, additional factors (Table 23.5):
  o Lack of sleep.
  o Receiving dental treatment on an empty stomach.
  o Excess heat and humidity.

### Clinical Manifestations

Vasovagal syncope occurs in 75% of cases during administration of the local anesthetic or shortly after during dental treatment (Table 23.6) and can progress through several phases:

1) Early phase, presyncope, or prodrome. This phase lasts several minutes and is characterized by the following:
    - The patient is ill at ease, dizzy, and weak, with facial flushing.
    - The first typical cutaneous signs appear, especially on the face, with pallor and cold sweat, sometimes accompanied by nausea (rarely vomiting) (McGimpsey 1977).
    - Occasionally, palpitations resulting from the increase in heart rate, as well as respiratory abnormalities

Table 23.5 Factors predisposing to vasovagal syncope.

| Factor | Harrington-Kiff (1969) (%) | McGimpsey (1977) (%) | Edmondson et al. (1978) (%) | Salins et al. (1992) (%) | Rounded average (%) |
|---|---|---|---|---|---|
| **Main factors** | | | | | |
| Younger age | 82 | 81 | 83 | — | 80 |
| Male sex | 76 | 81 | 70 | — | 75 |
| Previous history | 50 | 28 | 48 | — | 45 |
| **Additional factors** | | | | | |
| Lack of sleep | — | — | 0, 7 | 12 | 5 |
| Empty stomach | 28 | 80 | 8 | 19 | 35 |
| Heat | 24 | — | 23 | — | 25 |

Data expressed as percentages for main and additional factors.

Table 23.6 Time of onset of vasovagal syncope.

| Reference | Sample size | During anesthesia (%) | During extraction (%) | Total: anesthesia and extraction (%) |
|---|---|---|---|---|
| Hannington-Kiff (1969) | 50 | — | — | 84 |
| McGimpsey (1977) | 100 | 31 | 47 | 78 |
| Edmondson et al. (1978) | 139 | 45 | 22 | 67 |
| | | | Mean | 75 |

with more frequent, superficial, or deep breathing (hyperventilation).
- Less frequently, ringing in the ears (tinnitus), blurred vision, and mouth opening, such as when yawning.
- Examination of cardiovascular parameters at the onset of this phase reveals increased blood pressure and heart rate due to anxiety (Campbell et al. 1976), although this all changes radically during the next phase.

2) Late phase or syncope (faint). The main characteristic of this phase is loss of consciousness (syncope or fainting) due to *severe hypotension and bradycardia*. It is important to point out that this does not occur in all patients who experience vasovagal syncope: if the patient realizes what is happening and starts treatment during the first phase, it can be avoided relatively easily. In older studies on extractions, 30% of patients fainted (Hannington-Kiff 1969; McGimpsey 1977), although today, and with the patient lying down, this percentage is much lower. Thus, we can observe the following:
- Loss of consciousness (fainting or syncope). If timely measures are taken, as we will see, the fainting episode lasts less than 1 minute and rarely more than 2 minutes (Hannington-Kiff 1969; McGimpsey 1977).
- The faint may be accompanied by dilation of the pupils (mydriasis).
- Trembling or shaking is relatively common.
- The cardiovascular examination reveals the biphasic response. *Low blood pressure*, which may fall to lower than 50–60 mmHg (systolic) and at which point the patient faints (Harrison 1973; Campbell et al. 1976; Kuster and Udin 1985), and *bradycardia* (under 50–60 beats per minute).

3) Recovery phase, which is characterized by recovery of consciousness, accompanied by confusion, disorientation, weakness, and, occasionally, headache.

**Management by the Dentist**

When the patient is conscious, it is essential to apply the initial measures we saw in the section on basic management of complications, as follows:

1) Place the patient lying down (supine decubitus) with the head at the same height as the heart so that the blood can reach the brain and raise the legs 15–30° to facilitate venous return.
2) Unfasten tight clothing, belts, ties, and shirt collars so as not to interfere with blood flow.

Note: Some professionals tend to place the patient in a seated position with the head between the legs at the level of the heart to help blood reach the head. This posture is not recommended because it prevents us from monitoring the patient's breathing and consciousness and from raising the patient's legs to favor venous return (McCarthy 1982).

Most patients recover with these measures and therefore do not reach the next phase:
- When the patient is already unconscious, we apply the basic PABC or PCAB management protocol. However, it is important to implement the following:
   1) Maintain the posture: patient lying down with the legs raised.
   2) Provide 100% oxygen through a mask (Hannington-Kiff 1969; Verrill 1975; McCarthy 1982; Milan et al. 1986).
   3) Initiate support measures:
      - Inhalation of ammonia salts arousal and consciousness (McCarthy 1982; Kuster and Udin 1985).
      - Placement of cold towels on the patient's head and forehead (McCarthy 1982; Kuster and Udin 1985).
      - If the patient is cold, cover him/her with a blanket (McCarthy 1982; Kuster and Udin 1985).
      - If possible, check blood glucose.
      If the patient does not recover within 30–60 seconds of applying these measures, call the emergency services: the patient may have a more severe underlying problem (i.e. myocardial infarction, cardiac arrhythmia, cerebrovascular accident, hypoglycemia) (Greenwood 2008; Sambrook et al. 2011).
- When the patient has recovered:
   1) Do not allow him/her to stand up until total resolution of symptoms.
   2) Provide a sugary drink to raise the low sugar levels resulting from the vasovagal syncope (Edmondson

et al. 1978; Salins et al. 1992). Hypoglycemia may also be a contributing factor to the syncopal episode, which often occurs as patients may skip a meal and come to the dental appointment.

3) Decide whether the patient should continue with the treatment. We suggest the following:
   - If the loss of consciousness lasts less than 10–15 seconds, the total recovery time takes less than 15 minutes, and the patient is less than 35 years old, treatment can be continued if the patient agrees.
   - If the loss of consciousness lasts more than 1 minute, the total recovery time takes more than 30 minutes, and the patient is older than 40 years of age, suspend treatment, recommend the patient to see a doctor and not to drive, and ask a relative or friend to take the patient home.
   - If in doubt, suspend treatment.

**Prevention**

Although vasovagal syncope is easily controlled in healthy patients, in ASA III patients with cardiovascular abnormalities, who tolerate anxiety and pain poorly, the situation may become life-threatening:

1) **Position during treatment**
   Ever since the contour dental chair was introduced in the 1960s, we have been working with the patient lying back, the dentist seated (Golden 1959; Anderson 1960), and a high aspiration rate (Thompson 1967). Not only does this form of working improve precision dental work, but with the patient lying back, cerebral blood flow is better. In addition, the risk of vasovagal syncope is higher with the patient seated and the dentist standing (Bourne 1957, 1970).
   
   Table 23.4 shows that the frequency of vasovagal syncope in the pre-1980, when patients were seated while the dentist stood, was higher than when dental work was carried out with the patient lying down and the dentist seated (1.5% vs. 0.5%).

2) **Control of anxiety**
   Patients with high levels of anxiety should be offered techniques to reduce anxiety and approaches that are beyond the scope of this book (conscious sedation, intravenous sedation). To determine the level of anxiety, we propose two key questions in the health questionnaire (Chapter 8):
   1) How frightened/anxious are you about dental treatment?
      Not at all ☐   A little ☐   Some ☐   Quite a lot ☐   A lot ☐
      If the patient selects the last two options (quite a lot or a lot), and especially the last, we should obtain more detailed information.
   2) Have you ever had an abnormal reaction, felt dizzy, or fainted at the dentist's or doctor's office when receiving a local anesthetic or vaccination or giving blood?
      Yes ☐   No ☐
      An answer in the affirmative should lead us to question the patient, given that a previous history is a major predisposing factor (see above) (Table 23.5).

## Hyperventilation Syndrome

Hyperventilation syndrome or reaction, which is also known as psychogenic dyspnea (Gardner 2000), was first described in 1937 (Kerr et al. 1937). Its definition should be refined since many of its components are confusing (Gardner 2000; Malmberg et al. 2001). Nevertheless, doctors frequently use it. The signs and symptoms of hyperventilation syndrome are often associated with vasovagal syncope, with some overlap between both conditions, although the vasovagal components are usually much more predominant than the respiratory components.

We can define hyperventilation syndrome as rapid and continuous respiration caused by anxiety that leads to a reduction in carbon dioxide ($CO_2$) in blood (hypocapnia) and causes vasoconstriction of the cerebral vessels. This in turn leads to reduced blood flow in the central nervous system (CNS) and respiratory alkalosis, which decreases ionized calcium concentration and causes musculoskeletal reactions.

Hyperventilation syndrome is estimated to account for *8% of general complications* (Matsuura 1989; Malamed 1993) and rarely appears in children for the same reasons as vasovagal reaction.

**Pathophysiology**

The main cause of the syndrome is the patient's emotional status (anxiety, fear, hysteria, phobia), which increases the respiratory rate, thus reducing the level of carbon dioxide in blood and leading to hypocapnia, also known as hypocarbia. $CO_2$ is a basic factor in the self-regulation of cerebral blood flow that is independent of arterial blood pressure, with the result that the constriction of the cerebral vessels reduces the quantity of blood in the brain (Campbell et al. 1976; Noble 1977; Chapman 1984; Milan et al. 1986; Salins et al. 1992; Gardner 2000) and leads to peripheral vasodilation (Noble 1977).

The reduction in the pressure of $CO_2$ in blood reduces carbonic acid levels, therefore blood pH increases (respiratory alkalosis) from 7.4 (normal) to 7.55, leading to two phenomena:

- The Bohr effect, which describes the effect of changes in blood pH on the avidity with which hemoglobin binds oxygen. In acidic conditions, the hemoglobin binds

oxygen with less affinity and makes it more available to the tissues. In alkaline conditions, such as with hypocarbia, the hemoglobin binds oxygen with more affinity, thus making it more difficult to release and worsening oxygenation of the brain (Chapman 1984).
- Reduction in ionized calcium, leading to musculoskeletal irritation, which manifests as cramps, shaking, and tetany (muscle spasms) (Harrison 1973; Chapman 1984).

Anxiety also leads to increased activity of the sympathetic nervous system and release of epinephrine and norepinephrine, which in turn produces cardiovascular manifestations in the form of increased arterial pressure and heart rate (tachycardia) (Harrison 1973; Chapman 1984; Milan et al. 1986). Finally, a vicious cycle is created: anxiety leads to hyperventilation, which in turn increases anxiety (Compernolle et al. 1979).

**Clinical Manifestations**
Clinical manifestations can be classified as follows:

1) Manifestations due to anxiety.
   - 80% with dizziness, disorientation, weakness that rarely progresses to loss of consciousness (syncope/fainting) (Compernolle et al. 1979; Chapman 1984); in 60% accompanied by anxiety, nervousness, and agitation (Compernolle et al. 1979).
   - 60% with palpitations owing to the increased heart rate (Compernolle et al. 1979).
   - 60% with pallor and excessive sweating (diaphoresis) (Compernolle et al. 1979; Chapman 1984).
   - Other manifestations are headache, blurred vision, ringing in the ears (tinnitus), nausea, and, more rarely, vomiting (Harrison 1973; Compernolle et al. 1979).
   - During the examination, the state of agitation reveals an increase in heart rate (tachycardia) and arterial blood pressure.
   - Sometimes the patient feels a sensation of chest tightness (distress) that may be made worse by breathing, although it is neither serious nor irradiated (Harrison 1973; Chapman 1984). The sensation is caused by irritation of the intercostal muscles and diaphragm due to increased respiratory effort (Chapman 1984).
2) Respiratory manifestations.
   - *Increased respiratory rate (tachypnea) in 75% of cases*, which reaches 25–30 breaths per minute instead of the normal rate (9–16). The breaths are deep or superficial. This is a basic sign (Harrison 1973; Noble 1977; Chapman 1984; Milan et al. 1986).
   - Sensation of asphyxia and difficulty breathing (dyspnea), occasionally with a "lump in one's throat" (globus sensation) in 50% of cases (Compernolle et al. 1979).
   - Frequent movements to open the mouth and dry mouth sensation caused by anxiety and continuous breathing with the mouth open.
3) Musculoskeletal manifestations (caused by reduced ionized calcium levels). Typical findings for this manifestation include the following:
   - Feeling of numbness, tingling, and dullness (paresthesia) in the fingers and hands in 80% of cases, feet in 50% of cases, and face (tongue and lips) in 40% of cases, with muscle cramps and pain that can lead to muscle stiffness.
   - *Tetany (50% of cases)*, which is characterized by muscle spasms in the hands and feet (carpopedal spasm) involving the following:
     - Stiffness of the hands (fingers and wrists) in flexion or extension, which is often painful (Geffner and Murgatroyd 1980).
     - Feet (less common), with stiffness of the toes and ankles in flexion.

**Differential Diagnosis**
- Vasovagal syncope. Hyperventilation syndrome does not involve loss of consciousness or reduced heart rate/arterial blood pressure; in addition, it does not improve with the patient lying down.
- Asthma or allergic respiratory manifestations (Gardner 2000). Hyperventilation syndrome does not involve breath sounds (wheezing) because there is no constriction of the bronchioles. In addition, it improves with treatment.
- Heart attack (angina pectoris or myocardial infarction). The chest pain is not severe and does not irradiate to the arms or shoulders. Furthermore, it improves with treatment.

**Management by the Dentist**
We apply the basic measures (initial measures) seen above, although here we place emphasis on the patient's position. As the patient experiences difficulty breathing, *he/she should be seated*, not lying horizontally (in contrast with the approach to a vasovagal syncope) (Harrison 1973; Chapman 1984). Furthermore, specific measures for these cases are presented in increasing order of importance, as follows:

1) Explain to the patient what is happening to reassure him/her and ask him/her to breathe more slowly (six to eight breaths per minute) and thus reduce the respiratory rate (Harrison 1973; Chapman 1984). This measure is usually successful.
2) Breathe into a paper or plastic bag. This approach should only be applied when the previous measure has failed. The patient is asked to place a paper bag over his/her nose and mouth and breathe into the bag (a plastic

bag is also suitable, although as it is softer, it collapses easily over the nose and mouth). Thus, by breathing his/her own air, $CO_2$ re-enters the patient's lungs and the signs and symptoms tend to improve (Harrison 1973; Compernolle et al. 1979; McCarthy 1982; Chapman 1984).

Today, paper bag rebreathing should never recommended unless myocardial ischemia can be ruled out and the patient's oxygenation has been directly measured by arterial blood gases or pulse oximetry: since these conditions are impossible to achieve outside the hospital this method is not recommended (Callaham 1989).

3) Medication. If the previous measure fails because the patient is very nervous, then this last alternative must be applied. This situation is very unusual because the previous measures are usually successful. In this case, intramuscular midazolam 5 ml (5 mg) is injected, and in 5–15 minutes the patient relaxes and recovers. Midazolam can also be given orally, although its effect takes more than 30 minutes.

A classic alternative is to inject diazepam (Valium®) 2 ml (10 mg) intramuscularly, although as it is not water-soluble, this is more painful (Chapman 1984).

Patients who experience hyperventilation syndrome generally recover very well, do not lose consciousness, and can continue with their dental treatment.

## Allergic-like Reactions

These are also known as anaphylactoid reactions (Baldo et al. 2008) or allergic-like reactions because they are non-immune reactions caused by emotional tension that can lead to release of compounds such as histamine (Ring 1985) and reactions such as the following:

- Urticaria associated with anxiety (Milan et al. 1983; Tauberg et al. 1983).
- Angioedema associated with anxiety (Barclay and Edwards 1971; Chue 1976).

Note: The clinical description of these conditions is provided in this chapter (see below) in the section on allergy, where such conditions are typical.

Fortunately, this type of reaction is very rare and, logically, is confused with allergic reactions, since it is characterized by similar manifestations, but can be distinguished from allergic reactions by the negative result in allergy tests. Patients who experience reactions can be treated at the dentist's office with anxiolytics and sedation (Milan et al. 1983; Tauberg et al. 1983).

## Toxicity Induced by Sympathomimetic Vasoconstrictors

*Approximately 3% of the general adverse reactions* that occur during administration of local anesthetic are to epinephrine (Fast et al. 1986; Matsuura 1989). Interestingly, these reactions are usually confused with vasovagal syncope.

### Pathophysiology

Initially, it was thought that the signs and symptoms were caused by the action of catecholamines (epinephrine and norepinephrine) in the brain. However, it has been shown that this is not the case because the low lipid solubility of these substances makes it difficult for the drugs to penetrate the CNS and intraventricular or intracisternal injections (direct administration to the brain) lead to sedation (Marley and Stephenson 1972).

The real cause of these actions is via the cardiovascular system, metabolic action, and neuromuscular transmission caused by these same adrenergic amines (Jastak et al. 1995). *The reactions appear immediately* as a result of an inadvertent intravascular injection, overdose, or severe interactions with other drugs (Pogrel et al. 2014). In any case, *the effect is usually short*, since catecholamines are inactivated after a few minutes (less than 5) (Lund 1951).

### Symptoms of Reaction to Epinephrine

As we have seen, onset is rapid, occurring shortly after injection or even during injection. The reaction lasts only a few minutes and is characterized by the symptoms set out below (Dick 1953; Holroyd et al. 1960; Jastak et al. 1995; Malamed 2004):

- Patient-reported symptoms:
  - *Sensation of anxiety, nervousness*, fear, and apprehension.
  - *Palpitations (tachycardia)* resulting from the force and speed at which the heart contracts. This is the main symptom.
  - Dizziness, vertigo, and weakness.
  - Occasionally, nausea, which rarely progresses to vomiting, difficulty breathing (dyspnea) caused by anxiety and, more rarely, headache, which is sometimes throbbing owing to the force with which the heart pumps blood, thus increasing pressure in the head.
- The signs are as follows:
  - Pale and cold skin, mainly on the face, and sweating (diaphoresis).
  - Occasionally, trembling in the lips and hands.

- The cardiovascular examination reveals *increased heart rate*, with frequent premature ventricular contraction, increased systolic arterial pressure and increased blood pressure.

### Symptoms of Reaction to Norepinephrine

As seen above, onset of the reaction is rapid, shortly after the injection or even during the injection, generally at high concentrations, such as 1:25 000 (40 µg/ml) or 1:30 000 (33 µg/ml) (Boakes et al. 1972; New Zealand Committee on Adverse Drug Reactions 1974), and the reaction lasts a few minutes. The symptoms are set out below (Boakes et al. 1972; Meyer 1986; Van der Bijl and Victor 1992):

- Patient-reported symptoms:
  - *Headache is the main symptom* and the most frequent. Onset is immediate or within a few minutes. It is usually severe (often so intense that patients press their hands to their head). It generally affects the temporal or occipital area (nape of the neck), although there have been reports of frontal headache. The headache may be throbbing, although not always, and rarely may persist for hours or days, albeit with less intensity. This is due to involvement of the CNS.
  - Other symptoms include anxiety, nervousness, apprehension, nausea (although rarely vomiting), and difficulty breathing (dyspnea) caused by anxiety.
- The signs are as follows:
  - Pale and cold skin, mainly on the face, and sweating (diaphoresis).
  - In contrast, the skin of the face is sometimes flushed.
- The cardiovascular examination reveals *reduced heart rate (bradycardia)*, which is a very characteristic sign, and *increased arterial pressure* (both systolic and diastolic).

The general cause of reaction to norepinephrine is the encephalopathy caused by the hypertensive crisis.

### Management by the Dentist

- The usual approach is as follows:
  1) Interrupt the dental procedure in progress.
  2) Wait and see if the reaction resolves itself, given that it is usually mild or moderate and disappears after a few minutes (less than 5), and continue with treatment.
- If the reaction does not resolve within a few minutes:
  1) Place the patient in a comfortable position, generally erect or seated/semiseated (never lying down). This position minimizes the effect of hypertension on brain tissue.
  2) Monitor the patient every 5 minutes, recording heart rate and blood pressure.
  3) If the situation persists:
     - Administer oxygen through a mask. However, it is important not to confuse this situation with hyperventilation, in which case oxygen worsens the situation.
     - Administer a sedative (diazepam or midazolam) parenterally (intramuscular); however, when these drugs take effect, the reaction has generally resolved.
  4) Wait until the patient has completely recovered, seated in the dental chair, from the fatigue resulting from the adrenergic excitation and only allow him/her to leave when fully recovered. When in doubt of any resolution of symptoms, activate emergency medical response services.
- Exceptionally, in predisposed patients, these situations (owing to the increased heart rate and/or increased blood pressure) can cause a heart attack (angina pectoris or myocardial infarction) or cerebrovascular accident. In these cases, and although beyond the scope of this book, the support measures set out at the beginning of this chapter should be followed and the emergency services called (911 in the United States, 112 in the European Union, and 999 in the UK).

## Systemic Toxicity Induced by Local Anesthetics

Approximately 1.5% of all general complications occurring during administration of local anesthetics are caused by toxicity (Malamed 1993). It is important to remember that many such complications are mistaken for allergy and vasovagal syncope, when allergic reactions are usually very different from local anesthetic-induced toxicity (see below).

### Pathophysiology

Local anesthetics block sodium channels indiscriminately in excitable membranes (Covino 1987; Lai et al. 2004), the main targets being the nervous system and the muscles, especially the heart and cardiovascular system. In the case of toxicity, it is important to take into account the plasma level of the local anesthetic: venous concentrations are 20–50% lower than arterial levels (Eriksson et al. 1966; Moore et al. 1977; Knudsen et al. 1997), but physicians use the venous plasma values (expressed as micrograms per milliliter, µg/ml) (Annex 13).

Despite marked individual variability, toxic manifestations begin to appear when the local anesthetic exceeds a specific concentration (Annex 13). In addition, toxicity increases with the greater relative potency of the anesthetic and therefore is observed at lower plasma levels (Covino 1987; Garfield and Gugino 1987).

Local anesthetics first attack the CNS, which is more vulnerable, therefore lower plasma concentrations should be sought. Thus, as local anesthetic concentrations in blood increase, the drug can easily cross the blood–brain barrier owing to its high lipid solubility (Garfield and Gugino 1987) and low molecular weight (Covino 1987), affecting the CNS and leading to seizures. Subsequently, as plasma levels gradually increase, the cardiovascular system, which is more resistant, becomes involved, thus initiating the collapse that leads to death (Covino 1987; Garfield and Gugino 1987). The areas affected are as follows:

- CNS. In the delicate balance between inhibition and excitation, initial excitation is the predominant initial characteristic. The inhibitory neurons are blocked and the patient may have shaking, tremors, diplopia, tinnitus, and seizures. As toxicity advances, both inhibition and excitation are depressed, resulting in loss of consciousness (Garfield and Gugino 1987).
- Heart. Contractility is reduced, as is heart rate (bradycardia) (Covino 1987).
- Vessels. The direct action of the anesthetic leads to vasodilation as a result of relaxation of the vascular muscle tissue, and blood pressure falls (hypotension). In addition, as the sympathetic preganglionic nerve fibers are anesthetized, thus blocking the vasoconstrictor effect, both the vasodilator effect and hypotension become more pronounced.

During the convulsion phase, breathlessness is accompanied by a marked increase in oxygen consumption owing to the effort of muscular contractions. We therefore observe the following:

- The amount of oxygen reaching the tissues decreases (hypoxia), thus aggravating cerebral depression.
- $CO_2$ levels increase (hypercarbia), with two effects:

1) $CO_2$ is a basic feature of self-regulation of cerebral blood flow. Increased $CO_2$ levels lead to increased blood flow, with the result that the amount of local anesthetic reaching the brain also increases (Covino 1987).
2) The increase in $CO_2$ also increases carbonic acid levels and therefore decreases pH (respiratory acidosis). The free fraction of the local anesthetic increases as the fraction bound to plasma proteins decreases. The free fraction exerts the pharmacologic and toxic effect, and thus increases toxicity (Tucker and Mather 1979; Scott 1975a; Covino 1987; Garfield and Gugino 1987; Knudsen et al. 1997).

## Causes of Local Anesthetic-induced Toxicity

### Inadvertent Intravascular Injection

Inadvertent intravascular injection is the most common cause of local anesthetic-induced toxicity (Covino 1978; Scott 1986). It acts through two pathways:

1) Passage to the bloodstream. In this case, the intravascular injection sends the local anesthetic into the bloodstream. However, passage is not slow and gradual, as is the case with subcutaneous injection. Consequently, the high concentration of drug can reach the target organs, and lower doses can reach toxic levels in the CNS and cardiovascular system.

   It has been estimated that rapid intravascular injection of a 1.8-ml cartridge of 2% anesthetic (e.g. lidocaine 2%), which is equivalent to 36 mg of drug, reaches the same concentration in blood as a 1080-mg dose injected subcutaneously (equivalent to 30 cartridges) (Scott 1986).

   Slow injection, even if it is intravascular, partially reduces this risk since passage of the drug into the bloodstream is slightly slower, thus enabling it to dilute (Campbell and Adriani 1958; Forrest 1959). In addition, slow injection enables the lungs to retain the drug – albeit for a short period – thus attenuating its toxic effect (Tucker and Mather 1979; Scott 1986).

2) Direct passage to the brain. Retrograde arterial flow has been demonstrated in experiments (Aldrete et al. 1977, 1978) and enables intraorally injected anesthetic to reach branches of the superior alveolar artery (maxillary) or inferior alveolar artery (mandibular) and reverse the flow of blood with the force of the injection, to the extent that it reaches the maxillary artery and, from there, the external carotid artery and even the internal carotid artery, where normal flow returns and the drug is transported to the brain (Figure 22.6, Chapter 22). Thus, 2 mg of injected anesthetic can reach the cerebral bloodstream at a concentration of 20 μg/ml (Aldrete et al. 1977, 1978), although, fortunately, for a short time.

Intravascular injection therefore has a series of specific characteristics that can be summarized as follows:

1) The toxic *reaction occurs within a few minutes* (if the drug passes into the bloodstream) or *even immediately* (if the drug passes directly to the brain), with rapid onset of symptoms and even convulsions (Scott 1986).
2) The toxic reaction *is short-lived*, fortunately, because, as the blood in the CNS passes into the bloodstream, its toxic concentration in the brain decreases rapidly.

Furthermore, not all techniques for administering local anesthetics are equally likely to inject the drug into the bloodstream. Table 13.2 (Chapter 13) summarizes the percentages of positive aspirations in the different techniques for administering dental local anesthesia. It is very important to aspirate before injection and to inject the drug slowly.

**Overdose**

Administration of excess local anesthetic is a less common cause of toxicity, although it is more frequent in the following situations:

1) Children, especially preschool children and those aged under 6–8 years (Goodson and Moore 1983; Hersh et al. 1991; Virts 1999).
2) Low-weight adults and adults with low body mass. This is very often the case with elderly people.
3) Administration of topical anesthetics (Weisel and Tella 1951; Adriani and Campbell 1956; Wehner and Hamilton 1984; Mehra et al. 1998). It is important to remember that topical anesthetics contain much higher concentrations of anesthetic and their quantity must be added to the quantity of anesthetic already injected.

Toxicity by overdose is characterized by a series of specific factors, as follows:

1) *The toxic reaction appears much later, generally 5–20 minutes after the injection*, although rarely more than 30 minutes later (Weisel and Tella 1951; Adriani and Campbell 1956; Wehner Hamilton 1984; Mehra et al. 1998; Goodson and Moore 1983; Hersh et al. 1991; Virts 1999).
2) The reaction is *much more severe and long-lasting* than that caused by intravascular injection. In a case series of pediatric sedation and local anesthetic overdoses by Goodson et al., a distinct separation of fatal and nonfatal overdoses was demonstrated when the maximum recommended dose (MRD) was *exceeded by threefold*. This meant that any combination of adding the relative MRDs of the sedatives and the MRD of the local anesthetic administered was highly likely to lead to death or significant morbidity (irreversible brain damage). This study demonstrated that any combination of the following would be very likely to result in serious morbidity or mortality: (1) an overdose of local anesthetic by three times its MRD, (2) an overdose of a sedative agent by three times its MRD, or (3) a combination of dosing of the local anesthetic and the sedative that exceeds the sum of their respective MRDs by threefold (Goodson and Moore 1983; Hersh et al. 1991).

To avoid this complication, every attempt should be made not to exceed the MRDs of dental anesthetic according to body weight (Annex 10). It must also be remembered that the dose of topical anesthetic administered should be added to the injected dose (Cannell 1996; Meechan 1998).

**Rapid Absorption**

Rapid absorption may result from injection into very vascularized tissue (Scott 1986), for example inflamed areas, as is the case with patients receiving dental treatment. This situation is very rare in dentistry because of the low doses and local anesthetic solutions we apply.

## Clinical Manifestations

Much has been learned about the clinical manifestations of toxicity by local anesthetics from clinical trials with volunteers who received intravascular infusions (Foldes et al. 1960, 1965; Eriksson et al. 1966; Usubiaga et al. 1966; de Jong and Bonin 1966; Jorfeldt et al. 1968; Scott 1975a,b; Friedman et al. 1982; Knudsen et al. 1997), from published cases of toxicity (Weisel and Tella 1951; Adriani and Campbell 1956; Goodson and Moore 1983; Wehner and Hamilton 1984; Mehra et al. 1998; Hersh et al. 1991; Virts 1999), and from updated reviews (Gitman et al. 2019).

We divided clinical manifestations into four phases, from lesser to greater severity, although there may be numerous overlaps and presentation may vary widely from one patient to another (Eriksson et al. 1966).

**First Phase: Initial**

The initial phase is characterized by symptoms that may go unnoticed by the physician if the patient does not report them. The manifestations include the following:

- Dizziness, vertigo, somnolence, disorientation, and confusion. Patients sometimes complain of feeling drunk or, much more rarely, excited and euphoric.
- *Sensation of heat that spreads throughout the body.* Patients may also feel cold, although this is much rarer.
- *Sensation of numbness or paresthesia in the area of the mouth* (lips, tongue) and face that can spread to the extremities and throughout the body. The effect is thought to occur when the local anesthetic leaves the vessels and blocks the sensory nerve endings (Scott 1986). It is important to note that in a local anesthetic systemic toxicity or overdose, the patient will note perioral numbness and tingling, and not just numbness on the side anesthetized.
- Other less common manifestations include a metallic taste and headache (cephalea) resulting from cerebral vasodilation.

## Second Phase: Advanced

The advanced phase is characterized, in addition to new symptoms, by objective signs of toxicity that are observed by the physician and can be considered very typical.

- Ocular abnormalities, which may be subjective (symptoms) or objective (signs):
  - Subjective. Visual abnormalities such as blurred vision, double vision (diplopia), color blindness, and seeing lights or flashes and moving objects.
  - Objective. Involuntary eye movements up and down or side to side (nystagmus), which may first be slow in one direction and then rapid in the opposite direction. Dilation of the pupils (mydriasis) in the more advanced phases. Subtle movements of the eyelashes and eyelids, with occasional difficulty opening the eyes.
- Hearing abnormalities, such as sounds or metallic echoes (tinnitus) or, on the contrary, loss of auditory acuity.
- *Difficulty speaking*, saying unrecognizable words (slurred speech). In some cases, this sign must be differentiated from those observed in neurotic or hysterical patients (Scott 1986).
- *Involuntary muscle activity*, such as shaking, spasms, muscle twitch, and trembling affecting the muscles of the face, fingers, hands, and extremities. This type of muscle activity must be distinguished from trembling caused by cold or nervousness (Scott 1986).
- Other, less frequent manifestations include difficulty swallowing and the feeling of "a lump in one's throat," anxiety with a sensation of chest tightness (distress), nausea (rarer), and vomiting (very rare).

## Third Phase: Convulsions

The third phase is characterized only by objective signs of toxicity. Symptoms are no longer present. The signs are as follows:

- Loss of consciousness (almost always).
- *Convulsions*, which usually appear after loss of consciousness, although this is not always the case (Usubiaga et al. 1966).
  - Convulsions take the form of tonic and clonic contractions. In tonic (static) convulsions, the whole body is rigid, with the arms stretched or flexed but stiff and the legs stretched and stiff. Clonic (dynamic) convulsions are characterized by movements of the head and flexion, stretching, and violent shaking of the limbs.
  - Tonic and clonic contractions frequently alternate for several seconds, then stop for a few seconds before entering a new cycle.
  - Foaming at the mouth as a result of air entering and mixing with saliva and blood (from biting the edge of the tongue or lips).
  - Convulsions are violent movements that can be differentiated from the trembling (which is much softer) that often occurs during vasovagal syncope (Scott 1986).
- Respiratory difficulty or inability to breath (apnea), especially during the convulsion. Hyperventilation is rare.
- The end of the convulsion may be accompanied by involuntary urination owing to relaxation of the sphincters (de Jong and Bonin 1966).

Note: In the early phases, cardiovascular examination reveals moderate involvement with increased and decreased arterial blood pressure and heart rate, although moderate increases are more common. The acute phase is characterized by increased arterial blood pressure (Rutten et al. 1989).

## Fourth Phase: Final

The final phase is characterized by two possibilities: (i) toxicity is not controlled and the patient develops cardiovascular depression, and (ii) the patient recovers.

1) Cardiovascular depression. The patient always loses consciousness and toxicity affects the cardiovascular system, with a marked reduction in heart rate (bradycardia) and arterial blood pressure (hypotension), and peripheral vasodilation (red and hot skin). If the condition is not controlled the patient dies of cardiorespiratory failure.
2) Recovery. Clinical trials with volunteers show that recovery time after the patient presents signs and symptoms of toxicity (without reaching the final phase) and the intravenous infusion of local anesthetic has ceased is somewhat less than 20 minutes (Table 23.7). However,

Table 23.7 Average recovery time among clinical trial volunteers who received local intravenous anesthetics.

| Local anesthetic | Recovery time (min) | Reference |
|---|---|---|
| Procaine | 26 | Usubiaga et al. (1966) |
| Lidocaine | 18 | Foldes et al. (1960), (1965) |
|  | 10 | De Jong and Walts (1966) |
|  | 10–15 | Eriksson et al. (1966) |
|  | 38 | Usubiaga et al. (1966) |
|  | 5–20 | Knudsen et al. (1997) |
| Mepivacaine | 29 | Foldes et al. (1965) |
| Prilocaine | 10–15 | Eriksson et al. (1966) |
| Bupivacaine | 20 | Knudsen et al. (1997) |
| Ropivacaine | 13 | Knudsen et al. (1997) |
| Mean | 17.6 ≈ **20** |  |

recovery may take 40 minutes in some cases. Short periods of toxicity leave no permanent neurological abnormalities or sequelae (Garfield and Gugino 1987).

## Clinical Variations

Some local anesthetics present specific characteristics in the clinical manifestations of toxicity.

1) Tetracaine and toxicity without convulsions.
   Tetracaine is a local ester-type anesthetic that is currently used as a topical anesthetic. Toxicity is characterized by the following: (i) greater frequency than with other local anesthetics, (ii) rapid and sudden onset with no initial signs, and (iii) no convulsions in 70–80% of cases (Weisel and Tella 1951; Adriani and Campbell 1956). Tetracaine-induced toxicity progresses rapidly to cardiovascular depression, with loss of consciousness, which can prove fatal (Weisel and Tella 1951; Carabelli 1952; Adriani and Campbell 1956; Adriani et al. 1959); furthermore, owing to its high degree of vasodilation, tetracaine is the only topical anesthetic that enters the bloodstream quicker than by subcutaneous injection (Adriani and Campbell 1956).
2) Bupivacaine and cardiotoxicity.
   All local anesthetics are toxic for the central nervous and cardiovascular systems, and bupivacaine is no exception. However, this local anesthetic is characterized by being the most cardiotoxic (Covino 1987). Cardiotoxicity has already been addressed (Chapter 9), therefore the maximum dose in dentistry is 90 mg.

## Management by the Dentist

Onset of the signs and symptoms of local anesthetic-induced toxicity should be addressed using the basic initial measures seen above (e.g. suspend treatment, placing the patient in the supine position). However, a series of more specific measures should also be taken, as follows:

1) Remove the anesthetic and/or stop the injection
   If the manifestations of toxicity appear during the injection (immediate manifestations), then the reaction has resulted from intravascular passage directly to the brain and the injection should be stopped immediately. If topical anesthetic has been applied and the manifestations of toxicity appear after a few minutes, then the dose is excessive and the remaining anesthetic should be removed from the mouth (Wehner and Hamilton 1984).
2) Administer oxygen ($O_2$)
   It has been shown that $O_2$ (Daos et al. 1962; Englesson and Matousek 1975) and hyperventilation (Englesson and Matousek 1975) protect against the toxicity of local anesthetics, since higher doses were needed to kill experimental animals. Therefore, when necessary, oxygen 100% should be administered through a facemask and the patient should be asked to breathe more quickly (hyperventilation) to reduce $CO_2$ levels.
3) Prevention of lesions caused by convulsions
   If the patient begins to experience convulsions, we should *remove the dental unit* to prevent the patient from knocking against it. One member of the dental team should *support the upper part of the body* (head, arms, and trunk), while the other *holds the patient's legs* to avoid contact with the cuspidor or falling from the chair. The support should not be rigid, but rather should leave the patient with some freedom while preventing extreme movements (hyperextension), which can lead to dislocations and fractures.

   *Never place anything into the patient's mouth.* Many dentists and nurses have been trained to prevent intraoral lesions by introducing handkerchiefs, towels, or napkins into the patient's mouth. This maneuver is dangerous during convulsions owing to the strong contractions of the mouth. In addition, forcing the mouth open could lead to injury of the soft tissue, dental fractures, or injury to the fingers of the person involved (never insert your fingers into the mouth of a patient experiencing convulsions). Clinical studies report mild oral lesions in around half of cases. These almost all affect the border of the tongue, and only 2% require surgery (Roberge and Maceira-Rodriguez 1985).

   If the patient has fallen to the floor, the approach set out above is followed, although in this case, it is useful to *remove chairs and objects that the patient might come into contact with*. The patient's head should be protected by placing a pillow, blanket, towel, or jacket underneath to prevent violent contact with the floor.

   In the absence of intense overdose, these measures are generally sufficient and the convulsions resolve within 10 minutes (Scott 1986). However, if the convulsions last more than 2–5 minutes, we should move on to the next stage and administer an anticonvulsant.
4) Injection of an anticonvulsant (midazolam)
   The currently used medication is midazolam hydrochloride, a benzodiazepine that is three to four times stronger than diazepam. As it is water soluble (diazepam is not), it can be injected intramuscularly, sublingually, or submentally. It is less irritant than other drugs and has 90% bioavailability and absorption (Blumer 1998). In addition, its half-life is short (2 hours), its plasma peak is rapid, and its metabolites are not active, thus making it faster acting, safer, and more efficacious than diazepam (de Jong and Bonin 1981).

As dentists generally find it difficult to insert an intravenous line, an option is intramuscular administration. The drug can be injected into the deltoid muscle (shoulder), gluteus muscle (upper lateral quadrant so as not to inject the sciatic nerve or the vessels of the leg), or the vastus lateralis muscle of the leg (medial-lateral area of the thigh).

Convulsions were previously treated with barbiturates; however, these can lead to respiratory depression, thus aggravating the situation (Goodson and Moore 1983). Convulsions were later treated with diazepam (2 ml with 10 mg), a benzodiazepine that is as efficacious but does not lead to respiratory depression. Today, the preferred drug is another benzodiazepine, midazolam, because of the advantages set out above.

### Recovery and Discharge

If the signs and symptoms are mild and the patient does not experience convulsions and recovers well in a few minutes, then dental treatment can continue.

If, on the other hand, the clinical manifestations are very severe and recovery is slow, he/she should be sent home accompanied by a relative. In cases of doubt, a detailed report of the incident should be made and the patient should see his/her doctor for a check-up.

If the patient requires a benzodiazepine (midazolam or diazepam) for the convulsions, the patient loses consciousness, or it is necessary to call the emergency services because of severe cardiovascular depression, then he/she should be taken to a hospital for observation during the recovery phase. A detailed report of the incident should be made (e.g. time of onset, anesthetic solution and quantity injected, technique used, patient's reaction, onset of reaction, signs, and symptoms, patient's progress, etc.).

It is important to remember that severe systemic intoxication by local anesthetics in clinical practice may be fatal in 4% of cases. Consequently, advanced life support and intravenous lipid emulsion are necessary (Gitman et al. 2019).

### Prevention

The main measures for preventing local anesthetic-induced toxicity were addressed at the start of the chapter and include the following: (i) aspirate before injection, (ii) inject slowly, and (iii) do not exceed the maximum dental dose for body weight.

## Toxic Methemoglobinemia

Hemoglobin (Hb) is a stable, tetrameric iron-containing protein that is found in red cells (erythrocytes) and that binds reversibly to oxygen ($O_2$), which is released in body tissue. Each molecule of Hb has four iron atoms, each of which binds to an $O_2$ molecule. Iron has to be in its ferrous form ($Fe^{++}$ or $Fe^{2+}$) for gas exchange with tissue to take place. However, the ferrous form is unstable, and small amounts transfer to the ferric form ($Fe^{+++}$ or $Fe^{3+}$), in which $O_2$ binds so firmly that it cannot be released, with the result that gas exchange does not take place. Hb with iron in the $Fe^{3+}$ form is known as methemoglobin (MHb) (Curry 1982; Rodriguez et al. 1994; Coleman and Coleman 1996) or, albeit more rarely, hemoglobin (Hi) (Olson and McEvoy 1981).

Erythrocytes can reduce MHb to Hb via two pathways (Curry 1982; Rodriguez et al. 1994; Coleman and Coleman 1996):

- The nicotinamide-adenine-dinucleotide methemoglobin reductase (NADH-MHb-reductase) system or NADH-cytochrome $b_5$-reductase or diaphorase because it depends on cytochrome $b_5$ (Olson and McEvoy 1981; Jackobson and Nilsson 1985; Coleman and Coleman 1996; Aalfs et al. 2000). This system is responsible for recycling 95% of MHb to Hb.
- The nicotine-adenine-dinucleotide-phosphate-methemoglobin reductase (NADPH-MHb-reductase) system, which requires the enzyme glucose-6-phosphate-dehydrogenase (G-6-P-D) and is responsible for reducing the remaining 5% of MHb to Hb.

Under normal conditions, less than 1–2% of Hb is in the form of MHb (Hjelm and Holmdahl 1964; Lund and Cwick 1965; Curry 1982; Anderson et al. 1988; Rodriguez et al. 1994; Wilburn-goo and Lloyd 1999), although this may increase for two reasons:

1) Hereditary abnormalities:
   - Hemoglobin M. Altered Hb that is a poor transporter of $O_2$ (Anderson et al. 1988).
   - NADH-MHb-reductase deficiency caused by an alteration in chromosome 22 (Aalfs et al. 2000).
   - NADPH-MHb-reductase deficiency.
   - G-6-P-D deficiency.
2) Acquired (toxic) factors. Around 100 chemical compounds and medications can produce MHb (Coleman and Coleman 1996), including two local anesthetics, prilocaine and benzocaine (Coleman and Coleman 1996; Wilburn-goo and Lloyd 1999), therefore the condition is also called acquired or toxic methemoglobinemia. It is interesting to note that of 100 scientific reports on toxic methemoglobinemia in the twentieth century, nine were dental cases (Wilburn-goo and Lloyd 1999).

The earliest sign of toxic methemoglobinemia is cyanosis or a bluish color to the skin, nails, and lips (Lund and Cwick 1965). The toxicity stems from the fact that toxic methemoglobinemia can reduce the capacity to transport oxygen to the tissues, leading, in extreme cases, to death by hypoxia.

## Local Anesthetics Involved

A review of 242 cases of local anesthetic-induced toxic MHb collected between 1947 and 2007 revealed that 65% were caused by benzocaine and 30% by prilocaine; both anesthetics were clearly the most frequently involved (Guay 2009).

### Benzocaine

Benzocaine is a rapid and safe topical anesthetic, which, because it is scarcely water soluble, is absorbed poorly. However, cases of benzocaine-induced toxic methemoglobinemia have been appearing since the middle of the twentieth century (Ocklitz 1949; Bernstein 1950). In 1979, the United States Food and Drug Administration (FDA) reported this complication to be rare, with one case for every 140 000 applications of topical anesthetic (Wilburn-goo and Lloyd 1999). However, the number of cases published gradually increased, even in dental practice (Townes et al. 1977; Potter and Hillman 1979; Klein et al. 1983; Anderson et al. 1988).

Although benzocaine is not normally absorbed, it can enter the bloodstream through the gastrointestinal tract (Berstein 1950; Townes et al. 1977; Potter and Hillman 1979; Rodriguez et al. 1994) or via eroded and inflamed skin or mucosa (Severinghaus et al. 1991; Rodríguez et al. 1994).

The mechanism underlying toxic methemoglobinemia is not well known (Rodriguez et al. 1994), although the condition seems to involve a metabolite resulting from oxidation of benzocaine (Coleman and Coleman 1996), especially nitrobenzene-like (Singh and Al 2019).

There is no official figure for the maximum dose of benzocaine (Beutlich 1991); however, several authors agree that there is a clear risk of toxic methemoglobinemia with doses greater than 15–25 mg/kg (Potter and Hillman 1979; Rodriguez et al. 1994). This criterion is increasingly accepted (Klein et al. 1983; Severinghaus et al. 1991; Wilburn-goo and Lloyd 1999). In addition, the risk is elevated in small children (Townes et al. 1977; Kellet and Copeland 1983; Severinghaus et al. 1991), especially in those under one year old. In fact, one review of 44 cases showed that almost half involved children in this age group (Rodriguez et al. 1994). It is important to remember that the concentration of benzocaine in topical anesthetic is very high (20%).

In conclusion, we can say that benzocaine should be avoided in children aged less than 2 years (Singh and Al 2019) and that doses of more than 15–25 mg/kg should be avoided, given their association with toxic methemoglobinemia, but it is not possible to predict who will be at risk. Finally, after the 242 cases review, in susceptible individuals, there is no "therapeutic window" between the doses required to produce a therapeutic effect and those producing toxicity (Guay 2009).

### Prilocaine

Since the first reports of cases of methemoglobinemia caused by prilocaine (Daly et al. 1964; Scott et al. 1964), a direct association has been established between the amount of anesthetic administered and the level of MHb (Onji and Tyuma 1965; Hjelm and Holmdahl 1964; Lund and Cwick 1965; Spoerel et al. 1967), although considerable individual variations have been reported (Spoerel et al. 1967).

MHb reaches peak values at 1.5–4 hours after administration of prilocaine (Onji and Tyuma 1965; Lund and Cwick 1965; Spoerel et al. 1967) and tends to disappear spontaneously at 8–14 hours (Daly et al. 1964; Spoerel et al. 1967), although occasionally it can last 5–72 hours depending on the level reached in blood (Lund and Cwick 1965; Kreutz and Kini 1983).

The cause of methemoglobinemia is not prilocaine (Scott et al. 1964), but its metabolite orthotoluidine (o-toluidine) or 2-methylaniline (Onji and Tyuma 1965; Lund and Cwick 1965; Spoerel et al. 1967). Another metabolite of prilocaine 4-hydroxy-o-toluidine has been shown to cause methemoglobinemia (Frayling et al. 1990).

Clinical research has shown that onset of cyanosis is usually at 400 mg (Daly et al. 1964; Lund and Cwick 1965) and that it tends to become generalized at ≥900 mg of injected prilocaine (Scott et al. 1964; Lund and Cwick 1965). Thus, the absolute maximum recommended adult (≥70 kg) dose in medical practice is 600 mg (8.5 mg/kg) (Lund and Cwick 1965; Spoerel et al. 1967). According to the prudent 1984 recommendation of the Council on Dental Therapeutics of the American Dental Association, the maximum recommended adult dose in dental practice is 400 mg (5.7 mg/kg) (American Dental Association 1984).

It is interesting to note that most cases of cyanosis in dental practice occurred when the maximum medical dose (8.5 mg/kg) was exceeded (Anonymous 1994; Hardwick and Beaudreau 1995) or when the dose was close to the limit (Kreutz and Kini 1983; Duncan and Kobrinsky 1983; Johnson 1994). However, there is one report of a child with idiopathic toxic methemoglobinemia induced by low-dose prilocaine (Ludwig 1981).

### Other Anesthetics

Table 23.8 shows local anesthetics for which studies have *found no association* with toxic methemoglobinemia after

Table 23.8 Local anesthetics and studies showing that they do not produce toxic methemoglobinemia.

| Anesthetic | Reference |
| --- | --- |
| Lidocaine | Onji and Tyuma (1965) |
|  | Hjelm and Holmdahl (1964) |
|  | Lund and Cwick (1965) |
|  | Muschaweck and Rippel (1974) |
|  | Weiss et al. (1987) |
| Articaine | Muschaweck and Rippel (1974) |
|  | Rupieper et al. (1978) |
|  | Rupieper and Stocker (1981) |
| Bupivacaine | Rupieper and Stocker (1981) |
| Etidocaine | Lund et al. (1973) |
|  | Rupieper and Stocker (1981) |
| Procaine | Hjelm and Holmdahl (1964) |

intravenous administration or other types of parenteral administration. The main anesthetics involved are lidocaine, articaine, bupivacaine, etidocaine, and procaine.

However, the review of 242 cases includes 12 (5%) that are associated with lidocaine, although lidocaine was the trigger *in only three of these cases* since the remaining cases involved other drugs (oxidative drugs) that were administered concomitantly (nitrate therapy, benzocaine, dapsone, phenazopyridine, phenacetin, etc.) (Deas 1956; Burne and Doughty 1964; O'Donohue et al. 1980; Olson and McEvoy 1981; Hall et al. 2004), therefore the literature suggests a less clear association with lidocaine (Guay 2009).

The review addresses tetracaine in an even more limited fashion (Guay 2009) since there was only one case in which the anesthetic was the only trigger (Levergne et al. 2006). Consequently, the association is even weaker.

Nevertheless, it seems prudent to avoid both lidocaine and tetracaine in patients taking other oxidative drugs and especially in patients with congenital methemoglobinemia (Guay 2009).

## Aggravating Factors

Patients with diseases or abnormalities that alter or hamper transport of oxygen to tissues are more vulnerable to prilocaine- and benzocaine-induced toxic methemoglobinemia. These conditions include the following.

1) Cardiovascular disease
   - Any heart disease (e.g. heart failure, coronary artery disease, arrhythmias, etc.) because these reduce the flow of blood to the liver, where local anesthetics are metabolized (Spoerel et al. 1967; Wilburn-goo and Lloyd 1999), or reduce transport of oxygen to tissue (Olson and McEvoy 1981; Duncan and Kobrinsky 1983; Rodriguez et al. 1994).
   - Anemia (abnormalities of and/or reductions in red cells). Patients with anemia have less healthy hemoglobin in circulation, and the reduced hemoglobin caused by methemoglobinemia aggravates the situation (Lund and Cwick 1965; Spoerel et al. 1967; Olson and McEvoy 1981; Duncan and Kobrinsky 1983; Severinghaus et al. 1991; Anonymous 1994; Rodriguez et al. 1994; Wilburn-goo and Lloyd 1999).
   - Insufficient blood supply to the brain or periphery since transport of oxygen to the brain is more seriously compromised (Spoerel et al. 1967).
2) Severe respiratory diseases
   In patients with severe respiratory diseases, oxygen exchange in the lungs decreases and toxic methemoglobinemia aggravates this situation (Anonymous 1994; Wilburn-goo and Lloyd 1999).
3) Extreme age groups (children aged less than 1 year and elderly patients)
   - Newborns, infants, and, to a lesser extent, children aged less than 1 year have a greater proportion of MHb in blood owing to the immaturity of their enzymatic system (Kunzer and Schneider 1953; Ross and Desforges 1959; Ross 1963), seen mainly in the form of reduced activity of the methemoglobinemia reductase system (Ross 1963; Lo and Agar 1986). This situation is more severe during the first months of life (Kunzer and Schneider et al. 1953), although it is considered to involve a certain degree of risk until the patient is 1 year old (Severinghaus et al. 1991; Kellet and Copeland 1983; Rodriguez et al. 1994).
   - Elderly patients are more vulnerable to toxic methemoglobinemia because many have diseases that impair oxygen transport (i.e. cardiovascular disease, respiratory disease, anemia) and are on medication, some of which exerts oxidative action on hemoglobin (Wilburn-goo and Lloyd 1999).
4) Hereditary methemoglobinemia
   A few hundred cases have been reported of patients with genetic diseases that involve abnormalities of hemoglobin or of its metabolic pathways (Olson and McEvoy 1981; Curry 1982; Coleman and Coleman 1996; Wilburn-goo and Lloyd 1999). Most cases are diagnosed by pediatricians during the patient's first year of life (Wilburn-goo and Lloyd 1999).

## Clinical Manifestations

Onset of symptoms is late, generally within 2–4 hours after administration of the anesthetic, and usually coincides with the peaks of MHb (Malamed 2004; Esteban‐Sanchez et al. 2013). Anesthetics are metabolized during this interval, which is when toxic metabolites are generated. Furthermore, clinical manifestations are associated with the amount of MHb, that is, the greater the amount of MHb, the greater the severity, as follows:

- MHb 10–15%. Onset of cyanosis (Curry 1982; Kreutz and Kini 1983; Anderson et al. 1988; Wilburn‐goo and Lloyd 1999), which is characterized by the following:
  - Bluish‐colored or brown‐gray‐bluish‐colored skin (Lund and Cwick 1965; Townes et al. 1977; Curry 1982; Coleman and Coleman 1996; Wilburn‐goo and Lloyd 1999), although the condition is best observed in the nails (nail bed), lips, and oral mucosa. In persons with black skin, cyanosis is also detected in the nail bed and oral mucosa (Wilburn‐goo and Lloyd 1999).
  - Blood is dark in color (chocolate brown) (Daly et al. 1964; Olson and McEvoy 1981; Kreutz and Kini 1983; Anderson et al. 1988; Rodriguez et al. 1994; Coleman and Coleman 1996).
  - The patient's urine is dark (Curry 1982).
- MHb 30–40%. Symptoms of hypoxia (Spoerel et al. 1967; Curry 1982; Duncan and Kobrinsky 1983; Kellet and Copeland 1983; Anderson et al. 1988; Rodriguez et al. 1994; Coleman and Coleman 1996), which involve the following:
  - Sensation of weakness, fatigue, and dizziness.
  - Headache (cephalea).
  - Difficulty breathing, sensation of breathlessness (dyspnea).
  - On occasion, nausea, and even vomiting.
  - Physical examination reveals increased heart rate (tachycardia).
- MHb 55–60%. Onset of CNS depression (Curry 1982; Duncan and Kobrinsky 1983; Rodriguez et al. 1994; Anonymous 1994; Coleman and Coleman 1996):
  - Signs of lethargy and stupor that progress to loss of consciousness and coma.
  - The cardiovascular examination reveals arrhythmia, reduced heart rate (bradycardia), and progress to heart failure.
- MHb 70%. Death by hypoxia‐induced heart failure (Curry 1982; Anderson et al. 1988; Rodriguez et al. 1994; Coleman and Coleman 1996).

Some authors have reported that the signs of cyanosis first appear when MHb levels are 5–6% (Hjelm and Holmdahl 1964; Jakobson and Nelson 1985), although in healthy patients, malaise starts at 10–15% (Coleman and Coleman 1996).

Finally, it is important to bear in mind that the severity of symptoms depends on two factors simultaneously (Wilburn‐goo and Lloyd 1999): (i) the amount of MHb in blood depends on the amount of benzocaine or prilocaine administered and absorbed, and (ii) the risk the patient is at owing to his/her general health (e.g. cardiovascular disease, respiratory disease, extreme age groups).

### Management by the Dentist

If the first signs of cyanosis appear at the dentist's office (unusual because they usually appear hours after administration of the anesthetic), then the steps to be taken are as follows:

- Remove topical anesthetic from the mouth (Benzocaine, EMLA, Oraqix) or stop administering injectable prilocaine (Potter and Hillman 1979; Curry 1982; Anderson et al. 1988).
- Administer 100% oxygen through a facemask to facilitate the transport of $O_2$ to tissue (Olson and McEvoy 1981; Jakobson and Nelson 1985; Hardwick and Beaudreau 1995; Coleman and Coleman 1996). It should be noted that cyanosis does not resolve despite administration of oxygen (Jakobson and Nelson 1985).
- Send the patient to the emergency department for observation and determination of MHb in blood (Wilburn‐goo and Lloyd 1999). If the situation worsens, call the emergency services (911 in the United States, 112 in the European Union, and 999 in the UK).

At the medical center, the first step is to evaluate the patient's situation and determine the level of MHb in blood. The appropriate measures can then be taken. Data from modern pulse oximeters are not valid as they cannot detect methemoglobin and will often read out a false reading of 85% or 86% saturation (Pogrel et al. 2014). In severe cases, the patient receives a very slow (5 minutes) intravenous injection of methylene blue (methylthioninium chloride) (Curry 1982), which boosts the NADPH‐MHb‐reductase system and resolves cyanosis in 15–60 minutes (Wendel 1939; Ludwig 1981; Klein 1983; Klein et al. 1983; Kreutz and Kini 1983; Curry 1982; Rodriguez et al. 1994; Hardwick and Beaudreau 1995).

## Allergy

Allergies to local anesthetic solutions are adverse drug reactions triggered by an immune mechanism (Becker 1995). They account for *fewer than 1%* of all general complications in the dentist's office (Table 23.9), although many patients report any adverse effect as being allergic (Batinac et al. 2013). Table 23.10 shows some of the basic terms used in allergology. The substances that trigger

Table 23.9 Allergic reactions as a percentage of general complications in the dentist's office.

| Reference | Origin | No. of emergencies studied | Years of study | Allergic reactions (%) |
|---|---|---|---|---|
| Fast et al. (1986) | United States | 16 773 | 10 | 0.8 |
| Malamed (1993) | United States | 13 835 | 10 | 1.3 |
| Chapman (1997) | Australia | 2743 | 15 | 0.3 |
| Girdler and Smith (1999) | United Kingdom | 814 | 15 | 0.9 |
| | | | Mean | 0.8 ≈ 1 |

Table 23.10 Basic allergy terminology.

| | |
|---|---|
| Anaphylactic reaction or anaphylaxis | Severe systemic reaction (life-threatening) caused by an IgE-mediated immunological reaction |
| Anaphylactoid reaction | Severe systemic reaction (life-threatening) allergic type caused by a nonimmune mechanism or a reaction that has not been shown to be allergic |
| Allergic-like reaction | Reaction similar to allergic reactions but caused by a nonimmune mechanism |
| Reagin | Mainly, but not exclusively, immunoglobulin E (IgE) |
| Atopy | Hereditary predisposition to production high levels of IgE to common allergens |
| Sensitization | Process by which a person who does not react to an allergen comes to react to an allergen |
| Hypersensitivity | Exaggerated response of a target organ to specific stimuli (allergens) or nonspecific stimuli (physical exercise) |
| Idiosyncrasy | Exaggerated nonimmune response not due to pharmacologic effect |
| Intolerance | Exaggerated nonimmune response due to a pharmacologic effect |
| Skin tests | Prick test, intradermal test, patch test, subcutaneous test |

an allergic hypersensitivity reaction are known as *allergens* and may be of two types:

- Antigens, which are high-molecular-weight polysaccharides or proteins that stimulate the immune system directly to trigger an allergic reaction.
- Haptens (incomplete antigens), which are low-molecular-weight compounds that do not stimulate an immune response by themselves, but combine with a host protein to form new compounds that have sufficient antigenic capacity to trigger the allergic response (Giovannitti and Bennett 1979). Local anesthetics or products derived from their metabolism act as haptens (Giovannitti and Bennett 1979; Schatz 1984; Schatz and Fung 1986).

As adverse drug reactions, allergic reactions have a series of specific characteristics:

1) *Previous contact* with the drug and a latency (or incubation) period are necessary for the immune system to become sensitized.
2) *They are dose-independent.* The allergic reaction starts with very low doses of allergen. In contrast, toxicity is directly associated with dose (dose–response relationship). Although there is a certain association between dose and response in allergic reactions, the response is always disproportionate to the dose.
3) Once a patient has had allergy to a drug, then the patient is allergic *for an indefinite period*, given that the immune system has memory, therefore the drug is absolutely contraindicated (De Nova et al. 1996).

Allergic reactions can be classified into four types, as established by Gell and Coombs in 1963 (Coombs and Gell 1968):

- Type I or humoral or anaphylactic reaction or immediate type, which is mediated by immunoglobulin E (IgE) and includes anaphylaxis, bronchial asthma, and urticaria.
- Type II or cytotoxic reaction, such as autoimmune hemolytic anemia and fetal erythroblastosis.
- Type III or immune complex reaction, such as Arthus reaction and serum sickness.
- Type IV or delayed-type immune reaction, which is cell-mediated and includes contact dermatitis.

Local anesthetic solutions cause type I and IV allergic reactions (Germishuys and Anderson 1982; Canfield and Gage 1987; Assem and Punnia-Moorthy 1988; Doyle and Goepferd 1989; Ball 1999; Wilson et al. 2000; Fuzier et al. 2009; Batinac et al. 2013) and very rarely type III reactions (Lederman et al. 1980), although it is not always clear that a reaction is type III (see Chapter 22, "Localized Late-Onset Skin Lesion").

- Type I or humoral reaction. This IgE-mediated antigen–antibody reaction develops as a *systemic reaction* that manifests in a few minutes, although it often takes longer (generally less than 1 hour to a few hours) if the hapten is a metabolite resulting from the breakdown of a local anesthetic compound and takes time to catabolize. This type of reaction accounts for *20% of all allergies* to local anesthetics.

- Type IV or delayed-type immune reaction. This T lymphocyte-mediated reaction occurs at the contact site, although it may have systemic effects, as is the case with type I reactions (Campbell et al. 2001). It manifests after *hours or days* (generally more than 6 hours or 1 or 2 days) and is *the most frequent reaction (80%)* to local anesthetic solutions (Aldrete and Jonhson 1970; Larson 1977; Giovannitti and Bennett 1979; Johnson and DeStigter 1983; Ball 1999).

Finally, the most common causes of allergy in the dentist's office are (in order of frequency) latex, penicillin, non-steroidal anti-inflammatory drugs (NSAIDs), and, albeit much more rarely, local anesthetics (Greenwood 2008). Therefore, allergy to local anesthetics is very rare.

## Allergy to the Components of Local Anesthetic Solution

As we saw in Chapter 7, local anesthetic solutions have various components, and a patient may become sensitized to each of them. We analyze these components below.

### Local Anesthetic

As we saw in Chapter 5, the intermediate chain determines the type of biotransformation and catabolism of anesthetics, therefore, there are two groups that have clearly different allergic manifestations.

### Esters

Esters, or amino-esters, are anesthetics that are metabolized rapidly through hydrolysis by plasma cholinesterases or pseudocholinesterases and form compounds such as para-aminobenzoic acid (PABA). This compound has marked sensitizing potency (Giovannitti and Bennett 1979) and was reported in 1920 in the first cases of allergic dermatitis in dentists (Guptill 1920; Klauder 1922). Allergic reactions to the ester group are frequent and take the form of cross-reactions between the different ester anesthetics (Adler and Simon 1949; Aldrete and Jonhson 1970; Giovannitti and Bennett 1979; Johnson and DeStigter 1983; Schatz 1984; Adriani et al. 1986).

The frequency of allergic reactions to ester drugs has fallen dramatically since 1950 for various reasons (Adriani et al. 1986): (i) they have been replaced by new injectable amide anesthetics and are currently used only as topical anesthetics (benzocaine and tetracaine) and (ii) the use of gloves by dental staff prevents direct contact with drugs and the subsequent risk of sensitization. However, benzocaine is still used in some sunscreens (Bruze et al. 1990) and can therefore sensitize the patient before the dental topical anesthetic is administered (Kaidbey and Allen 1981).

### Amides

Amide or amino-amide anesthetics are the most widely used type today. The frequency of allergy to these drugs is unknown, although it seems to be very low, accounting for approximately <1% of all adverse reactions caused by local anesthetics (Verrill 1975; Giovannitti and Bennett 1979). This frequency is widely accepted (deShazo and Nelson 1979; Schatz 1984; Schatz and Fung 1986; Schwartz and Sher 1985; Chandler et al. 1987; Wilson et al. 2000). Table 23.11 shows the results of various series that only examined suspected cases of allergic reaction to local anesthetics from the amide group and in which only 5% of cases were true allergies.

Although some people are allergic to various amide anesthetics, allergy to this group is quite rare (Table 23.12), and in many cases, the patient has multiple allergies to other compounds. Allergy to amides is very rare because the chemical structure of the anesthetics in the group

Table 23.11 Studies of allergy tests in cases of suspected allergy to local anesthetic in which allergy is confirmed.

| Reference | No. of suspicious cases studied | No. of allergic cases proven | Allergic cases proven (%) |
| --- | --- | --- | --- |
| Incaudo et al. (1978) | 70 | 2 | 2.8 |
| deShazo and Nelson (1979) | 90 | 1 | 1.1 |
| Babajews and Ivanyi (1982) | 37 | 3 | 8.1 |
| Adriani et al. (1986) | 450 | 41 | 9.1 |
| Chandler et al. (1987) | 58 | 0 | 0 |
| Ruzicka et al. (1987) | 104 | 9 | 8.6 |
| Assem Punnia-Moorthy (1988) | 22 | 4 | 18 |
| Hodgson et al. (1993) | 90 | 22 | 25 |
| De Nova et al. (1996) | 20 | 1 | 5 |
| Fisher and Bowey (1997) | 205 | 8 | 3.9 |
| Wildsmit et al. (1998) | 25 | 2 | 8 |
| Ball (1999) | 702 | 73 | 10.4 |
| Ball (1999) | 217 | 27 | 12.4 |
| Rood (2000) | 44 | 0 | 0 |
| Rood (2000) | 97 | 0 | 0 |
| Nettis et al. (2001) | 105 | 0 | 0 |
| Malamed (2004) | 210 | 0 | 0 |
| Jacobsen et al. (2005) | 48 | 3 | 6.3 |
| Harboe et al. (2010) | 135 | 2 | 1.5 |
| Batinac et al. (2013) | 331 | 3 | 0.9 |
| | | Mean | 6.1 ≈ 5 |

Table 23.12 Cases of patients with allergy to several local anesthetics simultaneously (multiple allergies).

| Group | Reference | Anesthetics causing allergy in the same patient |
|---|---|---|
| Ester | Adler and Simon (1949) | Procaine, tetracaine |
|  | Sidon and Aldrete (1971) | Procaine, tetracaine |
|  | Johnson and DeStigter (1983) | Procaine, tetracaine |
| Amide | Waldman and Binkley (1967) | Lidocaine, prilocaine |
|  | Brown et al. (1981) | Lidocaine, prilocaine, bupivacaine |
|  | Hodgson et al. (1993) | Lidocaine, prilocaine, mepivacaine |
|  | Warrington and McPhillips (1997) | Lidocaine, prilocaine, bupivacaine, articaine |
|  | Fuzier et al. (2009) | Lidocaine, mepivacaine |

Table 23.13 Cases of allergy to a local anesthetic, mainly in dentistry.

| Group | Local anesthetic | Reference |
|---|---|---|
| Esters | Procaine | Guptil (1920) |
|  |  | Klauder (1922) |
|  |  | Adler and Simon (1949) |
|  |  | Rickles (1953) |
|  | Benzocaine | Magnuson et al. (1970) |
|  |  | Kaidbey and Allen (1981) |
|  |  | Wildsmith et al. (1998) |
|  | Tetracaine | Adler and Simon (1949) |
|  |  | Aldrete and Jonhson (1970) |
|  |  | Sidon and Aldrete (1971) |
|  |  | Johnson and DeStigter (1983) |
| Amides | Lidocaine | Waldman and Binkley (1967) |
|  |  | Wellis (1969) |
|  |  | Walker (1971) |
|  |  | Rood (1973) |
|  |  | Ravindranathan (1975) |
|  |  | Burguess (1987) |
|  |  | De Nova et al. (1996) |
|  |  | Ball (1999) |
|  |  | Al-Dosary et al. (2014) |
|  | Articaine | MacColl and Young (1989) |
|  |  | Malanin and Kalimo (1995) |
|  |  | Davila-Fernández et al. (2012) |
|  | Mepivacaine | Seskin (1978) |
|  |  | deShazo and Nelson (1979) |
|  |  | Johnson and DeStigter (1983) |
|  |  | Sambrook et al. (2011) |
|  | Prilocaine | Waldman and Binkley (1967) |
|  |  | Yeoman (1982) |
|  | Bupivacaine | Brown et al. (1981) |
|  |  | Wildsmith et al. (1998) |

differs from one drug to another (Aldrete and Jonhson 1970), therefore cross-reactions are rare and it is always easy to find alternatives within the group (Ball 1999; Batinac et al. 2013).

Of note, there are no cross-reactions between local anesthetics from the ester and amide groups, since these are different chemical families (Incaudo et al. 1978; Schatz 1984), therefore a patient who is allergic to an ester anesthetic can receive an amide anesthetic. Table 23.13 summarizes proven cases of allergy to various local anesthetics.

**Vasoconstrictor**
Vasoconstrictors are addressed in Chapter 10 under absolute contraindications. Epinephrine and norepinephrine are natural neurotransmitters and hormones, with the result that there are no cases of allergy to their base forms since this would be incompatible with life. However, the exogenous vasoconstrictors in local anesthetics take the form of bitartrates or hydrochlorides. Two cases of allergy to epinephrine have been reported (Kohase and Umino 2004).

Felypressin (octapressin) and levonordefrin are artificial vasoconstrictors, therefore they may cause allergic sensitization. In fact, there has been one case of allergy to levonordefrin (Germishuys and Anderson 1982).

Although the cases reported may lead us to consider these drugs to be absolutely contraindicated, we must remember that the reactions are extremely rare, with only three cases reported after many years using the drugs (more than a century in some cases).

**Antioxidants (Sulfites)**
Sulfites are addressed in Chapter 7, under the composition of local anesthetic solutions, and in Chapter 10, under absolute contraindications of sympathomimetic vasoconstrictors. The main sulfites are sodium or potassium bisulfite or metabisulfite, which are added to local anesthetic solutions with sympathomimetic vasoconstrictors (epinephrine, norepinephrine, and levonordefrin) to lengthen their self-life. The antioxidant captures the oxygen before it inactivates the vasoconstrictor (Milano et al. 1982; Klein 1983; Huang and Fraser 1984; Schwartz and Sher 1985; Seng and Gay 1986).

Sulfites are also added in the form of antimicrobials, reducing agents, and bleaches to foods such as fruit, vegetables, salads, mushrooms, pasta, wine, and beer, as well as to other medications (Bush et al. 1986; Seng and Gay 1986; Simon 1986; Ban et al. 2014). Consequently, allergic sensitization may occur before local anesthetic solutions are administered, although the FDA considers sulfites a safe additive (Bush et al. 1986; Seng and Gay 1986; Simon 1986) because they rarely produce allergic reactions (Bush et al. 1986). However, there have been rare cases of intolerance to dental local anesthetic solution with sympathomimetic vasoconstrictors caused by sulfites (Huang and Fraser 1984; Schwartz and Sher 1985; Schwartz et al. 1989; Dooms-Goossens et al. 1989; Campbell et al. 2001).

It is important to point out that sensitization to sulfites is difficult to evaluate using skin tests (Bush et al. 1986), and it may be necessary to use oral tests (Bush et al. 1986; Simon 1986; Ban et al. 2014) or challenge tests (Schwartz and Sher 1985; Schwartz et al. 1989). In the case of severe allergy to dental local anesthetic (Schwartz and Sher 1985) or in cases of unexplainable asthmatic reactions that are very resistant to treatment, we must evaluate the possibility of sensitization to sulfites, which may even be in anti-asthma medications (Bush et al. 1986). There have been proposals to replace sulfites with other antioxidants in these cases (Seng and Gay 1986), although the alternatives are less effective, more costly, and risky (Bush et al. 1986). At present, there are no antioxidants other than sulfites in local dental anesthetic solutions with sympathomimetic vasoconstrictors, therefore these solutions are absolutely contraindicated in patients with reaction to sulfites.

### Preservative (Methylparaben)

Parabens were addressed in Chapter 7. They have been used to keep local dental anesthetic cartridges free from contamination by bacteria (Latronica et al. 1969; Larson 1977; Luebke and Walker 1978), owing to their considerable bacteriostatic and fungistatic effects (Schorr 1968; Latronica et al. 1969; Nagel et al. 1977; Larson 1977; Luebke and Walker 1978). In addition, they are effective at low doses (Larson 1977; Luebke and Walker 1978) and have low toxicity (Luebke and Walker 1978). The most widely used preservative in dentistry is methylparaben or 4-(hydroxymethyl) benzoate.

Parabens are also used as additives in skin creams, ointments, lotions, toothpastes, cosmetics, and some foods (Schorr 1968; Nagel et al. 1977; Larson 1977; Luebke and Walker 1978; Lederman et al. 1980; Giovannitti and Bennett 1979), therefore they can cause allergic sensitization before anesthetic solutions are applied.

The main problem with these compounds is that they are the acid alkyl ester for aminobenzoate (Latronica et al. 1969; Nagel et al. 1977; Larson 1977; Luebke and Walker 1978; Giovannitti and Bennett 1979) and their chemical structure is similar and shared with ester-type anesthetics, therefore allergic reactions to anesthetic solutions caused by these compounds are common (Aldrete and Jonhson 1969; Latronica et al. 1969; Luebke and Walker 1978; Giovannitti and Bennett 1979; Johnson and DeStigter 1983), as is cross-sensitivity with ester-type local anesthetics (Aldrete and Jonhson 1969; Latronica et al. 1969; Larson 1977; Luebke and Walker 1978). Consequently, in 1984, the FDA banned these compounds in dental local anesthetic cartridges. Since then, they have been removed almost everywhere, with a dramatic reduction in associated adverse reactions (Malamed 2004; Pogrel et al. 2014).

### Confusion with Other Reactions

Administration of local anesthetic may be followed by other reactions whose signs and symptoms overlap with those of allergic reactions to the compounds in local anesthetic solutions, thus causing confusion and favoring the false criterion that many reactions are due to allergic responses to local anesthetic. Below we provide some examples:

1) Psychogenic reactions

    As seen at the beginning of this chapter, psychogenic reactions caused by factors such as emotional tension, anxiety (Aldrete and Jonhson 1970; Doyle and Goepferd 1989), and needle phobia can overlap with the allergic response and account for 40% of confusing cases (Table 23.14). This group includes vasovagal reactions and even rare cases of urticaria caused by the anxiety associated with dental local anesthetic (Milan et al. 1983; Tauberg et al. 1983) or, even more rarely, anxiety-induced angioedema (Barclay and Edwards 1971; Chue 1976). It is important to remember that adverse reactions have also been reported after administration of placebo (Batinac et al. 2013).

2) Toxicity reactions

    In this case, we include both reactions caused by toxicity to local anesthetics and reactions to sympathomimetic vasoconstrictors caused by intravascular injection, overdose, and rapid absorption. This situation can occur in 25% of cases (Table 23.14).

3) Allergic reactions to other compounds

    Allergic reactions to compounds that are not local anesthetic solutions (Rood 2000), as follows:
    - Allergy to latex in rubber dams or gloves (Wildsmith et al. 1998; Brown et al. 2002; Greenwood 2008; Harboe et al. 2010) is the most frequent allergy in the dentist's office (Greenwood 2008).
    - Allergy to drugs such as antibiotics (penicillin), disinfectants (chlorhexidine), and NSAIDs that were being taken when local anesthetic is administered (Wildsmith et al. 1998; Greenwood 2008; Harboe et al. 2010).

Table 23.14 Percentage of cases of psychogenic reaction and toxicity that were initially classified as allergy to local anesthetic.

| Reference | Sample size | Psychogenic reaction N | Psychogenic reaction % | Toxicity reaction N | Toxicity reaction % |
|---|---|---|---|---|---|
| Incaudo et al. (1978) | 71 | 4 | 5.6 | 29 | 42 |
| Adriani et al. (1986) | 450 | 91 | 20 | 175 | 39 |
| Fisher and Bowey (1997) | 205 | 92 | 45 | — | — |
| Wildsmith et al. (1998) | 25 | 8 | 32 | 3 | 12 |
| Rood (2000) | 44 | 26 | 59 | 7 | 16 |
| Rood (2000) | 97 | 75 | 77 | 22 | 23 |
| Nettis et al. (2001) | 17 | 9 | 53 | 2 | 12 |
| | Mean | | 42 | | 23 |
| | Rounded mean | | **40** | | **25** |

- Allergy to other materials used during dental treatment, such as endodontic products (Wilson et al. 2000).

It is easy to understand why confusion arises. The signs and symptoms of the reaction are almost the same as those of allergy, although the cause is totally different. In addition, we tend to think that any allergic reaction occurring during dental treatment is caused by the local anesthetic.

Of note, although the diaphragm of the mouth of the cartridge of dental local anesthetic and the plunger are made of latex and a similar reaction could occur during injection, there have been no reports of this type of latex allergy to date (Shojaei and Haas 2002).

4) Other factors leading to confusion

Other situations that have nothing to do with allergy but that may be confused with an allergic reaction and, in this case, are caused by or associated with local anesthetic solution include the following:
- Swelling and hematoma caused by needle injury (Milgrom and Fiset 1986; Fisher and Bowey 1997; Wildsmith et al. 1998; Rood 2000).
- Bacteremia and sialometaplasia (Wildsmith et al. 1998).
- Infection (Fisher and Bowey 1997).
- Angioedema or hereditary angioneurotic edema (Fisher and Bowey 1997).
- Unknown or idiopathic factors (Adriani et al. 1986; Levy and Baker 1986; Jackson et al. 1994; Wildsmith et al. 1998; Rood 2000).

## Clinical Manifestations

Allergic reactions can occur minutes after administration of local anesthetic, although they may also take hours or sometimes a few days. The manifestations are classed as minor and major according to their severity for the patient's life, although it is interesting to note that *the clinical manifestations that most commonly lead us to suspect an allergic reaction are cutaneous reactions and difficulty breathing* (Kelly and Patterson 1974).

Below, we describe the various manifestations in separate sections. Although several may occur simultaneously and overlap with others in clinical practice, *their course is very variable* (Kelly and Patterson 1974).

### Minor Manifestations

These are the most frequent and, fortunately, the least severe. They are usually cutaneous reactions.

1) Cutaneous reactions, mainly affecting the face, neck, and chest. Less frequently affecting the abdomen and arms. This is the main type of response.
    - Maculopapular rash. This appears suddenly on the skin (rash) and is characterized by reddish patches (erythematous macules) and solid circumscribed elevations that are swollen by local edema (papules).
    - Itching (pruritus), which may occur alone or accompany skin lesions.
    - Urticaria, which is a mix of the conditions described above. Urticaria comprises wheals or hives accompanied by itching. The welts are solid edematous elevations (papules) that are swollen and reddish (erythematous) and in which the raised center may be pale and the surrounding skin reddish. They form large plaques that are always itchy (pruritus).
2) Gastrointestinal reactions. These are caused by involvement of the digestive mucosa and are much less frequent.
    - Nausea and vomiting.
    - Abdominal pain caused by spasms of the digestive tract.
    - In severe cases, diarrhea and urinary incontinence.

### Major Manifestations

These responses may be serious and life-threatening, as they affect the respiratory and/or cardiovascular system.

1) Angioedema or angioneurotic edema or Quincke edema. This type is noninflammatory edema of the subcutaneous and/or submucosal tissue characterized by the following (Barclay and Edwards 1971; Megerian et al. 1992):
    - *Edema or swelling* is the basic sign, *affecting the face in 70% of cases*, with compromise of the lips, tongue, periorbital area, and/or neck in 40% of cases and generally

asymmetric involvement of the throat and pharynx. Involvement of the tongue and pharynx can cause obstruction of the upper airway with the following:
- Symptoms:
  - Difficulty breathing (dyspnea), with a sensation of breathlessness and asphyxia.
  - Difficulty swallowing (dysphagia).
  - Anxiety and nervousness.
- Signs:
  - Occasionally, breath sounds owing to difficulty breathing (stridor).
  - Hoarseness (dysphonia).

Note: Swelling is not accompanied by fever, pain, or itching and usually resolves spontaneously in 1–2 days once the contact with the antigen disappears (in this case, local anesthetic solution).

- *Occasionally, reddening of the skin on the neck and face (erythema).*
- *Sw*elling of the feet, hands, and genitals in 10% of cases. In some cases, swelling of the abdominal viscera, which may cause abdominal pain.

2) Bronchospasm or asthmatic reaction. Affects the lower airway (bronchioles):
- *Symptoms*:
  - Difficulty breathing (dyspnea), with a sensation of breathlessness or asphyxia.
  - Anxiety and nervousness.
- Signs:
  - Breath sounds, mainly on expiration, that are prolonged and have a musical tone (wheezing).
  - Cough and sneezing.
  - Rapid breathing (tachypnea) involving use of the accessory breathing muscles (neck muscles).
  - Sweating (diaphoresis).
- Examination reveals increased heart rate (tachycardia) and arterial pressure.

3) Cardiovascular. Typically, hypotension, which, if very marked, leads to anaphylactic shock.
- Malaise, dizziness, and vertigo, which may lead to loss of consciousness.
- Palpitations caused by increased heart rate (tachycardia) to compensate the hypotension.
- Pale skin with cold sweat.
- Examination reveals increased heart rate (tachycardia) and a considerable reduction in arterial blood pressure that can progress in the final phases to severely reduced heart rate and arterial blood pressure.

## Diagnosis

The diagnosis of drug allergy is based on clinical opinion. As we have seen, cutaneous reactions and difficulty breathing are the manifestations that provide the most information (Kelly and Patterson 1974). The reaction is confirmed using specific tests, mainly skin tests, with the suspect drug (pure anesthetics without vasoconstrictors, sulfites, additives, and preservatives tested independently against saline solution), which is not easy (Riedl and Casillas 2003). In any case, diagnostic suspicion must be confirmed by a specialist.

## Management by the Dentist

As we saw at the beginning of this chapter, once the signs and symptoms of allergy have started, basic measures must be taken (e.g. suspend dental treatment, consider the patient's position, i.e. place the patient in a seated position if he/she has difficulty breathing, place the patient supine if he/she is dizzy and about to lose consciousness, etc.). If the patient loses consciousness, start the PABC or PCAB protocol. Specific measures for major and minor manifestations are set out below.

### Treatment of Minor Manifestations

First, administer *antihistamines* orally, subcutaneously, or intramuscularly. Itching disappears 10–30 minutes after intramuscular injection, although this approach has little effect on skin lesions (Malamed 1993). Continue with oral administration for 24 hours (Kelly and Patterson 1974) or up to 3 days (Ravindranathan 1975; Malamed 1993). The most commonly used antihistamines are:

- Oral or intramuscular hydroxyzine at 25–50 mg (MacColl and Young 1989).
- Oral or intramuscular diphenhydramine at 25–50 mg (MacColl and Young 1989).
- Oral or intramuscular dexchlorpheniramine at 4–10 mg.

### Treatment of Major Manifestations

This treatment involves the most potent drugs because these act rapidly and in the most severe conditions.

1) *Epinephrine* (Malamed 1993; Ball 1999).
   Injected from 1-ml ampoules at a concentration of 1:1000 (1000 µg/ml), with a dose of 0.3–0.5 ml for adults and 0.15 mg (0.15 ml) for children.

   Action is very rapid with intramuscular injection. The drug acts before 30 seconds (Sklar and Schwartz 1965; Nichols and Cutright 1971), although the effect is short (approximately 10 minutes) (Sklar and Schwartz 1965; Greenwood 2008), therefore it is sometimes necessary to repeat the injection at 10–20 minutes until bronchospasm and hypotension have resolved (Malamed 1993).

Epinephrine is the most important drug because not only it is very fast-acting (essential feature), but it also acts on the basic components of the disease (Kelly and Patterson 1974; MacColl and Young 1989), as follows: (i) by increasing heart rate through the $\beta_1$ effect; (ii) by contracting the vessels and thus diminishing permeability (reduces edema) and increasing arterial blood pressure owing to the $\alpha$ adrenergic effect; (iii) by relaxing the bronchi through the $\beta_2$ effect; and (iv) by stabilizing the mastocyte membrane to prevent the cells from releasing histamine through the $\beta$ adrenergic effect.

2) *Oxygen 100%* through a facemask (Giovannitti and Bennett 1979; Malamed 1993; Becker 1995) at 6–10 l/min in adults.

3) *Cortisol* or hydrocortisone (Ball 1999).
   Injected intramuscularly or intravenously at 7–10 mg/kg for adults and half this amount for children (generally 100-, 300-, or 500-mg ampoules). While cortisol is not the most potent corticosteroid, it is the fastest acting (essential feature), and onset is within 1 hour (Haas 2014). It controls delayed inflammatory effects and improves hypotension and bronchospasm (Kelly and Patterson 1974).

   It is important to remember that a massive dose of cortisol over a short period, as is the case here, has very few complications. Classic complications (i.e. stomach ulcer, hyperglycemic diabetic coma, superinfection, psychosis) are not relevant here, therefore it can be administered in very severe reactions (CINIME 1979).

**Support Measures for Major Manifestations**
- In the case of severe bronchospasm with breathing difficulties that does not resolve with epinephrine, several inhalations of aerosolized bronchodilators ($\beta_2$ agonists) should be administered. Their effects are almost immediate (a few minutes) and last 4–6 hours (Haas 2014). However, they are subject to unpredictable cardiovascular effects with worsening of hypotension (Kelly and Patterson 1974). The most widely used bronchodilators are albuterol or salbutamol.
- Severe angioedema with obstruction of the upper airway should be treated using tracheotomy or cricothyroidotomy (Giovannitti and Bennett 1979; Becker 1995).

**Recovery and Discharge**
Any patient who experiences an allergic reaction should undergo an allergy work-up. Furthermore, if the reaction is severe, the patient may have to be admitted to hospital for observation (24–48 hours) (Malamed 1993). A detailed report should be provided (including time of onset of the reaction, anesthetic administered and dose, clinical manifestations, medication administered, and duration of effects).

## Prevention

When an allergic reaction to a local anesthetic solution is suspected and the component the patient is allergic to is unknown and/or allergy tests results are not yet available (relatively common, as this can take months or years; Harboe et al. 2010; Batinac et al. 2013), the options are as follows:

1) Provide only emergency treatments with drugs such as antibiotics and analgesics. Do not carry out a therapeutic procedure with local anesthesia.
2) Use alternatives to local anesthetic solutions:
   - Electronic dental anesthesia because this technique does not involve drugs (Jedrychowski and Duperon 1993; Yap and Ong 1996; Burke 1997; Munshi et al. 2000), although it is less effective than conventional anesthetic solutions (Chapter 20). Electronic dental anesthesia may be accompanied by sedation with nitrous oxide to increase effectiveness.
   - Use injected antihistamines as local anesthetics, although they are less effective and more irritant for tissue (Annex 38). These agents may be combined with nitrous oxide to increase their effect.
   - Provide treatment under general anesthetic.

When the component causing the allergy is known, it should be avoided for life since it is absolutely contraindicated (immune memory). The available options are as follows:

- If the allergy is to a specific local anesthetic, then we can use other drugs that are known to be safe for the patient based on the results of the allergy test.
- If the allergy is to the preservative (methylparaben), then we can use cartridges that do not contain this medication (almost no cartridges used today contain methylparaben). Of course, never use multidose vials because they frequently contain methylparaben (the component has not yet been withdrawn from these vials) (Graham and Hirshman 1986; Malamed 2004).
- If the allergy is to the antioxidant (sulfites), then we can use anesthetic solutions without sympathomimetic vasoconstrictors (epinephrine, norepinephrine, levonordefrin), such as prilocaine 3% with felypressin 0.03 IU or mepivacaine 3% without vasoconstrictor. However, the effectiveness of these solutions is lower than that of those containing epinephrine (Chapters 7 and 10).

# References

Aalfs, C.M., Salieb-Beugelaar, G.B., Wanders, R.J.A. et al. (2000). A case of methemoglobinemia type II due to NADH-cytochrome b5 reductase deficiency: determination of the molecular basis. *Hum. Mutat.* 16 (1): 18–22.

Abasi, E.G. (1987). A cardiac arrest in the dental chair. *Br. Dent. J.* 163 (6): 199–200.

Adler, P. and Simon, M. (1949). Contribution to the problem of allergy to local anesthetics. *Oral Surg. Oral Med. Oral Pathol.* 2 (8): 1029–1036.

Adriani, J. and Campbell, D. (1956). Fatalities following topical application of local anesthetics to mucous membranes. *JAMA* 162 (17): 1527–1530.

Adriani, J., Campbell, D., and Yarberry, D.H. Jr. (1959). Influence of absorption on systemic toxicity of local anesthetic agents. *Anesth. Analg.* 38 (5): 370–377.

Adriani, J., Coffman, V.D., and Naraghi, M. (1986). The allergenicity of lidocaine and other amide and related local anesthetics. *Anesthesiol. Rev.* 13 (6): 30–36.

Al-Dosary, K., Al-Qahtani, A., and Alangari, A. (2014). Anaphylaxis to lidocaine with tolerance to articaine in a 12 year old girl. *Saudi. Pharm. J.* 22 (3): 280–282.

Aldrete, J.A. and Johnson, D.A. (1970). Evaluation of intracutaneous testing for investigation of allergy to local anesthetic agents. *Anesth. Analg.* 49 (1): 173–183.

Aldrete, J.A. and Jonhson, D.A. (1969). Allergy to local anesthetics. *JAMA* 207 (2): 356–357.

Aldrete, J.A., Narang, R., Sada, T. et al. (1977). Reverse carotid blood flow – a possible explanation for some reactions to local anesthetics. *J. Am. Dent. Assoc.* 94 (6): 1142–1145.

Aldrete, J.A., Romo-Salas, F., Arora, S. et al. (1978). Reverse arterial blood flow as a pathway for central nervous system toxic responses following injection of local anesthetics. *Anesth. Analg.* 57 (4): 428–433.

American Dental Association (1984). Accepted dental therapeutics. In: *Council on Dental Therapeutics*, 40e. Chicago: American Dental Association. 185

Anderson, J.A. (1960). Dental office design and layout. *J. Am. Dent. Assoc.* 60 (3): 344–353.

Anderson, S.T., Hajduczek, J., and Barker, S.J. (1988). Benzocaine – induced methemoglobinemia in an adult: accuracy of pulse oximetry with methemoglobinemia. *Anesth. Analg.* 67 (11): 1099–1101.

Anonymous (1994). Prilocaine-induced methemoglobinemia – Wisconsin, 1993. *MMWR* 43 (35): 655–657.

Annex 1. Frequency of use of local anesthesia in dentistry.

Annex 10. Maximum doses of dental local anesthetics solutions.

Annex 13. Toxic plasma levels of local anesthetics.

Annex 17. Epinephrine III. Cardiovascular patients.

Assem, E.S.K. and Punnia-Moorthy, A. (1988). Allergy to local anaesthetics: an approach to definitive diagnosis. A review with an illustrative study. *Br. Dent. J.* 264 (2): 44–47.

Ayer, A.A., Domoto, P.K., Gale, E.N. et al. (1983). Overcoming dental fear: strategies for its prevention and management. *J. Am. Dent. Assoc.* 107 (1): 18–27.

Babajews, A.V. and Ivanyi, L. (1982). The relationship between in vivo and in vitro reactivity of patients with a history of allergy to local anesthetics. *Br. Dent. J.* 152 (11): 385–387.

Baldo, B.A., Zhao, Z., and Pham, N.H. (2008). Antibiotic allergy: immunochemical and clinical considerations. *Curr. Allergy Asthma Rep.* 8 (1): 49–55.

Ball, I.A. (1999). Allergy reactions to lignocaine. *Br. Dent. J.* 186 (5): 224–226.

Ban, G.-Y., Kim, M.-A., Yoo, H.-S. et al. (2014). Two major phenotypes of sulfite hypersensitivity: asthma and urticaria (letter). *Yonsei Med. J.* 55 (2): 542–544.

Barclay, J.K. and Edwards, J.L. (1971). Angioneurotic edema. *Oral Surg. Oral Med. Oral Pathol.* 32 (4): 552–556.

Batinac, T., Tokmadzic, V.S., Peharda, V., and Brajac, I. (2013). Adverse reactions and alleged allergy to local anesthetics: analysis of 331 patients. *J. Dermatol.* 40 (7): 522–527.

Becker, D.E. (1995). Management of immediate allergic reactions. *Dent. Clin. N. Am.* 39 (3): 577–586.

Bennett, J.D. and Rosenberg, M.B. (2002). *Medical Emergencies in Dentistry*. Philadelphia: Saunders Co.

Bernstein, B.M. (1950). Cyanosis following use of anesthesin (ethyl-amino-benzoate). (case report). *Rev. Gastroenterol.* 17 (2): 123–124.

Beutlich, F.W. (1991). Benzocaine and methemoglobin: recommended actions (letter). *Anesthesiology* 74 (2): 387.

Blair, G.S. and Meechan, J.G. (1985). Local anaesthesia in dental practice I. a clinical study of a self-aspirating system. *Br. Dent. J.* 159 (3): 75–77.

Blumer, J.L. (1998). Clinical pharmacology of midazolam in infants and children. *Clin. Pharmacokinet.* 35 (1): 37–47.

Boakes, A.J., Laurence, D.R., Lovel, K.W. et al. (1972). Adverse reactions to local anaesthetic/vasoconstrictor preparations. A study of the cardiovascular responses to Xylestesin and Hostacain- with- noradrenaline. *Br. Dent. J.* 133 (4): 137–140.

Bourne, J.G. (1957). Fainting and cerebral damage. Danger in patients kept upright during dental gas anaesthesia and after surgical operations. *Lancet* 273 (6994): 499–505.

Bourne, J.G. (1970). Deaths with dental anaesthetics. *Anaesthesia* 25 (4): 473–481.

Bourne, J.G. (1980). The common fainting attack. Its danger in dentistry. *Br. Dent. J.* 149 (4): 101–104.

Brown, D.T., Beamish, D., and Wildsmith, J.A.W. (1981). Allergic reaction to an amide local anaesthetic. *Br. J. Anaesth.* 53 (4): 435–437.

Brown, R.S., Paluvoi, S., Choksi, S. et al. (2002). Evaluating a dental patient for local anesthesia allergy. *Compend. Contin. Educ. Dent.* 23 (2): 125–138.

Bruze, M., Gruvberger, B., and Thulin, I. (1990). PABA, benzocaine, and other PABA esters in sunscreens and after-sun products. *Photodermatol. Photoimmunol. Photomed.* 7 (3): 106–108.

Burguess, J.O. (1987). Preventing local anesthetic reactions: the use of the skin tests. *Special Care Dent.* 7 (3): 135–136.

Burke, F.J.T. (1997). Dentist and patient evaluation of an electronic dental analgesia system. *Quintessence Int.* 28 (9): 609–613.

Burne, D. and Doughty, A. (1964). Methaemoglobinaemia following lignocaine. *Lancet* 2 (7366): 971.

Bush, R.K., Taylor, S.L., and Busse, W. (1986). A critical evaluation of clinical trials in reactions to sulfites. *J. Allergy Clin. Immunol.* 78 (1 Pt 2): 191–202.

Callaham, M. (1989). Hypoxic hazards of traditional paper bag rebreathing in hyperventilating patients. *Ann. Emerg. Med.* 18 (6): 622–628.

Campbell, D. and Adriani, J. (1958). Absorption of local anesthetics. *JAMA* 168 (7): 873–877.

Campbell, R.L., Gregg, J.M., Levin, K.J., and Elliott, R.A. (1976). Vasovagal response during oral surgery. *J. Oral Surg.* 34 (8): 698–701.

Campbell, J.R., Maestrello, C.L., and Campbell, R.L. (2001). Allergy response to metabisulfite in lidocaine anesthetic solutions. *Anesth. Prog.* 48 (1): 21–26.

Canfield, D.W. and Gage, T.W. (1987). A guideline to local anesthetic allergy testing. *Anesth. Prog.* 34 (5): 157–163.

Cannell, H. (1996). Evidence of safety margins of lignocaine local anaesthetics for perioral use. *Br. Dent. J.* 181 (7): 243–249.

Carabelli, A.A. (1952). The use of pontocaine in subposologic quantities for bronchoscopy and bronchography. *Anesthesiology* 13 (2): 169–183.

Cawson, R.A., Curson, I., and Whittington, D.R. (1983). The hazards of dental local anaesthetics. *Br. Dent. J.* 154 (8): 253–258.

Chandler, M.J., Grammer, L.C., and Patterson, R. (1987). Provocative challenge with local anesthetics in patients with a prior history of reaction. *J. Allergy Clin. Immunol.* 79 (6): 883–886.

Chapman, P.J. (1984). The hyperventilation (overbreathing) syndrome. *Aust. Dent. J.* 29 (5): 321–323.

Chapman, P.J. (1997). Medical emergencies in dental practice and choice of emergency drugs and equipment. A survey of Australian dentists. *Aust. Dent. J.* 42 (2): 103–108.

Chue, P.W.Y. (1976). Acute angioneurotic edema of the lips and tongue due to emotional stress. *Oral Surg. Oral Med. Oral Pathol.* 41 (6): 734–738.

CINIME (1979). Comisión de Farmacia y Terapéutica. Esteroides y shock. *Inf. Ter. SS (Madrid)* 3 (4): 78.

Coleman, M.D. and Coleman, N.A. (1996). Drug-induced methaemoglobinamia. Treatment issues. *Drug Safety* 14 (6): 394–405.

Compernolle, T., Hoogduin, K., and Joele, L. (1979). Diagnosis and treatment of the hyperventilation syndrome. *Psychosomatics* 20 (9): 612–625.

Coombs, R.R.A. and Gell, P.G.H. (1968). Classification of allergic reactions responsible for clinical hypersensitivity and disease (chapter 20). In: *Clinical Aspects of Immunology*, 2e (ed. Gell, P.G.H. and Coombs, R.R.A.). Oxford and Edinburgh: Blackwell Scientific Publications. 575–596.

Coplans, M.P. and Curson, I. (1982). Deaths associated with dentistry. *Br. Dent. J.* 153 (10): 357–362.

Covino, B.G. (1978). Systemic toxicity of local anesthetic agents (editorial). *Anesth. Prog.* 57 (4): 387–388.

Covino, B.G. (1987). The toxicity and systemic effects of local anesthetic agents (chapter 6). In: *Local Anesthetics. Handbook of Experimental Pharmacology*, vol. 81 (ed. G.R. Strichartz). Berlin: Springer-Verlag. 187–212.

Curry, S. (1982). Methemoglobinemia. *Ann. Emerg. Med.* 11 (4): 214–221.

Daly, D.J., Davenport, J., and Newland, M.C. (1964). Methaemoglobinaemia following the use of prilocaine (Citanest). A preliminary report. *Br. J. Anaesth.* 36 (11): 737–739.

Daos, F., Lopez, L., and Virtue, R.W. (1962). Anesthetic toxicity modified by oxygen and by combination of agents. *Anesthesiology* 23 (6): 755–761.

Daubländer, M., Müller, R., and Lipp, M.D.W. (1997). The incidence of complications associated with local anesthesia in dentistry. *Anesth. Prog.* 44 (4): 132–141.

Davila-Fernández, G., Sánchez-Morillas, L., Rojas, P., and Laguna, J.J. (2012). Urticaria due to an intradermal test with articaine hydrochloride (letter). *J. Investig. Allergol. Immunol.* 22 (5): 373–374.

De Jong, R.H. and Bonin, J.D. (1981). Benzodiazepines protect mice from local anesthetic convulsions and death. *Anesth. Analg.* 60 (6): 385–389.

De Jong, R.H. and Walts, L.F. (1966). Lidocaine-induced psychomotor seizures in man. *Acta Anaesthesiol. Scand.* 25 (Suppl): 598–604.

De Nova, M.J., Vaello, V., Bartolome, B., and Costa, F. (1996). Reacciones alérgicas a anestésicos locales en niños. *Odontol. Pediatr.* 5 (2): 59–66.

Deas, T.C. (1956). Severe methemoglobinemia following dental extractions under lidocaine anesthesia. *Anesthesiology* 17 (1): 204.

D'Eramo, E.M. (1992). Mortality and morbidity with outpatient anesthesia: the Massachusetts experience. *J. Oral Maxillofac. Surg.* 50 (7): 700–704.

D'Eramo, E.M. (1999). Mortality and morbidity with outpatient anesthesia: the Massachusetts experience. *J. Oral Maxillofac. Surg.* 57 (5): 531–536.

D'Eramo, E.M., Bookless, S.J., and Howard, J.B. (2003). Adverse events with outpatient anesthesia in Massachusetts. *J. Oral Maxillofac. Surg.* 61 (7): 793–800.

deShazo, R.D. and Nelson, H.S. (1979). An approach to patient with a history of local anesthetic hypersensibility: experience with 90 patients. *J. Allergy Clin. Immunol.* 63 (6): 387–394.

Dick, S.P. (1953). Clinical toxicity of epinephrine anesthesia. *Oral Surg. Oral Med. Oral Pathol.* 6 (6): 724–728.

Dooms-Goossens, A., de Alam, A.G., Degreef, H., and Kochuyt, A. (1989). Local anesthetic intolerance due to metabisulfite. *Contact Dermatitis* 20 (2): 124–126.

Doyle, K.A. and Goepferd, S.J. (1989). An allergy to local anesthetics? The consequences of a misdiagnosis. *J. Dent. Child.* 56 (2): 103–106.

Driscoll, E.J. (1974). ASOS anesthesia morbidity and mortality survey. *J. Oral Surg.* 32 (10): 733–738.

Duncan, P.G. and Kobrinsky, N. (1983). Prilocaine-induced methemoglobinemia in a newborn infant. *Anesthesiology* 59 (1): 75–76.

Edmondson, H.D., Gordon, P.H., Lloyd, J.M. et al. (1978). Vasovagal episodes in the dental surgery. *J. Dent.* 6 (3): 189–195.

Englesson, S. and Matousek, M. (1975). Central nervous system effects of local anaesthetic agents. *Br. J. Anaesth.* 47 (Suppl): 241–246.

Eriksson, E., Englesson, S., Wahlqvist, S., and Örtengren, B. (1966). Study of the intravenous toxicity in man and some in vitro studies on the distribution and adsorbability. *Acta Chir. Scand.* Suppl 358: 25–36.

Esteban-Sanchez, M., Izquierdo-Gil, A., and Hurtado-Gomez, M.F. (2013). Methaemoglobinaemiadue to topical administration of a local anaesthetic for laser depilation. *Farm. Hosp.* 37 (6): 558–561. (Text in Spanish).

European Resuscitation Council (2020). European Resuscitation Council COVID-19 guidelines. www.erc.edu (accessed 7 July 2023).

Fast, T., Martin, M.D., and Ellis, T.M. (1986). Emergency preparedness: a survey of dental practitioners. *J. Am. Dent. Assoc.* 112 (4): 499–501.

Field, J.M., Hazinski, M.F., Sayre, M.R. et al. (2010). Part 1: Executive summary: 2010 American Heart Association guidelines for cardiopulmonary resuscitation and emergency cardiovascular care. *Circulation* 122 (18 Suppl 3): S640–S645.

Fisher, M.M. and Bowey, C.J. (1997). Alleged allergy to local anaesthetics. *Anaesth. Intensive Care* 25 (6): 611–614.

Foldes, F.F., Molloy, R., and McNall, P.G. (1960). Comparison of toxicity of intravenously given local anesthetic agents in man. *JAMA* 172 (14): 1493–1498.

Foldes, F.F., Davidson, G.M., Duncalf, D., and Kuwabara, S. (1965). The intravenous toxicity of local anesthetic agents in man. *Clin. Pharmacol. Ther.* 6 (3): 328–335.

Forrest, J.O. (1959). Notes on aspiration before injection of local anesthetics using dental cartridges. *Br. Dent. J.* 107 (3): 259–262.

Frayling, I.M., Addison, G.M., Chattergee, G.M.A., and Meakin, G. (1990). Methaemoglobinaemia in children treated with prilocaine-lignocaine cream. *Br. Med. J.* 301 (6744): 153–154.

Friedman, G.A., Rowlingson, J.C., DiFazio, C.A., and Donegan, M.F. (1982). Evaluation of the analgesic effect and urinary excretion of systemic bupivacaine in man. *Anesth. Analg.* 61 (1): 23–27.

Fuzier, R., Lapeyre-Mestre, M., Mertes, P.-M. et al. (2009). Immediate- and delayed-type allergic reactions to amide anesthetics: clinical features and skin testing. *Pharmacoepidemiol. Drug Saf.* 18 (7): 595–601.

Gardner, W. (2000). Orthostatic increase of respiratory gas exchange in hyperventilation syndrome. *Thorax* 55 (4): 257–259.

Garfield, J.M. and Gugino, L. (1987). Central effects of local anesthetic agents (chapter 8). In: *Local Anesthetics. Handbook of Experimental Pharmacology*, vol. 81 (ed. G.R. Strichartz). Berlin: Springer-Verlag. 253–284.

Geffner, I. and Murgatroyd, J. (1980). Tetany. A case induced by hysterical hyperventilation. *Br. Dent. J.* 148 (11–12): 264.

Germishuys, P.J. and Anderson, R. (1982). Allergy to vasoconstrictor in a local anaesthetic solution: a case report. *J. Dent. Assoc. S. Afr.* 37 (4): 233–235.

Giovannitti, J.A. and Bennett, C.R. (1979). Assessment of allergy to local anesthetics. *J. Am. Dent. Assoc.* 98 (5): 701–706.

Girdler, N.M. and Smith, D.G. (1999). Prevalence of emergency events in British dental practice and emergency management skills of British dentists. *Resuscitation* 41 (2): 159–167.

Gitman, M., Fettiplace, M.R., Weinberg, G. et al. (2019). Local anesthetic systemic toxicity: a narrative literature review and clinical update on prevention, diagnosis and management. *Plast. Reconstr. Surg.* 144 (3): 783–795.

Golden, S.S. (1959). Human factors applied to study of dentist and patient in dental environment: a static appraisal. *J. Am. Dent. Assoc.* 59 (1): 17–28.

Goldman, V. and Gray, W. (1963). A clinical trial of a new local analgesic agent. *Br. Dent. J.* 115 (2): 59–65.

Goodson, J.M. and Moore, P.A. (1983). Life-threatening reactions after pedodontic sedation: an assessment of narcotic, local anesthetic, and antiemetic drug interaction. *J. Am. Dent. Assoc.* 107 (2): 239–245.

Graham, T. and Hirshman, C.A. (1986). Local anesthetic allergy (letter). *JAMA* 256 (19): 2737.

Greenwood, M. (2008). Medical emergencies in the dental practice. *Periodontol.* 2000 (46): 27–41.

Grimes, E.B. (2013). *Medical Emergencies: Essentials for the Dental Professional*, 2e. Upper Saddle River (New Jersey): Pearson Education Inc.

Guay, J. (2009). Methemoglobinemia related to local anesthetics: a summary of 242 episodes. *Anesth. Analg.* 108 (3): 837–845.

Guptill, A.E. (1920). Novocain as a skin irritant. *Dent. Cosmos.* 62 (12): 1460–1461.

Haas, D.A. (2010). Preparing dental office staff members for emergencies. Developing a basic action plan. *J. Am. Dent. Assoc.* 141 (Suppl 1): 8S–13S.

Haas, D.A. (2014). Emergency drugs (chapter 29). In: *Anesthesia Complications in the Dental Office* (ed. R.C. Bosack and S. Lieblich). Ames (Iowa): Willey Blackwell. 189–198.

Hall, D.L., Moses, M.K., Weaver, J.M. et al. (2004). Dental anesthesia management of methemoglobinemia-susceptible patients: a case report and review of literature. *Anesth. Prog.* 51 (1): 24–27.

Hannington-Kiff, J.G. (1969). Fainting and collapse in dental practice. *Dent. Pract. Dent. Rec.* 20 (1): 2–7.

Harboe, T., Guttormsen, A.B., Aarebrot, S. et al. (2010). Suspected allergy to local anaesthetics: follow-up in 135 cases. *Acta Anaesthesiol. Scand.* 54 (5): 536–542.

Hardwick, F.K. and Beaudreau, R.W. (1995). Methemoglobinemia in a renal transplant patient: case report. *Pediatric Dent.* 17 (7): 460–463.

Harrison, J.B. (1973). Faints and spells. *Dent. Clin. N. Am.* 17 (3): 461–472.

Hersh, E.V., Helpin, M.L., and Evans, O.B. (1991). Local anesthetic mortality: report of case. *J. Dent. Child.* 58 (6): 489–491.

Hidding, J. and Khoury, F. (1991). Allgemein Komplikationen bei der zahnärztlichen Lokalanästhesie. *Dtsch Zahnärztl Z* 46 (12): 834–836.

Hjelm, M. and Holmdahl, M.H. (1964). Methaemoglobinaemia following lignocaine. *Lancet* 1 (7375): 53–54.

Hodgson, T.A., Shirlaw, P.J., and Challacombe, S.J. (1993). Skin testing after anaphylactoid reactions to dental local anesthetics. *Oral Surg. Oral Med. Oral Pathol.* 75 (6): 706–711.

Holroyd, S.V., Watts, D.T., and Welch, J.T. (1960). The use of epinephrine in local anesthetics for dental patients with cardiovascular disease: a review of the literature. *J. Oral Surg. Anesth. Hosp. Dent. Surv.* 18: 492–503.

Horowitz, J., Almong, Y., Wolf, A. et al. (2005). Ophthalmic complications of dental anesthesia: three new cases. *J. Neuroophthalmol.* 25 (2): 95–100.

Huang, A.S. and Fraser, W.M. (1984). Are sulfite additives really safe? *N. Engl. J. Med.* 311 (8): 542.

Hughes, C.L., Leach, J.K., Allen, R.E., and Lambson, G.O. (1966). Cardiac arrhythmias during oral surgery with local anesthesia. *J. Am. Dent. Assoc.* 73 (5): 1095–1102.

Incaudo, G., Schatz, M., Patterson, R. et al. (1978). Administration of local anesthetics to patients with a history of prior adverse reaction. *J. Allergy Clin. Immunol.* 61 (5): 339–345.

Jackson, D., Chen, A.H., and Bennett, C.R. (1994). Identifying true lidocaine allergy. *J. Am. Dent. Assoc.* 125 (10): 1362–1366.

Jacobsen, R.B., Borch, J.E., and Bindslev-Jensen, C. (2005). Hypersensitivity to local anaesthetics. *Allergy* 60 (2): 262–264.

Jakobson, B. and Nilsson, A. (1985). Methemoglobinemia associated with a prilocaine-lidocaine cream and trimetroprim-sulphamethoxazole. A case report. *Acta. Anaesthesiol. Scand.* 29 (4): 453–455.

Jastak, J.T., Yagiela, J.A., and Donaldson, D. (1995). *Local Anesthesia of the Oral Cavity*. Philadelphia: WB Saunders Co. 78–79, 297.

Jedrychowski, J.R. and Duperon, D.F. (1993). Effectiveness and acceptance of electronic dental anesthesia by pediatric patients. *J. Dent. Child.* 60 (3): 186–192.

Johnson, P.L. (1994). Pulse oximetry signals local anesthetic-induced methemoglobinemia. *Anesth. Prog.* 41 (1): 11–12.

Johnson, W.T. and DeStigter, T. (1983). Hypersensitivity to procaine, tetracaine, mepivacaine, and methylparaben: report of a case. *J. Am. Dent. Assoc.* 106 (1): 53–56.

Jorfeldt, L., Löfström, B., Pernow, B. et al. (1968). The effect of local anaesthetics on the central circulation and respiration in man and dog. *Acta Anaesthesiol. Scand.* 12 (4): 153–169.

Kaidbey, K.H. and Allen, H. (1981). Photocontact allergy to benzocaine. *Arch. Dermatol.* 117 (2): 77–79.

Kaufman, E., Goharian, S., and Katz, Y. (2000). Adverse reactions triggered by dental local anesthetics: a clinical survey. *Anesth. Prog.* 47 (4): 134–138.

Kellet, P.B. and Copeland, C.S. (1983). Methemoglobinemia associated with benzocaine- containing lubricant. *Anesthesiology* 59 (5): 463–464.

Kelly, J.T. and Patterson, R. (1974). Anaphylaxis, course, mechanisms and treatment. *JAMA* 227 (12): 1431–1435.

Kerr, W.J., Dalton, J.W., and Gliebe, P.A. (1937). Some physical phenomena associated with the anxiety states and their relation to the hyperventilation. *Ann. Intern. Med.* 11 (5): 961–992.

Klauder, J.V. (1922). Novocain dermatitis. *Dent. Cosmos.* 64 (3): 305–309.

Klein, R.M. (1983). Components of local anesthetic solutions. *Gen. Dent.* 31 (6): 460–465.

Klein, S.L., Nustad, R.A., Feinberg, S.E., and Fonseca, R.J. (1983). Acute toxic methemoglobinemia caused by topical anesthetic. *Pediatr. Dent.* 5 (2): 107–108.

Kleinknecht, R.A. and Bernstein, D.A. (1978). The assessment of dental fear. *Behavior. Therap.* 9 (4): 626–634.

Knudsen, K., Suurküla, B., Blomberg, S. et al. (1997). Central nervous and cardiovascular effects of i.v. infusions of ropivacaine, bupivacaine and placebo in volunteers. *Br. J. Anaesth.* 78 (5): 507–514.

Kohase, H. and Umino, M. (2004). Allergy reaction to epinephrine preparation in 2% lidocaine. Two reports. *Anesth. Prog.* 51 (4): 134–137.

Kreutz, R.W. and Kini, M.E. (1983). Life-threatening toxic methemoglobinemia induced by prilocaine. *Oral Surg. Oral Med. Oral Pathol.* 56 (5): 480–482.

von Künzer, W. and Schneider, D. (1953). Zur Aktivität der reduzierenden Fermetsysteme in der Erythrozyten junger Säuglinge. *Acta Haematol.* 9 (6): 346–353.

Kuster, C. and Udin, R.D. (1985). Vasopressor syncope in children: incidence and treatment. *J. Pedod.* 9 (3): 210–217.

Lai, J., Porreca, F., Hunter, J.C., and Gold, M.S. (2004). Voltage-gated sodium channels and hyperalgesia. *Annu. Rev. Pharmacol. Toxicol.* 44: 371–397.

Larson, C.E. (1977). Methylparaben – an overlooked cause of local anesthesia hypersensitivity. *Anesth. Prog.* 34 (3): 72–74.

Latronica, R.J., Goldberg, A.F., and Wightman, J.R. (1969). Local anesthetic sensitivity. Report of a case. *Oral Surg. Oral Med. Oral Pathol.* 28 (3): 439–441.

Lederman, D.A., Freedman, P.D., Kerpel, S.M., and Lumerman, H. (1980). An unusual skin reaction following local anesthesia injection. Review of the literature and report of four cases. *Oral Surg. Oral Med. Oral Pathol.* 49 (1): 28–33.

Lemay, H., Albert, G., Hélie, P. et al. (1984). Ultracaine en dentisterie opératoire conventionnelle. *J. Can. Dent. Assoc.* 50 (9): 703–708.

Levergne, S., Darmon, M., Levy, V., and Azoulay, E. (2006). Methemoglobinemia and acute hemolysis after tetracaine lozenge use. *J. Crit. Care* 21 (1): 112–114.

Levy, S.M. and Baker, K.A. (1986). Considerations in differential diagnosis of adverse reactions to local anesthetic: report of case. *J. Am. Dent. Assoc.* 113 (2): 271–273.

Lipp, M.D.W., Dick, W.F., Daubländer, M. et al. (1988). Examination of the central-nervous epinephrine level during local dental infiltration and block anesthesia using tritium-marked epinephrine as vasoconstrictor. *Anesthesiology* 69. (3A-Suppl): A371.

Lloyd, J.M. (1992). Aspiration in dental local anaesthesia (letter). *Br. Dent. J.* 172 (4): 136.

Lo, S.C.-L. and Agar, N.S. (1986). NADH-methemoglobin reductase activity in the erythrocytes of newborn and adult mammals. *Experientia* 42 (11–12): 1264–1265.

Ludwig, S.C. (1981). Acute toxic methemoglobinemia following dental analgesia. *Ann. Emerg. Med.* 10 (5): 265–266.

Luebke, N.H. and Walker, J.A. (1978). Discussion of sensitivity to preservatives in anesthetics. *J. Am. Dent. Assoc.* 97 (4): 656–657.

Lund, A. (1951). Elimination of adrenaline and noradrenaline from the organism. *Acta. Pharmacol. Toxicol. (Copenhagen)* 7 (4): 297–308.

Lund, P.C. and Cwick, J.C. (1965). Citanest . . . a clinical and laboratory study. Part 2. *Anesth. Analg.* 44 (6): 712–721.

Lund, P.C., Cwick, J.C., and Pagdanganan, R.T. (1973). Etidocaine – a new long-acting local anesthetic agent: a clinical evaluation. *Anesth. Analg.* 52 (3): 482–494.

Lustig, J.P. and Zusman, S.P. (1999). Immediate complications of local anesthesia administered to 1,007 consecutive patients. *J. Am. Dent. Assoc.* 130 (4): 496–499.

Lytle, J.J. and Stamper, E.P. (1989). The 1988 anesthesia survey of the Southern California Society of Oral and Maxillofacial Surgeons. *J. Oral Maxillofac. Surg.* 47 (8): 834–842.

MacColl, S. and Young, E.R. (1989). An allergic reaction following injection of local anesthetic: a case report. *J. Can. Dent. Assoc.* 55 (12): 981–984.

Magnusson, B., Koch, G., and Nyquist, G. (1970). Contact allergy to medicaments and materials used in dentistry (I). *Odontol. Revy* 21 (3): 287–299.

Malamed, S.F. (1993). Managing medical emergencies. *J. Am. Dent. Assoc.* 124 (8): 40–53.

Malamed, S.F. (2004). *Handbook of Local Anesthesia*, 5e. Louis (Missouri): Elsevier-Mosby. 111, 155, 166-167, 310-311, 317-318, 324.

Malamed, S.F. (2007). *Medical Emergencies in the Dental Office*, 6e. Louis (Missouri): Mosby-Elsevier. 119–136.

Malanin, K. and Kalimo, K. (1995). Hypersensitivity to the local anesthetic articaine hydrochloride. *Anesth. Prog.* 42 (2–3): 144–145.

Malmberg, L.P., Tamminen, K., and Sonijärvi, A.R.A. (2001). Hyperventilation syndrome (letter). *Thorax* 56 (1): 85–86.

Marley, E. and Stephenson, J.D. (1972). Central actions of catecholamines (chapter 12). In: *Catecholamines. Handbook of Experimental Pharmacology (New Series)*, vol. 33 (ed. U. Blaschko and E. Muscholl). Berlin: Springer-Verlag. 436–573.

Matsuura, H. (1989). Analysis of systemic complications and deaths during dental treatment – Japan. *Anesth. Prog.* 36 (4–5): 223–225.

McCarthy, F.M. (1982). *Medical Emergencies in Dentistry. An Abridged Edition of Emergencies in Dental Practice*, 3e. Philadelphia: WB Saunders Co. 282–285.

McGimpsey, J.G. (1977). Fainting in the dental surgery. *Br. Dent. J.* 143 (2): 53–57.

Meechan, J. (1998). How to avoid local anaesthesia toxicity. *Br. Dent. J.* 184 (7): 334–335.

Meechan, J.G. and Blair, G.S. (1989). Clinical experience in oral surgery with 2 different automatic aspirating syringes. *Int. J. Oral Maxillofac. Surg.* 18 (2): 87–89.

Meechan, J.G. and Rood, J.P. (1992). Aspiration in dental local anaesthesia. *Br. Dent. J.* 172 (2): 40.

Megerian, C.A., Arnold, J.E., and Berger, M. (1992). Angioedema: 5 years' experience, with a review of the disorder's presentation and treatment. *Laryngoscope* 102 (3): 256–260.

Mehra, P., Caiazzo, A., and Maloney, P. (1998). Lidocaine toxicity. *Anesth. Prog.* 45 (1): 38–41.

Mercurio, J.P. (1967). Emergency submental injection. *J. Am. Dent. Assoc.* 74 (4): 717–719.

Meyer, F.-U. (1986). Hemodynamic changes of local dental anesthesia in normotensive and hypertensive subjects. *Int. J. Clin. Pharmacol. Ther. Toxicol.* 24 (9): 477–481.

Milan, S.B., Giovannetti, J.A., and Bright, D. (1983). Hypersensitivity to amide local anesthetics? Report of a case. *Oral Surg. Oral Med. Oral Pathol.* 56 (6): 593–596.

Milan, S.B., Giovannetti, J.A., and Israelson, H. (1986). Faint in the supine position. Selective review of the literature and a case report. *J. Periodontol.* 57 (1): 44–47.

Milano, E.A., Waraszkiewicz, S.M., and Dirubio, R. (1982). Aluminium catalysis of epinephrine degradation in lidocaine hydrochloride with epinephrine solutions. *J. Parenter. Sci. Technol.* 36 (6): 232–236.

Milgrom, P. and Fiset, L. (1986). Local anaesthetic adverse effects and other emergency problems in general dental practice. *Int. Dent. J.* 36 (2): 71–76.

Monsieurs, K.G., Nolan, J.P., Bossaert, L.L. et al. (2015). European Resuscitation Council Guidelines for Resuscitation 2015. Section I. Executive summary. *Resuscitation* 95: 1–80. http://dx.doi.org/10.1016/j.resuscitation.2015.07.038.

Moore, D.C., Mather, L.E., Bridenbaugh, L.D. et al. (1977). Bupivacaine (Marcain®): an evaluation of its tissue and systemic toxicity in humans. *Acta Anaesthesiol. Scand.* 21 (2): 109–121.

Moore, P.A., Boynes, S.G., Hersh, E.V. et al. (2006). The anesthetic efficacy of 4% articaine 1:200,000 epinephrine. Two controlled clinical trials. *J. Am. Dent. Assoc.* 137 (11): 1572–1581.

Moose, S. (1959). Clinical evaluation of levo-nordefrin in local anesthetics. *Oral Surg. Oral Med. Oral Pathol.* 12 (7): 838–845.

Munshi, A.K., Hegde, A., and Bashir, N. (2000). Clinical evaluation of the efficacy of anesthesia and patient preference using the needle-less jet syringe in pediatric dental practice. *J. Clin. Pediatr. Dent.* 25 (2): 131–136.

Muschaweck, R. and Rippel, R. (1974). Ein neues Lokalanästhetikum (Carticain) aus der Thiophenreihe. *Prakt Anästh* 9 (3): 135–146.

Nagel, J.E., Fuscaldo, J.T., and Fireman, P. (1977). Paraben allergy. *JAMA* 237 (15): 1594–1595.

Nettis, E., Napoli, G., Ferramini, A., and Tussi, A. (2001). The incremental challenge test in the diagnosis of adverse reactions to local anesthetics. *Oral Surg. Oral Med. Oral Pathol.* 91 (4): 402–405.

New Zealand Committee on Adverse Drug Reactions (1974). Eighth annual report. *N. Z. Dent. J.* 70 (319): 50–56.

Nichols, W.A. and Cutright, D.E. (1971). Intralingual injection site for emergency drugs. *Oral Surg. Oral Med. Oral Pathol.* 32 (4): 677–684.

Nkansha, P.J., Haas, D.A., and Saso, M.A. (1997). Mortality incidence in outpatient anesthesia for dentistry in Ontario. *Oral Surg. Oral Med. Oral Pathol.* 83 (6): 646–651.

Noble, R.J. (1977). The patient with syncope. *JAMA* 237 (13): 1372–1376.

Ocklitz, H.-W. (1949). Anaesthesinvergiftung beim Säugling. *Med. Klin.* 44 (25): 806–809.

O'Donohue, W.J. Jr., Moss, L.M., and Angelillo, V.A. (1980). Acute methemoglobinemia induced by topical benzocaine and lidocaine. *Arch. Intern. Med.* 140 (11): 1508–1509.

Olson, M.L. and McEvoy, G.K. (1981). Methemoglobinemia induced by local anesthetics. *Am. J. Hosp. Pharm.* 38 (1): 89–93.

Onji, Y. and Tyuma, I. (1965). Methemoglobinemia formation by a local anesthetic and some related compounds. *Acta Anaesthesiol. Scand.* Suppl 16: 151–159.

Panchal, A.R., Bartos, J.A., Cabañas, J.G. et al. (2020). On behalf of the adult basic and advanced life support writing group. Part 3: adult basic and advanced life support: 2020 American Heart Association guidelines for cardiopulmonary resuscitation and emergency cardiovascular care. *Circulation* 142 (Suppl 2): S366–S468.

Perea-Pérez, B., Labajo-González, E., Santiago-Sáez, A. et al. (2014). Analysis of 415 adverse events in dental practice in Spain from 2000 to 2010. *Med. Oral Patol. Oral Cir. Bucal.* 19 (5): e500–e505.

Persson, G. (1969). General side-effects of local anesthesia with special reference to catecholamines as vasoconstrictor and to the effect of some premedicants. *Acta Odontol. Scand.* 27 (Suppl 53): 1–141.

Persson, G., Keskitalo, E., and Evers, H. (1974). Clinical experiences in oral surgery using a new self-aspirating injection system. *Int. J. Oral Surg.* 3 (6): 428–434.

Pogrel, M.A., Stevens, R.L., Bosack, R.C., and Orr, T. (2014). Complications with the use of local anesthetics (chapter 31). In: *Anesthesia Complications in the Dental Office* (ed. R.C. Bosack and S. Lieblich). Ames (Iowa): Wiley–Blackwell. 207–218.

Potter, J.L. and Hillman, J.V. (1979). Benzocaine – induced methemoglobinemia. *J. Am. Coll. Emerg. Physicians* 8 (1): 26–27.

Ravindranathan, N. (1975). Allergic reaction to lignocaine. A case report. *Br. Dent. J.* 138 (3): 101–102.

Rickles, N.H. (1953). Procaine allergy in dental patients: diagnosis and management. *Oral Surg. Oral Med. Oral Pathol.* 6 (3): 375–382.

Riedl, M.A. and Casillas, A.M. (2003). Adverse drug reactions: types and treatment options. *Am. Fam. Physician* 68 (9): 1781–1790.

von Ring, J. (1985). Pseudo-allergische Arzneimittelreaktionen: Überlegungen zur Pathophysiologie, Klinik und Diagnostik am Beispiel von Röntgenkontrastmitteln und Lokalanästhetika. *Allergologie* 8 (8): S 342-350.

Roberge, R.J. and Maceira-Rodriguez, L. (1985). Seizure-related oral lacerations: incidence and distribution. *J. Am. Dent. Assoc.* 111 (2): 279–280.

Rodriguez, L.F., Smolik, L.M., and Zbehlik, A.J. (1994). Benzocaine-induced methemoglobinemia: report of a severe reaction and review of the literature. *Ann. Pharmacother.* 28 (5): 643–649.

Rood, J.P. (1973). A case of lignocaine hypersensibility. *Br. Dent. J.* 135 (9): 411–412.

Rood, J.P. (2000). Adverse reaction to dental local anesthetic injection – "allergy" is not the cause. *Br. Dent. J.* 189 (7): 380–384.

Ross, J.D. (1963). Deficient activity of DPMH-dependent methemoglobin diaphorase in cord blood erythrocytes. *Blood* 21 (1): 51–62.

Ross, J.D. and Desforges, J.F. (1959). Reduction of methemoglobin by erythrocytes from cord blood. Further evidence of deficient enzyme activity in the newborn period. *Pediatrics* 23 (4): 718–726.

Rosso, R. (2015). Percepción ciudadana: clínica dental tradicional frente a los nuevos modelos empresariales. *Gaceta Dental (Madrid)* 269: 190–194.

Rupieper, N. and Stocker, L. (1981). Met-Hb Bildung und Lokalanästhesie mit Bupivacain, Carticain und Etidocain. *Anaesthesist* 30 (5): 23–25.

Rupieper, N., Montel, H., and Stocker, L. (1978). Metahemoglobinverhalten unter Anwendung von Carticain (=Ultracain®). *Anaesthesist* 27 (10): 83–85.

Rutten, A.J., Nancarrow, C., Mather, L.E. et al. (1989). Hemodynamic and central nervous system effects of intravenous bolus of lidocaine, bupivacaine, and ropivacaine in sheep. *Anesth. Analg.* 69 (3): 291–299.

Ruzicka, T., Gerstmeier, R.M., and Ring, J. (1987). Lokalanästhetika-allergie. *Z. Hautkr.* 62 (6): 455–460.

Salins, P.C., Kuriakose, M., Sharma, S.M., and Tauro, D.P. (1992). Hypoglycemia as a possible factor in the induction of vasovagal syncope. *Oral Surg. Oral Med. Oral Pathol.* 74 (5): 544–549.

Sambrook, P.J., Smith, W., Elijah, J., and Gors, A.N. (2011). Severe adverse reactions to dental local anaesthetics in systemic reactions. *Aust. Dent. J.* 56 (2): 148–153.

Schatz, M. (1984). Skin testing and incremental challenge in the evaluation of adverse reactions to local anesthetics. *J. Allergy Clin. Immunol.* 74 (4-part 2): 606–616.

Schatz, M. and Fung, D.L. (1986). Anaphylactic and anaphylactoid reactions due to anesthetic agents. *Clin. Rev. Allergy* 4 (2): 215–227.

Schorr, W.F. (1968). Paraben allergy. A case of intractable dermatitis. *JAMA* 204 (10): 859–866.

Schwartz, H.J. and Sher, T.H. (1985). Bisulfite sensitivity manifesting as allergy to local dental anesthesia. *J. Allergy Clin. Immunol.* 75 (4): 525–527.

Schwartz, H.J., Gilbert, I.A., Lenner, K.A. et al. (1989). Metabisulfite sensitivity and local dental anesthesia. *Ann. Allergy* 62 (2): 83–86.

Scott, D.B. (1975a). Evaluation of clinical tolerance of local anesthetic agents. *Br. J. Anaesth.* 47 (Suppl): 328–333.

Scott, D.B. (1975b). Evaluation of the toxicity of local anesthetic agents in man. *Br. J. Anaesth.* 47 (1): 56–61.

Scott, D.B. (1986). Toxic effects of local anesthetic agents on the central nervous system. *Br. J. Anaesth.* 58 (7): 732–735.

Scott, D.S. and Hirschman, R. (1982). Psychological aspects of dental anxiety in adults. *J. Am. Dent. Assoc.* 104 (1): 27–31.

Scott, D.B., Owen, J.A., and Richmond, J. (1964). Methaemoglobinaemia due to prilocaine. *Lancet* 2 (7362): 728–729.

Scott, D.S., Hirschman, R., and Schroder, K. (1984). Historical antecedents of dental anxiety. *J. Am. Dent. Assoc.* 108 (1): 42–45.

Selding, H.M. and Recant, B.S. (1955). The safety of anesthesia in the dental office. *J. Oral Surg.* 13 (3): 199–208.

Seng, G.F. and Gay, B.J. (1986). Dangers of sulfites in dental local anesthetic solutions: warning and recommendations. *J. Am. Dent. Assoc.* 113 (5): 769–770.

Seskin, L. (1978). Anaphylaxis due to local anesthesia hypersensitivity: report of case. *J. Am. Dent. Assoc.* 96 (5): 841–843.

Severinghaus, J.W., Xu, F.-D., and Spellman, M.J. Jr. (1991). Benzocaine and methemoglobin: recommended actions (letter). *Anesthesiology* 74 (2): 385–386.

Shojaei, A.R. and Haas, D.A. (2002). Local anesthetic cartridges and latex allergy: a literature review. *J. Can. Dent. Assoc.* 68 (10): 622–626.

Sidon, M.A. and Aldrete, J.A. (1971). A patient with multiple allergies: what anesthetic to use? *J. Am. Dent. Assoc.* 82 (2): 366–368.

Simon, R.A. (1986). Sulfite sensitivity. *Ann. Allergy* 56 (4): 281–291.

Singh, R. and Al, K.Y. (2019). *Benzocaine. StatPearls* [Internet]. Treasure Island (FL): StatPearls Publishing.

Sklar, E. and Schwartz, M. (1965). The ventral surface of the tongue: an emergency site of injection. *Oral Surg. Oral Med. Oral Pathol.* 19 (1): 28–31.

Spoerel, W.E., Adamson, D.H., and Eberhard, R.S. (1967). The significance of methaemoglobinaemia induced by prilocaine (Citanest). *Can. Anaesth. Soc. J.* 14 (1): 1–10.

Taggart, P., Hedworth-Whitty, R., Carruthers, M., and Gorden, P.D. (1976). Observations on electrocardiogram and plasma catecholamines during dental procedures: the forgotten vagus. *Br. Med. J.* 2 (6039): 787–789.

Tauberg, J.A.H., Nique, T.A., and Giovannetti, J.A. (1983). Stress-induced urticaria associated with local anesthetic administration. *Anesth. Prog.* 30 (6): 199–200.

Thompson, E.O. (1967). Principles of efficient dental equipment use. *J. Am. Dent. Assoc.* 74 (4): 708–716.

Tomlin, P.J. (1974). Death in outpatient dental anesthesia practice. *Anaesthesia* 29 (4): 551–570.

Topjian, A.A., Raymond, T.T., Atkins, D. et al. (2020). On behalf of the pediatric basic and advanced life support collaborators. Part 4: pediatric basic and advanced life support: 2020 American Heart Association guidelines for cardiopulmonary resuscitation and emergency cardiovascular care. *Circulation* 142 (Suppl 2): S469–S523.

Townes, P.L., Geertsma, M.A., and White, M.R. (1977). Benzocaine – induced methemoglobinemia. *Am. J. Dis. Child.* 131 (6): 697–698.

Tucker, G.T. and Mather, L.E. (1979). Clinical pharmacokinetics of local anesthetics. *Clin. Pharmacokinet.* 4 (4): 241–278.

Usubiaga, J.E., Wikinski, J., Ferrero, R. et al. (1966). Local anesthetic-induced convulsions in man. *Anesth. Analg.* 45 (5): 611–620.

Van der Bijl, P. and Victor, A.M. (1992). Adverse reactions associated with norepinephrine in dental local anesthesia. *Anesth. Prog.* 39 (3): 87–89.

Verrill, P.J. (1975). Adverse reactions to local anaesthetics and vasoconstrictor drugs. *Practitioner* 214 (1281): 380–387.

Virts, B.E. (1999). Local anesthesia toxicity review. *Pediatr. Dent.* 21 (6): 375.

Waldman, H.B. and Binkley, G. (1967). Lidocaine hypersensitivity: report of case. *J. Am. Dent. Assoc.* 74 (4): 747–749.

Walker, R.T. (1971). Hypersensitivity reaction of local anesthetic (letter). *Br. Dent. J.* 130 (1): 2.

Warrington, R.J. and McPhillips, S. (1997). Allergic reaction to local anesthetic agents of the amide group. *J. Allergy Clin. Immunol.* 100 (6 Pt 1): 855.

Weaver, J.M. (2011). The fallacy of a life saving sublingual injection of flumazenil (editorial). *Anesth. Prog.* 58 (1): 1–2.

Wehner, D. and Hamilton, G.C. (1984). Seizures following topical application of local anesthetics to burn patients. *Ann. Emerg. Med.* 13 (6): 456–458.

Weisel, W. and Tella, R.A. (1951). Reaction to tetracaine (Pontocaine®) used as a topical anesthetic in bronchoscopy. *JAMA* 147 (3): 218–222.

Weiss, L.D., Generalovich, T., Heller, M.B. et al. (1987). Methemoglobinemia levels following intravenous lidocaine administration. *Ann. Emerg. Med.* 16 (3): 323–325.

Wellis, S.L. (1969). Hypersensitivity to lidocaine hydrochloride. *Oral Surg. Oral Med. Oral Pathol.* 28 (5): 761–763.

Wendel, W.B. (1939). The control of methemoglobinemia with methylene blue. *J. Clin. Invest.* 18 (2): 179–185.

Wilburn-Goo, D. and Lloyd, L.M. (1999). When patients become cyanotic: acquired methemoglobinemia. *J. Am. Dent. Assoc.* 130 (6): 826–831.

Wildsmith, J.A.W., Mason, A., McKinnon, R.P., and Rae, S.M. (1998). Alleged allergy to local anaesthetic drugs. *Br. Dent. J.* 184 (10): 507–510.

Wilson, A.W., Deacock, S., Downie, I.P., and Zaki, G. (2000). Allergy to local anaesthetic: the importance of thorough investigation. *Br. Dent. J.* 188 (3): 120–122.

Yap, A.U.J. and Ong, G. (1996). An introduction to dental electronic anesthesia. *Quintessence Int.* 27 (5): 325–331.

Yeoman, C.M. (1982). Hypersensitivity to prilocaine. *Br. Dent. J.* 153 (2): 69–70.

Yjipaavalniemi, P. and Sane, J. (1981). Changes in heart rate during injection of local anesthetics. *Proc. Finn. Dent. Soc.* 77 (6): 346–349.

# Index

## a

A-Airway   436–437
Abel, John Jacob   4
absolute contraindications   149
accessory branch, for wisdom teeth   35, 352
accessory foramina   41
accessory mandibular foramen   349
action potentials   56–58
Adams, H. J.   6
adapter, for needles   174
adrenaline, vasoconstrictive effect and   4–5
adrenergic amines   87
adrenergic receptors   88–90
adverse effects, of felypressin (Octapressin®)   100
aerosols, observations of   223
Akinosi, J. O.   7–8
Aldrich, Thomas Bell   4
alkalinization system (pH Onset System®)   186–188
allergic reactions
 about   453–455
 as an absolute contraindication for vasoconstrictors   157–158
 clinical manifestations   458–459
 to components of local anesthetic solution   455–457
 confusion with other reactions   457–458
 dentist management   459–460
 diagnosis   459
 to novocaine   6
 prevention   460
 as a relevant contraindication   148
allergic-like reactions   444
amide anesthetics and malignant hyperthermia, as a minor contraindication   151
amides   455–456
amino terminus   67
amphetamines, as a relative contraindication for vasoconstrictors   161
anatomic boundaries, of pterygomandibular space   42–43
anesthesia. See local anesthesia/anesthetics
anesthetic parameter   72
anesthetic/anesthesia. See local anesthesia/anesthetics
anesthetized area
 for buccal nerve block   315
 for greater palatine nerve block   274–275
 for intraosseous technique   331–332
 for intraseptal technique   328
 for lingual nerve block   312
 for nasopalatine nerve block   271
 for P-AMSA   371
 for P-ASA   373
 for periodontal ligament technique   324
 for QuickSleeper   377
angioedema, as a clinical manifestation of allergy   458–459
angioneurotic edema, as a clinical manifestation of allergy   458–459
Anrep, Vassily von   2, 3
anterior cap, of needles   175
anterior division, mandibular nerve and   31
anterior loop   35, 38
anterior part
 of cartridges   178
 of cartridge-type syringes   181–182
anterior superior alveolar nerve   19, 23
anterior/ventral boundaries, of pterygomandibular space   42–43
anti-adrenergic drugs   162
anticoagulants   141
antioxidants (sulfites)   107–108, 456–457
antiplatelet agents   140–141
antipsychotic drugs, as a contraindication for vasoconstrictors   163–164
anxiety, lack of patient cooperation and   135–136
aromatic ring   67
articaine
 about   6, 74–75, 113–115, 452, 456
 for children   390
 indications   116–117
 metabolism   115
 remarks   115–116
ASA III patients with cardiovascular conditions, as a relative contraindication for vasoconstrictors   160
ASA IV physical status   137–140
aspiration
 during injections   226–228
 needle gauge and   176
assessment, of local anesthetics   70–72

*Local Anesthesia in Dentistry: A Locoregional Approach*, First Edition. Jesús Calatayud and Mana Saraghi.
© 2024 John Wiley & Sons Ltd. Published 2024 by John Wiley & Sons Ltd.
Companion website: www.wiley.com/go/Calatayud/local

asthma controlled with corticosteroids, as an absolute contraindication for vasoconstrictors 156
aural complications
    about 423
    clinical manifestations 423–424
    dentist management 424
    techniques 423
auriculotemporal nerve 33, 352
axonotmesis 402
axons 50–51

## b

barbed needles 177
basic injection technique
    about 219
    causes of pain during 232–253
    phases of
        application of topical anesthetic 222–223
        aspiration 226–228
        evaluation of anesthesia 230–231
        final phase 229–230
        initial preparation 219–220
        injection 228–229
        insertion of needle 225–226
        post-treatment phase 231–232
        preparation phase 220–222
        transfer of syringe 223–225
    retraction 219
    terminology 234–255
basic management
    about 435
    administration of drugs 438
    calling emergency services 439
    initial measures 435–436
    unconscious patient 436–438
basic membrane proteins, for peripheral nerve
    about 54
    potassium channels 55–56
    sodium channels 54–55
    sodium-potassium pump 54
B-Breathing 437–438
behavioral problems, approach to 136–137
benzocaine
    about 5, 451, 456
    as a relevant contraindication 148–149
    as a topical anesthetic 197–199
Berling, Cläes 7

bevel, of needles 176
bilateral mandibular blocks 284
bitartrate salts 87
Björn, Hilding 6
Bochdalek's ganglion 23
body of the mandible
    about 36
    cortical bone thickness 36–37
    mandibular canal 37–38
    mental foramen 38–39
    retromolar zone (trigone and fossa) 37
Bohr effect 442–443
Braun, Heinrich 4–5
breakage, of needles 177
Brettauer, Josef 3
buccal anesthesia, of upper molars 241–242
buccal approach, to double infiltration in anterior teeth 305
buccal infiltration
    about 242
    in children 392
    complications of 245
    efficacy of 245
    modified cotton roll approach 245
    success factors of 245
    technique 242–245
    zones anesthetized 242
buccal nerve 31–33, 351–352
buccal nerve block
    about 314–315
    anesthetized area 315
    complications of 316
    technique 315–316
bupivacaine
    about 123, 452, 456
    indications and contraindications 125–126
    metabolism 123
    as a minor contraindication 150–151
    remarks 123–125

## c

*canalis sinuosus* 23
cardiotoxicity, as a minor contraindication 150–151
cardiovascular abnormalities 98–99, 328
cardiovascular disease

patients with amphetamines/psychostimulants, as an absolute contraindication for vasoconstrictors 157
    toxic methemoglobinemia and 149
Carrea, Juan Ubaldo 8
cartridge breakage in mouth 423
cartridge heaters 190
cartridge system, for needles 7
cartridges
    about 177–178
    components 178–179
    degradation of drugs in 180–181
    for periodontal ligament technique 324
    problems affecting 180
    storage of 179–180
cartridge-type syringes, variants of 184–185
Cassamani, C. 8
catecholamines
    about 87–88
    adrenergic receptors 88–90
    cartridges containing 179–180
    epinephrine 92–93
    isomers and 88
    levonordefrin 94–95
    metabolism of 92
    norepinephrine 93–94
    systemic effects 90–91
    vasoconstrictive effect 91
caudal/inferior boundaries, of pterygomandibular space 43
causes
    of facial blanching 399
    of local anesthetic-induced toxicity 446–447
    of localized late-onset skin lesion 400–401
    of needle breakage 420
    of nerve lesions 402–403
    of post-injection mucosal ulceration 419
    of psychogenic reactions 439
    of trismus 408
C-Circulation 438
cellulitis, as a clinical manifestation of needle-induced infection 418
central nervous system (CNS), local anesthetics and 150–151
central processing unit (CPU), in The Wand® 369

central/middle region, of
   pterygomandibular space   44
Charles V, Emperor   1–2
chemical structure, of local
   anesthetics   67
chemical tourniquet   4–5
Chenaux, G.   8
children
   about   389
   maximum doses of local anesthetics
      for   75–76
   primary mandibular molars
      391–392
   problem with   389
   solutions for   389–390
   technique in   390–391
   transpapillary technique in
      276–277
cholinesterase deficiency, as a relevant
   contraindication   149
chorda tympani nerve   33, 34, 44
circulatory system, effect of
   catecholamines on   91
cleaning syringes   183
clinical manifestations
   of allergies   458–459
   of aural complications   423–424
   of facial blanching   399
   of facial hematomas   401
   of facial palsy   410
   of hyperventilation syndrome   443
   of localized late-onset skin
      lesion   400
   of needle breakage   421
   of needle-induced infection   418
   of ocular complications   412–413
   of post-injection mucosal
      ulceration   419
   of psychogenic reactions   440–441
   of systemic toxicity induced by local
      anesthetics   447–449
   of toxic methemoglobinemia
      452–453
clinical variations, for systemic toxicity
   induced by local
   anesthetics   449
closed-mouth mandibular block
   technique   7–8
clotting abnormalities
   about   140
   alternatives and recommendations
      142

high-risk anesthetic techniques   140
   systemic causes of risk of
      hemorrhage   140–142
Cobo, Bernabé   2
coca leaf   1–2
cocaine
   as an absolute contraindication for
      vasoconstrictors   157
   dangers of   4
   development of   2–3
   as a topical anesthetic   203
   vasodilation and   70
cold aerosols   206–207
collateral branches   18–19
comfort control syringe from
   Midwest   376–377
complementary anesthesia
   about   312
   buccal nerve block
      about   314–315
      anesthetized area   315
      complications of   316
      technique   315–316
      indications   312
   lingual nerve block
      about   312
      anesthetized area   312
      complications of   314
      partial variant as   314
      technique   312–314
complementary anesthesia of
   the palate
   about   267
   anesthesia of palate
      without   267–268
   greater palatine nerve block
      area anesthetized   274–275
      complications of   276
      partial variant of the palate   276
      technique   275–276
   indications   268–269
   methods for reducing pain
      about   269
      minimal intervention
         technique   271
      periodontal ligament
         technique   270–271
      pressure techniques   270
      topical anesthesia   269
      topical cooling   270
   nasopalatine nerve   267
   nasopalatine nerve block

      about   271
      anesthetized area   271
      complications of   273–274
      intranasal variant   274
      technique   271–273, 274
   potency of anesthetic   267
   transpapillary technique in children
      about   276–277
      technique   277
complementary devices   185–186
complications
   about   397, 433, 434
   allergy
      about   453–455
      clinical manifestations   458–459
      to components of local anesthetic
         solution   455–457
      confusion with other
         reactions   457–458
      dentist management   459–460
      diagnosis   459
      prevention   460
   aural
      about   423
      clinical manifestations   423–424
      dentist management   424
      techniques   423
   basic management of
      about   435
      administration of drugs   438
      calling emergency services   439
      initial measures   435–436
      unconscious patient   436–438
   of buccal infiltration   245
   of buccal nerve block   316
   cartridge breakage in mouth   423
   of double infiltration in anterior
      teeth   306
   of electronic dental anesthesia
      (EDA)   368
   facial blanching
      about   398–399
      causes and   399
      clinical manifestations   399
      pathophysiology and   400
      techniques for   399
   facial hematomas
      about   401
      clinical manifestations   401
      dentist management   402
      factors contributing to   401
   facial palsy

complications (cont'd)
    about 409
    associated with mandibular block 410–412
    associated with maxillary infiltration 412
    clinical manifestations 410
  of greater palatine nerve block 276
  of high tuberosity approach 256
  of infraorbital nerve block 249–250
  of intranasal maxillary local anesthesia (Kovanaze®) 381–383
  of intraosseous technique 336–338
  of intraseptal technique 329
  of jet injection 363–364
  of lingual nerve block 314
  localized late-onset skin lesion
    about 400
    causes and pathophysiology 400–401
    clinical manifestations 400
  of mandibular block
    conventional/direct technique 291–292
    Gow-Gates technique 299–300
    Laguardia-Akinosi technique 303–304
  of nasopalatine nerve block 273–274
  needle breakage
    about 419–420
    causes of 420
    clinical manifestations 421
    decision to retrieve 421
    dentist management 421–422
    factors of interest 420
    preventive measures 422–423
    techniques 420
  needle-induced infection
    about 418
    clinical manifestations 418
    dentist management 419
  nerve lesions
    about 402
    anatomical 402
    electric shock sensation 403–404
    general causes 402–403
    hoarseness 407
    long-term paresthesia 404–407
    sense of taste alterations 407
  ocular
    about 412
    clinical manifestations 412–413
    dentist management 414
    onset and duration 413
    pathophysiology of 414–418
    predictors of sequelae 414
    techniques for 412
  of P-AMSA 373
  of P-ASA 375
  of periodontal ligament technique 326–328, 376
  persistent post-injection pain 397
  of posterior superior alveolar nerve block 253
  post-injection mucosal ulceration
    about 419
    clinical manifestations 419
    dentist management 419
    proposed causes 419
  preventive measures 435
  psychogenic reactions
    about 439
    allergic-like reactions 444
    general causes 439
    hyperventilation syndrome 442–444
    vasovagal syncope 439–442
  self-inflicted injury 397–398
  systemic toxicity induced by local anesthetics
    about 445
    causes of local anesthetic-induced toxicity 446–447
    clinical manifestations 447–449
    clinical variations 449
    dentist management 449–450
    pathophysiology 445–446
    prevention 450
    recovery and discharge 450
  toxic methemoglobinemia
    about 450–451
    aggravating factors 452
    clinical manifestations 452–453
    dentist management 453
    local anesthetics involved 451–452
  toxicity induced by sympathomimetic vasoconstrictors
    about 444
    dentist management 445
    pathophysiology 444
    symptoms of reaction to epinephrine 444–445
    symptoms of reaction to norepinephrine 445
  of transpalatal technique 261–262
  trismus
    about 407
    causes of 408
    clinical types of 408
    techniques implicated in development of 407–408
    treatment of 408–409
compounds, as a topical anesthetic 203–205
computer-controlled injection systems (The Wand®)
  about 368–369
  conventional techniques and 375–376
  device description 369–371
  P-AMSA 371–373
  P-ASA 373–375
computer-controlled injection techniques 185
COMT inhibitor-type antiparkinson drugs, as a relative contraindication for vasoconstrictors 160
concentration
  of local anesthetic
    about 60
    anesthetic potency and 73
    safety and 73
    tissue irritation and 73–74
    volume and 72
  of vasoconstrictors 87
congenital methemoglobinemia, toxic methemoglobinemia and 149
contents
  of pterygomandibular space 44–45
  pterygopalatine fossa and 27
contraindications
  absolute 149
  of bupivacaine 125–126
  of electronic dental anesthesia (EDA) 366–367
  of felypressin (Octapressin®) 100
  of intranasal maxillary local anesthesia (Kovanaze®) 380
  of intraosseous technique 330
  of intraseptal technique 328

of periodontal ligament
technique   320
of prilocaine
(propitocaine)   122–123
contraindications, for local anesthetic
techniques
about   135
ASA IV physical status   137–140
clotting abnormalities
about   140
alternatives and
recommendations   142
high-risk anesthetic
techniques   140
systemic causes of risk of
hemorrhage   140–142
impossible physical access   143
injection site infection   142–143
lack of cooperation from patient
about   135
approach to behavioral
problems   136–137
evaluation or risk   136
predisposing factors   135–136
contraindications, for local anesthetics
about   148
minor
amide anesthetics and malignant
hyperthermia   151
bupivacaine and
cardiotoxicity   150–151
lidocaine and cimetidine   150
lidocaine and propranolol   150
lidocaine and
succinylcholine   150
procaine and sulfonoamides   149
relevant
allergy to local anesthetics   148
benzocaine   148–149
cholinesterase deficiency   149
esther anesthetics   149
long-acting anesthetics   148
methemoglobinemia   148–149
myasthenia gravis and
esters   149
prilocaine   148–149
contraindications, for vasoconstrictors
about   155
absolute
allergy to   157–158
asthma controlled with
corticosteroids   156

cardiovascular disease patients
with amphetamines/
psychostimulants   157
intolerance to sulfites   156
pheochromocytoma-induced
arterial hypertension   156–157
recent consumption of
cocaine   157
uncontrolled insulin-dependent
Diabetes Mellitus   155–156
felypressin (Octapressin®)   164
little relevance
about   163
phenothiazines and antipsychotic
drugs   163–164
uncontrolled hyperthyroidism   163
vasoconstrictors and
osteoradionecrosis   164
relative
about   158
amphetamines and
psychostimulants   161
ASA III patients with
cardiovascular conditions   160
COMT inhibitor-type
antiparkinson drugs   160
digitalis glycosides (digoxin)
160–161
interaction involving drugs no
longer in use   162
nonselective beta-blockers
158–160
tricyclic antidepressants   161–162
conventional techniques
for anesthesia   7
computer-controlled injection
systems (The Wand®)
and   375–376
as a pressure technique   270
conventional techniques,
alternatives to
about   360
comfort control syringe from
Midwest   376–377
computer-controlled injection
systems (The Wand®)
about   368–369
conventional techniques
and   375–376
device description   369–371
P-AMSA   371–373
P-ASA   373–375

electronic dental anesthesia (EDA)
about   364
advantages   366
complications of   368
contraindications   366–367
disadvantages   366
equipment   367
indications   364–365
mechanism of action   364
technique   367–368
intranasal maxillary local anesthesia
(Kovanaze®)
about   379
advantages of   383–384
complications of   381–383
contraindications   380
disadvantages of   384
efficacy of   381
equipment   380
indications   379
solution composition   379
technique   380–381
zone anesthetized   379
jet injection
about   360
advantages   361
complications of   363–364
disadvantages   361
distribution of solution   360–361
equipment   361–362
indications   361
technique   362–363
QuickSleeper   377–379
conventional/direct technique
(mandibular block)
about   285
complications of   291–292
distribution of anesthetic
solution   285–286
efficacy of   291
technique   286–291
zone anesthetized   286
convulsions   448
Cook, Harvey S.   7
Corning, Leonard   4
coronoid notch   41
cortical bone, thickness of   25, 36–37
cranial/high region, of
pterygomandibular space   44
cranial/superior boundaries, of
pterygomandibular space   43
critical length   59–60

cutaneous reactions, as a clinical manifestation of allergy 458
Cybulski, Napoleon 4
cylindrical body, of cartridges 178–179

### d
Davis, Parke 5
deep tendon of the temporal muscle 42
deflection, of needles 176–177
degradation of drugs, in cartridges 180–181
dendrites 50
Dental Electronic Anesthesia System, 8670 3M Dental 8
DentalVibe® 188, 189–190
dentist management
 of allergies 459–460
 of aural complications 424
 of facial hematomas 402
 of hyperventilation syndrome 443–444
 of needle breakage 421–422
 of needle-induced infection 419
 of ocular complications 414
 of post-injection mucosal ulceration 419
 of psychogenic reactions 441–442
 of systemic toxicity induced by local anesthetics 449–450
 of toxic methemoglobinemia 453
 of toxicity induced by sympathomimetic vasoconstrictors 445
depolarization 57
dermojet 8
diagnosis
 for allergy 459
 of hyperventilation syndrome 443
differential nerve block 58–59
diffusion of the solution, for periodontal ligament technique 320–321
digitalis glycosides (digoxin), as a relative contraindication for vasoconstrictors 160–161
dilutions, of vasoconstrictors 87
direct approach, from buccal area 273
direct oral anticoagulants 141–142
direct technique, for anesthesia 7
disposable antineedle stick syringes 184–185
dissociation constant (pKa) 68–69
distribution of anesthetic solution
 in mandibular block: conventional/direct technique 285–286
 for mandibular block: Laguardia-Akinosi technique 301
divergent angle, of the ramus of the mandible 39
dorsal/posterior boundaries, of pterygomandibular space 43
double infiltration in anterior teeth
 about 304
 complications of 306
 efficacy of 306
 success factors for 304
 technique 304–306
 zone anesthetized 304
double (Bifid) mandibular canal and/or foramen 350
drug addiction and alcoholism, as a cause of local anesthesia failure 346
drugs, administration of 438
Du Vigneaud, V. 7
dysesthesia, as a clinical manifestation of long-term paresthesia 404, 406

### e
EDA (electronic dental anesthesia). See electronic dental anesthesia (EDA)
efficacy
 of buccal infiltration 245
 of double infiltration in anterior teeth 306
 of high tuberosity approach 256
 of infraorbital nerve block 249
 of intranasal maxillary local anesthesia (Kovanaze®) 381
 of intraosseous technique 336
 of mandibular block
  conventional/direct technique 291
  Gow-Gates technique 299
  Laguardia-Akinosi technique 303
 of P-AMSA 373
 of P-ASA 375
 of periodontal ligament technique 321–322, 326
 of phentalomine (OraVerse®) 97
 of posterior superior alveolar nerve block 252–253
 of prilocaine (propitocaine) 122
 of QuickSleeper 378–379
 of transpalatal technique 260–261
Einhorn, Alfred 5
Eisleb, Otto 6
Ekenstam, Bo af 6
electric pulp tester (EPT) 70–71
electric shock sensation 403–404
electronic dental anesthesia (EDA)
 about 8, 142, 364
 advantages 366
 complications of 368
 contraindications 366–367
 disadvantages 366
 equipment 367
 indications 364–365
 mechanism of action 364
 technique 367–368
emergency services, calling 439
endocrine system and metabolism, effect of catecholamines on 91
endoneurium 52
epinephrine
 about 4, 6–7, 76
 catecholamines and 92–93
 symptoms of reaction to 444–445
epineurium 53
EPT (electric pulp tester) 70–71
equipment. See also instrument set and equipment
 for electronic dental anesthesia (EDA) 367
 for intranasal maxillary local anesthesia (Kovanaze®) 380
 for jet injection 361–362
 for QuickSleeper 377
esters 455, 456
esther anesthetics, as a relevant contraindication 149
ethyl aminobenzoate. See benzocaine
etidocaine 452
Euler, Ulf Svante von 7
Eutectic Mixture of Local Anesthetic (EMLA) cream 200–201
Everett, Frank 6
excitation threshold 57
excited membrane 56–58
external/lateral boundaries, of pterygomandibular space 42

extraocular manifestations, as a clinical manifestation of ocular complications   413
extraoral technique, for infraorbital nerve block   248–249
extreme age groups, toxic methemoglobinemia and   149
eye disorders, as a clinical manifestation of ocular complications   413

## f

facial blanching
  about   398–399
  causes and   399
  clinical manifestations   399
  pathophysiology and   400
  techniques for   399
facial branches   19
facial hematomas
  about   401
  clinical manifestations   401
  dentist management   402
  factors contributing to   401
facial palsy
  about   409
  associated with mandibular block   410–412
  associated with maxillary infiltration   412
  clinical manifestations   410
failure, of local anesthesia. *See also* supplementary techniques
  about   344
  after mandibular blocks   349–354
  after maxillary infiltration   348–349
  consequences of   344–345
  frequency   344
  general causes
    drug addiction and alcoholism   346
    highly anxious patients   345–346
    irreversible acute pulpitis   346–348
    resistance to local anesthetics   348
failure rate   283
Falcon, Francisco   2
Falker, Mic   9
false positives/negatives   226–227
fascicle   52
felypressin (Octapressin®)
  about   7, 98
  advantages and disadvantages   100
  adverse effects   100
  cardiovascular effects   98–99
  contraindications of   100, 164
  maximum doses   100–101
  vasoconstrictive effect   99–100
Ferguson, James   8
fibrous band formation, chronic late-onset trismus due to   408
Figge, Frank   8
Fischer, Guido   5, 6, 7, 8
flexible stainless steel needles   173
floor of the mouth, lingual nerve and   33–34
foot control, in The Wand®   370
foramen ovale   31, 34
forced opening, under general anesthesia   409
Francis, Jerome B.   8
Franck, François   3
Freud, Sigmund   2, 3, 4
Fürth, Otto Ritter von   4

## g

gag reflex   209
Gasca, Pedro de la   1–2
gastrointestinal reactions, as a clinical manifestation of allergy   458
gate control theory   8, 189
general anesthesia   162, 409
Gow-Gates, George Albert Edward   8
Gow-Gates technique (mandibular block)
  about   292
  advantages, disadvantages and non-advantages   294–296
  complications of   299–300
  efficacy of   299
  mechanism   292–294
  remarks on   300
  technique   296–299
  zone anesthetized   296
greater palatine canal and foramen   24
greater palatine foramen technique, for anesthesia   8
greater palatine nerve   19, 20
greater palatine nerve block
  area anesthetized   274–275
  complications of   276
  partial variant of the palate   276
  technique   275–276
guanethidine   162
Guptill, Arthur   6

## h

Hall, Richard John   3
halothane   162
Halsted, William Stewart   3, 4, 7
handpiece, in The Wand®   370
heart, effect of catecholamines on   90
heart attack patients, as a contraindication of felypressin   164
hemophilia   142
high tuberosity approach, for pulpal anesthesia
  about   253
  complications of   256
  efficacy of   256
  remarks   256
  technique   254–255
  uses   253–254
  zone anesthetized   254
high/cranial region, of pterygomandibular space   44
highly anxious patients, as a cause of local anesthesia failure   345–346
high-pressure jet injection   8
high-pressure jet injectors   185
high-pressure syringes   185
high-risk anesthetic techniques, clotting abnormalities and   140
hoarseness   407
Hochman, Mark   8
hub, of needles   174
Huldt, Sven   6
Hunter, Charles   4
hyperpolarization   57–58
hyperventilation syndrome   442–444
hypospray   8

## i

indications
  for articaine   116–117
  for bupivacaine   125–126
  for complementary anesthesia   312
  for complementary anesthesia of palate   268–269
  for electronic dental anesthesia (EDA)   364–365
  for intranasal maxillary local anesthesia (Kovanaze®)   379
  for intraosseous technique   330
  for jet injection   361
  for lidocaine (lignocaine)   111–113
  for mepivacaine   119–120

indications (*cont'd*)
  for periodontal ligament technique  320
  for phentalomine (OraVerse®)  96
  for prilocaine (propitocaine)  122–123
  for topical anesthesia  208–209
indirect approach, from buccal area  272–273
induction stage, of peripheral nerve block  60
infection, chronic late-onset trismus due to  408
inferior alveolar nerve  34–36
inferior/caudal boundaries, of pterygomandibular space  43
infiltrative techniques, variants of  254–255
infraorbital foramen  25–26
infraorbital nerve block
  about  245–246
  complications of  249–250
  efficacy of  249
  extraoral technique  248–249
  intraoral technique  246–248
  remarks  250–251
  uses  246
  zones anesthetized  246
infraorbital zone, as a collateral branch  19
injectable anesthetic solutions
  articaine
    about  113–115
    indications  116–117
    metabolism  115
    remarks  115–116
  bupivacaine
    about  123
    indications and contraindications  125–126
    metabolism  123
    remarks  123–125
  lidocaine (lignocaine)
    about  109–111
    indications  111–113
    metabolism  111
    remarks  111
  mepivacaine
    about  117
    indications  119–120
    metabolism  117–119
    remarks  119

  prilocaine (propitocaine)
    about  120
    indications and contraindications  122–123
    metabolism  120
    remarks  120–122
  procaine (novocaine)  109
  solution composition
    antioxidants (sulfites)  107–108
    local anesthetic  107
    other compounds  109
    pH adjustment  108–109
    preservatives (methylparaben)  108
    vasoconstrictor  107
injection site infection  142–143
injections  228–229
Injex®, for jet injection  362
INR index  141
instrument set and equipment
  about  7
  alkalinization system (pH Onset System®)  186–188
  cartridge heaters  190
  cartridges
    about  177–178
    components  178–179
    degradation of drugs in  180–181
    problems affecting  180
    storage of  179–180
  complementary devices  185–186
  for intraosseous technique  330–331
  needles
    about  173
    components  173–175
    criteria for selecting  177
    critical aspects  175–177
    lengths and gauges  175
  for periodontal ligament technique  322–324
  syringes
    about  181
    components of cartridge-type  181–183
    self-aspirating  183–184
    variants of cartridge-type  184–185
  vibrating devices  188–190
interaction involving drugs no longer in use, as a relative contraindication for vasoconstrictors  162

intermediate aliphatic chain  67
internal branch  21
internal/medial boundaries, of pterygomandibular space  42
intolerance to sulfites, as an absolute contraindication for vasoconstrictors  156
intracranial zone, as a collateral branch  18
intraligamentary injection, for anesthesia  8
intramuscular route, for drugs  438
intranasal maxillary local anesthesia (Kovanaze®)
  about  9, 379
  advantages of  383–384
  complications of  381–383
  contraindications  380
  disadvantages of  384
  efficacy of  381
  equipment  380
  indications  379
  solution composition  379
  technique  380–381
  zone anesthetized  379
intranasal variant, nasopalatine nerve block  274
intraoral technique, for infraorbital nerve block  246–248
intraosseous technique
  about  329–330, 332–336
  anesthetic solutions  331
  anesthetized area  331–332
  complications of  336–338
  efficacy  336
  indications, contraindications, and disadvantages  330
  instrument set  330–331
intra-pulp technique, for anesthesia  8
intrapulpal anesthesia
  about  318
  topical anesthetic technique  319
  traditional technique  318–319
intraseptal technique
  about  328
  anesthetized area  328
  complications of  329
  contraindications  328
  success factors for  328
  technique  328–329
intravascular injection, inadvertent  446–447

intravenous route, for drugs  438
irreversible acute pulpitis, as a cause of local anesthesia failure  346–348
ischemia, as a cause of post-injection mucosal ulceration  419
ischemic necrosis, due to vasospasm  400–401
isomers
 about  78–79
 catecholamines and  88

## j

jaw-thrust technique  436–437
jet injection
 about  360
 advantages  361
 complications of  363–364
 disadvantages  361
 distribution of solution  360–361
 equipment  361–362
 indications  361
 technique  362–363
Jorgensen, Niels Bjorn  7

## k

Kneucker of Vienna, Alfred  5
Koller, Carl  3

## l

labial plexus  35, 353
lack of cooperation from patient
 about  135
 approach to behavioral problems  136–137
 evaluation or risk  136
 predisposing factors  135–136
lactation, local anesthetics and  77
Lafarge, Robert  8
Laguardia, H. J.  7–8
Laguardia-Akinosi technique (mandibular block)
 about  300
 advantages and disadvantages  300–301
 complications of  303–304
 distribution of anesthetic solution  301
 efficacy of  303
 technique  301–303
 zone anesthetized  301
Largus, Scribonius  8
lateral nasal branches  19

lateral/external boundaries, of pterygomandibular space  42
lengths and gauges, of needles  175
León, Pedro Cieza de  2
lesions
 caused by barbed needles  177
 on mucosa  209
lesser palatine nerves  19
Levitt, Boris  7
levonordefrin  7, 94–95
lidocaine (lignocaine)
 about  6, 74–75, 109–111, 452, 456
 for children  389–390
 cimetidine and, as a minor contraindication  150
 indications  111–113
 metabolism  111
 propranolol and, as a minor contraindication  150
 remarks  111
 succinylcholine and, as a minor contraindication  150
 for topical anesthesia  199
lidocaine adhesive patches, for topical anesthesia (DentiPatch®)  199–200
lingual approach, to double infiltration in anterior teeth  305
lingual nerve  33–34
lingual nerve block
 about  312
 anesthetized area  312
 complications of  314
 high-risk anesthetic techniques and  140
 partial variant as  314
 technique  312–314
lingula  39, 350
lipid solubility  69–70
local anesthesia/anesthetics
 about  67
 anesthetic parameter  72
 assessment of  70–72
 chemical structure  67
 in children (See children)
 complications of (See complications)
 composition of  107
 concentration
  anesthetic potency and  73
  safety and  73
  tissue irritation and  73–74
  volume and  72

 contraindications for (See contraindications)
 degradation of in cartridges  181
 development of  5–6
 development of in dentistry  5–9
 effect of articaine  116
 evaluation of  230–231
 frequency of use of  9
 history of  1–9
 for intraosseous technique  331
 isomers  78–79
 lactation  77
 local anesthetic potency
  articaine  115–116
  of local anesthetics  73
 lower lip  283
 maximum doses  74–75
 maximum doses for children  75–76
 mechanisms of
  about  58
  critical length  59–60
  differential nerve block  58–59
  tonic and phase block  59
  transient receptor potential channel  60
 mixing  77–78
 of palate, without complementary anesthesia of palate  267–268
 peripheral nerve and (See peripheral nerve)
 physical-chemical characteristics of
  about  67–68
  dissociation constant (pKa)  68–69
  lipid solubility  69–70
  partition coefficient  69–70
  protein binding  70
  vasodilation  70
 potency of  267
 pregnancy  76–77
 topical (See topical anesthesia)
local anesthesia/anesthetics, failure of
 about  344
 after mandibular blocks  349–354
 after maxillary infiltration  348–349
 consequences of  344–345
 frequency  344
 general causes
  drug addiction and alcoholism  346
  highly anxious patients  345–346
  irreversible acute pulpitis  346–348
  resistance to local anesthetics  348

localized late-onset skin lesion
  about  400
  causes and pathophysiology  400–401
  clinical manifestations  400
Löfgren, Nils Isak  6
long-acting anesthetics, as a relevant contraindication  148
long-term paresthesia, nerve lesions and  404–407
Lossen, Wilhelm  2
low platelet counts  142
lower lip anesthesia  283
lower region, of pterygomandibular space  44
lumen, of needles  174
Lundqvist, Bengt  6

## m

Maïz, Thomas Moreno y  2
mandibular anesthesia. *See* complementary anesthesia; pulpal anesthesia
mandibular arch
  about  31
  body of the mandible
    about  36
    cortical bone thickness  36–37
    mandibular canal  37–38
    mental foramen  38–39
    retromolar zone (trigone and fossa)  37
  mandibular nerve ($V_3$)
    about  31
    auriculotemporal nerve  33
    buccal nerve  31–33
    inferior alveolar nerve  34–36
    lingual nerve  33–34
    mylohyoid nerve  36
  pterygomandibular space
    about  41–42
    anatomic boundaries of the  42–43
    contents of  44–45
    open/closed mouth and  44
    positive aspirations and hematomas  45
  ramus of the mandible
    accessory foramina  41
    coronoid notch  41
    divergent angle  39
    lingula  39
    mandibular foramen  39–40
    ramus width  39
    sulcus colli  40–41
mandibular block
  about  7
  in children  392
  conventional/direct technique
    about  285
    complications of  291–292
    distribution of anesthetic solution  285–286
    efficacy of  291
    technique  286–291
    zone anesthetized  286
  facial palsy associated with  410–412
  failure of local anesthesia after  349–354
  in general
    about  281
    factors to consider for  282–285
    zone anesthetized  282
  Gow-Gates technique
    about  292
    advantages, disadvantages and non-advantages  294–296
    complications of  299–300
    efficacy of  299
    mechanism  292–294
    remarks on  300
    technique  296–299
    zone anesthetized  296
  high-risk anesthetic techniques and  140
  Laguardia-Akinosi technique
    about  300
    advantages and disadvantages  300–301
    complications of  303–304
    distribution of anesthetic solution  301
    efficacy of  303
    technique  301–303
    zone anesthetized  301
  The Wand® and  376
mandibular canal  37–38
mandibular foramen  39–40
mandibular incisive nerve  35
mandibular nerve ($V_3$)
  about  31
  auriculotemporal nerve  33
  buccal nerve  31–33
  inferior alveolar nerve  34–36
  lingual nerve  33–34
  mylohyoid nerve  36
Margetis, P. M.  8
margins, pterygopalatine fossa and  26
maxilla, pulpal anesthesia and  241
maxillary anesthesia. *See* complementary anesthesia of the palate; pulpal anesthesia
maxillary arch
  about  17
  cortical bone thickness  25
  greater palatine canal and foramen  24
  infraorbital foramen  25–26
  maxillary nerve ($V_2$)
    about  17–18
    collateral branches  18–19
    palatine nerves  19–21
    superior alveolar nerves  22–23
    superior dental plexus  23
  nasopalatine canal and foramen  24–25
  pterygoid venous plexus  25
  pterygopalatine fossa  26–27
  trigeminal ganglion  17
  trigeminal nerve  17
maxillary block, high-risk anesthetic techniques and  140
maxillary infiltration
  facial palsy associated with  412
  failure of local anesthesia after  348–349
maxillary nerve ($V_2$)
  about  17–18
  collateral branches  18–19
  palatine nerves  19–21
  pulpal anesthesia and  241
  superior alveolar nerves  22–23
  superior dental plexus  23
maximum doses
  about  74–75
  of articaine  115
  for children  75–76
  of felypressin (Octapressin®)  100–101
  of mepivacaine  119
Mayer, E.  6
mechanical therapy, for trismus  408–409

mechanisms
  for electronic dental anesthesia
      (EDA)   364
  of local anesthesia
      about   58
      critical length   59–60
      differential nerve block   58–59
      tonic and phase block   59
      transient receptor potential
          channel   60
  for mandibular block: Gow-Gates
      technique   292–294
medial/internal boundaries, of
      pterygomandibular space   42
membrane at rest (polarized)   56
membrane potentials   56
membranes   51
mental conditions, lack of patient
      cooperation and   135
mental foramen   38–39
mental nerve   35
mepivacaine
  about   6, 117, 456
  indications   119–120
  metabolism   117–119
  remarks   119
  vasodilation and   70
metabolism
  articaine   115
  bupivacaine   123
  of catecholamines   92
  lidocaine (lignocaine)   111
  mepivacaine   117–119
  prilocaine (propitocaine)   120
methemoglobinemia, as a relevant
      contraindication   148–149
methylparaben (preservative)   457
microanatomy, of peripheral nerve
  axons   50–51
  membranes   51
  nerve fibers and myelin   51–52
  neurons   50
  peripheral nerve structure   52–54
  sensory neurons   50
middle nasal branches   19
middle superior alveolar nerve
      (MSAN)   19, 22–23
middle/central region, of
      pterygomandibular space   44
minimal intervention technique, for
      complementary anesthesia of
      palate   271

mixing local anesthetics   77–78
mixing pen   187–188
modified adatia technique, for
      posterior superior alveolar
      nerve block   253
modified cotton roll approach, for
      buccal infiltration   245
Mortn, William Thomas Green
      (dentist)   1
MSAN (middle superior alveolar
      nerve)   19, 22–23
mucosa, lesions and ulcers on   209
Muschaweck, Roman   6
myasthenia gravis and esters, as a
      relevant contraindication   149
myelinated fibers   51–52
mylohyoid nerve   34, 36, 350–351

## n

nasopalatine canal and
      foramen   24–25
nasopalatine nerve   19, 20–21, 267
nasopalatine nerve block
  about   271
  anesthetized area   271
  complications of   273–274
  intranasal variant   274
  technique   271–273, 274
Nathalang, B.   6
neck, of cartridges   178
needle adapter
  for cartridges   178
  for cartridge-type syringes
      181–182
needle-induced infection
  about   418
  clinical manifestations   418
  dentist management   419
needles
  about   7, 173
  breakage of
      about   419–420
      causes of   420
      clinical manifestations   421
      decision to retrieve   421
      dentist management   421–422
      factors of interest   420
      preventive measures   422–423
      techniques   420
  for children   392
  components   173–175
  criteria for selecting   177

critical aspects   175–177
  gauge of   175
  insertion of   225–226
  length of   175, 284–285
  for periodontal ligament
      technique   324
  retraction of   219
  in The Wand®   370
nerve block kinetics, peripheral nerve
  about   60
  induction stage   60
  recovery stage   60–61
  re-injection   61
  resistance to local anesthetics   61
  tachyphylaxis   61
nerve blocks   254
nerve fibers, classification of   52
nerve fibers and myelin   51–52
nerve lesions
  about   402
  anatomical   402
  electric shock sensation   403–404
  general causes   402–403
  hoarseness   407
  long-term paresthesia   404–407
  sense of taste alterations   407
nerve trunk thickness   60
Neuner, Von   3
neurons   50
neurophysiology, peripheral nerve
  about   56
  action potentials   56–58
  fundamentals   56
  membrane potentials   56
  propagation of action potential   58
neuropraxia   402
neurotmesis   402
Nevin, Mendel   8
Niemann, Albert   2
nodes of Ranvier   52, 59
nonselective beta-blockers, as a
      relative contraindication
      for vasoconstrictors
      158–160
noradrenaline   7
nordefrin hydrochloride   7
norepinephrine
  about   7
  catecholamines and   93–94
  symptoms of reaction to   445
novocaine (procaine)   5, 6, 452, 456
Noyes, Henry D.   3

## o

Oberst of Hale, Maximilian  4
ocular complications
　about  412
　　clinical manifestations  412–413
　　dentist management  414
　　onset and duration  413
　　pathophysiology of  414–418
　　predictors of sequelae  414
　　techniques for  412
1-2-3 technique, for anesthesia  7
open/closed mouth, pterygomandibular space and  44
oral vitamin K antagonists  141
Oraqix® gel  8–9
OraVerse®  9
orbital branches  19
osteomyelitis, as a clinical manifestation of needle-induced infection  418
overdose  447

## p

pain
　during injections  232–253
　needle gauge and  176
　from tooth decay  209
pain reduction methods, for complementary anesthesia of palate
　about  269
　minimal intervention technique  271
　periodontal ligament technique  270–271
　pressure techniques  270
　topical anesthesia  269
　topical cooling  270
palatine nerves  19–21
P-AMSA  371–373
Pantocaine  6
paresthesia
　as a clinical manifestation of long-term paresthesia  404, 406
　as a clinical manifestation of needle-induced infection  418
partial variant
　as lingual nerve block  314
　of the palate  276
partition coefficient  69–70
P-ASA  373–375
passive diffusion to the orbit  417

pathophysiology
　of facial blanching  400
　of hyperventilation syndrome  442–443
　of localized late-onset skin lesion  400–401
　of ocular complications  414–418
　of systemic toxicity induced by local anesthetics  445–446
　of toxicity induced by sympathomimetic vasoconstrictors  444
periapical infiltration  142
perilemma  53
perineurium  52–53
periodontal abnormalities  326–327
periodontal ligament technique
　about  142, 320
　anesthetized area  324
　for complementary anesthesia of palate  270–271
　complications of  326–328
　diffusion of the solution  320–321
　efficacy factors  321–322
　efficacy of  326
　indications and contraindications  320
　instrument set  322–324
　technique  324–326
　The Wand® and  375–376
periodontal Oraqix® gel, for topical anesthesia (DentiPatch®)  209–211
periosteum, classification of anesthesia with respect to  254
peripheral nerve
　basic membrane proteins
　　about  54
　　potassium channels  55–56
　　sodium channels  54–55
　　sodium-potassium pump  54
　mechanisms of local anesthesia
　　about  58
　　critical length  59–60
　　differential nerve block  58–59
　　tonic and phase block  59
　　transient receptor potential channel  60
　microanatomy
　　axons  50–51
　　membranes  51
　　nerve fibers and myelin  51–52

　　neurons  50
　　peripheral nerve structure  52–54
　　sensory neurons  50
　nerve block kinetics
　　about  60
　　induction stage  60
　　recovery stage  60–61
　　re-injection  61
　　resistance to local anesthetics  61
　　tachyphylaxis  61
　peripheral nerve neurophysiology
　　about  56
　　action potentials  56–58
　　fundamentals  56
　　membrane potentials  56
　　propagation of action potential  58
peripheral nerve structure  52–54
Pernice, Ludwig  4
persistent post-injection pain  397
Pfender, Charles  3–4
pH  188
pH adjustment  108–109
pH Onset System  9
pharyngeal nerve  19
phenothiazines, as a contraindication for vasoconstrictors  163–164
phentalomine (OraVerse®)
　about  95–96
　advantages and indications  96
　clinical efficacy  97
　technique and dose  96–97
　tolerance, toxicity, and adverse side effects  97–98
phentolamine mesylate  9
phenylephrine  7
pheochromocytoma-induced arterial hypertension, as an absolute contraindication for vasoconstrictors  156–157
physical access, impossible  143
physical-chemical characteristics, of local anesthetics
　about  67–68
　dissociation constant (pKa)  68–69
　lipid solubility  69–70
　partition coefficient  69–70
　protein binding  70
　vasodilation  70
piston, for cartridge-type syringes  182
Pizarro, Francisco  1–2
plastic syringes  184

plunger, for cartridges  179
Pöppig, Eduard Friedrich  2
positive aspirations and hematomas, pterygomandibular space and  45
posterior cap, of needles  175
posterior division, mandibular nerve and  31
posterior part
  of cartridges  179
  of cartridge-type syringes  182
posterior superior alveolar nerve  22
posterior superior alveolar nerve block (PSA)
  about  251
  complications of  253
  efficacy of  252–253
  modified adatia technique  253
  technique  251–252
  zones anesthetized  251
posterior/dorsal boundaries, of pterygomandibular space  43
post-injection mucosal ulceration
  about  419
  clinical manifestations  419
  dentist management  419
  proposed causes  419
potassium channels (K⁺ channels)  55–56
power-driven injection systems, for anesthesia  8
power-operated injection systems, for anesthesia  8
power-operated syringes  185
P-Posture  436–437
Pravaz, Charles Gabriel  4
predisposing factors  135–136
pre-division, mandibular nerve and  31
pregnancy
  as a contraindication of felypressin  164–165
  local anesthetics and  76–77
pregnancy and lactation labeling rule (PLLR)  76
preschool children, lack of patient cooperation and  135
preservatives (methylparaben)  108, 457
press and roll technique  270
pressure techniques, for complementary anesthesia of palate  270

prevention
  for allergies  460
  for systemic toxicity induced by local anesthetics  450
preventive measures  435
prilocaine (propitocaine)
  about  120, 451, 456
  indications and contraindications  122–123
  metabolism  120
  as a relevant contraindication  148–149
  remarks  120–122
primary mandibular molars, anesthesia of in children  391–392
Prinz, Hermann  5
procaine (novocaine)
  about  5, 6, 109, 452, 456
  sulfonoamides and, as a minor contraindication  149
propagation of action potential  58
protective disk  185
protein binding  70
pseudo-unipolar neurons  50
psychiatric disorders, lack of patient cooperation and  135
psychogenic reactions
  about  439
  allergic-like reactions  444
  general causes  439
  hyperventilation syndrome  442–444
  vasovagal syncope  439–442
psychostimulants, as a relative contraindication for vasoconstrictors  161
pterygoid venous plexus  25
pterygomandibular depression  42
pterygomandibular raphe/ligament  42
pterygomandibular space
  about  41–42
  anatomic boundaries of the  42–43
  contents of  44–45
  lingual nerve and  33
  open/closed mouth and  44
  positive aspirations and hematomas  45
pterygomaxillary space. See pterygomandibular space
pterygopalatine fossa  26–27
pterygopalatine fossa zone, as a collateral branch  18–19

pulpal abnormalities  327, 338
pulpal anesthesia
  about  241, 263, 281
  buccal anesthesia of upper molars  241–242
  buccal infiltration
    about  242
    complications of  245
    efficacy of  245
    modified cotton roll approach  245
    success factors of  245
    technique  242–245
    zones anesthetized  242
  double infiltration in anterior teeth
    about  304
    complications of  306
    efficacy of  306
    success factors for  304
    technique  304–306
    zone anesthetized  304
  high tuberosity approach
    about  253
    complications of  256
    efficacy of  256
    remarks  256
    technique  254–255
    uses  253–254
    zone anesthetized  254
  infraorbital nerve block
    about  245–246
    complications of  249–250
    efficacy of  249
    extraoral technique  248–249
    intraoral technique  246–248
    remarks  250–251
    uses  246
    zones anesthetized  246
  mandibular block: conventional/direct technique
    about  285
    complications of  291–292
    distribution of anesthetic solution  285–286
    efficacy of  291
    technique  286–291
    zone anesthetized  286
  mandibular block: Gow-Gates technique
    about  292
    advantages, disadvantages and non-advantages  294–296
    complications of  299–300

pulpal anesthesia (cont'd)
   efficacy of   299
   mechanism   292–294
   remarks on   300
   technique   296–299
   zone anesthetized   296
mandibular block: in general
   about   281
   factors to consider for   282–285
   zone anesthetized   282
mandibular block: Laguardia-Akinosi technique
   about   300
   advantages and disadvantages   300–301
   complications of   303–304
   distribution of anesthetic solution   301
   efficacy of   303
   technique   301–303
   zone anesthetized   301
maxilla   241
maxillary nerve ($V_2$)   241
posterior superior alveolar nerve block
   about   251
   complications of   253
   efficacy of   252–253
   modified adatia technique   253
   technique   251–252
   zones anesthetized   251
transpalatal technique
   about   256–257
   complications of   261–262
   efficacy of   260–261
   success factors of   263
   technique   257–260
   uses   257
   zone anesthetized   257
pupillary disorders, as a clinical manifestation of ocular complications   413
Puterbaugh, Pliny Guy   8

## q
QuickSleeper   377–379
Quincke edema, as a clinical manifestation of allergy   458–459

## r
ramus of the mandible
   accessory foramina   41
   coronoid notch   41
   divergent angle   39
   lingula   39
   mandibular foramen   39–40
   ramus width   39
   sulcus colli   40–41
ramus width   39
rapid absorption   447
rebound vasodilation   91
Reclus, Paul   4
recovery and discharge, for systemic toxicity induced by local anesthetics   450
recovery stage, of peripheral nerve block   60–61
refrigerants   207
Regitine®   9
re-injection, for peripheral nerve block   61
relative anesthetic potency   69
relative refractory period   57
relative toxicity   69
remarks
   for articaine   115–116
   for bupivacaine   123–125
   for high tuberosity approach   256
   for infraorbital nerve block   250–251
   for lidocaine (lignocaine)   111
   for mepivacaine   119
   for prilocaine (propitocaine)   120–122
repolarization   57
reserprine   162
resistance to local anesthetics   61, 348
respiratory diseases, toxic methemoglobinemia and   149
respiratory tract, effect of catecholamines on   91
retraction, of needle   219
retrograde arterial flow   414
retrograde venous flow   414–417
retromolar zone (trigone and fossa)   37
Riethmüller, Richard   5
rigid recipient   186
risk of hemorrhage, clotting abnormalities and systemic causes of   140–142
Ritsert, Eduard   5
Rynd, Francis   3–4

## s
safety
   of local anesthetics   73
   prilocaine (propitocaine)   120–122
saltatory conduction   52
Sauvez, Emilie   8
scale   186
Scarpa's nerve   20–21
Schleich, Carl Ludwig   4
Schley, W. S.   5
Schwann cells   50, 51–52
selective serotonin reuptake inhibitors (SSRIs)   162
self-aspirating syringes   183–184
self-inflicted injury   397–398
sense of taste alterations, nerve lesions and   407
sensory neurons   50
sequelae, predictors of   414
sequential nature   283
shaft, of needles   173
shank, of needles   173
sheath, of needles   175
silicone lubricant, in cartridges   179
skin discoloration, as a clinical manifestation of facial hematomas   401
Smith, Arthur Ervin   8
socket, of needles   174
sodium channels ($NA^+$ channels)   54–55
sodium-potassium pump ($Na^+/K^+$ pump)   54
solution composition
   antioxidants (sulfites)   107–108
   local anesthetic   107
   other compounds   109
   pH adjustment   108–109
   preservatives (methylparaben)   108
   vasoconstrictor   107
somatotopic   60
sphenomandibular ligament   44–45, 350
Stabident®   330–335
sterilization, of syringes   183
Stolz, Friedrich   4
storage, of cartridges   179–180
structure, of peripheral nerve   52–54
subcutaneous route, for drugs   438
sublingual route, for drugs   438
submandibular zone, lingual nerve and   33–34
success factors
   of buccal infiltration   245
   of transpalatal technique   263
sulcus colli   40–41

sulfites (antioxidants)
    about   87, 456–457
    degradation of in cartridges   181
superior alveolar nerves   22–23
superior dental plexus   23
superior/cranial boundaries, of pterygomandibular space   43
supplementary techniques
    about   318, 338
    intraosseous technique
        about   329–330, 332–336
        anesthetic solutions   331
        anesthetized area   331–332
        complications of   336–338
        efficacy   336
        indications, contraindications, and disadvantages   330
        instrument set   330–331
    intrapulpal anesthesia
        about   318
        topical anesthetic technique   319
        traditional technique   318–319
    intraseptal technique
        about   328
        anesthetized area   328
        complications of   329
        contraindications   328
        success factors for   328
        technique   328–329
    periodontal ligament technique
        about   320
        anesthetized area   324
        complications of   326–328
        diffusion of the solution   320–321
        efficacy factors   321–322
        efficacy of   326
        indications and contraindications   320
        instrument set   322–324
        technique   324–326
suprarenin   4
surgical drainage, for trismus   409
swelling, as a clinical manifestation of facial hematomas   401
sympathetic system, irritation of the   417–418
sympathetic system block (Horner-like Syndrome)   418
sympathomimetic vasoconstrictors (epinephrine), degradation of in cartridges   181
sympathomimetics. See catecholamines
Syrijet®   8, 361–362

syringe barrel, of cartridge-type syringes   182
syringe body, of cartridge-type syringes   182
syringes
    about   181
    components of cartridge-type   181–183
    development of   3–4
    for periodontal ligament technique   322–324
    self-aspirating   183–184
    transfer of   223–225
    variants of cartridge-type   184–185
systemic effects, of catecholamines   90–91
systemic toxicity induced by local anesthetics
    about   445
    causes of local anesthetic-induced toxicity   446–447
    clinical manifestations   447–449
    clinical variations   449
    dentist management   449–450
    pathophysiology   445–446
    prevention   450
    recovery and discharge   450

## t

tachyphylaxis, for peripheral nerve block   61
Tainter, M. L.   6
Takamine, Jokichi   4, 5
techniques
    for anesthesia   7–8
    for aural complications   423
    for buccal infiltration   242–245
    for buccal nerve block   315–316
    for double infiltration in anterior teeth   304–306
    for electronic dental anesthesia (EDA)   367–368
    for facial blanching   399
    for greater palatine nerve block   275–276
    for high tuberosity approach   254–255
    for intranasal maxillary local anesthesia (Kovanaze®)   380–381
    for intraseptal technique   328–329
    for jet injection   362–363
    for lingual nerve block   312–314
    for local anesthetic in children   390–391
    for mandibular block: conventional/direct technique   286–291
    for mandibular block: Gow-Gates technique   296–299
    for mandibular block: Laguardia-Akinosi technique   301–303
    for nasopalatine nerve block   271–273, 274
    for needle breakage   420
    for ocular complications   412
    for P-AMSA   371–373
    for P-ASA   374–375
    for periodontal ligament technique   324–326
    for phentalomine (OraVerse®)   96–97
    for posterior superior alveolar nerve block   251–252
    for transpalatal technique   257–260
    for trismus   407–408
Tegner, Cläes   6
temporal crest   42
TENS (transcutaneous electrical nerve stimulation)   8
tensor veli palatini   42
terminal zone   19
terminology, for injections   234–255
tetracaine (amethocaine)
    about   6, 456
    for topical anesthesia (DentiPatch®)   201–202
thiopental   162
Thoma, Kurt Hermann   5
timer   185–186
tip, of needles   173–174
tissue irritation, from local anesthetics   73–74
tolerance, toxicity, and adverse side effects, of phentalomine (OraVerse®)   97–98
tonic and phase block   59
topical anesthesia/anesthetics
    about   195
    application of   222–223
    benzocaine   197–199
    cocaine   203
    for complementary anesthesia of palate   269
    compounds   203–205
    effect of   197
    effectiveness of   69–70

topical anesthesia/anesthetics (cont'd)
   Eutectic Mixture of Local Anesthetic (EMLA) cream 200–201
   experimental formulations 205–206
   factor affecting with local anesthesia
     amount administered 196
     application time 195
     area of the mouth 197
     local anesthetic 195
     method of application 195–196
     types of pain 196
   indications for 208–209
   for intrapulpal anesthesia 319
   lidocaine 199
   lidocaine adhesive patches (DentiPatch®) 199–200
   periodontal Oraqix® gel 209–211
   tetracaine (amethocaine) 201–202
   topical cooling
     about 206
     cold aerosols 206–207
     refrigerants 207
     topical ice 207–208
topical cooling
   about 206
   cold aerosols 206–207
   for complementary anesthesia of palate 270
   refrigerants 207
   topical ice 207–208
topical ice 207–208
toxic methemoglobinemia
   about 450–451
   aggravating factors 452
   clinical manifestations 452–453
   dentist management 453
   local anesthetics involved 451–452
toxicity
   articaine 115
   induced by sympathomimetic vasoconstrictors
     about 444
     dentist management 445
     pathophysiology 444
     symptoms of reaction to epinephrine 444–445
     symptoms of reaction to norepinephrine 445
   prilocaine (propitocaine) 120–122
traditional technique, for intrapulpal anesthesia 318–319

transcortical technique, for QuickSleeper 377–378
transcutaneous electrical nerve stimulation (TENS) 8
transient receptor potential channel 60
transpalatal technique
   electric shock sensation after 403–404
   pulpal anesthesia and
     about 256–257
     complications of 261–262
     efficacy of 260–261
     success factors of 263
     technique 257–260
     uses 257
     zone anesthetized 257
transpapillary technique in children 276–277
tricyclic antidepressants, as a relative contraindication for vasoconstrictors 161–162
trigeminal ganglion 17
trigeminal nerve 17
trismus
   about 407
   causes of 408
   as a clinical manifestation of needle-induced infection 418
   clinical types of 408
   techniques implicated in development of 407–408
   treatment of 408–409
tunica adventitia 88
twenty-first century developments 8–9
Type III allergic reaction 401

## U

Uhlfelder, Emil 5
ulcers, on mucosa 209
Ultracalm 8
Unanúe, José Hipólito 2
unconscious patients 436–438
uncontrolled hyperthyroidism, as a contraindication for vasoconstrictors 163
uncontrolled insulin-dependent Diabetes Mellitus, as an absolute contraindication for vasoconstrictors 155–156
uniject-type syringes 184
unipolar neurons 50

unmyelinated fibers 52
upper molars, buccal anesthesia of 241–242
Urech, E. 9
uterus, effect of catecholamines on 91

## V

Valentin's ganglion 23
Valverde, Vicente de 1–2
vasoconstrictive effect
   about 91
   adrenaline and 4–5
   of felypressin (Octapressin®) 99–100
vasoconstrictors
   about 6–7, 85, 456
   advantages 85
   catecholamines
     about 87–88
     adrenergic receptors 88–90
     epinephrine 92–93
     isomers and 88
     levonordefrin 94–95
     metabolism of 92
     norepinephrine 93–94
     systemic effects 90–91
     vasoconstrictive effect 91
   combinations of 101
   composition of 107
   concentrations 87
   contraindications for (See contraindications, for vasoconstrictors)
   dilutions 87
   disadvantages 85–87
   felypressin (Octapressin®)
     about 98
     advantages and disadvantages 100
     adverse effects 100
     cardiovascular effects 98–99
     contraindications 100
     maximum doses 100–101
     vasoconstrictive effect 99–100
   osteoradionecrosis and, as a contraindication for vasoconstrictors 164
   phentalomine (OraVerse®)
     about 95–96
     advantages and indications 96

clinical efficacy 97
technique and dose 96–97
tolerance, toxicity, and adverse side effects 97–98
vasodilation 70
vasospasm, ischemic necrosis due to 400–401
vasovagal syncope 439–442
ventral/anterior boundaries, of pterygomandibular space 42–43
VibraJect® 188, 189
vibrating devices 188–190
visual disorders, as a clinical manifestation of ocular complications 412
volume, of local anesthetics 72

## W
Walton, Richard 8
the Wand 8
Wells, Horace (dentist) 1
Wesley, John 8
Willstätter, Richard 2
Winther, J. E. 6
wisdom teeth, accessory branch for 35, 352
Wood, Alexander 4

## X
X-Tip® 331–335

## Z
zone of the second premolar apex 38, 39
zones anesthetized
  for buccal infiltration 242
  for double infiltration in anterior teeth 304
  for high tuberosity approach 254
  for infraorbital nerve block 246
  for intranasal maxillary local anesthesia (Kovanaze®) 379
  for mandibular block
    conventional/direct technique 286
    in general 282
    Gow-Gates technique 296
    Laguardia-Akinosi technique 301
  for posterior superior alveolar nerve block 251
  for transpalatal technique 257